AACN Procedure Manual for Critical Care

AMERICAN ASSOCIATION *of* CRITICAL-CARE NURSES

AACN

Procedure Manual for Critical Care

FOURTH EDITION

Edited by:

Debra J. Lynn-McHale, *RN, MSN, CS, CCRN*

Predoctoral Fellow
University of Pennsylvania
Philadelphia, Pennsylvania

Staff Nurse
Surgical Cardiac Care Unit
Thomas Jefferson University Hospital
Philadelphia, Pennsylvania

Karen K. Carlson, *RN, MN, CCRN*

Critical Care Clinical Nurse Specialist
Carlson Consulting Group
Bellevue, Washington

Clinical Faculty
Department of Biobehavioral Nursing
University of Washington
Seattle, Washington

W.B. SAUNDERS COMPANY
An Imprint of Elsevier Science
Philadelphia   London   New York   St. Louis   Sydney   Toronto

W.B. SAUNDERS COMPANY
An Imprint of Elsevier Science

The Curtis Center
Independence Square West
Philadelphia, Pennsylvania 19106

Library of Congress Cataloging-in-Publication Data

AACN procedure manual for critical care / edited by Debra J. Lynn-McHale, Karen K. Carlson.—4th ed.

p. cm.

Includes bibliographical references and index.

ISBN 0–7216–8268–5

1. Intensive care nursing—Handbooks, manuals, etc. I. Lynn-McHale, Debra J. II. Carlson, Karen K. III. American Association of Critical-Care Nurses. [DNLM: 1. Critical Care—Methods—Handbooks. 2. Critical Illness—Nursing—Handbooks. WY 49 A111 2001]

RT120.15 A17 2001 616'.028—dc21
DNLM/DLC 98–19200

Vice President, Nursing Editorial Director:	Sally Schrefer
Acquisitions Editor:	Barbara Cullen Nelson
Editorial Assistant:	Adrienne Simon
Production Manager:	Frank Polizzano
Manuscript Editor:	Jennifer Ehlers
Illustration Specialist:	Lisa Lambert
Book Designer:	Ellen Zanolle

AACN PROCEDURE MANUAL FOR CRITICAL CARE ISBN 0–7216–8268–5

Printed in the United States of America.

Last digit is the print number: 9 8 7 6 5 4 3 2

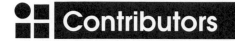 Contributors

Mary G. Adams, RN, MS

Nurse Educator, Critical Care, University of California, San Francisco, California

ST Segment Monitoring

Andrei V. Alexandrov, MD, RVT

Assistant Professor of Neurology, Department of Neurology, University of Texas–Houston, Houston, Texas

Transcranial Doppler Monitoring

Marie Arnone, RN, MA, CCRN

Clinical Development Specialist, Cardiac Services and Critical Care, Providence Seattle Medical Center, Seattle, Washington

Central Venous/Right Atrial Pressure Line Removal; Central Venous/Right Atrial Pressure Line Site Care; Central Venous/Right Atrial Pressure Monitoring; Single and Multiple Pressure Transducer Systems; Central Venous Catheter Insertion (Assist)

William Barefoot, RN, MSN, ACNP

Clinical Skills Laboratory Instructor, School of Nursing, University of Pennsylvania, Philadelphia, Pennsylvania

Performing Thoracentesis; Assisting with Thoracentesis

Deborah E. Becker, MSN, CRNP, CS, CCRN, RN

Assistant Program Director, Adult Acute/Tertiary and Critical Care Nurse Practitioner Program, University of Pennsylvania School of Nursing, Philadelphia, Pennsylvania

Temporary Transvenous Pacemaker Insertion (Perform); Arterial Catheter Insertion (Perform)

Barbara A. Brown, RN, BSN, CCRN

Nursing Program Manager, Critical Care Nursing, The Ohio State University Medical Center, Columbus, Ohio

Calculating Doses, Flow Rates, and Administration of Continuous Intravenous Infusions

Linda Bucher, RN, DNSc

Associate Professor, Department of Nursing, University of Delaware, College of Health and Nursing Sciences, Newark, Delaware; Staff Nurse, Emergency Department, Virtua Memorial Hospital of Burlington County, Mount Holly, New Jersey

Arterial Puncture; Peripheral Intravenous Line Insertion; Peripherally Inserted Central Catheter; Venipuncture

Suzanne M. Burns, RN, MSN, RRT, ACNP-CS, CCRN

Associate Professor of Nursing, University of Virginia, Charlottesville, Virginia; Clinician V, University of Virginia Health Systems, Charlottesville, Virginia

Arterial-Venous Oxygen Difference Calculation; Auto-PEEP Calculation; Measurement of Compliance and Resistance; Manual Self-Inflating Resuscitation Bag; Indices of Oxygenation: Alveolar-Arterial Oxygen Difference, Partial Pressure of Arterial Oxygenation to Fraction of Inspired Oxygen Ratio, Partial Pressure of Arterial Oxygen to Alveolar Oxygen Ratio; Shunt Calculation; Ventilatory Management—Volume and Pressure Modes; Standard Weaning Criteria: Negative Inspiratory Pressure, Positive Expiratory Pressure, Spontaneous Tidal Volume, and Vital Capacity; Weaning Procedure

Karen K. Carlson, RN, MN, CCRN

Clinical Faculty, Department of Biobehavioral Nursing, University of Washington, Seattle, Washington; Critical Care Clinical Nurse Specialist, Carlson Consulting Group, Bellevue, Washington

Assisting with Thoracentesis; Orogastric and Nasogastric Tube Insertion, Care, and Removal; Assisting with Abdominal Paracentesis; Assisting with Percutaneous Peritoneal Lavage; Automated External Defibrillation

Marianne Chulay, RN, DNSc, FAAN

Consultant, Critical Care Nursing and Clinical Research, Chapel Hill, North Carolina; Director, Nursing Research and Practice, Moses Cone Health System, Greensboro, North Carolina

Endotracheal or Tracheostomy Tube Suctioning

Michael W. Day, RN, MSN, CCRN

Clinical Nurse Specialist/Outreach Educator, Northwest MEDSTAR, Spokane, Washington

Esophagogastric Tamponade Tube

Robyn Dealtry, RN

Distance Education Tutor, NSW College of Nursing, Sydney, Australia; Registered Nurse/Clinical Nurse Consultant, Westmead Hospital, Sydney, Australia

Pain Management Using Epidural Catheters

Julianne M. Deutsch, RN, BAN, CCRN

Heart/Lung Leader, United Hospital, St. Paul, Minnesota

Assisting with Endotracheal Intubation; Endotracheal Tube Care; Autotransfusion

Mary Donahue, RN, BSN, CCRN

Director of Nursing, Rochester General Hospital, Rochester, New York

Parenteral Nutrition

Barbara J. Drew, PhD, RN, FAAN

Associate Professor, University of California–San Francisco, San Francisco, California

Extra Electrocardiographic Leads: Right Precordial and Left Posterior Leads

Phyllis Dubendorf, RN, MSN, CRNP

Lecturer, Adult Acute/Tertiary and Critical Care Nurse Practitioner Program, University of Pennsylvania, Philadelphia, Pennsylvania; Neuroscience Nurse Practitioner, Thomas Jefferson University Hospital, Philadelphia, Pennsylvania

Cerebrospinal Fluid Drainage Assessment; Iced Caloric Testing for Vestibular Function (Assist); Lumbar and Cisternal Punctures (Assist)

Margaret M. Ecklund, MS, RN, CCRN, CS

Advanced Practice Nurse–Clinician IV, Rochester General Hospital, Rochester, New York

Gastrostomy or Jejunostomy Tube Care; Small-Bore Feeding Tube Insertion

Desiree A. Fleck, MSN, CRNP, CCRN, RN

Nurse Practitioner, Temple University Hospital, Philadelphia, Pennsylvania

Pulmonary Artery Catheter Insertion (Perform); Central Venous Catheter Insertion (Perform)

Mary Beth Flynn, RN, MS, CCRN

Faculty, University of Colorado Health Science Center, School of Nursing, Denver, Colorado; Clinical Nurse Specialist, University of Colorado Hospital, Denver, Colorado

Cleansing, Irrigating, Culturing, and Dressing Open Wounds; Dressing Wounds with Drains; Drain Removal; Dressing and Pouching Draining Wounds

Janet G. Whetstone Foster, RN

Assistant Professor of Nursing, Houston Baptist University, Houston, Texas; President, Nursing Inquiry and Intervention, The Woodlands, Texas

Peripheral Nerve Stimulators

John J. Gallagher, RN, MSN, RRT

Trauma Program Coordinator, Crozer-Chester Medical Center, Upland, Pennsylvania; Staff Nurse, Shock/Trauma Unit, Cooper Hospital/University Medical Center, Camden, New Jersey

Intra-abdominal Pressure Monitoring; Intracompartment Pressure Monitoring

Karen K. Giuliano, RN, MSN, CCRN, ACNP

Critical Care Clinical Nurse Specialist, Baystate Medical Center, Springfield, Massachusetts

Continuous Renal Replacement Therapies; Hemodialysis; Peritoneal Dialysis; Assisting with Plasmapheresis

Margaret T. Goldberg, RN, MSN, CWOCN

Wound Care Consultant, Wound Treatment Center, Delray Medical Center, Delray Beach, Florida

Pressure-Reducing Devices: Lateral Rotation Therapy

Vicki S. Good, MSN, RN, CCRN

Director of Education, All Saints Health System, Fort Worth, Texas

Continuous End-Tidal Carbon Dioxide Monitoring

Cindy Goodrich, RN, MS, CCRN

Clinical Faculty, University of Washington, Seattle, Washington; Flight Nurse, Airlift Northwest, Seattle, Washington

Performing Endotracheal Intubation; Performing Needle Thoracostomy

Kathleen Ahern Gould, RN, MSN, CCRN

Critical Care Instructor, St. Elizabeth's Medical Center, Boston, Massachusetts

Cardiac Output Measurement Techniques (Invasive)

Charlotte A. Green, RN, CCRN, BSN

Staff Nurse, Critical Care, Group Health Cooperative of Puget Sound, East Side Hospital, Redmond, Washington

Automated External Defibrillation

Kay Knox Greenlee, MSN, RN, CCRN, CS

Clinical Nurse Specialist, Surgical/Special Care Services, St. Cloud Hospital, St. Cloud, Minnesota

Performing Extubation and Decannulation; Assisting with Extubation and Decannulation; Nasopharyngeal Airway Insertion; Oropharyngeal Airway Insertion; Tracheal Tube Cuff Care; Tracheostomy Tube Care

Dolores Grosso, RN, MSN, CRNP

Certified Registered Nurse Practitioner, Bone Marrow Transplant Program, Thomas Jefferson University Hospital, Philadelphia, Pennsylvania

Bone Marrow Biopsy and Aspiration (Perform); Bone Marrow Biopsy and Aspiration (Assist)

Cynthia Hambach, RN, MSN, CCRN

Clinical Nurse Specialist, Intermediate Cardiac Care Unit, Thomas Jefferson University Hospital, Philadelphia, Pennsylvania

Cardioversion

Colette Hartigan, BSN, MBA, CCRN, RN

Clinical Nurse I/Charge Nurse, St Elizabeth's Medical Center, Boston, Massachusetts

Cardiac Output Measurement Techniques (Invasive)

Jan M. Headley, RN, BS

Critical Care Education Consultant, Datex-Ohmeda, Tewksbury, Massachusetts

Continuous Mixed Venous Oxygen Saturation Monitoring

Joanne V. Hickey, PhD, RN, ACNP, CS, FAAN, FCCM

Professor, Clinical Nursing, and Clinical Associate Professor, Neurology, University of Texas, Health Science Center, School of Nursing, and School of Medicine, Houston, Texas

External Fixation Device Insertion (Assist); Halo Traction Care; Tong and Pin Care; Traction Maintenance

June Hinkle, MSN, RN

Program Manager, Bereavement Services, The Ohio State University Medical Center, Columbus, Ohio

Care of the Organ Donor; Identification of Potential Organ Donors; Request for Organ Donation

Carol Jacobson, RN, MN

Clinical Faculty, University of Washington School of Nursing, Seattle, Washington; Critical Care/Cardiology Clinical Specialist, Swedish Medical Center, Seattle, Washington

Overdrive Atrial Pacing

Ann Louise Jones, MSN, RN

United Surgical Associates, Surgical Associates of Lexington Division, Lexington, Kentucky

Pericardiocentesis (Assist)

Suzanne Farley Keane, RN

Clinical Nurse/Charge Nurse, St. Elizabeth Medical Center, Boston, Massachusetts

Cardiac Output Measurement Techniques (Invasive)

Eileen M. Kelly, RN, CCRN, MSN

Clinical Nurse Specialist, Medical and Surgical Cardiac Care Units, Thomas Jefferson University Hospital, Philadelphia, Pennsylvania

External Warming/Cooling Devices

Peggy Kirkwood, RN, MSN, ACNP

Cardiovascular Outcomes Manager, Mission Hospital, Mission Viejo, California

Chest Tube Removal; Performing Abdominal Paracentesis; Assisting with Abdominal Paracentesis; Performing Percutaneous Peritoneal Lavage; Assisting with Percutaneous Peritoneal Lavage; Suturing

Deborah G. LaMarr, RN, MSN, APRN

Nurse Practitioner, Surgical Critical Care, Hartford Hospital, Hartford, Connecticut

Emergent Open Sternotomy (Perform); Emergent Open Sternotomy (Assist)

Denise M. Lawrence, MS, RN, CS

Acute Care Nurse Practitioner, Trauma Surgery, Hartford Hospital, Hartford, Connecticut

Performing Chest Tube Placement; External Counterpressure with Pneumatic Antishock Garments

Debra J. Lynn-McHale, RN, MSN, CS, CCRN

Predoctoral Fellow, University of Pennsylvania, Philadelphia, Pennsylvania; Staff Nurse, Surgical Cardiac Unit, Thomas Jefferson University Hospital, Philadelphia, Pennsylvania

Blood Sampling from Pulmonary Artery Line; Atrial Electrogram; Intra-aortic Balloon Pump Management; Pulmonary Artery Catheter Insertion (Assist) and Pressure Monitoring; Pulmonary Artery Pressure Line, Removal; Pulmonary Artery Pressure Lines, Troubleshooting; Withholding/Withdrawing Life-Sustaining Treatment

Margaret M. Mahon, RN, PhD

Advanced Practice Nurse, Ethics and End-of-Life Care, Hospital of the University of Pennsylvania, Philadelphia, Pennsylvania

Withholding/Withdrawing Life-Sustaining Treatment

Marc Malkoff, MD

Associate Professor of Neurology, University of Texas–Houston, Houston, Texas

Lumbar Puncture (Perform)

Cathy M. Martin, RN, MS

Head Nurse, Trauma/Surgical Intensive Care Unit, Brooke Army Medical Center, Fort Sam Houston, Texas

Implantable Cardioverter-Defibrillator

Shawn McCabe, RN, MSN, CCRN, CNSC

Associate Professor, Columbia University, New York, New York; Clinical Nurse Specialist, Trauma, University of Medicine and Dentistry of New Jersey–University Hospital, Newark, New Jersey

Intracompartment Pressure Monitoring

Kathy McCloy, RN, MSN, ACNP-CS

Lecturer, University of California–Los Angeles School of Nursing, Acute Care Nurse Practitioner Tract, Los Angeles, California; Nurse Practitioner, University of California–Los Angeles Medical Center, Los Angeles, California

Pericardial Catheter Management

Ellen Strauss McErlean, MSN, RN, CCRN

Project Manager, Cardiology Research, The Cleveland Clinic Cardiovascular Coordinating Center, The Cleveland Clinic Foundation, Cleveland, Ohio

Permanent Pacemaker (Assessing Function); Temporary Transcutaneous (External) Pacing; Temporary Transvenous and Epicardial Pacing

Mary G. McKinley, RN, MSN

Clinical Nurse Specialist for Critical Care, Ohio Valley Medical Center, Wheeling, West Virginia

Electrophysiologic Monitoring: Hardwire and Telemetry; Twelve-Lead Electrocardiogram

Christine Moriarty, RN

Staff Nurse, Postanesthesia Care Unit, St. Elizabeth's Medical Center, Boston, Massachusetts

Defibrillation (Internal)

Patricia Gonce Morton, RN, PhD, ACNP, FAAN

Associate Professor and Coordinator, Clinical Nurse Specialist and Acute Care Nurse Practitioner, Master's Program in Trauma, Critical Care, and Emergency Nursing, University of Maryland School of Nursing, Baltimore, Maryland; Acute Care Nurse Practitioner, Preadmission Testing Center, St. Joseph Medical Center, Towson, Maryland

Implantable Cardioverter-Defibrillator

Michael A. Nace, RN, MS, CEN

Emergency Department Manager, Naval Hospital, Camp Pendleton, California

Implantable Cardioverter-Defibrillator

Barbara B. Ott, RN, PhD

Assistant Professor, Villanova University, Villanova, Pennsylvania

Advance Directives

Francine E. Paschall, RN, MSN

Vice President of Nursing/Chief Nurse Executive, Lakewood Hospital, Lakewood, Ohio

Permanent Pacemaker (Assessing Function); Temporary Transcutaneous (External) Pacing; Temporary Transvenous and Epicardial Pacing

Michele M. Pelter, RN, PhD

Project Director for the Ischemia Monitoring Laboratory, University of California–San Francisco, San Francisco, California

ST Segment Monitoring

Teresa Preuss, RN, MSN, CCRN

Staff Nurse, Medical Cardiac Care Unit, Thomas Jefferson University Hospital, Philadelphia, Pennsylvania

Atrial Electrogram; Blood Sampling from Pulmonary Artery Line; Pulmonary Artery Catheter Insertion (Assist) and Pressure Monitoring; Pulmonary Artery Pressure Line, Removal; Pulmonary Artery Pressure Lines, Troubleshooting

Eileen E. Pysznik, RN, BS, CCRN

Educator, Intensive Care Unit, Baystate Medical Center, Springfield, Massachusetts

Care of Donor Sites; Care of Burn Wounds; Care of Skin Grafts

Catherine Freismuth Robinson, RN, MS, CEN, CCRN

Clinical Nurse Specialist, Emergency Services/Trauma, Ohio Valley Medical Center, Wheeling, West Virginia

Assisting with Chest Tube Placement; Assisting with Chest Tube Removal; Closed Chest Drainage System

Donna M. Rosborough, MS, RN

Care Coordination Manager, Cardiology/Cardiac Surgery, Brigham and Women's Hospital, Boston, Massachusetts

Left Atrial Pressure Line, Care and Assisting with Removal

Lee Ann Ruess, MS, RN, CCRN, NP

Adjunct Faculty, The Ohio State University College of Nursing, Columbus, Ohio; Clinical Nurse Specialist, Surgical Intensive Care Unit and Burn Center, The Ohio State University Medical Center, Columbus, Ohio

Ventricular Assist Devices

Amy L. Schueler, MS, RN, CCRN

Clinical Nurse Specialist, The Ohio State University Medical Center, Columbus, Ohio

Arterial and Venous Sheath Removal

Christine S. Schulman, RN, MSN, CCRN

Clinical Nurse Specialist, Trauma and Surgery, Harborview Medical Center, Seattle, Washington

Continuous Arteriovenous Rewarming; Rapid Infuser for Massive Fluid Resuscitation

Sandra L. Schutz, RN, MSN, CCRN

Clinical Nurse Specialist, Swedish Medical Center–Ballard, Seattle, Washington

Oxygen Tank Preparation and Setup; Oxygen Saturation Monitoring by Pulse Oximetry

Rose B. Shaffer, RN, MSN, ACNP-CS, CCRN

Cardiology Nurse Practitioner, Thomas Jefferson University Hospital, Philadelphia, Pennsylvania

Arterial Catheter Insertion (Assist), Care, and Removal; Blood Sampling from Arterial Pressure Lines; Arterial and Venous Sheath Removal

Kellie Smith, RN

Clinical Leader, Surgical Intensive Care Unit, Saint Elizabeth's Medical Center, Boston, Massachusetts

Defibrillation (Internal)

Deborah C. Stamps, BSN, RN

Administrative Clinical Leader–Clinician III, Rochester General Hospital, Rochester, New York

Enteral Nutrition

Jacqueline Sullivan, RN, PhD, CCRN, CNRN

Clinical Assistant Professor, Thomas Jefferson University School of Nursing, Philadelphia, Pennsylvania; Clinician Researcher, Neuroscience and Critical Care Nursing, Thomas Jefferson University Hospital, Philadelphia, Pennsylvania

Intracranial Bolt Insertion (Assist), Monitoring, Care, Troubleshooting, and Removal; Intraventricular Catheter Insertion (Assist), Monitoring, Care, Troubleshooting, and Removal; Jugular Venous Oxygen Saturation Monitoring: Insertion (Assist), Care, Troubleshooting, and Removal; Lumbar Subarachnoid Catheter Insertion (Assist) for Cerebral Spinal Fluid Pressure Monitoring and Drainage; Determination of Death

Robin H. Thomas, RN, MN, ARNP

Medical-Surgical Clinical Development Specialist, Providence Seattle Medical Center, Seattle, Washington

Gastric Lavage in Hemorrhage and in Overdose; Scleral Endoscopic Therapy

Nancy L. Tomaselli, RN, MSN, CS, CRNP, CWOCN

President and Chief Executive Officer, Premier Health Solutions, Cherry Hill, New Jersey

Pressure-Reducing Devices: Lateral Rotation Therapy

Joan M. Vitello-Cicciu, MSN, MA, RN

Patient Care Manager of Emergency Services, St. Elizabeth's Medical Center, Brighton, Massachusetts

Defibrillation (Internal); Left Atrial Pressure Line, Care and Assisting with Removal

Kathleen M. Vollman, MSN, RN, CCNS, CCRN

Clinical Nurse Specialist, Medical Critical Care, Henry Ford Hospital, Detroit, Michigan

Manual Pronation Therapy

Kathryn T. Von Rueden, RN, MS, FCCM, CCRN

Adjunct Faculty, University of Maryland School of Nursing Graduate Program, Baltimore, Maryland; Senior Clinical Consultant, APACHE/National Health Advisors, McLean, Virginia

Noninvasive Hemodynamic Monitoring: Impedance Cardiography

Virginia Wilson, RN, MSN, CEN

Adjunct Faculty, Gwynedd-Mercy College, Gwynedd Valley, Pennsylvania; Education Specialist, Critical Care, Thomas Jefferson University Hospital, Philadelphia, Pennsylvania

Defibrillation (External)

Sandi Wind, RN, CWOCN

Enterostomal Nurse, Tenet Hospital, Philadelphia, Pennsylvania

Pressure-Reducing Devices: Lateral Rotation Therapy

Anne W. Wojner, MSN, RN, CCRN

Assistant Professor of Clinical Nursing and Clinical Nurse Specialist/Nurse Researcher, Department of Neurology, University of Texas–Houston School of Nursing and Medical School, Houston, Texas; President, Health Outcomes Institute, Inc., The Woodlands, Texas

Transcranial Doppler Monitoring; Lumbar Puncture (Perform)

Maribeth Wooldridge-King, MS, CNAA, OCN, RN

Clinical Supervisor, Memorial Sloan-Kettering Cancer Center, New York, New York

Blood and Blood Component Administration; Blood Pump Use; Transfusion Reaction Management; Determination of Microhematocrit via Centrifuge

Shu-Fen Wung, PhD, RN

Assistant Professor, College of Nursing, University of Illinois at Chicago, Chicago, Illinois

Extra Electrocardiographic Leads: Right Precordial and Left Posterior Leads

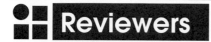
Reviewers

Debra R. Abraham, MSN, RN
Clinical Faculty/Lecturer, School of Nursing, University of Pennsylvania, Philadelphia, Pennsylvania

Nancy M. Albert, MSN, RN, CCRN, CNA
Clinical Outcomes Researcher/Clinical Specialist Nurse, The Kaufman Center for Heart Failure, The Cleveland Clinic Foundation, Cleveland, Ohio

Elizabeth Brady Avis, RN, MSN, CCRN, FNP
Clinical Nurse Specialist, Intermediate Cardiac Care Unit, Thomas Jefferson University Hospital, Philadelphia, Pennsylvania

Kristine A. Benvenuto, RN, MN, CCRN
Clinical Nurse Specialist—Critical Care/Emergency, Group Health Cooperative, Eastside Hospital, Redmond, Washington

Susan A. Bethel, RN, MS, CNRN
Director, Stroke Center and Neuroscience Program, St Joseph's Hospital, Atlanta, Georgia

Margaret F. Bevans, RN, MS, AOCN
Clinical Nurse Specialist in Bone Marrow Transplantation, National Institutes of Health, Bethesda, Maryland

Donna Zimmaro Bliss, PhD, RN, CCRN
Assistant Professor, University of Minnesota School of Nursing, Minneapolis, Minnesota

Cathryn D. Boardman, RN, MSN, CCRN
Clinical Nurse Specialist and Outcomes Manager, Medical Center East, Birmingham, Alabama

Susan Bonini, RN, MSN
University of Colorado Hospital, Denver, Colorado

Mitzi Chenault, RN, CPT
Clinical Nurse I, Coronary Intensive Care Unit, University of Michigan Health System, Ann Arbor, Michigan

Marie E. Colaianne-Wolfer, RN, BSN, CCRN
Staff Nurse, Thoracic Intensive Care Unit, University of Michigan Medical Center, Ann Arbor, Michigan

Lisa Consiglio, RN, MSN, APRN, CCRN, CS
Acute Care Nurse Practitioner, Bridgeport Hospital, Bridgeport, Connecticut

Elsie B. Croom, RN, BSN, CCRN
Nurse Consultant, Lafayette General Medical Center, Lafayette, Louisiana

Leigh F. Dangerfield, RN, MSN, CCRN
Clinical Nurse Specialist, Roper Heart Center, Carealliance Health Services, Charleston, South Carolina

Mary Ann Ducharme, RN, MSN, CS, CCRN
Clinical Nurse Specialist, Harper Hospital, Detroit Medical Center, Detroit, Michigan

Cameron Poston Evers, RN, MSN
Continuum of Care Manager, Medical University of South Carolina, Charleston, South Carolina

Susan Ezzone, RN, MSN, CNP
Ohio State University Medical Center, James Cancer Hospital, Columbus, Ohio

Eleanor R. Fitzpatrick, RN, MSN, CCRN
Clinical Nurse Specialist, Surgical and Intermediate Surgical Intensive Care Units, Thomas Jefferson University Hospital, Philadelphia, Pennsylvania

Susan K. Frazier, PhD, RN, CCRN
Assistant Professor, College of Nursing, Ohio State University, Columbus, Ohio

Polly E. Gardner, ARNP, ACNP, MN, CS, RN
Swedish Heart Institute, Seattle, Washington

Anna Gawlinski, RN, DNSc, CS-ACNP, CCRN
Clinical Nurse Specialist, University of California–Los Angeles Medical Center, Los Angeles, California; Associate Adjunct Professor, University of California–Los Angeles School of Nursing, Los Angeles, California

Karen K. Giuliano, RN, MSN, CCRN, ACNP
Critical Care Clinical Nurse Specialist, Baystate Medical Center, Springfield, MassachusettsDirector of Education, All Saints Health System, Forth Worth, Texas

Vicki Good, RN, MSN, CCRN
Director of Education, All Saints Health System, Fort Worth, Texas

Cynthia A. Goodrich, RN, MS, CCRN
Flight Nurse, Airlift Northwest, Seattle, Washington

Julie Gorveatt, RN, CCRN
Staff Nurse, Critical Care, Virginia Mason Medical Center, Seattle, Washington

Sheryl A. Greco, RN, MN, CCRN
Advanced Practice Nurse, Critical Care/Cardiac Services, Providence General Medical Center, Everett, Washington

Louise Grondin, MS, RN, CS
Clinical Nurse Specialist, Critical Care Medicine/Pulmonary, University of Michigan Hospitals and Health System, Ann Arbor, Michigan

Denise M. Guaglianone, RN, MSN, CCRN, APRN
Acute Care Nurse Practitioner for Cardiac Specialist, Yale University School of Nursing, Fairfield, Connecticut

Patricia Hanlon-Peña
International Product Manager, Arrow International, Everett, Massachusetts

Maureen Harrahill, RN, MS, ACNP-CS
Trauma Coordinator and Trauma Nurse Practitioner, Oregon Health Sciences University, Portland, Oregon

Robin Havrda, RN, CCRN
Principal Partner, Pacific Rim Health Care Consultants, Bellevue, Washington

Ann Marie Hayden, MSN, MBA, FNP, CCTC, RN
Education and Research Manager, Heart Valves, Medtronic, Inc, Minneapolis, Minnesota

Elizabeth I. Helvig, MS, RN, CWOCN
Burn-Plastic Clinical Nurse Specialist, Harborview Medical Center, Seattle, Washington

Lori Hendrickx, RN, EdD, CCRN
Associate Professor of Nursing, South Dakota State University, Brookings, South Dakota

Willemine Suzanne Hennessy, RN, MSN
Medical University of South Carolina, Charleston, South Carolina

Kathleen S. Hobson, RN, MS
Critical Care Clinical Nurse Specialist/Clinical Manager, Stevens Hospital, Edmonds, Washington

Jill T. Jesurum, RN, CCRN, CS
Cardiovascular Clinical Nurse Specialist, Swedish Medical Center and University of Washington School of Nursing, Seattle, Washington

Terry L. Jones, MS, RN
Nursing Education, Parkland Health and Hospital System, Dallas, Texas

Debra L. Joseph, RN
Vice President, Clinical Services, Datascope Corporation, Fairfield, New Jersey

Kathleen L. Julian, RN, MSN, MA, CCRN
Staff Nurse, Critical Care, Harborview Medical Center, Seattle, Washington

Gwen Emiko Kearly, RN, BSN, CCRN
Case Coordinator, University of Michigan Health System, Ann Arbor, Michigan

Mary Jo Kocan, RN, MSN, CNRN, CCRN
Clinical Nurse Specialist, Neurology/Neurosurgery, University of Michigan Health System, Ann Arbor, Michigan

Cheryl A. Koch, RN, ADN
St Joseph Hospital Medical Center, Reading, Pennsylvania

Julene B. Kruithof, MSN, RN, CCRN
Spectrum Health, Grand Rapids, Michigan

Barbara J. H. Kusisto, RN, BSN, CCRN
Case Manager, CHF Program, University of Michigan Health System, Ann Arbor, Michigan

Denise M. Lawrence, MS, ACNP, RN
Trauma/Surgery Acute Care Nurse Practitioner, Hartford Hospital, Hartford, Connecticut

Barbara Leeper, MN, RN, CCRN
Clinical Nurse Specialist, Cardiovascular Services, Baylor University Medical Center, Dallas, Texas

Marianne C. Lyons, RN, MS, CCRN
Clinical Manager, Georgetown University Medical Center, Washington, DC

Karen March, RN, MN, CNRN, CCRN
Director of Clinical Development, Integra Neurosciences, Plainsboro, New Jersey

Rhonda K. Martin, RN, MS, MLT (ASCP), CCRN, CNS/ANP-C
Nurse Practitioner/CNS—Abdominal Organ Transplant, University of California–San Diego Medical Center, San Diego, California

Suzanne A. Meader, ARNP, MN, CCRN, RN
Cardiovascular Nurse Practitioner, Overlake Hospital Medical Center, Bellevue, Washington

Carin Lea Mehan, RN, MS, ACNP
U.S. Education and Research Manager—Minimally Invasive Cardiac Surgery, Adjunct Faculty, University of Minnesota School of Nursing, Minneapolis, Minnesota

Debra K. Moser, DNSc, RN
Associate Professor, Ohio State University, Columbus, Ohio; Co-Editor, *The Journal of Cardiovascular Nursing*, Gaithersburg, Maryland

Donna Mower, RN, MS, CNRN, CS
Trauma Advanced Practice Nurse, Christiana Care Health Services, Newark, Delaware

Christopher Mroz, RN, RSN, CRNA
Veterans Administration Hospital, Grand Junction, Colorado

Nancy Munro, RN, MN, CCRN, ACNP
Acute Care Nurse Practitioner, Surgical Critical Care Services, Washington Hospital Center, Washington, DC

Alice M. Natke, RN, MS, CCRN
Clinical Nurse Specialist, Surgical Intensive Care Unit, Illinois Masonic Medical Center, Chicago, Illinois

Elizabeth M. Nolan, MS, RN, CS
Clinical Nurse Specialist, University of Michigan Health System, Ann Arbor, Michigan

Bianca L. Norman, RN
Case Manager, Nephrology Clinic, Group Health Cooperative, Seattle, Washington

Valerie Novotny-Dinsdale, RN, MSN, CEN
Clinical Nurse Specialist, Emergency Services, Northwest Hospital, Seattle, Washington

June Elizabeth Oliver, RN, BSN, CCRN
Clinical Nurse Specialist, Pain Management and Medical-Surgical Nursing, Illinois Masonic Medical Center, Chicago, Illinois

Maria Teresa Palleshi, RN, MSN, CCRN
Clinical Nurse Specialist, Harper Hospital, Detroit Medical Center, Detroit, Michigan

Mary O. Palazzo, RN, MS, CCRN
Director of Cardiovascular Services, Georgetown University Hospital, Washington, DC

Phyllis M.C. Patterson, MS, RN, CS, AOCN
Clinical Nurse Specialist, Hematology/Oncology, University of Michigan Health System, Ann Arbor, Michigan

Eileen E. Pysznik, RN, BS, CCRN
Educator, Intensive Care Unit, Baystate Medical Center, Springfield, Massachusetts

Patricia Jamison Reilly, MSN, RN
Regional Clinical Coordinator, Central Atlantic Region, Cardiovascular Division, Genentech, Inc.

Marti Reiser, RN, MSN, CCRN, CNS, NP-C
Nurse Practitioner, Patricio Aycinena, MD, Inc., Lorain, Ohio

Helen T. Roach, RN, MSN, CRNI, CCRN
Critical Care Clinical Educator, Georgetown University Medical Center, Washington, DC

Robert M. Rothwell, RN, MN, CCRN
Clinical Nurse Specialist/Surgical, VA Puget Sound Health Care System–Seattle, Seattle, Washington

Hildy Schell, RN, MS, CCRN
Clinical Nurse Specialist, Adult Critical Care, University of California–San Francisco Medical Center, UCSF Stanford Health Care; Assistant Clinical Professor, UCSF School of Nursing, San Francisco, California

Janice Schuette, RN, BSN, CCRN
Clinical Nurse III, University Hospital, University of Michigan, Ann Arbor, Michigan

Susan S. Scott, RN, BSN, CCRN
Critical Care Educator, Intensive Care Unit, Baystate Medical Center, Springfield, Massachusetts

Laura A. Shakarjian, BSN, RN
Educational Nurse Coordinator, University of Michigan Health System, Ann Arbor, Michigan

Robert E. St. John, RN, RRT, MSN, CCRN, CS
Respiratory Division, Mallinckrodt, Inc., St. Louis, Missouri

Debra Haas Stavarski, RN, MS
Manager, Clinical Support Services, Arrow International, Inc.

Karen Steffen, RN, MSN, CCRN, CNRN
Clinical Nurse Specialist, Neurosensory Intensive Care Unit, Intermediate Neurosensory Care Unit, Acute Stroke Unit, Thomas Jefferson University Hospital, Philadelphia, Pennsylvania

Diana May Studnick, MSN, RN, CCRN, CS
Acute Care Nurse Practitioner—Cardiac Surgery, University of Michigan, Ann Arbor, Michigan

Anne Marie Tallmadge, BSN, CCRN, RN
Clinical Nurse II, Coronary Intensive Care Unit, University of Michigan Health System, Ann Arbor, Michigan

Hilaire J. Thompson, RN, MSN, ACNP, CNRN
Clinical Nurse IV, Neuroscience Center of the Medical College of Virginia Hospitals, Richmond, Virginia

Barbara A. Todd, RN, MSN, CRNP
Director of Clinical Services, Temple University Hospital, Philadelphia, Pennsylvania

Marion Tolch, RN, BSN, CETN
Case Manager/Skin and Wound Care Nurse, University Hospital, Denver, Colorado

Barbara Ward, RN, MSN, CCRN
Manager, Intermountain Burn Center, University of Utah Hospital and Clinics, Salt Lake City, Utah

Janice M. Whitman, MSN, RN, CCRN
Advanced Practice Nurse, Providence Everett Medical Center, Everett, Washington

Michael L. Williams, MSN, RN, CCRN
Eastern Michigan University, Ypsilanti, Michigan

Sue Wingate, RN, DNSc, CS, CRNP
Cardiology Nurse Practitioner, Kaiser Permanente,
Rockville, Maryland

Charlene Adrienne Winters, DNSc, RN, CS
Assistant Professor, Montana State University, Bozeman
College of Nursing, Missoula Campus, Missoula,
Montana

Susan M. Wright, RN, BSN, CCRN
Educational Nurse Coordinator for the Thoracic and
Cardiac Intensive Care Units, University of Michigan
Health System, Ann Arbor, Michigan

Karen Yarbrough, MS, RN, CS, CCRN,
ACNP
Surgical Trauma Clinical Nurse Specialist, Christiana
Care Health Services, Newark, Delaware

Preface

As we begin the new millennium and a time of dramatic change in health care, it is with great pleasure that we present the fourth edition of the *AACN Procedure Manual for Critical Care*. The changes that our colleagues will find in this edition are a direct reflection of the knowledge and technology explosion that is rocketing us into the new century. Although we have made every attempt to capture current clinical practice, we recognize that critical care clinical practice is dynamic, and, therefore, any resource to support that practice must be considered a work in progress.

AACN is dedicated to the care of patients experiencing critical illness or injury and to the support of their families. AACN's vision is of a health care system driven by the needs of patients and their families, in which critical care nurses make their optimal contribution. Toward that vision, it is our hope that this edition of the *AACN Procedure Manual for Critical Care* will be a useful resource for critical care nurses in providing quality patient care.

The fourth edition of the *AACN Procedure Manual for Critical Care* will be an asset to practitioners across the spectrum of acute and critical care practice. The manual includes a comprehensive review and state-of-the-art information on acute and critical care procedures. In a significant change from the third edition, procedures not related specifically to critical care have been deleted, whereas procedures related to new and emerging advances in patient care have been added. With the increased presence of advanced practice nurses in critical care units, this edition of the *AACN Procedure Manual for Critical Care* contains not only procedures commonly performed by critical care nurses, but also procedures performed by advanced practice nurses. Because we recognize that the procedures included in this manual are only a portion of the repertoire needed by today's critical care practitioner to skillfully care for critically ill patients, we recommend that this manual be used in conjunction with *AACN Protocols for Practice*, *AACN's Clinical Reference for Critical Care Nurses*, and *AACN's Core Curriculum for Critical Care Nursing*.

This edition of the *AACN Procedure Manual for Critical Care* was redesigned to make it easier for the reader to locate and use procedures and the sections within each procedure. In an effort to provide high-quality care to seriously ill patients, we need resources that provide us with readily available "need to know" information. With that in mind, this edition has been organized using the following framework. The manual is organized in units, with most of the units having several sections. All procedures are designed using the same style, starting with a purpose. Following the purpose is the prerequisite nursing knowledge section, which includes information the nurse needs to know before performing the procedure. The equipment list includes equipment necessary to perform the procedure. Some of the procedures identify additional equipment that may be necessary based on individual patient situations. A patient and family education section identifies essential information that should be taught to patients and their families. The patient assessment and preparation section includes the specific assessment criteria that should be obtained before the procedure and discusses how the patient should be prepared for the procedure. The step-by-step procedure follows; it includes the rationale for each step and any special considerations. Associated research and appropriate figures and tables are included to enhance understanding of the procedure. Following the procedure is a list of expected and unexpected outcomes. The expected outcomes include the anticipated results of the procedure; the unexpected outcomes include potential complications or untoward outcomes of the procedure. The next section, patient monitoring, includes information related to assessments and interventions that should be completed. The rationale for each item is described, and conditions that should be reported if they persist despite nursing interventions are identified. A documentation section follows that describes what should be documented after the procedure is performed. Lastly, references used within the procedures and recommended additional readings are included.

Given the nature of critical care, many of the included procedures use electrical equipment. This manual makes the assumption that all equipment is maintained by your institution's bioengineering department according to accepted national and state regulations for individual pieces of equipment.

As nursing professionals, our quest to have our practice driven by research has never been greater. For the first time, this edition of the *AACN Procedure Manual for Critical Care* includes a research-based leveling system. As available, this information is provided to indicate the research-based strength of recommendation for various interventions. The research-based leveling system is the same one used for *AACN's Protocols for Practice* and includes

Level I: Manufacturer's recommendations only

Level II: Theory based, no research data to support recommendations; recommendations from expert consensus group may exist

Level III: Laboratory data only, no clinical data to support recommendations

Level IV: Limited clinical studies to support recommendations

Level V: Clinical studies in more than one or two different patient populations and situations to support recommendations

Level VI: Clinical studies in a variety of patient populations and situations to support recommendations

Although we believe that this leveling system is a major step forward in promoting research-based practice, the paucity of research available in many procedures also speaks loudly to the need for further investigation.

Acknowledgments

This text could not have been designed or developed without help from a number of people. First, we would like to thank AACN for giving us the opportunity to coedit this endeavor. We would especially like to thank Ellen French, AACN's director of publications, for believing in us and dedicating incredible energy to making this book a success. Ellen made numerous essential contributions to the development of the fourth edition of the *AACN Procedure Manual for Critical Care.*

We would also like to thank a number of key people at W.B. Saunders for their support and hard work through this entire project. We are extremely grateful to have worked closely with Thomas Eoyang, our editor at W.B. Saunders. Thomas has been a driving force behind many of AACN's publications, and we appreciate the opportunity to have worked with a man of his leadership in the publishing field. We also would like to thank our editorial assistants, Adrienne Simon and her predecessor, Gina Hopf, for keeping the progress of the text so organized. Adrienne's attention to detail and enthusiasm enhanced the publishing process. We extend a grateful thank-you to Frank Polizzano, our production manager; to Jennifer Ehlers for her excellent work in copy editing; and to Lisa Lambert for coordinating the text's illustrations. A special thank-you is owed to Ellen Zanolle, who designed the book and our cover. Without the creative, hard-working team at W.B. Saunders, our text would not have been possible.

A simple thank-you is inadequate for our clinical care colleagues, the experts in our field, who made this book a reality. Their hard work and efforts to produce high-quality, well-researched procedures will have a long-lasting effect on critical care practice for years to come. As well, we are indebted to our colleagues who served as procedure reviewers. We thank you for taking the time to critically review each procedure and to support our efforts to promote excellence. In addition, we would like to thank the AACN volunteers and volunteer groups who provided early reviews of our Table of Contents.

Lastly, yet very importantly, we would like to thank those close to us who provided personal support. Debra would like to thank her mother and father for their solid foundation and love, thank Jim for his everlasting love and support, and thank Michael for keeping her grounded in life's priorities. Karen would like to thank her mom, whose years of compassionate bedside nursing helped her to see what being a nurse is really all about; thank her critical care colleagues and friends across the country, especially in the Pacific Northwest, for their incredible support when personal trials attempted to overshadow this professional endeavor; thank Sandy Schutz for her friendship and willingness to do whatever was needed to make this book happen; thank Jim, whose love and support makes every day a better day; and thank Daniel and Katie, who helped her remember that whatever life brings is a God-given blessing.

DEBRA J. LYNN-MCHALE
KAREN K. CARLSON

Contents

UNIT **1**

Pulmonary System 1

SECTION **1**
Airway Management   1

1 Performing Endotracheal Intubation **AP**   1
Cindy Goodrich

2 Assisting with Endotracheal Intubation   11
Julianne M. Deutsch

3 Endotracheal Tube Care   17
Julianne M. Deutsch

4 Performing Extubation and Decannulation **AP**   21
Kay Knox Greenlee

5 Assisting with Extubation and Decannulation   24
Kay Knox Greenlee

6 Nasopharyngeal Airway Insertion   27
Kay Knox Greenlee

7 Oropharyngeal Airway Insertion   31
Kay Knox Greenlee

8 Oxygen Tank Preparation and Setup   37
Sandra L. Schutz

9 Endotracheal or Tracheostomy Tube
Suctioning   41
Marianne Chulay

10 Tracheal Tube Cuff Care   49
Kay Knox Greenlee

11 Tracheostomy Tube Care   56
Kay Knox Greenlee

SECTION **2**
Special Pulmonary Procedures   64

12 Continuous End-Tidal Carbon Dioxide
Monitoring   64
Vicki S. Good

13 Continuous Mixed Venous Oxygen Saturation
Monitoring   71
Jan M. Headley

14 Oxygen Saturation Monitoring by Pulse
Oximetry   77
Sandra L. Schutz

15 Manual Pronation Therapy   83
Kathleen M. Vollman

SECTION **3**
Thoracic Cavity Management   95

16 Autotransfusion   95
Julianne M. Deutsch

17 Performing Chest Tube Placement **AP**   99
Denise M. Lawrence

18 Assisting with Chest Tube Placement   109
Catherine Freismuth Robinson

19 Chest Tube Removal **AP**   117
Peggy Kirkwood

20 Assisting with Chest Tube Removal   123
Catherine Freismuth Robinson

21 Closed Chest Drainage System   127
Catherine Freismuth Robinson

22 Performing Needle Thoracostomy **AP**   141
Cindy Goodrich

23 Performing Thoracentesis **AP**   145
William Barefoot

24 Assisting with Thoracentesis   151
William Barefoot and Karen K. Carlson

SECTION **4**
Ventilatory Management   155

25 Arterial-Venous Oxygen Difference
Calculation   155
Suzanne M. Burns

26 Auto-PEEP Calculation   158
Suzanne M. Burns

27 Measurement of Compliance and Resistance   161
Suzanne M. Burns

28 Manual Self-Inflating Resuscitation Bag   164
Suzanne M. Burns

29 Indices of Oxygenation: Alveolar-Arterial Oxygen Difference, Partial Pressure of Arterial Oxygenation to Fraction of Inspired Oxygen Ratio, Partial Pressure of Arterial Oxygen to Alveolar Oxygen Ratio   170
Suzanne M. Burns

30 Shunt Calculation   175
Suzanne M. Burns

31 Ventilatory Management—Volume and Pressure Modes   178
Suzanne M. Burns

32 Standard Weaning Criteria: Negative Inspiratory Pressure, Positive Expiratory Pressure, Spontaneous Tidal Volume, and Vital Capacity   191
Suzanne M. Burns

33 Weaning Procedure   196
Suzanne M. Burns

UNIT II

Cardiovascular System 205

SECTION **5**
Cardiac Emergencies   205

34 Automated External Defibrillation   205
Charlotte A. Green and Karen K. Carlson

35 Cardioversion   211
Cynthia Hambach

36 Defibrillation (External)   219
Virginia Wilson

37 Defibrillation (Internal)   224
Joan M. Vitello-Cicciu, Christine Moriarty, and Kellie Smith

38 Emergent Open Sternotomy (Perform) **AP**   229
Deborah G. LaMarr

39 Emergent Open Sternotomy (Assist)   234
Deborah G. LaMarr

40 Pericardiocentesis (Assist)   238
Ann Louise Jones

SECTION **6**
Cardiac Pacemakers   243

41 Atrial Electrogram   243
Teresa Preuss and Debra J. Lynn-McHale

42 Overdrive Atrial Pacing **AP**   251
Carol Jacobson

43 Implantable Cardioverter-Defibrillator   257
Cathy M. Martin, Patricia Gonce Morton, and Michael A. Nace

44 Permanent Pacemaker (Assessing Function)   264
Francine E. Paschall and Ellen Strauss McErlean

45 Temporary Transcutaneous (External) Pacing   271
Francine E. Paschall and Ellen Strauss McErlean

46 Temporary Transvenous Pacemaker Insertion (Perform) **AP**   278
Deborah E. Becker

47 Temporary Transvenous and Epicardial Pacing   285
Francine E. Paschall and Ellen Strauss McErlean

SECTION **7**
Circulatory Assist Devices   299

48 Intra-aortic Balloon Pump Management   299
Debra J. Lynn-McHale

49 External Counterpressure with Pneumatic Antishock Garments   315
Denise M. Lawrence

50 Ventricular Assist Devices   320
Lee Ann Ruess

SECTION **8**
Electrocardiographic Leads and Cardiac Monitoring   329

51 Electrophysiologic Monitoring: Hardwire and Telemetry   329
Mary G. McKinley

52 Extra Electrocardiographic Leads: Right Precordial and Left Posterior Leads   338
Shu-Fen Wung and Barbara J. Drew

53 ST Segment Monitoring   349
Michele M. Pelter and Mary G. Adams

54 Twelve-Lead Electrocardiogram   354
Mary G. McKinley

SECTION **9**
Hemodynamic Monitoring   361

55 Arterial Catheter Insertion (Perform) **AP**   361
Deborah E. Becker

56 Arterial Catheter Insertion (Assist), Care and Removal   367
Rose B. Shaffer

57 Blood Sampling from Arterial Pressure Lines   379
Rose B. Shaffer

58 Blood Sampling from Pulmonary Artery Line   385
Teresa Preuss and Debra J. Lynn-McHale

59 Cardiac Output Measurement Techniques (Invasive)   389
Kathleen Ahern Gould, Colette Hartigan, and Suzanne Farley Keane

60 Central Venous/Right Atrial Pressure Line
Removal 401
Marie Arnone

61 Central Venous/Right Atrial Pressure Line
Site Care 405
Marie Arnone

62 Central Venous/Right Atrial Pressure
Monitoring 408
Marie Arnone

63 Left Atrial Pressure Line, Care and Assisting
with Removal 415
Joan M. Vitello-Cicciu and Donna Rosborough

64 Noninvasive Hemodynamic Monitoring:
Impedance Cardiography 421
Kathryn T. Von Rueden

65 Pulmonary Artery Catheter Insertion
(Perform) **AP** 431
Desiree A. Fleck

66 Pulmonary Artery Catheter Insertion (Assist)
and Pressure Monitoring 439
Debra J. Lynn-McHale and Teresa Preuss

67 Pulmonary Artery Pressure Line, Removal 457
Teresa Preuss and Debra J. Lynn-McHale

68 Pulmonary Artery Pressure Lines,
Troubleshooting 461
Debra J. Lynn-McHale and Teresa Preuss

69 Single and Multiple Pressure Transducer
Systems 472
Marie Arnone

SECTION **10**
Special Cardiac Procedures 484

70 Arterial and Venous Sheath Removal **AP** 484
Amy L. Schueler and Rose B. Shaffer

71 Pericardial Catheter Management 490
Kathy McCloy

SECTION **11**
Vascular Access 496

72 Arterial Puncture **AP** 496
Linda Bucher

73 Central Venous Catheter Insertion
(Perform) **AP** 503
Desiree A. Fleck

74 Central Venous Catheter Insertion (Assist) 514
Marie Arnone

75 Peripheral Intravenous Line Insertion 522
Linda Bucher

76 Peripherally Inserted Central Catheter **AP** 533
Linda Bucher

77 Venipuncture 543
Linda Bucher

UNIT **III**
Neurologic System 551

SECTION **12**
Neurologic Monitoring 551

78 Intracranial Bolt Insertion (Assist),
Monitoring, Care, Troubleshooting, and
Removal 551
Jacqueline Sullivan

79 Intraventricular Catheter Insertion (Assist),
Monitoring, Care, Troubleshooting, and
Removal 561
Jacqueline Sullivan

80 Jugular Venous Oxygen Saturation
Monitoring: Insertion (Assist), Care,
Troubleshooting, and Removal 570
Jacqueline Sullivan

81 Transcranial Doppler Monitoring **AP** 580
Anne W. Wojner and Andrei V. Alexandrov

SECTION **13**
Special Neurologic Procedures 588

82 Cerebrospinal Fluid Drainage Assessment 588
Phyllis Dubendorf

83 External Warming/Cooling Devices 591
Eileen M. Kelly

84 Iced Caloric Testing for Vestibular Function
(Assist) 598
Phyllis Dubendorf

85 Lumbar Puncture (Perform) **AP** 602
Anne W. Wojner and Marc Malkoff

86 Lumbar and Cisternal Punctures (Assist) 608
Phyllis Dubendorf

87 Lumbar Subarachnoid Catheter Insertion
(Assist) for Cerebral Spinal Fluid Pressure
Monitoring and Drainage 613
Jacqueline Sullivan

SECTION **14**
Traction Management 620

88 External Fixation Device Insertion (Assist) 620
Joanne V. Hickey

89 Halo Traction Care 625
Joanne V. Hickey

90 Tong and Pin Care 631
Joanne V. Hickey

91 Traction Maintenance 634
Joanne V. Hickey

SECTION **15**
Pain Management   639

92 Pain Management Using Epidural Catheters   639
        Robyn Dealtry
93 Peripheral Nerve Stimulators   647
        Janet G. Whetstone Foster

UNIT **IV**
Gastrointestinal System   655
94 Esophagogastric Tamponade Tube   655
        Michael W. Day
95 Gastric Lavage in Hemorrhage and in
        Overdose   664
        Robin H. Thomas
96 Intra-abdominal Pressure Monitoring   674
        John J. Gallagher
97 Orogastric and Nasogastric Tube Insertion,
        Care, and Removal   681
        Karen K. Carlson
98 Performing Abdominal Paracentesis **AP** 689
        Peggy Kirkwood
99 Assisting with Abdominal Paracentesis   694
        Peggy Kirkwood and Karen K. Carlson
100 Performing Percutaneous Peritoneal
        Lavage **AP**   698
        Peggy Kirkwood
101 Assisting with Percutaneous Peritoneal
        Lavage   705
        Peggy Kirkwood and Karen K. Carlson
102 Scleral Endoscopic Therapy   711
        Robin H. Thomas

UNIT **V**
Renal System   717

SECTION **16**
Renal Replacement   717

103 Continuous Renal Replacement Therapies   717
        Karen K. Giuliano
104 Hemodialysis   733
        Karen K. Giuliano
105 Peritoneal Dialysis   746
        Karen K. Giuliano

SECTION **17**
Special Renal Replacement   753

106 Assisting with Plasmapheresis   753
        Karen K. Giuliano

UNIT **VI**
Hematologic System   757

SECTION **18**
Fluid Management   757

107 Blood and Blood Component
        Administration   757
        Maribeth Wooldridge-King
108 Blood Pump Use   765
        Maribeth Wooldridge-King
109 Continuous Arteriovenous Rewarming   768
        Christine S. Schulman
110 Rapid Infuser for Massive Fluid
        Resuscitation   777
        Christine S. Schulman
111 Transfusion Reaction Management   786
        Maribeth Wooldridge-King

SECTION **19**
Special Hematologic Procedures   791

112 Bone Marrow Biopsy and Aspiration
        (Perform) **AP**   791
        Dolores Grosso
113 Bone Marrow Biopsy and Aspiration
        (Assist)   797
        Dolores Grosso
114 Determination of Microhematocrit via
        Centrifuge   801
        Maribeth Wooldridge-King

UNIT **VII**
Integumentary System   805

SECTION **20**
Burn Wound Management   805

115 Care of Donor Sites   805
        Eileen E. Pysznik
116 Care of Burn Wounds   811
        Eileen E. Pysznik
117 Care of Skin Grafts   822
        Eileen E. Pysznik

SECTION **21**
Special Integumentary Procedures   828

118 Intracompartment Pressure Monitoring   828
        John J. Gallagher and Shawn McCabe

119 Pressure-Reducing Devices: Lateral
Rotation Therapy   837
*Nancy L. Tomaselli, Margaret T. Goldberg, and
Sandi Wind*

120 Suturing **AP**   843
Peggy Kirkwood

SECTION **22**
Wound Management   851

121 Cleansing, Irrigating, Culturing, and
Dressing Open Wounds   851
Mary Beth Flynn

122 Dressing Wounds with Drains   859
Mary Beth Flynn

123 Drain Removal   863
Mary Beth Flynn

124 Dressing and Pouching Draining Wounds   865
Mary Beth Flynn

UNIT **VIII**

Nutrition   868

125 Enteral Nutrition   868
Deborah C. Stamps

126 Parenteral Nutrition   877
Mary Donahue

127 Gastrostomy or Jejunostomy Tube Care   883
Margaret M. Ecklund

128 Small-Bore Feeding Tube Insertion   888
Margaret M. Ecklund

UNIT **IX**

End of Life   892

129 Advance Directives   892
Barbara B. Ott

130 Determination of Death **AP**   897
Jacqueline Sullivan

131 Care of the Organ Donor   907
June Hinkle

132 Indentification of Potential Organ Donors   910
June Hinkle

133 Request for Organ Donation   914
June Hinkle

134 Withholding/Withdrawing Life-Sustaining
Treatment   917
Debra J. Lynn-McHale and Margaret M. Mahon

UNIT **X**

Calculating Medication Doses   922

135 Calculating Doses, Flow Rates, and
Administration of Continuous Intravenous
Infusions   922
Barbara A. Brown

Index   927

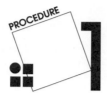

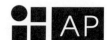

Performing Endotracheal Intubation

P U R P O S E: Endotracheal intubation is performed to establish and maintain a patent airway, facilitate oxygenation and ventilation, reduce the risk of aspiration, and assist with the clearance of secretions.

Cindy Goodrich

PREREQUISITE NURSING KNOWLEDGE

- Anatomy and physiology of the pulmonary system should be understood.
- Indications for endotracheal intubation include the following[1]:
  ❖ Upper airway obstruction (eg, secondary to swelling, trauma, tumor, bleeding)
  ❖ Apnea
  ❖ Ineffective clearance of secretions (eg, inability to adequately maintain airway)
  ❖ High risk of aspiration
  ❖ Respiratory distress
- Pulse oximetry should be used during intubation so that oxygen desaturation can be quickly detected.
- Preoxygenation with 100% oxygen using a bag-valve-mask device with a tight-fitting face mask should be performed for 3 to 5 minutes before intubation.
- Intubation attempts should take no longer than 15 to 30 seconds.
- Applying cricoid pressure (Sellick maneuver) may decrease the incidence of pulmonary aspiration and gastric distention. This procedure is accomplished by applying firm, downward pressure on the cricoid ring, pushing the vocal cords downward so they are more easily visualized. Once begun, cricoid pressure must be maintained until intubation is completed (Fig. 1–1).[2]

- Two types of laryngoscope blades exist, straight and curved. The straight blade (Miller blade) is designed so that the tip extends below the epiglottis, lifting and exposing the glottic opening. It is recommended for use in obese patients and in those with short necks because their tracheas may be more anteriorly located. When a curved blade (Macintosh blade) is used, the tip is advanced into the vallecula (the space between the epiglottis and the base of the tongue), exposing the glottic opening.
- Endotracheal tube size reflects the size of the internal diameter of the tube. Tubes range in size from 2.0 mm

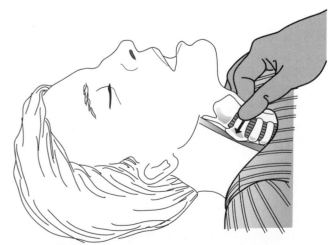

■ ● FIGURE 1–1. Cricoid pressure. Firm downward pressure on the cricoid ring pushes the vocal cords downward toward the field of vision while at the same time sealing the esophagus against the vertebral column.

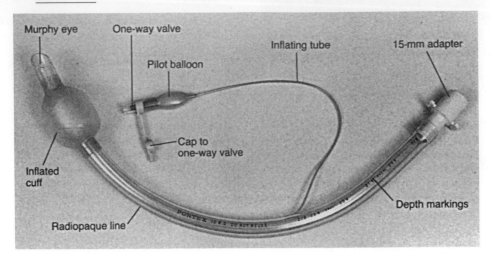

■ ● FIGURE 1–2. Parts of the endotracheal tube (soft-cuffed tube by Smiths Industries Medical Systems, Co., Valencia, Ca). (From Kersten LD. *Comprehensive Respiratory Nursing.* Philadelphia, Pa: WB Saunders; 1989:637.)

Labels on figure: Murphy eye, One-way valve, Pilot balloon, Inflating tube, 15-mm adapter, Cap to one-way valve, Inflated cuff, Radiopaque line, Depth markings

for neonates to 9.0 mm for large adults; the correct size is based on patient weight. 7.5- to 8.0-mm tubes are commonly used for average-sized adult women, while average-sized adult men receive an 8.0- to 9.0-mm tube (Fig. 1–2).[1] The tube with the largest clinically acceptable internal diameter should be used to minimize airway resistance and assist with suctioning.

- Endotracheal intubation can be done via nasal or oral routes. The skill of the practitioner performing intubation, as well as the patient's clinical condition, determines the route used.
- Nasal intubation is relatively contraindicated in the trauma patient with facial fractures or suspected fractures at the base of the skull.
- In patients with suspected spinal cord injuries, in-line cervical immobilization of the head must be maintained during endotracheal intubation.
- Improper intubation technique may result in trauma to the teeth, the soft tissues of the mouth or nose, the vocal cords, and the posterior pharynx.
- A disposable end-tidal carbon dioxide (CO_2) detector may be used to assist with identification of proper endotracheal tube placement. This device is chemically treated with a nontoxic indicator that changes color in the presence of CO_2, indicating that the endotracheal tube has been successfully placed into the trachea.
- Double-lumen endotracheal tubes are used for independent lung ventilation in situations where there is bleeding of one lung or a large air leak that would impair ventilation of the good lung.
- The endotracheal tube also provides a route for the administration of emergency medication (ie, lidocaine, epinephrine, atropine, and naloxone).

EQUIPMENT

- Personal protective equipment
- Endotracheal tube with intact cuff and 15-mm connector (Adult female 7.5- to 8.0-mm tube, adult male 8.0- to 9.0-mm tube)[1]
- Laryngoscope handle with fresh batteries
- Laryngoscope blades (straight or curved)
- Spare bulb for laryngoscope blades

- Flexible stylet
- Self-inflating resuscitation bag with mask connected to 100% oxygen
- Oxygen source and connecting tubes
- Swivel adapter
- Nonsterile gloves
- Luer-tip 10-mL syringe for cuff inflation
- Water-soluble lubricant
- Rigid pharyngeal suction-tip (Yankauer) catheter
- Suction apparatus (portable or wall)
- Suction catheters
- Bite-block or oropharyngeal airway
- Endotracheal tube–securing apparatus or appropriate tape
  ❖ Adhesive tape (6 to 8 in long)
  ❖ Twill tape (cut into 30-in lengths)
- Stethoscope

Additional equipment (to have available depending on patient need or practitioner preference) includes the following:

- Anesthetic spray (nasal approach)
- Local anesthetic jelly (nasal approach)
- Sedating or paralyzing medications
- Magill forceps (to remove foreign bodies obstructing the airway)
- Ventilator

PATIENT AND FAMILY EDUCATION

- Assess level of understanding about condition and rationale for endotracheal intubation. ➤*Rationale:* Identifies patient and family knowledge deficits concerning patient condition, procedure, expected benefits, and potential risks; allows time for questions to clarify information and voice concerns. Explanations decrease patient anxiety and enhance cooperation.
- Explain the procedure and the reason for intubation. ➤*Rationale:* Enhances patient and family understanding and decreases anxiety.
- If indicated, explain patient's role in assisting with insertion of endotracheal tube. ➤*Rationale:* Assists with insertion by eliciting patient's cooperation.

- Explain that patient will be unable to speak while the endotracheal tube is in place but that other means of communication will be provided. ➤*Rationale:* Enhances patient and family understanding and decreases anxiety.
- Explain that the patient's hands are often immobilized to prevent accidental dislodgment of the tube. ➤*Rationale:* Enhances patient and family understanding and decreases anxiety.

PATIENT ASSESSMENT AND PREPARATION
Patient Assessment

- Immediate history of trauma when spinal cord injury is suspected. ➤*Rationale:* Knowing pertinent patient history will allow for selection of the most appropriate method for intubation, helping reduce the risk for secondary injury.
- Nothing-by-mouth (NPO) status or signs of gastric distension, or both. ➤*Rationale:* Increased risk of aspiration and vomiting occurs with accumulation of air, food, or secretions. If a patient who has gastric distention or who has recently eaten needs to be intubated, use of cricoid pressure will decrease the risk of aspiration.
- Level of consciousness, level of anxiety, and respiratory difficulty. ➤*Rationale:* Determines need for sedation or use of paralytic agents and patient's ability to lie flat and supine for intubation.
- Patency of nares (for nasal intubation). ➤*Rationale:* Selection of the most appropriate nare will facilitate insertion and may improve patient tolerance of tube.
- Need for premedication. ➤*Rationale:* Various medications will allow for sedation or paralysis of the agitated patient.

Patient Preparation

- Ensure that patient understands preprocedural teaching. Answer questions as they arise, and reinforce information as needed. ➤*Rationale:* Evaluates and reinforces understanding of previously taught information.
- Before intubation, initiate intravenous (IV) access. ➤*Rationale:* Readily available IV access may be necessary if the patient needs to be sedated or paralyzed or needs other medications should the patient have a negative response to the intubation procedure.

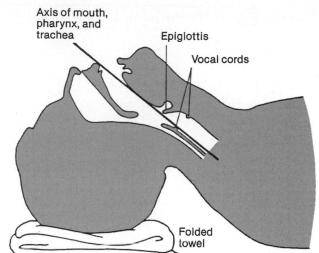

■ ● FIGURE 1–3. Neck hyperextension in the sniffing position aligns the axis of the mouth, pharynx, and trachea before endotracheal intubation. (From Kersten LD. *Comprehensive Respiratory Nursing.* Philadelphia, Pa: WB Saunders; 1989:642.)

- Position the patient appropriately.
  ❖ Positioning of the nontrauma patient is as follows: Place patient supine with head in sniffing position, in which the head is extended and the neck is flexed. Placement of a small towel under the occiput will elevate it several inches, allowing for proper flexion of the neck (Fig. 1–3). ➤*Rationale:* Placing the head in the sniffing position will allow for visualization of the larynx and vocal cords by aligning the axes of the mouth, pharynx, and trachea.
  ❖ Positioning of the trauma patient is as follows: In-line cervical spinal immobilization must be maintained during the entire process of intubation. ➤*Rationale:* Because cervical spinal cord injury must be suspected in all trauma patients until proven otherwise, this position will help prevent secondary injury should a cervical spine injury be present.
- Premedicate as indicated. ➤*Rationale:* Appropriate premedication will allow for more controlled intubation, reducing the incidence of insertion trauma, aspiration, laryngospasm, and improper tube placement.

Procedure for Performing Endotracheal Intubation		
Steps	**Rationale**	**Special Considerations**
General Setup		
1. Wash hands, and don personal protective equipment.	Reduces transmission of microorganisms and body secretions; standard precautions.	Protective eyewear should be worn to avoid exposure to secretions. *Procedure continued on following page*

Procedure	for Performing Endotracheal Intubation *Continued*

Steps	Rationale	Special Considerations
2. Insert oropharyngeal airway (see Procedure 7).	Assists in maintaining upper airway patency.	Use only in unconscious patients.
3. Set up suction apparatus, and connect rigid suction-tip catheter to tubing.	Prepares for oropharyngeal suctioning as needed.	
4. Check equipment.		
A. Use syringe to inflate cuff on tube, assessing for leaks. Completely deflate cuff.	Verifies that equipment is functional and that tube cuff is patent without leaks. Prepares tube for insertion.	Stylet must be recessed by at least 0.5 in from the distal end of the tube so that it does not protrude beyond the end of the tube, resulting in damage to the vocal cords and trachea.
B. Insert the stylet into the endotracheal tube, ensuring that the tip of the stylet does not extend past the end of the endotracheal tube.		
C. Check the laryngoscope batteries.		
5. Position the patient's head by flexing the neck forward and extending the head (sniffing position) (only if neck trauma is not suspected) (see Fig. 1–3).	Will allow for visualization of the vocal cords by aligning the three axes of the mouth, pharynx, and trachea.	Placement of a small towel under the occiput will elevate it, allowing for proper neck flexion. Do not flex or extend neck of patient with suspected spinal cord injury; the head must be maintained in a neutral position with in-line cervical spine immobilization.
6. Check the mouth for dentures and remove if present. Suction the mouth as needed.	Dentures should be removed before oral intubation is attempted but may remain in place for nasal intubation.	
7. Preoxygenate using a self-inflating bag-valve-mask (see Procedure 28) device attached to 100% oxygen for 3 to 5 minutes. Provide frequent and gentle breaths.	Helps prevent hypoxemia. Gentle breaths reduce incidence of air entering stomach (leading to gastric distention), decrease airway turbulence, and more evenly distribute ventilation within the lungs.	
8. Premedicate patient as indicated. For nasotracheal intubation, proceed to step 28.		

Orotracheal Intubation

Steps	Rationale	Special Considerations
9. Grasp laryngoscope (with blade in place and illuminated light on) in left hand.	Prepares for efficient blade placement.	Grasp handle as low as possible and keep wrist rigid to prevent using upper teeth as a fulcrum.
10. Open the patient's mouth using the crossed-finger technique.	Provides access to oral cavity.	
11. Slowly insert the blade into the right side of the patient's mouth, using it to push the tongue to the left (Fig. 1–4). Advance the blade inward and toward midline past the base of the tongue.	Displaces the tongue to the left, increasing visualization of the glottic opening (Fig. 1–5).	Avoids pressure on the teeth and lips.
12. Advance the blade.		
A. Using a curved blade, advance tip into vallecula and exert outward and upward gentle traction at a 45-degree angle to the bed (Fig. 1–6).	Exposes the glottic opening.	Keep left arm and back straight when pulling upward, allowing for use of shoulders when lifting patient's head (will decrease use of teeth as a fulcrum).
B. Using a straight blade, advance tip just beneath the epiglottis and exert gentle traction outward and upward at a 45-degree angle to the bed.	Exposes the glottic opening.	Keep left arm and back straight when pulling upward, allowing for use of shoulders when lifting patient's head (will decrease use of teeth as a fulcrum).

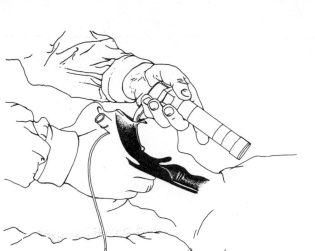

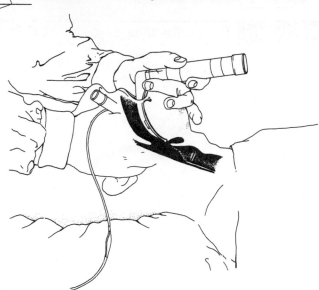

■ ● **FIGURE 1–4.** Technique of orotracheal intubation. Laryngoscope blade is inserted into oral cavity from the right, pushing tongue to the left as it is introduced.

■ ● **FIGURE 1–5.** Blade is advanced into oropharynx, and laryngoscope is lifted to expose the epiglottis.

Procedure | **for Performing Endotracheal Intubation** *Continued*

Steps	Rationale	Special Considerations
13. Lift the laryngoscope handle until the vocal cords are visualized.	Allows for correct placement of tube into trachea.	Gentle cricoid pressure (see Fig. 1–1) may assist in visualization of vocal cords and decrease risk of gastric distention and subsequent pulmonary aspiration. Once cricoid pressure is begun, it must be continued until the tube is correctly placed.
14. Hold end of tube in right hand with the curved portion downward.	Tube is placed by the right hand.	

Procedure continued on following page

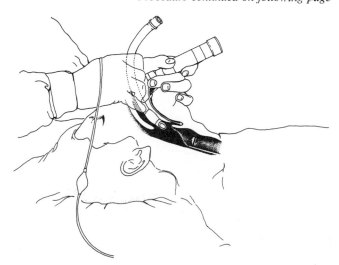

■ ● **FIGURE 1–6.** Tip of blade is placed in vallecula, and laryngoscope is lifted further to expose glottis. The tube is inserted through the right side of the mouth.

▦ AP This procedure should be performed only by physicians, advanced practice nurses, and other health care professionals (including critical care nurses) with additional knowledge, skills, and demonstrated competence per professional licensure or institutional standard.

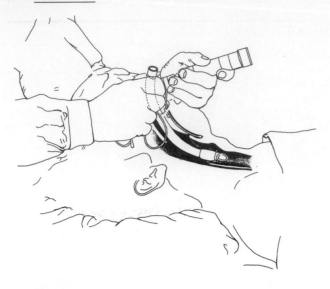

■ ● **FIGURE 1–7.** Tube is advanced through vocal cords into trachea.

Procedure	for Performing Endotracheal Intubation *Continued*

Steps	Rationale	Special Considerations
15. Under direct vision, gently insert tube from right corner of mouth through the vocal cords (Fig. 1–7) until the cuff is no longer visible (Fig. 1–8).	Must see tube pass through the vocal cords to ensure proper placement.	If intubation is unsuccessful within 30 seconds, remove the tube. Ventilate with 100% oxygen using a bag-valve-mask device before another intubation attempt is made (repeat steps 9 through 15).
16. Once tube is correctly placed, continue to hold it securely in place with right hand while withdrawing the laryngoscope blade and the stylet using left hand.	Firmly holding tube provides stabilization and prevents inadvertent extubation.	
17. Inflate cuff with 5 to 10 mL of air depending on the manufacturer's recommendation (see Procedure 10). *(Level IV: Limited clinical studies to support recommendations)*	Inflation volumes will vary depending on manufacturer and size of tube. Keep cuff pressures between 20 and 25 mm Hg to decrease risk of aspiration and prevent ischemia and decreased blood flow.[1-3]	Capillary blood flow in the tracheal mucosa is approximately 18 to 30 mm Hg. Mucosal ischemia may occur when lateral wall pressure exceeds capillary blood flow.
18. Confirm endotracheal tube placement while manually bagging with 100% oxygen.	Ensures correct placement of the endotracheal tube.	
A. Attach disposable CO_2 detector (if available). Watch for color change, indicating the presence of CO_2. *(Level IV: Limited clinical studies to support recommendations)*	Disposable CO_2 detectors may be used to assist with identification of proper tube placement.[2, 4, 5]	CO_2 detectors are usually placed between the self-inflating bag and the endotracheal tube. CO_2 detectors should be used in conjunction with physical assessment findings.

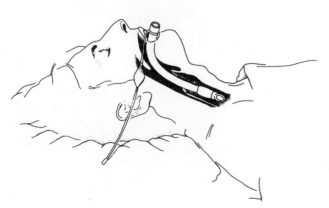

■ ● **FIGURE 1–8.** Tube is positioned so that cuff is below vocal cords, and laryngoscope is removed.

Procedure **for Performing Endotracheal Intubation** *Continued*

Steps	Rationale	Special Considerations
B. Auscultate over epigastrium. *(Level II: Theory based, no research data to support recommendations; recommendations from expert consensus group may exist)*	Allows for identification of esophageal intubation.[2, 4, 5]	If air movement or gurgling is heard, esophageal intubation has occurred. The tube must be pulled and intubation reattempted. Improper insertion may result in hypoxemia, gastric distention, vomiting, and aspiration.
C. Auscultate lung bases and apices for bilateral breath sounds. *(Level II: Theory based, no research data to support recommendations; recommendations from expert consensus group may exist)*	Assists in verification of correct tube placement into the trachea. A right main stem bronchus intubation will result in diminished left-sided breath sounds.[2, 4, 5]	Equal breath sounds will indicate proper placement of the endotracheal tube.
D. Observe for symmetric chest wall movement. *(Level II: Theory based, no research data to support recommendations; recommendations from expert consensus group may exist)*	Assists in verification of correct tube placement.[2, 4, 5]	Absence may indicate right main stem or esophageal intubation.
E. Evaluate oxygen saturation (SpO_2) by noninvasive pulse oximetry. *(Level II: Theory based, no research data to support recommendations; recommendations from expert consensus group may exist)*	SpO_2 will fall if the esophagus has been inadvertently intubated. It may or may not change in a right main stem bronchus intubation.[2, 4, 5]	SpO_2 findings should be used in conjunction with physical assessment findings.
19. If CO_2 detection, assessment findings, or SpO_2 reveals that the tube has not been correctly positioned, deflate cuff and remove tube immediately. Hyperoxygenate with 100% oxygen for 3 to 5 minutes, and then reattempt intubation, beginning with the first step. *(Level II: Theory based, no research data to support recommendations; recommendations from expert consensus group may exist)*	Esophageal intubation results in gas flow diversion and hypoxemia.[2, 3]	
20. If breath sounds are absent on the left, deflate the cuff and withdraw tube 1 to 2 cm. Reevaluate for correct tube placement (step 18).	Absence of breath sounds on the left may indicate right main stem intubation, which is common because of the anatomic position of the right main stem bronchi. When correctly positioned, the tube tip should be 1.0 to 2.5 cm below the trachea.[4]	
21. Connect endotracheal tube to oxygen source or mechanical ventilator, using swivel adapter.	Reduces motion on tube and mouth or nares.	
22. Insert a bite block or oropharyngeal airway (to act as a bite block) along the endotracheal tube.	Prevents the patient from biting down on the endotracheal tube.	The bite block should be secured separately from the tube to prevent dislodgment of the tube. *Procedure continued on following page*

Steps	Rationale	Special Considerations
23. Secure the endotracheal tube in place (according to institutional standard). *(Level II: Theory based, no research data to support recommendations; recommendations from expert consensus group may exist)*	Prevents inadvertent dislodgment of tube.[1-3, 6]	Various methods are used for securing endotracheal tubes including the use of specially manufactured tube holders, twill tape, or adhesive tape.
Use of Twill Tape		
A. Double over a 2-ft length of twill tape; tie the tape around the tube, pulling the frayed ends of tape through the looped end; and tie where tube emerges from the lips.	Allows for secure stabilization of the tube, decreasing the likelihood of inadvertent extubation.	
B. Pull the tape ends in opposite directions around the patient's neck.		
C. Tie the two ends of the tape at the side of the patient's neck securely.	Secures tube and prevents direct pressure on back of neck.	
Use of Adhesive Tape		
A. Prepare tape as shown in Figure 1–9.	Use of a hydrocolloid membrane (eg, Duoderm) on the patient's cheeks will help protect the skin.	
B. Secure tube by wrapping double-sided tape around patient's head and torn tape edges around endotracheal tube.		

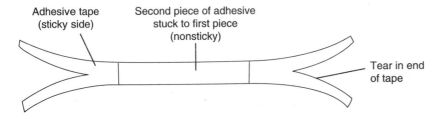

Adhesive tape (sticky side)

Second piece of adhesive stuck to first piece (nonsticky)

Tear in end of tape

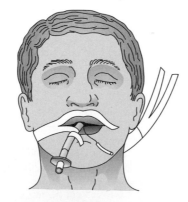
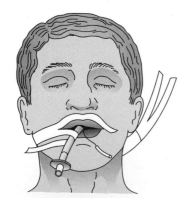
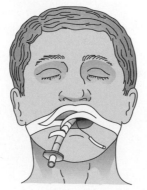
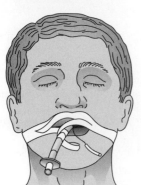

■ ● FIGURE 1–9. Methods for securing adhesive tape.

Example of protocol for securing endotracheal tube using adhesive tape:

1. Clean the patient's skin with mild soap and water.

2. Remove oil from the skin with alcohol and allow to dry.

3. Apply a skin adhesive product to enhance tape adherence. (When tape is removed, an adhesive remover will be necessary.)

4. Place a hydrocolloid membrane over the cheeks to protect friable skin.

5. Secure with adhesive tape as shown here.

(From Henneman E, Ellstrom K, St. John RE. *AACN Protocols for Practice: Care of the Mechanically Ventilated Patient Series.* Aliso Viejo, Ca: American Association of Critical-Care Nurses; 1999.)

Procedure for **Performing Endotracheal Intubation** *Continued*

Steps	Rationale	Special Considerations
24. Reconfirm tube placement (step 18).	Verifies that the tube was not inadvertently repositioned during the securing of the tube.	
25. Note position of tube at teeth (use centimeter markings on tube).	Common tube placement at the teeth is 21 cm for women and 23 cm for men.[7]	
26. Hyperoxygenate and suction endotracheal tube and pharynx (see Procedure 9) as needed.	Removes secretions that may obstruct tube or accumulate on the top of the cuff.	
27. Confirmation of correct tube position should be verified by a chest x-ray. *(Level II: Theory based, no research data to support recommendations; recommendations from expert consensus group may exist)*	Chest x-ray documents actual tube location (distance from the carina). Because chest x-ray is not immediately available, it should not be used as the primary method of tube assessment.[1-4]	Endotracheal tubes placed bronchoscopically may not require chest x-ray verification (check institutional standard).

Nasotracheal Intubation

Steps	Rationale	Special Considerations
28. Follow steps 1 through 8 under General Setup and steps 9 through 14.	Steps necessary to initiate nasal intubation. Dentures may be left in place for nasotracheal intubation.	
29. Spray nasal passage with anesthetic and vasoconstrictor, as indicated.	Anesthetizes and vasoconstricts nasal mucosa to decrease the incidence of trauma and bleeding.	
30. Lubricate tube with local anesthetic jelly.	Allows for smooth passage of tube.	
31. Slowly insert tube into selected nare, and guide tube up from the nostril and then backward and down into the nasopharynx.	Tube is introduced into airway channel.	
32. Gently advance the tube until maximal sound of moving air is heard through the tube.	Tube is located at opening of trachea.	Breath sounds become maximal just before entering the glottis.
33. While listening, continue to advance tube during inspiration.	Facilitates movement of tube through glottic opening.	Magill forceps may assist with advancement of tube. Cricoid pressure may help align the glottic opening.
34. Follow steps 18 through 21 and 23 through 27 to evaluate tube placement and secure tube in place.		

Expected Outcomes

- Placement of patent artificial airway
- Properly positioned and secured airway
- Improved oxygenation and ventilation
- Facilitation of secretion clearance

Unexpected Outcomes

- Intubation of esophagus or right main stem bronchus (improper tube placement)
- Accidental extubation
- Cardiac dysrhythmias because of hypoxemia and vagal stimulation
- Broken or dislodged teeth
- Leaking of air from endotracheal tube cuff
- Tracheal injury at tip of tube or at cuff site
- Laryngeal edema
- Vocal cord trauma
- Suctioning of gastric contents or food from endotracheal tube (aspiration)
- Obstruction of endotracheal tube

 This procedure should be performed only by physicians, advanced practice nurses, and other health care professionals (including critical care nurses) with additional knowledge, skills, and demonstrated competence per professional licensure or institutional standard.

Patient Monitoring and Care

Patient Monitoring and Care	Rationale	Reportable Conditions
		These conditions should be reported if they persist despite nursing interventions.
1. Auscultate breath sounds on insertion and every 2 to 4 hours.	Allows for detection of tube movement or dislodgment.	• Absent, decreased, or unequal breath sounds
2. Maintain tube stability, using specially manufactured holder, twill tape, or adhesive tape.	Prevents movement and dislodgment of tube.	• Unplanned extubation • Tube movement from original position
3. Monitor and record position of tube at teeth or nose (in reference to centimeter markings on tube).	Provides for identification of tube migration.	• Tube movement from original position
4. Maintain tube cuff pressure at 20 to 25 mm Hg. *(Level IV: Limited clinical studies to support recommendations)*	Provides adequate inflation to decrease aspiration risk and prevents overinflation of cuff to avoid tracheal damage.[1–3]	• Cuff pressure $\leq$20 to $\geq$25 mm Hg
5. Hyperoxygenate and suction endotracheal tube, as needed.	Prevents obstruction of tube and resulting hypoxemia.	• Inability to pass a suction catheter • Copious, frothy, or bloody secretions • Significant change in amount or character of secretions
6. Inspect nares or oral cavity once per shift while patient is intubated.	Will allow for the detection of skin breakdown and necrosis.	• Redness, necrosis, skin breakdown

Documentation

Documentation should include the following:

- Patient and family education
- Vital signs before, during, and after intubation, including oxygen saturation
- Type of intubation—oral or nasal
- Use of any medications
- Size of endotracheal tube
- Depth of endotracheal tube insertion—centimeters at teeth or nose
- Measurement of cuff pressure

- Assessment of breath sounds
- Confirmation of tube placement including chest radiograph (how placement was confirmed)
- Occurrence of unexpected outcomes
- Nursing interventions
- Secretions
- Patient response to procedure

References

1. Henneman E, Ellstrom K, St. John RE. Airway management. In: *AACN Protocols for Practice: Care of the Mechanically Ventilated Patient Series.* Aliso Viejo, Ca: American Association of Critical-Care Nurses; 1999.
2. Cummins RO, ed. Adjuncts for airway control, ventilation, and oxygenation. In: *Textbook of Advanced Cardiac Life Support.* Dallas, Tx: American Heart Association; 1997:2.5–2.6.
3. Wilson DJ, Shepherd KE. Modern airway appliances and their long-term complications. In: Robert JT, ed. *Clinical Management of the Airway.* Philadelphia, Pa: WB Saunders; 1994:461.
4. American Association of Respiratory Care Clinical Practice Guidelines. Resuscitation in acute care hospitals. *Respir Care.* 1993;38:1179–1188.
5. American Society of Anesthesiology. *1995 Standards for Basic Anesthetic Monitoring.* 60th ed. Dallas, Tx: Author; 1995: 384–385.
6. Barnason S, Graham J, Wild C, Jensen LB, Rasmussen D, Schulz P, Woods S, Carder B. Comparison of two endotracheal tube securement techniques on unplanned extubation, oral mucosa, and facial skin integrity. *Heart Lung.* 1998;27:409–417.
7. Holleran RS. *Flight Nursing: Principles and Practice.* 2nd ed. St. Louis, Mo: Mosby; 1996.

PROCEDURE 2

Assisting with Endotracheal Intubation

PURPOSE: Endotracheal intubation is performed to establish and maintain a patent airway, facilitate oxygenation and ventilation, reduce the risk of aspiration, and assist with the clearance of secretions.

Julianne M. Deutsch

PREREQUISITE NURSING KNOWLEDGE

- Anatomy and physiology of the pulmonary system should be understood.
- Indications for endotracheal intubation include the following[1]:
  - ❖ Upper airway obstruction (eg, secondary to swelling, trauma, tumor, bleeding)
  - ❖ Apnea
  - ❖ Ineffective clearance of secretions (eg, inability to adequately maintain airway)
  - ❖ High risk of aspiration
  - ❖ Respiratory distress
- Pulse oximetry should be used during intubation so that oxygen desaturation can be quickly detected.
- Preoxygenation with 100% oxygen using a bag-valve-mask device with a tight-fitting face mask should be performed for 3 to 5 minutes before intubation.
- Intubation attempts should take no longer than 15 to 30 seconds.
- Applying cricoid pressure (Sellick maneuver) may decrease the incidence of pulmonary aspiration and gastric distension. This procedure is accomplished by applying firm, downward pressure on the cricoid ring, pushing the vocal cords downward so they are more easily visualized. Once begun, cricoid pressure must be maintained until intubation is completed (see Fig. 1–1).[2]
- Two types of laryngoscope blades exist, straight and curved. The straight blade (Miller blade) is designed so that the tip extends below the epiglottis, lifting and exposing the glottic opening. It is recommended for use in obese patients and in those with short necks because their tracheas may be more anteriorly located. When a curved blade (Macintosh blade) is used, the tip is advanced into the vallecula (the space between the epiglottis and the base of the tongue), exposing the glottic opening.
- Endotracheal tube size reflects the size of the internal diameter of the tube. Tubes range in size from 2.0 mm for neonates to 9.0 mm for large adults; the correct size is based on patient weight. 7.5-mm to 8.0-mm tubes are commonly used for average-sized adult women, whereas average-sized adult men receive an 8.0-mm to 9.0-mm tube (see Fig. 1–2).[1] The tube with the largest clinically acceptable internal diameter should be used to minimize airway resistance and assist with suctioning.

- Endotracheal intubation can be done via nasal or oral routes. The skill of the practitioner performing the intubation as well as the patient's clinical condition determines the route used.
- Nasal intubation is relatively contraindicated in the trauma patient with facial fractures or suspected fractures at the base of the skull.
- In patients with suspected spinal-cord injuries, in-line cervical immobilization of the head must be maintained during endotracheal intubation. Nasotracheal intubation is often the preferred intubation route in these patients.
- Improper intubation technique may result in trauma to teeth, soft tissues of the mouth or nose, vocal cords, and posterior pharynx.
- A disposable end-tidal carbon dioxide (CO_2) detector may be used to assist with identification of proper endotracheal tube placement. This device is chemically treated with a nontoxic indicator that changes color in the presence of CO_2, indicating that the endotracheal tube has been successfully placed into the trachea.
- Double-lumen endotracheal tubes are used for independent lung ventilation in situations where there is bleeding of one lung or a large air leak that would impair ventilation of the good lung.
- The endotracheal tube also provides a route for the administration of emergency medication (eg, lidocaine, epinephrine, atropine, naloxone).

EQUIPMENT

- Personal protective equipment
- Endotracheal tube with intact cuff and 15-mm connector
  - ❖ Adult female, 7.5- to 8.0-mm tube; adult male, 8.0- to 9.0-mm tube[1]
- Laryngoscope handle with fresh batteries
- Laryngoscope blades (straight or curved)
- Spare bulb for laryngoscope blades
- Flexible stylet
- Self-inflating resuscitation bag with mask connected to 100% oxygen

- Oxygen source and connecting tubes
- Swivel adapter
- Nonsterile gloves
- Luer-Lok 10-mL syringe for cuff inflation
- Water-soluble lubricant
- Rigid pharyngeal suction-tip (Yankauer) catheter
- Suction apparatus (portable or wall)
- Suction catheters
- Bite-block or oropharyngeal airway
- Endotracheal tube–securing apparatus or appropriate tape
  - ❖ Adhesive tape (6 to 8 in long)
  - ❖ Twill tape (cut into 30-in lengths)
- Stethoscope

Additional equipment (to have available depending on patient need or practitioner preference) includes the following:

- Anesthetic spray (nasal approach)
- Local anesthetic jelly (nasal approach)
- Sedating or paralyzing medications
- Magill forceps (to remove foreign bodies obstructing the airway)
- Ventilator

PATIENT AND FAMILY EDUCATION

- Assess level of understanding about condition and rationale for endotracheal intubation. ➻*Rationale:* Identifies patient and family knowledge deficits concerning patient condition, procedure, expected benefits, and potential risks; allows time for questions to clarify information and to voice concerns. Explanations decrease patient anxiety and enhance cooperation.
- Explain the procedure and reason for intubation. ➻*Rationale:* Enhances patient and family understanding and decreases anxiety.
- If indicated, explain patient's role in assisting with insertion of endotracheal tube. ➻*Rationale:* Assists with insertion by eliciting patient's cooperation.
- Explain that patient will be unable to speak while the endotracheal tube is in place but that other means of communication will be provided. ➻*Rationale:* Enhances patient and family understanding and decreases anxiety.
- Explain that the patient's hands are often immobilized to prevent accidental dislodgment of the tube. ➻*Rationale:* Enhances patient and family understanding and decreases anxiety.

PATIENT ASSESSMENT AND PREPARATION
Patient Assessment

- Determine immediate history of trauma when spinal cord injury is suspected. ➻*Rationale:* Knowing pertinent pa-

tient history will allow for selection of the most appropriate method for intubation, helping to reduce the risk for secondary injury.

- Determine NPO (nothing by mouth) status or signs of gastric distention, or both. ➻*Rationale:* Increased risk of aspiration and vomiting occurs with accumulation of air, food, or secretions. If a patient who has gastric distention or has recently eaten needs to be intubated, use of cricoid pressure will decrease the risk of aspiration.
- Assess level of consciousness, level of anxiety, and respiratory difficulty. ➻*Rationale:* Determines need for sedation or use of paralytic agents and the ability to have patient flat and supine for intubation.
- Identify need for premedication. ➻*Rationale:* Various medications will allow for sedation or paralysis of the agitated patient.

Patient Preparation

- Ensure that patient understands preprocedural teaching. Answer questions as they arise and reinforce information as needed. ➻*Rationale:* Evaluates and reinforces understanding of previously taught information.
- Before intubation, initiate intravenous (IV) access. ➻*Rationale:* Readily available IV access may be necessary if the patient needs to be sedated or paralyzed or needs other medications if he or she has a negative response to the intubation procedure.
- Position the patient appropriately.
  - ❖ Positioning of nontrauma patients: Place patient supine with head in sniffing position, where the head is extended and the neck is flexed. Placement of a small towel under the occiput will elevate it several inches, allowing for proper flexion of the neck (see Fig. 1–3). ➻*Rationale:* Placing the head in the sniffing position will allow for visualization of the larynx and the vocal cords by aligning the axes of the mouth, pharynx, and trachea.
  - ❖ Positioning of trauma patients: In-line cervical spinal immobilization must be maintained during entire process of intubation. ➻*Rationale:* Because a cervical spinal cord injury must be suspected in all trauma patients until proven otherwise, this position will help prevent secondary injury should a cervical spinal cord injury be present.
- Premedicate as indicated. ➻*Rationale:* Appropriate premedication will allow for more controlled intubation, reducing the incidence of insertion trauma, aspiration, laryngospasm, and improper tube placement.

Procedure ▪ for Assisting with Endotracheal Intubation

Steps	Rationale	General Setup
1. Wash hands, and don personal protective equipment.	Reduces transmission of microorganisms and body secretions; standard precautions.	Protective eyewear should be worn to avoid exposure to secretions.
2. Insert oropharyngeal airway (see Procedure 7).	Assists in maintaining upper airway patency.	Used only in unconscious patients.

Procedure **for Assisting with Endotracheal Intubation** *Continued*

Steps	Rationale	Special Considerations
3. Set up suction apparatus and connect rigid suction-tip catheter to tubing.	Prepares for oropharyngeal suctioning as needed.	
4. Assist in positioning the patient's head by flexing the neck forward and extending the head (sniffing position).	Will allow for visualization of the vocal cords by aligning the three axes of the mouth, pharynx, and trachea.	Placement of a small towel under the occiput will elevate it, allowing for proper neck flexion. Do not flex or extend the neck of a patient with suspected spinal cord injury; the head must be maintained in a neutral position with in-line cervical spine immobilization.
5. Check the mouth for dentures, and remove if present. Suction the mouth as needed.	Dentures should be removed before oral intubation is attempted but may remain in place for nasal intubation.	
6. Preoxygenate using a self-inflating bag-valve-mask device (see Procedure 28) attached to 100% oxygen for 3 to 5 minutes. Provide frequent and gentle breaths.	Helps prevent hypoxemia. Gentle breaths reduce incidence of air entering stomach (leading to gastric distention), decrease airway turbulence, and more evenly distribute ventilation within the lungs.	
7. Premedicate patient as indicated.		
8. Apply cricoid pressure as requested.	Gentle cricoid pressure (see Fig. 1–1) may assist in visualization of vocal cords and decrease the risk of gastric distention and subsequent pulmonary aspiration. Once cricoid pressure is begun, it must be continued until the tube is correctly placed.	
9. Have manual resuscitation bag connected to 100% oxygen source and face mask ready for hyperoxygenation and manual ventilation.	Intubation attempts should not take longer than 30 seconds. Patients will need to be hyperoxygenated and ventilated between intubation attempts.[2]	
10. Once the endotracheal tube has been placed, confirm tube placement while bagging with 100% oxygen.	Confirms placement of the endotracheal tube.	
A. Attach disposable CO_2 detector (if available). Watch for color change indicating the presence of CO_2. *(Level IV: Limited clinical studies to support recommendations)*	Disposable CO_2 detectors may be used to assist with identification of proper tube placement.[2, 4, 5]	CO_2 detectors are usually placed between the self-inflating bag and the endotracheal tube. CO_2 detectors should be used in conjunction with physical assessment findings.
B. Auscultate over epigastrium. *(Level II: Theory based, no research data to support recommendations; recommendations from expert consensus group may exist)*	Allows for identification of esophageal intubation.[2, 4, 5]	If air movement or gurgling is heard, esophageal intubation has occurred. The tube must be pulled and intubation reattempted. Improper insertion may result in hypoxemia, gastric distention, vomiting, and aspiration.
C. Auscultate lung bases and apices for bilateral breath sounds. *(Level II: Theory based, no research data to support recommendations; recommendations from expert consensus group may exist)*	Assists in verification of correct tube placement into the trachea. A right main stem bronchus intubation will result in diminished left-sided breath sounds.[2, 4, 5]	Equal breath sounds will indicate proper placement of the endotracheal tube.
D. Observe for symmetric chest wall movement. *(Level II: theory based, no research data to support recommendations; recommendations from expert consensus group may exist)*	Assists in verification of correct tube placement.[2, 4, 5]	Absence may indicate right main stem or esophageal intubation.

Procedure continued on following page

Procedure for Assisting with Endotracheal Intubation *Continued*

Steps	Rationale	Special Considerations
E. Evaluate oxygen saturation (SpO₂) by noninvasive pulse oximetry. *(Level II: Theory based, no research data to support recommendations; recommendations from expert consensus group may exist)*	SpO₂ will fall if the esophagus has been inadvertently intubated. It may or may not change in a right main stem bronchus intubation.[2, 4, 5]	SpO₂ findings should be used in conjunction with physical assessment findings.
11. If CO_2 detection, assessment findings, or SpO₂ level reveals that the tube has not been correctly positioned, deflate cuff and remove tube immediately. Hyperoxygenate with 100% oxygen for 3 to 5 minutes and reattempt intubation, beginning with the first step. *(Level II: Theory based, no research data to support recommendations; recommendations from expert consensus group may exist)*	Esophageal intubation results in gas flow diversion and hypoxemia.[2, 3]	
12. If breath sounds are absent on the left, the cuff should be deflated and the tube pulled 1 to 2 cm. Reevaluate for correct tube placement (step 10).	Absence of breath sounds on the left may indicate right main stem intubation, which is common as a result of the anatomic position of the right main stem bronchi. When correctly positioned, the tube tip should be 1.0 to 2.5 cm below the trachea.[4]	
13. Connect endotracheal tube to oxygen source or mechanical ventilator, using swivel adapter.	Reduces motion on tube and mouth or nares.	
14. Insert a bite block or oropharyngeal airway (to act as a bite block) along the endotracheal tube.	Prevents the patient from biting down on the endotracheal tube.	The bite block should be secured separately from the tube to prevent dislodgment of the tube.
15. Secure the endotracheal tube in place (according to institutional standard). *(Level II: Theory based, no research data to support recommendations; recommendations from expert consensus group may exist)*	To prevent inadvertent dislodgment of tube.[1–3, 6]	Various methods are used for securing endotracheal tubes, including use of specially manufactured tube holders, twill tape, or adhesive tape.

Use of Twill Tape

A. Double over a 2-ft length of twill tape; tie the tape around the tube, pulling frayed ends of tape through the looped end; and tie where tube emerges from the lips.	Allows for secure stabilization of the tube, decreasing the likelihood of inadvertent extubation.	
B. Pull the tape ends in opposite directions around the patient's neck.		
C. Tie the two ends of the tape at the side of the patient's neck securely.	Secures tube and prevents direct pressure on back of neck.	

Use of Adhesive Tape

A. Prepare tape as shown in Figure 1–9.	Use of a hydrocolloid membrane (eg, Duoderm) on the patient's cheeks will help protect the skin.	
B. Secure tube by wrapping double-sided tape around patient's head and torn tape edges around endotracheal tube.		
16. Reconfirm tube placement (step 10).	Verifies that the tube was not inadvertently repositioned during the securing of the tube.	
17. Note position of tube at teeth (use centimeter markings on tube).	Common tube placement at the teeth is 21 cm for women and 23 cm for men.	

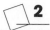

Procedure for Assisting with Endotracheal Intubation *Continued*

Steps	Rationale	Special Considerations
18. Hyperoxygenate and suction endotracheal tube and pharynx (see Procedure 9) as needed.	Remove secretions that may obstruct tube or accumulate on top of cuff.	
19. Confirmation of correct tube position should be verified by a chest x-ray. *(Level II: Theory based, no research data to support recommendations; recommendations from expert consensus group may exist)*	Chest x-ray documents actual tube location (distance from the carina). Because chest x-ray is not immediately available, it should not be used as the primary method of tube assessment.[1-4]	Endotracheal tubes placed bronchoscopically may not require chest x-ray verification (check institutional standard).

Expected Outcomes

- Placement of patent artificial airway
- Properly positioned and secured airway
- Improved oxygenation and ventilation
- Facilitation of secretion clearance

Unexpected Outcomes

- Intubation of esophagus or right main stem bronchus (improper tube placement)
- Accidental extubation
- Cardiac dysrhythmias as a result of hypoxemia and vagal stimulation
- Broken or dislodged teeth
- Leaking of air from endotracheal tube cuff
- Tracheal injury at tip of tube or at cuff site
- Laryngeal edema
- Vocal cord trauma
- Suctioning of gastric contents or food from endotracheal tube (aspiration)
- Obstruction of endotracheal tube

Patient Monitoring and Care

Patient Monitoring and Care	Rationale	Reportable Conditions
		These conditions should be repeated if they persist despite nursing interventions.
1. Auscultate breath sounds on insertion and every 2 to 4 hours.	Allows for detection of tube movement or dislodgment.	• Absent or unequal breath sounds
2. Maintain tube stability, using specially manufactured holder, twill tape, or adhesive tape.	Prevents movement and dislodgment of tube.	• Unplanned extubation • Tube movement from original position
3. Monitor and record position of tube at teeth or nose (in reference to centimeter markings on tube).	Provides for identification of tube migration.	• Tube movement from original position
4. Maintain tube cuff pressure at 20 to 25 mm Hg. *(Level IV: Limited clinical studies to support recommendations)*	Provides adequate inflation, decreases aspiration risk, and prevents overinflation of cuff to avoid tracheal damage.[1-3]	• Cuff pressure ≤20 to ≥25 mm Hg
5. Hyperoxygenate and suction endotracheal tube as needed.	Prevents obstruction of tube and resulting hypoxemia.	• Inability to pass a suction catheter • Copious, frothy, or bloody secretions • Significant change in amount or character of secretions
6. Inspect nares or oral cavity once per shift while patient is intubated.	Will allow for the detection of skin breakdown and necrosis.	• Redness, necrosis, skin breakdown

▌ D o c u m e n t a t i o n

Documentation should include the following:

- Patient and family education
- Vital signs before, during, and after intubation, including oxygen saturation
- Type of intubation—oral or nasal
- Use of any medications
- Size of endotracheal tube
- Depth of endotracheal tube insertion (centimeters at teeth or nose)
- Measurement of cuff pressure

- Assessment of breath sounds
- Confirmation of tube placement, including chest radiograph (how placement was confirmed)
- Occurrence of unexpected outcomes
- Nursing interventions
- Secretions
- Patient response to procedure

References

1. Henneman E, Ellstrom K, St. John RE. Airway management. In: *AACN Protocols for Practice: Care of the Mechanically Ventilated Patient Series.* Aliso Viejo, CA: American Association of Critical-Care Nurses; 1999.
2. Cummins RO, ed. Adjuncts for airway control, ventilation, and oxygenation. In: *Textbook of Advanced Cardiac Life Support.* Dallas, Tx: American Heart Association; 1997:2.5–2.6.
3. Wilson DJ, Shepherd KE. Modern airway appliances and their long-term complications. In: Robert JT, ed. *Clinical Management of the Airway.* Philadelphia, Pa: W.B. Saunders; 1994;461.
4. AARC Clinical Practice Guidelines. Resuscitation in acute care hospitals. *Respir Care.* 1993;38:1179–1188.
5. American Society of Anesthesiology. *1995 Standards for Basic Anesthetic Monitoring.* 60th ed. Dallas, Tx: Author; 1995:384–385.
6. Barnason S, Graham, J, Wild C, et al. Comparison of two endotracheal tube securement techniques on unplanned extubation, oral mucosa, and facial skin integrity. *Heart Lung.* 1998;27:409–417.
7. Holleran RS. *Flight Nursing: Principles and Practice.* 2nd ed. St. Louis, Mo: Mosby–Year Book; 1996.

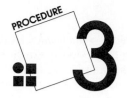

Endotracheal Tube Care

P U R P O S E: Endotracheal tube care is performed to prevent buccal, oropharyngeal, and tracheal trauma from the tube and cuff, to provide oral hygiene, and to promote ventilation.

Julianne M. Deutsch

PREREQUISITE NURSING KNOWLEDGE

- Anatomy and physiology of the pulmonary system should be understood.
- Endotracheal (ET) tubes are used to maintain a patent airway or to facilitate mechanical ventilation. Presence of these artificial airways, especially ET tubes, prevents effective coughing and secretion removal, requiring periodic removal of pulmonary secretions with suctioning. In acute care situations, suctioning is always performed as a sterile procedure to prevent nosocomial pneumonia.
- Suctioning of airways should be performed only for a clinical indication and not as a routine, fixed-schedule treatment.
- Adequate systemic hydration and supplemental humidification of inspired gases assist in thinning secretions for easier aspiration from airways.
- Appropriate cuff care will help prevent major pulmonary aspirations, prepare for tracheal extubation, decrease the risk of inadvertent extubation, provide a patent airway for ventilation and removal of secretions, and decrease the risk of iatrogenic infections.
- Constant pressure from the ET tube on the mouth or nose can cause skin breakdown.
- If the patient is anxious or uncooperative, using two caregivers when retaping or repositioning the ET tube will help prevent accidental dislodgment of the tube.

EQUIPMENT

- Suction catheter of appropriate size (see Table 9–1)
- Sterile, water-soluble lubricant or sterile saline solution
- Sterile gloves
- Sterile solution container or sterile basin
- Source of suction (wall mounted or portable)
- Connecting tube, 4 to 6 ft long
- Goggles or glasses and mask
- Bite block or oral airway if needed
- Adhesive or twill tape; commercial ET tube holder
- 4 × 4 gauze pads or cotton swabs
- Normal saline solution
- Toothettes
- Mouthwash
- Self-inflating manual resuscitation bag connected to an oxygen flowmeter, set at 15 L/min (not required if using the ventilator to deliver hyperoxygenation breaths)
- Stethoscope
- 10-mL syringe

PATIENT AND FAMILY EDUCATION

- Explain procedure to patient and family, including purpose of ET tube care. ➥*Rationale:* Identifies patient and family knowledge deficits concerning patient condition, procedure, expected benefits, and potential risks and allows time for questions to clarify information and voice concerns. Explanations decrease patient anxiety and enhance cooperation.
- If indicated, explain patient's role in assisting with ET tube care. ➥*Rationale:* Assists with care by eliciting patient's cooperation.
- Explain that patient will be unable to speak while the ET tube is in place but that other means of communication will be provided. ➥*Rationale:* Enhances patient and family understanding and decreases anxiety.
- Explain that the patient's hands are often immobilized to prevent accidental dislodgment of the tube. ➥*Rationale:* Enhances patient and family understanding and decreases anxiety.

PATIENT ASSESSMENT AND PREPARATION
Patient Assessment

- Signs and symptoms indicating that ET tube care is required are as follows:
  ❖ Excessive secretions (oral or tracheal)
  ❖ Soiled tape or ties
  ❖ Patient biting or kinking tube
  ❖ Pressure areas on naris, corner of mouth, or tongue
  ❖ Tube moving in and out of mouth
  ❖ Patient able to verbalize

➥*Rationale:* Assessment provides for early recognition that ET tube care needs to be done.

- Level of consciousness and level of anxiety should be assessed. ➤➤*Rationale:* Determines need for sedation during ET tube care.

Patient Preparation

Ensure that patient understands preprocedural teaching. Answer questions as they arise and reinforce information as needed. ➤➤*Rationale:* Evaluates and reinforces understanding of previously taught information.

Assist the patient to a position that is comfortable for the patient and the nurse, generally semi-Fowler or Fowler. ➤➤*Rationale:* Promotes comfort, oxygenation, and ventilation and reduces strain.

Procedure for Endotracheal Tube Care

Steps	Rationale	Special Considerations
1. Wash hands, and don personal protective equipment.	Decreases transmission of microorganisms and body secretions; standard precautions.	
2. Ensure that ET tube is connected to the ventilator using a swivel adapter.	Decreases pressure exerted by ventilator tubing on the ET tube, thereby minimizing risk of pressure ulceration.	
3. Support the ET tube and tubing as needed.		
4. Hyperoxygenate and suction ET tube and pharynx (see Procedure 9) as needed.	Removes secretions that may obstruct tube or accumulate on the top of the cuff.	
5. Loosen and remove old tape and ties.		
6. If patient is nasally intubated, clean around ET tube using saline-soaked gauze of cotton swabs. Proceed to step 8.	Removes secretions that could cause pressure and subsequent skin breakdown.	
7. If patient is intubated orally, remove bite block or oropharyngeal airway (acting as bite block).	Prevents the patient from biting down on the ET tube and occluding air flow.	The bite block should be secured separately from the tube to prevent dislodgment of the ET tube.
8. Perform oral hygiene, using Toothettes and mouthwash. Brush patient's teeth.	Good oral hygiene decreases the risk of the patient's developing sinusitis or otitis media.	
9. Move oral tube to the other side of the mouth. Replace bite block or oropharyngeal airway (to act as bite block) along the ET tube.	Prevents or minimizes pressure areas on lips, tongue, and oral cavity.	
10. Ensure proper cuff inflation (see Procedure 10) using minimum leak volume or minimum occlusion volume.	Decreases risk of aspiration; ensures airflow to lungs rather than to stomach.	
11. Reconfirm tube placement (see Procedure 1), and note position of tube at teeth or naris.	Common tube placement at the teeth is 21 cm for women and 23 cm for men.[1]	
12. Secure the ET tube in place (according to institutional standard) (see Procedure 2). *(Level II: Theory based, no research data to support recommendations; recommendations from expert consensus group may exist)*	Prevents inadvertent dislodgment of the tube.[2–5]	Various methods are used for securing ET tubes, including use of specially manufactured tube holder, twill tape, or adhesive tape.

Expected Outcomes	Unexpected Outcomes
• Patent airway	• Dislodged ET tube
• Secured ET tube	• Occluded ET tube
• Control of secretions	• Cuff leak
• Intact oral and nasal mucous membranes	• Pressure sores in mouth, lip, or naris

Patient Monitoring and Care

Patient Monitoring and Care	Rationale	Reportable Conditions
		These conditions should be reported if they persist despite nursing interventions.
1. Suction ET tube as needed.	Maintains patent airway.	• Inability to pass suction catheter
2. Monitor amount, type, and color of secretions.		• Change in quantity or characteristics of secretions
3. If patient is nasally intubated, monitor for nasal drainage.		• Purulent drainage
4. Assess oral cavity and lips, and perform oral care every 2 hours and as needed.	Early recognition of pressure or drainage allows for prompt intervention.	• Breakdown of lip, tongue, or oral cavity • Presence of mouth sores
5. Retape or secure ET tube every 24 hours and as needed for soiled or loose securing devices.	Ensures secured tube.	• Tube moving in and out of mouth

Documentation

- Patient and family education
- Patient tolerance to suctioning
- Aspirate amount, type, and color
- Presence of nasal drainage
- Repositioning of ET tube
- Retaping of ET tube
- Mouth care
- Condition of lips, mouth, and tongue
- Presence of cuff leak
- Amount of air used to inflate cuff
- Centimeter mark on ET tube
- Which naris ET tube is in

References

1. Holleran RS. *Flight Nursing: Principles and Practice.* 2nd ed. St. Louis, Mo: Mosby–Year Book; 1996.
2. Henneman E, Ellstrom K, St. John RE. Airway management. In: *AACN Protocols for Practice: Care of the Mechanically Ventilated Patient Series.* Aliso Viejo, Ca: American Association of Critical-Care Nurses; 1999.
3. Cummins RO, ed. Adjuncts for airway control, ventilation, and oxygenation. In: *Textbook of Advanced Cardiac Life Support.* Dallas, Tx: American Heart Association; 1997:2.5–2.6.
4. Wilson DJ, Shepherd KE. Modern airway appliances and their long-term complications. In: Robert JT, ed. *Clinical Management of the Airway.* Philadelphia, Pa: W.B. Saunders; 1994:461.
5. Barnason S, Graham J, Wild C, et al. Comparison of two endotracheal tube securement techniques on unplanned extubation, oral mucosa, and facial skin integrity. *Heart Lung.* 1998;27:409–417.

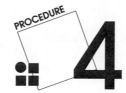

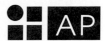

Performing Extubation and Decannulation

PURPOSE: The purpose of extubation and decannulation is to remove the artificial airway to allow the patient to breathe independently.

Kay Knox Greenlee

PREREQUISITE NURSING KNOWLEDGE

- Extubation refers to removal of an endotracheal tube, whereas decannulation refers to removal of a tracheostomy tube.
- Indications for extubation and decannulation include the following:[1]
  - ❖ Underlying condition that led to the need for an artificial airway is reversed or improved.
  - ❖ Hemodynamic stability is achieved, with no new reasons for continued artificial airway support.
  - ❖ Patient is able to clear pulmonary secretions.
  - ❖ Airway problems have resolved; there is minimal risk for aspiration.
  - ❖ Mechanical ventilatory support is no longer needed.
- Most extubations or decannulations are planned. Planning allows for preparation of the patient, both physically and emotionally, and decreases the likelihood of reintubation and hypoxic sequelae. Unintentional or unplanned extubation complicates a patient's overall recovery.[2]
- Extubation usually occurs within 24 hours of successful weaning from mechanical ventilatory support, whereas decannulation occurs much later. The patient with a tracheostomy tube is gradually weaned from the tracheostomy tube using a combination of techniques, including downsizing the tube diameter, using fenestration, and capping the tracheostomy. The tracheostomy tube is removed when the patient is able to comfortably breathe and maintain adequate ventilation and oxygenation, as well as manage secretions.

EQUIPMENT

- Suctioning equipment
- Sterile suction catheter or suction kit
- Endotracheal intubation supplies
- Stethoscope

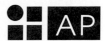

- Self-inflating resuscitation bag connected to 100% oxygen source
- Scissors
- Sterile gloves
- Supplemental oxygen with aerosol
- 10-mL syringe
- Emergency cart
- Rigid pharyngeal suction-tip (Yankauer) catheter
- Sterile dressing for tracheal stoma

PATIENT AND FAMILY EDUCATION

- Explain the procedure and the reason the endotracheal tube or tracheostomy tube is no longer needed. ➻*Rationale:* Identifies patient and family knowledge deficits concerning patient condition, procedure, and expected benefits and allows time for questions to clarify information and voice concerns. Explanations decrease patient anxiety and enhance cooperation.
- Explain the purpose and necessity of extubation. ➻*Rationale:* Communication and explanation for therapy encourage cooperation and minimize anxiety.
- Discuss the suctioning process and the importance of coughing and deep breathing. ➻*Rationale:* Understanding therapy encourages cooperation with the follow-up procedures necessary to maintain a patent airway.
- Explain that the patient's voice may be hoarse following extubation or decannulation. For patients who have a tracheostomy tube removed, occlusion of the stoma may be necessary to facilitate normal speech and coughing. ➻*Rationale:* Knowledge minimizes patient and family fear and anxiety.
- Explain that the patient may need continued oxygen or humidification support. ➻*Rationale:* Many patients continue to require oxygen support for some time following extubation. Continued humidification often helps decrease hoarseness and liquefy secretions.

PATIENT ASSESSMENT AND PREPARATION

Patient Assessment

- Desired level of consciousness has been achieved (for most patients, patient is awake and able to follow commands).[2]

- Signs and symptoms associated with independent breathing are as follows:[1, 3]
  ❖ Stable respiratory rate of <25 breaths per minute
  ❖ Absence of dyspnea
  ❖ Absence of accessory muscle use
  ❖ Negative inspiratory pressure ≤ -20 cm H_2O
  ❖ Positive expiratory pressure $\geq +30$ cm H_2O
  ❖ Spontaneous tidal volume ≥ 5 mL/kg
  ❖ Vital capacity ≥ 10–15 mL/kg
  ❖ Minute ventilation ≤ 10 L/min
  ❖ F_{IO_2} (fraction of inspired oxygen) $\leq 50\%$
  ❖ Stable pulse and blood pressure and absence of serious cardiac dysrhythmias[3] **➤Rationale:** Evaluation of the patient's respiratory status identifies that intubation is no longer necessary.

- Assess patient's ability to cough. **➤Rationale:** The ability to cough and clear secretions is important for successful airway management following extubation.

Patient Preparation

- Ensure that patient understands preprocedural teaching. Answer questions as they arise, and reinforce information as needed. **➤Rationale:** Evaluates and reinforces understanding of previously taught information.
- Place patient in semi-Fowler position. **➤Rationale:** Respiratory muscles are more effective in an upright position versus a prone position. This position facilitates coughing and minimizes the risk of vomiting and consequent aspiration.

Procedure   for Performing Extubation and Decannulation

Steps	Rationale	Special Considerations
1. Wash hands, and don personal protective equipment.	Reduces transmission of microorganisms and body secretions; standard precautions.	
2. Hyperoxygenate and suction endotracheal tube and pharynx (see Procedure 9).		
3. Cut twill tape or remove tape to free tube.		
4. Insert syringe into one-way valve in pilot balloon.	Prepares for cuff deflation.	
5. Instruct patient to deep breathe.	Promotes hyperinflation.	A manual resuscitation bag can assist in hyperinflation.
6. At the peak of a deep inspiration, deflate the cuff and remove the tube in one motion on inspiration.	Assists in a smooth, quick, less traumatic removal. Vocal cords are maximally abducted at peak inspiration. Additionally, initial cough response expected following extubation should be more forceful if started from maximal inspiration versus expiration.[1]	Alternative methods to facilitate removal of secretions while tube is removed include application of positive pressure while the cuff is deflated; insertion of suction catheter 1 to 2 in (5 cm) below distal end of tube; and application of suction while cuff is deflated and tube removed.[4]
7. Encourage the patient to deep breathe and cough.	Promotes hyperinflation; helps remove secretions.	
8. Suction the pharynx.	Removes secretions.	
9. Apply supplemental oxygen and aerosol, as appropriate.	Promotes warmth and moisture and prevents oxygen desaturation. Cool humidification is usually preferred after extubation to help minimize upper airway swelling.[1]	
10. Place a dry, sterile, 4 × 4 dressing over stoma when tracheostomy tube is removed.	Contains secretions that leak out of stoma.	Tracheostomy stoma closure usually occurs within a few days.

Expected Outcomes

- Smooth, atraumatic extubation or decannulation
- Stable respiratory status

Unexpected Outcomes

- Fatigue and respiratory failure
- Persistent hoarseness
- Tracheal stoma narrowing
- Aspiration
- Laryngospasm
- Trauma to soft tissue

Patient Monitoring and Care

Patient Monitoring and Care	Rationale	Reportable Conditions
		These conditions should be reported if they persist despite nursing interventions.
1. Monitor vital signs, respiratory status, and oxygenation immediately following extubation, within 1 hour, and per institutional standard.	Change in vital signs and oxygenation following extubation or decannulation may indicate respiratory compromise, necessitating reintubation.	• Tachycardia • Tachypnea • Blood pressure >110% baseline • Spo$_2$ (oxygen saturation) ≤90% • Stridor • Breathing difficulty • Chest-abdominal asynchrony
2. Promote optimal oxygenation by providing supplemental oxygen as needed.	Decreases incidence of oxygen desaturation immediately following extubation.	• Spo$_2$ ≤90%
3. Monitor for aspiration related to pooled secretions.	Failure to suction or ineffective suctioning of the pharynx allows accumulated secretions to further advance into the trachea on cuff deflation.	• Patient unable to handle secretions
4. Encourage coughing and deep breathing.	Prevents atelectasis and secretion accumulation.	• Ineffective cough
5. Assess swallowing ability.	Presence of tube over extended periods may result in impaired swallow.	• Inability to handle secretions • Inability to swallow without coughing

Documentation

Documentation should include the following:

- Patient and family education
- Respiratory and vital signs assessment before and after procedure
- Date and time when procedure is performed
- Patient response
- Unexpected outcomes
- Nursing interventions taken

References

1. Henneman E, Ellstrom K, St. John R. Airway management. In: *AACN Protocols for Practice: Care of the Mechanically Ventilated Patient Series.* Aliso Viejo, Ca: American Association of Critical-Care Nurses; 1999.
2. Longnecker DE, Murphy FL. *Introduction to Anesthesia.* Philadelphia, Pa: W.B. Saunders; 1997.
3. Burns SM, Fahey SA, Barton DM, Slack D. Weaning from mechanical ventilation: A method for assessment and planning. *AACN Clin Issues.* 1991;2:372–387.
4. Davies N. Nurse initiated extubation following cardiac surgery. *Intensive Crit Care Nurs.* 1997;1:77–79.

Additional Readings

Bach JR, Saporito LR. Criteria for extubation and tracheostomy tube removal for patients with ventilatory failure. *Chest.* 1996;110:1566–1571.

Boulain T, Association des Reanimateurs du Centre–Quest. Unplanned extubations in the adult intensive care unit. *Am J Respir Care Med.* 1998;157(4 pt 1):1131–1137.

Chiang AA, Lee KC, Lee JC, Wei CH. Effectiveness of a continuous quality improvement program aiming to reduce unplanned extubation: a prospective study. *Intensive Care Med.* 1996; 22:1269–1271.

Durbin CG, Campbell RS, Branson RD. AARC clinical practice guideline: removal of the endotracheal tube. *Respir Care.* 1999;44:85–90.

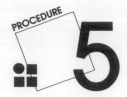

PROCEDURE

5

Assisting with Extubation and Decannulation

P U R P O S E: The purpose of extubation and decannulation is to remove the artificial airway to allow the patient to breathe independently.

Kay Knox Greenlee

PREREQUISITE NURSING KNOWLEDGE

- Extubation refers to removal of an endotracheal tube, whereas decannulation refers to removal of a tracheostomy tube.
- Indications for extubation or decannulation include the following:[1]
  ❖ Underlying condition that led to the need for an artificial airway is reversed or improved.
  ❖ Hemodynamic stability is achieved, with no new reasons for continued artificial airway support.
  ❖ Patient is able to clear pulmonary secretions.
  ❖ Airway problems have resolved; there is minimal risk for aspiration.
  ❖ Mechanical ventilatory support is no longer needed.
- Most extubations or decannulations are planned. Planning allows for preparation of the patient, both physically and emotionally, and decreases the likelihood of reintubation and hypoxic sequelae. Unintentional or unplanned extubation complicates a patient's overall recovery.[2]
- Extubation usually occurs within 24 hours of successful weaning from mechanical ventilatory support, whereas decannulation occurs much later. The patient with a tracheostomy tube is gradually weaned from the tracheostomy tube using a combination of techniques including downsizing the tube diameter, using fenestration, and capping the tracheostomy. The tracheostomy tube is removed when the patient is able to comfortably breathe and maintain adequate ventilation and oxygenation, as well as manage secretions.

EQUIPMENT

- Suctioning equipment
- Sterile suction catheter or suction kit
- Self-inflating resuscitation bag connected to 100% oxygen source
- Scissors
- Endotracheal intubation supplies
- Stethoscope
- 10-mL syringe
- Emergency cart
- Rigid pharyngeal suction-tip (Yankauer) catheter
- Sterile gloves
- Supplemental oxygen with aerosol
- Sterile dressing for tracheal stoma

PATIENT AND FAMILY EDUCATION

- Explain the procedure and the reason the endotracheal tube or tracheostomy tube is no longer needed. ➥*Rationale:* Identifies patient and family knowledge deficits concerning patient condition, procedure, and expected benefits and allows time for questions to clarify information and voice concerns. Explanations decrease patient anxiety and enhance cooperation.
- Explain the purpose and necessity of extubation. ➥*Rationale:* Communication and explanation for therapy encourage cooperation and minimize anxiety.
- Discuss the suctioning process and the importance of coughing and deep breathing. ➥*Rationale:* Encourages cooperation with the follow-up procedures necessary to maintain a patent airway.
- Explain that the patient's voice may be hoarse following extubation or decannulation. For patients who have a tracheostomy tube removed, occlusion of the stoma may be necessary to facilitate normal speech and coughing. ➥*Rationale:* Minimizes patient and family fear and anxiety.
- Explain that the patient may need continued oxygen or humidification support. ➥*Rationale:* Many patients continue to require oxygen support for some time following extubation. Continued humidification often helps decrease hoarseness and liquefy secretions.

PATIENT ASSESSMENT AND PREPARATION

Patient Assessment

- Desired level of consciousness has been achieved (for most patients; patient is awake and able to follow commands).[2]
- Signs and symptoms associated with independent breathing are as follows:[1, 3]
  ❖ Stable respiratory rate of <25 breaths per minute

❖ Absence of dyspnea
❖ Absence of accessory muscle use
❖ Negative inspiratory pressure ≤ -20 cm H_2O
❖ Positive expiratory pressure $\geq +30$ cm H_2O
❖ Spontaneous tidal volume ≥ 5 mL/kg
❖ Vital capacity $\geq 10–15$ mL/kg
❖ Minute ventilation ≤ 10 L/min
❖ FiO_2 (fraction of inspired oxygen) $\leq 50\%$
❖ Stable pulse and blood pressure and absence of serious cardiac dysrhythmias.[3] *➻Rationale:* Identifies that intubation is no longer necessary.

• Assess patient's ability to cough. *➻Rationale:* The abil-ity to cough and clear secretions is important for success-ful airway management following extubation.

Patient Preparation

• Ensure that the patient understands preprocedural teach-ing. Answer questions as they arise, and reinforce infor-mation as needed. *➻Rationale:* Evaluates and rein-forces understanding of previously taught information.
• Place patient in the semi-Fowler position. *➻Rationale:* Respiratory muscles are more effective in an upright position versus a prone position. This position facilitates coughing and minimizes the risk of vomiting and conse-quent aspiration.

Procedure   **for Assisting with Extubation and Decannulation**

Steps	Rationale	Special Considerations
1. Wash hands, and don personal protective equipment.	Reduces transmission of microorganisms and body secretions; standard precautions.	
2. Hyperoxygenate and suction endotracheal tube and pharynx (see Procedure 9).	Removes secretions, including those above the cuff.	
3. Cut twill tape, or remove tape to free tube.	Removes means for securing above the cuff.	
4. Instruct patient to deep breathe.	Promotes hyperinflation.	A manual resuscitation bag can assist in hyperinflation.
5. While the tube is being removed, at the peak of inspiration, monitor and support the patient.	Provides reassurance and possibly distraction as patient experiences removal of the tube.	Alternative methods to facilitate removal of secretions while tube is removed include application of positive pressure while the cuff is deflated; insertion of suction catheter 1 to 2 in (5 cm) below distal end of tube, and application of suction while cuff is deflated and tube removed.[4]
6. Encourage the patient to deep breathe and cough.	Promotes hyperinflation; helps remove secretions.	
7. Suction the pharynx.	Removes secretions.	
8. Apply supplemental oxygen and aerosol, as appropriate.	Promotes warmth and moisture and prevents oxygen desaturation. Cool humidification is usually preferred after extubation to help minimize upper airway swelling.[1]	
9. Place a dry, sterile, 4 × 4 dressing over stoma when tracheostomy tube is removed.	Contains secretions that leak out of stoma.	Tracheostomy stoma closure usually occurs within a few days.

Expected Outcomes

• Smooth, atraumatic extubation or decannulation
• Stable respiratory status

Unexpected Outcomes

• Fatigue and respiratory failure
• Persistent hoarseness
• Tracheal stoma narrowing
• Aspiration
• Laryngospasm
• Trauma to soft tissue

Patient Monitoring and Care

Patient Monitoring and Care	Rationale	Reportable Conditions
		These conditions should be reported if they persist despite nursing interventions.
1. Monitor vital signs, respiratory status, and oxygenation immediately following extubation, within 1 hour, and per institutional standard.	Change in vital signs and oxygenation following extubation or decannulation may indicate respiratory compromise, necessitating reintubation.	• Tachycardia • Blood pressure >110% baseline • SpO_2 (oxygen saturation) ≤90% • Stridor • Breathing difficulty • Chest-abdominal asynchrony
2. Promote optimal oxygenation by providing supplemental oxygen as needed.	Decreases incidence of oxygen desaturation immediately following extubation.	• SpO_2 ≤90%
3. Monitor for aspiration related to pooled secretions.	Failure to suction or ineffective suctioning of the pharynx allows accumulated secretions to further advance into the trachea upon cuff deflation.	• Patient unable to handle secretions
4. Encourage coughing and deep breathing.	Prevents atelectasis and secretion accumulation.	• Ineffective cough
5. Assess swallowing ability.	Presence of tube over extended periods may result in impaired swallow.	• Inability to handle secretions • Inability to swallow without coughing

Documentation

Documentation should include the following:

- Patient and family education
- Respiratory and vital signs assessment before and after procedure
- Date and time when procedure is performed
- Patient response
- Unexpected outcomes
- Nursing interventions taken

References

1. Henneman E, Ellstrom, K, St. John R. Airway management. In: *AACN Protocols for Practice: Care of the Mechanically Ventilated Patient Series.* Aliso Viejo, Ca: American Association of Critical-Care Nurses; 1999.
2. Longnecker DE, Murphy FL. *Introduction to Anesthesia.* Philadelphia, Pa: W.B. Saunders; 1997.
3. Burns SM, Fahey SA, Barton DM, Slack D. Weaning from mechanical ventilation: a method for assessment and planning. *AACN Clin Issues.* 1991;2:372–387.
4. Davies N. Nurse initiated extubation following cardiac surgery. *Intensive Crit Care Nurs.* 1997;1:77–79.

Boulain T, Association des Reanimateurs du Centre–Quest. Unplanned extubations in the adult intensive care unit. *Am Respir Care Med.* 1998;157(4 pt 1):1131–1137.

Chiang AA, Lee KC, Lee JC, Wei CH. Effectiveness of a continuous quality improvement program aiming to reduce unplanned extubation: A prospective study. *Intensive Care Med.* 1996;22:1269–1271.

Durbin CG, Campbell RS, Branson RD. AARC clinical practice guideline: Removal of the endotracheal tube. *Respir Care.* 1999;44:85–90.

Additional Readings

Bach JR, Saporito LR. Criteria for extubation and tracheostomy tube removal for patients with ventilatory failure. *Chest.* 1996;110:1566–1571.

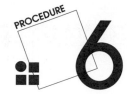

6 Nasopharyngeal Airway Insertion

PURPOSE: Nasopharyngeal airways are used to maintain a patent airway to the hypopharynx and to facilitate the removal of tracheobronchial secretions by directing the catheter and by averting tissue trauma that is associated with repeated suction attempts.[1, 2, 3]

Kay Knox Greenlee

PREREQUISITE NURSING KNOWLEDGE

- The nasopharyngeal airway is a flexible piece of rubber. It is passed through the nose and follows the posterior nasal and oropharyngeal walls to the base of the tongue (Fig. 6–1).
- The nasopharyngeal airway has three parts: the flange, cannula, and bevel, or tip. The flange is the wide, trumpetlike end that prevents further slippage into the airway. The hollow shaft of the cannula permits airflow into the hypopharynx. The bevel, or tip, is the opening at the distal end of the tube. When properly inserted, the tip can be seen resting posterior to the base of the tongue.
- The external diameter of the nasopharyngeal airway should be slightly smaller than the patient's external naris opening. The length of the nasopharyngeal airway is determined by measuring the distance between the naris and the tip of the ipsilateral earlobe and adding 1 in (2.5 cm) (Fig. 6–2). Improperly sized nasopharyngeal airways may result in increased airway resistance, limited airflow (if the airway is too small), kinking and mucosal trauma, gagging, vomiting, and gastric distention (if the airway is too large). Some manufacturers provide nasopharyngeal airways shaped specifically for the right and left nares.
- The advantages of the nasopharyngeal airway include increased comfort and tolerance in the conscious and pediatric patient, stable airway positioning for long periods, decreased incidence of gag reflex stimulation, and minimal incidence of mucosal trauma during frequent suctioning.
- Nasopharyngeal airways are especially useful for relieving airway obstruction associated with mandibular-type injuries that result in jaw immobility or soft-tissue obstruction. Examples of these injuries include jaw wiring, trismus, pain, edema, jaw spasms, or mechanical impairment such as temporomandibular joint fractures and zygomatic fractures.[4, 5] In selected patient situations, a nasopharyngeal airway may be used to facilitate the passage of a fiberoptic bronchoscope and to tamponade small, bleeding blood vessels in the nasal mucosa.
- Insertion of the nasopharyngeal airway in an alert patient may stimulate the gag reflex, causing retching and vomiting.
- The nasopharyngeal airway is most commonly used in the postanesthesia recovery period to facilitate pulmonary toileting and in situations when the patient is semiconscious.
- Contraindications to use of a nasopharyngeal airway include
  - ❖ Patients with a history of taking warfarin or heparin
  - ❖ Patients prone to epistaxis
  - ❖ Patients with obstructed nasal passageways
  - ❖ Patients with facial or head trauma where basilar skull fracture or cranial vault communication is suspected

EQUIPMENT

- Appropriately sized nasal airway (Table 6–1)
- Nonsterile gloves
- Water-soluble lubricant
- Tape
- Safety pin
- Suction equipment
- Flashlight
- Tongue depressor

Additional equipment (to have available depending on patient need) includes the following:

- Cotton swabs
- Topical anesthetic

PATIENT AND FAMILY EDUCATION

- Explain the purpose of the airway and the necessity of the procedure to conscious patients or to the family of the unconscious patient. ➼*Rationale:* Communication and explanation for therapy are cited as an important need

Table 6–1 ●■■	Nasopharyngeal Airway Sizing	
Approximate Body Weight	Size (mm)
<100 lb	5–6 (small)
101–150 lb	7–8 (medium)
>151 lb	9–10 (large)

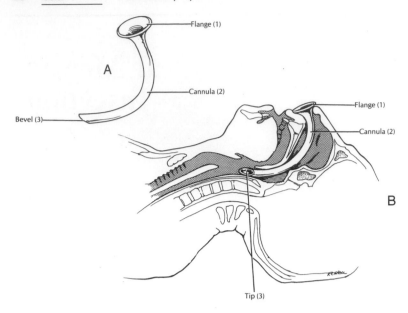

■ ● **FIGURE 6–1.** Nasopharyngeal airways. *A,* Airway parts. *B,* Proper placement. (From Eubanks DH, Bone RC. *Comprehensive Respiratory Care.* 2nd ed. St. Louis, Mo: Mosby; 1990:548.)

of patients and families; relieves anxiety and encourages communication.

• Explain the patient's role in assisting with insertion of the airway.   ➤*Rationale:* Elicits patient cooperation and facilitates tube insertion.

• Discuss the sensory experiences associated with nasal airway insertion, including the presence of a rubber airway in the nose and possible gagging.   ➤*Rationale:* Knowledge of anticipated sensory experiences reduces anxiety and distress.

PATIENT ASSESSMENT AND PREPARATION
Patient Assessment

• Cardiopulmonary status.   ➤*Rationale:* Evaluation of the patient's cardiopulmonary status will assist in determining the need for an artificial airway.

• Patent nasal passageway. With finger pressure, occlude one nostril. Feel for air movement under the open nostril. Patency also can be assessed by inspection of each naris with a flashlight.   ➤*Rationale:* Promotes smooth, quick, unobstructed airway insertion.

Patient Preparation

• Ensure that patient understands preprocedural teaching. Answer questions as they arise and reinforce information as needed.   ➤*Rationale:* Evaluates and reinforces understanding of previously taught information.

• Position patient. Unless contraindicated, a supine or high Fowler position is acceptable.   ➤*Rationale:* Promotes patient and nurse comfort and provides easy access to external nares.

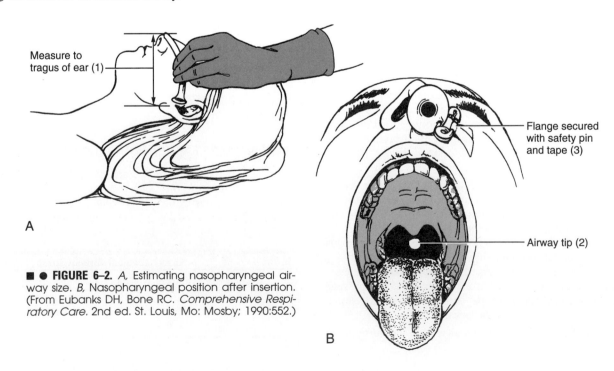

■ ● **FIGURE 6–2.** *A,* Estimating nasopharyngeal airway size. *B,* Nasopharyngeal position after insertion. (From Eubanks DH, Bone RC. *Comprehensive Respiratory Care.* 2nd ed. St. Louis, Mo: Mosby; 1990:552.)

Procedure	for Nasopharyngeal Airway Insertion

Steps	Rationale	Special Considerations
1. Wash hands; don personal protective equipment.	Reduces transmission of microorganisms and body secretions; standard precautions.	For copious secretions, don protective eyewear or face mask or both.
2. Prepare the nasopharyngeal airway. A. Inspect for smooth edges. B. Generously lubricate the tip and outer cannula with water-soluble lubricant.	Decreases chances of mucosal trauma during insertion. Decreases incidence of trauma by preventing friction against dry mucosal membrane.[5]	
3. Remove excess secretions from naris.	Allows for visual inspection of naris; removes possible source of obstruction; removes medium for organism growth.	Nasopharyngeal and nasotracheal suction are contraindicated in patients with actual or suspected maxillofacial and skull injuries.
4. When difficult insertion is anticipated (eg, with nasal polyps, septal deviation), apply topical anesthetic to cotton swabs, insert as far as possible, and coat the nasal passageway.	Topical anesthetics with a vasoconstrictor help shrink nasal mucosa and decrease the incidence of trauma and bleeding. Vasoconstrictor property acts on capillaries to decrease bleeding.	Check with physician, nurse practitioner, or institutional standards for topical anesthetic usage and indications.
5. Gently slide airway into nostril. Guide it medially and downward along the nasal passage.	Following the natural contour of the nasal passage will decrease the incidence of trauma.	If resistance is encountered, rotate the tube and continue gentle forward pressure. Do not force the tube. Should resistance continue, withdraw the tube and try the other nostril. While inserting, if the patient experiences increasing dyspnea or respiratory distress, consider removing the tube.
6. Ask patient to open his or her mouth, or hold patient's mouth open. Control tongue with a tongue depressor. Illuminate oral cavity and visualize tip of nasopharyngeal airway behind uvula (see Fig. 6–2)	Verifying location of airway in pharynx verifies proper airway positioning. Allows for inspection of posterior pharynx for excessive bleeding or mucus.	
7. Verify patency of airway. Feel for air movement over the flange. Auscultate breath sounds bilaterally.	Optimal airway positioning allows for forward gas flow, removal of secretions, and possible prevention of airway occlusion.	The conscious patient will need to exhale with his or her mouth closed.
8. Secure airway with a safety pin through the flange, and tape it in place (see Fig. 6–2).	Minimizes dislodgment, removal, and deeper penetration into the nasopharynx.	Make sure the safety pin remains closed to avoid pricking and trauma.
9. Suction secretions as needed.	Maintains patent airway.	Recheck flange for proper position.
10. Reassess patient's respiratory status.	Indicates effectiveness of the nasal airway.	

Expected Outcomes	Unexpected Outcomes
• Improvement of respiratory status • Long-term patent airway • Diminished mucosal edema and trauma related to frequent suction passes	• Inability to pass nasopharyngeal airway • Airway obstruction • Head or ear pain • Epistaxis • Naris and nasal mucosal ulceration

Patient Monitoring and Care

Patient Monitoring and Care	Rationale	Reportable Conditions
		These conditions should be reported if they persist despite nursing interventions. • Redness • Swelling • Drainage • Bleeding • Skin breakdown
1. Assess skin that is in contact with oral airway.		
2. Facilitate removal of secretions. Hyperoxygenate and suction as needed.	Retained secretions increase the potential for airway obstruction and pulmonary infections. Aging results in diminishing mucociliary clearance.	• Change in character or amount of secretions
3. Monitor respiratory status every 2 to 4 hours.	Change in respiratory status may indicate displacement of oral airway or worsening respiratory condition.	• Change in respiratory status not corrected with repositioning of airway or suctioning
4. Provide meticulous mouth care every 4 to 8 hours or as needed.	Prevents secretions, encrustations, mouth infections, and airway port occlusions.	• Lacerations • Ulcerations • Areas of necrosis

Documentation

Documentation should include the following:

- Patient and family education
- Insertion of nasopharyngeal airway
- Size of nasopharyngeal airway
- Any difficulties with insertion
- Patient tolerance, including respiratory and vital signs assessment before and after procedure
- Verification of proper placement
- Appearance and thickness of tracheal secretions, if present
- Skin integrity around tube
- Unexpected outcomes
- Nursing interventions

References

1. Eubanks DH, Bone RC. *Comprehensive Respiratory Care: A Learning System.* St. Louis, Mo: C.V. Mosby; 1990: 491–495.
2. Kersten LD. *Comprehensive Respiratory Nursing: A Decision-Making Approach.* Philadelphia, Pa: W.B. Saunders; 1989:630–635.
3. Miracle VA, Allnutt DR. How to perform basic airway management. *Nursing.* 1990;20(4):55–60.
4. Gotta A. Airway management for maxillofacial trauma. *Curr Rev Resp Crit Care.* 1988;10:114–120.
5. Cummins RO, ed. *Textbook of Advanced Cardiac Life Support.* Dallas, Tex: American Heart Association; 1997:2.2–2.3.

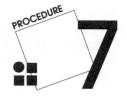

7 Oropharyngeal Airway Insertion

P U R P O S E: Oropharyngeal airways are inserted to relieve airway obstruction, provide short-term maintenance of an airway, and facilitate removal of tracheobronchial secretions.

Kay Knox Greenlee

PREREQUISITE NURSING KNOWLEDGE

- Oropharyngeal airways are usually disposable and made of hard, curved plastic.
- Oral airways are inserted through the open mouth with the posterior tip resting in the patient's pharynx. The oral airway is placed over the tongue. The curvature or body of the airway displaces the tongue forward from the posterior pharyngeal wall, a common site of airway obstruction.
- An oral airway has four parts: flange, body, tip, and channel (Fig. 7–1). The flange, or flat surface, protruding from the mouth rests against the lips. This design protects against aspiration into the airway. The body of the airway curves over the tongue. The tip is the distalmost part of the airway toward the base of the tongue. The channel enables passage of a suction catheter.
- The Guedel airway is tubular with a flattened-oval inner diameter. A suction catheter passes through the central lumen or channel.
- The Berman airway has a channel on either side that guides the catheter along the edge of the airway into the pharyngeal space.
- Oral airways are manufactured in a variety of lengths and widths for adults, children, and infants. Sizing is dependent on the age and size of the patient (Table 7–1). An alternative method used to select the size of an oral airway is to measure the airway by placing the flange alongside the patient's lips and the oral airway tip alongside the angle of the jaw (Fig. 7–2). Improperly sized airways can cause airway obstruction (if they are too small) and tongue displacement against the oropharynx (if they are too large).

- Oropharyngeal airways are most commonly used in unconscious patients because they may stimulate vomiting in the conscious or semiconscious patient.[1]
- Oral airways facilitate suctioning of the pharynx and prevent patients from biting their tongues, grinding their teeth, or occluding their endotracheal or oral gastric tubes. Additionally, an oropharyngeal airway may be used in conjunction with an oral endotracheal tube to facilitate artificial ventilation, to stimulate the effect of a bite block, and to prevent damage to the tongue and soft tissues of the mouth.
- Improper or rough insertion techniques can result in tooth damage or loss and lacerations to the roof of the mouth. Improper lip, mouth, and tube care can result in pressure sores, cracked lips, and stomatitis.
- Oropharyngeal airway placement should never be attempted in a patient who is actively seizing. If the patient has an aura preceding his or her seizure, an airway may be placed prophylactically.

EQUIPMENT

- Appropriately sized oral airway
- Nonsterile gloves
- Tongue depressor
- Tape

Additional equipment (to have available based on patient need) includes the following:

- Suction equipment
- Goggles, glasses, or face mask

PATIENT AND FAMILY EDUCATION

- Explain the procedure (if patient condition and time allow) and the reason for the airway insertion. **➤Rationale:** Identifies patient and family knowledge deficits about the patient's condition, the procedure, its expected benefits, and its potential risks and allows time for questions to clarify information and voice concerns. Explanations decrease patient anxiety and enhance cooperation.
- Explain the patient's role in assisting with insertion of

Table 7–1	Oral Airway Sizes	
Size of Patient	Diameter of Oral Airway (mm)	Size of Oral Airway
Large adult	100	5
Medium adult	90	4
Small adult	80	3

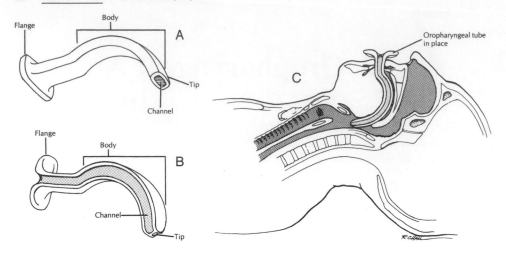

■ ● FIGURE 7–1. Oropharyngeal airways. *A,* Guedel airway. *B,* Berman airway. *C,* Properly inserted oropharyngeal tube. (From Eubanks DH, Bone RC. *Comprehensive Respiratory Care.* 2nd ed. St. Louis, Mo: Mosby; 1990:548.)

the airway. ➤*Rationale:* Elicits patient cooperation and facilitates tube insertion.

- Discuss the sensory experiences associated with oral airway insertion, including the inability to clench teeth together, the presence of a hard plastic airway in the mouth, the inability to freely move tongue, and the possibility of gagging. ➤*Rationale:* Knowledge of anticipated sensory experiences reduces anxiety and distress.

PATIENT ASSESSMENT AND PREPARATION

Patient Assessment

- Patient's need for long-term airway maintenance. ➤*Rationale:* Oropharyngeal airways are generally used for temporary airway maintenance.[2, 3]
- Condition of oral mucosa, dentition, and gums. ➤*Rationale:* Preprocedural assessment provides baseline information for later comparison.
- Remove loose-fitting dentures and any foreign objects

from the mouth. ➤*Rationale:* Removal ensures that objects will not be advanced farther into the airway during insertion.

Patient Preparation

- Ensure that patient understands preprocedural teaching. Answer questions as they arise and reinforce information as needed. ➤*Rationale:* Evaluates and reinforces understanding of previously taught information.
- Position patient. Semi-Fowler or supine position is preferred for the conscious patient. ➤*Rationale:* Promotes patient and nurse comfort and provides easy access to oral cavity.
- Hyperextend the patient's neck using the head-tilt, chin-lift technique; use the jaw-thrust technique for the unconscious patient. ➤*Rationale:* Airway obstructions can result from posterior displacement of the tongue and epiglottis.

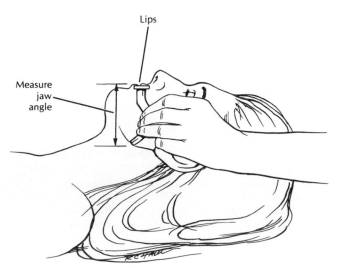

■ ● FIGURE 7–2. Alternative method for selecting size of an oropharyngeal airway. (From Eubanks DH, Bone RC. *Comprehensive Respiratory Care.* 2nd ed. St. Louis, Mo: Mosby; 1990:552.)

Procedure	for Oropharyngeal Airway Insertion

Steps	Rationale	Special Considerations
1. Wash hands, and don personal protective equipment.	Reduces transmission of microorganisms and body secretions; standard precautions.	Protective eyeware or face masks should be worn in the presence of copious secretions.
2. Suction the mouth and pharynx using a rigid pharyngeal suction-tip (Yankauer) catheter.	Clears airway of secretions, blood, and vomit so they do not enter into the airway with airway insertion.	
3. Open the mouth using the crossed finger technique (Fig. 7–3). Remove dentures, if present.	Provides access to oral cavity and leverage to open a tightly closed mouth.	
4. Insert oral airway. A. Hold oral airway with curved end up (Fig. 7–4).	Provides patent upper airway and prevents posterior tongue displacement.	
B. Advance oral airway over the base of the tongue until the flange is parallel with the patient's nose.	Positions airway appropriately.	Remove the airway immediately if the patient gags, gasps for air, or begins breathing irregularly.
C. Rotate the tip 180 degrees to point down (see Fig. 7–4).	Provides for open pathway from the mouth to the pharynx.	A tongue depressor may assist in tongue control during insertion.
5. Recheck the size and position of the oral airway. Verify airway patency.	Proper placement and size are essential for securing and maintaining a patent airway.	When the oral airway is properly sized, the flange should rest against the patient's lips (see Fig. 7–2). Gagging may indicate that the airway is too long. Make sure the lips and tongue are not between the teeth and airway.[1]
6. Consider securing the airway.	Taping is indicated to prevent expulsion of the airway. Leaving the airway untaped is indicated in patients who need to be able to cough out the airway if gagging should occur, because gagging may stimulate vomiting and aspiration (ie, in the postanesthesia or semiconscious patient).	Follow institutional standards. Use care not to tape over air channel.
7. Hyperoxygenate and suction pharynx as needed (see Procedure 9).	Maintains patent airway; pooled secretions provide a medium for bacterial growth.	
8. Reassess patient's respiratory status.	Validates the effectiveness of the oral airway.	

Expected Outcomes	Unexpected Outcomes
• Improvement of respiratory status • Short-term patent airway	• Airway obstruction • Pulmonary aspiration • Trauma to the lips and oral cavity • Inability to insert oral airway because patient is combative or seizing or patient's mouth cannot be opened

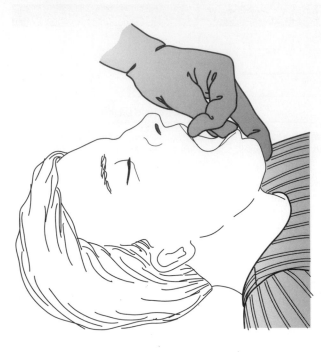

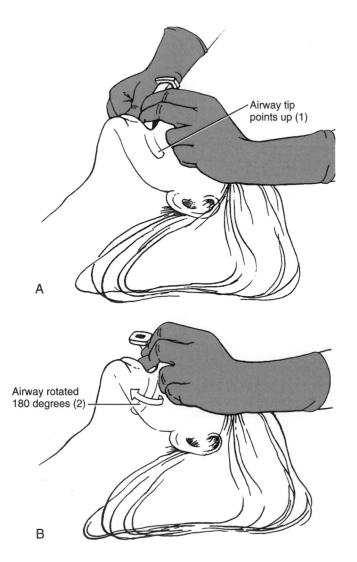

Airway tip
points up (1)

A

Airway rotated
180 degrees (2)

B

■ ● **FIGURE 7–3.** Crossed-finger technique for opening the mouth. (From Kersten LD. *Comprehensive Respiratory Nursing.* Philadelphia: WB Saunders; 1989:631.)

■ ● **FIGURE 7–4.** Insertion of an oropharyngeal airway. *A,* Advance airway with curved end up. *B,* Rotate airway 180 degrees. (From Eubanks DH, Bone RC. *Comprehensive Respiratory Care.* 2nd ed. St. Louis, Mo: Mosby; 1990:551.)

Patient Monitoring and Care

Patient Monitoring and Care	Rationale	Reportable Conditions
		These conditions should be reported if they persist despite nursing interventions.
1. Reposition the oral airway every 1 to 2 hours, assessing the lips, tongue, and mouth with each position change.	Pressure of the flange on the lips may produce ulcers and necrosis.	• Lacerations • Ulcerations • Areas of necrosis
2. Apply water-soluble jelly, petrolatum, or lip balm to the lips.	Prevents mucosal drying and cracking.	• Cracked and bleeding lips
3. Provide meticulous oral care every 4 to 8 hours or as needed.	Decreases secretions, encrustations, oral infections, and airway port occlusions.	• Lacerations • Ulcerations • Areas of necrosis • Drainage
4. Remove the oral airway every 24 hours or as needed. Clean airway and reinsert, as needed.	Allows for more complete inspection of the lips and oral cavity; enables complete oral hygiene.	
5. Monitor respiratory status every 2 to 4 hours.	Change in respiratory status may indicate displacement of oral airway or worsening respiratory condition.	• Stridor • Crowing • Gasping respirations • Snoring

Documentation

Documentation should include the following:

- Patient and family education
- Insertion of oropharyngeal airway
- Type and size of oral airway
- Any difficulties in insertion
- Patient tolerance, including respiratory and vital signs assessments before and after procedure
- Verification of proper placement
- Appearance and thickness of tracheal or oral secretions, if present
- Oral care
- Skin integrity around tube
- Unexpected outcomes
- Nursing interventions

References

1. Cummins RO, ed. *Textbook of Advanced Cardiac Life Support.* Dallas, Tex: American Heart Association; 1997:2.2.
2. Eubanks DH, Bone RC. *Comprehensive Respiratory Care: A Learning System.* St. Louis, Mo: C.V. Mosby; 1990:491–495.
3. Kersten LD. *Comprehensive Respiratory Nursing: A Decision-Making Approach.* Philadelphia, Pa: W.B. Saunders; 1989:630–635.

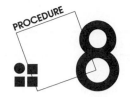

8

Oxygen Tank Preparation and Setup

P U R P O S E: Oxygen tank preparation and setup may be required to deliver supplemental oxygen therapy for patient transportation and in emergency situations outside the critical care unit.

Sandra L. Schutz

PREREQUISITE NURSING KNOWLEDGE

- Medical gas cylinders are color coded according to the gas contained in the cylinder. Cylinder color and labeling are the primary ways to identify the type of gas in a cylinder. All oxygen cylinders in the United States are green in color and are labeled with the symbol O_2.
- Cylinders of oxygen contain high-pressure compressed gas and require special handling techniques for management during use and transport.
- The most common oxygen gas cylinder used is an E cylinder, which, when full, contains approximately 5 hours of available oxygen at a delivery rate of 2 L/min.
- The effectiveness of oxygen delivered from a portable system is affected by all the physiologic variables that affect oxygenation from piped systems. Physiologic variables affecting oxygenation include patency of the airway, depth and rate of respiration, gas exchange at the alveolar level, oxygen-carrying capacity, oxygen delivery and uptake at the cellular level, and rate of oxygen consumption.

EQUIPMENT

- Oxygen tank
- Oxygen flowmeter and regulator or pressure relief valve
- Nipple adapter
- Slotted wrench or regulator knob
- Wheeled or portable carrier or basket
- Appropriate oxygen-delivery system

Additional equipment (to allow use of the oxygen tank at an extended distance from the patient, such as in diagnostic testing situations) includes the following:

- Oxygen extension tubing
- Straight connector

PATIENT AND FAMILY EDUCATION

- Explain the need for supplemental oxygen. ➤*Rationale:* Decreases patient anxiety.
- Explain patient's need to remain still while oxygen tank is used for transport. ➤*Rationale:* Patient movement could dislodge the oxygen tank from the bed and cause pressurized displacement of the flowmeter and regulator.
- Restrict smoking to at least 10 feet or farther from the oxygen source. ➤*Rationale:* Oxygen supports combustion and is highly volatile in the presence of an open flame or ignition source.

PATIENT ASSESSMENT

- Ensure that patient understands preprocedural teaching. Answer questions as they arise, and reinforce information as needed. ➤*Rationale:* Evaluates and reinforces understanding of previously taught information.
- Determine need for oxygen or adequacy of existing oxygen flow rate and delivery system. ➤*Rationale:* Evaluation of the patient's continued need for oxygen therapy will determine the need for use of an oxygen tank.

Procedure **for Oxygen Tank Preparation and Setup**

Steps	Rationale	Special Considerations
1. Obtain and prepare all necessary equipment and supplies for proper tank setup.	Ensures quick and efficient assembly of tank and availability of use.	
2. Inspect tank and cylinder valve for damage. If damage is present, do not use.	A damaged tank may cause malfunction and inadequate oxygen delivery to the patient.	

Procedure continued on following page

Procedure	**for Oxygen Tank Preparation and Setup** *Continued*

Steps	Rationale	Special Considerations
3. Place oxygen tank in portable carrier in the upright position.	Prevents oxygen tank from falling or being dropped or dragged.	Oxygen tanks have the potential to become dangerous or lethal missiles if dropped or mishandled.
4. Ensure that the environment is safe for portable oxygen use.	Oxygen supports and accelerates the combustion of other materials, making fire a potential hazard of concentrated oxygen flow.	Other gases, dirt, dust, oil, grease, hydrocarbons, and fuel or potential ignition sources must be kept away from the oxygen regulator and cylinder valve.
5. If the tank has a regulator or pressure relief valve on it, proceed to step 8.		
6. Before attaching the regulator or pressure relief valve, "crack" or "bleed" the oxygen tank. Remove the plastic cap over the outlet opening (if present). With the tank secured in the upright position, point the outlet opening on the stem of the tank away from any person and stand to one side away from the opening. Slowly open the valve clockwise with the knob or a wrench. A hissing sound should be heard. When the hissing sound is heard, immediately close the valve. Ensure that the tank is fully turned off by turning the valve stem counterclockwise with the knob or wrench.	Cracking the tank clears the outlet valve of the regulator of any particulate matter. An oxygen tank should never be fully opened without a regulator in place. The tank is at full pressure between 1800 and 2400 pounds per square inch (psi), and the valve stem end can become a missile when opened without a pressure relief valve or regulator.	This ensures that there is no dust or other combustible material in the valve itself. If the tank can't be cracked, return it with a note stating, "Do Not Use, Unable to Crack."
7. Place the yoke attachment over the stem valve and line up the "O" ring surrounding the regulator nipple-pin system with the outlet opening before tightening the yoke to the stem valve. Ensure that there is only one O ring present.	A regulator or pressure relief valve is needed to properly regulate the flow of oxygen in L/min and to determine the volume of oxygen in the tank. Insertion of a regulator through a plastic cap or presence of debris in the outlet may severely damage the regulator, rendering it unusable. More than one O ring will cause leakage of oxygen from the outlet valve.	Inspect and identify the regulator for signs of damage or a missing O ring. If damage is present or if the O ring is missing, do not use. Do not attempt repairs. Check with the appropriate hospital department handling oxygen supplies for repair.
8. Attach a green nipple onto the regulator (if not already present). This is usually screwed in just below the pressure gauge.	Allows attachment of the oxygen tubing–oxygen-delivery system.	
9. Attach all necessary tubing. Before turning on oxygen, note the pressure gauge reading.	A tank is full at 2000 psi and needs refilling at 500 psi or ¼ full. It is important to know the amount of oxygen available in the cylinder before use. This will ensure sufficient oxygen supply for the anticipated duration of need of the portable system.	Never use a cylinder if it contains less than 500 psi or is less than ¼ full. Particles settle in the bottom of the cylinder and may be pulled into the patient's airway if a tank less than ¼ full is used.
10. To start the flow of oxygen, slowly turn the valve stem clockwise one full 360-degree turn and then back one-quarter turn.		
11. Turn the flowmeter to the desired oxygen flow rate appropriate for the oxygen-delivery system and patient oxygen need.	Be certain the flow rate is appropriate for the oxygen-delivery system. Insufficient flow rates can result in hypoxia.	
12. Check the system for visual and audible indications of leakage.	A leaking system is a hazard and can result in more rapid use of the oxygen supply than anticipated.	If the cylinder is leaking, move it to an isolated, well-ventilated area. Mark the cylinder as leaking. Do not continue using the cylinder, and notify the appropriate department immediately.

Procedure	**for Oxygen Tank Preparation and Setup** *Continued*

Steps	Rationale	Special Considerations
13. To turn the cylinder off or replace the cylinder, close the oxygen outlet valve. Turn the valve with a wrench or the knob counterclockwise until it is tightly sealed. Turn the flowmeter off and then on again. This will bleed the remaining oxygen from the regulator. When the flow ceases, turn the flowmeter off completely.	This prevents pressure buildup in the regulator.	

Expected Outcomes	Unexpected Outcomes
• Oxygen tank set up correctly	• Inappropriate setup of oxygen tank or malfunction of oxygen tank, resulting in inappropriate oxygen delivery, worsening of patient hypoxia, or oxygen toxicity

Patient Monitoring and Care

Patient Monitoring and Care	Rationale	Reportable Conditions
		These conditions should be reported if they persist despite nursing interventions.
1. Monitor the patient's respiratory status and response to oxygen therapy on an ongoing basis.	Ensures that oxygen therapy is appropriate to support oxygenation needs at the tissue level.	• Decline in patient oxygenation or worsening respiratory status, or both
2. Monitor the cylinder for supply of available oxygen during the duration of use.	Ensures that a continuous supply is available and that the supply will not end, leaving the patient subject to hypoxia.	• Tank $<\frac{1}{4}$ full; psi <500
3. Monitor the patient for signs of retention of carbon dioxide (CO_2).	As patients retain CO_2, their level of consciousness will decrease until they are unarousable. This may be related to excess oxygen eliminating the patient's hypoxic drive to breathe (as in patients with chronic obstructive pulmonary disease). Immediately decrease the oxygen flow rate or remove the oxygen entirely while reporting the change. Decreasing the source of the excess oxygen will return the patient to the baseline hypoxic state and reestablish the drive to breathe.	• Decreased level of consciousness
4. Monitor the cylinder's stability every time the patient is moved.	This ensures the cylinder will not be overturned or fall unexpectedly.	
5. Observe for proper function of the oxygen-delivery system (nasal cannula tips are correctly in both nares, oxygen mask is secured tightly to the face, or the non-rebreather reservoir is fully expanded).	Proper setup of the cylinder and oxygen-delivery system will be defeated if the oxygen-delivery system is not properly secured.	

Documentation

Documentation should include the following:

- Patient and family education
- Oxygen-delivery system
- Oxygen flow rate
- Ongoing clinical assessment of patient

- Unexpected outcomes
- Nursing interventions

Additional Readings

Perry AG, Potter PA. *Clinical Nursing Skills and Techniques.* 4th ed. St. Louis, Mo: Mosby–Year Book; 1998:442–446.

Ryerson GG, Block A. Oxygen as a drug: clinical properties, benefits, modes and hazards of administration. In: Burton GG, Hodgkin JE, Ward JJ eds. *Respiratory Care: A Guide to Clinical Practice.* 3rd ed. Philadelphia, Pa: J.B. Lippincott; 1991:319–339.

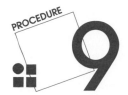

Endotracheal or Tracheostomy Tube Suctioning

P U R P O S E: Endotracheal or tracheostomy tube suctioning is performed to maintain the patency of the artificial airway and to improve gas exchange, decrease airway resistance, and reduce infection risk by removing secretions from the trachea and main stem bronchi. Suctioning may also be performed to obtain samples of tracheal secretions for laboratory analysis.

Marianne Chulay

PREREQUISITE NURSING KNOWLEDGE

- Endotracheal and tracheostomy tubes are used to maintain a patent airway and to facilitate mechanical ventilation. Presence of these artificial airways, especially endotracheal tubes, prevents effective coughing and secretion removal, requiring periodic removal of pulmonary secretions with suctioning. In acute care situations, suctioning is always performed as a sterile procedure to prevent nosocomial pneumonia.
- Suctioning is performed using one of two basic methods. In the open-suction technique, following disconnection of the endotracheal or tracheostomy tube from any ventilatory tubing or oxygen sources, a single-use suction catheter is inserted into the open end of the tube. In the closed-suction technique, also referred to as in-line suctioning, a multi-use suction catheter inside a sterile plastic sleeve is inserted through a special diaphragm attached to the end of the endotracheal or tracheostomy tube (Fig. 9–1). The closed-suction technique allows for the maintenance of oxygenation and ventilation support, which may be beneficial when high levels of inspired oxygen or positive end-expiratory pressure (PEEP) are required during mechanical ventilation. In addition, the closed-suction technique decreases the risk for aerosolization of tracheal secretions during suction-induced coughing. Consider use of the closed-suction technique in patients who develop cardiopulmonary instability during suctioning with the open technique, who have high levels of PEEP (>10 cm H_2O) or inspired oxygen ($>80\%$) or both, or who have grossly bloody pulmonary secretions or when active tuberculosis is suspected.
- Indications for suctioning include the following:
  - ❖ Secretions in the artificial airway
  - ❖ Suspected aspiration of gastric or upper airway secretions
  - ❖ Auscultation of adventitious lung sounds over the trachea or main stem bronchi or both

- ❖ Increase in peak airway pressures when patient is on mechanical ventilation
- ❖ Increase in respiratory rate or sustained coughing or both
- ❖ Gradual or sudden decrease in arterial blood oxygen (Pao$_2$), arterial blood oxygen saturation (Sao$_2$), or arterial saturation levels via pulse oximetry (Spo$_2$) levels
- ❖ Sudden onset of respiratory distress, when airway patency is questioned
- Suctioning of airways should be performed only for a clinical indication and not as a routine, fixed schedule treatment.
- Contraindications to suctioning are as follows: Suctioning is a necessary procedure for patients with artificial airways. When clinical indicators of the need for suctioning exist, there is no absolute contraindication to suctioning. In situations where the development of a suctioning complication would be poorly tolerated by the patient, very strong evidence of a clinical need for suctioning should exist.
- Complications associated with suctioning of artificial airways include the following:
  - ❖ Respiratory arrest
  - ❖ Cardiac arrest
  - ❖ Cardiac dysrhythmias
  - ❖ Hypertension or hypotension
  - ❖ Decreases in mixed venous oxygen saturation (Svo$_2$)
  - ❖ Increased intracranial pressure
  - ❖ Bronchospasm
  - ❖ Pulmonary hemorrhage or bleeding
- Tracheal mucosal damage (epithelial denudement, hyperemia, loss of cilia, edema) occurs during suctioning when tissue is pulled into the catheter tip holes. These areas of damage increase the risk of infection and bleeding. Use of special-tipped catheters, low levels of suction pressure, or intermittent suction pressure has not been shown to decrease tracheal mucosal damage with suctioning.
- Postural drainage and percussion may improve secretion

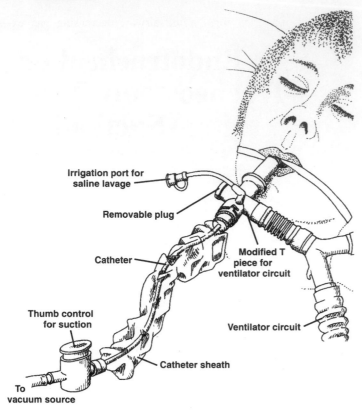

Irrigation port for
saline lavage

Removable plug

Catheter

Modified T
piece for
ventilator circuit

Thumb control
for suction

Ventilator circuit

Catheter sheath

To
vacuum source

■ ● **FIGURE 9–1.** Closed-suction technique. (From Sills JR. *Respiratory Care Certification Guide.* St. Louis, Mo: CV Mosby; 1991:283.)

mobilization from small to large airways in large mucus-production types of disease (eg, cystic fibrosis, bronchitis).

• Adequate systemic hydration and supplemental humidification of inspired gases assist in thinning secretions for easier aspiration from airways. Instillation of bolus normal saline (5 to 10 mL) does not thin secretions and may cause decreases in arterial oxygenation.

• The suction catheter should not be any larger than one half of the internal diameter of the endotracheal or tracheostomy tube.

EQUIPMENT—OPEN TECHNIQUE

• Suction catheter of appropriate size (Table 9–1)
• Sterile water-soluble lubricant or sterile saline solution
• Sterile gloves
• Sterile solution container or sterile basin
• Source of suction (wall mounted or portable)
• Connecting tube, 4 to 6 ft
• Self-inflating manual resuscitation bag (MRB) connected to an oxygen flowmeter, set at 15 L/min (not required if using the ventilator to deliver hyperoxygenation breaths)
• Goggles or glasses and mask

Additional equipment (to have available depending on patient need) includes the following:

• PEEP valve (for patients on >5 cm H_2O PEEP)

EQUIPMENT—CLOSED TECHNIQUE

• Closed-suction setup with a catheter of appropriate size (see Table 9–1)
• Source of suction (wall mounted or portable)
• Connecting tube, 4 to 6 ft

• Sterile saline lavage containers (5 to 10 mL)
• Suction catheter (individually packaged) for oral and nasal suctioning
• Nonsterile gloves
• Goggles or glasses and mask

PATIENT AND FAMILY EDUCATION

• Explain the procedure for endotracheal or tracheostomy tube suctioning.   ➤*Rationale:* Reduces anxiety.
• Explain that suctioning may be uncomfortable, causing the patient to experience shortness of breath.   ➤*Rationale:* Reduces anxiety and elicits patient cooperation.
• Explain the patient's role in assisting with secretion removal by coughing during the procedure.   ➤*Rationale:*

Table 9–1 ● ■ ■	Guideline for Catheter Size for Endotracheal and Tracheostomy Tube Suctioning*		
Patient Age	Endotracheal Tube Size (mm)	Tracheostomy Tube Size (mm, inner diameter)	Suction Catheter Size (Fr)
Small child (2 to 5 years)	4.0 to 5.0	3.5 to 4.5	6 to 8
School-aged child (6 to 12 years)	5.0 to 6.0	4.5 to 5.0	8 to 10
Adolescent to adult	7.0 to 9.0	5.0 to 9.0	10 to 16

*This guide should be used as an estimate only. Actual sizes depend on the size and individual needs of the patient.

From Henneman E, Ellstrom K, St. John R. Airway management. In: *AACN Protocols for Practice: Care of the Mechanically Ventilated Patient Series.* Aliso Viejo, Ca: American Association of Critical-Care Nurses; 1999.

Encourages cooperation and facilitates removal of secretions.

PATIENT ASSESSMENT AND PREPARATION

Patient Assessment

Signs and symptoms of airway obstruction are as follows:

- Secretions in the airway
- Inspiratory wheezes
- Expiratory crackles
- Restlessness
- Ineffective coughing
- Decreased level of consciousness
- Decreased breath sounds
- Tachypnea
- Tachycardia or bradycardia
- Cyanosis
- Hypertension or hypotension
- Shallow respirations ➤*Rationale:* Physical signs and symptoms result from inadequate gas exchange associated with airway obstruction.
- Note peak airway pressures on the ventilator. ➤*Rationale:* Indicates potential secretions in the airway, increasing resistance to gas flow.
- Evaluate SaO_2 and SpO_2 levels. ➤*Rationale:* Indicates

potential secretions in the airway, decreasing gas exchange.

Signs and symptoms of inadequate breathing patterns are as follows:

- Dyspnea
- Shallow respirations
- Intercostal and suprasternal retractions
- Frequent triggering of ventilator alarms
- Increased respiratory rate ➤*Rationale:* Respiratory distress is a late sign of lower airway obstruction.

Patient Preparation

- Ensure that patient understands preprocedural teaching. Answer questions as they arise, and reinforce information as needed. ➤*Rationale:* Evaluates and reinforces understanding of previously taught information.
- Assist the patient in achieving a position that is comfortable for the patient and nurse, generally semi-Fowler or Fowler. ➤*Rationale:* Promotes comfort, oxygenation, and ventilation and reduces strain.
- Secure additional personnel to assist with hyperoxygenation with the MRB bag to provide hyperoxygenation (open-suction technique only). ➤*Rationale:* Two hands are necessary to inflate the MRB for adult tidal volume levels (>600 mL).

Procedure for Endotracheal or Tracheostomy Tube Suctioning

Steps	Rationale	Special Considerations
1. Wash hands, and don personal protective equipment.	Reduces transmission of microorganisms and body secretions; standard precautions.	
2. Turn on suction apparatus and set vacuum regulator to 100 to 120 mm Hg. *(Level II: Theory based, no research data to support recommendations; recommendations from expert consensus group may exist)* Follow manufacturer's directions for suction pressure levels when using closed-suction catheter systems. *(Level I: Manufacturer's recommendation only)*	The amount of suction applied should be only enough to effectively remove secretions. High negative-pressure settings may increase tracheal mucosal damage.[1-3]	
3. Secure one end of the connecting tube to the suction machine, and place the other end in a convenient location within reach.	Prepares suction apparatus.	
4. Monitor patient's cardiopulmonary status before, during, and after the suctioning period. *(Level II: Theory based, no research data to support recommendations; recommendations from expert consensus group may exist)*	Observes for signs and symptoms of complications: decreased arterial oxygen saturation, cardiac dysrhythmias, bronchospasm, respiratory distress, cyanosis, increased blood pressure or intracranial pressure, anxiety, agitation, or changes in mental status.[1, 2, 4-14]	Development of cardiopulmonary instability, particularly cardiac dysrhythmias or arterial desaturation, requires immediate termination of the suctioning procedure.
5a. **Open-Suction Technique Only** A. Open sterile catheter package on a clean surface, using the inside of the wrapping as a sterile field.	Prepares catheter and prevents transmission of microorganisms.	

Procedure continued on following page

Procedure	**for Endotracheal or Tracheostomy Tube Suctioning** *Continued*

Steps	Rationale	Special Considerations
B. Set up the sterile solution container or sterile field. Be careful not to touch the inside of the container. Fill with approximately 100 mL of sterile normal saline solution or water.	Prepares catheter flush solution.	
C. Don sterile gloves.	Maintains sterility and standard precautions.	In the event that one sterile glove and one nonsterile glove are used, apply the nonsterile glove to the nondominant hand and the sterile glove to the dominant hand. Handle all nonsterile items with the nondominant hand.
D. Pick up suction catheter, being careful to avoid touching nonsterile surfaces. With the nondominant hand, pick up the connecting tubing. Secure the suction catheter to the connecting tubing.	Maintains catheter sterility. Connects the suction catheter and the connecting tubing.	The dominant hand should not come in contact with the connecting tubing. Wrapping the suction catheter around the sterile dominant hand will help prevent inadvertent contamination of the catheter.
E. Check equipment for proper functioning by suctioning a small amount of sterile saline solution from the container. Proceed to step 6.	Ensures equipment function.	
5b. **Closed-Suction Technique Only**		
A. Connect the suction tubing to the closed system suction port, according to manufacturer's guidelines.		
6. Hyperoxygenate the patient for at least 30 seconds by one of the following three methods. *(Level V: Clinical studies in more than one patient population and situation)*	Hyperoxygenation with 100% oxygen is used to prevent a decrease in arterial oxygen levels during the suctioning procedure.[1, 2, 5–7, 11, 15–18]	Limited data indicate that use of a ventilator to deliver the hyperoxygenation may be more effective in increasing arterial oxygen levels.[19, 20]
A. Press the suction hyperoxygenation button on the ventilator with the nondominant hand. OR		
B. Increase the baseline fraction of inspired oxygen (FIO_2) level on the mechanical ventilator.		When using this method, caution must be used to return the FIO_2 to baseline levels following completion of suctioning.
C. Disconnect the ventilator or gas delivery tubing from the end of the endotracheal or tracheostomy tube, attach the MRB to the tube with the nondominant hand, and administer 5 to 6 breaths over 30 seconds.	Attach a PEEP valve to the MRB for patients on >5 cm H_2O PEEP. Verify 100% oxygen delivery capabilities of MRB by checking manufacturer's guidelines or with direct measurement with an in-line oxygen analyzer when baseline ventilator oxygen delivery to the patient is >60%. Some models of MRB entrain room air and deliver less than 100% oxygen.	Use of a second person to deliver hyperoxygenation breaths with the MRB will significantly increase tidal volume delivery. One-handed "bagging" rarely achieves adult tidal volume breaths (>500 mL).[19, 21–23]
7. With the suction off, gently but quickly insert the catheter with the dominant hand into the artificial airway until resistance is met; then pull back 1 cm. *(Level II: Theory based, no research data to support recommendations; recommendations from expert consensus group may exist)*	Suction should be applied only as needed to remove secretions and for as short a time as possible to minimize decreases in arterial oxygen levels.[1, 2]	Directional or Coude catheters are available for selective right or left main stem bronchus placement. Straight catheters usually enter the right main stem bronchus.[24, 25]

Steps	Rationale	Special Considerations
8. Place the nondominant thumb over the control vent of the suction catheter and apply continuous or intermittent suction. *(Level III: Laboratory data; no clinical data to support recommendations)* Rotate the catheter between the dominant thumb and forefinger as you withdraw the catheter over 10 seconds or less into the sterile catheter sleeve (closed-suction technique) or out of the open airway (open-suction technique). *(Level II: Theory based, no research data to support recommendations; recommendations from expert consensus group may exist)*	Tracheal damage from suctioning is similar with intermittent or continuous suction.[26–29] Decreases in arterial oxygen levels during suctioning can be kept to a minimum with brief suction periods.[1, 2, 30]	
9. Hyperoxygenate for 30 seconds as described in step 6. *(Level V: Clinical studies in more than one patient population and situation)*		
10. One or two more passes of the suction catheter, as delineated in steps 7 and 8, may be performed if secretions remain in the airway and the patient is tolerating the procedure. *(Level II: Theory based, no research data to support recommendations; recommendations from expert consensus group may exist)* Provide 30 seconds of hyperoxygenation before and after each pass of the suction catheter. *(Level V: Clinical studies in more than one patient population and situation)*	Arterial oxygen desaturation and cardiopulmonary complications increase with each successive pass.[1, 2, 3, 31]	If secretions remain in the airways following 2 to 3 suction catheter passes, allow the patient to rest before additional suctioning passes. Saline should not be routinely instilled into the artificial airway before suctioning. *(Level V: Clinical studies in more than one patient population and situation)*[1, 32–37]
11. If the patient does not tolerate suctioning despite hyperoxygenation, try the following steps. *(Level II: Theory based, no research data to support recommendations; recommendations from expert consensus group may exist)* A. Ensure that 100% O_2 is being delivered. B. Maintain PEEP during suctioning. Check that the PEEP valve is attached properly to the MRB if using that method for hyperoxygenation. C. Switch to another method of suctioning (eg, closed-suctioning technique). D. Allow longer recovery intervals between suction passes. E. Hyperventilation may be used in situations where the patient does not tolerate suctioning with hyperoxygenation alone, using either the MRB or the ventilator.	Use of a different suctioning technique may be physiologically less demanding.[1]	

Procedure continued on following page

Procedure for Endotracheal or Tracheostomy Tube Suctioning *Continued*

Steps	Rationale	Special Considerations
12. Rinse the catheter and connecting tubing with sterile saline solution until clear.	Removes buildup of secretions in the connecting tubing and, when using the closed-suction catheter system, in the in-line suction catheter.	
13. Once the lower airway has been adequately cleared of secretions, perform nasal or oral pharyngeal suctioning. *(Level II: Theory based, no research data to support recommendations; recommendations from expert consensus group may exist)* A separate suction catheter must be opened for this step when using the closed-suction technique.	Prevents contamination of the lower airways with upper airway organisms, particularly gram-negative bacilli.[38]	Care should be taken to avoid nasal or oropharyngeal tissue trauma and gagging during suctioning.
14. Open-suction technique only: On completion of upper airway suctioning, wrap the catheter around the dominant hand. Pull glove off inside out. Catheter will remain in glove. Pull off other glove in same fashion, and discard. Turn off suction device.	Reduces transmission of microorganisms.	
15. Reposition patient.		
16. Wash hands.		
17. Discard remaining normal saline solution and solution container. If basin is nondisposable, place in soiled utility room. Suction collection tubing and canisters may remain in use for multiple suctioning episodes. *(Level II: Theory based, no research data to support recommendations; recommendations from expert consensus group may exist)*	Solutions and catheters, which come in direct contact with the lower airways during suctioning, must be sterile to decrease the risks for nosocomial pneumonia. Devices that are not in direct contact have not been shown to increase infection risk.[38]	Check institutional standards for equipment removal.

Expected Outcomes

- Removal of secretions from the large airways
- Improved gas exchange
- Airway patency
- Amelioration of clinical signs or symptoms of need for suctioning (eg, adventitious breath sounds, coughing, high airway pressures)
- Sample for laboratory analysis

Unexpected Outcomes

- Cardiac dysrhythmias (premature contractions, tachycardias, bradycardias, heart blocks, asystole)
- Hypoxemia
- Bronchospasm
- Excessive increases in arterial blood pressure or intracranial pressure
- Nosocomial infections
- Cardiopulmonary distress
- Decreased level of consciousness
- Airway obstruction

Patient Monitoring and Care	Rationale	Reportable Conditions
1. Monitor patient's cardiopulmonary status before, during, and after the suctioning period. *(Level II: Theory based, no research data to support recommendations; recommendations from expert consensus group may exist)*	Observes for signs and symptoms of complications.[1, 2, 4–14]	*These conditions should be reported if they persist despite nursing interventions.* • Decreased arterial oxygen saturation • Cardiac dysrhythmias • Bronchospasm • Respiratory distress • Cyanosis • Increased blood pressure or intracranial pressure • Anxiety, agitation, or changes in mental status
2. Reassess patient for signs of suctioning effectiveness. *(Level II: Theory based, no research data to support recommendations; recommendations from expert consensus group may exist)*		• Diminished breath sounds • Decreased oxygenation • Increased peak airway pressures • Coughing • Increased work of breathing

Documentation

Documentation should include the following:

- Patient and family education
- Presuctioning assessment, including clinical indication for suctioning
- Suctioning of endotracheal or tracheostomy tube
- Size of suction catheter
- Type of hyperoxygenation method used
- Number of passes of the suction catheter
- Volume, color, consistency, and odor of secretions obtained
- Any difficulties during catheter insertion or hyperoxygenation
- Tolerance of suctioning procedure, including development of any unexpected outcomes during or after the procedure
- Nursing interventions
- Postsuctioning assessment

References

1. Henneman E, Ellstrom K, St. John R. Airway management. In: *AACN Protocols for Practice: Care of the Mechanically Ventilated Patient Series.* Aliso Viejo, Ca: American Association of Critical-Care Nurses; 1999.
2. AARC Clinical Practice Guideline. Endotracheal suctioning of mechanically ventilated adults and children with artificial airways. *Respir Care.* 1993;38:500–504.
3. Kersten L. *Comprehensive Respiratory Nursing: A Decision-Making Approach.* Philadelphia, Pa: W.B. Saunders; 1989.
4. Chase D, Campbell G, Byram D, et al. Hemodynamic changes associated with endotracheal suctioning. *Heart Lung.* 1989;18:292–293.
5. Lookinkind S, Appel PL. Hemodynamic and oxygen transport changes following endotracheal suctioning in trauma patients. *Nurs Res.* 1991;40:133–139.
6. Clark A, Winslow E, Tyler D, White K. Effects of endotracheal suctioning on mixed venous oxygen saturation and heart rate in critically ill adults. *Heart Lung.* 1990;19:552–557.
7. Preusser B, Stone K, Broch K, Karl J. The effect of two methods of preoxygenation (manual versus ventilator) on mean arterial pressure, peak airway pressure and postsuctioning hypoxemia. *Heart Lung.* 1987;16:317–322.
8. Brown B, Peeples D. The effects of hyperventilation and lidocaine on intracranial pressure. *Heart Lung.* 1991;21:286.
9. Campbell V. Effects of controlled hyperoxygenation and endotracheal suctioning on intracranial pressure in head-injured adults. *Appl Nurs Res.* 1991;4:138–140.
10. Hepburn D, Chulay M, Byram D, et al. Electrocardiographic changes associated with endotracheal suctioning [abstract]. *Circulation.* 1990;82(suppl 4):210.
11. McCauley C, Boller L. Bradycardiac responses to endotracheal suctioning. *Crit Care Med.* 1986;16:1165–1166.
12. Rudy E, Baun M, Stone K, Turner B. The relationship between endotracheal suctioning and changes in intracranial pressure: A review of the literature. *Heart Lung.* 1986; 15:488–493.
13. Rudy E, Turner B, Baun M, Stone K, Brucia J. Endotracheal

suctioning in adults with head injury. *Heart Lung.* 1991; 20:667–674.

14. Gunderson L, Stone K, Hamlin R. Endotracheal suctioning-induced heart rate alterations. *Nurs Res.* 1991;40:139–143.

15. Chulay M, Graeber G. Efficacy of a hyperinflation and hyperoxygenation suctioning intervention. *Heart Lung.* 1988; 17:15–22.

16. Stone K, Preusser B, Grouch K, Karl J. Effect of lung hyperinflation on cardiopulmonary hemodynamics and post suctioning hypoxemia. *Heart Lung.* 1988;17:309.

17. Walsh J, Vanderwarf C, Hoscheit D, Fahey P. Unsuspected hemodynamic alterations during endotracheal suctioning. *Chest.* 1989;95:162–165.

18. Mancinelli-Van Atta J, Beck S. Preventing hypoxemia and hemodynamic compromise related to endotracheal suctioning. *Am J Crit Care.* 1991;1(3):62–79.

19. Grap MJ, Glass C, Corley M, Parks T. Endotracheal suctioning: ventilator versus manual delivery of hyperoxygenation breaths. *Am J Crit Care.* 1996;5(3):192–197.

20. Anderson K. Effects of manual bagging vs mechanical ventilatory sighing on oxygenation during the suctioning procedure. *Heart Lung.* 1989;18:301–302.

21. Glass C, Grap J, Corley M, Wallace D. Nurse performance of hyperoxygenation. *Heart Lung.* 1991;20:299.

22. Glass C, Grap MJ, Corley M, Wallace D. Nurses' ability to achieve hyperinflation and hyperoxygenation with a manual resuscitation bag during endotracheal suctioning. *Heart Lung.* 1993;22:158–165.

23. Hess D, Goff G. The effects of two-hand versus one-hand ventilation on volumes delivered during bag-valve ventilation at various resistances and compliances. *Respir Care.* 1987;32:1025–1028.

24. Kirimili B, King J, Pfaeffle H. Evaluation of tracheal bronchial suction techniques. *J Cardiovasc Surg.* 1970;59:340–344.

25. Kubota Y, Toyoda Y, Kubota H, et al. Is a straight catheter necessary for selective bronchial suctioning in the adult? *Cr Care Med.* 1986;14:755–756.

26. Kuzenski B. Effect of negative pressure on tracheobronchial trauma. *Nurs Res.* 1978;27:260–263.

27. Ogburn-Russell L. The effect of continuous and intermittent suctioning on the tracheal mucosa of dogs. *Heart Lung.* 1987;16:297.

28. Czarnik R, Stone K, Everhardt C, Preusser B. Differential effects of continuous versus intermittent suction on tracheal tissue. *Heart Lung.* 1991;20:144–151.

29. Kleiber C, Krutzfield N, Rose E. Acute histologic changes in the tracheobronchial tree associated wih different suction catheter insertion techniques. *Heart Lung.* 1988;17:10–14.

30. Neagley S. The pulmonary system. In: Alspach J, ed. *Core Curriculum for Critical Care Nursing.* Philadelphia, Pa: W.B. Saunders; 1991:1–131.

31. Stone KS, Bell SD, Preusser BA. The effect of repeated endotracheal suctioning on arterial blood pressure. *Appl Nurs Res.* 1991;4:152–158.

32. Rutula W, Stiegel M, Sarubbi F. A potential infection hazard associated with the use of disposable saline vials. *Infect Control.* 1984;5:170–172.

33. Chulay M. Why do we keep putting saline down endotracheal tubes? It's time for a change in the way we suction! *Capsules Comments.* 1994;2(4):7–11.

34. Ackerman M. The effect of saline lavage prior to suctioning. *Am J Crit Care.* 1993;2:326–330.

35. Bostick J, Wendelgass S. Normal saline instillation as part of the suctioning procedure: effects on PaO_2 and amount of secretions. *Heart Lung.* 1986;16:532–537.

36. Hanley M, Rudd T, Butler J. What happens to intratracheal instillations? [abstract]. *Am Rev Respir Dis.* 1978; 177(suppl): 124.

37. Raymond S. Normal saline instillation before suctioning: helpful or harmful? A review of the literature. *Am J Crit Care.* 1995;4(4):267–271.

38. Tablan O, Anderson L, Arden N, et al. Guideline for prevention of nosocomial pneumonia. *Infect Control Hosp Epidemiol.* 1994;15(9):588–623.

Additional Readings

Birdsall C. How do you use a closed suction adapter? *Am J Nurs.* November 1986;86(11):1222–1223.

Redick E. Closed-system, in-line endotracheal suctioning. *Crit Care Nurse.* August 1993;13(4):47–51.

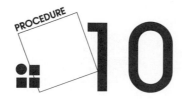

10

Tracheal Tube Cuff Care

P U R P O S E: The tracheal tube cuff helps stabilize the tracheal tube and maintain an adequate airway seal so air moves through the tube into the lungs. The cuff may also decrease the risk of aspiration of large food particles, but it does not protect against aspiration of liquid.

Kay Knox Greenlee

PREREQUISITE NURSING KNOWLEDGE

- The tracheal tube cuff is an inflatable "balloon" that surrounds the shaft of the tracheal tube near its distal end. When inflated, the cuff presses against the tracheal wall to prevent air leakage and pressure loss from the lungs.
- Appropriate cuff care will help prevent major pulmonary aspirations, prepare for tracheal extubation, decrease the risk of inadvertent extubation, provide a patent airway for ventilation and removal of secretions, and decrease the risk of iatrogenic infections.
- Although a variety of cuffs exists, the most desirable cuff provides a maximum airway seal with minimal tracheal wall pressure. The most widely used cuff is the high-volume, low-pressure cuff (Fig. 10–1). This cuff has a relatively large inflation volume requiring lower filling pressure to obtain a seal (less than 25 mm Hg or 34 cm H_2O).
- High-volume, low-pressure cuffs allow a large surface area to come into contact with the tracheal wall, thus distributing the pressure over a much greater area. The older cuff design (low volume, high pressure) can require as much as 40 mm Hg (54.4 cm H_2O) to obtain an effective seal and is therefore undesirable.
- The amount of pressure and volume necessary to obtain a seal and prevent mucosal damage depends on tube size and design, cuff configuration, mode of ventilation, and the individual's arterial blood pressure.
- A variety of devices are available to measure cuff pressures. These include bedside sphygmomanometers, special aneroid cuff manometers, and electronic cuff pressure devices. Ideally, most tubes seal at pressures between 14 and 20 mm Hg (19 to 27 cm H_2O). Tracheal capillary pressure lies between 20 and 30 mm Hg, with impairment in tracheal blood flow seen at 22 mm Hg and total obstruction seen at 37 mm Hg.[1]
- Two techniques, minimum leak volume (MLV) and minimum occlusion volume (MOV), are employed to inflate and monitor air in the cuff.
  - ❖ MLV involves air inflation of the tube cuff until any leak stops, and then a small amount of air is slowly removed until the leak is observed at peak inflation pressure.[2]
  - ❖ MOV is air inflation of the tube cuff until the airflow heard escaping around the cuff during positive pressure breath ceases.[2]
- Each technique has distinct advantages. MLV decreases mucosal injury and assists in mobilizing secretions forward into the pharynx. MOV decreases the incidence of aspirations and is most effective for patients who are changing position frequently and are at increased risk for tube movement.[3]
- Although rare since the use of high-volume, low-pressure devices became common, the adverse effects of tracheal tube cuff inflation include tracheal stenosis, necrosis, tracheoesophageal fistulas, and tracheomalacia. These complications may be more likely to occur in conditions that adversely affect tissue response to mucosal injury (eg, malnutrition, dehydration, infection, metastatic cancer, hypotensive states, hypoxemia) and in patients receiving corticosteroids.[4]
- Routine cuff deflation is unnecessary but may be indicated to evaluate cuff leak, clear upper airway secretions, and allow the patient to vocalize and, after intubation, cardiopulmonary resuscitation (CPR), and surgery, to re-evaluate the number of milliliters of air in the cuff.[5]
- Unintentional extubation and tube manipulation can occur with ineffective patient restraint, inadequate securing of the tube, inadequate sedation, incorrect tube size and length, improper support or respiratory underinflation of endotracheal cuff, and prolonged intubation.[6]

EQUIPMENT

- 10-mL syringe
- Pressure manometer with extension line
- Three-way stopcock
- Stethoscope
- Manual resuscitation bag connected to oxygen

Additional equipment (for cuff inflation with faulty inflating device) includes the following:

SOFT CUFF
■ High volume
■ Exerts low and equal lateral tracheal wall pressure (TWP) (*arrows*)
■ Minimizes tracheal injury

HARD CUFF
■ Low volume
■ Exerts high and unequal lateral TWP (*arrows*)
■ Causes tracheal injury

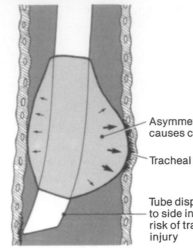

Cuff conforms to trachea

Centrally positioned tube

Asymmetric inflation causes cuff herniation

Tracheal erosion

Tube displacement to side increases risk of tracheal injury

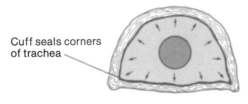

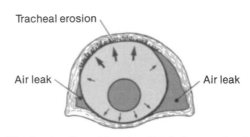

Cuff seals corners of trachea

Tracheal erosion

Air leak   Air leak

■ ● **FIGURE 10–1.** Cross-sectional view in D-shaped trachea. Effects of soft and hard cuff inflation on the tracheal wall. (From Kersten LD. *Comprehensive Respiratory Nursing: A Decision-Making Approach.* Philadelphia, Pa: WB Saunders; 1989:648.)

- Scissors
- Padded hemostats
- Short 18- or 23-G blunt needle
- Tongue depressor
- Tape, 1 in wide

- Reintubation equipment, in case of accidental extubation
- Suction supplies (see Procedure 9)

PATIENT AND FAMILY EDUCATION

- Explain the procedure (if patient condition and time allow) and the reason for tracheal tube cuff care. ➞*Rationale:* Identifies patient and family knowledge deficits concerning patient condition, procedure, expected benefits, and potential risks and allows time for questions to clarify information and voice concerns. Explanations decrease patient anxiety and enhance cooperation.
- Explain the patient's role in assisting with cuff care. ➞*Rationale:* Elicits patient cooperation.
- Explain that the procedure can be uncomfortable and cause the patient to cough.   ➞*Rationale:* Elicits patient cooperation.

PATIENT ASSESSMENT AND PREPARATION
Patient Assessment

- Presence of bilateral breath sounds.   ➞*Rationale:* Assists in verifying tube placement.

- Signs and symptoms of cuff leakage, as follows:
  ❖ Audible or auscultated inspiratory leak over larynx
  ❖ Patient able to audibly vocalize
  ❖ Pilot balloon deflation
  ❖ Loss of inspiratory and expiratory volume on mechanically ventilated patient

  ➞*Rationale:* Adequate seal of cuff to tracheal wall will not permit air to flow past the cuff.

- Signs and symptoms of inadequate ventilation, as follows:
  ❖ Rising arterial carbon dioxide tension
  ❖ Chest-abdominal dyssynchrony
  ❖ Patient-ventilator dyssynchrony
  ❖ Dyspnea
  ❖ Headache
  ❖ Restlessness
  ❖ Confusion
  ❖ Lethargy
  ❖ Rising (early sign) or falling (late sign) arterial blood pressure
  ❖ Activation of expiratory or inspiratory volume alarms on mechanical ventilator

  ➞*Rationale:* Inadequate ventilation results when cuff seal is improper or cuff leak is extensive.

- Amount of air or pressure previously used to inflate the cuff. ➤*Rationale:* The amount of air previously used to inflate the cuff can be used as guideline to determine changes in volume or pressure, or both.
- Size of tracheal tube and size of patient. ➤*Rationale:* Volume and pressure of air needed to seal the airway is dependent on the relationship of tube and trachea diameters.

Patient Preparation

- Ensure that the patient understands preprocedural teaching. Answer questions as they arise and reinforce information as needed. ➤*Rationale:* Evaluates and reinforces understanding of previously taught information.
- Place patient in semi-Fowler position. ➤*Rationale:* Promotes general relaxation, oxygenation, and ventilation. Reduces stimulation of gag reflex and risk of aspiration.

Procedure **for Tracheal Tube Cuff Care**

Steps	Rationale	Special Considerations
Deflation and Inflation		
1. Wash hands, and don personal protective equipment.	Reduces transmission of microorganisms and body secretions; standard precautions.	
2. Remove oxygen tubing attached to the endotracheal or tracheostomy tube.	Accesses tube opening.	
3. Hyperoxygenate and suction tracheobronchial tree (see Procedure 9) and pharynx before cuff deflation.	Clears secretions in the lower airway and decreases incidence of aspiration.	A fresh sterile catheter is necessary.
MOV Technique		
4. Deflate cuff while applying positive pressure.	Prepares for measurement of cuff pressure and prevents aspiration of pharyngeal secretions.	Instruct the alert, cooperative patient to cough.
5. Insert air-filled, 10-mL syringe tip into inflating tube valve.	Provides a pathway between air source and cuff.	Most cuffs are sufficiently inflated with less than 10 mL of air.
6. Slowly inject air on inhalation until sounds cease over larynx.	The trachea dilates during inhalation. The cuff needs to seal the airway during inhalation so air is directed toward the lung. Cessation of air movement on auscultation indicates that the cuff is sealed against the tracheal mucosal wall.	Hazards of cuff inflation include cuff overinflation, distention, and rupture.
7. Apply positive pressure with manual resuscitation bag.	The cuff is inflated when an audible leak is not heard.	The alert, cooperative patient may be asked to speak. If the trachea is sealed, vocalization is not possible.
8. Proceed to step 11.		
MLV Technique		
9. Place a stethoscope over larynx.	Indirectly assesses inflation of cuff.	
10. Slowly withdraw air (in 0.1-mL increments) from the cuff until a small leak is heard by auscultation on inspiration.	Auscultation of air movement indicates air escaping through the larynx.	
11. Remove syringe tip, check inflation of pilot balloon.	A firm pilot balloon indicates air placement into cuff.	Pilot balloon serves as a rough estimate of intracuff pressure through feeling the give or compliance of the balloon. It does not replace more accurate volume or pressure recordings.[7]
12. Replace any oxygen or humidity tubing. Check and secure ventilator connections, as needed.	Allows for oxygen flow and prevents oxygen desaturation.	
13. Reassess patient's airway and respiratory status.	Identifies effects of tracheal cuff care.	

Procedure continued on following page

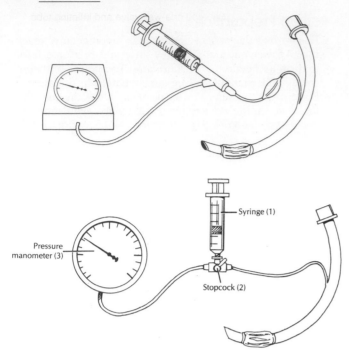

■ ● **FIGURE 10–2.** Measuring cuff pressure by way of home-made pressure monitor. (From Eubanks DH, Bone RC. *Comprehensive Respiratory Care: A Learning System.* 2nd ed. St. Louis, Mo: Mosby; 1990:559.)

Procedure	**for Tracheal Tube Cuff Care** *Continued*

Steps	Rationale	Special Considerations

Cuff Pressure Measurement

14. Wash hands, and don personal protective equipment.	Reduces transmission of microorganisms; standard precautions.	
15. Connect the manometer line to the patient inflation system with a three-way stopcock (turned "off" to the patient) (Fig. 10–2).	Develops an intracuff pressure-monitoring device.	This device is easily made using parts of the blood pressure cuff (eg, aneroid manometer device).
16. With your thumb, occlude the open port, and, with an air-filled syringe, inject air into the tubing leading to the manometer until the needle of the manometer reads between 20 and 25 mm Hg.	Measures the pressure of the air applied from the system.	Pressure should be kept at a level to maintain a seal between cuff and tracheal wall. The volume necessary to create the seal depends on tube size and cuff configuration.
17. Turn the stopcock off to the open port (syringe). Read the cuff pressure now shown on the aneroid face.	The connecting channel is now between the manometer and the patient's inflation line, allowing evaluation of pressure in the patient's cuff.	
18. Turn the stopcock off to the inflating tube. Disconnect the manometer line from the patient's inflation line.	The connecting channel to the inflating tube is now closed maintaining air in the cuff.	
19. Detach the manometer line with three-way stopcock from the patient's inflation system.	Removes apparatus to monitor cuff pressure.	

Troubleshooting Tracheal Cuff Problems

Faulty Inflating Valve

| 20. Identify faulty inflating valve. | Determines need for repair. | When inflating line becomes faulty and reintubation is undesirable, consider instituting an emergency cuff-inflation technique (Fig. 10–3). |

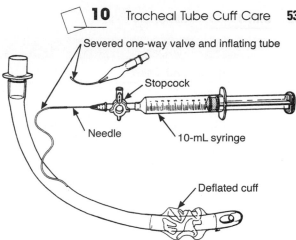

Severed one-way valve and inflating tube

Stopcock

Needle

10-mL syringe

Deflated cuff

■ ● **FIGURE 10–3.** Attachments for emergency cuff inflation for faulty inflating line. (From Sills J. An emergency cuff inflation technique. *Respir Care.* 1986;31(3):200.)

Procedure	**for Tracheal Tube Cuff Care** *Continued*

Steps	Rationale	Special Considerations
Cuff Pressure Measurement		
21. Insert three-way stopcock into the distal opening of the inflating balloon.	Provides access to cuff.	
22. Inflate the cuff using MOV (steps 6–8, 11) or MLV (steps 9–11) technique.	Allows for cuff inflation; restores tracheal wall and cuff seal.	
23. Clamp the inflating tube by applying a padded hemostat distal to the pilot balloon.	Maintains air in cuff; provides a quick occlusion of the inflating tube.	
24. Turn the stopcock off to the inflating tube; remove clamp.	Provides for temporary use of the tracheal tube while maintaining cuff pressure.	
Faulty Inflating Line		
25. Identify malfunctioning of inflating line.	Determines need for and method of repair.	
26. Cut off faulty end of inflation line with scissors (see Fig. 10–3).	Prepares inflation line for repair.	
27. Insert short 18- to 23-G blunt needle into inflation line.	Provides inflation access.	Maintain care to avoid puncture or severing of inflation line or skin.
28. Attach a three-way stopcock to a blunt needle.	Provides control of airflow in and out of inflating line.	
29. Using a 10-mL syringe, inflate the cuff with air using MOV (steps 6–8, 11) or MLV (steps 9–11) technique.	Allows cuff inflation; restores tracheal wall and cuff seal.	
30. Turn the stopcock off to the inflating tube.	Provides for temporary use of the tracheal tube while maintaining cuff pressure.	
31. Secure assembled device with tape to a tongue depressor.	Provides for stabilization and protection.	

Expected Outcomes	Unexpected Outcomes
• Tracheal tube remains in correct position. • Cuff pressure is kept at a level to maintain a seal between cuff and tracheal wall (usually between 20 and 25 mm Hg). • Cuff remains intact.	• Extubation or tube dislodgment • Mucosal ischemia • Faulty cuff and inflating line • Cuff overinflation and distention over the end of the tube • Cuff rupture

Patient Monitoring and Care

Patient Monitoring and Care	Rationale	Reportable Conditions
		These conditions should be reported if they persist despite nursing interventions.
1. Assess respiratory status for optimal ventilation.	Inadequate interface between tracheal cuff and tracheobronchial mucosa decreases inspiratory flow.	• Rising arterial carbon dioxide tension • Chest-abominal dysynchrony • Patient-ventilator dysynchrony • Dyspnea • Headache • Restlessness • Confusion • Lethargy • Rising (early sign) or falling (late sign) arterial blood pressure • Activation of expiratory or inspiratory volume alarms on the mechanical ventilator
2. Measure cuff pressure every 8–12 hours, maintaining cuff pressure between 20 and 25 mm Hg. *(Level IV: Limited clinical studies to support recommendations)*	Prevents tracheal injury and aspiration. Excessive cuff pressure is cited as the most frequent problem of tracheal intubation and the best predictor of tracheolaryngeal injury.[2, 3, 8]	• Cuff pressure <20 mm Hg or >25 mm Hg
3. Maintain tracheal tube cuff integrity.	Manipulation of the tracheal tube increases the likelihood of cuff disruption. Cuff leak or rupture is evident when the pressure on the manometer continues to fall.	• Inability to maintain cuff inflation • Audible air through the patient's nose or mouth • Low-pressure or low-volume alarm sounds on the mechanical ventilator • Audible or auscultated inspiratory leak over larynx • Patient able to audibly vocalize • Pilot balloon deflation • Loss of inspiratory and expiratory volume on mechanically ventilated patients
4. Hyperoxygenate and suction patient based on assessment (see Procedure 9).	Removal of secretions reduces the chance for partial or complete airway obstruction.	
5. Reinflate cuff using MOV or MLV whenever deflation is necessary. *(Level II: Theory based, no research data to support recommendations; recommendations from expert consensus group may exist)*	Cuff should be deflated only when problems arise[1] or every 48 to 72 hours.[2] If the number of milliliters needed to seal the airway increases, evaluate patient for tracheal dilation using chest radiography of cuff diameter to tracheal diameter ratio. Increasing number of milliliters may also indicate leak in cuff or pilot balloon valve. Hypoxemia, overinflation of the cuff on reinflation, and pulmonary aspiration occur with periodic cuff deflation.[7]	
6. Compare patient's cardiopulmonary status before and after tracheal tube cuff care.	Identifies the effects of tracheal tube cuff care.	• Decreased arterial oxygen saturation • Cardiac dysrhythmias • Bronchospasm • Respiratory distress • Cyanosis • Increased blood pressure or intracranial pressure • Anxiety, agitation, or changes in level of consciousness

Patient Monitoring and Care *Continued*

Patient Monitoring and Care	Rationale	Reportable Conditions
7. Reassess cuff pressure and volume when transporting patient from one altitude to another (ie, air transport) or during hyperbaric therapy without environmental pressurization.	Changes in altitude will change the volume of gas in the cuff; therefore, volume and pressure need to be reevaluated during and after transport.	

Documentation

Documentation should include the following:

- Patient and family education
- Cardiopulmonary and vital sign assessment before and after procedure
- Method of cuff inflation
- Cuff inflation volume and cuff pressure
- Patient tolerance
- Appearance and characteristics of tracheal secretions, if present
- Unexpected outcomes
- Use of medications
- Use of restraints
- Date, time, and frequency with which procedure is performed
- Nursing interventions

References

1. Guyton D, Banner MJ, Kirgby RR. High-volume, low-pressure cuffs: are they always low pressure? *Chest.* 1991;100:1076–1081.
2. Henneman E, Ellstrom K, St. John R. Airway management. In: *AACN Protocols for Practice: Care of the Mechanically Ventilated Patient Series.* Aliso Viejo, Ca: American Association of Critical-Care Nurses; 1999.
3. Crimlisk JT, Horn MH, Wilson DJ, Marino B. Artificial airways: a survey of cuff management practices. *Heart Lung.* 1996;25:225–235.
4. Ignatavicius DD, Workman ML, Mishler MA. Interventions for clients with upper airway problems. In: *Medical Surgical Nursing: A Nursing Process Approach.* Philadelphia, Pa: W.B. Saunders; 1995:657–666.
5. Powaser MM, Brown MC, Chezem J, et al. The effectiveness of hourly cuff deflation in minimizing tracheal damage. *Heart Lung.* 1976;5:734–741.
6. Pesiri AJ, Stewar K, Kobe E, Parrilo JE. Protocol for prevention of unintentional exubation. *Crit Care Nurs Q* 1990:12(4):87–90
7. Longnecker DE, Murphy FL. *Introduction to Anesthesia.* Philadelphia, Pa: W.B. Saunders; 1997:156–157.
8. Wilson DJ, Shepherd KE. Modern airway appliances and their long term complications. In: Robert JT, ed. *Clinical Management of the Airway.* Philadelphia, Pa: W.B. Saunders; 1994:461.

Additional Readings

MacKenzie C. Compromises in the choice of orotracheal or nasotracheal intubation and tracheostomy. *Heart Lung.* 1983;12:485–492.
Tyler DO, Clark AP, Ogburn-Russell L. Developing a standard for endotracheal tube cuff care. *DCCN.* 1991;10:54–61.

11

Tracheostomy Tube Care

P U R P O S E : Tracheostomy tube care is performed to maintain airway patency and to decrease infection risk by removing secretions accumulating within the inner cannula.

Kay Knox Greenlee

PREREQUISITE NURSING KNOWLEDGE

- Tracheotomy refers to the surgical procedure where an incision is made below the cricoid cartilage through the second to fourth tracheal rings (Fig. 11–1). Tracheostomy refers to the opening, or stoma, made by the incision. The tracheostomy tube is the artificial airway inserted into the trachea during tracheotomy (Fig. 11–2).
- Tracheostomy tubes have a variety of parts (Fig. 11–3) and are available in various types. A tracheostomy tube is shorter than but similar in diameter to an endotracheal tube and has a squared-off distal tip for maximizing airflow. The outer cannula forms the body of a tracheostomy tube with a cuff. The neck flange, attached to the outer cannula, assists in stabilizing the tube in the trachea and provides the small holes necessary for proper securing of the tube. Some tracheostomy setups have an inner cannula inserted into the outer cannula. The inner cannula is removable for easy cleaning without compromising the airway. The cuff is a balloon inflated with air to maintain a seal around the tube. As the air flows through the one-way inflation valve, the pilot balloon inflates, indicating the volume of air present in the cuff.
- A cuffed tube is appropriate for use in patients who require mechanical ventilation or when aspiration is a problem. The cuff prevents or limits aspiration of oral and gastric secretions. Uncuffed tubes are commonly used in children, in adult patients with laryngectomies, and during decannulation of the tracheostomy.
- A tracheostomy is performed as either an elective procedure or an emergency procedure for a variety of reasons (Table 11–1). Most often, the procedure is elective and performed in the operating room under sterile conditions. An emergency tracheotomy is performed at the bedside under aseptic technique or before arrival in the critical care unit when swelling, injury, or other upper airway obstruction prevents intubation with an endotracheal tube. Percutaneous tracheostomies are also performed at the bedside. This procedure consists of passing a needle into the trachea, placing a J-tipped guidewire, progressively dilating the trachea, and placing the tracheostomy tube. The percutaneous procedure has achieved outcomes comparable to those of the surgical technique.[1]

- Protocols for emergency tracheotomy vary among institutions. Often, nurses at the bedside take an active role in assisting with tracheotomy and insertion of a tracheostomy tube; however, some institutions have surgical personnel at the bedside to assist with the procedure.
- During insertion, the obturator replaces the inner cannula. Its smooth surface protrudes from the outer cannula, minimizing tracheal trauma. Once the tracheostomy tube is inserted, the obturator is removed and replaced with the inner cannula, which locks in place. The obturator should be placed in a plastic bag and kept at the bedside in case the tube must be reinserted emergently.
- The decision for a tracheostomy in long-term mechanically ventilated patients is based on patient situation and physician or nurse practitioner preference. Studies completed to compare length of stay and complications, including nosocomial pneumonia, for early and late tracheostomies have demonstrated mixed results.[2, 3]
- When compared with an endotracheal tube, tracheostomy tubes provide added benefit to patients. These include the following:
  - ❖ Prevention of further laryngeal injury from the translaryngeal tube
  - ❖ Improved patient comfort
  - ❖ Decreased work of breathing
  - ❖ Provision of a speech mechanism
  - ❖ Increased patient mobility
- A fenestrated tracheostomy tube has an opening in the curvature of the posterior wall of the outer cannula. Fenestration allows for speech with cuff deflation, removal of inner cannula, and occlusion of outer cannula

Table 11–1 ● ■ ■ **Indications for Tracheostomy**

Bypass acute upper airway obstruction
Prolonged need for artificial airway
Prophylaxis for anticipated airway problems
Reduction of anatomic dead space
Prevention of pulmonary aspiration
Retained tracheobronchial secretions
Chronic upper airway obstruction

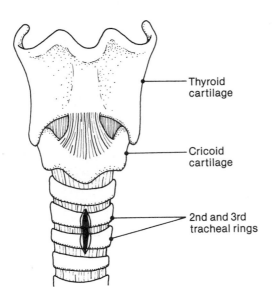

Thyroid cartilage

Cricoid cartilage

2nd and 3rd tracheal rings

■ ● FIGURE 11–1. Vertical tracheal incision during a tracheotomy procedure. (From Kersten LD. *Comprehensive Respiratory Nursing: A Decision-Making Approach.* Philadelphia, Pa: W.B. Saunders; 1989:654.)

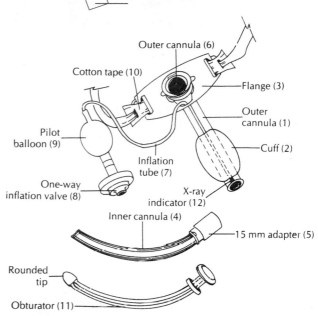

Outer cannula (6)

Cotton tape (10)

Flange (3)

Pilot balloon (9)

Outer cannula (1)

Cuff (2)

Inflation tube (7)

One-way inflation valve (8)

X-ray indicator (12)

Inner cannula (4)

15 mm adapter (5)

Rounded tip

Obturator (11)

■ ● FIGURE 11–3. Parts of a tracheostomy tube. (From Eubanks DH, Bone RC. *Comprehensive Respiratory Care: A Learning System.* 2nd ed. St. Louis, Mo: Mosby–Year Book; 1990:570.)

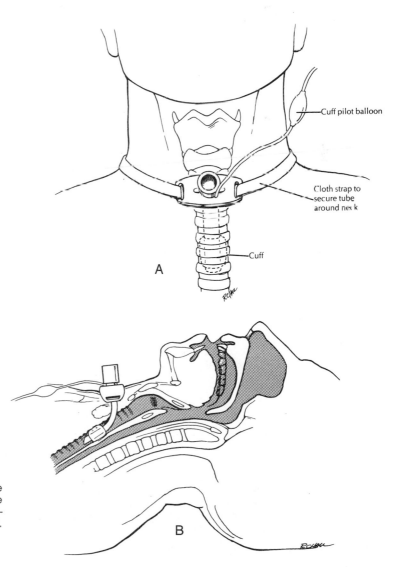

Cuff pilot balloon

Cloth strap to secure tube around neck

Cuff

A

B

■ ● FIGURE 11–2. *A,* Anterior view of tracheostomy tube after insertion. *B,* Lateral view of tracheostomy tube after insertion. (From Eubanks DH, Bone RC, *Comprehensive Respiratory Care: A Learning System.* 2nd ed. St. Louis, Mo: Mosby–Year Book; 1990:554.)

because air is permitted to flow through the upper airway and tracheostomy opening.

- A tracheostomy is viewed by the body as foreign material. The body responds by increasing mucus production. Additionally, ciliary movement is impaired, limiting the forward movement of the mucociliary escalator. Because the tracheostomy bypasses the upper airway and its protective and hydrating mechanisms, patients are at increased risk of infection. Inadequate tracheostomy care and prolonged tracheostomy are associated with a 60% to 100% colonization of the tracheobronchial tree.[4] As well, lack of hydration by the upper airway can lead to very thick mucus, increasing the risk of airway obstruction.
- The tracheostomy creates a more stable airway, making it feasible for the patient to transfer out of the critical care unit when the patient's overall condition warrants. Additionally, care of the patient, such as suctioning, mouth care, and ability to meet nutritional needs, is simplified.
- A stoma less than 48 hours old has not fully formed a tracheostomy tract. If the tracheostomy tube is accidentally dislodged, the tracheostomy may close, compromising the patient's airway.
- A small amount of bleeding is expected for the first few days following a tracheotomy. Bright, frank bleeding or constant oozing is not expected and should be brought to the attention of the physician or nurse practitioner.
- Consideration should be given to obtaining assistance with tracheostomy care, especially when changing tracheal ties or with the agitated patient. An extra pair of hands can minimize the risk for accidental dislodgment.

EQUIPMENT

Some institutions may use tracheostomy care kits, which include some or all of the following items:

- Hydrogen peroxide (H_2O_2)
- Sterile normal saline (NS) or water
- Twill tape or tracheal ties
- Sterile cotton swabs
- Sterile basin
- Small, sterile brush
- Scissors
- Sterile, disposable inner cannula (if disposable setup is used)
- Suction supplies

- Towel
- Sterile 4 × 4 gauze pad
- Sterile precut tracheostomy dressing
- Two sterile gloves
- Self-inflating manual resuscitation bag and mask

Additional equipment (to have available based on patient need) includes the following:

- Second practitioner (if changing tracheal ties)

PATIENT AND FAMILY EDUCATION

- Explain the purpose and the necessity of tracheotomy or tracheostomy care. ➥*Rationale:* Communication and explanation for therapy encourage cooperation, minimize anxiety, and are a continually stated patient and family need.

PATIENT ASSESSMENT AND PREPARATION

Patient Assessment

- Increased production of secretions. ➥*Rationale:* Tube irritation to mucosa results in increased production of secretions.
- Cardiopulmonary status.
  - ❖ Decreased arterial oxygen saturation
  - ❖ Cardiac dysrhythmias
  - ❖ Bronchospasm
  - ❖ Respiratory distress
  - ❖ Cyanosis
  - ❖ Increased blood pressure or intracranial pressure
  - ❖ Anxiety, agitation, or changes in level of consciousness

➥*Rationale:* Evaluation of the patient's cardiopulmonary status provides valuable information about need for and tolerance of tracheostomy tube care.

Patient Preparation

- Ensure that patient understands preprocedural teaching. Answer questions as they arise, and reinforce information as needed. ➥*Rationale:* Evaluates and reinforces understanding of previously taught information.

Procedure **for Tracheostomy Tube Care**

Steps	Rationale	Special Considerations
1. Wash hands, and don personal protective equipment.	Reduces transmission of microorganisms and body secretions; standard precautions.	Protective eyewear or face masks should be worn when secretions are copious.
2. Hyperoxygenate and suction trachea and pharynx as needed (see Procedure 9).	Reduces risk of hypoxemia; removes secretions and diminishes patient's need to cough during the procedure.	
3. Remove soiled dressing.		
4. Remove soiled gloves, and set up sterile saline solution container on sterile field. Be careful not to touch the inside of the container. Fill with equal parts sterile NS or water or H_2O_2, totaling approximately 100 mL.		

| Procedure | **for Tracheostomy Tube Care** *Continued* |

Steps	Rationale	Special Considerations
5. Don sterile gloves.	Reduces transmission of microorganisms; standard precautions.	
6. Remove oxygen source and inner cannula, placing it in a 1:1 solution of H_2O_2 and NS or water.	Removes inner cannula for cleaning. H_2O_2 loosens debris from inner cannula.	This is not required when patient has a disposable inner cannula.
7. Apply tracheostomy collar oxygen source over outer cannula, or, if ventilator assistance is needed, attach outer cannula to connector on ventilator.	Maintains oxygen supply. Maintains mechanical ventilation, as appropriate.	
8. Clean inner cannula with pipe cleaners or small brush.	Assists in the removal of debris and thick secretions.	
9. Rinse inner cannula by pouring NS over the cannula.	Removes H_2O_2 and debris.	
10. Remove oxygen source from over outer cannula.	Allow access to opening of outer cannula.	
11. Insert inner cannula and lock into place.	Secures inner cannula.	
12. Reapply oxygen or ventilator oxygen source.	Reestablishes oxygen supply.	
13. Moisten swabs and 4×4 gauze pads with H_2O_2. Clean stoma site and outer cannula surface by wiping with cotton-tipped swabs and 4×4 gauze pads.	Removes debris and secretions from the stoma area.	
14. Rinse stoma site and outer cannula with NS-soaked cotton-tipped swabs and 4×4 gauze pad.	Rinses H_2O_2 and removes additional debris.	
15. Pat dry the skin area surrounding the stoma site.	Dry surface decreases likelihood of microorganism growth and skin breakdown.	
16. To make new ties, cut twill tape at a length that will wrap around the patient's neck two times.	Provides length for circumferential wrapping around the patient's neck.	Premade Velcro tracheal ties may also be used. The tracheostomy tube may be sutured in place and no ties used (eg, for patients with new laryngectomy and flap).
17. Have assistant hold neckplate securely.	Decreases the incidence of tracheal tube decannulation.	
18. Cut and remove current twill tape.	Prepares for new twill tape.	Assistant must maintain hold while ties are not secure.

Procedure continued on following page

Procedure for Tracheostomy Tube Care *Continued*

Steps	Rationale	Special Considerations
19. Insert one tie end through the faceplate and pull until one half of the tape is through the eyelet. (Tape will not be "doubled.") Slide the doubled tie around the back of neck, insert through the second eyelet, bring one tie around neck, pull snug, and tie in double square knot on the side of the neck (Fig. 11–4).	Reestablishes secure tracheal faceplate. Knot should be visible on side of neck to be able to observe that it remains tied.	Allow one finger space between twill tape and neck to allow for venous outflow

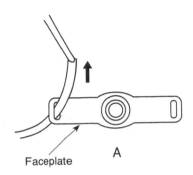

Faceplate A

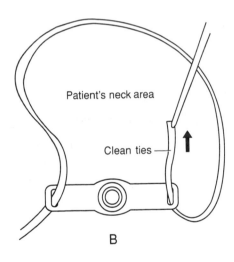

Patient's neck area

Clean ties

B

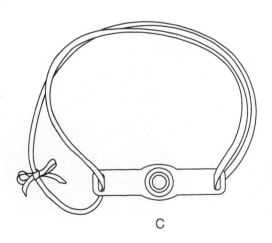

C

■ ● **FIGURE 11–4.** Placement of tracheostomy twill tape. *A,* Faceplate with threading of twill tape (to prevent decannulation, an additional person will need to stabilize faceplate); *B,* advancing of the twill tape around the back of the neck and looping through the other side of faceplate; *C,* doubling of the twill tape and securing in a knot.

Procedure **for Tracheostomy Tube Care** *Continued*

Steps	Rationale	Special Considerations
20. Apply clean, precut tracheostomy dressing under faceplate.	Promotes drainage absorption.	Never cut a 4 × 4 gauze pad because cut edges fray and provide a potential source for infection.

Expected Outcomes	Unexpected Outcomes
• Airway patency • Infection prevention • Healing promotion	• Prolonged apnea, increasing hypoxemia, or cardiopulmonary arrest • Hemorrhage • Interstitial air: subcutaneous emphysema, pneumothorax, pneumopericardium, and pneumoperitoneum • Thyroid gland injury • Cardiac dysrhythmias • Tube-tip erosion into the tracheal innominate artery • Stoma infection • Bronchopulmonary infection • Displacement or dislodgment out of trachea • Excessive cuff pressure • Leaking airway cuff • Airway obstruction from misalignment, cuff overinflation, and dried or excessive secretions • Agitation • Tracheal stenosis, malacia, or tracheoesophageal fistula • Tracheal ischemia, necrosis, or dilation • Laryngeal disorders • Dysphasia

Patient Monitoring and Care

Patient Monitoring and Care	Rationale	Reportable Conditions
		These conditions should be reported if they persist despite nursing interventions.
1. Check proper placement by auscultation.	Displacement into the bronchus or at the carina is very rare with tracheostomy tube because of the short length. However, because of the variety of tracheal tube lengths and patient sizes, the potential for displacement does exist. Improper placement may lead to inadequate ventilation and complications.	• Decreased or delayed chest motion • Unilateral breath sounds • Excessive coughing • Localized expiratory wheeze • Bilateral decreased breath sounds
2. Inspect and palpate for air under skin.	Air may escape into the incision, causing subcutaneous emphysema. *Special Note: Subcutaneous emphysema will not usually harm patients with an airway already in place. However, puffiness of the soft tissue may result and, if significant, can change the patient's appearance, alarming the patient and the family.*	• Subcutaneous emphysema
3. Assess for frank bleeding or constant oozing of blood.	Surgical procedures increase the risk of potential injury to adjacent tissues and structures. Stoma placement below the second and third cartilaginous rings results in an increased incidence of innominate artery erosion.	• Frank bleeding or constant oozing of blood

Continued on following page

Patient Monitoring and Care *Continued*

Patient Monitoring and Care	Rationale	Reportable Conditions
4. Palpate the tube for pulsation.	If pulsations are felt in the tracheal tube, it is suggestive of impending erosion of major blood vessels.	• Pulsation of the tracheal tube
5. Assess for presence of pain.	Pain and discomfort increase the incidence of anxiety and disorientation.	• Uncontrolled pain
6. Maintain mucosal tissue integrity using appropriate cuff care procedures (see Procedure 10).	Constant pressure and irritation of the mucosal tissue can result in blood vessel and cellular damage.	• Need for increasing pressure or volume to maintain tracheal cuff seal
7. Assess skin for signs of infection or inflammation.	Moisture promotes maceration and skin breakdown at stomal opening.	• Redness • Swelling • Purulent drainage
8. Maintain dry, clean dressing.	Decreases risk of skin breakdown. Moisture promotes maceration of the tracheal opening.	• Copious drainage • Change in characteristics of drainage
9. Monitor secretions (color, amount, and consistency). Hyperoxygenate and suction (see Procedure 9) based on assessment.	Suctioning should be based on patient need rather than on a standard frequency. Change in secretion characteristics may indicate infection or inadequate hydration.	• Excessively thick secretions • Copious or purulent secretions
10. Maintain head of bed at 30 degrees for approximately 24 hours and during enteral feedings. *(Level IV: Limited clinical studies to support recommendations)*	An elevated head of bed will promote oropharyngeal and nasopharyngeal drainage and minimize the risk of aspiration.[4, 5]	
11. Ensure that tube is securely in place (using twill tape or tracheal Velcro tie).	During the initial 48 hours following tracheostomy tube insertion, the tube should not be removed. If removed too early, the newly created stoma may collapse, making reintubation difficult.	
12. Perform oral hygiene every 2 to 4 hours. *(Level II: Theory based, no research data to support recommendations; recommendations from expert consensus group may exist)*	Prevents bacterial overgrowth and promotes patient comfort.	
13. Promote effective patient-provider communication (paper and pencil, letter or word boards, one-way speaking valves, if appropriate).	The patient cannot talk, which may result in fear and anxiety. Patients need an established communication mechanism.	

Documentation

Documentation should include the following:

- Patient and family education
- Respiratory and vital signs assessment before and after procedure
- Type and size of tube
- Nursing interventions taken
- Use of medications for sedation or pain
- Placement of inner cannula
- Expected and unexpected outcomes

- Patient response to procedure
- Date, time, and frequency with which procedure is performed
- Type and amount of secretions
- General condition of stoma and surrounding skin
- Nursing interventions
- Retaping of ET tube
- Mouth care

References

1. Henrich DE, Blyth WR, Weissler MC, Pillsbury HC. Tracheotomy and the ICU patient. *Laryngoscope.* 1997;107:844–847.
2. Kane TD, Rodriquez JL, Luchette FA. Early versus late tracheostomy in the trauma patient. *Respir Care Clin N Am* 1997;3:1–20.
3. Sugerman HJ, Wolfe L, Pasquale MD, et al. Multicenter, randomized, prospective trial of early tracheostomy. *J Trauma—Inj Infect Crit Care.* 1997;43:741–747.
4. Elpern EH, Scott MG, Petro L, Ries MG. Pulmonary aspiration in mechanically ventilated patients with tracheostomies. *Chest.* 1994;105:563–566.
5. Elpern EH, Jacobs RJ, Bone C. Incidence of aspiration in tracheally intubated adults. *Heart Lung* 1987;16:527–531.

Additional Readings

Kasper CL, Stubbs CR, Barton JA, Pieson DJ. Tracheostomy in the 1990s. *Respir Care.* 1996;41:37–42.
Pannunzio TG. Aspiration of oral feedings in patients with tracheostomies. *AACN Clin Issues.* 1996;7:560–569.

Continuous End-Tidal Carbon Dioxide Monitoring

P U R P O S E: End-tidal carbon dioxide (CO_2) monitoring is used to monitor a patient's ventilatory status and pulmonary blood flow, allowing the practitioner to detect changes in the ventilation-perfusion (V/Q) ratio of the lung.[1] The partial pressure of end-tidal CO_2 (PET_{CO_2}) is assumed to represent alveolar gas, which under normal V/Q matching in the lungs closely parallels arterial levels of CO_2.

Vicki S. Good

PREREQUISITE NURSING KNOWLEDGE

- The principles of ventilation. CO_2 is a byproduct of oxygen used by the cells after aerobic metabolism. Once the CO_2 reaches the lungs, the CO_2 of venous blood (Pv_{CO_2}) diffuses from the capillaries to the alveoli (PA_{CO_2}). The normal Pv_{CO_2} is equal to 45 mm Hg, and the normal PA_{CO_2} is 40 mm Hg. This pressure difference of 5 mm Hg causes the CO_2 to diffuse out of the capillaries into the alveoli for elimination. As the blood passes through the pulmonary capillaries, the Pv_{CO_2} will equal the PA_{CO_2} of 40 mm Hg.[2] In patients with normal ventilation-to-perfusion relationships, the PA_{CO_2}, partial pressure of CO_2 in arterial blood (Pa_{CO_2}), PA_{CO_2} and PET_{CO_2} will closely resemble one another. Thus, PET_{CO_2} can be used as an estimate of Pa_{CO_2}, with PET_{CO_2} generally 1 to 5 mm Hg lower than Pa_{CO_2}.[3]
- The principles of arterial blood gas sampling (see Procedure 72) and interpretation.
- Indications for continuous end-tidal CO_2 monitoring include the following:
  - ❖ Determine a baseline CO_2 waveform and PET_{CO_2}.
  - ❖ Continuously monitor the patency of the airway and the presence of breathing.
  - ❖ Provide mechanism for early detection of changes in waveform pattern or PET_{CO_2} value that may accompany a sudden or gradual change in CO_2 production or elimination (permissive hypercapnia, hyperthermia, hyperventilation therapy).[3]
  - ❖ Evaluate the patient's response to activities that may positively or negatively affect ventilation (eg, suctioning, repositioning, change in mechanical support, nutritional supplementation, cardiopulmonary resusci-

tation,[4] neuromuscular blockade,[3] verification of endotracheal tube placement[3]). *(Level VI recommendation: Clinical studies in a variety of patient populations and situations)*

- Basic principles of PET_{CO_2} monitoring. The end-tidal CO_2 monitor may be a standalone system or a module incorporated into the patient's bedside hemodynamic monitor. An infrared capnograph passes light through an expiratory gas sample and, using a photodector, measures absorption of that light by the gas. The capnograph determines the amount of CO_2 in the gas sample based on the absorption properties of CO_2. The capnograph also visually graphs the pattern in which CO_2 is exhaled and provides a display called a capnogram or PET_{CO_2} waveform.[5]
- The capnograph samples exhaled CO_2 by one of two methods: aspiration (sidestream) or nonaspiration (mainstream) sampling. In the sidestream method, a sample of gas is transported via small-bore tubing to the bedside monitor for analysis. In the mainstream system, analysis occurs directly at the patient-ventilator circuit.[2]
- The principles of normal capnographic waveform interpretation. The normal capnographic waveform has the following characteristics (Fig. 12–1):
  1. A zero baseline, which represents the beginning of exhalation of CO_2 free gas from anatomic dead space. This gas comes from the large airways, oropharynx, and nasopharynx (A–B).
  2. A rapid, sharp upstroke as the gas from the intermediate airways, containing a mixture of fresh gas and CO_2, begins to be exhaled from the lungs (B–C).
  3. A nearly flat alveolar plateau that occurs as exhaled

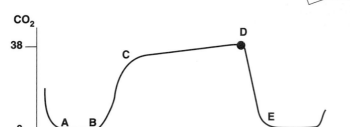

FIGURE 12–1. Essentials of the normal capnographic waveform. (From Mallinckrodt Nellcor Puritan Bennett, Pleasanton, CA.)

flow velocity slows and mixed gas is displaced by alveolar gas (C–D). Alveolar exhalation of CO_2 is nearing completion.

4. A distance end-tidal point that most closely reflects the maximum concentration of exhaled CO_2 and the end of exhalation (D).
5. A rapid downstroke as the patient begins the inspiration of gas that is essentially devoid of CO_2 (D–E).

Note that the positively deflected limb occurs with exhalation, whereas the negatively deflected limb occurs with inhalation. This is opposite from other respiratory waveforms, including the respigram, spirograms, and flow-volume loop. The capnogram will deviate from normal whenever there is a physiologic or mechanical disruption of the breath.

- Abnormalities between $PaCO_2$ and $PETCO_2$. The common physiologic basis for $PaCO_2$ and $PETCO_2$ abnormalities is incomplete alveolar emptying and increased alveolar dead space. This results in $PETCO_2$ values greater than 5 mm Hg below $PaCO_2$.
- (V/Q) relationship within the lung. The ideal gas exchanging unit has a V/Q ratio of 1.0. Practically speaking, V/Q ratio in the normal human lung is something other than 1.0 because areas of high V/Q and low V/Q exist within the normal physiologic realm. Under normal V/Q conditions, $PaCO_2$ and $PETCO_2$ values will be equal or nearly equal to the $PETCO_2$ values, an average of 2 to 5 mm Hg less than the $PaCO_2$. This difference is known as the a-ADCO$_2$ gradient. It is determined by subtracting the $PETCO_2$ value from the $PaCO_2$ value.

In conditions in which abnormally large numbers of alveolar-capillary units are underperfused in relation to their ventilation (high V/Q units) or in which lung units are ventilated but totally nonperfused (dead space units), transfer of CO_2 gas from blood to lung is impaired. When employing $PETCO_2$ monitoring, a lower exhaled CO_2 concentration than that measured in arterial blood (widened a-ADCO$_2$) will be observed. This occurs because the CO_2-free gas exhaled from nonperfused units mixes with CO_2-rich gas from perfused units, thereby diluting the overall concentration of CO_2 exhaled. At the opposite end of the V/Q spectrum are low V/Q units and shunt units. In these situations, perfusion exceeds ventilation. While low V/Q and shunt units are known contributors to the development of hypoxemia, they do not result in abnormal widening of the a-ADCO$_2$.

Caution should be taken when interpreting $PETCO_2$ in the presence of decreased pulmonary blood flow because the $PETCO_2$ may not accurately reflect $PaCO_2$.

EQUIPMENT

- Capnograph
- Airway adapter
- Arterial blood gas equipment

PATIENT AND FAMILY EDUCATION

- Discuss the rationale for implementing capnography. **Rationale:** Reduces anxiety for patient and family associated with an additional monitor, related interventions, and unfamiliar procedures.
- If the patient is alert, explain the procedure to the patient. **Rationale:** Informs the patient of the purpose of monitoring, improves cooperation with interventions, and reduces anxiety.

PATIENT ASSESSMENT AND PREPARATION
Patient Assessment

- Indications for $PETCO_2$ monitoring
  ❖ Acute airway obstruction or apnea (or potential for)
  ❖ Dead space ventilation (or potential for)
  ❖ Incomplete alveolar emptying (or potential for)
- **Rationale:** Assessment for initiation of $PETCO_2$ monitoring ensures that patients at risk for inadequate ventilation and gas exchange will receive monitoring for such occurrences, allowing for early institution of appropriate interventions.

Patient Preparation

- Ensure that patient understands preprocedural teaching. Answer questions as they arise, and reinforce information as needed. **Rationale:** Evaluates and reinforces understanding of previously taught information.

Procedure **for Continuous End-Tidal Carbon Dioxide Monitoring**

Steps	Rationale	Special Considerations
1. Obtain order for continuous $PETCO_2$ monitoring by capnography.	Order provides guideline for duration of monitoring, acceptable parameters for results, and appropriate interventions for abnormal results.	

Procedure continued on following page

Procedure for Continuous End-Tidal Carbon Dioxide Monitoring *Continued*

Steps	Rationale	Special Considerations
2. Assess for proper functioning of capnograph, including airway adapter, sensor, and display monitor; check electrical grounding and accurate setup; and secure connections.	Ensures reliability of PET_{CO_2} values and waveforms obtained.	
3. Wash hands, and don personal protective equipment.	Reduces transmission of microorganisms; standard precautions.	
4. Connect capnograph into grounded wall outlet, and connect appropriate patient cable into display monitor. Turn instrument on.	Decreases incidence of electrical interference.	Check capnograph's battery capacity and charging time, if applicable.
5. Perform calibration routine. Calibration procedure should occur daily or more often when instrument is in clinical use. *(Level I: Manufacturer's recommendation)*	Accurate measurement is dependent on proper calibration. Improper calibration may lead to erroneous PET_{CO_2} values.	All monitors have some type of calibration procedure; see operator's manual for exact steps.
6. Assemble airway adapter, sensor, and display monitor, and connect to patient circuit as close as possible to the patient's ventilation connection. *(Level I: Manufacturer's recommendation)*	Decreases incidence of improper gas sampling.	Sampling errors and gas leaks in system are major causes of inaccurate readings. Place adapter or sampling port as close as possible to the patient's airway to decrease response time to detect a change in CO_2.
7. Make sure that the sampling port is placed at the right angle to the endotracheal tube or ventilator circuit (applicable in sidestream sampling). *(Level I: Manufacturer's recommendation)*	Decreases secretion accumulation on CO_2 port where gas is drawn for sampling.	
8. Set appropriate alarms. Alarm limits should include respiratory rate, apnea default, high and low PET_{CO_2}, and minimal levels of inspiratory CO_2. *(Level VI: Clinical studies in a variety of patient populations and situations)*	Alerts the nurse to potentially life-threatening problems.	The PET_{CO_2} alarm is set 5% below acceptable parameter or per institutional standard. If monitor is interfaced with other equipment (electrocardiogram monitor, mechanical ventilator, pulse oximeter), make sure alarms are set consistently among all monitors.
9. Wash hands.	Reduces transmission of microorganisms.	

Expected Outcomes

- Significant changes in ventilatory status are detected.
- Alterations in the a-AD_{CO_2} gradient are identified.

Unexpected Outcomes

- Inaccurate measurements of PET_{CO_2} are displayed.
- Inaccurate measurements resulting from calibration drift or contamination of optics with moisture or secretions are displayed.
- Equipment malfunction occurs.

Patient Monitoring and Care

Patient Monitoring and Care	Rationale	Reportable Conditions
		These conditions should be reported if they persist despite nursing interventions.
1. Observe artificial airway for patency.	The airway adapter often adds weight to the airway and increases the risk of dislodgment or kinking. If kinking occurs, support the airway with an artificial support or towel.[2]	• Endotracheal or tracheal tube dislodgment
2. Observe waveform for quality.	If waveform is of poor quality, the numerical PET_{CO_2} value should not be accepted. If the PET_{CO_2} waveform is acceptable and the PET_{CO_2} numerical reading is questionable, obtain arterial blood gas measurement to confirm changes in PET_{CO_2}.	• Poor-quality waveform • Questionable PET_{CO_2} reading
3. Observe waveform for gradually increasing PET_{CO_2} (Fig. 12–2).	Increasing PET_{CO_2} will occur from absorption of CO_2 from exogenous sources and increased CO_2 production.[2, 3] Clinical conditions where increasing PET_{CO_2} will be found include increased metabolism, hyperthermia (usually indicated by a rapid rise in PET_{CO_2}), sepsis, hypoventilation or inadequate minute ventilation, neuromuscular blockade, decreased alveolar ventilation, partial obstruction of the airway, use of respiratory-depressant drugs, and conditions that cause metabolic alkalosis.	• PET_{CO_2} increase of >10% of baseline
4. Observe for a gradual increase in both baseline and PET_{CO_2} value (Fig. 12–3).	Reflects rebreathing of previously exhaled gas. Clinical conditions in which a gradual increase in both baseline and PET_{CO_2} levels will be found include defective exhalation valve on mechanical ventilator and excessive mechanical dead space in ventilator circuit.	• Malfunction of the ventilator

Continued on following page

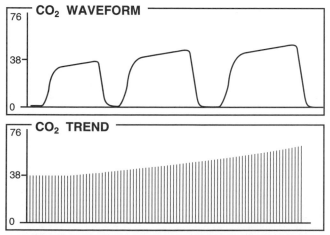

■ ● **FIGURE 12–2.** Gradually increasing PET_{CO_2}. (From Mallinckrodt Nellcor Puritan Bennett, Pleasanton, CA.)

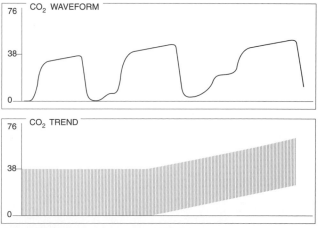

■ ● **FIGURE 12–3.** Gradual increase in baseline and PET_{CO_2} value. (From Mallinckrodt Nellcor Puritan Bennett, Pleasanton, CA.)

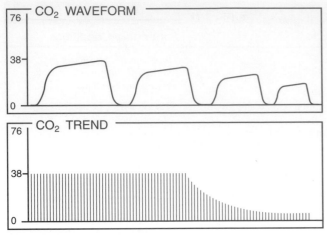

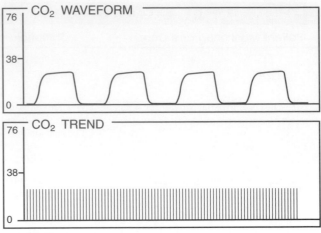

■ ● **FIGURE 12–4.** Exponential fall in PET_{CO_2}. (From Mallinckrodt Nellcor Puritan Bennett, Pleasanton, CA.)

■ ● **FIGURE 12–5.** Decreased PET_{CO_2}. (From Mallinckrodt Nellcor Puritan Bennett, Pleasanton, CA.)

Patient Monitoring and Care *Continued*

Patient Monitoring and Care	Rationale	Reportable Conditions
5. Observe for an exponential fall in PET_{CO_2} (Fig. 12–4).	Indicates a widening of the $a\text{-}AD_{CO_2}$ gradient from a sudden increase in dead space ventilation.[2,3] This is seen in such clinical conditions as cardiopulmonary bypass, cardiopulmonary arrest, pulmonary embolism, and severe pulmonary hypoperfusion.	• Cardiopulmonary arrest • Fall of >10% in baseline
6. Observe for decreased PET_{CO_2} (with a normal waveform) (Fig. 12–5).	Gradual decreases indicate a decrease in perfusion or a decrease in production of CO_2 and may be seen in patients with high minute volumes, hypothermia, metabolic acidosis, decreased cardiac output, and hypovolemia.	• PET_{CO_2} decreased >10% of baseline
7. Observe for a sudden decrease in PET_{CO_2} to low values (Fig. 12–6).	Incomplete sampling or full exhalation is not detected in the system.[2,3] This may be seen in patients with leak in airway system, partial airway obstruction, mechanical ventilator malfunction, or partial disconnection of ventilator circuit.	• PET_{CO_2} decreased >10% of baseline

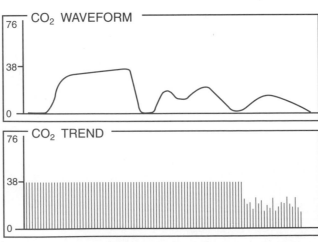

■ ● **FIGURE 12–6.** Sudden decrease in PET_{CO_2} values. (From Mallinckrodt Nellcor Puritan Bennett, Pleasanton, CA.)

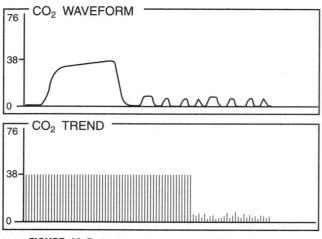

■ ● **FIGURE 12–7.** Sudden decrease in PETco₂ to near zero. (From Mallinckrodt Nellcor Puritan Bennett, Pleasanton, CA.)

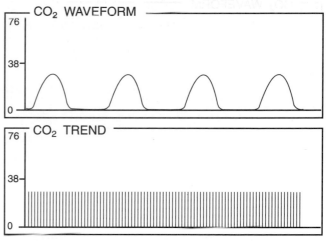

■ ● **FIGURE 12–8.** Low PETco₂ without alveolar plateau. (From Mallinckrodt Nellcor Puritan Bennett, Pleasanton, CA.)

Patient Monitoring and Care *Continued*

Patient Monitoring and Care	Rationale	Reportable Conditions
8. Observe for a sudden decrease in PETco₂ to near zero (Fig. 12–7).	Drop in waveform to baseline or near baseline (baseline equals zero) implies that no respirations are present.[3]	• Dislodged endotracheal tube • Complete airway obstruction • Mechanical ventilator malfunction • Airway disconnection • Esophageal intubation
9. Observe for a sustained low PETco₂ without alveolar plateau (Fig. 12–8).	Sustained low PETco₂ values are indicative of incomplete alveolar emptying such as in partially kinked endotracheal tube, bronchospasm, mucus plugging, improper exhaled gas sampling, or insufficient expiratory time on the ventilator.	• Complete airway obstruction requiring reintubation • PETco₂ decreased >10% of baseline
10. Routinely monitor the airway adapter or sampling port for signs of obstruction.	If the adapter or the port becomes obstructed, the quality of the capnographic waveform will be poor and PETco₂ will not be reliable.[3]	• Obstruction in the airway adapter or sampling port

Documentation

Documentation should include the following:

- Patient and family education
- Mechanical ventilator settings
- PETco₂ value and capnogram
- Paco₂-PETco₂ gradient
- Arterial blood gases
- Times of calibration
- Respiratory therapies

- Medications that may affect respiratory system, such as neuromuscular blockers, sedation, or bronchodilators
- Respiratory assessment (eg, respiratory rate, breathing patterns, adventitious sounds)
- Unexpected outcomes
- Nursing interventions

References

1. Sitzwohl C, Kettner SC, Reinprecht A, et al. The arterial to end-tidal carbon dioxide gradient increases with uncorrected but not with temperature-corrected $PaCO_2$ determination during mild to moderate hypothermia. *Anesth Analg.* 1998;85(5): 1131–1136.
2. La-Valle TL, Perry AG. Capnography: assessing end-tidal CO_2 levels. *DCCN.* 1995;14(2):70–77.
3. St. John RE. End tidal CO_2 monitoring. *American Association of Critical-Care Nurses Technology Series.* Aliso Viejo, Ca: American Association of Critical-Care Nurses; 1996:1–31.
4. Levine PD, Pizov R. End-tidal carbon dioxide and outcome of out-of-hospital cardiac arrest. *N Engl J Med.* 1997;337(5): 301–306.
5. Petterson, MT. Questions and answers on capnography. *Crit Care Choices.* 1990;1:12–17.

Additional Reading

Pierce LNB. *Mechanical Ventilation and Intensive Respiratory Care.* Philadelphia, Pa: W.B. Saunders; 1995.

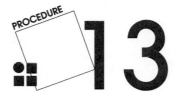

Continuous Mixed Venous Oxygen Saturation Monitoring

PURPOSE: Mixed venous oxygen saturation (SvO$_2$) monitoring is performed to measure the oxygen saturation of the venous blood in the pulmonary artery (PA). A continuous assessment of the balance between a patient's oxygen delivery and consumption is monitored by using a specialized fiber optic PA catheter and computer.

Jan M. Headley

PREREQUISITE NURSING KNOWLEDGE

- Anatomy and physiology of the cardiopulmonary system must be understood.
- Physiologic principles related to invasive hemodynamic monitoring should be known.
- Technical aspects of PA pressure monitoring should be understood.
- Physiologic concepts of oxygen delivery, oxygen demand, and tissue oxygen consumption should be known.
- Measured in the PA, SvO$_2$ is the percent of venous O$_2$ saturation. Because the blood in the PA is the mixture of all venous blood, it is believed to be representative of an average or overall venous oxygen saturation.
- Clinically, SvO$_2$ is a valuable index of the oxygen balance, a dynamic relationship between the patient's oxygen delivery (DO$_2$) and consumption (VO$_2$). Whenever there is a threat to the oxygen balance, the body's primary compensatory mechanisms are to increase delivery by increasing cardiac output (CO) or to increase extraction. In the critically ill patient, CO may be limited by poor cardiac reserve; thus, to meet the tissue's demand for oxygen, increased extraction occurs. This will result in decreased oxygen returning to the heart, thereby lowering SvO$_2$. Many factors can affect the requirements for oxygen and, subsequently, SvO$_2$[1-4] (Table 13–1).
- SvO$_2$ does not correlate directly with any of the determinants of DO$_2$ or VO$_2$. Because the critically ill patient is in a dynamic state with rapidly changing oxygen demand and VO$_2$, SvO$_2$ must be viewed in the light of these changing determinants and considered an index of oxygen balance.[1-4]
- A clinically significant change in SvO$_2$ (which is defined as a change of 5% to 10% from baseline) can be an early

indicator of physiologic instability. SvO$_2$ values of less than 60% may indicate either inadequate DO$_2$ or excess VO$_2$. SvO$_2$ monitoring is used in critically ill patients for earlier detection of oxygenation instability than that obtained through traditional PA monitoring.

- The proper setup and maintenance of the bedside computer or module is necessary for accurate monitoring.

Table 13–1 ● ■ ■ **Common Conditions and Activities Affecting SvO$_2$ Values**

Decreased SvO$_2$

Decreased oxygen delivery
    Decreased cardiac output
    Decreased hemoglobin
    Decreased arterial oxygen saturation
    Decreased arterial partial pressure of oxygen
Increased oxygen consumption
    Fever
    Pain
    Shivering
    Seizures
    Increased work of breathing
    Increased musculoskeletal activities

Increased SvO$_2$

Increased oxygen delivery
    Increased cardiac output
    Increased hemoglobin
    Increased arterial oxygen saturation
    Increased arterial partial pressure of oxygen
Decreased oxygen consumption
    Hypothermia
    Hypothyroidism
    Pharmacologic paralysis and sedation
    Anesthesia
    Cellular dysfunction
    Decreased work of breathing
    Decreased musculoskeletal activities

Additionally, proper blood sampling techniques from the distal port of the PA catheter are necessary for ensuring accurate values for calibration. There are two separate calibrations that must be done to ensure accurate SvO_2 monitoring. The light source must be electronically calibrated before catheter insertion (in vitro calibration). The second calibration is done by comparing SvO_2 values from a laboratory-analyzed sample with the SvO_2 monitor samples to ensure accuracy of continuous monitoring samples (in vivo calibration). This second calibration should be performed daily.

• Continuous monitoring is performed with a three-component system (Fig. 13–1)[2, 3, 5–7]:

❖ A fiber optic PA catheter, which contains two fiber optic filaments, exiting at the distal port. One filament serves as a sending fiber for the emission of light, the other a receiving fiber for the light reflected back from the blood in the PA.

❖ The optic module, which houses the light-emitting diodes (LEDs), which transmit various wavelengths of light, and a photodetector, which receives light back. Various wavelengths of lights are shone through a blood sample. Desaturated, saturated (oxyhemoglobin), and dyshemoglobins (carboxyhemoglobin, methemoglobin) have different light absorption characteristics. The ratio of hemoglobin to oxyhemoglobin is determined and reported as a percentage value.[2] All previous patient data, including calibration of SvO_2 values and patient identification information, are stored in this component. Therefore, this module should not be disconnected. If the module must be disconnected, refer to the manufacturer's instructions for a disconnection procedure that will not result in memory loss.

❖ An oximeter computer, which can be a stand-alone unit or module for a bedside monitor, has a microprocessor that converts the light information from the optic module into an electric display, updated every few seconds for continuous monitoring. This information is displayed either as a continuous graphic trend, a numeric display, or both, depending on the manufacturer.

EQUIPMENT

• Fiber optic PA catheter (7.5 or 8 Fr)
• Optic module
• Oximeter computer or bedside monitor module
• Equipment required for PA catheterization and pressure monitoring

Additional equipment (to have available depending on patient need) includes the following:

• Printer

PATIENT AND FAMILY EDUCATION

• Assess patient and family understanding of rationale for invasive hemodynamic monitoring. ➤**Rationale:** Pro-

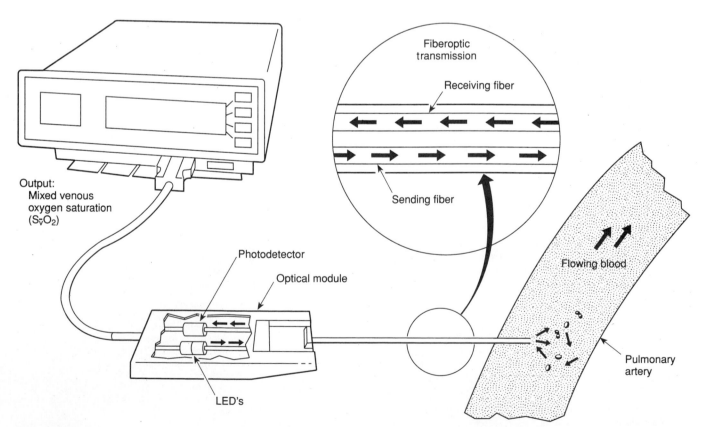

■ ● **FIGURE 13–1.** Example of a mixed venous oxygen saturation system using reflection spectrophotometry. (From American Edwards Laboratories. *Understanding Continuous Mixed Venous Oxygen Saturation (SvO₂) Monitoring with the Swan-Ganz Oximetry TD System.* Irvine, Ca: Author; 1987.)

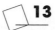

vides mechanism to assess level of patient and family understanding of need for advanced monitoring.

* Explain the continuous on-line nature of this monitoring system as well as the significance of the alarms. **➤➤*Rationale:*** Explanation of procedure to patient and family helps to alleviate fears and concerns. Additional monitors may produce increased anxiety in the patient and family.

PATIENT ASSESSMENT AND PREPARATION

Patient Assessment

* Indications for use of SvO$_2$ monitoring include the following[8]:
  * ❖ High-risk cardiovascular surgery

* ❖ Advanced-stage heart failure
* ❖ Myocardial infarction
* ❖ Acute hypoxemic respiratory failure
* ❖ Severe burns
* ❖ Multisystem organ dysfunction

➤➤*Rationale:* SvO$_2$ monitoring is useful in the early detection of oxygenation imbalance. Early detection can assist the health care team in early, appropriate interventions.

Patient Preparation

* Ensure that patient understands preprocedural teaching. Answer questions as they arise and reinforce information as needed. **➤➤*Rationale:*** Evaluates and reinforces understanding of previously taught information.

Procedure **for Continuous Mixed Venous Oxygen Saturation Monitoring**

Steps	Rationale	Special Considerations
1. Assemble necessary equipment and supplies for continuous monitoring. *(Level II: Theory based, no research data to support recommendations; recommendations from expert consensus group may exist)*	Ensures equipment is ready and available for the procedure.[7]	
2. Connect alternating current (AC) power cord to computer, turn on, and observe system check on the computer screen. *(Level I: Manufacturer's recommendation only)*	Allows electronics to warm up; confirms component function.	Warm-up times may vary by manufacturer.
3. Connect optics module to computer. *(Level I: Manufacturer's recommendation only)*	Light emitting diodes are housed in optics module. Approximately 20 minutes is required to sufficiently warm light source.[5, 6]	
4. Remove outer wrap of catheter package and aseptically peel back the inner wrap portion covering the optic connector of the catheter. *(Level I: Manufacturer's recommendation only)*	Provides access to inner package.[5, 6] Isolates connector from catheter tip to maintain sterility during in vitro calibration.[5, 6]	
5. Firmly connect the optic connector to the optic module. *(Level I: Manufacturer's recommendation only)*	Ensures connections are tight and properly aligned for light transmission.[5, 6]	
6. Perform in vitro calibration or standardization. *(Level I: Manufacturer's recommendation only)*	Standardizes or calibrates the light source to the catheter. Calibration is performed before catheter insertion. Catheter tip should be left in the calibration cup or container in the package during in vitro calibration.[5, 6]	Catheter lumens must be dry. Do not flush catheter before performing this step or in vitro calibration will be invalid.
7. Pull back remaining wrap convering catheter package using aseptic technique. *(Level I: Manufacturer's recommendation only)*	Prepares catheter for insertion.[5, 6]	

Procedure continued on following page

Procedure for Continuous Mixed Venous Oxygen Saturation Monitoring *Continued*

Steps	Rationale	Special Considerations
8. Carefully remove catheter from tray using sterile technique. Pull catheter tip up and out of the calibration cup. *(Level I: Manufacturer's recommendation only)*	Prevents transmission of microorganisms; prevents damage to the balloon.[5, 6]	Fiber optics in catheter and balloon are fragile and may be damaged if not handled properly.
9. Attach pressure tubing and prime lumens with flush solution (see Procedure 66).	Enables monitoring of chamber pressures during insertion. Maintains patency of lumens. Refer to institutional standards for use of heparinized flush solution.[8–10]	
10. Assist physician or nurse practitioner with catheter insertion (see Procedure 65).		
11. Observe waveforms during insertion.	Central PA catheter tip placement is necessary for optimal light reflection.[5, 6]	A light intensity or signal indicator verifies adequate reflection of the light signals after the catheter tip is correctly placed.
12. Note amount of air required to inflate balloon.	Inflation volume of 1.25 to 1.5 mL is recommended for proper catheter tip placement.[5, 6, 9]	Less than optimal inflation volume to obtain a wedge tracing may indicate distal catheter migration. A change in the intensity or signal indicator may also alert the clinician to this condition.
13. Set high and low alarm limits and activate alarms. *(Level II: Theory based, no research data to support recommendations; recommendations from expert consensus group may exist)*	Individualizes alarm settings according to patient baseline. Audible alarms notify the clinician of significant changes in SvO_2 values and trends.[7]	
14. Input patient height and weight data.	Allows for calculation of derived parameters.	
15. Apply a sterile dressing to insertion site (see Procedure 74).	Reduces transmission of microorganisms.	Use institutional standard for central venous catheter dressings.
16. Firmly secure the optic module near the patient.	Excessive tension on catheter or optic module may cause breakage of optic fibers.	
17. After calibration and insertion of catheter, obtain baseline set of hemodynamic and oxygenation indices (see Procedure 66).	Provides baseline information for comparison with patient's response to interventions.[5, 6]	
18. Continuously monitor PA pressure tracings and SvO_2 values. *(Level V: Clinical studies in more than one patient population and situation)*	Spontaneous catheter migration may occur after insertion. As a reflection of postcapillary arterialized blood and the vessel wall, the SvO_2 value may rise.[1, 3]	
Mixed Venous Blood Sampling Skill/In Vivo Calibration		
19. Draw mixed venous blood sample (see Procedure 58).	In vivo calibration is required to verify the accuracy of the computer and value displayed after insertion of the fiber optic PA catheter. Follow specific recommendations from the manufacturer about the frequency of calibration and specific steps to implement the process. Common to any monitoring system, the patient's hemodynamic and oxygenation status should be stable for optimal calibration.[1, 2, 5–7]	Sample not analyzed within 10 minutes should be iced for accurate values.

Procedure **for Continuous Mixed Venous Oxygen Saturation Monitoring** *Continued*

Steps	Rationale	Special Considerations
20. Perform a verification or in vivo calibration per institutional standard.	Typically, this is done every 24 hours or whenever the displayed value is in question. In vivo calibration verifies the accuracy of the SvO_2 being displayed.[5, 6]	
21. Ensure measurement is performed with a co-oximeter. *(Level V: Clinical studies in more than one patient population and situation)*	Co-oximetry measures saturation. Blood gas analyzers calculate saturation from measured partial pressure values. A calculated saturation value from a gas analyzer may not correlate with the actual patient value and, if used for calibration, will produce erroneous results.[9]	
22. Observe bedside oscilloscope for PA tracing and resume SvO_2 monitoring.	Reconfirms catheter tip placement in the PA.	

Expected Outcomes

- SvO_2 values and trends within normal range (60% to 80%)[1–3, 8]
- SvO_2 trends not fluctuating more than 5% to 10% of baseline value
- Hemodynamic and oxygenation parameters optimal for patient condition

Unexpected Outcomes

- SvO_2 values less than 60% or greater than 80%
- SvO_2 value trends $\pm 5\%$ to 10% from baseline
- Infection from presence of an indwelling PA catheter
- PA infarction or rupture

Patient Monitoring and Care

Patient Monitoring and Care	Rationale	Reportable Conditions
		These conditions should be reported if they persist despite nursing interventions.
1. Ensure that there are no kinks or bends in the catheter.	Fiber optics are fragile and can break if not handled carefully. Overtightening of the introducer connector can cause crimping of the fiber optics.[5, 6] Subclavian or internal jugular approaches for insertion may cause kinking in the vessel if the vessel is tortuous. Sending and receiving wavelengths may show either a change in light signal or values that do not reflect the patient's status.	- Change in PA waveform or SvO_2 value that does not correlate to patient condition
2. Monitor PA waveforms continuously.	Migration of the catheter tip may reflect postcapillary arterialized blood causing an elevation in the SvO_2 value. Uncorrected catheter migration places the patient at risk for PA infarction or rupture.	- Permanent wedge waveform
3. Observe SvO_2 value and trends.	Normal SvO_2 values range from 60% to 80%.[1, 2] Values outside this range may indicate an imbalance between oxygen delivery and consumption. A trending change of 5% to 10% over a 3- to 5-minute period may signify a clinically significant change. If the patient's clinical presentation differs from the observed SvO_2 value or trends, recheck the accuracy of the monitoring system.	- SvO_2 values >80% or <60%

Documentation

Documentation should include the following:

- Patient and family education
- SvO_2 whenever the hemodynamic profile is recorded
- Additional oxygenation indices as indicated
- Specific events, such as suctioning, turning the patient, or titrating a vasoactive drug, and the relationship of the event with the SvO_2, especially if the event produces a marked change in the value

- Hard copy printout (as available)
- Unexpected outcomes
- Nursing interventions

References

1. Nelson LD. Mixed venous oximetry. In: Snyder JV, Pinksy MR, eds. *Oxygenation Transport in the Critically Ill.* Chicago, Ill: Yearbook Medical Publishers; 1987:235–247.
2. Schweiss JF. Introduction and historical perspective. In: Schweiss JF, ed. *Continuous Measurement of Blood Oxygenation Saturation in the High Risk Patient.* Vol 1. San Diego, Calif: Beach International, 1983:1–12.
3. Headley JM. Strategies to optimize the cardiorespiratory status of the critically ill. *AACN Clin Issues Crit Care Nurs.* 1995;6(1):121–134.
4. Gawlinski A. Can measurement of mixed venous oxygen saturation replace measurement of cardiac output in patient with advanced heart failure? *Am J Crit Care.* 1998;7(5):374–380.
5. Baxter Healthcare Corporation. Vigilance: continuous cardiac output and SvO_2 monitoring system. In: *Operations Manual.* Irvine, Calif: Baxter Healthcare Corp; 1995.
6. Abbott Laboratories. *Oximetrix 3 System SO₂/CO Computer* (Operator's Manual). North Chicago, Ill: Abbott Laboratories; 1989.
7. Daily EK. Hemodynamic monitoring. In: Dolan J, ed. *Critical Care Nursing: Clinical Management Through the Nursing Process.* Philadelphia, F.A. Davis; 1991:828–854.
8. Jesurum JT. SvO_2 monitoring. In: *AACN Protocols for Practice: Hemodynamic Monitoring.* Aliso Viejo, Calif: American Association of Critical-Care Nurses; 1998.
9. Baxter Healthcare Corp. Swan-Ganz Thermodilution Catheters Product Information Data Sheet. Irvine, Calif: Baxter Healthcare; 1998.
10. Nierman DM, Schecter CB. Mixed venous O_2 saturation: measures by co-oximetry versus calculated from PvO_2. *J Clin Monit.* 1994;10:39–44.

Additional Readings

Keckeisen M. Pulmonary artery pressure monitoring. In: *AACN Protocols for Practice: Hemodynamic Monitoring.* Aliso Viejo, Calif: American Association of Critical-Care Nurses; 1998.
Shoemaker WC, guest ed. Mini-symposium: tissue perfusion and oxygenation. *Crit Care Med.* 1991;19(5):595–672.

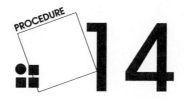

14 Oxygen Saturation Monitoring by Pulse Oximetry

P U R P O S E: Pulse oximetry is a noninvasive monitoring technique used to estimate the measurement of arterial oxygen saturation (SaO$_2$) of hemoglobin.

Sandra L. Schutz

PREREQUISITE NURSING KNOWLEDGE

- Oxygen saturation is an indicator of the percentage of hemoglobin saturated with oxygen at the time of the measurement. The reading, obtained through pulse oximetry, uses a light sensor containing two sources of light (red and infrared) that are absorbed by hemoglobin and transmitted through tissues to a photodetector. The amount of light transmitted through the tissue is then converted to a digital value representing the percentage of hemoglobin saturated with oxygen (Fig. 14–1).
- Oxygen saturation values obtained from pulse oximetry (SpO$_2$) are one part of a complete assessment of the patient's oxygenation status and are not a substitute for measurement of arterial partial pressure of oxygen (PaO$_2$) or of ventilation.
- The accuracy of SpO$_2$ measurements requires consideration of a number of physiologic variables. Such patient variables include the following:
  - ❖ Hemoglobin level
  - ❖ Arterial blood flow to the vascular bed
  - ❖ Temperature of the digit or the area where the oximetry sensor is located
  - ❖ Patient's oxygenation ability
  - ❖ Percentage of inspired oxygen
  - ❖ Evidence of ventilation-perfusion mismatch
  - ❖ Amount of ambient light seen by the sensor
  - ❖ Venous return at the probe location
- A complete assessment of oxygenation includes evaluation of oxygen content and delivery, which includes the following parameters: PaO$_2$, SpO$_2$, hemoglobin, cardiac output, and, when available, mixed venous oxygen saturation (SvO$_2$.)
- Normal oxygen saturation values are 97% to 99% in the healthy individual. An oxygen saturation value of 95% is clinically accepted in a patient with a normal hemoglobin level. Using the oxyhemoglobin dissociation curve, an oxygen saturation value of 90% is generally equated with a PaO$_2$ of 60 mm Hg.
- Tissue oxygenation is not reflected by oxygen saturation. The affinity of hemoglobin to oxygen may impair or enhance oxygen release at the tissue level.

- ❖ Decreased oxygen affinity—Oxygen is more readily released to the tissues when pH is decreased, body temperature is increased, arterial partial pressure of carbon dioxide (PaCO$_2$) is increased, and 2,3-DPG levels (a byproduct of glucose metabolism also found in stored blood products) are increased.
- ❖ Increased oxygen affinity—When the hemoglobin has greater affinity for oxygen, less is available to the tissues. Conditions such as increased pH, decreased temperature, decreased PaCO$_2$, and decreased 2,3-DPG will increase oxygen binding to the hemoglobin and limit its release to the tissue.
- Oxygen saturation values may vary with the amount of oxygen utilization by the tissues. For example, in some patients, there is a difference in SpO$_2$ values at rest compared with those during activity, such as ambulation or positioning.
- Oxygen saturation does not reflect the patient's ability to ventilate. Utilization of SpO$_2$ in a patient with obstructive pulmonary disease may be very misleading. As the de-

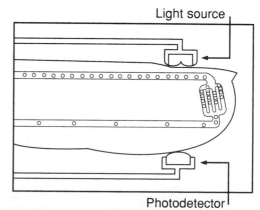

■ ● FIGURE 14–1. A sensor device that contains a light source and a photodetector is placed around a pulsating arteriolar bed, such as the finger, great toe, nose, or earlobe. Red and infrared wavelengths of light are used to determine arterial oxygen saturation. (Reprinted by permission of Mallinckrodt Inc., Pleasanton, California.)

In the figure: Light source, Photodetector

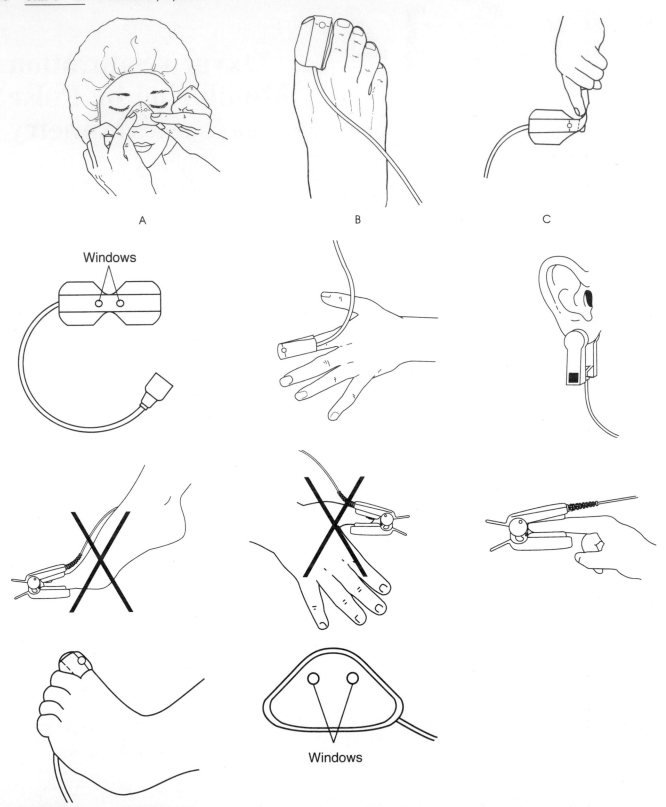

■ ● FIGURE 14–2. Sensor types and sensor sites for pulse oximetry monitoring. Use ''wrap'' style sensors on the fingers (including thumb), great toe, and nose. The windows for the light source and photodetector must be placed directly opposite each other on each side of the arteriolar bed to ensure accuracy of Spo₂ measurements. Choosing the correct size of the sensor will help decrease the incidence of excess ambient light interferences and optical shunting. ''Clip'' style sensors are appropriate for fingers (except the thumb) and the earlobe. Ensuring that the arteriolar bed is well within the clip with the windows directly opposite each other will decrease the possibility of excess ambient light interference and optical shunting. (Reprinted by permission of Mallinckrodt Inc., Pleasanton, California.)

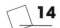

gree of lung disease increases, the patient's drive to breathe may shift from an increased carbon dioxide stimulus to a hypoxic stimulus. Therefore, enhancing the patient's SpO_2 may limit his or her ability to ventilate. The baseline SpO_2 for a patient with known severe restrictive disease needs to be considered.

- Any discoloration of the nail bed can affect the transmission of light through the digit. Dark nail polish and bruising under the nail can severely limit the transmission of light and result in an artificially decreased SpO_2 value.
- Pulse oximeters are unable to differentiate between oxygen and carbon monoxide bound to hemoglobin. Readings in the presence of carbon monoxide will be falsely elevated. Pulse oximetry should never be used in suspected cases of carbon monoxide exposure. An arterial blood gas reading should always be obtained.
- A pulse oximeter should never be used in a cardiac arrest situation because of the extreme limitations of blood flow.

EQUIPMENT

- Oxygen saturation meter and monitor
- Oxygen saturation cable and sensor

PATIENT AND FAMILY EDUCATION

- Explain the need for determination of oxygen saturation with a pulse oximeter. ➤➤*Rationale:* Informs patient of the purpose of monitoring, enhances patient cooperation, and decreases patient anxiety.
- Explain that the values displayed may vary by patient movement, amount of environmental light, patient level of consciousness (awake or asleep), and position of the sensor. ➤➤*Rationale:* Decreases patient and family anxiety over the constant variability of the values.
- Explain that the use of pulse oximetry is part of a much larger assessment of oxygenation status. ➤➤*Rationale:* Prepares patient and family for other possible diagnostic tests of oxygenation, such as an arterial blood gas test.
- Explain the equipment to the patient. ➤➤*Rationale:* Facilitates patient cooperation in maintaining sensor placement.
- Explain the need for an audible alarm system for determination of oxygen saturation values below a set acceptable limit. Demonstrate the alarm system, alerting the patient and family to the possibility of alarms, including causes

of false alarms. ➤➤*Rationale:* Providing an understanding of the use of an alarm system and its importance in the overall management of the patient, as well as of circumstances in which a false alarm may occur, assists in patient understanding of the values seen while at the bedside.

PATIENT ASSESSMENT AND PREPARATION

Patient Assessment

- Signs and symptoms of decreased ability to ventilate are as follows:
  - ❖ Cyanosis
  - ❖ Dyspnea
  - ❖ Tachypnea
  - ❖ Decreased level of consciousness
  - ❖ Increased work of breathing
  - ❖ Loss of protective airway (patients undergoing conscious sedation)

  ➤➤*Rationale:* Patient assessment will determine the need for continuous pulse oximetry monitoring. Anticipation of conditions in which hypoxia could be present allows earlier intervention before unfavorable outcomes occur.

- Conditions of the extremity (digit) or area where the sensor will be placed include the following:
  - ❖ Decreased peripheral pulses
  - ❖ Peripheral cyanosis
  - ❖ Decreased body temperature
  - ❖ Decreased blood pressure
  - ❖ Exposure to excessive environmental light sources (such as examination lights)
  - ❖ Excessive movement or tremor in the digit, presence of dark nail polish, or bruising under the nail

  ➤➤*Rationale:* Assessment of factors that may inhibit accuracy of the measurement of oxygenation before attempting to obtain an SpO_2 value will enhance the validity of the measurement.

Patient Preparation

- Ensure that patient understands preprocedural teaching. Answer questions as they arise, and reinforce information as needed. ➤➤*Rationale:* Evaluates and reinforces understanding of previously taught information.

Procedure **for Oxygen Saturation Monitoring by Pulse Oximetry**

Steps	Rationale	Special Considerations
1. Wash hands, and use personal protective equipment.	Reduces transmission of microorganisms and body secretions; standard precautions.	
2. Select the appropriate pulse oximeter sensor for the area with the best pulsatile vascular bed to be sampled (Fig. 14–2). Use of finger probes has been found to produce the best results over other sites.[1] *(Level VI: Clinical studies in a variety of patient populations and situations)*	The correct sensor optimizes signal capture and minimizes artifact-related difficulties.[1–4]	Several different types of sensors are available. These include disposable and nondisposable sensors that may be applied over a variety of vascular beds.

Procedure continued on following page

Procedure **for Oxygen Saturation Monitoring by Pulse Oximetry** *Continued*

Steps	Rationale	Special Considerations
3. Select desired sensor site. If using the digits, assess for warmth and capillary refill. Confirm the presence of an arterial blood flow to the area monitored.	Adequate arterial pulse strength is necessary for obtaining accurate SpO_2 measurements.	Avoid sites distal to indwelling arterial catheters, blood pressure cuffs, military antishock trousers (MAST), or venous engorgement (eg, arteriovenous fistulas, blood transfusions).
4. Plug oximeter into grounded wall outlet if the unit is not portable. If the unit is portable, ensure sufficient battery charge by turning it on before using. Plug patient cable into monitor.	When using electrical outlets, grounded outlets decrease the occurrence of electrical interference.	Portable systems have rechargeable batteries and are dependent on sufficient time plugged into an electrical outlet to maintain proper level of battery charge. When system is used in the portable mode, always check battery capacity.
5. Apply the sensor in a manner that allows the light source (light-emitting diodes) to be A. Directly opposite the light detector (photodetector) *(Level IV: Limited clinical studies to support recommendations)*	To properly determine a pulse oximetry value, the light sensors must be in opposing positions directly over the area of the sample.[1, 5–7]	
B. Shielded from excessive environmental light *(Level V: Clinical studies in more than one patient population and situation)*	Light from sources such as examination lights or overhead lights can cause elevated oximetry values.[5–7]	If the oximeter sensor fails to detect a pulse when perfusion seems adequate, excessive environmental light (overhead examination lights, phototherapy lights, infrared warmers) may be binding the light sensor. Troubleshoot by reapplying the sensor or shielding the sensor with a towel or blanket.
C. All sensor-emitted light comes in contact with perfused tissue beds and is not seen on the other side of the sensor without coming in contact with the area to be read.	If the light is seen directly from the sensor without coming in contact with the vascular bed, too much light can be seen by the sensor, resulting in either a falsely high reading or no reading.	Known as optical shunting, the light bypasses the vascular bed. Shielding the sensor will not eliminate this if the sensor is too large or not properly positioned.
D. The sensor does not cause restriction to arterial flow or venous return. *(Level IV: Limited clinical studies to support recommendations)*	The pulse oximeter is unable to distinguish between true arterial pulsations and fluid waves or fluid accumulation.[1–2, 8]	Restriction of arterial blood flow can cause a falsely low value as well as lead to vascular compromise, causing potential loss of viable tissues. Edema from restriction of venous return can cause venous pulsation. Elevating the site above the level of the heart will reduce the possibility of venous pulsations. Moving the sensor to another site on a routine schedule will also reduce tissue compromise.
6. Plug sensor into oximeter patient cable.	Connects the sensor to the oximeter, allowing SpO_2 measurement and analysis of waveforms.	
7. Turn instrument on with the power switch.		Allow 30 seconds for self-testing procedures and for detection and analysis of waveforms before values are displayed.

Procedure for Oxygen Saturation Monitoring by Pulse Oximetry *Continued*

Steps	Rationale	Special Considerations
8. Determine accuracy of detected waveform by comparing the numeric heart rate value to that of a monitored heart rate or an apical heart rate or both.	If there is insufficient arterial blood flow through the sensor, the heart rate values will vary significantly. If the pulse rate detected by oximeter does not correlate with the patient's heart rate, the oximeter is not detecting sufficient arterial blood flow for accurate values.	Consider moving the sensor to another area site, such as the earlobe or the nose. This problem occurs particularly with the use of the fingers and the toes in conditions of low blood flow.
9. Set appropriate alarm limits.	Alarm limits should be set appropriate to the patient's condition.	Oxygen saturation limits should be 5% less than patient acceptable baseline. Heart rate alarms should be consistent with the cardiac monitoring limits (if monitored).
10. Wash hands.	Reduces transmission of microorganisms to other patients.	

Expected Outcomes

- All changes in oxygen saturation are detected.
- The number of oxygen desaturation events is reduced.
- The need for invasive techniques for monitoring oxygenation is reduced.
- False-positive pulse oximeter alarms are reduced.

Unexpected Outcomes

- Accurate pulse oximetry is not obtainable because of movement artifact.
- Low perfusion states or excessive edema prevents accurate pulse oximetry measurements.
- Disagreements occur in Sao_2 and oximeter Spo_2.

Patient Monitoring and Care

Patient Monitoring and Care	Rationale	Reportable Conditions
		These conditions should be reported if they persist despite nursing interventions.
1. Evaluate the physical assessment, the laboratory data, and the patient.	Spo_2 values are one segment of a complete evaluation of oxygenation and supplemental oxygen therapy. Data should be integrated into a complete assessment to determine the overall status of the patient.	• Inability to maintain oxygen saturation levels as desired
2. Evaluate sensor site every 8 hours (if a disposable sensor is used) or every 4 hours (if a ridged encased nondisposable sensor is used).	Assessment of the skin and tissues under the sensor identifies skin breakdown or loss of vascular flow, allowing appropriate interventions to be initiated.	• Change in skin color • Loss of warmth of the tissue unrelated to vasoconstriction • Loss of blood flow to the digit
3. Monitor the site for excessive movement.	Excessive movement of the sampled site may result in unreliable saturation values. Moving the sensor to a less physically active site will reduce motion artifact. Using a lightweight sensor will also help. If the digits are used, ask the patient to rest the hand on a flat or secure surface.	
4. Compare and monitor the actual heart rate with the pulse rate value from the oximeter to determine accuracy of values.	The two numeric heart rate values should correlate closely. A difference in heart rate values may indicate excessive movement or a loss of pulsatile flow detection.	• Inability to correlate actual heart rate and pulse rate from oximeter

Documentation

Documentation should include the following:

- Patient and family education
- Indications for use of pulse oximetry
- Patient's pulse with SpO_2 measurements
- Fraction of inspired oxygen (FIO_2) delivered (if patient is receiving oxygen)
- Patient clinical assessment at the time of the saturation measurement

- Sensor site
- Simultaneous arterial blood gases (if available)
- Recent hemoglobin measurement (if available)
- Skin assessment at sensor site
- Oximeter alarm settings
- Events precipitating acute desaturation
- Unexpected outcomes
- Nursing interventions

References

1. Grap MJ. Pulse oximetry. In: *AACN Protocols for Practice: Technology Series.* Aliso Viejo, Ca: American Association of Critical-Care Nurses; 1996.
2. Grap MJ. Pulse oximetry. *Crit Care Nurse.* 1998;18:94–99.
3. Rutherford KA. Principles and application of pulse oximetry. *Crit Care Nurs Clin Am.* 1989;1:649–657.
4. Robertson RE, Kaplan RF. Another site for the pulse oximeter probe. *Anesthesiology.* 1991;74:198.
5. Siegel MN, Garvenstein N. Preventing ambient light from affecting pulse oximetry. *Anesthesiology.* 1987;67:280.
6. Zablocki AD, Rasch DK. A simple method to prevent interference with pulse oximetry by infrared heating lamps. *Anesth Analg.* 1987;66:915.
7. Hanowell L, Eisele JH, Downs D. Ambient light affects pulse oximeters. *Anesthesiology.* 1987;67:864–865.
8. Szarlarski NL, Cohen NH. Use of pulse oximetry in critically ill adults. *Heart Lung.* 1989;18:444–453.

Additional Readings

Carroll P. Using pulse oximetry in the home. *Home Healthc Nurse.* 1997;15:88–97.
Tittle M, Flynn MB. Correlation of pulse oximetry and co-oximetry. *Dimens Crit Care Nurs.* 1997;16:88–95.
Wahr JA, Tremper KK, Dlab M. Pulse oximetry. *Respir Care Clin N Am.* 1995;1:77–105.

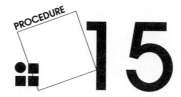

15

Manual Pronation Therapy

PURPOSE: The prone position may be used in conjunction with other supportive strategies in an attempt to improve oxygenation in patients with acute lung injury or acute respiratory distress syndrome (ARDS). The position also may be used for mobilization of secretions as a postural drainage technique, for posterior wound management that allows excellent visualization and management of the site, relief of pressure in the sacral region, positioning for operative or diagnostic procedures, and for therapeutic sleep for critically ill patients who normally sleep on their abdomen at home.

Kathleen M. Vollman

PREREQUISITE NURSING KNOWLEDGE

- Prone positioning is used as an adjunct short-term, supportive therapy in an attempt to improve gas exchange in the critically ill patient with severely compromised lungs. Based on recent studies, greater than 70% of all ARDS patients studied responded to prone positioning with an increased partial pressure of arterial oxygen (PaO_2).[1-7] To enhance an understanding of how prone positioning may impact gas exchange, it is important to understand the factors that influence the distribution of ventilation and perfusion within the lung.

- Distribution of ventilation: The volume of air distributed regionally throughout the lungs is jointly determined by regional pleural pressures and local lung compliance. There are three major factors, including gravity and weight of the lung, compliance, and heterogeneously diseased lungs, which influence regional distribution. In the upright individual, the pleural pressure next to the diaphragm is less negative than at the pleural apices. The weight of the lung and the effect of gravity on the lung and its supporting structures in the upright position create this difference in regional pleural pressures. This relationship results in a higher functional residual capacity (FRC) in the nondependent zone or the apices, thereby redirecting ventilation to the dependent zone.[8, 9] When body position changes, there are changes in regional pleural pressures, compliance, and volume distribution. In the supine position, distribution becomes more uniform from apex to base. However, it has been noted that dependent lung units' ventilation exceeds that of nondependent lung units, and a reduction in FRC is seen.[8, 9] The two factors contributing to the reduction in FRC seen when going from the upright to supine position include (1) the impact of the abdominal contents on the diaphragm,[10] and (2) the position of the heart, and the relationship of the

supporting structures to the lung and its influence on pleural pressure gradients.[11]

- ❖ The first factor to influence pleural pressure/regional volumes/FRC is the impact of the abdominal contents on the function of the diaphragm. In spontaneously breathing individuals in the supine position, the diaphragm acts as a shield against the pressure exerted by the abdominal contents, preventing those contents from interfering with dependent lung volume distribution. When patients are mechanically ventilated with positive-pressure breaths, sedated, or paralyzed, the active muscle tension in the diaphragm is lost, resulting in a cephalad displacement of the diaphragm and allowing abdominal pressures to impact dependent lung volume inflation and FRC.[10] The only way to modify this influence is to change the posture to a prone position with the abdomen unsupported.[10, 12]

- ❖ The second factor to influence pleural pressure/regional differences/FRC and compliance is the position of the heart and supporting structures. The heart and the diaphragm extend farther dorsally and rest against a rigid spine in the supine position, squeezing the lungs beneath them. This pressure on the lungs generates more positive pleural pressures, resulting in a greater propensity toward collapse of the alveoli at end expiration. In the prone position, the heart and upper abdomen rest against the sternum, exerting less weight on the lung tissue; therefore, less impact is provided on pleural pressure. This leaves the pleural pressures less positive, maintaining open alveoli.[11]

- ❖ A third factor that contributes to the distribution of volume is heterogeneously or unevenly distributed diseased lungs. The ARDS lung weight is increased two- to threefold from normal. The increased weight is due to edema and the resulting hydrostatic forces. This causes a progressive squeezing of gas along a vertical–dorsal axis. This decrease of regional inflation along the vertical axis results in dependent/dorsal lung collapse. In the prone position, these densities shift. The pattern almost completely reverts. The inflation gradient is less steep, and the difference results in a more homogenous regional inflation. This may be related to a redistribution of gas because of the change in hydrostatic forces caused by differences in pleural pressure, as described earlier.[13, 14]

- Distribution of perfusion: Similar to ventilation, regional distribution of perfusion is influenced by three factors, including cardiac output, pulmonary vascular resistance, and gravity or body position.
- In the upright individual, blood flow decreases as it moves from base to apex with virtually no flow at the apex. This is caused by the influence of gravity on pulmonary vascular pressures within the lung (Fig. 15–1). In zone 1, near the apex, alveolar pressure exceeds arterial pressure, creating little or no flow. In zone 2, the pulmonary artery pressure exceeds alveolar pressure, which in turn exceeds the venous pressure. Blood flow in this area occurs based on the differences in pressure between the arterial and alveolar. In zone 3, the arterial pressure is greater than the venous pressure, which is greater than the alveolar pressure. In this zone, the influence of the alveolar pressure on blood flow is reduced, resulting in freedom of flow in this region.[15] In supine and lateral positions, apical region blood flow changes. There is no real change in basalar units, but a greater dependent versus nondependent blood flow occurs. However, in the prone position there is a marked reduction in the gravitational perfusion gradient, suggesting no gravity-dependent benefit to flow in the prone position.[16]
- Based on the current available data as outlined here, it appears that changes in oxygenation may be related to differences in the regional inflation/ventilation of the lung while prone and are not necessarily related to a redistribution of blood flow.[6, 10, 11]

- Contraindications to pronation therapy include the following:[17]
  ❖ Unable to tolerate a head-down position
  ❖ Increased intracranial pressure
  ❖ Unstable spine
  ❖ Hemodynamically unstable patients (as defined by a systolic blood pressure of <90 mm Hg with fluid and vasoactive support in place)
  ❖ If using a support frame, a patient weight greater than 300 lb

EQUIPMENT

- Pillows or foam blocks
- Five or six staff members
- Lift sheet

  OR

- Vollman Prone Positioner® (VPP) (Fig. 15–2)
- Three staff members (with VPP)

Additional equipment (to have available depending on patient need) includes the following:

- Lateral rotation therapy bed
- Stryker Frame® for use in patients with unstable spines
- Capnography monitor

PATIENT AND FAMILY EDUCATION

- Assess the patient's and family's current understanding of the patient's lung/oxygenation problem and the reason for the use of the prone position. ➤*Rationale:* Decreases patient and family anxiety by providing information and clarification.
- Explain the standard of care to the patient and family, including positioning procedure, perceived benefit, fre-

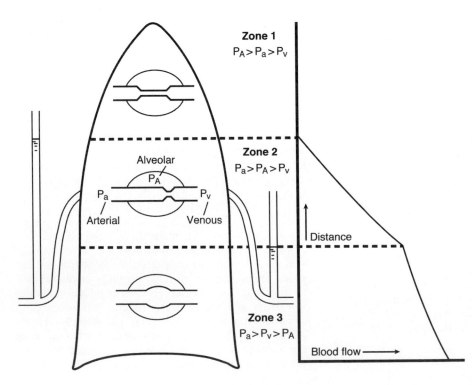

■ ● FIGURE 15–1. Zone model of the lung. (Three-zone model of the lung is used to explain distribution of blood flow based on pressure variations.) (From West JB, Dollery CT, Naimark A. *J Appl Physiol,* 1964; 19:713.)

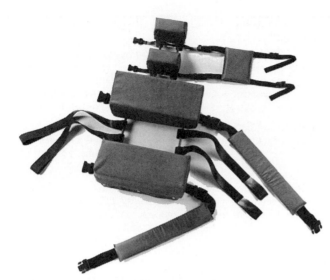

■ ● FIGURE 15–2. Diagram of Vollman Prone Positioner. (From Hill-Rom, Inc.)

quency of assessments, expected response, and parameters for discontinuation of the positioning technique and equipment (if special bed or frame is initiated). ➤*Rationale:* Provides an opportunity for the patient and family to verbalize concerns or ask questions about the procedure.

PATIENT ASSESSMENT AND PREPARATION
Patient Assessment

• Time interval from injury to position change. ➤*Rationale:* A trial of prone positioning should be performed early in the course of acute lung injury to assess the patient's level of response. However, if initial positioning does not elicit a positive response, this should not rule out periodic attempts to assess patient's responsiveness throughout the course of lung injury. Response to severe position change has been noted at all stages of acute lung injury.

• Hemodynamic status of the patient to identify ability to tolerate a position change. ➤*Rationale:* Imbalances between oxygen supply and demand must be addressed prior to the pronation procedure to offset any increases in oxygen demand that may be created by the physical turning. The final decision to place the hemodynamically unstable patient prone rests with the physician or nurse practitioner, who must weigh the risks against the potential benefits of using the prone position.

• Mental status before use of the prone position. ➤*Rationale:* Agitation—whether caused by delirium, anxiety, or pain—can have a negative effect when using the prone

position. Nevertheless, agitation is not a contraindication for use of the prone position. The health care team should strive to effectively manage the agitation in order to provide a safe environment for the use of the prone position.

• Size and weight load, to determine the ability to turn within the narrow critical care bed frame. ➤*Rationale:* When turning a patient prone in a hospital bed, with or without a frame, one must determine whether a 180-degree turn can be accomplished within the confines of the space available. Critical care bed frames are narrow, making it difficult to complete the turn on patients who weigh greater than 140 kg. One option may be to move the patient onto a stretcher while supine and then position him or her back onto the bed in the prone position if he or she exceeds the suggested weight limit.

Patient Preparation

• Ensure that patient understands preprocedural teaching. Answer questions as they arise and reinforce information as needed. ➤*Rationale:* Evaluates and reinforces understanding of previously taught information.

• Turn off the tube feeding 1 hour before the prone position turn. ➤*Rationale:* Assists with gastric emptying and reduces the risk of aspiration during the turning procedure.

• Prior to positioning the patient prone, the following care activities should be performed:
  ❖ Removal of electrocardiogram (ECG) leads from the anterior chest wall
  ❖ Eye care to include lubrication and taping of the eyelids closed in a horizontal fashion
  ❖ Ensure the tongue is inside the patient's mouth. If swollen or protruding, insert a bite block.
  ❖ Ensure the tape/ties of the endotracheal tube or tracheotomy tube are clean and secure. If adhesive tape is used to secure the endotracheal tube, double taping is recommended, because increased salivary drainage occurs in the prone position and may loosen the adhesive.
  ❖ If a wound dressing on the anterior body is due to be changed during the prone position sequence, perform the dressing change before the turn.
  ❖ Empty ileostomy/colostomy bags prior to positioning.
  ❖ Capnography monitoring is suggested to help ensure proper positioning of the tube during the turning procedure and while in the prone position.

➤*Rationale:* Prevents areas of pressure and potential breakdown, avoids complications related to injury or accidental extubation, and promotes the delivery of comprehensive care before, during, and after the pronation therapy.

Procedure for Manual Pronation Therapy

Steps	Rationale	Special Considerations
1. Wash hands, and don personal protective equipment.	Reduces risk of transmission of microorganisms and body secretions; standard precautions.	If using the frame, ensure it has been cleaned with an appropriate hospital-approved disinfectant.
2. Place a lift sheet under the patient to assist with the turning.	A lift sheet allows for the use of correct body alignment during the turning procedure.	A lift sheet is unnecessary if the patient is on a low air-loss surface and a support frame is being used.
3. Without a frame: two staff are positioned on each side of the bed, with another staff person positioned at the head of the bed. Proceed to step 5.	A total of five to six individuals are required to safely position a patient prone without a frame. Additional personnel may be required, based on the size of the patient.	The individual at the head of the bed is responsible for monitoring the stability and position of the endotracheal tube, ventilator tubing, and monitoring/intravenous lines located by the patient's head.
4. With a frame: one staff person is positioned on either side of the bed, with another staff member positioned at the head of the bed. *(Level IV: Limited clinical studies to support recommendations)*	A total of three staff members are required for the turn; two will perform the actual lifting and turning while the third is positioned at the head of the bed.[7, 17]	
5. Correctly position all tubes and invasive lines: A. Lines inserted in the upper torso will be aligned with either shoulder and the excess tubing will be placed at the head of the bed. The only exception to this rule is for chest tubes. B. Chest tubes and lines or tubes placed in the lower torso will be aligned with either leg and extend off the end of the bed.	All IV tubing and invasive lines are adjusted to prevent kinking, disconnection, or contact with the body during the turning procedure and while the patient remains in the prone position.	If the patient is in skeletal traction, one individual will need to apply traction to the leg while the lines and weights are removed for the turn. If a skeletal pin comes in contact with the bed, a pillow will need to be placed in the correct position to alleviate pressure points.
6. If on a low air-loss surface, maximally inflate.	Maximally inflating the air surface will firm up the mattress, making it easier to perform the turn.	
7. Always turn the patient in the direction of the mechanical ventilator. A. Turn the patient's head so it is facing away from the ventilator. Without disconnecting the ventilator tubing from the endotracheal tube (ET), place the portion of the tubing extending out from the ET on the side of the patient's face that is turned away from the ventilator. B. Loop the remaining ventilator tubing above the patient's head (Fig. 15–3). *(Level IV: Limited clinical studies to support recommendations)*	These maneuvers are performed to prevent disconnection of the ventilator tubing or kinking of the endotracheal tube during the turning procedure.[7, 17]	
8. If a frame is used, the straps, which secure the positioner to the body, are placed under the patient's head, chest (axillary area), and pelvic region at this time.		

Procedure	**for Manual Pronation Therapy** *Continued*

Steps	Rationale	Special Considerations

Placing Chest/Pelvic Support or the Vollman Prone Positioner®

1. When turning prone without a frame and using the abdomen unrestricted position, gather pillows at this time for manual placement under the head, upper chest, and pelvic region at a later phase in the procedure.

2. If using the VPP: Attach the frame to the patient while in the supine position. Lay the frame gently on top of the patient. Align the chest piece to rest between the clavicle and sixth rib. *(Level IV: Limited clinical studies to support recommendations)*

   The chest piece is the only nonmovable part and serves as the marker piece for proper placement/alignment of the device.[7, 17]

3. Adjust the pelvic piece to rest ½ inch above the iliac crest. *(Level IV: Limited clinical studies to support recommendations)*

   This prevents direct pressure over bony prominences, as well as providing sufficient distance between the chest and pelvis to allow the abdomen to be free of restriction while also preventing bowing of the back.[7, 17]

4. Adjust the forehead and chin pieces to provide full facial support in a face-down or a sidelying position without interfering with the ET tube.

   If the patient has limited neck range of motion or a short neck, the face-down position is optimal. However, because it will be difficult to readjust the head to relieve pressure points, it is recommended to move both headpieces up to the top of the frame. Therefore, only the head cushion supports the forehead and the chin is suspended to reduce the risk of skin breakdown from pressure.

   Procedure continued on following page

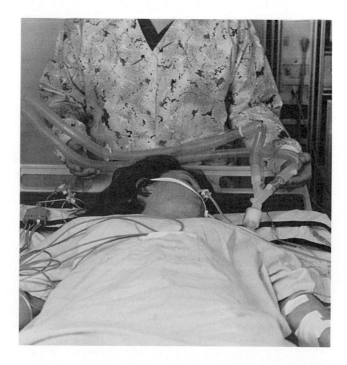

■ ● **FIGURE 15–3.** Positioning of ventilator tubing. (From Hill-Rom, Inc.)

Procedure **for Manual Pronation Therapy** *Continued*

Steps	Rationale	Special Considerations
5. Fasten the positioner to the patient using the soft adjustable straps. As the straps are tightened, the cushions will compress. Once fastened, lift the positioner to assess whether a secure fit has been obtained. Readjust as necessary. *(Level I: Manufacturer's recommendation only)*	If the device is not secured tightly, prior to the turn the patient may develop shear/friction injuries on the chest and pelvic area during the turning process.	When the device is secured correctly, it appears uncomfortable and possibly painful. As a result, the practitioner has a tendency not to fasten the device as tightly as is needed to prevent injury. When secured correctly, the device creates a feeling of pressure as well as a sense of security for the patient during the turning process.

Turning Prone Using the Half-step Technique

1. Using a draw sheet, move the patient to the edge of the bed farthest away from the ventilator in preparation for the prone turn. The individual closest to the patient maintains body contact with the bed at all times, serving as a side rail to ensure a safe environment. *(Level IV: Limited clinical studies to support recommendations)*	Provides sufficient room to rotate the body safely 180 degrees within the confines of a narrow critical care bed.[7, 17]	

2. Turning without a frame: turn the patient to a 45-degree angle toward the ventilator.
  A. Tuck the patient's arm and hand that now rest in the center of the bed under the buttocks after position alignment with the edge of the mattress is achieved.
  B. Cross the leg closest to the edge of the bed over the opposite leg at the ankle.
  C. The staff person on the ventilator side of the bed grasps onto the patient's body at the chest, pelvic, and leg areas.
  D. The staff on the opposite side reach under the patient at the same positions. The staff person at the head of the bed supports the head during the turn, while also ensuring that all tubes and lines are secure.
  E. Using a three count, the patient is then lifted and placed into a prone position.
  F. The patient can be placed in the abdomen-unrestricted position at this time by lifting and inserting pillows under the head, chest, and pelvic region.
	It is extremely important to use a wide base of support to improve balance and prevent self-injury during the turning procedure.	

Procedure **for Manual Pronation Therapy** *Continued*

Steps	Rationale	Special Considerations
3. Gently rotate the arms parallel to the body and then flex them into a position of comfort, so that they are lying adjacent to the head. Minor adjustments of the patient's body may be necessary to obtain correct alignment once in the prone position, whether using a frame or not.		Many patients have range-of-motion limitations to the shoulder area that may make it difficult to keep the arms in a flexed position. There are a number of ways to position the arms for comfort. The arms can be left in a sidelying position, aligned with the body, or one up and one down, similar to a swimmer position.
4. Turning with the VPP: A. Tuck the straps on the bar located between the chest and pelvic piece underneath the patient. B. Tuck the patient's arm and hand that now rest in the center of the bed under the buttocks, after position alignment with the edge of the mattress is achieved. C. Cross the leg closest to the edge of the bed over the opposite leg at the ankle. *(Level IV: Limited clinical studies to support recommendations)*	Helps with forward motion when the turning process begins.[7, 17]	
5. Turn the patient to a 45-degree angle toward the ventilator. A. The staff member on the ventilator side of the bed grips the upper steel bar. B. The staff person on the opposite side of the bed grasps the straps attached to the lower steel bar. C. Using a three count, lift the patient by the frame into a prone position. D. During the turning procedure, the individual at the head of the bed ensures that all tubes and lines are secure and patent (Fig. 15–4). *(Level IV: Limited clinical studies to support recommendations)*	It is extremely important to use a wide base of support to improve balance and prevent self-injury during the turning procedure.[7, 17]	
6. With the VPP: Loosen the straps at this time. If the patient is unstable, it is recommended to keep the straps fastened securely to facilitate a safe, quick return to the supine position in the event of an emergency (Fig. 15–5).	The procedure for returning to the supine position takes less than 1 minute if the straps are fastened and a support frame is used.	
7. If on a low air-loss surface, release the maximal inflation.	A return to normal pressures on the surface will help to alleviate pressure at various bony prominences while in the prone position.	If on a standard hospital mattress, the thigh-knee-calf area must be supported to minimize the risk of pressure and prevent discomfort. *Procedure continued on page 91*

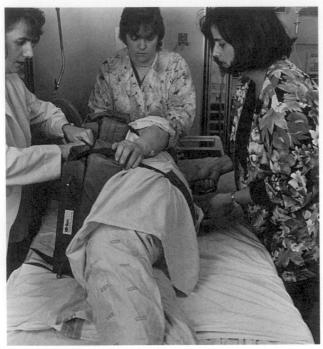

■ ● **FIGURE 15–4.** Patient lying prone on Vollman Prone Positioner. (From Hill-Rom, Inc.)

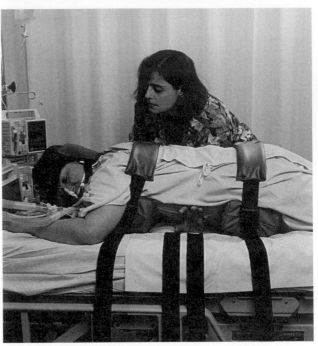

■ ● **FIGURE 15–5.** Turning patient prone on Vollman Prone Positioner. (From Hill-Rom, Inc.)

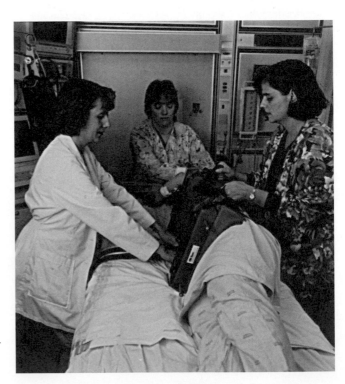

■ ● **FIGURE 15–6.** Patient returning to supine position. (From Hill-Rom, Inc.)

Steps	Rationale	Special Considerations
8. Place a support or other pillow under the ankle area.	A support in this area will allow for correct body alignment and prevent tension on the tendons in the feet and ankle region.	If the patient is tall enough, dangling the feet over the edge of the mattress may be a sufficient alternative to support the ankles and feet in correct alignment.
Returning to the Supine Position		
9. Align the patient with the edge of the mattress closest to the ventilator.		The patient will be turning toward the center of the mattress, away from the ventilator.
10. Arrange the ventilator tubing to provide sufficient mobility and length to prevent pulling during the turning procedure.	The staff member at the head of the bed is responsible for monitoring placement of the ventilator tubing, monitoring wires, and invasive lines.	
11. Straighten the patient's arms from a flexed position and bring them to rest on either side of the head. Remove leg and ankle pillow supports. If on a low air-loss surface, maximally inflate.		
12. Cross the leg closest to the edge of the bed over the opposite leg at the ankle.		
13. Without a frame: turn the patient to a 45-degree angle using the lift sheet and the patient's body, and then roll the patient onto his or her back.	Lifting and realignment in the center of the bed may be necessary when returning to the supine position if a support frame is not used.	
14. Stretch the arms parallel to the body and bring them into a downward position.		
15. With the VPP: fasten the straps tightly before repositioning.		
16. Turn the patient to a 45-degree angle using the steel bars and then roll the patient onto his or her back (Fig. 15–6).	The steel bars on the positioning frame allow lifting as the patient is realigned into the center of the bed.	
17. Unfasten the positioner and remove from the patient. The straps may be left under the patient in preparation for the next turn.		

Expected Outcomes

- Increased oxygenation
- Improved secretion clearance
- Improved compliance of the lungs

Unexpected Outcomes

- Agitation
- Disconnection/dislodgment of tubes and lines
- Peripheral arm nerve injury
- Periorbital and conjunctival edema
- Skin injuries or pressure ulcers
- Eye pressure

Patient Monitoring and Care	Rationale	Reportable Conditions
		These conditions should be reported if they persist despite nursing interventions.
1. Assess patient's tolerance to the turning procedure: ○ Respiratory rate and effort ○ Heart rate and blood pressure	Oxygen saturation is not used as a measure of intolerance to the turning procedure because patients often experience desaturation with a deep lateral turn; however, if a responder to the prone position, the patient will stabilize quickly once settled into the prone position. The lateral turn decrease in oxygen saturation may deter the health care team from trying the prone position. If respiratory rate and effort, heart rate, and blood pressure do not return to normal within 10 minutes of the turn, the patient may be displaying initial signs of intolerance.[18, 19]	• Failure of the respiratory rate, respiratory effort, heart rate, and blood pressure to return to normal 5 to 10 minutes after the turn
2. Assess the patient's response to the prone position: ○ Pulse oximetry (SpO_2) ○ Mixed venous oxygenation saturation (SvO_2) ○ Arterial blood gases (ABGs) ½ hour after position change	Greater than 70% of all acute lung injury patients turned prone improved their oxygenation.[1-7] The time response varies among patients. Some patients immediately respond, whereas others may take up to 6 hours to demonstrate maximal response to the position change.	• Decrease from baseline in the SpO_2 or failure of the SvO_2 to return to baseline after 5 to 10 minutes
3. Reposition the patient's head on an hourly basis while in the prone position to prevent facial breakdown. While one staff member lifts the patient's head, the second staff member moves the headpieces to provide support for the head in a different position.	The face and ears have minimal structural padding to reduce the risk of skin breakdown. Patients with short necks or limited neck range of motion have difficulty assuming a head sidelying position. Therefore, these patients are more likely to develop facial breakdown, making it necessary to turn the patient more frequently to prevent breakdown or use the technique described in procedure step 4, Special Considerations.	• Skin breakdown
4. Assess skin frequently for areas of nonblanchable redness or breakdown. Place a hydrocolloid dressing over areas where shearing and friction injuries are likely to occur (ie, chest, pelvis, elbows, and knees). *(Level I: Manufacturer's recommendation only)*	Greater than 2 hours on a standard surface without changing position increases a patient's risk for breakdown. If on a pressure-reduction surface, the time remaining in a stationary position can be lengthened. The use of a hydrocolloid may serve as a protective barrier, reducing the risk of shearing and friction injuries.[20] If using the VPP® and a skin injury occurs on the chest or pelvis, reassess tightness of the device prior to the prone position turn. The injury is most likely related to a loose-fitting apparatus.	• Nonblanchable redness • Shearing and friction injuries
5. Provide frequent oral care and suctioning of the airway as needed.	The prone position promotes postural drainage through the natural use of gravity. Drainage from the nares may be a clinical sign of an undetected sinus infection.	• Drainage from the nares • Change in amount or character of secretions

Patient Monitoring and Care *Continued*

Patient Monitoring and Care	Rationale	Reportable Conditions
6. Maintain tube feeding as tolerated.	The risk for aspiration is minimal in the prone position because the patient is already in a head-down, sidelying position that maximizes the use of gravity to move vomited matter safely. A reverse Trendelenberg position will change that relationship and increase the risk of aspiration.	• Evidence of tube feeding material when suctioning
7. Scheduling frequency: The positioning schedule is based on whether the patient is able to sustain improvements in PaO_2 made while in the prone position. A schedule of every 6 hours in the prone position is suggested.[18] Time spent in the supine position is based on the length of time the patient is able to sustain or maintain the improvement in gas exchange that occurred while prone. ○ If the patient maintains the improvement in PaO_2 when repositioned supine, the patient can remain in the supine to lateral position for 4 to 6 hours maximum or return to the prone position when or if a decrease in PaO_2 is seen. *(Level V. Clinical studies in more than one patient population and situation)* ○ If the patient is unable to maintain the improvement in gas exchange seen with the prone position when returned to a supine position, the patient should remain in the supine/lateral position for only 1 hour before being repositioned prone. ○ The use of the prone position is discontinued when the patient no longer demonstrates a positive response to the position change.	Without a clear direction from the literature on frequency of position change, the health care team must weigh other physiologic factors when a patient remains in a stationary position for an extended period of time. The potential for skin injury and edema formation can be minimized by following the principles of pressure relief used when positioning patients laterally or supine. Longer time spent in a single position requires that the support surface provide greater pressure reduction or relief than a standard hospital mattress. Combining the literature on the prone position and surface interface pressure, a safe suggestion for frequency of repositioning is between 4 and 6 hours.[1–7, 18, 20] It is suggested to use lateral rotation therapy in conjunction with prone positioning so that when the patient is returned to a supine position, he or she is laterally rotated. The use of continuous lateral rotation therapy has been associated with a reduction in pulmonary complications.[18, 21]	• Clinically significant drops in oxygenation (>10 mm Hg) or oxygen saturation $<88\%$

Documentation

Documentation should include the following:

- Patient and family education
- Ability to tolerate the turning procedure
- Length of time in the prone position
- Maximal oxygenation response while in the prone position
- Oxygenation response when returned to the supine position
- Positioning schedule used
- Complications noted during or after the procedure
- Use of continuous lateral rotation therapy
- Amount and type of secretions
- Unexpected outcomes
- Nursing interventions

References

1. Brussel T, Hachenberg T, Roos N, Lemzem H, Konertz W, Lawin P. Mechanical ventilation in the prone position for acute respiratory failure after cardiac surgery. *J Cardiothorac Vasc Anesth.* 1993;7:541–546.

2. Chatte G, Sab JM, Dubois JM, Sirodot M, Gaussorgues P, Robert D. Prone position in mechanically ventilated patients with severe acute respiratory failure. *Am J Respir Crit Care Med.* 1997;155:473–478.

3. Douglas WW, Rehder K, Beynen FM, Sessler AD, Marsh HM. Improved oxygenation in patients with acute respiratory failure: the prone position. *Am Rev Respir Dis.* 1977; 115:559–566.

4. Pappert D, Rossaint R, Slama K, Gruning T, Falke KJ. Influence of positioning on ventilation-perfusion relationships in severe adult respiratory distress syndrome. *Chest.* 1994;106:1511–1516.

5. Fridrich P, Krafft P, Hochleuthner H, Mauritz W. The effects of long-term prone positioning in patients with trauma induced adult respiratory distress syndrome. *Anesth Analg.* 1996;83:1206–1211.

6. Pelosi P, Yubiolo D, Mascheroni D, et al. Effects of the prone position on respiratory mechanics and gas exchange during acute lung injury. *Am J Respir Crit Care Med.* 1998;157:387–393.

7. Vollman KM, Bander JJ. Improved oxygenation utilizing a prone positioner in patients with acute respiratory distress syndrome. *Intens Care Med.* 1996;22:1105–1111.

8. Kaneko K, Milic-Emili J, Polovich MB, Danson A, Bates DV. Regional distribution of ventilation and perfusion as a function of body position. *J Appl Physiol.* 1966;21:767–777.

9. West JB. *Respiratory Physiology: The Essentials.* 3rd ed. Baltimore, Md: Williams & Wilkins; 1985:11–66.

10. Froese AB, Bryan AC. Effects of anesthesia and paralysis on diaphragmatic mechanics in man. *Anesthesiology.* 1974; 41:242–255.

11. Mutoh T, Guest RJ, Lamm WJE, Albert RK. Prone position alters the effect of volume overload on regional pleural pressures and improves hypoxemia in pigs in vivo. *Am Rev Respir Dis.* 1992;146:300–306.

12. Douglas WW, Rehder K, Beynen FM, Sessler AD, Marsh HM. Improved oxygenation in patients with acute respiratory failure: the prone position. *Am Rev Respir Dis.* 1977; 115:559–566.

13. Gattinoni L, Presenti A, Bombino M, et al. Relationships between lung computed tomographic density, gas exchange and PEEP in acute respiratory failure. *Anesthesiology.* 1988;69:824–832.

14. Gattinoni L, Pelosi P, Vitale G, Presenti A, D'Andrea L, Mascheroni D. Body position changes redistribute lung computed tomographic density in patients with acute respiratory failure. *Anesthesiology.* 1991;74:15–23.

15. West JB, Dollery CT, Naimark A. Distribution of blood flow in isolated lung: relation to vascular and alveolar pressures. *J Appl Physiol.* 1964;19:713–724.

16. Wiener CM, Kir W, Albert RK. Prone position reverses gravitational distribution of perfusion in dog lungs with oleic acid induced injury. *J Appl Physiol.* 1990;68:1386–1392.

17. Vollman KM. The effect of suspended prone positioning on PaO$_2$ and A-a gradients in adult patients with acute respiratory failure. Masters Thesis, California State University, Long Beach; 1989.

18. Vollman KM. Prone positioning for the ARDS patients. *Dimen Crit Care Nurs.* 1997;16:184–193.

19. Winslow EH, Clark AP, White KM, Tyler DO. Effects of a lateral turn on mixed venous oxygen saturation and heart rate in critically ill adults. *Heart Lung.* 1990;19:555–561.

20. Glavis C, Barbara S. Pressure ulcer prevention in critical care: state of the art. *AACN Clin Issues.* 1990;1:602–613.

21. Basham KR, Vollman KM, Miller A. To everything turn turn turn: an overview of continuous lateral rotation therapy. *Respir Care Clin North Am.* 1997;3:109–134.

Additional Readings

Albert RE, Leasa D, Sanderson M, Robertson T, Hlastala M. The prone position improves arterial oxygenation and reduces shunt in oleic acid induced acute lung injury. *Am Rev Respir Dis.* 1987;135:628–633.

Bryan AC, Bentivoglio LG, Beerel F, MacLeish M, Zidulka A, Bates DV. Factors affecting regional distribution of ventilation and perfusion in the lung. *J Appl Physiol.* 1964;19:395–402.

Langer M, Mascheroni D, Marcolin R, Gattinoni L. The prone position in ARDS patients: a clinical study. *Chest.* 1988; 91:103–107.

Schmitz TM. The semiprone position in ARDS: five case studies. *Crit Care Nurse.* 1991;11:22–33.

Vollman KM, Aulbach RK. Acute respiratory distress syndrome. In: Kinney MG, Dunbar SB, Brooks-Brunn JA, Molter N, Vitello-Cicciu JM, eds. *AACN Clinical Reference for Critical Care Nursing.* 4th ed. St. Louis, Mo: Mosby; 1998:529–564.

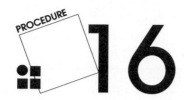

16 Autotransfusion

PURPOSE: Autotransfusion is the collection of blood from an active bleeding site and reinfusion of that blood into the same patient for the maintenance of blood volume.

Julianne M. Deutsch

PREREQUISITE NURSING KNOWLEDGE

- Understanding of transfusion and intravenous (IV) therapy and fluid balance is necessary.
- Autotransfusion is commonly used for trauma victims and for patients undergoing cardiovascular and orthopedic procedures, reducing the need for banked blood transfusions and thus reducing the risk of transfusion reactions and disease transmission.
- A variety of autotransfusion devices are available. An autotransfusion system may be a standard water-seal chest drainage system (see Fig. 21–1A), a separate autotransfusion setup, or a modified chest drainage autotransfusion system. Additionally, both continuous and intermittent systems are available. A continuous system has an IV line connected directly from the drainage unit collection chamber to the patient. An intermittent system uses a blood collection bag in-line between the chest tube and the collection chamber.
- Many of the disposable systems available today have the ability to act as a reservoir for autotransfusion, should the need arise. To initiate autotransfusion, the autotransfusion bag is disconnected from the disposable system and connected to the saline-filled blood administration tubing. Nurses should gain familiarity with their institution's autotransfusion system.
- Indications for autotransfusion in the appropriate patient populations include active bleeding (>100 mL/h) and the accumulation of >300 mL of drainage in the collection chamber.
- Contraindications to autotransfusion include the following:
  - ❖ Active infection or contamination of shed blood
  - ❖ Malignant cells in shed blood
  - ❖ Renal or hepatic insufficiency
  - ❖ Established coagulopathies
  - ❖ Blood that has been in the autotransfusion system for more than 6 hours

- Any contraindications to autotransfusion are overruled in the presence of exsanguinating hemorrhage in the absence of an adequate supply of banked blood.
- As with banked blood, patients may refuse to receive blood based on their religious beliefs.

EQUIPMENT

- Personal protective equipment
- Autotransfusion collection system
- Autotransfusion system replacement bag
- Blood administration set
- 40-micron micro-emboli filter
- Normal saline (NS)

PATIENT AND FAMILY EDUCATION

- Explain procedure to patient, if appropriate, and to the family, including the benefits of using patient's own blood. ➥*Rationale:* Information enhances patient and family understanding and decreases anxiety.

PATIENT ASSESSMENT AND PREPARATION

Patient Assessment

- Signs and symptoms of hypovolemia and associated hypoperfusion include the following:
  - ❖ Pale, clammy skin
  - ❖ Hypotension
  - ❖ Tachycardia
  - ❖ Dyspnea
  - ❖ Decreased pulmonary artery pressure (PAP) or pulmonary artery wedge pressure (PAWP)
  - ❖ Decreased cardiac output or index
  - ❖ Oliguria
  - ❖ Decreased hemoglobin or hematocrit

➥*Rationale:* Significant blood loss, related systemic hypoperfusion, and the associated decrease in oxygen-carrying capacity, with its impact on hypoxemia, will often require the replacement of blood with whole blood or packed cells. In appropriate patient populations (trauma, cardiovascular, or orthopedic surgical patients), autotransfusion should be considered as the need to replace blood becomes apparent.

Patient Preparation

- Ensure that patient understands preprocedural teaching. Answer questions as they arise and reinforce information as needed. **➤Rationale:** Evaluates and reinforces understanding of previously taught information.

Procedure **for Autotransfusion**

Steps	Rationale	Special Considerations
1. Wash hands, and don personal protective equipment.	Decreases transmission of microorganisms; standard precautions.	
2. Assemble equipment.		
3. Set up autotransfusion unit. (See manufacturer's instructions.)	Suction is required to drain blood into drainage unit.	
4. Inject anticoagulant into the autotransfusion bag before collecting blood from the patient. *(Level IV: Limited clinical studies to support recommendations)*	Several different anticoagulants may be used. Citrate phosphate dextrose (CPD) is commonly used, 1 mL per 7 mL blood.[1, 2]	Use of anticoagulants remains controversial.
5. Connect the patient's drainage or chest tube to the collection bag directly or via a water-seal setup.	Allows for collection of shed blood in preparation for autotransfusion.	Although autotransfusion is often performed with blood drained from the thoracic cavity, it can also be done after orthopedic procedures.
6. Before disconnecting the filled collection bag for patient infusion, a new collection system should be prepared.	Allows for the collection of additional blood as well as keeping the system closed and sterile.	
7. Clamp the tubes (attached to the tubing by the manufacturer) on the new collection bag.	Clamping eliminates the risk of air entering the system.	
8. Close the clamp on the patient drainage tubing	Stops further drainage into the bag.	
9. If the collection bag is part of the water-seal system (see Fig. 21–1A), close the clamps on the tubing connected to the water-seal drainage unit.	Prepares the system for disconnection.	
10. Disconnect the filled bag from the patient system, maintaining sterility at all times.		
11. Take the previously prepared new collection bag; attach it to the water-seal unit or to the patient's chest tube or drainage tube.	Allows for continued collection of blood.	
12. Ensure that all connections are secure; open clamps on autotransfusion bag and patient drainage tubing.	Connections must be secured to create suction for drainage.	
13. Prime the blood administration tubing with NS. Connect filled collection bag to blood administration set with microfilter. *(Level IV: Limited clinical studies to support recommendations)*	Filters should be used to reduce the danger of microembolization.[1, 2]	A 40-micron filter is commonly used for autotransfusion.
14. Initiate infusion as prescribed (see Procedure 107).	Restores blood volume.	Reinfuse blood within 6 hours of collection.[1]
15. Repeat procedure as needed.		

Procedure	**for Autotransfusion** *Continued*

Steps	Rationale	Special Considerations
16. Discard disposable supplies with blood in infectious waste.	Prevent exposure to blood; standard precautions.	

Expected Outcomes	Unexpected Outcomes
• Patient infused with own blood in a timely manner • Improved hemoglobin and hematocrit • Improved oxygenation through increased oxygen-carrying capacity of blood • Hemodynamic stability	• Blood transfusion reaction • Fluid overload

Patient Monitoring and Care

Patient Monitoring and Care	Rationale	Reportable Conditions
		These conditions should be reported if they persist despite nursing interventions.
1. Assess cardiopulmonary status and vital signs every hour and as needed.	Provides baseline and ongoing assessment of patient's condition.	• Tachypnea • Decreased or absent breath sounds • Hypoxemia • Tracheal deviation • Subcutaneous emphysema • Neck vein distention • Muffled heart tones • Tachycardia • Hypotension • Dysrhythmias • Fever
2. Evaluate and maintain drainage tube patency every 2 to 4 hours.	In chest tubes, obstruction of drainage interferes with lung reexpansion.	• Inability to establish patency
3. Monitor amount and type of drainage from collection system hourly for 8 hours and then every 2 hours.	Volume loss can cause patients to become hypovolemic. Decreased or absent drainage associated with respiratory distress may indicate obstruction; decreased or absent drainage without respiratory distress may indicate lung reexpansion.	• Bloody drainage >200 mL/h • New onset of clots • Sudden decrease or absence of drainage
4. Mark the drainage level on the outside of the drainage-collection chamber in hourly or shift increments and document in patient record.	Provides reference point for future measurements and assists in monitoring how quickly blood is accumulating for possible autotransfusion. Sudden flow of dark, bloody drainage occurring with position change is often old blood that finds its way into the chest tube.	• Drainage >200 mL/h • Sudden decrease or absence of drainage • Change in characteristics of drainage
5. Monitor for blood transfusion reaction (see Procedure 111).	It is extremely unlikely that a patient receiving autotransfusion will experience a blood transfusion reaction.	• Temperature spike • Chills • Tachycardia • Abdominal pain or back pain • Hypotension • Hematuria

D o c u m e n t a t i o n

- Patient and family education
- Amount of drainage system loss
- Amount of blood autotransfused
- Date and time when collection of blood started

- Patient tolerance
- Unexpected outcomes
- Nursing interventions

References

1. American Association of Blood Banks. *Guidelines for Blood Salvage and Reinfusion in Surgery and Trauma.* Bethesda, Md: American Association of Blood Banks; 1998.

2. Purcell TB. Autotransfusion (autologous blood transfusion). In: Roberts JR, Hedges JR, eds. *Clinical Procedures in Emergency Medicine.* Philadelphia, Pa: W. B. Saunders; 1998:410–426.

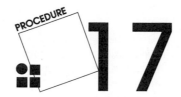
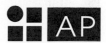
17

Performing Chest Tube Placement

P U R P O S E: Chest tubes are placed for the removal or drainage of air, blood, or fluid from the intrapleural or mediastinal space. They are also used to introduce sclerosing agents into the pleural space, thereby preventing a reaccumulation of fluid.

Denise M. Lawrence

PREREQUISITE NURSING KNOWLEDGE

- The thoracic cavity, under normal conditions, is a closed air space. Any disruption results in the loss of negative pressure within the intrapleural space; air or fluid entering the space competes with the lung, resulting in collapse of the lung. Associated conditions are the result of disease, injury, surgery, or iatrogenic causes.
- Chest tubes are sterile, flexible vinyl, silicone nonthrombogenic catheters approximately 20 inches (51 cm) long, varying in size from 12 to 40 French (Fr). The size of the tube placed is determined by the condition. Chest tubes inserted for traumatic hemopneumothorax or hemothorax (blood) should be large (36 to 40 Fr). Medium tubes (26 to 36 Fr) should be used for fluid accumulation (pleural effusions). Tubes inserted for pneumothorax (air) should be small (12 to 26 Fr).
- Indications for chest tube insertion include the following:
  - ❖ Pneumothorax (the collection of air in the pleural space)
  - ❖ Hemothorax (the collection of blood)
  - ❖ Hemopneumothorax (the accumulation of air and blood in the pleural space)
  - ❖ Tension pneumothorax
  - ❖ Thoracostomy (eg, open heart surgery, pneumonectomy)
  - ❖ Pyothorax or empyema (the collection of pus)
  - ❖ Chylothorax (the collection of chyle from the thoracic duct)
  - ❖ Cholothorax (the collection of fluid containing bile)
  - ❖ Hydrothorax (the collection of noninflammatory serous fluid)
  - ❖ Pleural effusion
- A pneumothorax may be classified as open, closed, or a tension pneumothorax:
  - ❖ Open pneumothorax: both the chest wall and the pleural space are penetrated, allowing air to enter the pleural space, as in penetrating injury or trauma; surgical incision in the thoracic cavity (ie, thoracotomy); or iatrogenic: occurs as complication of surgical treatment (eg, unintentional puncture during invasive procedures such as thoracentesis or central venous catheter insertion).
  - ❖ Closed pneumothorax: the pleural space is penetrated, but the chest wall is intact, allowing air to enter the pleural space from within the lung, as in spontaneous pneumothorax: occurs without apparent injury and is often seen in individuals with chronic lung disorders (eg, emphysema, cystic fibrosis, tuberculosis, necrotizing pneumonia) and in young, tall males who have a greater than normal height-to-width chest ratio; following blunt traumatic injury; or iatrogenic: occurs as a complication of medical treatment (eg, intermittent positive-pressure breathing [IPPB], mechanical ventilation with positive end-expiratory pressure [PEEP]).
  - ❖ Tension pneumothorax: air leaks into the pleural space through a tear in the lung and has no means to escape from the pleural cavity, creating a one-way valve effect. With each breath the patient takes, air accumulates, pressure within the pleural space increases, and then the lung collapses. This causes the mediastinal structures (ie, the heart, great vessels, and the trachea) to shift to the opposite or unaffected side of the chest. Venous return and cardiac output are impeded, along with the possibility of collapse of the unaffected lung. This is a life-threatening emergency that requires prompt recognition and intervention.
  - ❖ Special applications (anesthesia, sclerosing agents).
- There are no absolute contraindications to chest tube therapy. Use of chest tubes in patients with multiple adhesions, giant blebs, or coagulopathies are carefully considered; however, these relative contraindications are superseded by the need to re-inflate the lung.
- The insertion site selected for chest tube insertion is determined by the indication. If draining air, the tube is placed near the apex of the lung (second intercostal space); if draining fluid, the tube is placed near the base of the lung (fifth or sixth intercostal space) (Fig. 17–1).

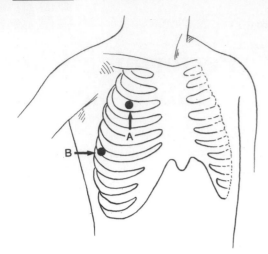

■ ● FIGURE 17–1. Standard sites for tube thoracostomy. *A,* The second intercostal space, midclavicular line. *B,* The fourth or fifth intercostal space, midaxillary line. Most clinicians prefer midaxillary line placement for all chest tubes, regardless of pathology. Note that placing the tube too far posteriorly will not allow the patient to lie down comfortably. (From Roberts JR, Hedges JR. *Clinical Procedures in Emergency Medicine.* 3rd ed. Philadelphia, Pa: WB Saunders; 1998:156.)

- Mediastinal tubes are generally placed in the operating room by a surgeon after cardiac surgery.

EQUIPMENT

- Antiseptic solution
- Sterile gloves, caps, gowns, masks, drapes
- Protective eyewear (goggles)
- Local anesthetic: 1% lidocaine solution
- Tube thoracotomy tray
  - ❖ Sterile towels, 4 × 4 sterile gauze
  - ❖ Scalpel with no. 11 blade
  - ❖ Two Kelly clamps, curved clamps
  - ❖ Needle holder
  - ❖ 2-0, 3-0 silk suture with cutting needle
  - ❖ Suture scissors
  - ❖ Two hemostats
  - ❖ 10-mL syringe with 20-G, 1½-in needle
  - ❖ 5-mL syringe with 25-G, 1-in needle
  - ❖ Thoracostomy tube (choose size appropriate to condition)
  - ❖ Closed chest drainage system
  - ❖ Suction source
  - ❖ Suction connector and connecting tubing (usually 6 feet for each tube)
  - ❖ Y connector
  - ❖ 1-in adhesive tape
  - ❖ Dressing materials (4 × 4 gauze pads, slit drain sponges, petroleum gauze, tape)

PATIENT AND FAMILY EDUCATION

- Explain the procedure (if patient condition and time allows) and the reason for the chest tube insertion. ➤*Rationale:* Identifies patient and family knowledge deficits concerning the patient's condition, procedure, expected benefits, and potential risks, and allows time for questions to clarify information and to voice concerns. Explanations decrease patient anxiety and enhance cooperation.
- Explain that the patient's participation during the procedure is to remain as immobile as possible and do relaxed breathing. ➤*Rationale:* Facilitates insertion of the chest tube and prevents complications during insertion.
- After the procedure, instruct the patient to sit in a semi-Fowler position (unless contraindicated). ➤*Rationale:* Facilitates drainage from the lung by allowing air to rise and fluid to settle in order to be removed via the chest tube. This position also makes breathing easier.
- Instruct the patient to turn and change position every 2 hours. The patient may lie on the side with the chest tube but should keep the tubing free of kinks. ➤*Rationale:* Turning and positioning prevents complications related to immobility and retained pulmonary secretions. Keeping the tube free of kinks maintains patency of the tube, facilitates drainage, and prevents the accumulation of pressure within the pleural space that interferes with lung reexpansion.
- Instruct the patient to cough and deep breath, splinting the affected side. ➤*Rationale:* Coughing and deep breathing raises pressure within the pleural space, thus facilitating drainage, promoting lung reexpansion, and preventing respiratory complications associated with retained secretions. The application of firm pressure over the chest tube insertion site (ie, splinting) decreases pain and discomfort.
- Encourage active or passive range-of-motion exercises of the arm on the affected side. ➤*Rationale:* The patient may limit movement of the arm on the affected side to decrease the discomfort at the insertion site, resulting in joint discomfort and potential joint contractures.
- Instruct the patient and family about activity as prescribed while maintaining the drainage system below the level of the chest. ➤*Rationale:* Facilitates gravity drainage and prevents backflow and potential infectious contamination into the pleural space.
- Instruct the patient about the availability of prescribed analgesic medication and other pain relief strategies. ➤*Rationale:* Pain relief ensures comfort, facilitates coughing, deep breathing, positioning, range of motion, and recuperation.

PATIENT ASSESSMENT AND PREPARATION

Patient Assessment

- Significant medical history or injury, including chronic lung disease, spontaneous pneumothorax, hemothorax, pulmonary disease, therapeutic procedures, mechanism of injury. ➤*Rationale:* Medical history or injury may provide the etiologic basis for the occurrence of the pneumothorax, empyema, pleural effusion, or chylothorax.
- Baseline cardiopulmonary status for signs and symptoms requiring chest tube insertion.
  - ❖ Tachypnea
  - ❖ Decreased or absent breath sounds on the affected side
  - ❖ Crackles adjacent to the affected area

- ❖ Shortness of breath, dyspnea
- ❖ Asymmetrical chest excursion with respirations
- ❖ Cyanosis
- ❖ Decreased oxygen saturation
- ❖ Hyperresonance in the affected side (pneumothorax)
- ❖ Subcutaneous emphysema (pneumothorax)
- ❖ Dullness or flatness in the affected side (hemothorax, pleural effusion, empyema, chylothorax)
- ❖ Sudden, sharp chest pain
- ❖ Anxiety, restlessness, apprehension
- ❖ Tachycardia
- ❖ Hypotension
- ❖ Dysrhythmias
- ❖ Tracheal deviation to the unaffected side (tension pneumothorax)
- ❖ Neck vein distention (tension pneumothorax)
- ❖ Muffled heart sounds (tension pneumothorax)

➡*Rationale:* Accurate assessment of signs and symptoms allows for prompt recognition and treatment. Baseline assessment provides comparison data for evaluating changes and outcomes of treatment.
- Diagnostic tests (if patient's condition does not necessitate immediate intervention), including chest x-ray and arterial blood gases. ➡*Rationale:* Diagnostic testing confirms the presence of air or fluid in the pleural space, a collapsed lung, hypoxemia, and respiratory compromise.

Patient Preparation

- Ensure that patient understands preprocedural teaching. Answer questions as they arise and reinforce information as needed. ➡*Rationale:* Evaluates and reinforces understanding of previously taught information.
- Obtain consent if circumstances allow. ➡*Rationale:* Invasive procedures, unless performed under implied consent in a life-threatening situation, require written consent of the patient or significant other.
- Determine insertion site. ➡*Rationale:* Insertion site is determined by the indication for the chest tube. Air: second intercostal space; fluid: fifth or sixth intercostal space.
- Assist the patient to the lateral, supine (for pneumothorax), or semi-Fowler position (for hemothorax). ➡*Rationale:* Enhances accessibility to the insertion site for positioning of the chest tube.
- Administer prescribed analgesics or sedatives as needed. ➡*Rationale:* Analgesics and sedatives reduce the discomfort and anxiety experienced, facilitating patient cooperation.

 This procedure should be performed only by physicians, advanced practice nurses, and other health care professionals (including critical care nurses) with additional knowledge, skills, and demonstrated competence per professional licensure or institutional standard.

Procedure **for Performing Chest Tube Placement**

Steps	Rationale	Special Considerations
1. Wash hands, and don sterile personal protective equipment.	Reduces the transmission of microorganisms and body secretions; standard precautions.	Chest tube insertion is a sterile procedure and requires full attire, unless performed in a life-threatening situation.
2. Open the chest tube insertion tray using sterile technique.	Reduces transmission of microorganisms.	

3. Prepare equipment:
  A. Check that all equipment is present.
  B. Pour antiseptic solution into basin using aseptic technique.
  C. Attach needle holder to suture.
  D. Apply a large Kelly clamp to proximal end of tube.
  E. Prepare syringe with lidocaine solution.
	Facilitates insertion of the tube.	

4. Identify insertion site and have assistant position the patient. *(Level V: clinical studies in more than one patient population and situation)*	Assists in preparing area for insertion and proper placement of tube.[1-3]	Air: right or left second intercostal space. Fluid: right or left fifth or sixth intercostal space, mid-axillary line. Incision site is one rib below insertion site (Fig. 17–1).
5. Surgically prepare the skin with antiseptic solution and drape the area surrounding the insertion site. *(Level VI: clinical studies in a variety of patient populations and situations)*	Inhibits growth of bacteria at insertion site. Maintains sterility.[1, 2, 4]	Prepare the area from the clavicle to umbilicus; mid-chest to anterior axillary line.

Procedure continued on following page

Procedure	**for Performing Chest Tube Placement** *Continued*

Steps	Rationale	Special Considerations
6. Anesthetize the skin, subcutaneous tissue, muscle, and periosteum with 1% lidocaine solution. 　A. Using a 5-mL syringe (25-G needle), inject a subcutaneous wheal of lidocaine at the insertion site. 　B. Using a 10-mL syringe (20-G, 1½-in needle), advance the needle/syringe, aspirating as you go, until air or pleural fluid confirmed. Inject the lidocaine deeper, and slowly withdraw the syringe, generously anesthetizing rib periosteum, subcutaneous tissue, and pleura (Fig. 17–2). *(Level V: clinical studies in more than one patient population and situation)*	Results in loss of sensation and decreased pain during insertion.[1, 3-5]	When infiltrating with lidocaine, aspirate as you go to confirm the presence of air or fluid. As much as 30 to 40 mL of lidocaine may be required for anesthesia.
7. Using a no. 11 blade, make a 3-cm transverse skin incision directly over the inferior aspect of the anesthetized rib below the insertion site (Fig. 17–3). *(Level V: clinical studies in more than one patient population and situation)*	Allows for the diameter of the chest tube.[1, 3-5]	When making the incision, incise down through the subcutaneous tissue. The space should be large enough to admit a finger.
8. Introduce the curved clamp through the incision, with the tips down, creating a tunnel through the subcutaneous tissue and muscle; use an opening and spreading maneuver; aim toward the superior aspect of the rib until the pleural space is reached (Fig. 17–4). *(Level V: clinical studies in more than one patient population and situation)*	Facilitates insertion of the tube. Blunt dissection minimizes trauma to the neurovascular bundle.[1, 3, 4]	Additional lidocaine is infiltrated as needed. The direction of the tunnel created through the subcutaneous tissue and muscle will determine the direction the chest tube will take after insertion. Make sure the clamp stays close to the ribs to avoid injury to the neurovascular bundle.

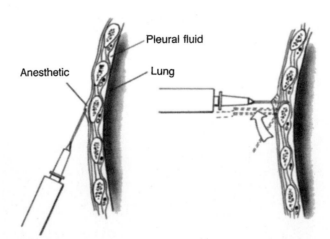

Anesthetic　Pleural fluid　Lung

■ ● **FIGURE 17–2.** Insertion of a chest tube can be relatively painless with proper infiltration of the skin and pleura with local anesthetic. The liberal use of *buffered* 1% lidocaine with epinephrine (maximum lidocaine dose, 5 mg/kg) is recommended. (From Roberts JR, Hedges JR. *Clinical Procedures in Emergency Medicine.* 3rd ed. Philadelphia, Pa: WB Saunders; 1998:156.)

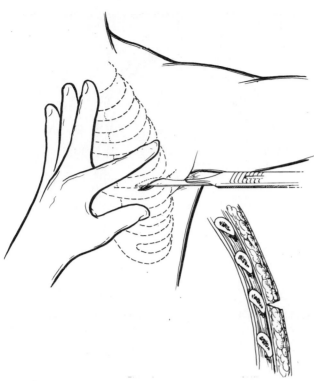

▪ ● **FIGURE 17–3.** Transverse skin incision is made directly over the inferior aspect of the anesthetized rib down to the subcutaneous tissue. (From Dumiro SM, Paris PM. *Atlas of Emergency Procedures.* Philadelphia, Pa: WB Saunders; 1994:61.)

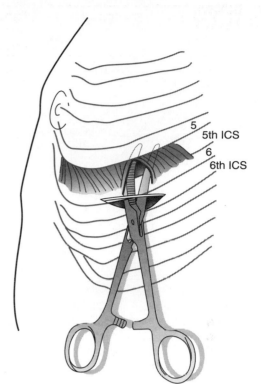

▪ ● **FIGURE 17–4.** Blunt dissection is accomplished by forcing a closed clamp through the incision and by using an opening-and-spreading maneuver, creating a tunnel to the pleura.

Procedure	**for Performing Chest Tube Placement** *Continued*	
Steps	**Rationale**	**Special Considerations**
9. When the clamp is just over the superior portion of the rib, close the clamp and push it with steady pressure through the parietal pleura and into the pleural space. Widen the hole in the pleural space by spreading the clamp (Fig. 17–5). *(Level V: clinical studies of more than one patient population and situation)*	Ensures opening is large enough for the chest tube. Steady, even, controlled pressure provides control of the clamp once the pleura is perforated.[1, 3, 4]	This maneuver requires more pressure than might be anticipated. A lunging motion or use of the trocar may cause hole in lung or injury to the liver or spleen.
10. Insert the index finger to dilate the tract and hole in the pleura. *(Level IV: limited clinical studies to support recommendations)*	Relieves air or fluid once penetration of the space is made. Ensures entry into the pleural space and not into a space inadvertently created between the parietal pleura and chest wall.[3, 4, 6]	Feel for lung tissue (lung should expand and meet finger on inspiration), diaphragm, or adhesions. Break up clot, if found.

Procedure continued on following page

▪▪ AP This procedure should be performed only by physicians, advanced practice nurses, and other health care professionals (including critical care nurses) with additional knowledge, skills, and demonstrated competence per professional licensure or institutional standard.

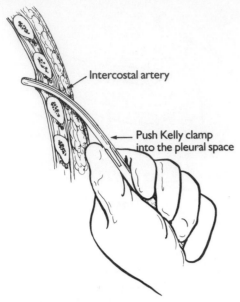

■ ● FIGURE 17–5. Just over the superior portion of the rib, close the clamp, and push with steady pressure into the pleura. (From Dumire SM, Paris PM. *Atlas of Emergency Procedures.* Philadelphia, Pa: WB Saunders; 1994:61.)

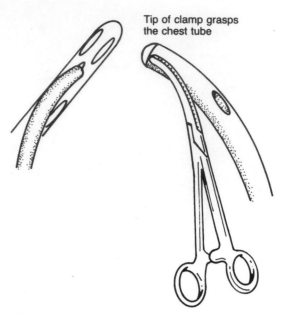

■ ● FIGURE 17–6. The tube is grasped with the curved clamp, with the tube tip protruding from the jaws. (From Roberts JR, Hedges JR. *Clinical Procedures in Emergency Medicine.* 3rd ed. Philadelphia, Pa: WB Saunders; 1998:159.)

Procedure **for Performing Chest Tube Placement** *Continued*

Steps	Rationale	Special Considerations
11. Insert the chest tube into the chest cavity using a curved Kelly clamp, holding the proximal end to guide the tip into the pleural space (Fig. 17–6). Remove the clamp and guide the tube, in a rotating motion, through the tract and into the space. The tube is advanced until the last hole is in the pleural space. Condensation of air or fluid in the tube should be noted. *(Level V: clinical studies in more than one patient population and situation)*	Confirms placement of the tube.	To drain air, aim the tube posteriorly and superiorly toward the apex of the lung; to drain fluid, aim the tube inferiorly and posteriorly. Do not allow any side holes of the tube to remain outside the thoracic cavity.
12. Connect the chest tube to the closed chest drainage system (see Procedure 21) and check for respiratory variation of the H_2O column. Have assistant apply ordered amount of suction. *(Level V: clinical studies of more than one patient population and situation)*	Ensures the tube is properly positioned.	
13. Suture the tube to the chest wall. Wrap the free ends of the suture around the tube (like lacing a shoe). Tie the ends of the suture snugly around the top of the tube (Fig. 17–7). *(Level V: clinical studies in more than one patient population and situation)*	Secures the position of the tube.[4, 6, 7] Secures the tube snugly to prevent subcutaneous air/emphysema.	Type of stitch used is dependent on the individual. The goal is to prevent displacement of the chest tube.

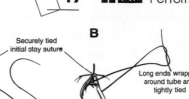

■ ● FIGURE 17–7. A "stay" suture is first placed next to the tube to close the skin incision. *A,* The knot is tied securely, and the ends, which will subsequently be wrapped around the chest tube, are left long. *B,* The ends of the suture are wound twice about the tube tightly enough to indent the tube slightly and are tied securely. (From Roberts JR, Hedges JR. *Clinical Procedures in Emergency Medicine.* 3rd ed. Philadelphia, Pa: WB Saunders; 1998:160.)

Procedure **for Performing Chest Tube Placement** *Continued*

Steps	Rationale	Special Considerations

14. Apply occlusive dressing.
  A. Petrolatum gauze is used around the chest tube or follow institutional standard.
  B. Split drain sponges are placed around the chest tube, one from top, one underneath.
  C. Cover with 4 × 4 gauze.
  D. Tape dressing.
  (Level IV: limited clinical studies to support recommendations)
	Provides airtight seal around the chest tube.[6, 7]	

15. Tape all connection points to the drainage system. *(Level V: clinical studies in more than one patient population and situation)*	Creates an airtight system. Airtight connections prevent air leaks into the pleural space.[6, 7]	Check that all holes are in the pleural space.
16. Obtain a chest x-ray. *(Level VI: clinical studies in a variety of patient populations and situations)*	Confirms placement of tube and reexpansion of lung and removal of fluid.[1, 2, 5, 7]	Document location, tube size, complications, and result of chest x-ray in the chart.
17. Dispose of equipment in receptacle.	Standard precautions.	

AP This procedure should be performed only by physicians, advanced practice nurses, and other health care professionals (including critical care nurses) with additional knowledge, skills, and demonstrated competence per professional licensure or institutional standard.

Expected Outcomes	Unexpected Outcomes
• Removal of air, fluid, or blood from the pleural space • Relief of respiratory distress • Reexpansion of the lung (validated by chest x-ray) • Restoration of negative pressure within the pleural space	• Hemorrhage/shock • Increasing respiratory distress • Infection • Damage to intracostal nerve resulting in neuropathy, neuritis • Incorrect tube placement • Chest tube kinking, clogging, or dislodgment from chest wall • Subcutaneous emphysema

Patient Monitoring and Care

Patient Monitoring and Care	Rationale	Reportable Conditions
		These conditions should be reported if they persist despite nursing interventions.
1. Assess cardiopulmonary and vital signs every 2 hours and as needed.	Provides baseline and ongoing assessment of patient's condition. Abnormalities can indicate reoccurrence of the condition that required chest tube insertion.	• Tachypnea • Decreased or absent breath sounds • Hypoxemia • Tracheal deviation • Subcutaneous emphysema • Neck vein distention • Muffled heart tones • Tachycardia • Hypotension • Dysrhythmias • Fever
2. Monitor output every 2 hours and record amount and color.	Provides data for diagnosis.	• Bloody drainage of 200 mL/hr or greater • Sudden cessation of drainage • Change in character of drainage
3. Assess for pain at the insertion site or for chest discomfort.	Interferes with adequate deep breathing. Pain at insertion site, particularly with inspiration, may indicate improper tube placement.	• Pain at insertion site
4. Evaluate the chest drainage system for fluctuation in water-seal chamber (see Procedure 21). Check connections.	Water level will normally rise and fall with respiration until lung is expanded. Bubbling immediately after insertion and with exhalation and coughing is normal. Persistent bubbling indicates an air leak and should be corrected.	• Absence of fluctuation in water-seal chamber • Persistent bubbling
5. Assess insertion site and surrounding skin for presence of subcutaneous air and signs of infection or inflammation with each dressing change, or every day.	Skin integrity is altered during insertion and can lead to infection.	• Fever • Redness around insertion site • Purulent drainage • Subcutaneous emphysema

Documentation

Documentation should include the following:

- Patient and family education
- Reason for chest tube insertion
- Respiratory and vital sign assessment before and after insertion
- Description of procedure, including the following: tube size, date and time of insertion, insertion site, and any complications associated with the procedure

- Results of procedure, type and amount of drainage
- Presence of fluctuation and bubbling
- Amount of suction
- Patient's tolerance to procedure
- Postinsertion chest x-ray results
- Unexpected outcomes
- Nursing interventions

References

1. Lewinter JR. Tube thoracostomy. In: Jastremski MS, Dumas M, Penalver L, eds. *Emergency Procedures*. Philadelphia, Pa: W.B. Saunders; 1992:391–397.
2. Kravis TC, Warner CG, Jacobs LM. *Emergency Medicine Procedures Manual*. New York, NY: Raven Press; 1994: 51–55.
3. Chen H, Sola JE, Lillemae KD. *Manual of Common Bedside Surgical Procedures*. Baltimore, Md: Williams & Wilkins; 1996:100–108.
4. Wright SW. Tube thoracostomy. In: Roberts JR, Hedges JR, eds. *Clinical Procedures in Emergency Medicine*. 3rd ed. Philadelphia, Pa: W.B. Saunders; 1998:148–171.
5. Dunmire SM, Paris PM. *Atlas of Emergency Procedures*. Philadelphia, Pa: W.B. Saunders; 1991:50–70.
6. Wilson RF. Thoracic trauma. In: Tininalli JE, Ruiz E, Krome RL, eds. *Emergency Medicine: A Comprehensive Guide*. 4th ed. New York, NY: McGraw Hill; 1996:1156–1182.
7. Iberti TJ, Stern PM. Chest tube thoracostomy. In: Krause JA, ed. *Critical Care Clinics*. Philadelphia, Pa: W.B. Saunders; 1998:879–892.

▪▪ AP This procedure should be performed only by physicians, advanced practice nurses, and other health care professionals (including critical care nurses) with additional knowledge, skills, and demonstrated competence per professional licensure or institutional standard.

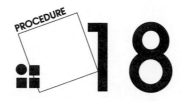

18 Assisting with Chest Tube Placement

P U R P O S E: Chest tubes are placed for the removal or drainage of air, blood, or fluid from the intrapleural or mediastinal space. They are also used to introduce sclerosing agents into the pleural space, preventing a reaccumulation of fluid.

Catherine Freismuth Robinson

PREREQUISITE NURSING KNOWLEDGE

- A chest tube is inserted when disease, injury, surgery, or iatrogenic etiology causes a loss of negative pressure within the pleural space. Air, fluid, or blood may collect, taking up space within the pleural cavity that impedes lung expansion, resulting in partial or total collapse of the lung.
- The insertion of a chest tube (also known as a thoracostomy tube or a thoracic catheter) assists with the removal of air, fluid, and blood from the pleural space. Negative pressure is thus reestablished, allowing the collapsed lung to reexpand. A mediastinal tube may also be indicated after cardiac surgery to drain fluid and blood from around the heart. Although the pleura usually remains intact in cardiac surgery cases and there is no pneumothorax, the blood and fluid, if allowed to accumulate postoperatively, would create enough pressure to compress the heart, causing cardiac tamponade.
- Indications for chest tube insertion include the following:
  - ❖ Pneumothorax (collection of air in the pleural space)
  - ❖ Hemothorax (collection of blood in the pleural space)
  - ❖ Hemopneumothorax (accumulation of air and blood in the pleural space)
  - ❖ Tension pneumothorax
  - ❖ Thoracostomy (eg, open heart surgery, pneumonectomy)
  - ❖ Pyothorax or empyema (collection of pus in the pleural space)
  - ❖ Chylothorax (collection of chyle from the thoracic duct)
  - ❖ Cholothorax (collection of fluid containing bile)
  - ❖ Hydrothorax (collection of noninflammatory serous fluid)
  - ❖ Pleural effusion
- A pneumothorax may be classified as open, closed, or a tension pneumothorax.
  - ❖ Open pneumothorax: Both the chest wall and the pleural space are penetrated, allowing air to enter the pleural space, as in the following: penetrating injury or trauma, surgical incision in the thoracic cavity (eg, thoracotomy) iatrogenic (occurs as complication of surgical treatment) (eg, unintentional puncture during invasive procedures such as thoracentesis or central venous catheter insertion)
  - ❖ Closed pneumothorax: The pleural space is penetrated, but the chest wall is intact, allowing air to enter the pleural space from within the lung, as in the following: spontaneous (occurs without apparent injury and is often seen in individuals with chronic lung disorders [eg, emphysema, cystic fibrosis, tuberculosis necrotizing pneumonia] and in young, tall males who have a greater than normal height-to-width chest ratio); following blunt traumatic injury; iatrogenic (occurs as a complication of medical treatment [eg, intermittent positive pressure breathing, mechanical ventilation with positive end-expiratory pressure]).
  - ❖ Tension pneumothorax: Air leaks into the pleural space through a tear in the lung and has no means to escape from the pleural cavity, creating a one-way valve effect. With each breath the patient takes, air accumulates, pressure within the pleural space increases, and the lung collapses. This causes the mediastinal structures (ie, heart, great vessels, and trachea) to shift to the opposite or unaffected side of the chest. Venous return and cardiac output are impeded, and collapse of the unaffected lung is possible. This is a life-threatening emergency that requires prompt recognition and intervention.
- The need for insertion of a chest tube depends on the size and severity of the pneumothorax. A small pneumothorax, occupying less than 15% of the pleural space, may not require the insertion of a chest tube. A moderate pneumothorax, occupying 15% to 60% of the pleural space, and a large pneumothorax, occupying greater than 60% of the pleural space, require placement of a chest tube.
- Chest tubes are sterile, flexible, vinyl, silicone, or latex nonthrombogenic catheters, approximately 20 in (51 cm) long, varying in size. Adults usually require a 12- to 26-G chest tube for a simple pneumothorax, whereas a 28- to 40-G tube is used to drain liquid accumulations. The end of the chest tube that rests in the patient's pleural

space has a number of drainage holes to facilitate ease of drainage and to prevent tip occlusion from clots and tissue. The distal end connects to a chest drainage system.
- The insertion site selected for chest tube insertion is determined by the indication. If draining air, the tube is placed near the apex of the lung (second intercostal space); if draining fluid, the tube is placed near the base of the lung (fifth to sixth intercostal space) (see Fig. 17–1). Two chest tubes may be inserted; one in the apex and one at the base of the lung, to remove both air and fluid (hemopneumothorax). Two chest tubes may also be inserted, one anteriorly and one laterally, following certain surgical procedures (eg, after heart surgery), to drain blood from behind and in front of the heart, decreasing the incidence of postoperative cardiac tamponade. When two chest tubes are used, they may be attached to a single chest drainage system by a Y connector or have separate drainage systems.
- The insertion site is locally anesthetized, and a small incision (2 to 3 cm) is made. Using the blunt dissection method (see Procedure 17), a forceps is passed through a skin incision to penetrate the pleural space. A finger is used to create a tract for the chest tube, to lyse adhesions, and to ensure placement of the chest tube within the pleural space. The chest tube, clamped to the forceps, is advanced into the pleural space so that the last eyelet rests 5 cm within the pleura.
- Once in place, the tube is sutured to the skin to prevent displacement and an occlusive dressing is applied (Fig. 18–1).
- Following insertion, the chest tube is connected to a chest drainage system to remove air and fluid from the pleural space and to prevent backflow into the pleural space. This facilitates reexpansion of the collapsed lung. All connection points are secured with tape or Parham bands to ensure that the system remains airtight (Fig. 18–2).

EQUIPMENT

- Antiseptic solution
- Sterile gloves, caps, gowns, masks, and drapes
- Protective eyewear (goggles)
- Local anesthetic—1% lidocaine solution
- Tube thoracotomy tray with the following:
  - ❖ Sterile towels, 4 × 4 sterile gauze pad
  - ❖ Scalpel with #11 blade

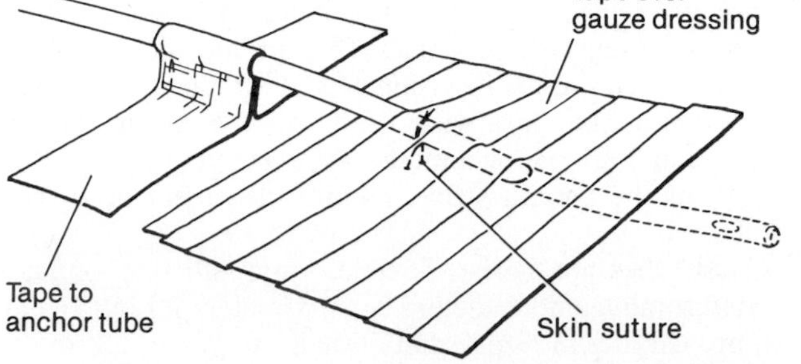

■ ● **FIGURE 18–1.** Occlusive chest tube dressing. (From Kerston LD. *Comprehensive Respiratory Nursing: A Decision-Making Approach.* Philadelphia, Pa: W.B. Saunders; 1989:772.)

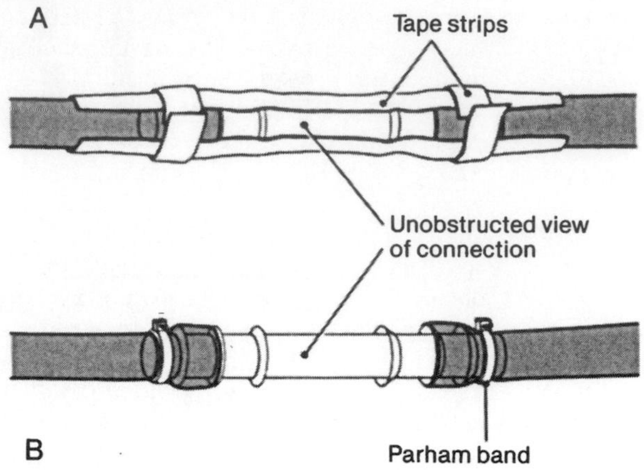

■ ● **FIGURE 18–2.** The securing of connection points. *A,* Tape; *B,* Parham bands. (From Kerston LD. *Comprehensive Respiratory Nursing: A Decision-Making Approach.* Philadelphia, Pa: W.B. Saunders; 1989:783.)

  - ❖ 2 Kelly clamps, curved clamps
  - ❖ Needle holder
  - ❖ 2-0, 3-0 silk suture with cutting needle
  - ❖ Suture scissors
  - ❖ 2 hemostats
  - ❖ 10-mL syringe with 20-G 1.5-in needle
  - ❖ 5-mL syringe with 25-G 1-in needle
  - ❖ Thoracostomy tube (choose size appropriate to condition)
  - ❖ Closed chest drainage system
  - ❖ Suction source
  - ❖ Suction connector and connecting tubing (usually 6 ft for each tube)
  - ❖ Y connector
  - ❖ Adhesive tape (1 in) or Parham bands
  - ❖ Dressing materials (4 × 4 gauze pads, split drain sponges, petroleum gauze, tape)

PATIENT AND FAMILY EDUCATION

- Explain the procedure (if patient condition and time allow) and the reason for the chest tube insertion. ➻***Rationale:*** Identifies patient and family knowledge deficits concerning patient condition, procedure, expected benefits, and potential risks and allows time for questions to clarify information and voice concerns. Explanations decrease patient anxiety and enhance cooperation.
- Explain the patient's participation during the procedure: to remain as immobile as possible and to do relaxed breathing. ➻***Rationale:*** To facilitate insertion of the chest tube and prevent complications during insertion.
- After the procedure, instruct the patient to sit in a semi-Fowler position (unless contraindicated). ➻***Rationale:*** Facilitate drainage from the lung by allowing air to rise and fluid to settle in order to be removed by the chest tube. This position also makes breathing easier.
- Instruct the patient to turn and change position every 2 hours. The patient may lie on the side with the chest tube but should keep the tubing free of kinks. ➻***Rationale:*** Turning and positioning prevent complications related to immobility and retained pulmonary secretions. Keeping

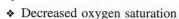

the tube free of kinks maintains patency of the tube, facilitates drainage, and prevents the accumulation of pressure within the pleural space that interferes with lung reexpansion.
- Instruct the patient to cough and deep breathe, splinting the affected side. ➤*Rationale:* Coughing and deep breathing raise pressure within the pleural space, thus facilitating drainage, promoting lung reexpansion, and preventing respiratory complications associated with retained secretions. The application of firm pressure over the chest tube insertion site (ie, splinting) decreases pain and discomfort.
- Encourage active or passive range-of-motion exercises of the arm on the affected side. ➤*Rationale:* The patient may limit movement of the arm on the affected side to decrease discomfort at the insertion site, resulting in joint discomfort and potential joint contractures.
- Instruct the patient and family about activity as prescribed while maintaining the drainage system below the level of the chest. ➤*Rationale:* Facilitates gravity drainage and prevents backflow and potential infectious contamination into the pleural space.
- Instruct the patient about the availability of prescribed analgesic medication and other pain-relief strategies. ➤*Rationale:* Pain relief ensures comfort and facilitates coughing, deep breathing, positioning, range of motion, and recuperation.

PATIENT ASSESSMENT AND PREPARATION

Patient Assessment

- Significant medical history or injury including chronic lung disease, spontaneous pneumothorax, pulmonary disease, therapeutic procedures, and mechanism of injury. ➤*Rationale:* Medical history or injury may provide the etiologic basis for the occurrence of pneumothorax, hemothorax, empyema, pleural effusion, or chylothorax.
- Baseline cardiopulmonary status for signs and symptoms requiring chest tube insertion, as follows:
  ❖ Tachypnea
  ❖ Decreased or absent breath sounds on the affected side
  ❖ Crackles adjacent to the affected area
  ❖ Shortness of breath, dyspnea
  ❖ Asymmetric chest excursion with respirations
  ❖ Cyanosis

  ❖ Decreased oxygen saturation
  ❖ Hyperresonance in the affected side (pneumothorax)
  ❖ Subcutaneous emphysema (pneumothorax)
  ❖ Dullness or flatness in the affected side (hemothorax, pleural effusion, empyema, chylothorax)
  ❖ Sudden sharp chest pain
  ❖ Anxiety, restlessness, apprehension
  ❖ Tachycardia
  ❖ Hypotension
  ❖ Dysrhythmias
  ❖ Tracheal deviation to the unaffected side (tension pneumothorax)
  ❖ Neck vein distention (tension pneumothorax)
  ❖ Muffled heart sounds (tension pneumothorax)

  ➤*Rationale:* Accurate assessment of signs and symptoms allows for prompt recognition and treatment. Baseline assessment provides comparison data for evaluating changes and outcomes of treatment.
- Diagnostic tests (if patient's condition does not necessitate immediate intervention), as follows:
  ❖ Chest x-ray
  ❖ Arterial blood gases

  ➤*Rationale:* Diagnostic testing confirms the presence of air or fluid in the pleural space, a collapsed lung, hypoxemia, and respiratory compromise.

Patient Preparation

- Ensure that patient understands preprocedural teaching. Answer questions as they arise, and reinforce information as needed. ➤*Rationale:* Evaluates and reinforces understanding of previously taught information.
- Ensure that consent of the patient (if able) or of the family has been obtained. ➤*Rationale:* Invasive procedures, unless performed under implied consent in a life-threatening situation, require the written consent of the patient or the family.
- Assist the patient to the lateral, supine (for pneumothorax), or semi-Fowler position (for hemothorax). ➤*Rationale:* Enhances accessibility to the insertion site for positioning of the chest tube.
- Administer prescribed analgesics or sedatives as needed. ➤*Rationale:* Analgesics and sedatives reduce the discomfort and anxiety experienced, facilitating patient cooperation.

Procedure	for Assisting with Chest Tube Placement

Steps	Rationale	Special Considerations
1. Wash hands, and don personal protective equipment.	Reduces the transmission of microorganisms and body secretions; standard precautions.	
2. Open the chest tube tray using sterile technique.	Reduces transmission of microorganisms.	

Procedure continued on following page

Procedure	for Assisting with Chest Tube Placement *Continued*	

Steps	Rationale	Special Considerations
3. Assist the physician or nurse practitioner with preparation of the insertion site.	Inhibits the growth of bacteria at the insertion site.	Determine that the patient has no allergies to the antiseptic solution.
A. Pour antiseptic solution into the basin using aseptic technique.	Used to saturate gauze pads for cleansing.	
B. Wipe the top of the vial of local anesthetic with an alcohol swab.	Disinfects the surface of the vial.	
C. Invert the vial so that the anesthetic can be withdrawn into the syringe.	Maintains sterility.	
4. Assist the patient to the lateral, supine (for pneumothorax), or semi-Fowler position (for hemothorax).	If draining air, the tube is placed near the apex of the lung (second intercostal space); if draining fluid, the tube is placed near the base of the lung (fifth to sixth intercostal space).	
5. Assist the physician or nurse practitioner with insertion (see Procedure 17) of the chest tube.		While the sterile procedure is performed, the nurse monitors and reassures the patient.
6. Remove the adapter from the end of the connecting tubing to the collection chamber of the drainage system, keeping the exposed end sterile. Connect to the chest tube.	Maintains the sterility and creates a closed system.	Length of connecting tube must be sufficient to allow patient movement and to decrease the chance that a patient's deep breath will draw chest drainage back into the pleural space. If two chest tubes are in place, a Y connector may be used to join them to a single drainage system.
7. Place the chest drainage system below the level of the patient's chest.	This position promotes gravity drainage and prevents backflow.	
8. Assist with suturing the chest tube in place. *(Level V: Clinical studies in more than one patient population and situation)*	Prevents displacement of the chest tube; the skin next to the tube is sutured and the ends of the suture are wrapped around the tube, anchoring the tube to che chest wall.[1–3]	
9. Tape all connection points in the chest drainage system (see Figure 18–2). *(Level V: Clinical studies in more than one patient population and situation)*	Airtight connections keep the tubes together and prevent air leaks into the pleural space.[2, 3]	Parham bands may be used to secure connections instead of tape.
A. One inch of tape is placed horizontally, extending over connections (a portion of the connector may be left unobstructed by the tape).	Secures connections but allows visualization of drainage.	
B. Reinforce the horizontal tape with tape placed vertically so that it encircles both ends of the connector.	Secures connections.	

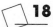

Steps	Rationale	Special Considerations
10. Instruct the patient to take a deep breath and exhale slowly.	Facilitates drainage and reexpansion of the lung.	
11. Apply an occlusive dressing (see Fig. 18–1). *(Level II: Theory based, no research data to support recommendations; recommendations from expert consensus group may exist)*	Provides for an airtight seal around the insertion site.	
A. Apply split drain sponges around the chest tube, one over the top and one from underneath the tube.		Petroleum gauze may be wrapped around the tube close to the insertion site if the air leak is large. However, this may cause maceration of the skin and is not routinely necessary.
B. Apply two to three gauze pads (4 × 4) on top of the split sponges.		
C. Tape the dressing to the skin.	Secures the dressing.	Determine that the patient is not allergic to the tape.
12. Tape the chest tube to the skin.	Prevents side-to-side movement of the chest tube and accidental dislodgment of the chest tube and reinforces the sutures.	
13. If prescribed, turn on suction source to the prescribed level.	Assists in pulling drainage from the pleural cavity.	
14. Obtain a stat portable chest x-ray per order or instructional standard.	Verifies correct placement and position of the chest tube.	
15. Dispose of equipment in appropriate receptacle.	Standard precautions.	
16. Wash hands.	Reduces transmission of microorganisms.	

Expected Outcomes

- Removal of air, fluid, or blood from the pleural space
- Relief of respiratory distress
- Reexpansion of the lung (validated by chest x-ray)
- Restoration of negative pressure within the pleural space

Unexpected Outcomes

- Tension pneumothorax
- Hemorrhagic shock
- Fever, purulent drainage, and redness around the insertion site, or purulent drainage in the chest tube

Patient Monitoring and Care

Patient Monitoring and Care*	Rationale	Reportable Conditions
		These conditions should be reported if they persist despite nursing interventions.
1. Assess cardiopulmonary and vital signs every 2 hours and as needed	Provides baseline and ongoing assessment of patient's condition. Abnormalities can indicate reccurrence of the condition that required chest tube insertion.	• Tachypnea • Decreased or absent breath sounds • Hypoxemia • Tracheal deviation • Subcutaneous emphysema • Neck vein distention • Muffled heart tones • Tachycardia • Hypotension • Dysrhythmias • Fever
2. Maintain and check tube patency every 2 to 4 hours. Maintain drainage tubing free of dependent loops. *(Level III: Laboratory data; no clinical data to support recommendations)*	Obstruction of drainage from the chest tube interferes with lung reexpansion. Drainage accumulating in dependent loops obstructs chest drainage into the collecting system and increases pressure within the lung.[4]	• Inability to establish patency
3. Monitor amount and type of drainage from chest tube.	Volume loss can cause patients to become hypovolemic. Decreased or absent drainage associated with respiratory distress may indicate obstruction. Decreased or absent drainage without respiratory distress may indicate lung reexpansion.	• Bloody drainage >200 mL/hr • Sudden decrease in or absence of drainage • Change in character of drainage
4. Milk the tubing when a visible clot or other obstructing drainage is present in the tubing. *(Level IV: Limited clinical studies to support recommendations)*	If drainage is bloody or thick, small segments of the tubing may need to be milked to keep it patent. This is done by manually squeezing and releasing the chest tubing between the fingers. Stripping the entire length of the chest tube is contraindicated because it results in transient high negative pressures in the pleural space and lung entrapment.[5] No significant differencs are reported between the amount of drainage when the tubing is milked versus when it is stripped.	• Inability to establish patency • Excessive drainage
5. Assess insertion site and surrounding skin for presence of subcutaneous air and signs of infection or inflammation with each dressing change, or every day.	Skin integrity is altered during insertion and can lead to infection.	• Fever • Redness around insertion site • Purulent drainage • Subcutaneous emphysema
6. Assess and treat pain that interferes with the patient's ability to cough, deep breathe, turn and position, and perform range-of-motion exercises.	Pain levels that interfere with the ability to cough, deep breathe, turn and position, and perform range-of-motion exercises place the patient at risk to develop complications related to immobility.	• Pain that is not managed or tolerable • Activity impairments as a result of pain

*Procedure 21 outlines the management of patients with closed chest drainage systems.

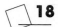

Documentation

Documentation should include the following:

- Patient and family education
- Cardiopulmonary and vital signs assessment before and after procedure
- Date and time procedure performed
- Who performed procedure, size of chest tube, insertion site
- Connection to either a bottle or a disposable chest drainage system, amount of suction, tidaling and fluctuation, type and amount of drainage

- Patient's tolerance of the procedure, medications given, complications, and interventions performed as a result of complications
- Completion and results of the postinsertion chest x-ray and any other ordered diagnostics
- Unexpected outcomes
- Nursing interventions

References

1. Wright SW. Tube thoracostomy. In: Roberts JR, Hedges JR. *Clinical Procedures in Emergency Medicine.* 3rd ed. Philadelphia, PA: W. B. Saunders; 1998:148–172.
2. Iberti TJ, Stern PM. Chest tube thoracostomy. In: Krause JA, ed. *Critical Care Clinics.* Philadelphia, PA: W. B. Saunders; 1998:879–892.
3. Wilson RF. Thoracic trauma. In: Tininalli JE, Ruiz E, Krome RL, ed. *Emergency Medicine: A Comprehensive Guide.* 4th ed. New York, NY: McGraw-Hill; 1996:1156–1182.
4. Gordon PA, Norton JM, Guerra JM, Perdu ST. Positioning of chest tubes: effects on pressure and drainage. *Am J Crit Care.* 1997;6:33–38.
5. Duncan C, Erickson R. Pressures associated with chest tube stripping. *Heart Lung.* 1982;11:166–171.
6. Gordon PA, Norton JM, Merrell R. Refining chest tube management: analysis of the state of practice. *Dimensions Crit Care Nur.* 1995;14:6–13.

Additional Reading

Gross SB. Current challenges, concepts and controversies in chest tube management. *AACN Clin Issues Crit Care Nur.* 1993;4:260–275.

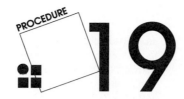

19

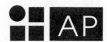

Chest Tube Removal

P U R P O S E: Chest tube removal is performed to discontinue a chest tube when it is no longer needed for the removal or drainage of air, blood, or fluid from the intrapleural or mediastinal space.

Peggy Kirkwood

PREREQUISITE NURSING KNOWLEDGE

- Chest tubes are placed in the pleural or the mediastinal space to evacuate an abnormal collection of air or fluid.
- Indications for removal are based on the reason for insertion and include the following:
    - ❖ Drainage has decreased to 50 to 100 mL in 24 hours if tube was placed for hemothorax, empyema, or pleural effusion.
    - ❖ Drainage has changed from bloody to serosanguineous, no air leak is present, and amount is less than 100 mL in the past 8 hours (if tube was placed after cardiac surgery).
    - ❖ Lungs are reexpanded (as shown on chest x-ray).
    - ❖ Respiratory status has improved (ie, nonlabored respirations, equal bilateral breath sounds, absence of shortness of breath, decreased use of accessory muscles, symmetric respiratory excursion, and respiratory rate less than 24 breaths per minute).
    - ❖ Fluctuations are absent in the water-seal chamber of the collection device, and the level of solution rises in the chamber.
    - ❖ Air leaks have resolved (assessed by the air-leak chamber or the absence of continuous bubbling in the water-seal chamber).
- The water-seal chamber should bubble gently immediately on insertion of the chest tube during expiration, and with coughing. Continuous bubbling in this chamber indicates a leak in the system. Fluctuations in the water level in the water-seal chamber of 5 to 10 cm, rising during inhalation and falling during expiration, should be observed with spontaneous respirations. If the patient is on mechanical ventilation, the pattern of fluctuation will be just the opposite. If suction is being applied, this must be temporarily disconnected to correctly assess for fluctuations in the water-seal chamber.
- Pleural tubes are placed after cardiac surgery if the pleural cavity has been entered. They are typically removed singly and within 24 to 48 hours after surgery.

- Mediastinal chest tubes are most often removed 24 to 36 hours after cardiac surgery.
- Pleural tubes placed for reasons other than post–cardiac-surgery necessity will remain until the patient no longer needs them (ie, no persistent airleak, patient is stable for >24 hours on water seal alone, ongoing fluid leak or bleeding has stopped, or lung is reexpanded on chest x-ray).
- Chest tubes that remain in place for more than 7 days increase the risk of infection along the chest tube tract.
- Chest x-rays are done periodically to determine whether the lung has reexpanded. Reexpanded lungs, along with respiratory assessments that demonstrate improvement in the patient's respiratory status, are the basis for the decision to remove the chest tube.
- The chest tube may be clamped 12 hours before its removal to assess patient tolerance.
- While the tubes are in place, patients may experience related discomfort. Therefore, prompt removal of chest tubes encourages patients to increase ambulation and respiratory measures to improve lung expansion after surgery (eg, coughing, deep breathing). Additionally, removal of the chest tube is a painful procedure for the patient[1-4] (*Level V: Clinical studies in more than one patient population and situation*).
- The types of sutures used to secure chest tubes vary according to the preference of the physician, the physician assistant, or the nurse practitioner. One common type is the horizontal mattress or "purse-string" suture, which is threaded around and through the wound edges in a U shape with the ends left unknotted until the chest tube is removed. Usually there are one or two anchor stitches accompanying the purse-string suture (Fig. 19–1).
- A primary goal of chest tube removal is to remove tubes without introducing air or contaminants into the pleural space.

EQUIPMENT

- Suture removal set
- Petrolatum gauze
- Kelly clamps (two per chest tube) or disposable umbilical clamps
- Wide, occlusive tape (2 in)
- Dry 4 × 4 gauze sponges (two to four)
- Towel or chux pad
- Personal protective equipment (goggles, sterile and nonsterile gloves, mask, gown)

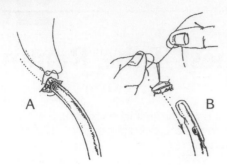

■ ● **FiGURE 19–1.** Purse-string suture. Removing the chest tube. *A,* First throw of a knot in the mattress suture; *B,* Removal of the chest tube and tying of purse-string suture. (From Thomson SC, Wells S, Maxwell M. Chest tube removal after cardiac surgery. *Crit Care Nurse.* 1997;17(1):35.)

Additional equipment (to have available depending on patient need) includes the following:

• Specimen collection cup (if catheter tip is to be sent to the laboratory for analysis)

PATIENT AND FAMILY EDUCATION

• Assess patient and family understanding of the procedure. ➥*Rationale:* Identifies patient and family knowledge deficits concerning patient condition, procedure, expected benefits, and potential risks and allows time for questions to clarify information.
• Explain the procedure and the reason for removal. ➥*Rationale:* Decreases patient anxiety and enhances cooperation.
• Explain the patient's role in assisting with removal. Explain that when prompted, she or he should take a deep breath and hold it. ➥*Rationale:* Elicits patient cooperation and facilitates removal.
• Instruct the patient to turn and reposition every 2 hours after the chest tube has been removed. ➥*Rationale:* Prevents complications related to immobility and retained secretions.
• Instruct the patient to cough and deep breathe after the chest tube has been removed, splinting the affected side or sternum (with mediastinal tubes). ➥*Rationale:* Prevents respiratory complications associated with retained secretions. The application of firm pressure over the insertion site (ie, splinting) decreases pain and discomfort.
• Instruct the patient as to the availability of prescribed

analgesic medication. ➥*Rationale:* Alleviates pain and facilitates coughing, deep breathing, and repositioning.
• Instruct the patient and family to report signs and symptoms of respiratory distress or infection immediately. ➥*Rationale:* Facilitates prompt intervention to relieve a recurrent pneumothorax or to treat an infection.

PATIENT ASSESSMENT AND PREPARATION

Patient Assessment

• Respiratory status

❖ Oxygen saturation within normal limits
❖ Nonlabored respirations
❖ Absence of shortness of breath
❖ Decreased use of accessory muscles
❖ Respiratory rate of less than 24 breaths per minute
❖ Equal bilateral breath sounds

➥*Rationale:* Ensures patient's readiness for removal.

• Chest tube drainage (less than 50 to 100 mL in 24 hours, or less than 100 mL in 8 hours after cardiac surgery)
• Absence of fluctuation in water-seal chamber and air leak indicator ➥*Rationale:* Indicates if lung is reexpanded and air leak is not present.
• Chest x-ray ➥*Rationale:* Lung reexpansion indicates that need for chest tube is resolved.
• Vital signs and (optional) arterial blood gases ➥*Rationale:* Indicates if patient can tolerate chest tube removal.

Patient Preparation

• Ensure that patient understands preprocedural teaching. Answer questions as they arise, and reinforce information as needed. ➥*Rationale:* Evaluates and reinforces understanding of previously taught information.
• Premedicate the patient with adequate analgesics at least 15 minutes before procedure. Intravenous morphine may be used, or, in conjunction with the cardiac surgeon, subfascial lidocaine may be injected into the chest tube track *(Level V: Clinical studies in more than one patient population and situation).* ➥*Rationale:* Pain medication reduces the discomfort and anxiety experienced, facilitating patient cooperation.[1-5]
• Place patient in the semi-Fowler position or on the unaffected side with the bed protector (towel or chux pad) underneath. ➥*Rationale:* Enhances accessibility to the insertion site of the chest tube and protects the bed from drainage removal.

Procedure	for Chest Tube Removal	
Steps	**Rationale**	**Special Considerations**
1. Wash hands, and don personal protective equipment.	Reduces transmission of microorganisms and body secretions; standard precautions.	
2. Open the sterile suture removal set and prepare petrolatum gauze dressing and two to four 4 × 4 gauze sponges.	Aseptic technique is maintained to prevent contamination of the wound. Removal of pleural chest tubes must be accomplished rapidly with the simultaneous application of an occlusive dressing to prevent air from entering the pleural space.	

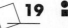

Procedure **for Chest Tube Removal** *Continued*

Steps	Rationale	Special Considerations
3. Discontinue suction from chest drainage system and check for air leakage in water-seal chamber. Observe the water-seal chamber while the patient coughs.	Bubbling in this chamber is associated with an air leak. When an air leak is present, removal of the chest tube can cause development of a pneumothorax.	If an air leak is present, the tube should not be removed. Consult with the physician to determine appropriate action.
4. Remove existing tape and determine type of suture that secures each chest tube. Clip appropriately. If a purse-string suture is present, leave the long suture ends intact.	Allows access to the chest tube at the skin level and prepares the sutures for removal.	
5. Confirm that the tube is free from the suture and the tape.		
6. Clamp each tube to be removed with two Kelly clamps or umbilical clamps.	Prevents air from being introduced into the pleural space.	
7. Instruct patient to take a deep breath and hold it for each tube removed. If the patient is receiving ventilator support, pause the ventilator.	Full inspiration is needed to guarantee positive pressure in the pleural cavity and does not allow an involuntary gasp by the patient when the tube is removed.	
8. Remove chest tubes rapidly and individually, each one while patient is in full inspiration. A. Hold sutures in hand closest to head of patient and apply mild pressure over exit site with folded 4 × 4 gauze pad. B. If tube was "Y" connected to another tube, cut the removed tube below the clamp to allow for easier manipulation when removing the remaining chest tubes.	Prevents accidental entrance of air into the pleural space.	Some resistance is expected; however, if strong resistance is encountered and rapid removal of the tube is not possible, stop the procedure and consult with the physician immediately. This may indicate that the tube was inadvertently sutured during surgery or sternal closure.
9. Tie purse-string suture using a square knot, if available (see Fig. 19–1).	Creates a firm closure of the chest tube site.	Avoid pulling the suture too tight to prevent tissue necrosis at the site and to facilitate easier removal later.
10. Cover pleural insertion sites with petrolatum gauze dressing and mediastinal insertion site with 4 × 4 gauze pads. Secure with tape.	Avoids the influx of air.	Sterile petrolatum gauze should be applied over the skin site immediately after removal if tube was in pleural space or if no purse-string suture was present.
11. Examine each chest tube to verify that all of the tube has been removed.	If portion of tube is not removed, resternotomy is necessary to remove it.	Consult with physician immediately.
12. Assess the patient after the procedure and compare the results with those of previous assessment.	Ensures stable respiratory status after the procedure.	Increased work of breathing, decreased oxygen saturation, increased restlessness, complaints of chest discomfort, and diminished breath sounds on the affected side are warning signs to be observed.
13. Obtain a stat portable chest x-ray per order or protocol.	Assesses that the lung has remained expanded.	

Procedure continued on following page

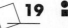 This procedure should be performed only by physicians, advanced practice nurses, and other health care professionals (including critical care nurses) with additional knowledge, skills, and demonstrated competence per professional licensure or institutional standard.

Procedure **for Chest Tube Removal** *Continued*

Steps	Rationale	Special Considerations
14. Dispose of equipment in appropriate receptacle.	Standard precautions.	
15. Wash hands.	Decreases transmission of microorganisms.	

Expected Outcomes

- Patient is comfortable and experiences no respiratory distress.
- Lung remains expanded following chest tube removal.
- Site remains free of infection.

Unexpected Outcomes

- Pneumothorax
- Bleeding
- Skin necrosis
- Retained chest tube
- Infected chest tube insertion site

Patient Monitoring and Care

Patient Monitoring and Care	Rationale	Reportable Conditions
		These conditions should be reported if they persist despite nursing interventions.
1. Ensure adequate respiratory status. Obtain chest x-ray if difficulties arise.	Diminished respiratory status could indicate a pneumothorax. This could be from removal of the chest tube before all the air, fluid, or blood in the pleural space had been drained, or it may recur following removal of the chest tube if air is accidentally introduced into the pleural space through the chest tube tract.	- Decreased oxygen saturation on pulse oximetry - Increased work of breathing - Diminished breath sounds on affected side - Increased restlessness and complaints of chest discomfort
2. Monitor insertion site for bleeding. Apply pressure at site. Place a tight occlusive dressing over site.	Persistent bleeding from insertion site could mean chest tube was against a vein or artery of chest wall before removal.	- Persistent bleeding
3. Monitor purse-string suture site for signs of skin necrosis. If seen, remove the suture and cleanse wound.	If purse-string suture was pulled too tightly closed when chest tube was removed, skin necrosis may be seen.	- Dark or inflamed skin with necrotic areas visible
4. Monitor site for signs of infection. If seen, prepare for wound cultures.	Prolonged insertion of a chest tube increases the risk that the tract created by the chest tube may become infected, or infection may occur following removal of the chest tube if the opening created by the removal beomes contaminated.	- Purulent drainage - Increased body temperature - Inflammation - Tenderness - Warmth at site

Documentation

Documentation should include the following:

- Patient and family education
- Respiratory and vital signs assessments before and after the procedure
- Date, time, and by whom procedure was performed
- Amount, color, and consistency of any drainage
- Application of a sterile, occlusive dressing
- Type of suture in place and what was done to it (cut or tied)
- Patient's tolerance of the procedure
- Completion and results of chest x-ray
- Specimens sent to lab (if applicable)
- Unexpected outcomes
- Nursing interventions

References

1. Carson MM, Barton DM, Morrison CC, Tribble CG. Managing pain during mediastinal chest tube removal. *Heart Lung.* 1994;23(6):500–505.
2. Kinney MR, Kirchhoff KT, Puntillo KA. Chest tube removal practices in critical care units in the United States. *Am J Crit Care.* 1995;4(6):419–424.
3. Gift AG, Bogiano CS, Cunningham J. Sensations during chest tube removal. *Heart Lung.* 1991;20:131–137.
4. Puntillo K. Dimensions of procedural pain and its analgesic management in critically ill surgical patients. *Am J Crit Care.* 1994;3:116–122.
5. Puntillo K. Effects of intrapleural bupivacaine on pleural chest tube removal pain: a randomized controlled sample. *Am J Crit Care.* 1996;5:102–108.

Additional Readings

Davis JW, Mackersie RC, Hoyt DB, Garcia J. Randomized study of algorithms for discontinuing tube thoracostomy drainage. *J Am Coll Surg.* 1994;179(5):553–557.
Otero NA. Chest tube insertion. In: Pfenninger JL, Fowler GC, eds. *Procedures for Primary Care Physicians.* St. Louis, Mo: Mosby–Year Book; 1994:444–451.
Thomson SC, Wells S, Maxwell M. Chest tube removal after cardiac surgery. *Crit Care Nurse.* 1997;17(1):34–38.

AP This procedure should be performed only by physicians, advanced practice nurses, and other health care professionals (including critical care nurses) with additional knowledge, skills, and demonstrated competence per professional licensure or institutional standard.

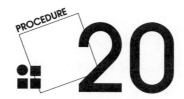

20 Assisting with Chest Tube Removal

PURPOSE: Chest tube removal is performed to discontinue a chest tube when it is no longer needed for removal or drainage of air, blood, or fluid from the intrapleural or mediastinal space.

Catherine Freismuth Robinson

PREREQUISITE NURSING KNOWLEDGE

- Chest tubes are placed in the pleural or the mediastinal space to evacuate an abnormal collection of air or fluid.
- Indications for removal are based on the reason for insertion and include the following:
  - ❖ Drainage has decreased to 50 to 100 mL in 24 hours if tube was placed for a hemothorax, empyema, or pleural effusion.
  - ❖ Drainage has changed from bloody to serosanguineous, no air leak is present, and amount of fluid is less than 100 mL for the past 8 hours (if tube was placed after cardiac surgery).
  - ❖ Lungs are reexpanded (as shown on chest x-ray).
  - ❖ Respiratory status has improved (ie, nonlabored respirations, equal bilateral breath sounds, absence of shortness of breath, decreased use of accessory muscles, symmetric respiratory excursion, and respiratory rate of less than 24 breaths per minute).
  - ❖ Fluctuations are absent in the water-seal chamber of the collection device, and the level of solution rises in the chamber.
  - ❖ Air leaks have resolved (assessed by the air-leak chamber or the absence of continuous bubbling in the water-seal chamber).
- The water-seal chamber should bubble gently immediately on insertion of the chest tube, during expiration, and with coughing. Continuous bubbling in this chamber indicates a leak in the system. Fluctuations in the water level in the water-seal chamber of 5 to 10 cm, rising during inhalation and falling during expiration, should be observed with spontaneous respirations. If the patient is on mechanical ventilation, the pattern of fluctuation will be just the opposite. If suction is being applied, it must be temporarily disconnected to correctly assess for fluctuations in the water-seal chamber.
- Pleural tubes are placed after cardiac surgery if the pleural cavity has been entered. They are typically removed singly and within 24 to 48 hours after surgery.
- Mediastinal chest tubes are most often removed 24 to 36 hours after cardiac surgery.
- Pleural tubes placed for reasons other than post–cardiac-surgery necessity will remain until the patient no longer

needs them (ie, no persistent airleak, patient is stable for >24 hours on water seal alone, ongoing fluid leak or bleeding has stopped, or lung is reexpanded on chest x-ray).
- Chest tubes that remain in place for more than 7 days increase the risk of infection along the chest tube tract.
- Chest x-rays are done periodically to determine whether the lung has reexpanded. Reexpanded lungs, along with respiratory assessments that demonstrate improvement in the patient's respiratory status, are the basis for the decision to remove the chest tube.
- The chest tube may be clamped 12 hours before its removal to assess patient tolerance.
- While the tubes are in place, patients may experience related discomfort. Therefore, prompt removal of chest tubes encourages patients to increase ambulation and respiratory measures to improve lung expansion after surgery (ie, coughing, deep breathing). Additionally, removal of the chest tube is a painful procedure for the patient[1-4] *(Level V: Clinical studies in more than one patient population and situation)*.
- The types of sutures used to secure chest tubes vary according to the preference of the physician, physician assistant, or nurse practitioner. One common type is the horizontal mattress or "purse-string" suture, which is threaded around and through the wound edges in a U shape with the ends left unknotted until the chest tube is removed. Usually one or two anchor stitches accompany the purse-string suture (see Fig. 19–1).
- A primary goal of chest tube removal is to remove tubes without introducing air or contaminants into the pleural space.

EQUIPMENT

- Suture removal set
- Petrolatum gauze
- Kelly clamps (two per chest tube) or disposable umbilical clamps
- Wide, occlusive tape (2 in)
- Dry 4 × 4 gauze sponges (2 to 4)
- Towel or chux pad
- Personal protective equipment (goggles, sterile and nonsterile gloves, mask, gown)

Additional equipment (to have available depending on patient need) includes the following:

- Specimen collection cup (if catheter tip is to be sent to the laboratory for analysis)

PATIENT AND FAMILY EDUCATION

- Assess patient and family understanding of procedure. ➠*Rationale:* Identifies patient and family knowledge deficits concerning patient condition, procedure, expected benefits, and potential risks and allows time for questions to clarify information.
- Explain the procedure and the reason for removal. ➠*Rationale:* Decreases patient anxiety and enhances cooperation.
- Explain the patient's role in assisting with removal. Explain that when prompted, she or he should take a deep breath and hold it. ➠*Rationale:* Elicits patient cooperation and facilitates removal.
- Instruct the patient to turn and reposition every 2 hours after the chest tube has been removed. ➠*Rationale:* Prevents complications related to immobility and retained secretions.
- Instruct the patient to cough and deep breathe after the chest tube has been removed, splinting the affected side or sternum (with mediastinal tubes). ➠*Rationale:* Prevents respiratory complications associated with retained secretions. The application of firm pressure over the insertion site (ie, splinting) decreases pain and discomfort.
- Instruct the patient as to the availability of prescribed analgesic medication. ➠*Rationale:* Alleviates pain and facilitates coughing, deep breathing, and repositioning.
- Instruct the patient and family to report signs and symptoms of respiratory distress or infection immediately. ➠*Rationale:* Facilitates prompt intervention to relieve a recurrent pneumothorax or to treat an infection.

PATIENT ASSESSMENT AND PREPARATION

Patient Assessment

- Respiratory status
  - ❖ Oxygen saturation within normal limits
  - ❖ Nonlabored respirations
  - ❖ Absence of shortness of breath
  - ❖ Decreased use of accessory muscles
  - ❖ Respiratory rate of less than 24 breaths per minute
  - ❖ Equal bilateral breath sounds ➠*Rationale:* Ensures patient's readiness for removal
- Chest tube drainage (less than 50 to 100 mL in 24 hours, or less than 100 mL in 8 hours after cardiac surgery)
- Absence of fluctuation in water-seal chamber and air-leak indicator ➠*Rationale:* Indicates if lung is reexpanded and air leak is not present.
- Chest x-ray ➠*Rationale:* Lung reexpansion indicates that need for chest tube is resolved.
- Vital signs and (optional) arterial blood gases ➠*Rationale:* Indicates if patient can tolerate chest tube removal.

Patient Preparation

- Ensure that patient understands preprocedural teaching. Answer questions as they arise, and reinforce information as needed. ➠*Rationale:* Evaluates and reinforces understanding of previously taught information.
- Premedicate the patient with adequate analgesics at least 15 minutes before procedure. Intravenous morphine is often used (*Level V: Clinical studies in more than one patient population and situation*). ➠*Rationale:* Pain medication reduces the discomfort and anxiety experienced, facilitating patient cooperation.[1-5]
- Place patient in the semi-Fowler position or on the unaffected side with the bed protector (towel or chux pad) underneath. ➠*Rationale:* Enhances accessibility to the insertion site of the chest tube and protects the bed from drainage on removal.

Procedure for Assisting with Chest Tube Removal

Steps	Rationale	Special Considerations
1. Wash hands, and don personal protective equipment.	Reduces transmission of microorganisms; standard precautions.	
2. Open the sterile suture removal set.	Aseptic technique is maintained to prevent contamination of the wound.	
3. Prepare a petroleum gauze dressing and two to four 4 × 4 gauze pads.	Removal of the chest tube must be accomplished rapidly, with the simultaneous application of an occlusive dressing to prevent air from entering the pleural space.	
4. Assist with chest tube removal.	Prevents the introduction of air into the pleural space.	
A. If two chest tubes are connected with a Y connector, clamp the remaining chest tube, placing Kelly clamps in opposite directions while the first tube is being removed.		
B. Loosen the dressing over the insertion site.	Allow access to the chest tube at the skin level.	

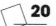

Procedure	**for Assisting with Chest Tube Removal** *Continued*

Steps	Rationale	Special Considerations
C. Cut the sutures that secure the chest tube in place, unless the suture is a purse-string type, which will be pulled into place to close the insertion site once the chest tube is removed.	Allows the chest tube to be removed without resistance.	
D. Instruct the patient to take a deep breath and hold it.	Increases the intrathoracic pressure to prevent air from entering the pleural space.	
5. Cover the entire dressing with 2 to 4 4 × 4 gauze pads, and secure with occlusive tape.	Creates an airtight dressing and absorbs any drainage that may seep from the insertion site.	
6. Obtain a stat portable chest x-ray after chest tube removal per order or institutional standards.	Assesses that the lung has remained expanded.	
7. Dispose of equipment in appropriate receptacle.	Standard precautions.	
8. Wash hands.	Decreases the transmission of microorganisms.	

Expected Outcomes	Unexpected Outcomes
• Patient will be comfortable and will experience no respiratory distress. • Lung will remain expanded following chest tube removal. • Site will remain infection free.	• Pneumothorax • Bleeding • Skin necrosis • Retained chest tube • Infected chest tube insertion site

Patient Monitoring and Care

Patient Monitoring and Care	Rationale	Reportable Conditions
		These conditions should be reported if they persist despite nursing interventions.
1. Ensure adequate respiratory status. Obtain chest x-ray if difficulties arise.	Diminished respiratory status could indicate a pneumothorax. This could be from removal of the chest tube before all the air, fluid, or blood in the pleural space has been drained, or it may recur following removal of the chest tube if air is accidentally introduced into the pleural space through the chest tube tract.	• Decreased oxygen saturation on pulse oximetry • Increased work of breathing • Diminished breath sounds on affected side • Increased restlessness and complaints of chest discomfort
2. Monitor insertion site for bleeding. Apply pressure at site. Place a tight occlusive dressing over site.	Persistent bleeding from insertion site could mean chest tube was against a vein or an artery of chest wall before removal.	• Persistent bleeding
3. Monitor purse-string suture site for signs of skin necrosis. If seen, remove suture and cleanse wound.	If purse-string suture is pulled too tightly closed when chest tube is removed, skin necrosis may be seen.	• Dark or inflamed skin with necrotic areas visible
4. Monitor site for signs of infection. If seen, prepare for wound cultures.	Prolonged insertion of a chest tube increases the risk that the tract created by the chest tube may become infected, or infection may occur following removal of the chest tube if the opening created by the removal becomes contaminated.	• Purulent drainage • Increased body temperature • Inflammation • Tenderness • Warmth at site

▌ Documentation

Documentation should include the following:

- Patient and family education
- Respiratory and vital signs assessments before and after procedure
- Date and time of procedure and who performed it
- Amount, color, and consistency of any drainage
- Application of sterile, occlusive dressing

- Type of suture in place and what was done to it (cut or tied)
- Patient's tolerance of procedure
- Completion and results of chest x-ray
- Specimens sent to laboratory (if applicable)
- Unexpected outcomes
- Nursing interventions

References

1. Carson MM, Barton DM, Morrison CC, Tribble CG. Managing pain during mediastinal chest tube removal. *Heart Lung.* 1994;23(6):500–505
2. Kinney MR, Kirchhoff KT, Puntillo KA. Chest tube removal practices in critical care units in the United States. *Am J Crit Care.* 1995;4(6):419–424.
3. Gift AG, Bogiano CS, Cunningham J. Sensations during chest tube removal. *Heart Lung.* 1991;20:131–137.
4. Puntillo K. Dimensions of procedural pain and its analgesic management in critically ill surgical patients. *Am J Crit Care.* 1994;3:116–122.
5. Puntillo K. Effects of intrapleural bupivacaine on pleural chest tube removal pain: a randomized controlled sample. *Am J Crit Care.* 1996;5:102–108.

Additional Readings

Davis JW, Mackersie RC, Hoyt DB, Garcia J. Randomized study of algorithms for discontinuing tube thoracostomy drainage. *J Am Coll Surgeons.* 1994;179(5):553–557.

Thomson SC, Wells S, Maxwell M. Chest tube removal after cardiac surgery. *Crit Care Nurse.* 1997;17(1):34–38.

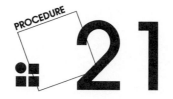

21

Closed Chest Drainage System

PURPOSE: Closed chest drainage systems are used to prevent the entrance of atmospheric air into the pleural space through the use of a water seal. Additionally, chest-drainage systems facilitate the removal of fluid, blood, and air from the pleural space or the mediastinum, restore negative pressure to the pleural space, and promote reexpansion of a collapsed lung.

Catherine Freismuth Robinson

PREREQUISITE NURSING KNOWLEDGE

- Closed chest drainage systems—single-, double-, triple-, and four-bottle setups, as well as disposable units (Fig. 21–1A–C)—use gravity or suction or both to restore negative pressure and remove air, fluid, and blood from the pleural space.
- A one-way mechanism created by a water seal allows air or fluid to exit the pleural space as a result of gravity while preventing it from being drawn back into the cavity.
- Closed chest drainage systems require that the pressure within the chest be greater than within the system. This is accomplished by keeping the drainage unit at least 1 ft below the chest-tube insertion site and the tubing free of dependent loops and obstructions.
- All connections must remain airtight for negative pressure to be reestablished in the pleural space.
- The addition of a suction source can enhance drainage when large volumes of air or fluid must be evacuated.
- Concerns with a bottle system include the risk for error during assembly because of multiple parts and connections, increased risk for contamination because of the multiple parts, the difficulty in transportation because of the weight and awkwardness of the system, and increased risk of breakage.
- Disposable chest-drainage units are an alternative to the traditional glass-bottle chest-drainage systems and correlate to the triple-bottle drainage system with collection, water-seal, and suction control chambers positioned side by side in a molded plastic disposable unit (Fig. 21–2). A positive pressure relief valve prevents a tension pneumothorax if the suction tubing is occluded or the suction source fails. Automatic and manual pressure relief valves vent excessive negative pressure. Some disposable chest-drainage units have replaceable collection chambers which, when filled, can be removed and replaced with a new one without changing the entire unit. Some disposable chest-drainage systems have accessories to convert them to an autotransfusion unit. Additionally, latex-free tubing is used in some disposable drainage units.

- Disposable systems can be converted easily to gravity drainage by disconnecting the suction source and leaving the tubing from the suction chamber on the disposable chest-drainage unit open to air.
- Disposable units have a tip-over design to keep water and drainage from spilling into other chambers.
- Some disposable chest-drainage systems are waterless, eliminating the need to fill any chambers. A valve opens on expiration allowing patient air to exit, then closes to prevent atmospheric air from entering during inspiration. This one-way valve feature allows the system to be used in the vertical or horizontal position without loss of the seal; thus, they are safe if accidentally tipped. The amount of suction delivered to the suction chamber is regulated by an adjustable dial or knob. Because the systems are waterless, they are quiet, are unaffected by evaporation, and carry no danger that water can accidentally be siphoned back into the pleural space. The presence of air leak can be assessed via an air-leak detection chamber.
- Disposable systems have self-sealing ports or collection tubes for aspiration of drainage samples.

EQUIPMENT
Disposable Setup

- Disposable chest-drainage unit
- Gloves
- Suction source
- Connecting tubing
- Tape (1 in), one roll, or Parham bands
- 1-L bottle of sterile water or normal saline (NS) (for systems that use water)
- 50-mL irrigation syringe (if not supplied with unit) for systems that use water

Bottle Setup
All Bottle Systems

- Gloves
- Sterile water or NS

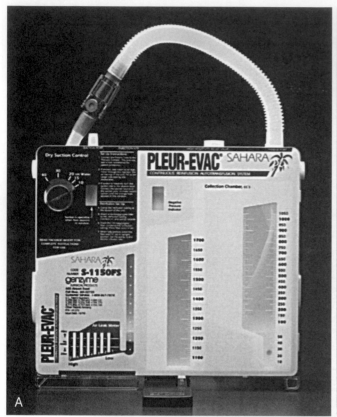
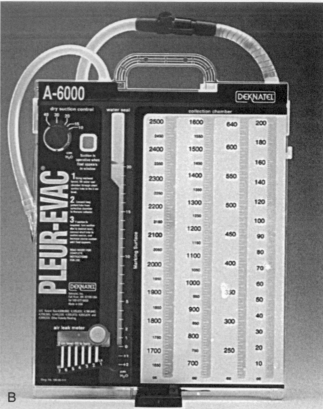
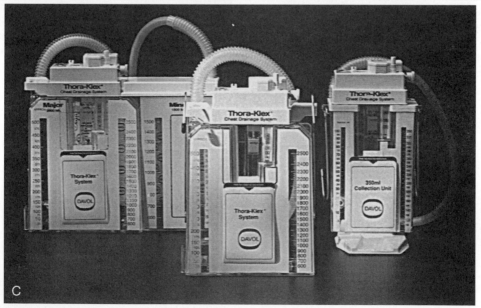

■ ● **FIGURE 21–1.** Disposable chest-drainage systems. (Courtesy of Genzyme Surgical Products, Fall River, MA.)

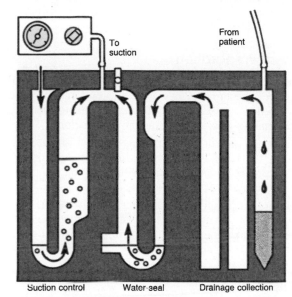

■ ● FIGURE 21–2. Disposable system correlates with triple-bottle system. (From Luce JM, Tyler ML, Pierson DJ. *Intensive Respiratory Care.* Philadelphia: WB Saunders; 1984:164.)

- Rack or holder for the bottles
- Tape (1 in), one roll
- Parham bands

Single-Bottle System

- Sterile 2-L bottle
- One short straw
- One long straw
- Sterile rubber stopper with two holes

Double-Bottle System

- Two sterile 2-L bottles
- Three short straws
- One long straw
- Two sterile rubber stoppers, one with two holes and the other with either two or three holes (depending on which type of double-bottle system is used)
- Sterile connecting tubing (6 ft)
- One short sterile connecting tubing
- Suction source, if prescribed

Triple-Bottle System

- Three sterile 2-L bottles
- Five short straws
- Two long straws
- Two sterile rubber stoppers with two holes
- One sterile rubber stopper with three holes
- Suction source
- Sterile connecting tubing (6 ft)
- Two short sterile connecting tubings
- Suction source

Four-Bottle System

- Four sterile 2-L bottles
- Seven short straws
- Three long straws
- Two sterile rubber stoppers with two holes
- Two sterile rubber stoppers with three holes
- Sterile connecting tubing (6 ft)
- Three short sterile connecting tubings
- Suction source

PATIENT AND FAMILY EDUCATION

- Explain the procedure and how the closed chest drainage system works. ➤*Rationale:* Identifies patient and family knowledge deficits about the patient's condition, procedure, expected benefits, and potential risks and allows time for questions to clarify information and to voice concerns. Explanations decrease patient anxiety and enhance cooperation.

- After the procedure, instruct the patient to sit in a semi-Fowler position (unless contraindicated). ➤*Rationale:* This position facilitates drainage from the lung, by allowing air to rise and fluid to settle, enhancing removal via the chest tube. This position also makes breathing easier.

- Instruct the patient to turn and reposition every 2 hours. The patient may lie on the side with the chest tube but should keep the tubing free of kinks. ➤*Rationale:* Turning and positioning prevents complications related to immobility and retained secretions. Keeping the tubing free of kinks maintains patency of the tube, facilitates drainage, and prevents the accumulation of pressure within the pleural space, which interferes with lung reexpansion.

- Instruct the patient to cough and deep breathe, splinting the affected side or sternum (if mediastinal tube is in place). ➤*Rationale:* Coughing and deep breathing raise pressure within the pleural pressure, thus facilitating drainage, promoting lung reexpansion, and preventing respiratory complications associated with retained secretions. Applying firm pressure over the chest tube insertion site (ie, splinting) decreases pain and discomfort.

- Encourage active or passive range-of-motion exercises of the arm on the affected side. ➤*Rationale:* The patient may limit the movement of the arm on the affected side to decrease the discomfort at the insertion site, resulting in joint discomfort and potential joint complications.

- Instruct the patient and family about activity as prescribed while maintaining the drainage system below the level of the chest.   ➤*Rationale:* To facilitate gravity drainage and to prevent backflow and potential infectious contamination into the pleural space.

- Instruct about the availability of prescribed analgesic medication and other pain relief strategies.   ➤*Rationale:* Pain relief ensures comfort and facilitates coughing, deep breathing, positioning, range-of-motion exercises, and recuperation.

PATIENT ASSESSMENT AND PREPARATION

Patient Assessment

- Significant medical history or injury, including chronic lung disease, spontaneous pneumothorax, pulmonary disease, therapeutic procedures, or mechanism of injury.   ➤*Rationale:* Medical history or injury may provide the etiologic basis for the occurrence of pneumothorax, hemothorax, empyema, pleural effusion, or chylothorax.

- Baseline cardiopulmonary status, as follows:
  - ❖ Tachypnea
  - ❖ Decreased or absent breath sounds on the affected side
  - ❖ Crackles adjacent to the affected area
  - ❖ Shortness of breath or dyspnea
  - ❖ Asymmetric chest excursion with respirations
  - ❖ Cyanosis
  - ❖ Decreased oxygen saturation
  - ❖ Hyperresonance in the affected side (pneumothorax)
  - ❖ Subcutaneous emphysema (pneumothorax)
  - ❖ Dullness or flatness in the affected side (hemothorax, pleural effusion, empyema, or chylothorax)
  - ❖ Sudden sharp chest pain
  - ❖ Anxiety, restlessness, or apprehension

- ❖ Tachycardia
- ❖ Hypotension
- ❖ Dysrhythmias
- ❖ Tracheal deviation to the unaffected side (tension pneumothorax)
- ❖ Neck vein distention (tension pneumothorax)
- ❖ Muffled heart sounds (tension pneumothorax)

➤*Rationale:* Accurate assessment of signs and symptoms allows for prompt recognition and treatment. Baseline assessment provides comparison data for evaluating changes and outcomes of treatment.

- Diagnostic tests (if patient's condition does not necessitate immediate intervention):
  - ❖ Chest x-ray
  - ❖ Arterial blood gases

➤*Rationale:* Diagnostic testing confirms the presence of air or fluid in the pleural space, a collapsed lung, hypoxemia, and respiratory compromise.

Patient Preparation

- Ensure that patient understands preprocedural teaching. Answer questions as they arise and reinforce information as needed.   ➤*Rationale:* Evaluates and reinforces understanding of previously taught information.

- Assist the patient to the lateral, supine (for pneumothorax), or semi-Fowler position (for hemothorax).   ➤*Rationale:* To enhance accessibility to the insertion site for positioning of the chest tube.

- Administer prescribed analgesics or sedatives as needed.   ➤*Rationale:* Analgesics and sedatives reduce the discomfort and anxiety experienced, facilitating patient cooperation.

Procedure **for Using Closed Chest Drainage Systems**		
Steps	**Rationale**	**Special Considerations**
These Steps Should Be Followed for Both Bottle and Disposable Units		
1. Wash hands, and don personal protective equipment.	Reduces transmission of microorganisms and body secretions; standard precautions.	
2. Open sterile packages.	Maintain aseptic technique whenever making changes to the system.	

Disposable Drainage System

Proceed to step 3.

Single-Bottle System

Proceed to step 10.

Double-Bottle System

Proceed to step 16.

Triple-Bottle System

Proceed to step 39.

Four-Bottle System

Proceed to step 55.

Procedure **for Using Closed Chest Drainage Systems** *Continued*

Steps	Rationale	Special Considerations

Disposable Chest-Drainage System (see Figs. 21–1 and 21–2)

Steps	Rationale	Special Considerations
3. Remove the connector cap from the short tubing of the water-seal chamber and use the funnel provided or a 50-mL syringe to add sterile water or NS to the 2-cm level, unless the system is waterless.	Depth of solution needed to establish the water seal.	Water-seal levels of more than 2 cm increase the work of breathing; less than 2 cm can expose the water seal to air and increase the risk for pneumothorax. Some systems color the solution for easy visibility of air-leak detection. Refill with water as necessary to the 2-cm level to replace water lost through evaporation.
4. For gravity drainage, leave the short tubing from the suction control chamber open to air.	Creates the exit vent for the escape of air.	Clamping or occlusion of the exit vent may cause collapse of the lung.
5. For suction drainage, fill the suction control chamber to the prescribed level (usually −20 cm H$_2$O suction level), unless the system is waterless. Connect the short tubing from the suction control chamber to the suction source.	Suction is regulated by the height of the solution level in this chamber.	Refill the solution level as necessary to the prescribed amount to replace solution lost through evaporation.
6. Hang drainage unit from bed frame or set it on a floor stand.	Drainage unit must be kept below the level of the chest to prevent backflow of drainage into the pleural space, which interferes with lung expansion.	
7. Connect the long tubing from the drainage-collection chamber to the chest tube.	Creates the drainage-collection system. Avoid dependent or fluid-filled loops.	
8. Turn on the suction source if prescribed, to elicit gentle, constant bubbling.	Activates suction.	Some systems have a suction control feature to automatically maintain the desired suction level despite fluctuations in the suction source.
9. Proceed to step 76.		

Single-Bottle Setup (Fig. 21–3)

Steps	Rationale	Special Considerations
10. Fill the water-seal bottle with sterile water or NS so that the bottom of the long straw is immersed approximately 2 cm.	Depth of solution required to establish a water seal and protect the patient from air leak or loss of water seal.	Water-seal levels more than 2 cm increase the work of breathing; less than 2 cm expose the water seal to air and increase the risk for pneumothorax.
11. Seal the bottle with the rubber stopper.	An airtight system is required to reestablish negative pressure in the pleural space.	
12. Insert the short straw through one of the openings in the stopper and leave open to air.	Creates the water seal and protects the patient against air leaks.	Clamping or occlusion of the exit vent may cause collapse of the lung.
13. Insert the long straw through the second opening, immersing it 2 cm (1 in) beneath the surface of the solution.	Creates the water seal and protects the patient against air leaks.	Immersing the straw deeper than 2 cm increases the work of breathing.
14. Stabilize the drainage bottle on the floor or in a special holder.	The bottle must be kept below the level of the chest to prevent backflow of drainage into the pleural space, which interferes with lung expansion.	Disruption of the system endangers the patient by allowing the entrance of atmospheric air into the pleural space, which may collapse the lung.
15. Connect the drainage tubing from the chest tube to the long straw of the water-seal bottle. Proceed to step 76.	This creates the water-seal drainage-collection bottle.	

Procedure continued on following page

Procedure for Using Closed Chest Drainage Systems *Continued*

Steps	Rationale	Special Considerations

Double-Bottle Setup with a Drainage-Collection Bottle and a Water-Seal Bottle (Fig. 21–4)

Steps	Rationale	Special Considerations
16. Seal one bottle with a rubber stopper with two openings.	An airtight system is required to reestablish negative pressure in the pleural space.	
17. Insert two short straws into the rubber stopper.	Creates the drainage-collection bottle.	
18. Fill the water-seal bottle with sterile water or NS so that the bottom of the long straw is immersed approximately 2 cm.	Depth of solution required to establish a water seal and protect the patient from air leak or loss of water seal.	Water-seal levels of more than 2 cm increase the work of breathing; less than 2 cm expose the water seal to air and increase the risk for pneumothorax.
19. Seal the bottle with a rubber stopper with two openings.	An airtight system is required to reestablish negative pressure in the pleural space..	
20. Insert the short straw through one of the openings in the stopper.	Creates the exit vent for the escape of air or for connection to the suction source.	
21. Insert the long straw through the second opening, immersing it 2 cm beneath the surface of the solution.	Creates the water seal and protects the patient from air leaks or loss of water seal.	Immersing the straw deeper than 2 cm increases the work of breathing.
22. Use the sterile tubing to connect one of the short straws of the drainage-collection bottle to the long straw of the water-seal bottle.	Connects the drainage collection bottle to the water-seal bottle.	
23. Stabilize the bottles on the floor or in a special holder.	The bottles must be kept below the level of the chest, to prevent backflow of drainage into the pleural space, which interferes with lung expansion.	Disruption of the system endangers the patient by allowing the entrance of atmospheric air into the pleural space, which may collapse the lung.
24. Connect the drainage tubing from the chest tube to the second short straw of the drainage-collection bottle.	Creates a drainage avenue.	

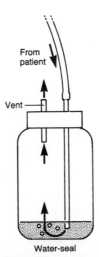

■ ● FIGURE 21–3. Single-bottle chest-drainage system. (From Luce JM, Tyler ML, Pierson DJ. *Intensive Respiratory Care.* Philadelphia: WB Saunders; 1984:164.)

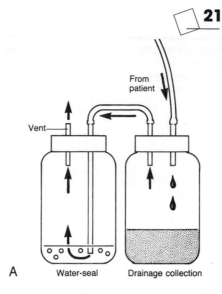

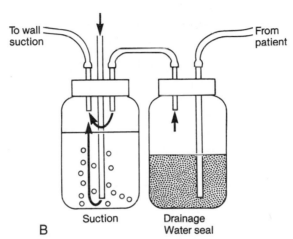

■ ● FIGURE 21–4. Double-bottle chest-drainage system. (From Luce JM, Tyler ML, Pierson DJ. *Intensive Respiratory Care.* Philadelphia: WB Saunders; 1984:164. Kerston LD. *Comprehensive Respiratory Nursing.* Philadelphia: WB Saunders, 1989.)

| Procedure | **for Using Closed Chest Drainage Systems** *Continued* |

Steps	**Rationale**	**Special Considerations**
25. Leave the exit vent of the water-seal bottle open to air, OR Connect the suction source to the exit vent and adjust to the prescribed level (usually -20 cm H_2O suction level). Proceed to step 76.	Increases pressure differences between the pleural space and drainage bottles, which facilitate drainage from the pleural space.	Surges in suction and accidental displacement of the control knobs are possible with this setup.

Double-Bottle Setup with a Water-Seal/Drainage-Collection Bottle and a Suction-Control Bottle (see Fig. 21–4)

26. Fill the water-seal/drainage-collection bottle with sterile water or NS so that the bottom of the long straw is immmersed approximately 2 cm.	Depth of solution required to establish a water seal and protect the patient from air leak or loss of water seal.	
27. Seal the bottle with a rubber stopper with two openings.	An airtight system is required to reestablish negative pressure in the pleural space.	

Procedure continued on following page

Procedure for Using Closed Chest Drainage Systems *Continued*

Steps	Rationale	Special Considerations
28. Insert the short straw through one of the openings in the stopper.	Initial step for connecting the drainage bottle to the water-seal bottle.	
29. Insert the long straw through the second opening, immersing it 2 cm beneath the surface of the solution.	Creates the water seal and protects the patient from air leaks or loss of water seal.	Immersing the straw deeper than 2 cm increases the work of breathing.
30. Add prescribed amount of sterile water or NS to the suction bottle (usually -20 cm H_2O suction level).	Creates at least -20 cm H_2O of suction.	The depth the straw is immersed in the solution determines the amount of suction delivered to the chest tube.
31. Seal the suction bottle with the rubber stopper with three openings.	An airtight system is required to reestablish negative pressure in the pleural space.	
32. Insert the long straw through the middle opening (leaving one end immersed in the solution and the other end open to the atmosphere).	Creates an air vent.	
33. Insert the two short straws into the remaining opening so the stopper.	Creates the setup for attachment to suction and to the overflow-drainage bottle.	
34. Use the sterile tubing to connect the short straw from the water-seal/drainage-collection bottle to one of the short straws of the suction bottle.	Connects the water-seal bottle to the suction source.	
35. Attach one end of the 6-ft connecting tubing to the second short straw of the suction bottle and the other end to the suction source.	Connects the suction bottle to the suction source.	
36. Stabilize the drainage bottles on the floor or in a special holder.	The bottles must be kept below the level of the chest to prevent backflow of drainage into the pleural space, which interferes with lung expansion.	Disruption of the system endangers the patient by allowing the entrance of atmospheric air into the pleural space, which may collapse the lung.
37. Connect the drainage tube from the chest tube to the long straw of the water-seal/drainage-collection bottle.	Creates the water-seal/drainage collection bottle.	
38. Turn on the suction source to elicit gentle, constant bubbling in the suction. Proceed to step 76.	Activates suction.	

Triple-Bottle Setup (Fig. 21–5)

Steps	Rationale	Special Considerations
39. Seal one of the bottles with the rubber stopper with two openings.	An airtight system is required to reestablish negative pressure in the pleural space.	
40. Insert two short straws into the rubber stopper.	This creates the drainage-collection bottle.	This bottle can be calibrated if it is not already by placing a piece of tape on the side so that drainage can be measured and recorded.
41. Fill the water-seal bottle with sterile water or NS so that the bottom of the long straw is immersed approximately 2 cm.	Depth of solution required to establish a water seal and protect the patient from air leak or loss of water seal.	Water-seal levels more than 2 cm increase the work of breathing; less than 2 cm expose the water seal to air and increase the risk for pneumothorax.
42. Seal the bottle with a rubber stopper with two openings.	An airtight system is required to reestablish negative pressure in the pleural space.	

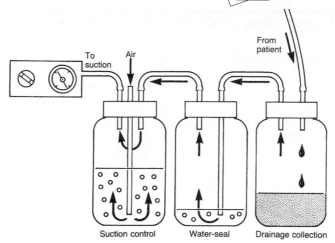

■ ● FIGURE 21–5. Triple-bottle chest-drainage system. (From Luce JM, Tyler ML, Pierson DJ. *Intensive Respiratory Care*. Philadelphia: WB Saunders; 1984:164.)

| Procedure | for Using Closed Chest Drainage Systems *Continued* |

Steps	Rationale	Special Considerations
43. Insert the short straw through one of the openings in the stopper.	Creates the exit vent for the escape of air or for connection to the suction source.	
44. Insert the long straw through the second opening, immersing it 2 cm beneath the surface of the solution.	Creates the water seal and protects the patient from air leaks or loss of water seal.	Immersing the straw deeper than 2 cm increases the work of breathing.
45. Add prescribed amount of sterile water or NS to the suction bottle (usually -20 cm H_2O suction level).	Creates a water seal.	The depth the straw is immersed in the solution determines the amount of suction delivered to the chest tube.
46. Seal the suction bottle with the rubber stopper with three openings.	An airtight system is required to reestablish negative pressure in the pleural space.	
47. Insert the long straw through the middle opening (leaving one end immersed in the solution and the other end open to the atmosphere).	Creates the suction bottle.	
48. Insert the two short straws into the remaining openings of the stopper.	Creates the setup for attachment to suction and to the overflow-drainage bottle.	
49. Use the sterile tubing to connect the short straw of the drainage-collection bottle to the long straw of the water-seal bottle.	Connects the water-seal bottle to the suction bottle.	
50. Use the sterile tubing to connect the short straw from the water-seal bottle to one of the short straws of the suction bottle.	Connects the water-seal bottle to the suction bottle.	
51. Attach one end of the 6-ft connecting tubing to the second short straw of the suction bottle and the other end to the suction source.	Connects the suction bottle to the suction source.	
52. Stabilize the drainage bottles on the floor or in a special holder.	The bottles must be kept below the level of the chest to prevent backflow of drainage into the pleural space, which interferes with lung expansion.	Disruption of the system endangers the patient by allowing the entrance of atmospheric air into the pleural space, which may collapse the lung.

Procedure continued on following page

Procedure for **Using Closed Chest Drainage Systems** *Continued*

Steps	Rationale	Special Considerations
53. Connect the drainage tube from the chest tube to the short straw of the drainage-collection bottle.	Provides a route for drainage to flow from the patient to the collection bottle.	
54. Turn the suction source on to elicit gentle, constant bubbling in the suction. Proceed to step 76.	Activates suction.	

Four-Bottle Setup (Triple-Bottle Setup with Vented Water-Seal Bottle) (Fig. 21–6)

55. Fill the vented water-seal bottle with sterile water or NS so that the bottom of the long straw will be immersed approximately 2 cm.	Depth of solution required to establish a water seal and protect the patient from air leak or loss of water seal.	
56. Seal the bottle with a rubber stopper with two openings.	An airtight system is required to reestablish negative pressure in the pleural space.	
57. Insert the long straw through one of the openings, immersing it 2 cm beneath the surface of the solution.	Creates the water seal and protects the patient from air leaks or loss of water seal.	Immersing the straw deeper than 2 cm increases the work of breathing.
58. Insert a short straw through the second opening in the stopper and leave open to air.	Creates the vented water seal that acts as a safety feature to allow the escape of positive pressure in case of problems with the suction source.	
59. Seal the drainage-collection bottle with a rubber stopper with three openings.	An airtight system is required to reestablish negative pressure in the pleural space.	
60. Insert three short straws into the rubbler stopper.	This creates the drainage-collection bottle.	This bottle can be calibrated if it is not already by placing a piece of tape on the side so that drainage can be measured and recorded.
61. Fill the water-seal bottle with sterile water or NS so that the bottom of the long straw is immersed approximately 2 cm.	Depth of solution required to establish a water seal and protect the patient from air leak or loss of water seal.	

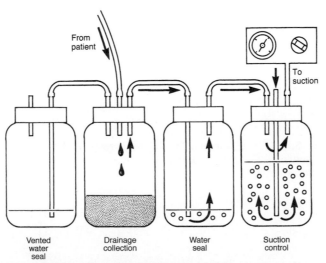

■ ● FIGURE 21–6. Four-bottle chest-drainage system. (From Luce JM, Tyler ML, Pierson DJ. *Intensive Respiratory Care.* Philadelphia: WB Saunders; 1984:164.)

Procedure for Using Closed Chest Drainage Systems *Continued*

Steps	Rationale	Special Considerations
62. Seal the bottle with a rubber stopper with two openings.	An airtight system is required to reestablish negative pressure in the pleural space.	
63. Insert the short straw through one of the openings in the stopper.	Creates the exit vent for the escape of air for connection to the suction source.	
64. Insert the long straw through the second opening, immersing it 2 cm beneath the surface of the solution.	Creates the water seal and protects the patient from air leaks or loss of water seal.	Immersing the straw deeper than 2 cm increases the work of breathing.
65. Add prescribed amount of sterile water or NS to the suction bottle (usually −20 cm H_2O suction level).	Creates a water seal.	The depth the straw is immersed in the solution determines the amount of suction delivered to the chest tube.
66. Seal the suction bottle with the rubber stopper with three openings.	An airtight system is required to reestablish negative pressure in the pleural space.	
67. Insert the long straw through the middle opening (leaving one end immersed in the solution and the other end open to the atmosphere).	Creates the manometer tube or air vent.	
68. Insert the two short straws into the remaining openings.	Creates the setup for attachment to suction and to the overflow-drainage bottle.	
69. Use the sterile tubing to connect the long straw of the vented water-seal bottle to one of the short straws of the drainage-collection bottle.	Provides for communication between the drainage system bottle and the vented water-seal bottle.	
70. Use the sterile tubing to connect the second straw of the drainage-collection bottle to the long straw of the water-seal bottle.	Connects the drainage collection bottle to the water-seal bottle.	
71. Use the sterile tubing to connect the short straw from the water-seal bottle to one of the short straws of the suction bottle.	Connects the water-seal bottle to the suction bottle.	
72. Attach one end of the 6-ft connecting tubing to the second short straw of the suction bottle and the other end to the suction source.	Connects the suction bottle to the suction source.	
73. Stabilize the drainage bottles on the floor or in a special holder.	The bottles must be kept below the level of the chest to prevent backflow of drainage into the pleural space, which interferes with lung expansion.	Disruption of the system endangers the patient by allowing the entrance of atmospheric air into the pleural space, which may collapse the lung.
74. Connect the drainage tube from the chest tube to the middle short straw of the drainage-collection bottle.	Provides a route for drainage to flow from the patient to the collection bottle.	
75. Turn the suction source on to elicit gentle, constant bubbling in the suction bottle.	Activates suction.	

Procedure continued on following page

Procedure for Using Closed Chest Drainage Systems *Continued*

Steps	Rationale	Special Considerations
76. Tape all connection points in the chest-drainage system (see Fig. 18–2). A. One-inch tape is placed horizontally extending over the connections (a portion of the connector may be left unobstructed by the tape). B. Reinforce the horizontal tape with tape placed vertically so it encircles both ends of the connector.	Maintains connections and prevents air leaks into the pleural space. This technique secures the connections but allows visualization of drainage in the connector.	Parham bands may be used to secure connections instead of tape.
77. Dispose of equipment in appropriate receptacle.	Standard precautions.	
78. Wash hands.	Reduces transmission of microorganisms.	

Expected Outcomes

- Removal of air, fluid, or blood
- Fluctuation or tidaling noted in the water-seal chamber
- Relief of respiratory distress
- Reexpansion of the collapsed lung validated by chest x-ray

Unexpected Outcomes

- Tension pneumothorax
- Hemorrhagic shock
- Absence of drainage and fluctuation or tidaling, or continuous bubbling in the water-seal chamber with continued respiratory distress
- Lung not showing evidence of reexpansion
- Fever, purulent drainage, and redness around the insertion site or purulent drainage in the chest tube

Patient Monitoring and Care

Patient Monitoring and Care	Rationale	Reportable Conditions
		These conditions should be reported if they persist despite nursing interventions.
1. Assess cardiopulmonary and vital signs every 2 hours and as needed.	Provides baseline and ongoing assessment of patient's condition.	• Tachypnea • Decreased or absent breath sounds • Hypoxemia • Tracheal deviation • Subcutaneous emphysema • Neck vein distention • Muffled heart tones • Tachycardia • Hypotension • Dysrhythmias • Fever
2. Maintain and check tube patency every 2 to 4 hours.	Obstruction of drainage from the chest tube interferes with lung reexpansion.	• Inability to establish patency
3. Monitor amount and type of drainage from chest tube.	Volume loss can cause patients to become hypovolemic. Decreased or absent drainage associated with respiratory distress may indicate obstruction; decreased or absent drainage without respiratory distress may indicate lung reexpansion.	• Bloody drainage >200 mL/h • New onset of clots • Sudden decrease or absence of drainage
4. Mark the drainage level on the outside of the drainage-collection chamber in hourly or shift increments and document.	Provides reference point for future measurements. Drainage should gradually decrease and change from bloody to pink to straw colored. Sudden flow of dark bloody drainage that occurs with position change is often old blood that finds its way into the chest tube.	• Drainage >200 mL/h • Sudden decrease or absence of drainage • Change in characteristics of drainage

Patient Monitoring and Care	Rationale	Reportable Conditions
5. Keep the drainage tubing free of dependent loops (ie, placing the tube horizontally on the bed and down into the collection chamber, coiling the tubing on the bed). *(Level III: Laboratory data, no clinical data to support recommendations)*	Drainage accumulating in dependent loops obstructs chest drainage into the collecting system and increases pressure within the lung[1, 3-4] Allow enough length for patient movement.	
6. Milk the tubing when a visible clot or other obstructing drainage is present in the tubing. *(Level IV: Limited clinical studies to support recommendations)*	If drainage is bloody or thick, small segments of the tubing may need to be milked to keep it patent. Milking is done by manually squeezing and releasing the chest tubing between the fingers. Stripping the entire length of the chest tube is contraindicated because it results in transient high negative pressures in the pleural space and lung entrapment.[2] No significant differences are reported between the amount of drainage when the tubing is milked as opposed to stripped.[3]	• Inability to establish patency • Excessive drainage
7. Refill the solution level as necessary to the prescribed amount to replace solution lost through evaporation.	To maintain prescribed water-seal and suction levels and prevent complications.	
8. Assess for fluctuations or tidaling in fluid level in the long straw of the water-seal bottle or the water-seal chamber with respiration.	Indicates effective communication between the pleural space and drainage system and provides an indication of lung expansion. Fluctuations or tidaling will stop when the lung is reexpanded or when the tubing is obstructed by a kink, a fluid-filled loop, the patient lying on the tubing, or a clot or tissue at the distal end. (If a suction source has been added, it must be temporarily disconnected to accurately assess for fluctuations or tidaling.)	• Absence of fluctuations or tidaling
9. Assess for air leaks in the system, as indicated by constant bubbling in the water-seal bottle or chamber. (Some disposable chest drainage systems have an air-leak assessment chamber.) ○ To assess location of a leak, intermittently occlude the chest tube or drainage tubing, beginning at the insertion site and progressing to the chest drainage unit.	An airtight system is required to reestablish negative pressure in the pleural space. Chest-tube drainage from a mediastinal tube should not cause bubbling in the water-seal chamber. Intermittent bubbling when suction is initially turned on occurs when air is displaced by fluid drainage in the collection chamber, or if the patient has a small leak in the pleural space, or if the patient exhales or coughs. If the bubbling in the water-seal chamber stops when the chest tube is occluded at the dressing site, the air leak is inside the patient's chest or under the dressing; reinforce the dressing. If the bubbling stops when the drainage tubing is occluded along its length, the air leak is between the occlusion and the patient's chest; check to make sure all connections are airtight. If the bubbling does not stop with occlusion, replace the chest-drainage unit.	• Air leak inside the patient's chest or under the dressing
10. Obtaining a drainage specimen with disposable chest drainage systems, use a syringe with an 18-G or 20-G needle to withdraw the specimen from the diaphragm on the back of the unit.	Obtains a specimen for analysis.	

Continued on following page

Patient Monitoring and Care

Patient Monitoring and Care	Rationale	Reportable Conditions
11. Monitor patient's pain and intervene appropriately.	Pain relief ensures comfort and facilitates coughing, deep breathing, positioning, range-of-motion exercises, and recuperation.	
12. Assess insertion site and surrounding skin for presence of subcutaneous air and signs of infection or inflammation with each dressing change or every day. Dressings should be changed when soiled, every two to three days, or when ordered by physician or nurse practitioner.	Skin integrity is altered during insertion and can lead to infection.	• Fever • Redness around insertion site • Purulent drainage • Subcutaneous emphysema

Documentation

Documentation should include the following:
- Patient and family education
- Cardiopulmonary and vital sign assessment
- Type of drainage system used
- Amount of suction, fluctuation or tidaling, the type and amount of drainage
- Patient's tolerance of the therapy
- Respiratory, thoracic, and vital sign assessment with changes in therapy
- Completion and results of the postinsertion chest x-ray and any other ordered diagnostic tests
- Unexpected outcomes
- Nursing interventions

References

1. Gordon PA, Norton JM, Guerra JM, et al: Positioning of chest tubes: effects on pressure and drainage. *Am J Crit Care.* 1997; 6:33–38.
2. Duncan C, Erickson R. Pressures associated with chest tube stripping. *Heart Lung.* 1982; 11:166–171.
3. Gordon PA, Norton JM, Merrell R. Redefining chest tube management: analysis of the state of practice. *Dimens Crit Care Nurs.* 1995; 14:6–13.
4. Gross SB. Current challenges, concepts and controversies in chest tube management. *AACN Clin Issues Crit Care Nurs.* 1993; 4:260–275.

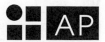
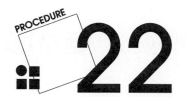

Performing Needle Thoracostomy

P U R P O S E: Needle thoracostomy is used to reduce a tension pneumothorax to a simple pneumothorax in a rapidly deteriorating patient. This is a temporary measure and is quickly followed by the insertion of a chest tube for more definitive management.

Cindy Goodrich

PREREQUISITE NURSING KNOWLEDGE

- Anatomy and physiology of the pulmonary system should be understood.
- The thoracic cavity, under normal conditions, is a closed air space. Any disruption results in the loss of negative pressure within the intrapleural space; air or fluid entering the space competes with the lung, resulting in collapse of the lung. Associated conditions are the result of disease, injury, surgery, or iatrogenic causes.
- A pneumothorax is classified as open, closed, or tension pneumothorax. In patients with tension pneumothorax, air leaks into the pleural space through a tear in the lung and, having no means to escape from the pleural cavity, creates a one-way valve effect. With each breath the patient takes, air accumulates, pressure within the pleural space increases, and the lung collapses. This causes the mediastinal structures (ie, the heart, great vessels, and the trachea) to shift to the opposite or unaffected side of the chest. Venous return and cardiac output are impeded, along with the possibility of collapse of the unaffected lung.
- Tension pneumothorax is a medical emergency, requiring immediate intervention. Accurate assessment of signs and symptoms allows for the prompt recognition and treatment:
  - ❖ Tracheal deviation to the unaffected side
  - ❖ Neck vein distention
  - ❖ Muffled heart sounds
  - ❖ Tachypnea
  - ❖ Decreased or absent breath sounds on the affected side
  - ❖ Shortness of breath, dyspnea
  - ❖ Asymmetric chest excursion with respirations
- Needle thoracostomy is performed by placing a needle into the pleural space to remove air and reestablish nega-

tive pressure in unstable patients with tension pneumothorax (Fig. 22–1).

EQUIPMENT

- 14- to 16-G hollow needle or catheter with one-way valve attached or commercially available (Heimlich) flutter valve
- Povidone-iodine solution
- 4 × 4 gauze dressing
- Tape

Additional equipment (to have available depending on patient need) includes the following:

- Scissors
- Sterile glove (powder free)
- Small rubber band

The above equipment can be used to create a one-way valve. Cut a finger off the glove and attach it to the needle using the rubber band. Sterilize before use.

- Oxygen
- Manual resuscitation bag with mask

PATIENT AND FAMILY EDUCATION

- Explain the procedure and reason for needle thoracostomy. ➤*Rationale:* Identifies patient and family knowledge deficits concerning the patient's condition, procedure, expected benefits, potential risks, and allows time for questions to clarify information and to voice concerns. Explanations decrease patient anxiety and enhance cooperation.
- If indicated, explain patient's role in assisting with needle thoracostomy. ➤*Rationale:* Assists with insertion of flutter valve by eliciting patient's cooperation.

PATIENT ASSESSMENT AND PREPARATION

Patient Assessment

- Signs and symptoms consistent with tension pneumothorax include the following:

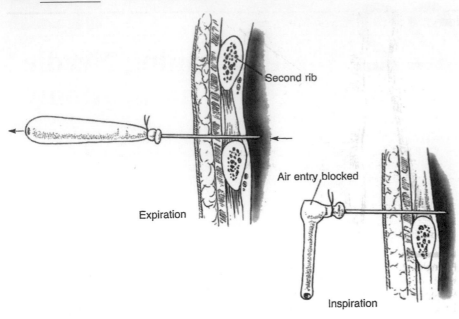

Expiration

Second rib

Air entry blocked

Inspiration

■ ● **FIGURE 22–1.** Use of a needle and a sterile finger cot or a finger from a sterile glove to fashion a one-way (flutter) valve for emergency evacuation of a tension pneumothorax. A small opening is made in the free end of the glove to allow air to escape during expiration. (From Cosgniff JH. *An Atlas of Diagnostic and Therapeutic Procedures for Emergency Personnel.* Philadelphia, Pa: JB Lippincott; 1978:243.)

- ❖ Tracheal deviation to the unaffected side
- ❖ Neck vein distention
- ❖ Muffled heart sounds
- ❖ Tachypnea
- ❖ Decreased or absent breath sounds on the affected side
- ❖ Shortness of breath, dyspnea
- ❖ Asymmetric chest excursion with respirations
- ❖ Cyanosis
- ❖ Decreased oxygen saturation
- ❖ Subcutaneous emphysema
- ❖ Sudden, sharp chest pain
- ❖ Anxiety, restlessness, apprehension
- ❖ Tachycardia
- ❖ Hypotension
- ❖ Dysrhythmias

➥*Rationale:* Accurate assessment of signs and symptoms allows for the prompt recognition and treatment. Baseline assessment provides comparison data for evaluating changes and outcomes of treatment. Tension pneumothorax is a medical emergency, requiring immediate intervention.

Patient Preparation

- Ensure that patient understands preprocedural teaching. Answer questions as they arise and reinforce information as needed.   ➥*Rationale:* Evaluates and reinforces understanding of previously taught information.
- Position patient in supine position with the head of the bed flat.   ➥*Rationale:* Allows for identification of landmarks for proper placement of needle and flutter valve.

Procedure   for Performing Needle Thoracostomy

Steps	Rationale	Special Considerations
1. Wash hands, and don personal protective equipment.	Reduces transmission of microorganisms and body secretions; standard precautions.	
2. Administer high-flow oxygen and ventilate as needed.	Allows for oxygenation and ventilation before needle insertion.	
3. Locate the second intercostal space at the midclavicular line on the side of the suspected tension pneumothorax (see Fig. 17–1).	Identification of landmarks for needle thoracostomy.	
4. Cleanse area with providone-iodine solution, using a circular motion.	Cleanses area before needle insertion.	
5. Locate the upper margin of the third rib with several fingers. Insert flutter valve into the second intercostal space at the midclavicular line, pointing the needle posterior but slightly upward and sliding it over the top of the third rib.	Allows the proper placement of the flutter valve into the pleural space. Insert flutter valve above third rib to avoid damaging the nerve, artery, and vein that lie just beneath each rib.	Flutter valve acts as a one-way valve to prevent reentry of air into pleural space during inspiration, but allowing for escape of air during expiration (see Fig. 22–1).

Procedure for Performing Needle Thoracostomy *Continued*

Steps	Rationale	Special Considerations
6. Puncture the parietal pleural. Listen for an audible escape of air as the needle enters the parietal pleural.	Although an audible rush of air indicates that needle decompression has been successful, a dramatic improvement in the patient's clinical condition is the best indicator of successful intervention.	
7. Apply a small dressing around the flutter valve or suture the valve in place.	Allows for temporary stabilization of flutter valve until a chest tube can be inserted.	
8. Prepare for immediate chest tube insertion (see Procedure 17).	Definitive treatment of tension pneumothrax.	

Expected Outcomes

- Removal of air from pleural space
- Reestablishment of negative intrapleural pressure
- Tension pneumothorax conversion to simple pneumothorax
- Improved oxygenation and ventilation

Unexpected Outcomes

- Resultant pneumothorax in patient without tension pneumothorax
- Damage to nerves, veins, or arteries because of improper flutter valve placement
- Local hematoma or cellulitis
- Pleural infection

Patient Monitoring and Care

Patient Monitoring and Care	Rationale	Reportable Conditions
		These conditions should be reported if they persist despite nursing interventions.
1. Stabilize flutter valve with dressing until chest tube is inserted.	Prevents movement and dislodgment flutter valve.	• Dislodged flutter valve
2. Constantly monitor for signs and symptoms of tension pneumothorax.	Determines if chest decompression has been successful and allows for early identification of new pneumothorax until chest tube has been placed.	• Tracheal deviation to the unaffected side • Neck vein distention • Muffled heart sounds • Tachypnea • Decreased or absent breath sounds on the affected side • Shortness of breath, dyspnea • Asymmetric chest excursion with respirations • Cyanosis • Decreased oxygen saturation • Subcutaneous emphysema • Sudden sharp chest pain • Anxiety, restlessness, apprehension • Tachycardia • Hypotension • Dysrhythmias

AP This procedure should be performed only by physicians, advanced practice nurses, and other health care professionals (including critical care nurses) with additional knowledge, skills, and demonstrated competence per professional licensure or institutional standard.

Documentation

Documentation should include the following:

- Patient and family education
- Vital signs before and after insertion of flutter valve
- Location of flutter valve
- Size of flutter valve used
- Response after flutter valve placement

- Unexpected outcomes
- Nursing interventions
- Occurrence of unexpected oucomes

Additional Readings

Dunmire SM, Paris PM. *Atlas of Emergency Procedures.* Philadelphia, Pa: W.B. Saunders; 1994.

Kraus TC, Warner CG, Jacobs LM. *Emergency Medicine Procedures Manual.* New York, NY: Raven Press; 1994.

Lewinter JR. Tube thoracostomy. In: Jastremski MS, Dumas M, Penalver L, eds. *Emergency Procedures.* Philadelphia, Pa: W.B. Saunders; 1992:391–398.

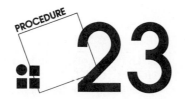
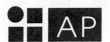

Performing Thoracentesis

PURPOSE: Thoracentesis is performed for diagnostic and therapeutic purposes in patients with pleural effusions.

William Barefoot

PREREQUISITE NURSING KNOWLEDGE

- Thoracentesis is performed by inserting a needle or a catheter into the pleural space, allowing for removal of pleural fluid.
- Thoracentesis is not used to verify the presence of pleural effusion. Pleural effusions are verified by chest x-ray, ultrasound, or computed tomography (CT) scan.
- Therapeutic thoracentesis is indicated to relieve the symptoms (eg, dyspnea) caused by a pleural effusion.
- Diagnostic thoracentesis is indicated for use in differential diagnosis for patients with pleural effusion of unknown etiology. A diagnostic thoracentesis may be repeated if initial results fail to yield a diagnosis.
- Samples of pleural fluid are analyzed and assist in distinguishing between exudative and transudative etiologies of effusion. Pleural fluid laboratory results alone do not establish a diagnosis; instead, the laboratory results must be correlated with the clinical findings and serum laboratory results.
- Exudative pleural effusions meet one of the following criteria:[1]
  - ❖ Pleural fluid lactate dehydrogenase (LDH)–serum LDH greater than 0.6 IU/mL
  - ❖ Pleural fluid LDH more than two thirds of the upper limit of normal for serum LDH
  - ❖ Pleural fluid protein–serum protein greater than 0.5 g/dL
- A transudative pleural effusion is considered when none of the exudative criteria are met.
- Transudative effusions are usually associated with systemic etiologies (eg, heart failure), whereas exudative effusions indicate a local etiology (eg, pulmonary embolus).
- Relative contraindications for performing a thoracentesis include the following:

- ❖ Patient anatomy that hinders the practitioner from clearly identifying the appropriate landmarks
- ❖ Patients receiving anticoagulants or having an uncorrectable coagulation disorder
- ❖ Patients receiving positive end-expiratory pressure (PEEP) therapy
- ❖ Patients with splenomegaly, elevated left hemidiaphragm, and left-sided pleural effusion
- ❖ Patients with only one lung as a result of a previous pneumonectomy
- ❖ Patients with known lung disease
- Ultrasonography-guided thoracentesis is thought to reduce complications, especially when used in the last four patient groups listed in the relative contraindications list.

EQUIPMENT

For Diagnostic Thoracentesis

- Sterile gloves
- Sterile drapes
- Sterile towels
- Adhesive bandage or adhesive strip
- Antiseptic solution
- Sterile 4 × 4 gauze pads
- Local anesthetic (1% or 2% lidocaine)
- One small needle (25 G, ⅝ in long)

- 5-mL syringe for local anesthetic
- Three large needles (18 to 22 G, 1½ to 2 in long)
- Sterile 20-mL syringe
- Sterile 50-mL syringe
- Two chemistry blood tubes
- Aqueous heparin (1:1000)

For Therapeutic Thoracentesis (in Addition to Equipment for Diagnostic Thoracentesis)

- 14-G needle
- 16-G catheter
- Three-way stopcock
- Sterile 50-mL syringe

- Vacutainers or evacuated bottles (1 to 2 L) with pressure tubing

Additional equipment (to have available depending on patient need) includes the following:

- Two complete blood count (CBC) tubes

- Sterile tubes for fungal and tuberculosis cultures

- One anaerobic and one aerobic media bottle for culture and sensitivity
- Hemostat or Kelly clamp
- Pulse oximetry equipment

PATIENT AND FAMILY EDUCATION

- Explain the procedure and purpose for thoracentesis, including potential complications such as pneumothorax, pain at insertion site, cough, infection, hypoxemia, and hypovolemia. Also, include an explanation of amount of fluid expected to be withdrawn, duration of time procedure may last, and expectation of and reason for coughing during or after thoracentesis. ➥*Rationale:* Identifies patient and family knowledge deficits concerning patient condition, procedure, expected benefits, and potential risks and allows time for questions to clarify information and voice concerns. Explanations decrease patient anxiety and enhance cooperation.
- Explain the patient's role in thoracentesis. ➥*Rationale:* Increases patient compliance, facilitates needle and catheter insertion, and enhances fluid removal.

PATIENT ASSESSMENT AND PREPARATION

Patient Assessment

- Signs and symptoms of pleural effusion include the following:
  - Trachea deviated away from the affected side
  - Affected side dull to flat by percussion
  - Absent or decreased breath sounds
  - Tactile fremitus ➥*Rationale:* Although the above physical findings may suggest a pleural effusion, radiography will confirm the presence of a pleural effusion.
- Chest x-ray findings ➥*Rationale:* If at least half the hemidiaphragm is obliterated on anterior-posterior x-ray, there is sufficient fluid in the pleural space to perform a thoracentesis. However, if there is a small amount of loculated fluid, a decubitus x-ray should be obtained. If the pleural effusion is greater than 10 mm on decubitus x-ray, a diagnostic thoracentesis can be performed. If the pleural effusion is less than 10 mm in diameter or loculated, ultrasonography is required to distinguish between pleural effusion and pleural lesion. Ultrasonography-guided thoracentesis may be necessary if a pleural effusion has been confirmed.
- Past medical history of pleuritic chest pain, cough, dyspnea, malignancy, or heart failure ➥*Rationale:* Past medical history may provide valuable clues to the cause of a patient's pleural effusion.
- Baseline vital signs, including pulse oximetry (if available) ➥*Rationale:* Having baseline assessment data provides information about patient status and allows for comparison during and following the procedure.
- Recent serum laboratory results, including the following:
  - CBC
  - Platelet count
  - Prothrombin time
  - Partial thromboplastin time ➥*Rationale:* These studies help determine if the patient is at increased risk for bleeding.

Patient Preparation

- Ensure that patient understands preprocedural teaching. Answer questions as they arise and reinforce information. ➥*Rationale:* Evaluates and reinforces understanding of previously taught information.
- Ensure that written informed consent for the procedure has been obtained. ➥*Rationale:* Invasive procedures, unless performed under implied consent in a life-threatening situation, require written consent of patient or significant other.
- Position the patient. Several alternative positions may be used, as follows:
  - ❖ If the patient is alert and able, position him or her on the edge of the bed with legs supported and arms resting on a pillow on the elevated bedside table (Fig. 23–1).
  - ❖ The patient may sit on a chair backward and rest arms on a pillow on the back of the chair.
  - ❖ If the patient is unable to sit, position him or her on the unaffected side, with the back near the edge of the bed and the arm on the affected side above the head. Elevate the head of the bed to 30 or 45 degrees, as tolerated. ➥*Rationale:* Enhances ease of withdrawal of pleural fluid.
- Have an additional member of the health care team positioned in front of the patient. ➥*Rationale:* Reassures or comforts the patient and provides additional assistance.
- Select appropriate site by percussing until dullness is heard. Dullness indicates the highest point of the pleural effusion. Mark this site with a pen. The insertion site is one intercostal space below this point. ➥*Rationale:* Provides the practitioner with an identified site.
- Consider sedation or paralysis. ➥*Rationale:* Sedation or paralysis may be necessary to maximize positioning.
- Have atropine available. ➥*Rationale:* Bradycardia, from a vasovagal reflex, is not an uncommon occurrence during thoracentesis.

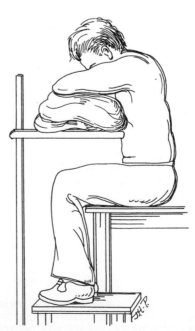

■ ● **FIGURE 23–1.** Ideal patient position for thoracentesis.

• Initiate pulse oximetry monitoring as appropriate. ➥*Rationale:* Pulse oximetry provides a noninvasive means for monitoring oxygenation at the bedside, allowing for prompt recognition of problems.

Procedure for Diagnostic and Therapeutic Thoracentesis

Steps	Rationale	Special Considerations
1. Wash hands, and don personal protective equipment.	Reduces transmission of microorganisms and body secretions; standard precautions.	
2. Percuss the affected side posteriorly to determine the highest point of the pleural effusion. Identify the intercostal space below this point.	This identifies the superior border of the pleural effusion and identifies and validates the planned site for thoracentesis.	Use the posterior axillary line as the insertion point to avoid the spinal cord. If the space identified for insertion is below the eighth intercostal space, ultrasonography should be done to mark the fluid level and its relationship to the diaphragm. This will help identify a safe point of entry to avoid solid-organ damage.
3. Heparinize the 50-mL syringe.	Prepares syringe for use in accessing pleural fluid.	
4. Prepare site with antiseptic. Don sterile gloves, and drape area with sterile drape.	Reduces skin contaminants, reducing the risk of infection.	
5. Anesthetize the skin with lidocaine (25-G, ⅝-in needle) in the typical wheal fashion around the insertion site.	Increases comfort for patient by anesthetizing the periosteum of the rib and pleura.	
6. Using 2% lidocaine and a 20- to 22-G, 1½- to 2-in needle, insert the needle through the wheal. Inject the lidocaine into the deep tissue and periosteum of the underlying rib superiorly and laterally.	To anesthetize the work area for optimal patient comfort.	Always aspirate before injecting to prevent lidocaine from entering a blood vessel or the pleural space.
7. After anesthetizing the periosteum of the underlying rib, gently advance the needle and alternately aspirate and inject lidocaine until pleural fluid is obtained in the syringe.	Anesthetizes the parietal pleura. The pleural space is identified by pleural fluid aspirate in the syringe.	
8. Once pleural fluid is obtained, place a sterile gloved finger on the needle at the point where the needle exits the skin. Withdraw the needle and syringe.	This approximates the length of insertion for the thoracentesis needle or catheter.	
For therapeutic thoracentesis, proceed to step 13.		
9. Attach a three-way stopcock and heparinized 50-mL syringe to a 20- to 22-G, 1½- or 2-in needle. Open the stopcock valve between the syringe and the needle.	The open stopcock valve will allow for aspiration of pleural fluid during needle insertion. The aqueous heparin will ensure accurate pH and blood cell counts.	
10. Insert the selected needle via the anesthetized tract and continually aspirate until pleural fluid is obtained, filling the 50-mL syringe.	The pleural fluid is used for laboratory testing to help delineate a differential diagnosis. A change in patient position can be attempted to facilitate fluid drainage.	It is possible that no fluid will be accessed (dry tap). A larger-gauge needle may be needed for thick or loculated fluid, or the needle may have been inserted above or below the pleural fluid. Once pleural fluid is aspirated, the needle may be stabilized by placing a hemostat or clamp on the needle at the skin site to keep the needle from advancing further into the pleural space, preventing lung puncture. *Procedure continued on following page*

Procedure	**for Diagnostic and Therapeutic Thoracentesis** *Continued*

Steps	Rationale	Special Considerations
11. Fill the specimen tubes from the pleural-fluid–filled syringe. Send the specimen tubes to the laboratory for appropriate analysis.	Analysis may aid in determining an etiology of the pleural effusion.	In order to interpret pleural fluid laboratory values, serum chemistry laboratory values must be obtained, such as pH, total protein, glucose, and LDH. When collecting pleural fluid for cytology or estrogen receptor analysis, add 10,000 units of heparin to the specimen sample.
12. On completion of diagnostic thoracentesis, withdraw the needle. Apply pressure to the puncture site for a few minutes and then apply an adhesive strip or adhesive bandage over the puncture site.		
13. Insert a 14-G needle attached to a 20-mL syringe, bevel down, into the anesthetized tract until pleural fluid is returned.	The 14-G needle is selected because it allows for insertion and passage of a 16-G catheter. A smaller-sized catheter may be unstable and fold or kink on itself.	
14. Once pleural fluid is obtained, remove the syringe from the needle, occluding the needle with an index finger.	Occluding the needle helps prevent the possible occurrence of a pneumothorax.	
15. Insert the 16-G catheter through the 14-G needle. Advance the catheter slowly through the needle, angling the catheter in a downward fashion toward the costodiaphragm until the catheter moves freely in the pleural space.	Advancing the catheter toward the costodiaphragm allows for optimal drainage of pleural fluid.	In therapeutic thoracentesis, a catheter is preferred instead of a needle because the lung is expected to reexpand. A needle could puncture the lung during reexpansion, causing a pneumothorax.
16. While advancing the catheter beyond the needle tip, remove the needle and leave the catheter in the pleural space. Attach a three-way stopcock with a 50-mL heparinized syringe to the end of the catheter.	Never pull the catheter back through the needle because the catheter may be cut or sheared by the needle tip.	
17. Fill the 50-mL heparinized syringe with pleural fluid. Fill the specimen tubes from the pleural-fluid–filled syringe. Send the specimen tubes to the laboratory for appropriate analysis.	When changing syringes, be certain the stopcock is positioned such that air does not enter the pleural space. Analysis may aid in determining an etiology of the pleural effusion.	In order to interpret pleural fluid chemistry laboratory values, serum chemistry lab values must also be obtained (eg, pH, total protein, glucose, LDH). When collecting pleural fluid for cytology or estrogen receptor analysis, add 10,000 units of heparin to the specimen sample.
18. Attach the vacutainer or evacuated bottles with tubing to the three-way stopcock. Open the valve to the vacutainer, and fill the vacutainer.	The vacutainer or evacuated bottles use negative pressure to withdraw pleural fluid from the pleural space, providing therapeutic relief. Reposition catheter if drainage stops to determine if fluid is still present.	Do not remove more than 1000 to 1500 mL of pleural fluid at one time. Removing more than this can cause hypovolemia, hypoxemia, or even reexpansion pulmonary edema. The patient may feel the need to cough as the lung reexpands.
19. On completion of thoracentesis, remove the catheter. Apply pressure to the puncture site for a few minutes, and then apply an adhesive strip or adhesive bandage over the puncture site.		

Expected Outcomes	Unexpected Outcomes

- Patient will be comfortable and will experience decreased respiratory distress.
- Lung reexpansion will occur.
- Site will remain infection free.
- Procedure will aid in diagnosing etiology of pleural effusion.

- Pneumothorax
- Vasovagal response
- Dyspnea
- Hypovolemia
- Hematoma
- Hemothorax
- Liver or splenic laceration
- Reexpansion pulmonary edema

Patient Monitoring and Care

Patient Monitoring and Care	Rationale	Reportable Conditions
		These conditions should be reported if they persist despite nursing interventions.
1. Monitor vital signs and cardiopulmonary status before and after thoracentesis and as needed.	Any change in vital signs may alert the practitioner of possible unexpected outcomes. Use of supplemental oxygen may be necessary in certain patient populations.	• Tachypnea • Decreased or absent breath sounds on the affected side • Shortness of breath, dyspnea • Asymmetric chest excursion with respirations • Decreased oxygen saturation • Subcutaneous emphysema • Sudden sharp chest pain • Anxiety, restlessness, apprehension • Tachycardia • Hypotension • Dysrhythmias • Tracheal deviation to the unaffected side • Neck vein distention • Muffled heart sounds
2. Obtain a postthoracentesis expiratory chest x-ray.	A chest x-ray is used to evaluate for lung reexpansion and evidence of a possible pneumothorax or hemothorax. If a pneumothorax or hemothorax is present, a chest tube may be necessary.	• Pneumothorax • Expanding pleural effusion • Catheter migration

Documentation

Documentation should include the following:

- Patient and family teaching
- Insertion of catheter or needle
- Catheter or needle size used
- Any difficulties in insertion
- Patient tolerance
- Pleural fluid aspirate characteristics
- Total amount of pleural fluid aspirated

- Site assessment
- Occurrence of unexpected outcomes
- Postthoracentesis x-ray results
- Laboratory test ordered and results as available
- Interpretation of laboratory results
- Nursing interventions

Reference

1. Qureshi N, Momin ZA, Brandstetter RD. Thoracentesis in clinical practice. *Heart Lung.* 1994;23(5):376–383.

Additional Readings

Heffner JE, Brown LK, Barbieri CA. Diagnostic value of tests that discriminate between exudative and transudative pleural effusions. *Chest.* 1997;111:970–980.

Klima LD, Benditt JO. Pulmonary procedures. In Goldstein RH, O'Connell JJ, Karlinsky JB, eds. *A Practical Approach to Pulmonary Medicine.* Philadelphia, Pa: Lippincott-Raven; 1997:39–54.

Light RW, Macgregor I, Luchsinger PC, Ball WC. Pleural effusion: the diagnostic separation of transudates and exudates. *Ann Intern Med.* 1992;77:507–513.

Quigley RL. Thoracentesis and chest tube drainage. *Crit Care Clinics.* 1995;11(1):111–126.

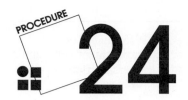

24

Assisting with Thoracentesis

P U R P O S E: Thoracentesis is performed for diagnostic and therapeutic purposes in patients with pleural effusions.

William Barefoot
Karen K. Carlson

PREREQUISITE NURSING KNOWLEDGE

- Thoracentesis is performed by inserting a needle or catheter into the pleural space, allowing for removal of pleural fluid.
- Thoracentesis is not used to verify the presence of pleural effusion. Pleural effusions are verified by chest x-ray, ultrasound, or computed tomography (CT) scan.
- Therapeutic thoracentesis is indicated to relieve the symptoms (eg, dyspnea) caused by a pleural effusion.
- Diagnostic thoracentesis is indicated for use in differential diagnosis for patients with pleural effusion of unknown etiology. A diagnostic thoracentesis may be repeated if initial results fail to yield a diagnosis.
- Samples of pleural fluid are analyzed and assist in distinguishing between exudative and transudative etiologies of effusion. Pleural fluid laboratory results alone do not establish a diagnosis; instead, the laboratory results must be correlated with the clinical findings and serum laboratory results.
- Exudative pleural effusions meet one of the following criteria:[1]
  - ❖ Pleural fluid lactate dehydrogenase (LDH)–serum LDH greater than 0.6 IU/mL
  - ❖ Pleural fluid LDH more than two thirds of the upper limit of normal for serum LDH
  - ❖ Pleural fluid protein–serum protein greater than 0.5 g/dL
- A transudative pleural effusion is considered when none of the exudative criteria are met.
- Transudative effusions are usually associated with systemic etiologies (eg, heart failure), whereas exudative effusions indicate a local etiology (eg, pulmonary embolus).
- Relative contraindications for performing a thoracentesis include the following:
  - ❖ Patient anatomy that hinders the practitioner from clearly identifying the appropriate landmarks
  - ❖ Patients receiving anticoagulants or having an uncorrectable coagulation disorder
  - ❖ Patients receiving positive end-expiratory pressure (PEEP) therapy
  - ❖ Patients with splenomegaly, elevated left hemidiaphragm, and left-sided pleural effusion
  - ❖ Patients with only one lung as a result of a previous pneumonectomy
  - ❖ Patients with known lung disease
- Using ultrasonography-guided thoracentesis is thought to reduce complications, especially when used in the last four patient groups listed in the relative contraindications list.

EQUIPMENT
For Diagnostic Thoracentesis

- Sterile gloves
- Sterile drapes
- Sterile towels
- Adhesive bandage or adhesive strip
- Antiseptic solution
- Sterile 4 × 4 gauze pads
- Local anesthetic (1% or 2% lidocaine)
- One small needle (25-G, ⅝ in long)
- 5-mL syringe for local anesthetic
- Three large needles (18- to 22-G, 1½ to 2 in long)
- Sterile 20-mL syringe
- Sterile 50-mL syringe
- Two chemistry blood tubes
- Aqueous heparin (1:1000)

For Therapeutic Thoracentesis (in Addition to Equipment for Diagnostic Thoracentesis)

- 14-G needle
- 16-G catheter
- Three-way stopcock
- Sterile 50-mL syringe
- Vacutainers or evacuated bottles (1 to 2 L) with pressure tubing

Additional equipment (to have available depending on patient need) includes the following:

- Two complete blood count (CBC) tubes
- One anaerobic and one aerobic media bottle for culture and sensitivity
- Sterile tubes for fungal and tuberculosis cultures
- Hemostat or Kelly clamp
- Pulse oximetry equipment

PATIENT AND FAMILY EDUCATION

- Explain the procedure and purpose for thoracentesis, including potential complications such as pneumothorax, pain at insertion site, cough, infection, hypoxemia, and hypovolemia. Also include an explanation of amount of fluid expected to be withdrawn, duration of time procedure may last, and expectation and reason for coughing during or after thoracentesis. ➠*Rationale:* Identifies patient and family knowledge deficits concerning patient condition, procedure, expected benefits, and potential risks and allows time for questions to clarify information and voice concerns. Explanations decrease patient anxiety and enhance cooperation.

- Explain the patient's role in thoracentesis. ➠*Rationale:* Increases patient compliance, facilitates needle and catheter insertion, and enhances fluid removal.

PATIENT ASSESSMENT AND PREPARATION
Patient Assessment

- Signs and symptoms of pleural effusion include the following:
  ❖ Trachea deviated away from the affected side
  ❖ Affected side dull to flat by percussion
  ❖ Absent or decreased breath sounds
  ❖ Tactile fremitus ➠*Rationale:* Although the above physical findings may suggest a pleural effusion, radiography confirms the presence of a pleural effusion.
- Chest x-ray findings ➠*Rationale:* If at least half the hemidiaphragm is obliterated on anterior-posterior x-ray, there is sufficient fluid in the pleural space to perform a thoracentesis. Chest x-ray findings may indicate that ultrasonography-guided thoracentesis should be performed.
- Past medical history of pleuritic chest pain, cough, dyspnea, malignancy, or heart failure ➠*Rationale:* Past medical history may provide valuable clues to the cause of a patient's pleural effusion.
- Baseline vital signs, including pulse oximetry (if available) ➠*Rationale:* Having baseline assessment data provides information about patient status and allows for comparison during and following the procedure.
- Recent serum laboratory results, as follows:
  ❖ CBC
  ❖ Platelet count

- ❖ Prothrombin time
- ❖ Partial thromboplastin time ➠*Rationale:* These studies help determine if the patient is at increased risk for bleeding.

Patient Preparation

- Ensure that patient understands preprocedural teaching. Answer questions as they arise, and reinforce information as needed. ➠*Rationale:* Evaluates and reinforces understanding of previously taught information.
- Obtain written informed consent for the procedure. ➠*Rationale:* Invasive procedures, unless performed under implied consent in a life-threatening situation, require written consent of patient or significant other.
- Position the patient. Several alternative positions may be used.
  ❖ If the patient is alert and able, position her or him on the edge of the bed with legs supported and arms resting on a pillow on the elevated bedside table (see Fig. 23–1).
  ❖ The patient may sit on a chair backward and rest arms on a pillow on the back of the chair.
  ❖ If the patient is unable to sit, position her or him on the unaffected side, with the back near the edge of the bed, the arm on the affected side above the head. Elevate the head of the bed to 30 or 45 degrees, as tolerated. ➠*Rationale:* Enhances ease of withdrawal of pleural fluid.
- Have an additional member of the health care team position in front of the patient. ➠*Rationale:* Reassures or comforts the patient and provides additional assistance.
- Consider sedation or paralysis. ➠*Rationale:* Sedation or paralysis may be necessary to maximize positioning.
- Have atropine available. ➠*Rationale:* Bradycardia, from a vasovagal reflex, is not an uncommon occurrence during thoracentesis.
- Initiate pulse oximetry monitoring as appropriate. ➠*Rationale:* Pulse oximetry provides a noninvasive means for monitoring oxygenation at the bedside, allowing for prompt recognition of problems.

| Procedure | for Diagnostic and Therapeutic Thoracocentesis |

Steps	Rationale	Special Considerations
1. Wash hands, and don personal protective equpment.	Reduces transmission of microorganisms and body secretions; standard precautions.	
2. Heparinize the 50-mL syringe.	Prepares syringe for use in accessing pleural fluid.	
3. Assist to prepare site with aneseptic, and drape area with sterile drape.	Reduces skin contaminants, reducing the risk of infection.	
4. Assist physician or nurse practitioner to draw up lidocaine for anesthetizing the site. *For therapeutic thoracentesis, proceed to step 8.*	Appropriate use of anesthetics increases comfort for patient by providing for anesthesia of the periosteum of the rib and pleura.	

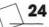

Procedure **for Diagnostic and Therapeutic Thoracocentesis** *Continued*

Steps	Rationale	Special Considerations
5. Attach a three-way stopcock and heparinized 50-mL syringe to a 20 to 22-G 1½- or 2-in needle. Open the stopcock valve between the syringe and neede.	The open stopcock valve will allow for aspiration of pleural fluid during needle insertion. The aqueous heparin will ensure accurate pH and blood cell counts.	
6. Fill the specimen tubes from the pleural-fluid–filled syringe. Send the specimen tubes to the laboratory for appropriate analysis.	Analysis may aid in determining an etiology of the pleural effusion.	In order to interpret pleural fluid laboratory values, serum chemistry laboratory values must be obtained, such as pH, total protein, glucose, and LDH. When collecting pleural fluid for cytology or estrogen receptor analysis, add 10,000 units of heparin to the specimen sample.
7. On completion of diagnostic thoracentesis, apply pressure to the puncture site for a few minutes and then apply an adhesive strip or an adhesive bandage over the puncture site.		
8. After the catheter has been inserted, fill the 50-mL heparinized syringe with pleural fluid. Fill the specimen tubes from the pleural-fluid–filled syringe. Send the specimen tubes to the laborabory for appropriate analysis.	When changing syringes, be certain the stopcock is positioned such that air does not enter the pleural space. Analysis may aid in determining an etiology of the pleural effusion.	In order to interpret pleural fluid chemistry laboratory values, serum chemistry laboratory values must also be obtained (eg, pH, total protein, glucose, LDH). When collecting pleural fluid for cytology or estrogen receptor analysis, add 10,000 units of heparin to the specimen sample.
9. Attach the vacutainer or evacuated bottles with tubing to the three-way stopcock. Open the valve to the vacutainer and fill the vacutainer.	The vacutainer or evacuated bottles use negative pressure to withdraw pleural fluid from the pleural space, providing therapeutic relief. Reposition catheter if drainage stops to determine if fluid is still present.	Do not remove more than 1000 to 1500 mL of pleural fluid at one time. Removing more than this can cause hypovolemia, hypoxemia, or even reexpansion pulmonary edema. The patient may feel the need to cough as the lung reexpands.
10. On completion of thoracentesis, remove the catheter. Apply pressure to the puncture site for a few minutes and then apply an adhesive strip or an adhesive bandage over the puncture site.		

Expected Outcomes

- Patient will be comfortable and will experience decreased respiratory distress.
- Lung reexpansion will occur.
- Site will remain infection free.
- Procedure will aid in diagnosing etiology of pleural effusion.

Unexpected Outcomes

- Pneumothorax
- Vasovagal response
- Dyspnea
- Hypovolemia
- Hypoxemia
- Hematoma
- Hemothorax
- Liver or splenic laceration
- Reexpansion pulmonary edema

Patient Monitoring and Care

Patient Monitoring and Care	Rationale	Reportable Conditions
		These conditions should be reported if they persist despite nursing interventions.
1. Monitor vital signs and cardiopulmonary status before and after thoracentesis and as needed.	Any change in vital signs may alert the practitioner of possible unexpected outcomes. Use of supplemental oxygen may be necessary in certain patient populations.	• Tachypnea • Decreased or absent breath sounds on the affected side • Shortness of breath, dyspnea • Asymmetric chest excursion with respirations • Decreased oxygen saturation • Subcutaneous emphysema • Sudden, sharp chest pain • Anxiety, restlessness, apprehension • Tachycardia • Hypotension • Dysrhythmias • Tracheal deviation to the unaffected side • Neck vein distention • Muffled heart sounds
2. Obtain a postthoracentesis expiratory chest x-ray.	A chest x-ray is used to evaluate for lung reexpansion and evidence of a possible pneumothorax or hemothorax. If a pneumothorax or hemothorax is present, a chest tube may be necessary.	• Pneumothorax • Expanding pleural effusion • Catheter migration

Documentation

Documentation should include the following:

- Patient and family teaching
- Insertion of catheter or needle
- Catheter or needle size used
- Any difficulties in insertion
- Patient tolerance
- Pleural fluid aspirate characteristics
- Total amount of pleural fluid aspirated

- Site assessment
- Occurrence of unexpected outcomes
- Postthoracentesis x-ray results
- Laboratory test ordered and results as available
- Interpretation of laboratory results
- Nursing interventions

Reference

1. Qureshi N, Momin ZA, Brandstetter RD. Thoracentesis in clinical practice. *Heart Lung.* 1994;23(5):376–383.

Additional Readings

Heffner JE, Brown LK, Barbieri CA. diagnostic value of tests that discriminate between exudative and transudative pleural effusions. *Chest.* 1997;111: 9701980.

Klima LD, Benditt JO. Pulmonary procedures. In Goldstein RH, O'Connell JJ, Karlinsky JB eds. *A Practical Approach to Pulmonary Medicine.* Philadelphia, Pa: Lippincott-Raven; 1997:39–54.

Light RW, Macgregor I, Luchsinger PC, Ball WC. Pleural effusion: the dignostic separation of transudates and exudates. *Ann Intern Med.* 1992;77:507–513.

Quigley RL. Thoracentesis and chest tube drainage. *Crit Care Clinics.* 1995;11(1): 111–126.

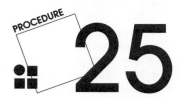

PROCEDURE

25

Arterial-Venous Oxygen Difference Calculation

P U R P O S E: The arterial-venous oxygen difference (a-vDO$_2$) is calculated in the mechanically ventilated patient to provide an indication of oxygen delivery, oxygen consumption, and adequacy of tissue oxygenation.

Suzanne M. Burns

PREREQUISITE NURSING KNOWLEDGE

- The majority of oxygen carried in the blood is bound to hemoglobin and is referred to as oxygen saturation. A very small percent is also dissolved in the plasma. The total blood *oxygen content* is then determined by adding the amount of oxygen bound to hemoglobin to that dissolved in the plasma. Oxygen content can be calculated for both the arterial blood (CaO$_2$) and the venous blood (CvO$_2$). By calculating the oxygen contents for arterial and venous blood and subtracting them, a rough estimate of oxygen utilization can be made. A normal a-vDO$_2$ is 5 vol% (range is 4 to 6 vol%). In general, because the contribution of dissolved oxygen is slight, it is not used clinically to calculate CaO$_2$.
- Mixed venous oxygen pressure (PvO$_2$) and mixed venous oxygen saturation (SvO$_2$) reflect tissue oxygenation under most conditions. When blood flow does not increase to meet higher tissue oxygen demands (re: hypotension), more oxygen is extracted from the arterial blood, and the PvO$_2$ and SvO$_2$ fall. The gradient between CaO$_2$ and CvO$_2$ widens. Conversely, when blood flow is increased (eg, hyperdynamic flow, as in sepsis), less oxygen is extracted from the arterial blood; PvO$_2$ and SvO$_2$ increase, and a-vDO$_2$ decreases.
- A major clinical goal of positive pressure ventilation (PPV) and positive end-expiratory pressure (PEEP) is improved oxygenation. One potential complication of these therapies is hypotension secondary to the effect of increased intrathoracic pressures on venous return.
- Calculation of a-vDO$_2$ may be reflective of tissue oxygenation in some cases; however, it is not a direct measurement and can be used only for approximation. The measurement of lactic acid is thought to be a more accurate assessment of tissue hypoxia; however, the formation of

lactic acid occurs quite late in the clinical course and is often irreversible.[1, 2]
- One of the most important variables affecting oxygen utilization is cardiac output (CO). When CO is low, more oxygen will be extracted from the arterial blood, thus lowering the CvO$_2$. Therefore, a drop in PvO$_2$ may be reflective of decreased perfusion.
- The product of CO and CaO$_2$ is oxygen delivery. Oxygen consumption may be calculated by determining the product of CO and a-vDO$_2$
- Measurement of CO is necessary for oxygen delivery and oxygen consumption calculations (see Procedures 59 and 64).
- Confirmation of pulmonary artery catheter placement is necessary (see Procedure 66).
- Sampling of arterial blood from indwelling catheter or arterial puncture should be done (see Procedure 57 or 72).
- Sampling of mixed venous blood from pulmonary artery catheter should be done (see Procedure 58).
- Interpretation of arterial blood gases is necessary.

EQUIPMENT

- Calculator and mathematical equations
- Arterial blood gas and saturation*
- Mixed venous blood gas and saturation*
- Hemoglobin level
- Hemodynamic profile (if calculating of oxygen delivery/consumption CO is required)

*Note: To obtain accurate arterial and venous saturations, a heparinized blood sample will need to be sent for analysis by co-oximeter. The saturation calculated from a blood gas is less accurate.

PATIENT AND FAMILY EDUCATION

- Inform the patient and the family of patient perfusion status and changes in therapy, and interpret the changes. If the patient or the family requests specific information about arterial venous oxygen content differences, explain the general relationship between a-vDO_2 and perfusion. ➻*Rationale:* Most patients and families are less concerned with the diagnostic and therapeutic details and more concerned with how the patient is progressing overall or in relation to a specific physiologic function.

PATIENT ASSESSMENT AND PREPARATION

Patient Assessment

- Signs and symptoms of inadequate tissue oxygenation include the following:
  - Thirst
  - Nausea
  - Anxiety
  - Apprehension
  - Skin temperature
  - Bounding pulse
  - Tachycardia
  - High CO with low systemic vascular resistance
  - Cool skin
  - Weak pulse
  - Tachycardia
  - Low cardiac output
  - Hypotension
  - Decreased mentation
  - Metabolic acidosis
  - Decreased pulse pressure
  - Increased systemic vascular resistance
  - Tachypnea
  - Decreased urine output ➻*Rationale:* Calculation of a-vDO_2 is indicated to provide a rough quantitative estimate of tissue perfusion and oxygenation.

Patient Preparation

- Ensure that patient understands preprocedural teaching. Answer questions as they arise, and reinforce information as needed. ➻*Rationale:* Evaluates and reinforces understanding of previously taught information.

Procedure for Arterial-Venous Oxygen Difference Calculation

Steps	Rationale	Special Considerations
1. Determine and record the value to be used for oxygen-carrying capacity (either 1.39 or 1.34). *(Level II: Theory based, no research data to support recommendations: recommendations from expert consensus group may exist)*	Consistently use the same oxygen-carrying capacity value for all a-vDO_2 calculations per patient. This prevents erroneous results.[1, 2]	
2. Calculate CaO_2 using the modified Fick equation: $CaO_2 = 1.39$ (or 1.34) $\times$ Hgb $\times$ $\%SaO_2$ (use decimal). *(Level V: Clinical studies in more than one patient population and situation)*	Only approximation is needed for clinical purposes.[1, 2]	If using dissolved oxygen, add ($0.003 \times PaO_2$). This is generally not necessary because it adds little to content.
3. Calculate CvO_2 using the modified Fick equation: $CvO_2 = 1.39$ (or 1.34) $\times$ Hgb $\times$ $\%SvO_2$ (use decimal). *(Level V: Clinical studies in more than one patient population and situation)*	Only approximation is needed for clinical purposes.[1, 2]	If using dissolved oxygen in the equation, add ($0.003 \times PvO_2$); this is not usually necessary.
4. Subtract CvO_2 from CaO_2.	Results in a-vDO_2 value.	
5. Consult with physician if needed changes in therapy exceed therapeutic guidelines.	Large changes in a-vDO_2 value may indicate the need for revising the therapeutic guidelines. Provides integrated trend data to evaluate tissue oxygenation in light of pulmonary function and ventilator parameters and demonstrates appropriate use of diagnostic and monitoring tests to evaluate therapy and alter therapy if needed.	

Expected Outcome	Unexpected Outcome
• Titration of PPV parameters (eg, tidal volume, PEEP, inspiratory-expiratory ratio) to maintain adequate perfusion and tissue oxygenation	• Hemodynamic instability

Patient Monitoring and Care

Patient Monitoring and Care	Rationale	Reportable Conditions
		These conditions should be reported if they persist despite nursing interventions.
1. Observe trend in a-vDO$_2$.	PPV, particularly with a large tidal volume and PEEP, can compromise hemodynamics from increased intrathoracic pressure. A narrowing difference may indicate hyperdynamic perfusion. A widening difference may indicate hypodynamic perfusion. The effect of PPV therapy on perfusion needs to be explored. (Unless a therapeutic plan has been predetermined, decisions related to interventions will need to be decided with each measurement. For example, although an increase in PEEP may be thought to have resulted in hypotension, and a widened a-vDO$_2$, the intervention may be to give fluid instead of lowering PEEP.)	• Acute changes in a-vDO$_2$

Documentation

Documentation should include the following:

- Patient and family education
- The a-vDO$_2$, arterial blood gas, and hemoglobin results with which it was calculated
- The time, the date, and the position of the patient (eg, supine, prone, semiprone)
- Ventilator parameters at the time the blood gas samples were drawn
- Changes in therapy based on the a-vDO$_2$ value
- Patient response to the interventions
- Unexpected outcomes

References

1. Silance PG, Simon C, Vincent JL. The relationship between cardiac index and oxygen extraction in acutely ill patients. *Chest.* 1994;105:1190–1197.
2. Barone JE. Maximization of oxygen delivery: a plea for moderation. II. *J Trauma.* 1994;37:337–338.

Ahrens TS, Powers CC. Pulmonary clinical physiology. In: Kinney MR, Dunbar SB, Brooks-Brunn J, Molter N, Vitello-Cicciu JM, eds. *AACN's Clinical Reference for Critical Care Nursing.* 4th ed. St. Louis, Mo: CV Mosby; 1998:491–516.
West JB. *Respiratory Physiology: The Essentials.* 5th ed. Baltimore, Md: Williams & Wilkins; 1994.

Additional Readings

Ahrens TS, Rutherford KA. *Essentials of Oxygenation.* Boston, Ma: Jones & Bartlett; 1993.

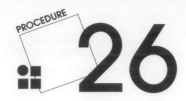

26

Auto-PEEP Calculation

P U R P O S E: Auto-PEEP (auto positive end-expiratory pressure) is measured in the mechanically ventilated patient to identify the presence of auto-PEEP, to quantify the level to assess patient risk and the need for changes in ventilator therapy, and to quantify the level to accurately calculate static compliance.

Suzanne M. Burns

PREREQUISITE NURSING KNOWLEDGE

- Auto-PEEP is often called *occult* because it is not set on the ventilator; instead, it is a result of inadequate exhalation time (Fig. 26–1).
- Auto-PEEP is associated with high minute ventilation requirements, small-diameter endotracheal tubes, bronchospasm, long inspiratory times, and high respiratory rates.
- Auto-PEEP may result in an increased work of breathing. The set sensitivity of the ventilator will not reflect the pressure required to initiate a breath; the patient will have to generate a pressure equal to the set sensitivity plus auto-PEEP.
- Auto-PEEP elevates static pressure (ie, plateau pressure). High plateau pressures can result in barotrauma and hemodynamic compromise.[1, 2]
- Auto-PEEP may be a desirable outcome of select ventilator settings (eg, pressure-controlled inverse ratio ventilation).[3] In these cases, auto-PEEP restores functional residual capacity (FRC) and reduces shunt.
- Interventions to offset auto-PEEP include the use of sedatives and narcotics, large-diameter endotracheal tubes, bronchodilators, short inspiratory times, and slower respiratory rates. Occasionally, the addition of set-PEEP is used to offset auto-PEEP. An example is in the case of the patient with chronic obstructive pulmonary disease (COPD), in whom early airway closure during exhalation results in gas trapping. The addition of set-PEEP serves as splint by keeping the airway open throughout exhalation, thereby decreasing auto-PEEP.

EQUIPMENT

Generally no additional equipment is necessary because most ventilators have an end-expiratory hold button to use for determining auto-PEEP. If the ventilator is an old one, auto-PEEP can be manually measured.

PATIENT AND FAMILY EDUCATION

- Inform the patient and family about the patient's respiratory status, changes in therapy, and how to interpret the changes. If the patient or family requests specific information about auto-PEEP measurements, explain the general relationship among auto-PEEP, the work of breathing, and complication risks. **➤➤Rationale:** Most patients and families are less concerned with the diagnostic and therapeutic details and more concerned with how the patient is progressing overall or in relation to a specific physiologic function.

PATIENT ASSESSMENT AND PREPARATION

Patient Assessment

- Assess for the presence of auto-PEEP; have a high index of suspicion if any of the following is noted:

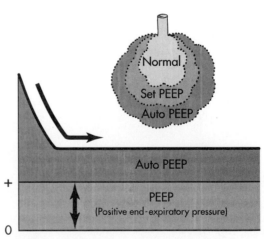

■ ● **FIGURE 26–1.** Auto-PEEP. Auto-PEEP is PEEP over and above the set PEEP. It can be measured by performing an end-expiratory hold maneuver and observing the airway pressure manometer. Auto-PEEP is caused by insufficient expiratory time (eg., high rates, inverse ratios, obstructions). Too much PEEP can increase pulmonary pressures, decrease systemic blood pressure, and risk diverting blood flow to poorly ventilated alveoli, thus increasing hypoxemia. PEEP, positive end-expiratory pressure. (From *AACN Clinical Reference for Critical Care Nursing.* St. Louis, Mo: Mosby–Year Book; 1998:615.)

❖ Minute ventilation requirements are greater than 10 L/min.
❖ The patient has COPD.
❖ The patient has bronchospasm.
❖ The respiratory rate is rapid (ie, ≥20/min).
❖ The inspiratory time is long (ie, >1 second).
❖ Any of the above is present in conjunction with bronchospasm.[4, 5]
❖ Dyssynchrony exists between patient and ventilator, especially when the ventilator does not cycle with patient inspiration.[4] ➡*Rationale:* Auto-PEEP increases the work of breathing by increasing the threshold load to trigger inspiration. The increased work of breathing may cause fatigue.
❖ Presence of auto-PEEP (when any of the above are present) and the patient is hypotensive or demonstrates signs of barotrauma.
❖ Patients in status asthmaticus (high risk). Consider the presence of auto-PEEP secondary to vigorous bagging, especially if hypotension is present.[6] ➡*Rationale:* Auto PEEP, like intentional PEEP, puts the patient at risk for barotrauma secondary to increased intra-alveolar pressures. In patients with asthma, for example, lung compliance is good but airway resistance is high, thus encouraging alveolar overdistention and potential barotrauma. Hemodynamic compromise occurs when the increased alevolar pressure collapses or squeezes the capillaries; decreased venous return and hypotension result.

Patient Preparation

• Ensure that the patient understands preprocedural teaching. Answer questions as they arise and reinforce information as needed. ➡*Rationale:* Evaluates and reinforces understanding of previously taught information.

Procedure	**for Auto-PEEP Calculation**	
Procedure	**Rationale**	**Special Considerations**
1. Identify the end-expiratory hold button on the ventilator. *(Level V: Clinical studies in more than one patient population or situation)* If no end-expiratory hold button is available, proceed to step 3.	Normally the pressure in the ventilator is exposed to atmospheric pressure during exhalation, and the airway pressure needle will fall to zero or the set PEEP level. End-expiratory hold buttons close the ventilator systems to atmospheric pressure at end-exhalation. Thus, the presence and degree of auto-PEEP can be measured because the maneuver allows for the equalization of pressure within the system.[1, 2]	
2. A. Push the end-expiratory hold button at the end of exhalation (right before the next inspiration). *(Level I: Manufacturer's recommendation)* B. Observe the baseline pressure level on the airway pressure manometer or on the digital readout. C. If auto-PEEP is present, the baseline (zero or set PEEP level) will increase to the level of auto-PEEP. *(Level IV: Limited clinical studies to support recommendation)* D. Record the total PEEP over the set PEEP level.	In patients with rapid respiratory rates and in agitated patients, auto-PEEP is difficult to accurately measure. Using sedatives or muscle relaxants or both may be necessary.[4–6]	
3. Occlude the expiratory port of the ventilator with a gloved hand at the end of expiration, just before initiation of the subsequent mechanical breath. While watching the airway pressure manometer during this maneuver, note where the needle rests. Immediately release the expiratory port.		

Expected Outcomes	Unexpected Outcomes
• Auto-PEEP will be identified, monitored, and eliminated (if undesirable). • Therapy will be titrated, if possible, to minimize or eliminate auto-PEEP.	• Pulmonary barotrauma • Cardiovascular depression

Patient Monitoring and Care

Patient Monitoring and Care	Rationale	Reportable Conditions
		These conditions should be reported if they persist despite nursing interventions.
1. Evaluate the presence of auto-PEEP in the conditions noted in patient assessment.	Prevent complications by determining the presence of auto-PEEP and intervening appropriately. This is especially important in patients with profound hyperinflation (ie, status asthmaticus). Interventions may need to be aggressive. For example, the patient may require paralytics and sedatives so that ventilatory support can be reduced to allow for more complete exhalation. Hypercarbia is expected and is called *permissive hypercarbia*. The clinical goal is to reduce dynamic hyperinflation and potential lung injury.	• Presence of auto-PEEP
2. Assess for signs and symptoms of barotrauma or hemodynamic compromise or both.	Barotrauma is a potential complication of auto-PEEP.	• Decreased breath sounds or absent breath sounds on one side • Respiratory distress • Unexplained vital sign changes

Documentation

Documentation should include the following:

- Patient and family education
- The presence and degree of auto-PEEP
- Any changes in ventilator parameters
- Unexpected outcomes
- Nursing interventions taken

References

1. Mercat A, Graini L, Teboul JL, Lenique F, Richard C. Cardiorespiratory effects of pressure-controlled ventilation with and without inverse ratio in the adult respiratory distress syndrome. *Chest.* 1993;101:871–875.
2. Chan K, Abraham E. Effects of inverse-ratio ventilation on cardiorespiratory parameters in severe respiratory failure. *Chest.* 1992;102:1556–1561.
3. Burns SM. Understanding, applying, and evaluating pressure modes of ventilation. *AACN Clin Issues.* 1996;7:495–506.
4. Burns SM. Auto-PEEP: A complication you can't afford to overlook. *Nurs 94.* 24:32U–32W.
5. Benson MS, Pierson DJ. Auto-PEEP during mechanical ventilation of adults. *Respir Care.* 1988;33:557–568.
6. Pepe PE, Marini JJ. Occult positive end-expiratory pressure in mechanically ventilated patients with airflow obstruction. *Am Rev Respir Dis.* 1994;126:166–173.

Additional Readings

MacIntyre NR. Complications of positive pressure ventilation. In: Dantzker DR, MacIntyre NR, Bakow ED, eds. *Comprehensive Respiratory Care.* Philadelphia, Pa: W.B. Saunders; 1995;447–450.

Rossei A, Ranieri MV. Positive end-expiratory pressure. In: Tobin MJ, ed. *Principles and Practice of Mechanical Ventilation.* New York, NY: McGraw-Hill; 1994:288–289.

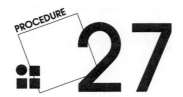

27

Measurement of Compliance and Resistance

P U R P O S E: Clinical measurements of compliance and resistance are performed to assess trends in respiratory status, to determine the effectiveness of therapy, and to titrate therapy.

Suzanne M. Burns

PREREQUISITE NURSING KNOWLEDGE

- *Compliance* is a measure of lung (and chest wall) distensibility. Conditions that decrease compliance include acute respiratory distress syndrome (ARDS), pulmonary edema, atelectasis, pneumonia, obesity, pulmonary fibrosis, and kyphoscoliosis. Compliance increases with emphysema.
- *Resistance* is a measure of how easy it is to move gases down the airways. Examples of conditions that adversely affect resistance include bronchospasm, secretions, and endotracheal tube size.
- Both compliance and resistance are reflected in the mechanically ventilated patient by changes in peak inspiratory and plateau pressures (ie, volume modes) or by changes in volume (ie, pressure modes) or both. Thus, by monitoring changes in volume per unit change in pressure (mL/cm H_2O), trends can be measured and therapies adjusted.
- Though spirometry or plethysmography or both are required for the exact measurement of airways flow resistance and lung compliance, two clinical measurements are frequently employed to estimate the contributions of each in the mechanically ventilated patient. They are commonly called *dynamic compliance* (C_{dyn}), which is more accurately called *dynamic characteristic*, and *static compliance* (C_{stat}).
  - ❖ The measurements of both C_{dyn} and C_{stat} are obtained on volume modes of ventilation. C_{dyn} requires that the delivered volume be divided by the peak inspiratory pressure (PIP) minus positive end-expiratory pressure (PEEP). Because gases are actively moving down the airways during volume breath delivery, PIP reflects the contribution of both airways resistance and lung compliance. Thus, *dynamic characteristic* is a more accurate term than *dynamic compliance*. The normal C_{dyn} on a mechanically ventilated patient is 35 to 50 mL/cm H_2O.
  - ❖ C_{stat}, in contrast, is measured during a breath hold maneuver (ie, end inspiration). By stopping gas flow, the pressure in the system equilibrates and the resultant pressure reflects the pressure required to distend the lungs separate from the pressure needed to move gases down the airways. The pressure measured during the breath hold is called *static pressure* (ie, plateau, alveolar, or distending pressure). By also subtracting PEEP, this number becomes the denominator for the calculation of C_{stat} (ie, tidal volume ÷ [plateau pressure − PEEP]). The normal gradient between PIP and static pressure is 10 to 15 cm H_2O. By comparing the difference between the two, the contribution of airways resistance is easily noted. Whereas using PIP and static pressure is very helpful for monitoring trends clinically, calculating C_{dyn} and C_{stat} is most useful for quantifying the degree of improvement or compromise over time.

- Static pressure is especially helpful to monitor when the lung is stiff (eg, in ARDS) and when there is great potential for barotrauma (eg, in air leak phenomena) and volu-pressure trauma (eg, in alveolar injury). In these cases, ventilatory goals often include ventilator pressure limits. Specifically, the goal is to maintain a plateau pressure (ie, static pressure) no higher than 35 cm H_2O.[1–6]
- Though the risk is low, measuring static pressure may increase the risk of barotrauma or cardiovascular compromise.

EQUIPMENT

- Calculator
- Values to be collected: Tidal volume (V_t), PIP, static pressure, PEEP, and auto-PEEP, if present (see Procedure 26).

PATIENT AND FAMILY EDUCATION

- Inform the patent and family about the patient's respiratory status, changes in therapy, and how to interpret the changes. If the patient or family requests specific information about C_{dyn} or C_{stat}, explain the relationship between the measurements and how easy it is to get air into the lungs and down the airway. ➥*Rationale:* Most patients and families are less concerned with diagnostic and therapeutic details and more concerned with how the patient is progressing overall.

PATIENT ASSESSMENT AND PREPARATION

Patient Assessment

- Determine PIP to assess gradual or acute changes. ➥*Rationale:* Given a constant tidal volume, a change in PIP indicates a change in airway resistance or lung compliance.
- Changes in ease or difficulty of compression of the manual self-inflating resuscitation bag. ➥*Rationale:* Compliance is change in volume for a change in pressure. If more pressure is required to inflate the lungs, ventilation will be affected.

Patient Preparation

- Ensure that patient understands preprocedural teaching. Answer questions as they arise and reinforce information as needed. ➥*Rationale:* Evaluates and reinforces understanding of previously taught information.
- Premedicate as needed. ➥*Rationale:* This measurement may be extremely difficult in a patient who is breathing rapidly or agitated. Sedation and paralytics are sometimes necessary.

Procedure **for Measurement of Compliance and Resistance**

Steps	Rationale	Special Considerations
Dynamic Characteristic (C_{dyn})		
(Level VI: Clinical studies in a variety of patient populations and situations)	Both C_{dyn} and C_{stat} have been extensively tested at bedside in many patient populations.[1-7]	
1. Identify the PIP.	PIP is used as a rough estimate of the mechanical properties of the lung and chest wall and airways resistance.	
2. Identify the delivered exhaled Vt.	Data collection for calculation.	Air leaks around the artificial airway or through chest tubes will prevent an accurate measurement of C_{dyn}. Make sure the cuff leak is minimal. Exhaled Vt will differ from inspired Vt with large leaks.
3. Identify the amount of PEEP and auto-PEEP.	Data collection for calculation.	If auto-PEEP is present, add to PEEP as total PEEP to ensure accurate calculation (see Procedure 26).
4. Record the PIP, Vt, and total PEEP (ie, PEEP plus auto-PEEP).	Data collection for calculation.	
5. Subtract total PEEP from PIP.	Reflects PIP without PEEP.	
6. Divide Vt by the number obtained in step 5. The result equals the C_{dyn}.	Compliance is defined as the unit change in volume per unit change in pressure.	
7. Record C_{dyn} in mL/cm H_2O.	Communicates data.	
Static Compliance (C_{stat})		
8. Observe several ventilator respiratory cycles.	Determines timing of the end of inspiration.	
9. Identify initiation of the ventilator inspiratory cycle.	Determines timing of the beginning of inspiration.	
10. At the end of inspiration, activate the inspiratory pause (inflation hold), while watching the pressure gauge. Note the drop and plateau of the PIP needle (plateau pressure), and immediately deactivate the inspiratory pause, allowing exhalation.	At this point, the flow of gas through the airway stops, causing the inspiratory pressure to drop.	This maneuver requires hand–eye coordination to ensure a short inspiratory pause (ie, less than 2 seconds). This measurement may be extremely difficult in a patient who is breathing rapidly or agitated. Administering sedation and paralytics is sometimes necessary.

Procedure **for Measurement of Compliance and Resistance** *Continued*

Steps	Rationale	Special Considerations
11. Record the plateau pressure.	Data collection for calculation.	
12. Subtract total PEEP (PEEP plus auto-PEEP) from plateau pressure.	Reflects pressure plateau without PEEP.	
13. Divide Vt by the number obtained in step 12.	C_{stat} is the relationship of the tidal volume to the plateau (static) pressure.	Air leaks around the artificial airway or through chest tubes will prevent an accurate measurement of static compliance. Ensure an intact cuff.

Expected Outcome

- Therapy titrated to patient response

Unexpected Outcomes

- Pulmonary barotrauma
- Cardiovascular depression

Patient Monitoring and Care

Patient Monitoring and Care	Rationale	Reportable Conditions
		These conditions should be reported if they persist despite nursing interventions.
1. Observe trends in C_{dyn} and C_{stat}.	Increasing values with a constant Vt indicate improvement in underlying disease process and effectiveness of interventions. Decreasing values with constant Vt indicate increased airway resistance (C_{dyn}) or progression of underlying disease process and ineffective interventions (C_{dyn} and C_{stat}).	• Bradycardia • Tachycardia • Drop in saturation to 90% or less • Changes or trends

Documentation

Documentation should include the following:

- Patient and family education
- C_{dyn} and C_{stat} calculations
- Patient toleration
- Unexpected outcomes
- Nursing interventions

References

1. Dreyfuss D, Solar P, Basset G, Saunon G. High inflation pressure pulmonary edema: respective effects of high airway pressure, high tidal volume, and positive end-expiratory pressure. *Am Rev Respir Dis.* 1988;137:1159–1164.
2. Gattinoni L, Pesanti A, Torresin A, et al. Pressure volume curve of total respiratory system in acute respiratory failure: computed tomographic scan study. *Am Rev Respir Dis.* 1987;136:730–736.
3. Fu Z, Costell ML, Tsukimoto K, et al. High lung volume increases stress failure in pulmonary capillaries. *J Appl Physiol.* 1992;73:123–133.
4. Lachmann B. Open up the lung and keep the lungs open. *Intensive Care Med.* 1992;18:319–321.
5. Parker JC, Hernandez LA, Deevy KJ. Mechanisms of ventilator-induced lung injury. *Crit Care Med.* 1993;21:131–143.
6. West JB, Tsukimoto K, Mathieu–Costello O, et al. Stress fracture in pulmonary capillaries. *J Appl Physiol.* 1991;70:1731–1742.
7. Truwit JD: Lung mechanics. In: Dantzker DR, MacIntyre NR, Bakow ED. *Comprehensive Respiratory Care.* Philadelphia, Pa: W.B. Saunders; 1997:20–26.

Additional Readings

Ahrens TS, Powers CC. Pulmonary clinical physiology. In: Kinney MR, Dunbar SB, Brooks–Brunn J, Molter N, Vitello–Cicciu JM, eds. *AACN's Clinical Reference for Critical Care Nursing.* 4th ed. St Louis, Mo: Mosby–Year Book; 1998:494–495.
Slutsky AS. Consensus conference on mechanical ventilation—January 28–30, 1993 at Northbrook, Illinois, USA, Parts 1 and 2. *Intensive Care Med.* 1994;20:64–79, 150–162.
Tobin MJ, Van De Graaff WB. Monitoring of lung mechanics and work of breathing. In: Tobin MJ, ed. *Principles and Practice of Mechanical Ventilation.* New York, NY: McGraw–Hill Book Co; 1994:978–984.

28 Manual Self-Inflating Resuscitation Bag

P U R P O S E: The manual self-inflating resuscitation bag is used to provide ventilation and oxygenation with or without an artificial airway in place and is called *bagging*.

Suzanne M. Burns

PREREQUISITE NURSING KNOWLEDGE

- Bagging is an essential skill used in emergency situations such as cardiopulmonary arrest. Bagging is also indicated for the following:
  - ❖ To provide oxygenation and ventilation before and after suctioning airway procedures and during patient transports
  - ❖ To assess airway patency and placement
  - ❖ To evaluate the interaction of patient and ventilator
  - ❖ To alter the ventilatory pattern
- Bagging should result in chest movement and auscultatory evidence of bilateral air entry.
- In patients without an artificial airway in place, effective bagging requires an unobstructed airway, slight head and neck hyperextension (ie, the same technique used for mouth-to-mouth ventilation), and firm placement of the face mask over the nose and mouth (Fig. 28–1). Effective bagging is best accomplished with two people: one to secure the mask and ensure head and neck placement and one to bag.
- In patients with artificial airways, such as endotracheal or nasotracheal tubes or tracheostomies, the nurse must understand the components of artificial airways and the relationship of the airways to the upper airway anatomy (see Procedures 1, 6, 7, or 11).
- When signs and symptoms of respiratory distress are noted in the mechanically ventilated patient, the patient should be bagged if troubleshooting does not immediately elucidate the problem.
- Large breaths and rapid rates provided during bagging may result in dynamic hyperinflation and resultant hypotension.[1, 2] Dynamic hyperinflation is most commonly associated with bronchospasm and in chronic obstructive pulmonary disease (COPD). This occurs when exhalation time is inadequate, which results in auto-PEEP and decreased venous return (see Procedure 26). Thus, a high index of suspicion is necessary if hypotension occurs with bagging. A brief disconnection from the bag or the provision of longer exhalation times or both will result in a rapid increase in blood pressure. Resume bagging at a slower rate and with longer expiratory times.

EQUIPMENT

- Manual self-inflating resuscitation bag (of appropriate size) and mask (Fig. 28–2)
- Oxygen source (flowmeter or needle valve) and tubing
- Positive end-expiratory pressure (PEEP) valve or PEEP attachment (if patient on higher than 5 cm H_2O of PEEP)

Additional equipment (to have available depending on patient need) includes the following:

- Oxygen analyzer when specific fraction of inspired oxygen (FIO_2) is desired
- Portable respirometer if accurate tidal volume (Vt) delivery on a breath-to-breath basis is required (eg, during patient transports)

PATIENT AND FAMILY EDUCATION

- Inform the patient and family that disconnection from the ventilator will occur and that bagging will be performed. The reason is also described (eg, suctioning, transporting,

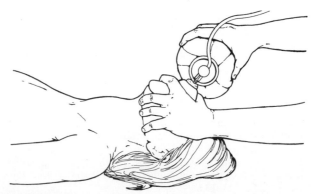

■ ● FIGURE 28–1. Proper technique for ventilation with manual self-inflating resuscitation bag and face mask. (From Scanlon CL, Spearman CB, Sheldon RL, eds. *Egan's Fundamentals of Respiratory Care.* 5th ed. St. Louis, Mo: Mosby; 1990:538.)

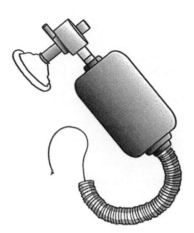
Bag-valve assembly with rear bag reservoir

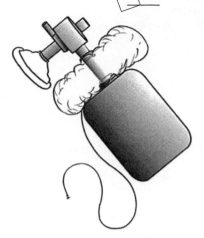
Bag-valve assembly with collar reservoir

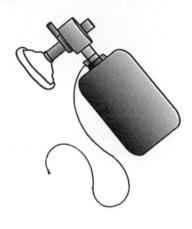
Bag-valve assembly without reservoir

■ ● **FIGURE 28–2.** Manual self-inflating bags: bag-valve assembly with and without reservoir.

making patient more comfortable). Explain that if the patient is dyspneic or otherwise distressed, it is important that bagging be done immediately. ➥*Rationale:* Information about the patient's therapy is an important need of patients and family members. Dyspnea is uncomfortable and frightening. It leads to anxiety, fear, and distrust. Failure to promptly diagnose and alleviate the cause of respiratory distress puts the patient at risk for further decompensation.

- Inform the patient and family that the patient may be in different positions during bagging (ie, side lying, prone, supine, Trendelenburg, reverse Trendelenburg, semi-Fowler). However, bagging may be more difficult if the diaphragm and abdominal contents are in positions that resist lung inflation. ➥*Rationale:* Positioning is not an impediment to bagging as long as an intact airway is in place. Bagging may be more difficult in some positions.
- Discuss the sensory experience associated with bagging. ➥*Rationale:* Knowledge of anticipated sensory experiences decreases anxiety and distress.
- Instruct the patient to communicate discomfort with breathing during bagging. ➥*Rationale:* The bagging technique can be altered to produce a comfortable breathing pattern.
- Offer the opportunity for both patient and family to ask questions about bagging. ➥*Rationale:* Being able to ask questions and to have questions answered honestly are cited consistently as the most important needs of patients and families.

PATIENT ASSESSMENT AND PREPARATION

Patient Assessment

- Determine oxygenation and ventilation status and observe for the following signs:
  ❖ Sudden drop in arterial oxygen saturation (SaO$_2$)
  ❖ Sudden change in mental status
  ❖ Tachycardia
  ❖ Tachypnea
  ❖ Respiratory distress ➥*Rationale:* Any acute change in patient status may indicate that bagging is indicated. Rapid response with 100% FIO$_2$ protects the patient

and allows for rapid evaluation of airways resistance, placement and function of artificial airway, and interaction of patient and ventilator.

- Determine airways resistance (how easy it is to move air down the airways) and lung compliance (how easy it is to distend the lungs and chest wall). ➥*Rationale:* Airways resistance and lung compliance can be assessed by bagging the patient with breaths that are similar in volume and rate to those provided by the ventilator. Focus on the degree of ease (or difficulty) with which the bag is compressed during inspiration. If it is difficult to bag the patient, look for causes of high airway resistance (eg, obstructed airway, bronchospasm) or low lung compliance (eg, pulmonary edema, pneumonia, acute respiratory distress syndrome [ARDS], pneumothorax). Compare findings to those following interventions such as suctioning and bronchodilator use. Changes in resistance and compliance can be confirmed by evaluating dynamic characteristic and static compliance when the patient is placed back on the ventilator (see Procedure 27).
- Ensure proper placement and function of the artificial airway (see Procedures 1, 6, and 7). ➥*Rationale:* Ensures the positioning and patency of the airway.
- Evaluate interaction of patient and ventilator, and specifically note dyssynchrony of patient and ventilator, by observing for the following:
  ❖ Breathing pattern not in synchrony with ventilator breaths
  ❖ Wheezing
  ❖ Restlessness
  ❖ Dyspnea
  ❖ Altered level of consciousness
  ❖ Agitation
  ❖ Decreased or unequal breath sounds
  ❖ Tachycardia or bradycardia
  ❖ Dysrhythmias
  ❖ Cyanosis
  ❖ Hypertension or hypotension ➥*Rationale:* Bagging may aid in the return of a synchronous breathing pattern and recognition of the cause (eg, obstruction). If signs and symptoms persist despite bagging, other causes, such as pulmonary embolus, should be consid-

ered. Therapeutic interventions to ensure synchrony and effective oxygenation and ventilation may be necessary and may include administering medications such as sedatives, narcotics, and bronchodilators. Additional diagnostic evaluations may also be required (eg, bronchoscopy, ventilation perfusion scans).

Patient Preparation

• Ensure that patient understands preprocedural teaching. Answer questions as they arise and reinforce information as needed. ➤*Rationale:* Evaluates and reinforces understanding of previously taught information.

Procedure	for Manual Self-Inflating Resuscitation Bag	

Steps	Rationale	Special Considerations
Using the Manual Self-Inflating Bag for Respiratory Distress or Evaluation of Pulmonary Status *(Level IV: Limited clinical studies to support recommendations)*[1,2]		
1. Check that bag is attached to oxygen source which is turned on.	Safety precaution. Allows oxygen to flow to the bag.	
2. If the patient is mechanically ventilated, disconnect patient from the ventilator. Connect bag to artificial airway.	Allows for manual ventilation.	
3. Observe patient's breathing pattern and rate. Attempt to synchronize manual breaths with the patient's spontaneous effort. Because it is difficult to provide larger breaths with manual ventilation compared with breaths provided by the ventilator, a higher manual rate may be required initially.	Helps patient gain control over breathing by ensuring ventilation and adequate oxygenation.[3]	
4. Encourage patient to relax as manual breaths are provided.	Provides synchrony between patient breaths and manual breaths.	
5. Gradually slow the rate of manual breaths to approximate the ventilator frequency (fx) or to a rate that meets the patient's demand.	Reestablishes synchrony. Once respiratory distress is relieved with a rate and volume comparable with that delivered by the ventilator, the patient can be reconnected. However, if the patient is on a low rate (eg, intermittent mandatory ventilation [IMV] of 4) or low pressure support level, common during weaning, the distress may be the result of fatigue. A return to higher ventilator support settings is required following bagging.	
6. Ascertain whether patient is comfortable with the manual breaths.	Promotes comfort.	If patient becomes distressed after reconnection, consider further assessment to determinine etiology and interventions. Additional steps are as follows: call for assistance while bagging, and look for additional confirmatory physical assessment findings, such as a tympanic percussion sound with pneumothorax or dull sound with consolidation to determine etiology of acute distress.
A. If signs and symptoms of distress are absent, the patient can be reconnected to the ventilator.	Indicates that respiratory distress is relieved.	
B. If distress is not eliminated with bagging, consider the following steps:	Indicates respiratory distress cannot be relieved without bagging. Further assessment is required.	

Procedure	**for Manual Self-Inflating Resuscitation Bag** *Continued*

Steps	**Rationale**	**Special Considerations**
Provide higher level of ventilator support if distress is evident on lower levels as in weaning trials; hyperoxygenate and suction (see Procedure 9); assess for the presence of bilateral breath sounds and symmetric chest expansion; assess the ease (or difficulty) with which the bag can be inflated; evaluate ventilator functioning. Obtain assistance (respiratory care or seasoned nurse) to determine adequacy of ventilator function; consider anxiety and discomfort as potential causes of dyspnea.	Distress may be a result of fatigue. Suction will provide information related to the presence of secretions or airway obstruction. By auscultating the lungs during bagging, essential information related to tube placement (eg, migration to right main stem) or patient status (eg, bronchospasm, pulmonary edema) can be obtained. Asymmetric chest expansion may be the result of a displaced artificial airway, pneumothorax, or obstruction. A change in ease of bagging provides gross data about increasing (improved) or decreasing (deteriorating) lung compliance. Alarms should automatically deactivate unless the problem has not been adequately addressed. A leak or other malfunction will result in patient distress and inadequate oxygenation and ventilation. Although psychologic reasons for respiratory distress are possible, rule out physiologic causes first.	This data should correlate with changes in positive inspiratory pressure (PIP; volume ventilation) or Vt (pressure ventilation) on the ventilator. In some situations, such as pulmonary embolus, no distinct physical assessment findings may be immediately evident. Whether or not distress is alleviated with bagging and returns with reconnection, the ventilator may be malfunctioning or the settings may be inadequate for the patient's acute change in physical status. Support the patient until appropriate interventions are accomplished. The use of anxiolytics or analgesics or both is appropriate to decrease pain and anxiety regardless of the etiology. It is essential, however, that a thorough evaluation of the cause of distress be undertaken following their administration.
7. Return patient to ventilator when respiratory distress is relieved. Reactivate and check ventilator alarms and settings. Observe breathing pattern, patient ventilator synchrony, PIP (volume ventilation), and Vt and frequency (pressure ventilation). Check that call bell is within patient reach, if appropriate.	Safety precautions. Ensures nurse is alerted to actual or potential life-threatening problems.	

Maintenance Ventilation

(It is highly recommended *that portable ventilators be used during transport instead of manual bagging. Regardless, it is possible that bagging will be required for long intervals in some cases. The following procedure is designed to provide a ventilatory pattern similar to that provided by the ventilator. Procedures may vary dependent on institutional standards.)*

1. Check that bag is attached to oxygen source that is turned on.	Safety precaution. Provides direct route for oxygen to flow into the bag.	
2. Disconnect patient from ventilator. Silence ventilator alarms.	Because the nurse is at the bedside and there is no problem with the patient or ventilator, there is no reason for the alarms to summon help or disturb other patients.	
3. Insert portable respirometer between bag and artificial airway.	Ensures that Vt delivery approximates that provided by ventilator.	
4. Bag patient at approximate rate depth and pattern as ventilator breaths.	Maintains ventilation pattern similar to that provided by ventilator.	

Procedure continued on following page

Procedure for Manual Self-Inflating Resuscitation Bag *Continued*

Steps	Rationale	Special Considerations
5. Analyze average Vt delivered manually. Adjust bag compressions as necessary to produce Vt that approximates ventilator Vt. Repeat until approximate Vt is reproducible.	Achieves reproducible manual breaths.	
6. Remove portable respirometer and insert portable oxygen analyzer between bag and artificial airway or use 1.0 flow of inspired oxygen (FIO_2).	Allows FIO_2 to be analyzed.	Policies vary among institutions. Generally, 1.0 FIO_2 is used during patient transports and analysis of oxygen level is not necessary.
7. Analyze FIO_2 delivered. Adjust liter flow of oxygen to produce same FIO_2 as ventilator breaths or to maintain SaO_2 at desired level.	Prevents hypoxia and maintains prescribed FIO_2.	FIO_2 delivered with bag depends on delivered oxygen liter flow and the type of manual resuscitation bag used. Reservoir tubing may be needed to ensure desired O_2 in some cases.
8. Remove oxygen analyzer and manually ventilate patient at Vt, fx, and FIO_2 that approximate ventilator settings.	Approximates baseline ventilation and oxygenation.	
9. Periodically ascertain that the patient is comfortable with the bagging technique. Adjustments may be needed to maintain patient comfort with manual ventilation.	Promotes patient comfort.	The patient who is being ambulated may require a larger minute ventilation than usual to match increased CO_2 production and oxygen consumption during activity.
10. Reconnect patient to ventilator. Reactivate ventilator alarms. Ensure that call bell is within patient reach.	Safety precautions. Ensures that the nurse will be alerted to actual or potential life-threatening problems.	

Expected Outcomes

- Maintenance of adequate oxygenation and ventilation
- Resolution of acute respiratory distress

Unexpected Outcomes

- Hemodynamic instability secondary to dynamic hyper-inflation
- Pulmonary barotrauma (eg, pneumothorax)
- Inability to restore adequate ventilation and oxygenation with bagging
- Inadvertent extubation during bagging
- Equipment failure and inability to bag

Patient Monitoring and Care

Patient Monitoring and Care	Rationale	Reportable Conditions
		These conditions should be reported if they persist despite nursing interventions.
1. Evaluate trends or sudden changes in lung compliance or airways resistance.	Improvement or deterioration in lung function can be approximated by evaluation of patient's response to bagging.	• Difficulty bagging (very stiff) • No observable chest movement • Agitation • Diaphoresis • Hypertension or hypotension • Tachycardia or bradycardia • Dyssynchronous breathing
2. Observe for signs and symptoms of patent upper and lower airways, including comfortable appearance, stable or improved level of consciousness, synchrony of patient and ventilator, symmetric breath sounds, stable heart rate, rhythm, and blood pressure, and absence of rhonchi, wheezes, and dyspnea.	Proper technique will result in a comfortable, synchronous breathing pattern.	
3. Observe the patient during bagging. The patient should look comfortable. The chest should rise and fall evenly with bagging deflations and inflations.	Proper technique will result in a comfortable, synchronous breathing pattern.	• Dyssynchronous breathing
4. Monitor SaO_2 for maintenance of adequate oxygenation during bagging. End-tidal carbon dioxide tension ($PETCO_2$) may be used to monitor adequacy of ventilation (eg, CO_2 with acceptable limits).	If adequate oxygen is being delivered and ventilation is adequate, SaO_2 and $PETCO_2$ should be unchanged or improve with bagging.	• Drop in SaO_2 greater than 10% • Increase of $PETCO_2$ greater than 10%

Documentation

Documentation should include the following:

- Patient and family education
- Reason for bagging (eg, to suction during transport)
- Frequency
- Response of the procedure
- Unexpected outcomes
- Nursing interventions

References

1. Wilmoth DF, Carpenter RM. Preventing complications of mechanical ventilation: permissive hypercapnia. *AACN Clin Issues.* 1996;7:473–481.
2. Tuxen DV. Permissive hypercapnic ventilation. *Am J Respir Crit Care Med.* 1994;150:870–874.
3. Henneman E, Ellstrom K, St John R. Airway management. In: *AACN Protocols for Practice: Care of the Mechanically Ventilated Patient Series.* Aliso Viejo, Ca: American Association of Critical-Care Nurses; 1999.
4. Chulay M. Airway and ventilatory management. In: Chulay M, Guzetta C, Dossey B, eds. *AACN Handbook of Critical Care Nursing.* Stamford, Conn: Appleton & Lange; 1997:119–153.
5. Grap MJ, Glass C, Corley M, Parks T. Endotracheal suctioning: ventilator vs manual delivery of hyperoxygenation breaths. *Am J Crit Care.* 1996;5:192–197.

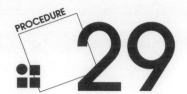

29

Indices of Oxygenation: Alveolar-Arterial Oxygen Difference, Partial Pressure of Arterial Oxygenation to Fraction of Inspired Oxygen Ratio, Partial Pressure of Arterial Oxygen to Alveolar Oxygen Ratio

PURPOSE: Alveolar-arterial oxygen difference (A-aDO$_2$), arterial partial pressure of oxygen to fraction of inspired oxygen (Pao$_2$:Fio$_2$) ratio, and arterial partial pressure of oxygen to alveolar partial pressure of oxygen (Pao$_2$: Pao$_2$) ratio are calculated to identify shunt as the primary mechanism of hypoxemia, to assess trends in oxygenation, and to determine effectiveness and titration of therapies.

Suzanne M. Burns

PREREQUISITE NURSING KNOWLEDGE

- Pao$_2$ is primarily determined by the concentration of inspired oxygen and the amount of carbon dioxide in the alveolus.
- In normal lungs, alveolar oxygen diffuses rapidly into the pulmonary capillaries and arterial oxygenation approximates that of the alveolus. The normal alveolar-to-arterial oxygen difference in a patient breathing 21% oxygen is 10 to 30 mm Hg (ie, Pao$_2$ [100] − Pao$_2$ [80]). When 100% oxygen is inspired, the normal gradient is 50 to 70 mm Hg.
- Trends in A-a gradient are most accurately evaluated when the Pao$_2$ and Pao$_2$ are measured following inspiration of 100% oxygen for 15 minutes.
- Other clinical indices of oxygenation that are commonly used include Pao$_2$:Pao$_2$ (a:A) ratio and the Pao$_2$:Fio$_2$ (P:F)

ratio. These indices are all relatively easy to use and also to estimate trends in shunt. The advantage of the a:A ratio and P:F ratio is that a more constant value, despite changes in Fio$_2$, can be calculated. A normal a:A ratio is 0.8 to 1.0. The smaller the number, the higher the degree of shunt. The normal value for P:F ratio is >300. A smaller P:F ratio reflects a higher degree of shunt. A P:F ratio of 200 to 300 is used to define acute lung injury, whereas a P:F ratio of <200 is associated with acute respiratory distress syndrome (ARDS).

- In patients with shunt (perfusion to unventilated lung units), venous blood is shunted past the closed alveoli without becoming oxygenated. Even though Pao$_2$ may be normal because of an increase in Fio$_2$, a shunt exists. The A-a gradient increases. Thus, A-a gradient is considered a useful, albeit crude, clinical estimate of shunt. It is helpful to trend changes in oxygenation status and the effect of therapies and other interventions.

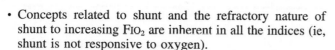

- Concepts related to shunt and the refractory nature of shunt to increasing FIO_2 are inherent in all the indices (ie, shunt is not responsive to oxygen).
- The gold standard for quantifying shunt is calculation of Qs:Qt (shunted blood flow to total blood flow ratio). Calculation of Qs:Qt (see Procedure 30) requires analysis of a mixed venous sample (from a pulmonary artery catheter or venous oxygen saturation [SvO_2] catheter); A-a gradient, PaO_2:FIO_2, and PaO_2:PAO_2 do not.
- Interpretation of arterial and mixed venous blood gas analysis.

EQUIPMENT

- Arterial blood gas (ABG) results (after 15 minutes of 100% FIO_2) for calculation of A-aDO_2. If other indices are used (ie, a:A ratio, P:F ratio), record the FIO_2 level when the ABG is drawn.
- Calculator

PATIENT AND FAMILY EDUCATION

- Inform the patient and family about the patient's oxygenation status and the rationale and implications for changes in therapy. If the patient or family requests specific information about alveolar-arterial oxygen differences, explain the general relationship between A-aDO_2 and hypoxemia. ➤*Rationale:* Most patients and families are less concerned with the diagnostic and therapeutic details and more concerned with how the patient is progressing overall.

PATIENT ASSESSMENT AND PREPARATION

Patient Assessment

- Assess for signs and symptoms of inadequate oxygenation:
  - ❖ Falling arterial oxygen tension
  - ❖ Tachypnea
  - ❖ Dyspnea
  - ❖ Central cyanosis
  - ❖ Restlessness
  - ❖ Confusion
  - ❖ Agitation
  - ❖ Tachycardia
  - ❖ Bradycardia
  - ❖ Dysrhythmias
  - ❖ Intercostal and suprasternal retractions
  - ❖ Rising or falling arterial blood pressure
  - ❖ Adventitious breath sounds
  - ❖ Falling urine output
  - ❖ Metabolic acidosis ➤*Rationale:* Clinical findings may indicate problems with oxygenation.
- Determine arterial oxygen tension or saturation. ➤*Rationale:* Hypoxemia is confirmed by a falling PaO_2 or SaO_2 or an absolute PaO_2 of less than 60 mm Hg and/or an absolute SaO_2 of less than 90% confirms oxygenation problems.
- Determine trend of indices and therapies. ➤*Rationale:* Improvement or deterioration can be quantified by monitoring indices over time.

Procedure **for Oxygenation Indices**

Steps	Rationale	Special Considerations
(Level V: Clinical studies in a variety of patient populations and situations to support recommendations)		

Calculation of Oxygenation Indices

1. Use the equation in Table 29–1 for calculation of A-aDO_2.

> **Table 29–1** ● ■ ■ **Calculation of A-aDO_2**
>
> $$PAO_2 = FIO_2 (P_{Bar} - PH_2O) - \frac{PaCO_2}{RQ}$$
> $$PAO_2 - PaO_2 = A\text{-}aDO_2$$
>
> Abbreviations: P_{Bar} = barometric pressure (713 mm Hg); PH_2O = pressure of water (vapor) (47 mm Hg); RQ = respiratory quotient (0.8).

2. Use the equation in Table 29–2 for calculation of PaO_2:PAO_2 ratio (a:A ratio).

> **Table 29–2** ● ■ ■ **Equation for Calculation of Arterial:Alveolar Ratio**
>
> PaO_2 (obtained from arterial blood gas) ÷ PAO_2 (see Table 29–1)

3. Use the equation in Table 29–3 for calculation of PaO_2:FIO_2 (P:F) ratio.

> **Table 29–3** ● ■ ■ **Equation for Calculation of PaO_2 : FIO_2 (P:F) Ratio**
>
> PaO_2 (obtained from arterial blood gas) ÷ FIO_2 (expressed as a decimal)

Procedure continued on following page

Procedure for Oxygenation Indices *Continued*

Steps	Rationale	Special Considerations
4. Document indices in patient record with the following data: A. Arterial blood gas (ABG) results.	All the data viewed together are needed for decision making regarding changes in therapy.	
B. Ventilator parameters, including FIO_2 at the time ABG was drawn.		
C. Position of patient at the time the blood was drawn.	Positioning (eg, placing patient in prone position) may be used as a means to improve shunt.	
D. Date and time ABG was drawn.		
E. Changes in therapy, if any, based on indices.		

Expected Outcomes

- Maintenance of adequate oxygenation (ie, SaO_2, PaO_2)
- Timely decrease in FIO_2 and titration of positive end-expiratory pressure (PEEP)

Unexpected Outcomes

- Hemodynamic instability
- Pulmonary barotrauma
- Oxygen toxicity

Patient Monitoring and Care

Patient Monitoring and Care	Rationale	Reportable Conditions
		These conditions should be reported if they persist despite nursing interventions.
1. Observe trends in oxygenation indices.	Oxygenation indices reflect the approximate degree of shunting as a mechanism of hypoxemia. Changes may reflect worsening of disease process or ineffective therapy or an improving disease process or effective therapy.	• Significant change in indices
2. Observe for increasing PaO_2 or SaO_2. When PaO_2 is >60 mm Hg or SaO_2 is >90% on an FIO_2 of less than 0.40, monitoring of the indices is rarely helpful.	Shunting, as a mechanism of hypoxemia, requires high oxygen concentrations to maintain marginal oxygenation. Shunting is not contributing significantly to hypoxemia if the patient has an adequate arterial oxygen tension on an FIO_2 of less than 0.40.	• Acceptable PaO_2 or SaO_2 with FIO_2 <0.40

Documentation

Documentation should include the following:

- Patient and family education
- Oxygenation index value, ABG results, Fio_2, and ventilator parameters at the time the blood was drawn
- The time, date, position of patient (eg, supine or left lateral)
- Changes in therapy based on the $A\text{-}aDO_2$
- Patient response to the interventions
- Unexpected outcomes
- Nursing interventions

Additional Readings

Ahrens TS, Powers CC. Pulmonary clinical physiology. In: Kinney MR, Dunbar SB, Brooks-Brunn J, Molter N, Vitello-Cicciu JM, eds. *AACN's Clinical Reference for Critical Care Nursing.* 4th ed. St Louis, Mo: CV Mosby–Year Book; 1998:496–503.

Ahrens TS, Rutherford KA. *Essentials of Oxygenation.* Boston, Ma: Jones & Barlett Publishers; 1993.

Dantzker DR. Pulmonary gas exchange. In: Dantzker DR, MacIntyre NR, Bakow ED, eds. *Comprehensive Respiratory Care.* Philadelphia, Pa: W.B. Saunders Co; 1995:98–118.

West JB. *Respiratory Physiology—The Essentials.* 5th ed. Baltimore, Md: Williams & Wilkins; 1994:54–57.

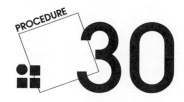

30

Shunt Calculation

P U R P O S E: Shunt calculation is performed to differentiate shunting from other mechanisms of hypoxemia, to quantify the shunt, to assess trends in progression or improvement of shunt, and to determine the effectiveness and duration of therapy.

Suzanne M. Burns

PREREQUISITE NURSING KNOWLEDGE

- *Right-to-left intrapulmonary shunting* (variously called *physiologic shunting, wasted blood flow,* and *venous admixture*) is the pathologic phenomenon whereby venous blood is shunted past the alveoli without taking up oxygen. This blood then returns to the left side of the heart as venous blood with a low oxygen tension.
- Right-to-left intrapulmonary shunting is expressed as a fraction or percentage of shunted blood flow to total blood flow (Qs/Qt). The normal physiologic shunt is less than 5% and is caused by venous blood from the bronchial and coronary veins returning to the left side of the heart as desaturated blood.
- Shunting of blood flow past the alveoli means that a certain percentage of the blood courses through an area of lung that receives no ventilation. Examples of conditions where shunt is present include acute respiratory distress syndrome (ARDS), atelectasis, pneumonia, pulmonary edema with fluid-filled alveoli, and total bronchial obstruction.
- As the percentage of the shunted cardiac output increases, the mixture of venous shunted blood with arterial blood increases with a concomitant fall in the arterial oxygen tension. The extent of the hypoxemia depends on the amount of the lung parenchyma that is not ventilated.
- The hallmark of right-to-left intrapulmonary shunting is that the hypoxemia cannot be corrected by high concentrations of inspired oxygen (referred to as *refractory* to oxygen).
- For evaluation of shunt, heparinized arterial and mixed venous blood samples are analyzed by co-oximeter. Use of the calculated saturation obtained in conjunction with blood gas analysis will not be as accurate.

EQUIPMENT

- Calculator
- Qs/Qt equation
- Mixed venous and arterial blood gases and saturations
- Pulmonary artery catheter, for drawing mixed venous blood samples, or venous oxygen saturation (SvO_2) catheter. If an SvO_2 catheter is used, the mixed venous saturation recorded on the monitor can be used for the calculation, (as long as in vitro and in vivo calibrations have been done according to manufacturer's recommendations).

PATIENT AND FAMILY EDUCATION

- Keep the patient and family informed about the patient's oxygenation status in general. Inform them of changes in therapy and how to interpret the changes. If the patient or family requests specific information about intrapulmonary shunting, explain the general relationship between Qs/Qt and hypoxemia. ➼*Rationale:* Most patients and families are less concerned with the diagnostic and therapeutic details and more concerned with how the patient is progressing overall or in relation to a specific physiologic function.

PATIENT ASSESSMENT AND PREPARATION

Patient Assessment

- Signs and symptoms of inadequate oxygenation include the following:
  - ❖ Falling arterial oxygen tension
  - ❖ Tachypnea
  - ❖ Dyspnea
  - ❖ Central cyanosis
  - ❖ Restlessness
  - ❖ Confusion
  - ❖ Agitation
  - ❖ Tachycardia
  - ❖ Bradycardia
  - ❖ Dysrhythmias
  - ❖ Intercostal and suprasternal retractions
  - ❖ Rising or falling arterial blood pressure
  - ❖ Adventitious breath sounds
  - ❖ Falling urine output
  - ❖ Metabolic acidosis ➼*Rationale:* Calculation of Qs/Qt is indicated to help differentiate between the mechanisms of hypoxemia.

Patient Preparation

• Determine arterial oxygen tension or saturation. ➤➤*Rationale:* Hypoxemia is confirmed by a falling arterial partial pressure of oxygen (PaO_2) or falling arterial oxygen saturation (SaO_2) or an absolute PaO_2 of less than 60 mm Hg or an absolute SaO_2 of less than 90%. A low PaO_2 and low SaO_2 with increasing supplemental oxygen confirm hypoxemia caused by right-to-left intrapulmonary shunting.

• Determine Qs/Qt trends with therapies and interventions. ➤➤*Rationale:* Calculation of Qs/Qt is indicated to help differentiate mechanisms of hypoxemia and to provide appropriate interventions. The effect of therapies such as positive end-expiratory pressure (PEEP) and proning on shunting and oxygenation can be quantified.

Procedure	**for Shunt Calculation**

Steps	Rationale	Special Considerations
1. Draw heparinized blood sample slowly from distal port of the pulmonary artery catheter. Be sure to discard the first 3 mL because it will contain flush solution. *(Level VI: Clinical studies in a variety of patient populations to support recommendations)*	If sample is drawn rapidly, it is possible to aspirate arterialized blood from the capillary bed; calculation of Qs/Qt will be inaccurate. The calculation of Qs/Qt has been used as the gold standard for clinical shunt measurement.	
2. Draw arterial blood sample within a few minutes of drawing mixed venous sample.	Ensures accuracy.	
3. Send the samples to be analyzed. Analysis of saturation is best done by co-oximeter.	Use of calculated saturation obtained via blood gas analysis is less accurate.	
4. Obtain Qs/Qt by using the equation in Table 30–1.		

Expected Outcomes	**Unexpected Outcomes**
• Maintenance of adequate PaO_2 • Timely titration of PEEP and fraction of inspired oxygen (FIO_2) as well as the application of other therapies such as proning	• Severe hypoxemia • Hemodynamic instability

---

Table 30–1 ●■■ **Qs/Qt Calculation**

$$Qs/Qt = \frac{C\bar{c}CO_2 - CaO_2}{C\bar{c}CO_2 - CvO_2}$$

Where Qs = intrapulmonary shunted blood flow
Qt = total lung blood flow
$C\bar{c}CO_2$ = end capillary O_2
$C\bar{c}CO_2$ = (Hgb × 1.34* × Sat† (1.0)) + (PaO_2‡ × 0.003)
CaO_2 = arterial oxygen content in mL/100 mL of blood
(Hgb × 1.34* × SaO_2) + (PaO_2 × 0.003)
CvO_2 = mixed venous oxygen content in mL/100 mL of blood
(Hgb × 1.34* × SvO_2) + (PvO_2 × 0.003)

For ease of calculation, the portion of the equation that determines the oxygen dissolved in plasma may be eliminated because the contribution of the dissolved portion of O_2 to oxygen content is extremely small. For continuity purposes, this should be determined by unit policy.

*Depending on institutional policy, either 1.34 or 1.39 is used.

†In this equation, saturation is assumed to be 100% as in an "ideal" capillary with no shunt.

‡PaO_2 = FIO_2 (713) − $\dfrac{PaCO_2}{0.8}$ (see Table 29–1 for calculation of PaO_2)

Patient Monitoring and Care

Patient Monitoring and Care	Rationale	Reportable Conditions
		These conditions should be reported if they persist despite nursing interventions.
1. Observe trend in Qs/Qt.	An increasing shunt indicates worsening of the disease process or ineffective therapy. A decreasing shunt indicates improving disease process or effective therapy. The greater the blood flow past unoxygenated alveoli, the greater the shunt and the greater the hypoxemia.	• A change in Qs/Qt of more than 5%
2. Observe for increasing PaO_2 or SaO_2 in conjunction with FIO_2 and PEEP levels.	Shunt, as a mechanism of hypoxemia, requires high oxygen concentrations to maintain marginal oxygenation. Shunting is not contributing significantly to hypoxemia if the patient has adequate arterial oxygen tension on an FIO_2 of 0.40 or less. When PaO_2 >60 mm Hg or SaO_2 >90% on an FIO_2 of 0.45 or less, monitoring of Qs/Qt is no longer necessary.	• PaO_2 <60 mm Hg • SaO_2 <90 mm Hg

Documentation

Documentation should include the following:

- Patient and family education
- Qs/Qt percent
- Date and time the Qs/Qt was performed
- The arterial and mixed venous blood gas results calculated
- The time, date, position of patient (eg, supine or left lateral)
- FIO_2 and ventilator parameters at the time the blood gases were drawn
- Changes in therapy based on the calculated Qs/Qt
- Patient response to the interventions
- Unexpected outcomes
- Nursing interventions

References

1. West J. *Pulmonary Pathophysiology: The Essentials.* 5th ed. Baltimore, Md: Williams & Wilkins; 1994:54–57.
2. Ahrens TS, Powers CC. Pulmonary clinical physiology. In: Kinney MR, Dunbar SB, Brooks-Brunn J, Molter N, Vitello-Cicciu JM, eds. *AACN's Clinical Reference for Critical Care Nursing.* 4th ed. St. Louis, Mo: Mosby–Year Book; 1998:491–516.

Additional Reading

Ahrens TS, Rutherford KA. *Essentials of Oxygenation.* Boston, Ma: Jones & Bartlett Publishers; 1993.

31

Ventilatory Management— Volume and Pressure Modes

P U R P O S E: Initiation and maintenance of positive pressure ventilation (PPV) maintains or improves oxygenation, maintains or improves ventilation, and provides respiratory muscle rest.

Suzanne M. Burns

PREREQUISITE NURSING KNOWLEDGE

- Indications for the initiation of mechanical ventilation include the following:
  - ❖ Apnea (eg, neuromuscular or cardiopulmonary collapse)
  - ❖ Acute ventilatory failure, which is generally defined as a pH of ≤7.25 with an arterial partial pressure of carbon dioxide ($PaCO_2$) ≥50 mm Hg.
  - ❖ Impending ventilatory failure
  - ❖ Severe hypoxemia. An arterial partial pressure of oxygen (PaO_2) of ≤50 mm Hg on room air indicates a critical level of oxygen in the blood. Though oxygen delivery devices may be employed before intubation, the refractory nature of shunt (perfusion without ventilation) may require that positive pressure be applied to reexpand closed alveoli. Restoration of functional residual capacity (lung volume that remains at the end of a passive exhalation) is the goal.
  - ❖ Respiratory muscle fatigue. The muscles of respiration can become fatigued if they are made to contract repetitively at high workloads. Fatigue occurs when the muscles' energy stores become depleted. Weakness, hypermetabolic states, and chronic lung disease are examples of conditions in which patients are especially prone to fatigue. Once fatigue occurs, the muscles no longer contract optimally, hypercarbia results,[1, 2] and 12 to 24 hours of rest are typically required to rest the muscles. Respiratory muscle rest requires that the workload of the muscles (or muscle *loading*) be offset so that mitochondral energy stores can be repleted.[1, 2] In general, once hypercarbia is present, mechanical ventilation is necessary to relieve the work of breathing.[3] Muscle *unloading* is accomplished differently, depending on whether the mode is a volume or pressure mode.

- Ventilators are categorized as either negative or positive pressure. Although negative pressure ventilation (eg, the iron lung) was used extensively in the 1940s, introduction of the cuffed endotracheal tube resulted in the dominance of positive pressure ventilation in clinical practice during the second half of the 20th century. Although there continues to be sporadic interest in negative pressure ventilation, the cumbersome nature of the ventilators and the lack of protection they give airways, and the ability of PPV to alter the ventilatory parameters preclude a serious resurgence of negative pressure ventilation.

- Positive pressure ventilators are categorized into volume and pressure ventilators.
  - ❖ As noted, with *volume ventilation*, a predetermined tidal volume (Vt) is delivered with each breath regardless of resistance and compliance. Thus, Vt is stable from breath to breath, but airway pressure may vary. To rest the respiratory muscles with volume ventilation, the ventilator rate must be increased until spontaneous respiratory effort ceases. When spontaneous effort is present, such as when initiating an assist control (AC) breath, respiratory muscle work continues throughout the breath.[4]
  - ❖ With *pressure ventilation*, the clinician selects the desired pressure level, and the Vt is determined by the selected pressure level, resistance, and compliance. This is an important characteristic to note when caring for an unstable patient on a pressure mode of ventilation. Careful attention to Vt is necessary to prevent inadvertent hyperventilation or hypoventilation. To ensure respiratory muscle rest on pressure support ventilation (PSV), workload must be offset with the appropriate adjustment of the pressure support (PS) level. To accomplish this, the PS level is increased to lower the spontaneous respiratory rate to ≤20/min and to attain a Vt of 8 to 12 mm/kg.[5, 6]

- For a description of volume and pressure ventilation modes, see Table 31–1.

  Volume ventilation has traditionally been the most popular form of positive-pressure ventilation, largely be-

Table 31–1 ● ■ ■ **Modes of Mechanical Ventilation**

Volume Modes

Control Ventilation (CV) or Controlled Mandatory Ventilation (CMV)

Description: With this mode, the ventilator provides all of the patient's minute ventilation. The clinician sets the rate, Vt, inspiratory time, and PEEP. Generally, this term is used to describe those situations in which the patient is chemically relaxed or is paralyzed from a spinal cord or neuromuscular disease and is therefore unable to initiate spontaneous breaths. The ventilator mode setting may be set on CMV, assist/control (A/C), or synchronized intermittent mandatory ventilation (SIMV) because all these options provide volume breaths at the clinician-selected rate.

Assist/Control (A/C) or Assisted Mandatory Ventilation (AMV)

Description: This option requires that a rate, Vt, inspiratory time, and PEEP be set for the patient. The ventilator sensitivity is also set, and when the patient initiates a spontaneous breath, a full volume breath is delivered.

Intermittent Mandatory Ventilation (IMV) and Synchronized Intermittent Mandatory Ventilation (SIMV)

Description: This mode requires that rate, Vt, inspiratory time, sensitivity, and PEEP are set by the clinician. In between "mandatory breaths," patients can spontaneously breath at their own rates and Vt. With SIMV, the ventilator synchronizes the mandatory breaths with the patient's own inspirations.

Pressure Modes

Pressure Support Ventilation (PSV)

Description: This mode provides an augmented inspiration to a spontaneously breathing patient. With PS, the clinician selects an inspiratory pressure level, PEEP, and sensitivity. When the patient initiates a breath, a high flow of gas is delivered to the preselected pressure level and pressure is maintained throughout inspiration. The patient determines the parameters of Vt, rate, and inspiratory time.

Pressure-Controlled/Inverse Ratio Ventilation (PC/IRV)

Description: This mode combines pressure-limited ventilation with an inverse ratio of inspiration to expiration. The clinician selects the pressure level, rate, inspiratory time (1:1, 2:1, 3:1, 4:1), and the PEEP level. With the prolonged inspiratory times, auto-PEEP may result. The auto-PEEP may be a desirable outcome of the inverse ratios. Some clinicians use PC without IRV. Conventional inspiratory times are used and rate, pressure level, and PEEP are selected.

Positive End-Expiratory Pressure (PEEP) and Continuous Positive Airway Pressure

PEEP

Description: This ventilatory option creates positive pressure at end exhalation. PEEP restores functional residual capacity (FRC). The term PEEP is used when end-expiratory pressure is provided during ventilator positive pressure breaths.

Continuous Positive Airway Pressure (CPAP)

Description: Similar to PEEP, CPAP restores FRC. However, this pressure is continuous during spontaneous breathing; no positive pressure breaths are present.

---

cause Vt and minute ventilation are ensured; this is an essential goal in the acutely ill patient. In contrast, with pressure ventilation, Vt can change drastically with changes in compliance or resistance. Initially, pressure ventilation was described for use only in stable weaning patients; however, pressure ventilation has become extremely popular in the 1990s for use in acutely ill patients as well. This change has occurred for three reasons:

❖ A decelerating flow pattern is associated with pressure ventilation. Pressure ventilation provides for an augmented inspiration (pressure is maintained throughout inspiration). The flow pattern (speed of the gas) is described as decelerating. That is, gas flow delivery is high at the beginning of the breath and tapers off towards the end of the breath. This is in contrast to volume ventilation, in which the flow rate is typically the same at the beginning of the breath as at the end of the breath. The decelerating flow pattern associated with pressure ventilation is thought to provide better gas distribution and therefore more efficient ventilation.[6, 7]

❖ The concept of volu-pressure trauma has evolved. Investigators have demonstrated that large volumes, traditionally used to ventilate the noncompliant lung (eg, in acute respiratory distress syndrome [ARDS]), result in high plateau pressures and lung injury. Plateau pressures of ≥ 35 cm H_2O for more than 48 to 72 hours have been associated with acute lung injury. Volu-

pressure trauma results in the loss of alveolar integrity (ie, alveolar fractures) and movement of fluids and proteins into the alveolar space. As a result, current recommendations are to limit volumes (and thus lower pressures) in patients with stiff lungs. With pressure ventilation, pressure is limited by definition, thus ensuring this clinical goal.[8–10]

❖ Increasingly sophisticated ventilator technology has developed with volume-assured pressure modes of ventilation. Ventilator manufacturers have responded rapidly to the request of clinicians that pressure modes of ventilation be designed in such a way that volume be guaranteed on a breath-to-breath basis. The potential value of such modes is obvious. The more desirable decelerating flow pattern may be provided and plateau pressures controlled while ensuring Vt and minute ventilation.

• Complications of positive-pressure ventilation include hemodynamic changes, pulmonary barotrauma, and volu-pressure trauma.

❖ The extent of hemodynamic changes depends on the level of positive pressure applied, the duration of positive pressure during different phases of the breathing cycle, the amount of pressure transmitted to the vascular structures, the patient's intravascular volume, and the adequacy of hemodynamic compensatory mechanisms. PPV can reduce venous return, shift the interventricular septum to the left, and increase right ventricular afterload as a result of increased pulmonary vascular resistance. The hemodynamic effects of PPV may be prevented or corrected by optimizing filling pressures to accommodate the PPV-induced changes in intrathoracic pressures; by minimizing the peak, plateau, and positive end-expiratory pressure (PEEP); and by optimizing the inspiratory-to-expiratory (I:E) ratio.

❖ Pulmonary barotrauma is damage to the lung from extrapulmonary air that may result from changes in intrathoracic pressures during PPV. Barotrauma is manifested by pneumothorax, pneumomediastinum, pneumopericardium, pneumoperitoneum, or subcutaneous emphysema. The risk of barotrauma in the patient receiving PPV is increased with preexisting lung lesions (eg, localized infections, blebs), high inflation pressure (ie, large Vts, PEEP, main stem bronchus intubation, patient-ventilator asynchrony), and invasive thoracic procedures (eg, subclavian catheter insertion, bronchoscopy, thoracentesis). Barotrauma from PPV may be prevented by controlling peak and plateau pressures, optimizing PEEP, preventing auto-PEEP, ensuring patient-ventilator asynchrony, and ensuring proper artificial airway position.

EQUIPMENT

- Endotracheal tube (see Procedures 1 and 2) or tracheostomy
- ECG and pulse oximetry
- Manual self-inflating resuscitation bag (with PEEP valve if PEEP level is above 5 cm H_2O)

- Appropriately sized resuscitation face mask
- Ventilator
- Suction equipment

Additional equipment to have available depending on patient need includes the following:

- End-tidal CO_2 monitor

PATIENT AND FAMILY EDUCATION

- Explain the procedure to the patient and family and why PPV is being initiated. ➤*Rationale:* Communication and explanations for therapy are cited as important needs of patients.
  - ❖ Discuss the potential sensations the patient will experience, such as relief of dyspnea, lung inflations, noise of ventilator operation, and alarm sounds. ➤*Rationale:* Knowledge of anticipated sensory experiences reduces anxiety and distress.
  - ❖ Encourage the patient to relax. ➤*Rationale:* Promotes general relaxation, oxygenation, and ventilation.
  - ❖ Explain that the patient will be unable to speak. Establish a method of communication in conjunction with the patient and family before initiating mechanical ventilation, if necessary. ➤*Rationale:* Ensuring the patient's ability to communicate is important to alleviate anxiety.
  - ❖ Teach the family how to perform desired and appropriate activities of direct patient care, such as pharyn-

geal suction with the tonsil sucker, range-of-motion exercises, and reconnection to ventilator if inadvertently disconnected. Demonstrate how to use call bell. ➤*Rationale:* Family members have identified the need and desire to help in the patient's care.

- ❖ Provide the patient and family with information on the critical nature of the patient's dependence on PPV. ➤*Rationale:* Knowing the prognosis, probable outcome, or chance for recovery is cited as an important need of patients and families.
- ❖ Offer the opportunity for both patient and family to ask questions about PPV. ➤*Rationale:* Asking questions and having questions answered honestly are cited consistently as the most important need of patients and families.

PATIENT ASSESSMENT AND PREPARATION
Patient Assessment

- Assess for the following signs and symptoms of acute ventilatory failure and fatigue:
  - ❖ Rising arterial carbon dioxide tension
  - ❖ Chest-abdominal dyssynchrony
  - ❖ Shallow or irregular respirations
  - ❖ Tachypnea, bradypnea, or dyspnea
  - ❖ Decreased mental status
  - ❖ Restlessness, confusion, or lethargy
  - ❖ Rising or falling arterial blood pressure
  - ❖ Tachycardia
  - ❖ Atrial or ventricular dysrhythmias ➤*Rationale:* Ventilatory failure indicates the need for initiation of PPV. While PPV is being considered and assembled, support ventilation via a manual self-inflating resuscitation bag, if necessary.
- Determine arterial carbon dioxide tension and pH. ➤*Rationale:* Acute ventilatory failure is confirmed by an uncompensated respiratory acidosis. Ventilatory failure is an indication for PPV.
- Assess for the following signs and symptoms of inadequate oxygenation:
  - ❖ Falling arterial oxygen tension
  - ❖ Tachypnea
  - ❖ Dyspnea
  - ❖ Central cyanosis
  - ❖ Restlessness
  - ❖ Confusion
  - ❖ Agitation
  - ❖ Tachycardia
  - ❖ Bradycardia
  - ❖ Dysrhythmias
  - ❖ Intercostal and suprasternal retractions
  - ❖ Rising or falling arterial blood pressure
  - ❖ Adventitious breath sounds
  - ❖ Falling urine output
  - ❖ Metabolic acidosis ➤*Rationale:* Hypoxemia may indicate the need for PPV. While PPV is being considered and assembled, provide 100% oxygen via manual resuscitation bag and mask or via oxygen delivery device such as a non-rebreather mask.
- Determine arterial oxygen tension or saturation. ➤*Rationale:* Hypoxemia is confirmed by a Pao_2 of less than 60 mm Hg or an arterial oxygen saturation (Sao_2)

of less than 90% on supplemental oxygen. Hypoxemia may indicate the need for PPV.

- Signs and symptoms of inadequate breathing pattern include the following:
  ❖ Dyspnea
  ❖ Chest-abdominal dyssynchrony
  ❖ Rapid-shallow breathing pattern
  ❖ Irregular respirations
  ❖ Intercostal or suprasternal retractions ➡️**Rationale:** Respiratory distress is an indication for PPV. A comfortable breathing pattern is a goal of PPV. An inadequate breathing pattern can be corrected by adjusting the ventilator parameters or by finding and treating the underlying acute cause (eg, malpositioned endotracheal tube, leak in the endotracheal tube cuff, improper assembly of ventilator components).

- Signs of atelectasis include the following:
  ❖ Localized changes in auscultation (decreased or bronchial breath sounds)
  ❖ Localized dullness to percussion
  ❖ Increased breathing effort
  ❖ Tracheal deviation toward the side of abnormal findings
  ❖ Increased peak and plateau pressures
  ❖ Decreased compliance
  ❖ Decreased PaO_2 or SaO_2 (with constant ventilator parameters)
  ❖ Localized consolidation ("white out," opacity) on chest radiograph ➡️**Rationale:** Early detection of atelectasis indicates the need for altering interventions to promote resolution (eg, hyperinflation techniques, PEEP adjustments).

- Signs and symptoms of pulmonary barotrauma (ie, pneumothorax) include the following:
  ❖ Acute, increasing, or severe dyspnea
  ❖ Restlessness
  ❖ Agitation
  ❖ Localized changes in auscultation (decreased or absent breath sounds)
  ❖ Localized hyperresonance or tympany to percussion
  ❖ Increased breathing effort
  ❖ Tracheal deviation away from the side of abnormal findings
  ❖ Increased peak and plateau pressures
  ❖ Decreased compliance
  ❖ Decreased PaO_2 or SaO_2
  ❖ Subcutaneous emphysema
  ❖ Localized increased lucency with absent lung markings on chest radiograph ➡️**Rationale:** Early detection of pneumothorax is essential to minimize progression and the adverse effects on the patient. Tension pneumothorax requires immediate emergency decompression with a large-bore needle (ie, 14-gauge) into the second intercostal space, midclavicular line on the affected side, or immediate chest tube placement (see Procedure 17).

- Signs of cardiovascular depression (particularly after an increase in Vt, PEEP, or continuous positive airway pressure [CPAP], or with hyperinflation) include the following:
  ❖ Acute or gradual fall in arterial blood pressure
  ❖ Tachycardia, bradycardia, or dysrhythmias

  ❖ Weak peripheral pulses, pulsus paradoxus, or decreased pulse pressure
  ❖ Acute or gradual increase in pulmonary capillary wedge pressure
  ❖ Decreased mixed venous oxygen tension ➡️**Rationale:** PPV can cause decreased venous return and afterload because of the increase in intrathoracic pressure. This mechanism is often manifested immediately after initiation of mechanical ventilation and with large Vts, increases in PEEP or CPAP levels, and with manual hyperinflation techniques. Cardiovascular depression associated with manual or periodic ventilator hyperinflation is immediately reversible with cessation of hyperinflation. Decreases in blood pressure with PPV may also be seen with hypovolemia.

- Signs and symptoms of inadvertent extubation include the following:
  ❖ Vocalization
  ❖ Activated low-pressure ventilator alarm
  ❖ Decreased or absent breath sounds
  ❖ Gastric distention
  ❖ Signs and symptoms of inadequate ventilation, oxygenation, and breathing pattern ➡️**Rationale:** Inadvertent extubation is sometimes obvious (eg, the endotracheal tube is in the patient's hand). Often, however, the tip of the endotracheal tube is in the hypopharynx or in the esophagus, and inadvertent extubation is not immediately apparent. Reintubation may be required; however, some patients may not require reintubation. If reintubation is necessary, ventilation and oxygenation are assisted with a self-inflating manual resuscitation bag and face mask.

- Signs and symptoms of malpositioned endotracheal tube include the following:
  ❖ Dyspnea
  ❖ Restlessness or agitation
  ❖ Unilateral decreased or absent breath sounds
  ❖ Unilateral dullness to percussion
  ❖ Increased breathing effort
  ❖ Asymmetric chest expansion
  ❖ Increased peak inspiratory pressure (PIP)
  ❖ Radiographic evidence of malposition ➡️**Rationale:** Early detection and correction of a malpositioned endotracheal tube can prevent inadvertent extubation, atelectasis, barotrauma, and problems with gas exchange.

- Evaluate the patient's need for long-term mechanical ventilation. ➡️**Rationale:** Allows nurse to anticipate patient and family needs for the patient's discharge to an extended care facility, rehabilitation center, or home on PPV.

Patient Preparation

- Ensure that patient understands preprocedural teaching. Answer questions as they arise and reinforce information as needed. ➡️**Rationale:** Evaluates and reinforces understanding of previously taught information.
- Premedicate as needed. ➡️**Rationale:** Administering sedatives, narcotics, or muscle relaxants may be necessary to provide adequate oxygenation and ventilation in some patients.

Procedure for Ventilatory Management—Volume and Pressure Modes

Steps	Rationale	Special Considerations
Volume Modes		
1. Select mode (see Table 31–1). *(Level V: Clinical studies in more than one patient population and situation)*	Mode selection will vary depending on the clinical goal and clinician preference. Either IMV or AC mode can be used to provide total ventilatory support. However, to do so requires that the rate be high enough or the patient sedated so that spontaneous effort is not present.[4, 10]	Intermittent mandatory ventilation (IMV) is often used in conjunction with PSV (to overcome circuit resistance and to decrease the work of breathing associated with spontaneous effort). If respiratory muscle rest is the goal, the level of PSV should be high enough to provide a Vt of 8–12 mL/kg and to maintain the total rate (IMV plus PSV breaths) of 20 or less.[5–7, 10]
2. Set Vt between 8 and 12 mL/kg. *(Level V: Clinical studies in one or more different populations. Expert consensus also exists)*	Vt is selected in conjunction with rate (fx) to attain a minute ventilation (MV) between 5 and 10 L/min with a $Paco_2$ between 35 and 45 mm Hg.[10] Large Vts have been associated with lung injury, especially in patients with ARDS. In patients with poor lung compliance, Vts may be set between 3 and 8 mL/kg to protect the lung from high distending pressures. Hypercarbia will result.[8–11, 13]	When lower Vts are used in an attempt to reduce lung injury, the patient will require heavy sedation and often muscle relaxants to prevent spontaneous effort. Hypercarbia is an expected outcome of low Vts. Permissive hypercarbia is generally well tolerated in patients if the pH is allowed to be reduced gradually (over 24–48 h). PHs around 7.2 are cited as an end point. Occasionally, bicarbonate infusions are used to keep the pH within an acceptable range. Permissive hypercarbia should not be attempted in patients with elevated intracranial pressure or patients with myocardial ischemia, injury, or dysrhythmias. Patients who are allowed to become hypercarbic will require sedation and often muscle relaxants (paralytic agents) to control ventilation.
3. Select respiratory frequency between 10 and 20 breaths/min.	Vt and fx are selected to maintain an acceptable $Paco_2$ with an MV between 5 and 10 L/min. Generally, once Vt is selected, fx is the parameter adjusted to attain a desired $Paco_2$. The rate selected will depend on whether or not the clinical goal is to rest or work the respiratory muscles.	
4. For I:E times, select inspiratory time (this parameter is different depending on the ventilator). Examples include percent inspiratory time, inspiratory time, flow rate, peak flow, etc. Adjust as necessary to attain patient ventilator synchrony. *(Level VI: Limited clinical studies to support recommendation)*	*Inspiratory flow* refers to the speed with which a Vt is delivered during inspiration. Achieves the desired I:E ratio and comfortable breathing patterns.[4, 14, 15]	Generally, flow rates of 50 L/min are used initially and adjusted to provide an inspiratory time that synchronizes with patient effort. I:E ratios are usually 1:2 or 1:3. Longer expiratory times are necessary in patients with obstructive lung diseases (eg, emphysema, asthma). A typical inspiratory time for an adult is 1 second.

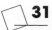

Procedure **for Ventilatory Management—Volume and Pressure Modes** *Continued*

Steps	Rationale	Special Considerations
5. Set the sensitivity (trigger sensitivity) between -1 and -2 cm H_2O pressure. *(Level VI: Clinical studies in a variety of patient populations and situations)* If the ventilator has a flow-triggering option, select the flow trigger in L/min. The smaller the number, the more sensitive the ventilator. Flow triggering is set in conjunction with a base flow (flow in L/min that is provided between ventilator breaths). Flow rate is monitored in the expiratory limb of the ventilator. When flow is disrupted during a spontaneous breath, a drop in flow downstream is sensed; additional flow is added to the inspiratory circuit.	The more negative the number, the less sensitive the ventilator will be to patient effort. This will increase the patient respiratory workload and may lead to dyssynchrony.[18] Flow triggering has been associated with faster ventilator response times and less work of breathing than pressure sensing.[14]	It is important to remember that when auto-PEEP is present, the patient has to generate a negative pressure equal to the set sensitivity plus the level of auto-PEEP.[16] This additional work may fatigue the patient.[14] Patient ventilator dyssynchrony is likely.
6. Set fraction of inspired oxygen (F_{IO_2}) to 0.60–1.0 (60%–100%) if Pao_2 is unknown. *(Level VI: Clinical studies in a variety of patient populations and situations)* Adjust down as tolerated using Sao_2 and arterial blood gas (ABG).	Initiating PPV with maximum oxygen concentration avoids hypoxemia while optimal ventilator settings are being determined and evaluated. Additionally, it permits measurement of the percentage of venous admixture (shunt), which provides an estimate of the severity of the gas-exchange abnormality (see Procedures 29 and 30). Goal is $F_{IO_2} \leq 0.5$. High levels of F_{IO_2} result in increased risk of oxygen toxicity, absorption atelectasis, and reduction of surfactant synthesis.[19–21]	
7. Select PEEP level. Initial setting is often 5 cm H_2O. PEEP may be adjusted as needed after evaluation of tolerance (eg, ABG, physical assessment). PEEP levels are increased to increase functional residual capacity (FRC) and allow for reduction of F_{IO_2} to safe levels (ie, ≤ 0.5) to decrease the risk of developing oxygen toxicity. *(Level V: Clinical studies in more than one patient population and situation)*	A PEEP level of 5 cm H_2O is considered physiologic (essentially the amount of pressure at end exhalation normally provided by the glottis). The work of breathing imposed by the artificial airway is thought to be offset by 5 cm H_2O.	High levels of PEEP ≥ 10 cm H_2O should rarely be interrupted because it may take hours to reestablish FRC (and Pao_2). Super PEEP levels (ie, ≥ 20 cm H_2O) may be necessary in patients with noncompliant lungs (eg, those with ARDS) to prevent lung injury. It is thought that the repetitive opening and closing of stiff alveoli result in alveolar damage. To that end, the use of high PEEP levels to maintain alveolar distention and to prevent injury during mechanical ventilation is considered a protective lung strategy.[8, 22–27] In general, when high PEEP levels are used, Vts will be lower than normal and hypercarbia is anticipated. Using muscle relaxants, sedatives, and narcotics is often necessary.

Pressure Modes

Steps	Rationale	Special Considerations
1. Select mode: PSV, pressure-controlled/inverse ratio ventilation (PC/IRV), volume-assured pressure option (VAPS). *(Level VI: Clinical studies in a variety of patient populations and situations)*	Mode selection depends on clinical goals and clinician preference. If spontaneous breathing is desired, PSV is selected. If a controlled rate and inspiratory time are desired, PC/IRV may be chosen.	PSV is sometimes used between IMV breaths to offset the work of breathing associated with artificial airways and circuits during spontaneous breathing.[6, 28] Some ventilators have VAPs (ie, pressure modes with volume guarantees). Refer to specific ventilator operating manuals for details. *Procedure continued on following page*

Procedure	for Ventilatory Management—Volume and Pressure Modes *Continued*	

Steps	Rationale	Special Considerations
2. For PSV, adjust to attain Vt between 8 and 12 mL/kg with spontaneous respiratory rate (RR) ≤20/min (if respiratory muscle rest is desired; called *PSV max*). Decrease PSV level during weaning trials as tolerated by patient. Tolerance criteria for trials may be predetermined by protocols or on an individual basis. Often during trials, Vts are allowed to be lower (ie, 5–8 mL/kg) and RR higher (ie, 25–30/min) than when rest is the goal. Follow these steps: A. Set sensitivity (as with volume ventilation). B. Set PEEP (as with volume ventilation). C. Set FiO_2 (as with volume ventilation).	Pressure level in conjunction with compliance and resistance determine delivered Vt.	PSV is generally considered a weaning mode of ventilation, thus necessitating patient stability. Regardless, PSV may be used in less stable patients provided close attention is given to changes in Vt and RR. With changes in resistance and compliance, Vt will be affected.
3. For PC/IRV, follow these steps: A. Select inspiratory pressure support level (IPS). In this pressure mode, the level of pressure support is often identified as IPS versus PSV (as in pressure support). B. Select rate.	Absolute pressure level is the sum of IPS level and PEEP. This is a controlled mode. Rate and IPS level determine MV.	If goal is to ensure plateau pressure of ≤35 cm H_2O, the pressure level may gradually be lowered over 24–48 hours to prevent sudden changes in $PaCO_2$ and pH.[10, 11, 13]
C. Select inverse I:E ratio.	I:E ratios are set at 1:1, 2:1, 3:1, or 4:1 by selecting the appropriate inspiratory time. Ratios are adjusted upward to improve shunt and thus oxygenation. Blood pressure may be adversely affected.	Generally, clinicians start with 1:1 ratios and increase as necessary to improve oxygenation. A limiting factor related to prolonged inspiratory times is hemodynamic compromise and hypotension. This is generally why the use of ratios >2:1 are rarely seen clinically. Auto-PEEP is common and often a desired outcome of PC/IRV.
D. Select PEEP level. When transitioning from volume ventilation to PC/IRV, the PEEP is initially maintained at the level used previously until the effect of the IRV is assessed.	Because IRV may result in auto-PEEP adjustments, set PEEP may not be necessary.	
E. Select FiO_2 (as with volume ventilation).		The goal of PC/IRV is to improve oxygenation and allow for reduction of FiO_2 to ≤0.50.[20]
F. Set sensitivity (as with volume ventilation).	Always set sensitivity so that the patient can get a breath if needed. If, however, controlled ventilation is the goal, chemical relaxation may be necessary in conjunction with sedatives and narcotics. It is unlikely that the patient will tolerate IRV (ie, the prolonged inspiratory times) without such interventions.	

Procedure	**for Ventilatory Management—Volume and Pressure Modes** *Continued*

Steps	Rationale	Special Considerations
4. For volume guaranteed pressure modes, parameter selection (ie, pressure, volume, rate, etc) is specific to the ventilator; however, selection of desired (or guaranteed) Vt is required. Some ventilators also require selection of the pressure level. Both spontaneous breathing modes and controlled modes are available. Parameters such as inspiratory time, rate, FIO$_2$, and PEEP are selected accordingly, but principles are similar to volume ventilation. *(Level III: Laboratory data, no clinical data to support recommendations)*	Specific names vary depending on ventilator manufacturer. Examples include Pressure Augmentation (Bear Medical Systems, Riverside, Ca), Volume Support, Pressure Regulated Volume Control (both VS and PRVC: Siemens Medical, Iselin, NJ).[29]	These modes are complex. Concurrent use of pressure, flow, and volume waveform displays may be necesary to accurately assess the modes. Please refer to specific ventilator operating manuals.
Ensure Activation of Alarms (Table 31–2).	Safety of patient is paramount.	
Humidity	Inspired gases may be humidified with the use of standard cascade or high-volume humidifiers. Some institutions use disposable heat and moisture exchanges (HMEs) in place of conventional ventilators.	
1. For conventional humidifiers, make sure humidifier has adequate fluid (sterile distilled water) and that the thermostat setting is adjusted according to manufacturer's recommendations. *(Level II: Theory based, no research data to support recommendations; recommendations from expert consensus group may exist)*	Gases must be humidified before entering the artificial airway. Temperature is measured at the patient wye. Temperatures between 35°C and 37°C (95°F and 98°F) are considered optimal.[30]	Cool circuits may be tolerated well in patients without secretions. However, in those with thick or tenacious secretions, attention to inspired temperature is important to prevent mucus plugging. Circuit temperatures may need to be closer to body temperature (37°C versus 35°C) in these cases.

Procedure continued on following page

Table 31–2 • ■ ■ **Ventilator Alarms**

Disconnect Alarms (Low-Pressure or Low-Volume Alarms)

It is essential that when disconnection occurs, the clinician is immediately notified. Generally, this alarm is a continuous one and is triggered when a preselected inspiratory pressure level or minute ventilation (MV) is not sensed. With circuit leaks, this same alarm may be activated even though the patient may still be receiving a portion of the preset breath. Physical assessment, digital displays, and manometers are helpful in troubleshooting the etiology of the alarms.

Pressure Alarms

- *High-pressure alarms* are set with volume modes of ventilation to ensure notification of pressures exceeding the selected threshold. These alarms are usually set 10–15 cm H$_2$O above the usual peak inspiratory pressure (PIP). Some causes for alarm activation (generally, an intermittent alarm) include secretions, condensate in the tubing, biting on the endotracheal tubing, increased resistance (ie, bronchospasm), decreased compliance (eg, pulmonary edema, pneumothorax), and tubing compression.
- *Low-pressure alarms* are used to sense disconnection, circuit leaks, and changing compliance and resistance. They are generally set 5–10 cm H$_2$O below the usual PIP or 1–2 cm H$_2$O below the PEEP level or both.
- *Minute ventilation* alarms may be used to sense disconnection or changes in breathing pattern (rate and volume). Generally, both low- and high-MV alarms are set (usually 5–10 L per minute above and below usual MV). When stand-alone pressure support ventilation (PSV) is in use, this alarm may be the only audible alarm available on some ventilators.
- FIO$_2$ alarms. Most new ventilators provide FIO$_2$ alarms that are set 5% to 10% above and below the selected FIO$_2$ level.
- *Alarm silence or pause.* Because it is essential that alarms stay activated at all times, ventilator manufacturers have built-in silence or pause options so that clinicians can temporarily silence alarms for short periods (ie, 20 seconds). The ventilators "reset" the alarms automatically. Alarms provide important protection for ventilated patients. However, inappropriate threshold settings decrease usefulness. When threshold gradients are set too narrowly, alarms occur needlessly and frequently. Conversely, alarms that are set too loosely (wide gradients) do not allow for accurate and timely assessments.

From Burns SM. Mechanical ventilation and weaning. In: Kinney MR, Dunbar SB, Brooks-Brun J, Molter N, Vitello-Cicciu JM, eds: *AACN Clinical Reference for Critical Care Nursing.* 4th ed. St. Louis, Mo: Mosby–Year Book; 1998:607–633. Used with permission.

Procedure	for Ventilatory Management—**Volume and Pressure Modes** *Continued*	
Steps	**Rationale**	**Special Considerations**
2. HMEs These humidifiers are placed between the airway and the patient wye. *(Level V: Clinical studies in more than one patient population and situation)*	The moisture in warmed, exhaled gases passes through the vast surface area of the HME and condenses. With inspiration, dry gases pass through the HME and become humidified. The use of HMEs has been associated with decreased incidence of ventilator-associated pneumonias in ventilated patients.[31–34]	
A. Change HMEs per manufacturer's instructions. *(Level IV: Limited clinical studies to support recommendations)*	The longer the HME is in line, the more efficient the humidification; however, inspiratory resistance increases over time. Thus, the HMEs are often changed every 2–3 days (refer to manufacturer's instructions). In weaning patients, the additional resistive load added by these humidifiers may preclude their use.[35–37]	
B. Do not use if secretions are copious or bloody.	Obstruction is possible. HMEs are not indicated in these conditions.	

Expected Outcomes	Unexpected Outcomes
• Maintenance of adequate pH and $Paco_2$ • Maintenance of adequate Pao_2 • Maintenance of adequate breathing pattern • Respiratory muscle rest	• Unacceptable pH, $Paco_2$, and Pao_2 • Hemodynamic instability • Pulmonary barotrauma • Inadvertent extubation • Malpositioned endotracheal tube • Nosocomial lung infection • Acid-base disturbance • Respiratory muscle fatigue

Patient Monitoring and Care

Patient Monitoring and Care	Rationale	Reportable Conditions
		These conditions should be reported if they persist despite nursing interventions.
1. Ensure activation of all alarms each shift (see Table 31–2).	Ensures patient safety.	• Continued activation of alarms
2. Check for secure stabilization, maintenance of endotracheal tube (see Procedure 3).	Reduces risk of inadvertent extubation.	• Unplanned extubation • Dislodgment of airway
3. Monitor in-line thermometer to maintain inspired gas temperature in the range 35–37°C (95–98°F).	Reduces risk of thermal injury from overheated inspired gas and risk of poor humidity from underheated inspired gas.	• Temperature <35°C or >37°C (<95°F or >98°F)
4. Keep ventilator tubing clear of condensation (drain tubing from clean to dirty).	Reduces risk of respiratory infection by decreasing inhalation of contaminated water droplets.	• Continued condensation
5. Ensure availability of manual self-inflating resuscitation bag with supplemental oxygen at the head of the bed. Attach or adjust PEEP valve if the patient is on PEEP >5 cm H_2O.	Provides capability for immediately delivering ventilation and oxygenation to relieve acute respiratory distress caused by hypoxemia or acidosis.	

Patient Monitoring and Care	Rationale	Reportable Conditions
6. Check ventilator for baseline FIO$_2$, PIP, Vt, and alarm activation with initial assessment and after removal of ventilator from patient for suctioning, bagging, or draining ventilator tubing.	Ensures that prescribed ventilator parameters are used (eg, 100% oxygen used for suctioning is not inadvertently delivered after suctioning procedure), provides diagnostic data to evaluate interventions (eg, PIP is reduced after suctioning or bagging), and ensures that the monitoring and warning functions of the ventilator are functional (ie, alarms).	• FIO$_2$, PIP, Vt, or fx settings different from prescribed
7. Explore any changes in peak inspiratory pressure greater than 4 cm H$_2$O or decreased (sustained) Vt on PSV. Immediately explore the cause of high-pressure alarms.	Acute changes in PIP or Vt may indicate mechanical malfunction such as tubing disconnection, cuff or connector leaks, tubing or airway kinks, or changes in resistance and compliance. Always consider possibility of tension pneumothorax. Have equipment readily available (see Procedure 17).	• Unexplained high-pressure alarms
8. Place bite block between the teeth if the patient is biting on the oral endotracheal tube (see Procedure 3).	An oral airway serves the same purpose but may not be tolerated as well as the bite block because it may induce gagging.	• Biting on tube
9. Change the patient's body position as often as possible, but at least every 2 hours.	Frequent position changes are indicated to reduce the potential for atelectasis and pneumonia caused by secretion stasis. Promotes airway clearance.	
10. Evaluate patient-ventilator dyssynchrony by manually ventilating the patient with a self-inflating resuscitation bag (see Procedure 28).	By taking the patient off the ventilator for manual ventilation, synchrony may be more quickly accomplished than on the ventilator. This intervention may reduce risk of barotrauma and cardiovascular depression. If patient breathes in synchrony with bagging, consider changes in ventilatory parameters. If patient does not breathe synchronously with bagging, explore differential diagnoses of problems distal to the airway. Physician consultation may be required.	• Patient-ventilator dyssynchrony
11. Observe for hemodynamic changes associated with increased Vt or PEEP.	May indicate functional changes in circulating volume caused by positive intrathoracic pressure. Always consider potential for pneumothorax with acute changes. Equipment used for rapid release of tension pneumothorax should be at bedside at all times (ie, 14-gauge needle). Chest tube insertion equipment should be readily available.	• Decreased blood pressure • Change in heart rate (increase or decrease of more than 10% of baseline) • Decreased cardiac output • Decreased mixed venous oxygen tension • Increased arterial-venous oxygen difference (see Procedure 25)
12. Monitor for signs and symptoms of acute respiratory distress, hypoxemia, hypercarbia, and fatigue	Respiratory distress indicates the need for changes in PPV. While troubleshooting the difficulties, support ventilation via a manual self-inflating resuscitation bag (see Procedure 28), if necessary.	• Rising arterial carbon dioxide tension • Chest-abdominal dyssynchrony • Shallow or irregular respirations • Tachypnea, bradypnea, or dyspnea • Decreased mental status • Restlessness, confusion, lethargy • Rising or falling arterial blood pressure • Tachycardia • Atrial or ventricular dysrhythmias • Significant changes in pH, PaO$_2$, PaCO$_2$, or SaO$_2$

Documentation

Documentation should include the following:

- Patient and family education
- Date and time ventilatory assistance was instituted
- Ventilator settings including the following: FIO_2, mode of ventilation, Vt, respiratory frequency (total and mandatory), PEEP level, I:E ratio or inspiratory time, PIP, C_{dyn}, and C_{stat}
- ABG results
- Sao_2 readings

- The reason for initiating PPV
- Patient responses to PPV (including the patient's indication of level of comfort and respiratory complaints)
- Hemodynamic values
- Vital signs
- Respiratory assessment findings
- Unexpected outcomes
- Nursing interventions

References

1. Bellemare F, Grassino A. Evaluation of human diaphragm fatigue. *J Appl Physiol.* 1982;53:1196–1206.
2. Cohen CA, Zagelbaum G, Gross D, Roussos CH, Macklem PT. Clinical manifestations of inspiratory muscle fatigue. *Am J Med.* 1982;73:308–316.
3. Tobin MJ, Geunther S, Perez W, et al. Konno-Mead analysis of ribcage-abdominal motion during successful and unsuccessful trials of weaning from mechanical ventilation. *Am Rev Respir Dis.* 1987;135:1320–1328.
4. Marini JJ, Rodriguez M, Lamb V. The inspiratory workload of patient-initiated mechanical ventilation. *Am Rev Respir Dis.* 1986;134:902–909.
5. Brochard L, Harf A, Lorino H, Lemaire F. Inspiratory pressure support prevents diaphragmatic fatigue during weaning from mechanical ventilation. *Am Rev Respir Dis.* 1989;139:513–521.
6. Brochard L, Pluskwa F, Lemaire R. Improved efficacy of spontaneous breathing with inspiratory pressure support. *Am Rev Respir Dis.* 1987;136:411–415.
7. MacIntyre NR. Respiratory function during pressure support ventilation. *Chest.* 1986;89:677–683.
8. Dreyfuss D, Soler P, Basset G, Saumon KG. High inflation pressure pulmonary edema: Respective effects of high airway pressure, high Vt, and positive end-expiratory pressure. *Am Rev Respir Dis.* 1988;137:1159–1164.
9. Parker JC, Hernandez LA, Peevy KJ. Mechanisms of ventilator-induced lung injury. *Crit Care Med.* 1993;21:131–143.
10. Slutsky AS. Consensus conference on mechanical ventilation, January 28–30, 1993 at Northbrook, Il, USA. Parts 1 & 2. *Intensive Care Med.* 1994;20:64–79, 150–162.
11. Hickling KG, Walsh J, Henderson S, Jackson R. Low mortality rate in acute respiratory distress syndrome using low volume, pressure limited ventilation with permissive hypercapnia: a prospective study. *Crit Care Med.* 1994;22:1568–1578.
12. Tang WC, Weil MH, Gazmuri RJ. Reversible impairment of myocardial contractility due to hypercapnic acidosis in the isolated perfused rat heart. *Crit Care Med.* 1991;19:218–224.
13. Bidani A, Tzouanakis AE, Cardenas VJ Jr, Zwischenberger JB. Permissive hypercapnia in acute respiratory failure. *JAMA.* 1994;272:957–962.
14. Sassoon CSH, Lodia R, Rheeman CH, Kuei JH, Light RW, Malhutte CK. Inspiratory muscle work of breathing during flow-by, demand-flow and continuous-flow systems in patients with chronic obstructive pulmonary disease. *Am Rev Respir Dis.* 1993;143:860–866.
15. Marini JJ, Smith TC, Lamb VJ. External work output and force generation during synchronized intermittent mechanical ventilation: effect of machine assistance on breath effort. *Am Rev Respir Dis.* 1998;138:1169–1179.
16. MacIntyre NR, Cheng K-CG, McConnell R. Applied PEEP during pressure support reduces the inspiratory threshold load of intrinsic PEEP. *Chest.* 1997;111:188–193.
17. Burns SM. Auto-PEEP: A complication you can't afford to overlook. *Nurs 94.* 1994;24:32U–32W.
18. Banner MJ, Blanch PB, Kirby RR. Imposed work of breathing and methods of triggering a demand-flow continuous positive airway system. *Crit Care Med.* 1993;21:183–190.
19. Fisher AB. Oxygen therapy. Side effects and toxicity. *Am Rev Respir Dis.* 1980;122:61–69.
20. Davis WB, Rennard SI, Bitterman PB, et al. Pulmonary oxygen toxicity. Early reversible changes in human alveolar structures induced by hyperoxia. *N Engl J Med.* 1983;309:878–883.
21. Holm BA, Notter RH, Siegle J, et al. Pulmonary physiological and surfactant changes during injury and recovery from hyperoxia. *J Appl Physiol.* 1985;59:1402–1409.
22. Chapman JJ. Adult respiratory distress syndrome: an update. *Anaesth Intensive Care.* 1994;22:255–261.
23. Haake R, Schlichtig R, Ulsted DR, Henschen RR. Barotrauma: pathophysiology risk factors and prevention. *Chest.* 1987;91:608–613.
24. Dreyfuss D, Saumon G. The role of V_T, FRC, and end-inspiratory volume in the development of pulmonary edema following mechanical ventilation. *Am Rev Respir Dis.* 1993;148:1194–1203.
25. Lachman B. Open up the lung and keep the lung open. *Intensive Care Med.* 1992;18:319–321.
26. Muscedere JG, Mullen JB, Gan K, Slutsky AS. Tidal ventilation at low airway pressure can augment lung injury. *Am J Respir Crit Care Med.* 1994;149:1327–1334.
27. Ranieri VM, Eissa NT, Corbeil C, et al. Effects of positive end-expiratory pressure on alveolar recruitment and gas exchange in patients with the adult respiratory distress syndrome. *Am Rev Respir Dis.* 1991;144:544–551.
28. Fiastro JF, Habib MP, Quan SF. Pressure support compensation for respiratory work due to endotracheal tubes and demand continuous positive airway pressure. *Chest.* 1998;93:499–505.
29. Amato MBP, Barbas CSV, Bonassa J, Saldiva PHN, Zin WA, deCarvalho CRR. Volume-Assured, Pressure Support Ventilation (VAPSV): A new approach for reducing muscle workload during acute respiratory failure. *Chest.* 1992;102:1225–1234.
30. McEvoy MT, Carey TJ. Shivering and rewarming after cardiac surgery: comparison of ventilator circuits with humidifier and heated wires to heat and moisture exchangers. *Am J Crit Care.* 1995;4:293–299.

31. Unal N, Kanhai JKK, Buijk SLCE, Pompe JC, Holland WPJ, Gultuna I, et al. A novel method of evaluation of three heat-moisture exchangers in six different ventilator settings. *Intensive Care Med.* 1998;24:138–146.

32. Boots RJ, Howe S, George N, Harris FM, Faoagali J. Clinical utility of hygroscopic heat and moisture exchanges in intensive care patients. *Crit Care Med.* 1997;25:1707–1712.

33. Djedaini K, Billiard M, Mier L, LeBourdelles G, Brun P, Markowicz P, et al. Changing heat and moisture exchanges every 48 hours rather than 24 hours does not alter their efficacy and the incidence of nosocomial pneumonia. *Am J Respir Crit Care Med.* 1995;152(1):1562–1569.

34. Iotti GA, Olivei MC, Palo A, Galbusera C, Veronesi R, Comelli A, et al. Unfavorable mechanical effects of heat and moisture exchangers in ventilated patients. *Intensive Care Med.* 1997;23:399–405.

35. Johnson PA, Raper RF, Fisher M. The impact of heat and moisture exchanging humidifiers on work of breathing. *Anaesth Intensive Care.* 1995;23:697–701.

36. Manthous CA, Schmidt GA. Resistive pressure of a condenser humifier in mechanically ventilated patients. *Crit Care Med.* 1994;22:1792–1795.

37. Nishimara M, Nishijima MK, Okadu T, Taenaka N, Yoshiya I. Comparison of flow-resistive work load due to humidifying devices. *Chest.* 1990;97:600–604.

Additional Readings

Burns SM. Advanced respiratory concepts. In: Chulay M, Guzzetta C, Dossey B, eds. *AACN Handbook of Critical Care Nursing.* Stamford, Ct: Appleton & Lange; 1997:487–498.

Burns SM. Mechanical ventilation and weaning. In: Kinney MR, Dunbar SB, Brooks-Brunn J, Molter N, Vitello-Cicciu JM, eds. *AACN Clinical Reference for Critical Care Nursing.* 4th ed. St. Louis, Mo: Mosby–Year Book; 1998:607–633.

Chulay M. Airway and ventilatory management. In: Chulay M, Guzzetta C, Dossey B, eds. *AACN Handbook of Critical Care Nursing.* Stamford, Ct: Appleton & Lange; 1997:135–147.

Pierce LNB. Traditional and non-traditional modes of mechanical ventilation. In: Chulay M, exec ed, Burns SM, series ed. *Protocols for Practice: Care of the Mechanically Ventilated Patient. AACN Critical Care.* Aliso Viejo, Ca: American Association of Critical-Care Nurses; 1998.

Pierce LNB. *Mechanical Ventilation and Intensive Respiratory Care.* Philadelphia, Pa: W.B. Saunders Co., 1995:147–242.

32

Standard Weaning Criteria: Negative Inspiratory Pressure, Positive Expiratory Pressure, Spontaneous Tidal Volume, and Vital Capacity

---

P U R P O S E: Standard weaning criteria are measured to evaluate *respiratory muscle strength* (negative inspiratory pressure (NIP) and positive expiratory pressure (PEP)) and *endurance* (spontaneous tidal volume (SVt) and vital capacity (VC)). The results may help determine the need for intubation, the ability of the patient to tolerate weaning trials, and the potential for extubation.

Suzanne M. Burns

PREREQUISITE NURSING KNOWLEDGE

- NIP is also called *negative inspiratory force* (NIF) or, sometimes, *maximal inspiratory pressure* (MIP). The measurement of NIP is *effort independent* (meaning that the patient does not have to actively cooperate), and thus, it is considered the most reliable of the standard weaning criteria (SWC). NIP is a measure of inspiratory respiratory muscle strength. It is a strong negative predictor but a poor positive predictor.[1-3] The most common threshold cited for NIP is ≤ -20 cm H_2O.
- PEP, also called *positive expiratory force* (PEF), is *effort dependent*, requiring that the patient cooperate fully to obtain a reliable value. PEP is a measure of expiratory muscle strength and ability to cough. The threshold for PEP is ≥ 30 cm H_2O.
- *Spontaneous tidal volume* (SVt) is a measure of respiratory muscle endurance. The threshold for SVt is ≥ 5 mL/kg. When muscles fatigue, the compensatory breathing pattern is rapid and shallow. As a result, investigators have combined SVt and spontaneous respiratory rate (fx) in a ratio called the rapid:shallow breathing index or fx:Vt.[2]
- *Vital capacity* (VC) is also a measure of respiratory muscle endurance or reserve or both. For example, in a fatigued patient, the patient will be unable to triple or even double the size of a breath. The threshold for VC is ≥ 15 mL/kg (at least three times SVt).

- All SWC are best used in combination with other assessment data to determine the need for intubation.[1-6]

EQUIPMENT*

- An aneroid manometer (called a *force meter*)
- A respirometer (to measure volumes)
- Appropriate adapters and one-way valves

PATIENT AND FAMILY EDUCATION

- Inform the patient and family about the patient's respiratory status, changes in therapy, and how to interpret the changes. If the patient or family requests specific information about the measurements, explain the relationship between these measurements and respiratory muscle strength and endurance. ➤*Rationale:* Most patients and families are less concerned with the diagnostic and therapeutic details and more concerned with how the patient is progressing overall. However, the concepts of muscle strength and endurance are readily grasped by patients and families. They may wish to follow the patient's

---

*Some ventilators allow for measurement of these parameters while the patient is on the ventilator. Please refer to specific ventilator guidelines for measurement.

NEGATIVE INSPIRATORY PRESSURE

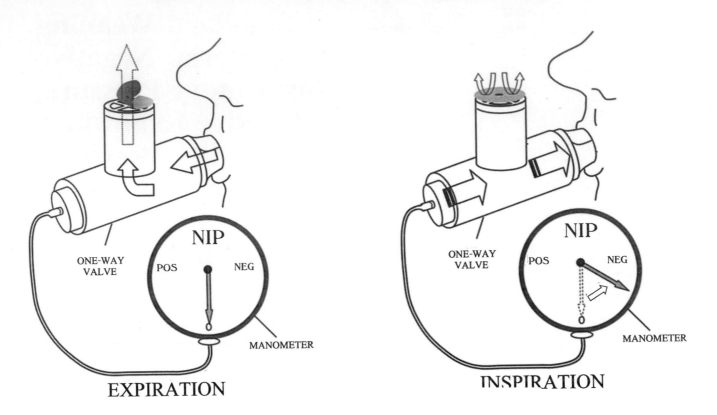

POSITIVE EXPIRATORY PRESSURE

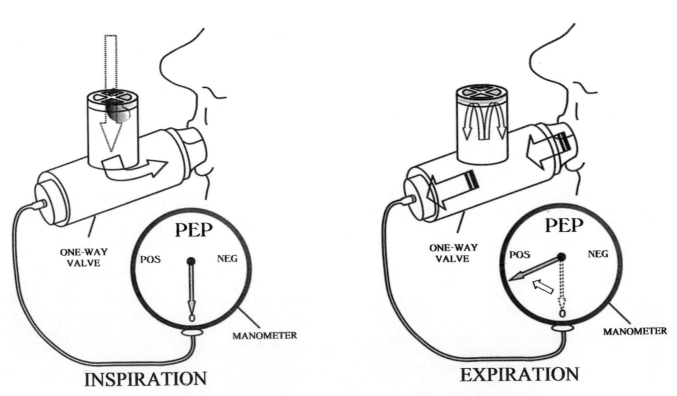

■ ● **FIGURE 32–1.** Negative inspiratory pressure and positive expiratory pressure.

progress in mechanical respiratory assistance with quantitative measurements. If so, the family can be recruited to help the patient provide a maximal effort during measurements.

- Discuss the sensations the patient may experience, such as transient shortness of breath and fatigue. ➛Rationale: Knowledge of anticipated sensory experiences reduces anxiety and distress.
- Explain to the patient the importance of cooperation and maximal effort to achieve valid and reliable measurements. ➛*Rationale:* Information about the patient's therapy, including its rationale, is cited consistently as an important need of patients and family members.

PATIENT ASSESSMENT AND PREPARATION

Patient Assessment

- Assess for the following signs and symptoms of inadequate ventilation:
  - ❖ Rising arterial carbon dioxide tension
  - ❖ Chest-abdominal dyssynchrony
  - ❖ Shallow or irregular respirations
  - ❖ Tachypnea or bradypnea
  - ❖ Dyspnea
  - ❖ Restlessness, confusion, lethargy
  - ❖ Rising or falling arterial blood pressure
  - ❖ Tachycardia
  - ❖ Atrial or ventricular dysrhythmias ➛*Rationale:* Inadequate ventilation may indicate the need for positive-pressure ventilation. If signs and symptoms suggest inadequate ventilation, measurement of SWC may be helpful for determining respiratory muscle strength and endurance and the potential need for positive-pressure ventilation. Conversely, if no signs and symptoms of inadequate ventilation are present in the patient on positive-pressure ventilation, SWC measurements (in conjunction with other patient data) are useful to determine the patient's ability to tolerate weaning trials and possibly extubation.
  - ❖ Assess patient's need for a long-term artificial airway and mechanical ventilatory assistance. ➛*Rationale:* Consistently low measurements in conjunction with overall patient status (eg, mental status, hemodynamics, fluid and electrolyte balance, comfort, mobility) may suggest the need for permanent complete or partial ventilator support.

Patient Preparation

- Ensure that patient understands preprocedural teaching. Answer questions as they arise and reinforce information as needed. ➛*Rationale:* Evaluates and reinforces understanding of previously taught information.

Procedure for Standard Weaning Criteria

Level IV: Limited clinical studies to support recommendations; problems with reproducibility of data obtained from measurement of SWC make attention to exact procedure essential.[7–11]

Steps	Rationale	Special Considerations
1. Wash hands.	Reduces transmission of microorganisms.	
2. Don examination gloves.	Standard precautions.	
3. Attach portable respirometer to airway via adapter and series of one-way valves.	Respirometer is used to measure SVt and VC. Depending on institutional standard and specific ventilator, volumes and pressures may be measured while patient is on the ventilator.	Generally, a series of one-way valves are used for attachment of the respirometer and aneroid manometer.
Note: If patient is on positive pressure ventilation (PPV), place patient's back on ventilator to rest for a few minutes between all measurements.		
4. SVt: Instruct the patient to breathe normally for 1 minute. Count the fx and record the MV. Divide MV by fx to obtain average SVt.		If patient's saturation drops or other signs of intolerance of the procedure emerge, the test is aborted or may be done for a shorter interval (ie, test for 15 seconds, multiply result by 4 for calculation of full minute).
5. For VC, instruct patient to inhale as deeply as possible, zero respirometer, and instruct patient to exhale as completely as possible. The VC may be tested more than once to obtain the best effort.	A good VC effort mandates a maximum inspiration followed by a maximum expiration.	

Procedure continued on following page

| Procedure | **for Standard Weaning Criteria** *Continued* |

Steps	Rationale	Special Considerations
6. Measure NIP as follows: A. The inspiratory one-way valve should be closed or capped, thus ensuring a closed system for measurement of inspiratory effort. Attach pressure manometer to airway with adapter and one-way valves.	Ensures best effort and evaluation reproducibility. Pressure manometer is used to measure NIP. Some ventilators allow for the measurement to be accomplished with the patient on the ventilator.	The pressure manometer is usually attached to the airway via a series of one-way valves (Fig. 32–1). The valves (one is for inspiration and one is for expiration) are capped as necessary to ensure a closed system and a clean measurement device for attachment to the patient's artificial airway.
B. Instruct the patient to inhale as deeply as possible. Observe the manometer needle during inspiration. This test can be done for 20 seconds with multiple attempts by patient.	The goal is to obtain the patient's best effort.	NIP can be frightening for patients because it is impossible to get a breath during the maneuver. Coaching should include warning the patient that this test will make them temporarily unable to take a breath. Watch the manometer as the 20 seconds elapse. Stop the procedure if the NIP measurements begin to get weaker as time elapses or if the patient does not tolerate the procedure (eg, experiences agitation, bradycardia, desaturation).
7. Measure PEP as follows: A. The expiratory valve should be closed or capped. This ensures that the patient is able to take a breath in but must exhale against a closed system. Attach the pressure manometer to the airway via adapter and one-way valves.		
B. Instruct the patient to exhale forcefully after taking a big breath. Do this a number of times (not to exceed 20 seconds). Take the greatest positive number.	Obtains patient's best effort.	As with NIP, any deterioration of the patient indicates that the test should be aborted.
8. Encourage the patient throughout all measurements.	Provides incentive.	
A. Document findings and discuss with team.	Decisions related to weaning trials, intubation, or extubation will be made with the results of these tests in conjunction with others.	

Expected Outcome	Unexpected Outcomes
• Valid and reliable measurements	• Invalid and unreliable measurements • Untoward physical, emotional, or hemodynamic changes

Patient Monitoring and Care

Patient Monitoring and Care	Rationale	Reportable Conditions
		These conditions should be reported if they persist despite nursing interventions.
1. Compare the SWC measurements to the desired patient goals.	If the measurements are less than anticipated, the patient may need either initiation of positive-pressure ventilation or continuance of mechanical ventilation. If the measurements equal or exceed the goals, initiation of weaning trials or extubation may be possible.	• NIP >20 cm H_2O (eg, −10 cm H_2O) • PEP < +30 cm H_2O (eg, +10 cm H_2O) • SVt <5 mL/kg • VC <10 mL/kg • Any deterioration of patient during measurements that does not immediately respond by returning to mechanical ventilator or bagging

Documentation

Documentation should include the following:

- Patient and family education
- The best values obtained
- How the patient tolerated the tests
- Unexpected outcomes
- Nursing interventions

References

1. Morganroth ML, Morganroth JL, Nett LM, Petty TL. Criteria for weaning from prolonged mechanical ventilation. *Arch Intern Med.* 1984;144:1012–1016.
2. Yang KL, Tobin MJ. A prospective study of indexes predicting the outcome of trials of weaning from mechanical ventilation. *N Engl J Med.* 1991;324:1445–1450.
3. Burns SM, Burns JE, Truwit JD. Comparison of five clinical weaning indices. *Am J Crit Care.* 1994;3:342–352.
4. Burns SM, Clochesy JM, Hanneman SK, Ingersoll GE, Knebel AR, Shekleton ME. Weaning from long term mechanical ventilation. *Am J Crit Care.* 1995;4:4–22.
5. Hanneman SK, Ingersoll GL, Knebel AR, Shekleton ME, Burns SM, Clochesy JM. Weaning from short term mechanical ventilation: a review. *Am J Crit Care.* 1994;3:421–443.
6. Hanneman SKG. Multidimensional predictors of success or failure with early weaning from mechanical ventilation after cardiac surgery. *Nurs Res.* 1994;43:4–10.
7. Yang KL. Reproducibility of weaning parameters: a need for standardization. *Chest.* 1992;102:1829–1832.
8. Mador MJ. Weaning parameters: are they clinically useful? *Chest.* 1992;102:1642.
9. Burns SM. Mechanical ventilation and weaning. In: MR Kinney, Dunbar SB, Brooks-Brunn J, Molter N, Vitello-Cicciu JM, eds. *AACN's Clinical Reference for Critical Care Nursing.* 4th ed. St. Louis, Mo: Mosby–Year Book; 1998:624–627.
10. Pierce LNB. Weaning from mechanical ventilation. In: Pierce LNB, ed. *Mechanical Ventilation and Intensive Respiratory Care.* Philadelphia, Pa: W.B. Saunders Co; 1995:292–298.
11. Burns SM. Weaning from long-term mechanical ventilation. In: Chulay M, exec. ed, Burns SM, series ed. *AACN Protocols for Practice: Care of the Mechanically Ventilated Patient.* Aliso Viejo, Ca: American Association of Critical-Care Nurses; 1998.

PROCEDURE 33

Weaning Procedure

PURPOSE: The purposes of weaning patients from mechanical ventilation (MV) are liberation from ventilatory support and removal of artificial airways.

Suzanne M. Burns

PREREQUISITE NURSING KNOWLEDGE

- Knowledge and skills related to the care of patients on MV (eg, airway management, suctioning, mechanical ventilator modes, blood gas interpretation) are necessary.
- The weaning process is markedly different between short-term MV (STMV) and long-term MV (LTMV).[1, 2] In short-term MV (≤3 days), the weaning progress is linear, whereas in long-term MV (>3 days), progress is generally manifested by peaks and valleys.[3]
- Weaning may be viewed as a continuum with three distinct stages: prewean phase, weaning phase, and outcome phase[3] (Fig. 33–1).
- Weaning readiness in STMV is determined by the patient's level of consciousness, hemodynamic stability, adequacy of gas exchange, and pulmonary mechanics.[4]
- LTMV weaning readiness is assessed with a wide variety of factors, including physiologic, psychologic, and pulmonary impediments. To date, no single factor or impediment has been identified that is responsible for ventilator dependence. Instead, a combination is responsible.[4–6]
- Weaning indices have proven disappointing predictors of a patient's ability to wean. Most predictors focus on pulmonary-specific factors. However, some investigators have combined indices and pulmonary factors to enhance the comprehensive nature of the indices, thus their predictive potential. In general, the indices are poor positive predictors (they do not tell us the patient *will* wean), but they are strong negative predictors (they do tell us the patient *will not* wean).[5–7] The weaning indices are best used to evaluate the components important to the weaning process and to track the patient over time. This type of approach prevents lapses in care and may result in shorter ventilator durations. Table 33–1 describes standard or traditional weaning parameters, whereas Tables 33–2 and 33–3 are examples of integrated weaning indices.
- Studies about weaning suggest that weaning progress in patients requiring prolonged ventilation is more likely when rigorous attention to the correction of impediments is paid and a standardized comprehensive approach is used.[6, 8–10]
- No weaning modes or methods of weaning appear to be superior[2]; however, attention to early testing of ability to wean combined with distinct trials that balance respiratory muscle work and rest may result in shorter weaning durations.[11–13]
- Protocols for weaning have been noted to improve weaning outcomes in both STMV and LTMV patients.[11–14] In general, these protocols consist of three components: entry criteria, definition of weaning trial tolerance (when to initiate and when to stop trials), and distinct steps for

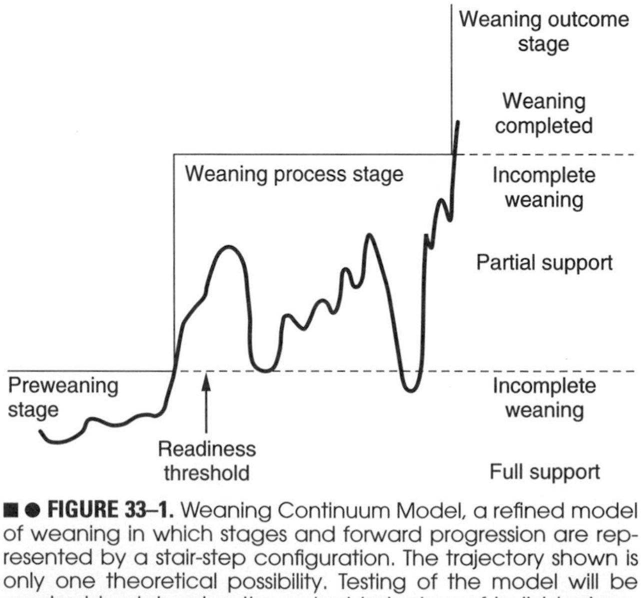

FIGURE 33–1. Weaning Continuum Model, a refined model of weaning in which stages and forward progression are represented by a stair-step configuration. The trajectory shown is only one theoretical possibility. Testing of the model will be required to determine the actual trajectory of individual patients. The length of the steps is not intended to represent the actual duration of each stage. For clarity, relevant elements of the original model (eg, factors affecting weaning, decisions about weaning) have been omitted. (From Knebel A, Shekleton M, Burns SM, Clochesy JM, Hanneman SK. Weaning from mechanical ventilatory support: refinement of a model. *Am J Crit Care.* 1998;7:151.)

Table 33–1 **Standard Weaning Criteria**

Negative inspiratory pressure (NIP) ≤ −20 cm H_2O
Positive expiratory pressure (PEP) ≥ +30 cm H_2O
Spontaneous tidal volume (STV) ≥5 mL/kg
Vital capacity (VC) ≥10–15 mL/kg
Fraction of inspired oxygen (FIO_2) ≤50%
Minute ventilation (MV) ≤10 L/min

From Burns SM. *AACN's Clinical Reference for Critical Care Nursing.* 4th ed. St. Louis, Mo: C. V. Mosby; 1998:626.

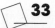

| Table 33–2 ●■■ | Rapid Shallow Breathing (fx/Vt) and Compliance, Rate, Oxygenation, and Pressure (CROP) Indices |

fx/Vt	CROP
Spontaneous respiratory frequency in 1 min divided by Vt in liters	Dynamic characteristic × NIP × (PaO_2/PAO_2) divided by respiratory rate
fx/Vt <105 = weaning success	>13 = weaning success
fx/Vt >105 = weaning failure	<13 = weaning failure

fx, frequency; NIP, negative inspiratory pressure; PaO_2, partial pressure of arterial oxygen; PAO_2, partial pressure of alveolar oxygen; Vt, tidal volume.
Data from Yang KL, Tobin JM. A prospective study of indexes predicting the outcome of trials of weaning from mechanical ventilation. *N Engl J Med.* 1991;324;1445–1450.

progression of the specific modes or methods to be used (Tables 33–4 and 33–5).
- The concepts of work, rest, and conditioning are integrated into many protocols. The use of two classifications—high-pressure, low-volume work and low-pressure, high-volume work—may help with practical applications of specific modes and methods.
  - ❖ High-pressure, low-volume work is found with the use of a T-piece, continuous positive airway pressure (CPAP), and low intermittent mandatory ventilation

| Table 33–3 ●■■ | Burns Weaning Assessment Program (BWAP)* |

Patient name _____ Patient history number _____

General Assessment

YES	NO	NOT ASSESSED	
____	____	____	1. Hemodynamically stable (pulse rate, cardiac output)?
____	____	____	2. Free from factors that increase or decrease metabolic rate (seizures, temperature, sepsis, bacteremia, hypo/hyperthyroid)?
____	____	____	3. Hematocrit >25% (or baseline)?
____	____	____	4. Systemically hydrated (weight at or near baseline, balanced intake and output)?
____	____	____	5. Nourished (albumin >2.5, parenteral/enteral feedings maximized)? (If albumin is low and anasarca or third spacing is present, score for hydration should be "No")
____	____	____	6. Electrolytes within normal limits (including Ca^{++}, Mg^+, PO_4)? *Correct Ca^{++} for albumin level
____	____	____	7. Pain controlled? (subjective determination)
____	____	____	8. Adequate sleep/rest? (subjective determination)
____	____	____	9. Appropriate level of anxiety and nervousness? (subjective determination)
____	____	____	10. Absence of bowel problems (diarrhea, constipation, ileus)?
____	____	____	11. Improved general body strength/endurance (ie, out of bed in chair, progressive activity program)?
____			12. Chest roentgenogram improving?

Respiratory Assessment

Gas Flow and Work of Breathing

____	____	____	13. Eupneic respiratory rate and pattern (spontaneous respiratory rate <25, without dyspnea, absence of accessory muscle use). †This is assessed off the ventilator while measuring #20–23.
____	____	____	14. Absence of adventitious breath sounds (rhonchi, rales, wheezing)?
____	____	____	15. Secretions thin and minimal?
____	____	____	16. Absence of neuromuscular disease/deformity?
____	____	____	17. Absence of abdominal distention/obesity/ascites?
____	____	____	18. Oral endotracheal tube >Fr 7.5 or trach >Fr 6.0

Airway Clearance

____	____	____	19. Cough and swallow reflexes adequate?

Strength

____	____	____	20. Negative inspiratory pressure < −20?
____	____	____	21. Positive expiratory pressure > +30?

Endurance

____	____	____	22. Spontaneous tidal volume >5 mL/kg?
____	____	____	23. Vital capacity >10 to 15 mL/kg?

Arterial Blood Gases

____	____	____	24. pH 7.30 to 7.45?
____	____	____	25. $PaCO_2$ approximately 40 mm Hg (or baseline) with minute ventilation <10 L/min (evaluated while on ventilator)?
____	____	____	26. PaO_2 60 or FIO_2 <40%?

*To score the BWAP: divide the number of "Yes" responses by 26.
Threshold: >65% = weaning probable.
         <65% = weaning improbable.
†If unsure how to obtain information, refer to tutorial menu for help.
Abbreviations: Ca^{++}, calcium; FIO_2, fraction of inspired oxygen; Fr, French; Mg^+, magnesium; $PaCO_2$, arterial partial pressure of carbon dioxide; PaO_2, arterial partial pressure of oxygen; PO_4, phosphate; trach, tracheotomy.
From Burns SM. Weaning from long-term mechanical ventilation. In: Chulay M, exec ed; Burns SM, series ed. *Protocols for Practice.* Aliso Viejo, Ca: American Association of Critical-Care Nurses; 1998.

Table 33–4 ■■■ **"Sprint" (or CPAP) Protocol**

A. Mode

CPAP (0, or level determined by team)

B. Entry Criteria

BWAP score ≥50%

FIO_2 ≤.5

PEEP ≤6 cm H_2O

C. Protocol Steps

1. Ensure complete rest the previous night and until the trial begins. (Complete respiratory muscle rest is defined as total cessation of respiratory effort when in assist-control or IMV modes; respiratory rate less than 20 with inspiratory tidal volumes of 8 to 12 mL/kg in PSV mode.)
2. Place the patient on a CPAP level of 0 (or level determined by team) at the same FIO_2 as when ventilated.
3. Maintain CPAP at 0 for up to 2 hours unless signs of intolerance develop. Trials will be done twice a day at approximately 10:00 and 16:00. (The second trial will begin after 6 hours of rest.)
4. If signs of intolerance develop at any time during the trials, place the patient back on the previous ventilator settings. Make adjustments as necessary to achieve complete respiratory muscle rest. Total rest continues until the next trial.
5. If the patient tolerates 2 hours of CPAP trial, consider extubation.

D. Intolerance Criteria

1. Respiratory rate increase to 30 BPM (sustained).
2. Heart rate increase by 20% (sustained).
3. Oxygen saturation falls to <91% or 2% below baseline (sustained).
4. Systolic blood pressure >180 mm Hg or <90 mm Hg.
5. Agitation.
6. Diaphoresis.
7. Anxiety.
8. Tidal volume <5 mL/kg (sustained).
9. Excessive dyspnea (new or unrelated to activity).
10. ABGs with respiratory acidosis (pH 7.31).

Abbreviations: ABGs, arterial blood gases; BPM, breaths per minute; BWAP, Burns Weaning Assessment Program; CPAP, continuous positive airway pressure; FIO_2, fraction of inspired oxygen; IMV, intermittent mechanical ventilation; PEEP, positive end-expiratory pressure; PSV, pressure support ventilation.

Adapted from University of Virginia, MICU Weaning Protocols.

From Burns SM. Weaning from long-term mechanical ventilation In: Chulay M, exec ed; Burns SM, series ed. *Protocols for Practice.* Aliso Viejo, Ca: American Association of Critical-Care Nurses; 1998.

(IMV) rates. Generally, any method that requires that the patient breathe spontaneously (without inspiratory support) results in high-pressure, low-volume work. This form of muscle conditioning is thought to build sarcomeres because it employs maximum muscle loading.[15, 16] Thus, conditioning episodes are generally of short duration with full muscle rest between episodes. This type of conditioning is referred to as *strengthening training.*

❖ Low-pressure, high-volume work is found with the use of pressure support ventilation (PSV) where inspiration is augmented. For any given pressure level, workload is less than if the patient were breathing spontaneously. At high levels of PSV, little work occurs, but as the level is reduced, muscle workload increases. Conditioning with PSV is often referred to as endurance conditioning; muscles are not worked to maximum effort. Instead, training focuses on maintaining a specific level of work for progressively longer intervals.[15, 16]

• With both types of conditioning, the goal is to progress

with the trials without inducing fatigue. Thus, noninvasive criteria that define intolerance (see Tables 33–4 and 33–5 section D) may result in cessation of the trial and a return to full rest. Rest and fatigue are described in Procedure 31 MV and in sample protocols (see Table 33–4 and 33–5, sections C-1 and D).

• Weaning is the process of gradual reduction of ventilatory support. To that end, a plan for weaning is essential. The plan, whether it means employing a protocol or consists of an individualized written plan, should be available to all health care workers involved in the weaning process.

Table 33–5 ■■■ **Gentle Work Protocol (PSV Protocol)**

A. Mode

Pressure support wean/pressure support rest

B. Entry Criteria

BWAP score ≥50%

FIO_2 ≤.5

PEEP ≤6 cm H_2O

C. Protocol Steps

1. The baseline (or resting) PSV level is set to achieve tidal volume of 8 to 12 mL/kg while assuring a respiratory rate of ≤20 breaths per minute.
2. The PSV level is decreased by 2–5 cm H_2O/day. If the patient successfully maintains the previous day's PSV level for the required 14 hours, the PSV level is decreased by 2 cm H_2O. This process is continued until the patient reaches a PSV level of 3 to 4 cm H_2O. (If the team wishes to advance the wean based on rapid improvements in the patient's physical status, the PSV level may be decreased twice daily.)
3. The patient is rested at night or with any acute events (see "baseline" definition).
4. If a patient exhibits signs of fatigue during a PSV trial, the patient is returned to the previous day's PSV level. After 30 minutes, if the patient continues to be fatigued, the patient is returned to the resting level of PSV.
5. The patient is progressed to a lower PSV level the following day only if 14 hours of PSV is achieved on the current setting.
6. When the patient reaches a PSV of 3 to 4 cm H_2O and can maintain this level for 14 hours, the patient may be rested that night and extubation considered on the following day, or the patient may be extubated that day if the team agrees. For some patients (eg, the obese), the lowest level of PSV may need to be higher.

D. Intolerance Criteria

1. Respiratory rate increases to 30 BPM (sustained).
2. Heart rate increases by 20% (sustained).
3. Oxygen saturation falls to <91% or 2% below baseline (sustained).
4. Systolic blood pressure >180 mm Hg or <90 mm Hg.
5. Agitation.
6. Diaphoresis.
7. Anxiety.
8. Tidal volume <5 mL/kg (sustained).
9. Excessive dyspnea (new or unrelated to activity).
10. Patients are also "rested" and the weaning process held if any of the following conditions apply:
    a. During acute events (hypotension, bronchospasm, etc).
    b. Intrahospital transports.
    c. Temperature spikes.
    d. Decreased weaning indices scores (BWAP <50%, WI >4.5).
    e. Trendelenburg position required (eg, for line placement).

Abbreviations: BWAP, Burns Weaning Assessment Program; FIO_2, fraction of inspired oxygen; PEEP, positive end-expiratory pressure; PSV, pressure support ventilation; WI, wean index.

From Burns SM. Weaning from long-term mechanical ventilation. In: Chulay M, exec ed; Burns SM, series ed. *Protocols for Practice.* Aliso Viejo, Ca: American Association of Critical-Care Nurses; 1998.

Assessment of weaning potential may include checklists of factors important to weaning, such as the Burns Weaning Assessment Program (BWAP) (see Table 33–3), and the measurement and application of various weaning indices, such as standard weaning criteria (see Procedure 32 and Table 33–1), frequency/tidal volume (Vt) (see Table 33–2) and BWAP (see Table 33–3).

EQUIPMENT

- If T-piece or tracheotomy collar setup is required, a flowmeter with functional heated aerosol humidifier for T-piece or tracheotomy collar trials is necessary. The setup should have an in-line thermometer and a water trap.

- Tracheotomy collar or T-piece adapters
- Pressure manometers
- Weaning protocol or wean plan
- Extubation equipment (see Procedure 4)

PATIENT AND FAMILY EDUCATION

- Explain the procedures and why weaning is being initiated. ➤**Rationale:** Anxiety is reduced when patients are prepared for the sensations they may experience during procedures.
- Reassure the patient of the nurse's or the therapist's presence during initiation of weaning (especially in the presence of a tracheotomy collar, a T-piece, and during CPAP trials). ➤**Rationale:** Dependence on the caregiver's support and monitoring decreases anxiety.
- Discuss the sensations the patient may experience, such as smaller lung inflations, dyspnea, change or absence of ventilator sounds, and so on. Describe that weaning trials are a form of conditioning and do take effort. Some dyspnea is to be expected. ➤**Rationale:** Patients (in particular those who have been on prolonged positive pressure ventilation [PPV] support) may report discomfort with resumption of spontaneous breathing.
- Encourage the patient to relax and breathe comfortably. ➤**Rationale:** Relaxation decreases muscle tension.
- Assure the patient and family that rapid return to ventilatory support will be accomplished if patient becomes excessively dyspneic, becomes anxious, or exhibits untoward physiologic changes (eg, desaturation; blood pressure, heart rate, and rhythm changes; diaphoresis). ➤**Rationale:** To develop trust, the patient and family must believe that the nurse will not allow the trials to harm the patient.

PATIENT ASSESSMENT AND PREPARATION

Patient Assessment

- Regular evaluation of factors that impede weaning in conjunction with those that measure respiratory muscle strength, endurance, and gas exchange are necessary to determine when to begin weaning trials (see Tables 33–1, 33–2, and 33–3). ➤**Rationale:** Premature attempts at weaning may be harmful physiologically and psychologically.

- Progress toward achievement of the individual short-term goals every 5 to 30 minutes, as appropriate. ➤**Rationale:** Successful weaning may be achieved within several hours if patient response is monitored closely and interventions are applied in tandem with patient response.
- In patients who are ventilator-dependent, daily progress toward achievement of the individual long-term goals, in collaboration with the physician, respiratory therapist, patient, and family, as appropriate ➤**Rationale:** Successful weaning may be achieved within days to weeks in these patients if patient response is methodically evaluated and interventions are applied in tandem with patient response.
- Observe breathing pattern, and note complaints of dyspnea in response to decrements in PPV support. Other signs of fatigue include the following:
  - ❖ Accessory muscle use
  - ❖ Chest or abdominal asynchrony
  - ❖ Retractions
  - ❖ Rapid shallow breathing pattern

  ➤**Rationale:** These are signs and symptoms of potential or actual respiratory muscle fatigue. Interventions to offset the work of breathing are necessary.
- Note if the patient experiences changes in level of consciousness or nonverbal behavior and complains of dyspnea or fatigue. ➤**Rationale:** Work of breathing may be such that the patient is maintaining adequate breathing pattern and gas exchange at the moment but does not have sufficient reserves to continue expending energy to breathe. Patient exhaustion during weaning results in psychologic and physiologic delays in the weaning progress.
- Arterial blood gases (ABGs) as needed ➤**Rationale:** Although frequent ABGs are rarely necessary during weaning if active attention is paid to signs and symptoms of intolerance, they are the only definitive method of evaluating efficiency of gas exchange. It is especially important to evaluate arterial carbon dioxide tension with spontaneous breathing if rapid return to increased ventilatory settings is not part of the plan or if there are dramatic changes in the patient's condition. Arterial partial pressure of carbon dioxide ($PaCO_2$) is the definitive indicator of the adequacy of ventilation. $PaCO_2$ within the patient's normal physiologic range indicates that the patient's ventilation is adequate with spontaneous breathing. The advantage to the use of weaning protocols is that criteria that identify intolerance are clearly defined and result in a return to ventilatory support. ABGs rarely need to be obtained with each trial.
- Oxygenation indices (see Procedure 29); arterial oxygen saturation (SaO_2) or arterial partial pressure of oxygen (PaO_2) during trials ➤**Rationale:** PaO_2 is the definitive indicator of the adequacy of oxygenation. A PaO_2 within the patient's normal physiologic range indicates that the patient's oxygenation is adequate with spontaneous breathing. Generally, $PaO_2 > 60$ mm Hg and $SaO_2 \geq 90\%$ on a fraction of inspired oxygen (FIO_2) of ≤ 0.4 is acceptable during trials.
- Patient anxiety level ➤**Rationale:** Resumption of spontaneous breathing may cause anxiety, particularly in patients who have been on prolonged PPV support. Encour-

agement is necessary in addition to assurance that prompt return to ventilatory support will be accomplished if the patient gets excessively tired, anxious, or otherwise distressed. Patients must trust that the health care workers will competently and rapidly address their concerns during weaning trials.

Patient Preparation

- Ensure that the patient understands preprocedural teaching. Answer questions as they arise and reinforce information as needed. ➤*Rationale:* Evaluates and reinforces understanding of previously taught information.
- Address all factors that are impeding wean potential. In STMV, this may be such factors as pH level, hemodynamic stability, electrolytes, strength, and endurance. In the patient who requires LTMV, other factors such as mobility, nutrition, and fluid status may be more of an issue. ➤*Rationale:* Weaning of both STMV and LTMV patients has been associated with the correction of a myriad of physiologic factors. Weaning is not solely dependent on respiratory muscle strength and endurance. Frequency and timing of measurement of weaning criteria are dependent on whether the patient requires STMV or LTMV.
- Establish weaning criteria. ➤*Rationale:* Weaning criteria (pulmonary and nonpulmonary) should be used to determine a patient's weaning potential, track progress, and determine when extubation is appropriate.

Procedure for Weaning

Steps	Rationale	Special Considerations
1. Communicate with the patient throughout the weaning process.	Attention is given to the patient's subjective response to weaning. The nurse remains with the patient (especially at the beginning of the trial); monitors frequently during trials; coaches the patient; reinforces the goals and desired outcomes; reminds the patient that talking, eating, self-care activities, and mobilization will be facilitated by successful weaning and extubation; and celebrates weaning progress with the patient.	
T-Piece or Tracheotomy Collar Trials		
1. Wash hands, and don gloves.	Reduces transmission of microorganisms; standard precautions.	
2. Connect patient to heated aerosol. Instruct patient to breathe normally, and monitor frequency, breathing pattern, heart rate, cardiac rhythm, SaO_2, and general appearance of patient. *(Level V: Clinical studies in more than one patient population and situation)*	Heated aerosol replaces water that normally would be added by the upper airway if it were not bypassed by the endotracheal or tracheostomy tube. This method of weaning employs high-pressure, low-volume work. Signs and symptoms of tolerance must be heeded if respiratory muscle fatigue is to be prevented.[11–14]	Abort weaning for any signs of patient intolerance and place patient back on PPV support.
3. After a predetermined time interval or with the emergence of signs of intolerance, place patient back on resting ventilator settings. *(Level V: Clinical studies in more than one patient population and situation)*	To ensure respiratory muscle conditioning and forward progress during weaning trials, the work of breathing must not be excessive. Do not exceed predetermined wean trial duration. Adequate rest between trials and at night offsets fatigue and encourages effective respiratory muscle conditioning. Patient is placed back on the ventilator to rest until all data regarding weaning response can be assessed.[11–14]	

| Procedure | for **Weaning** *Continued* |

Steps	Rationale	Special Considerations

4. If patient successfully meets full trial criteria, notify physician, nurse practitioner, or team of patient response and consider extubation. If protocol is in place, extubation may be the next step and will not require such notification.

CPAP Trials (Levels 0–10 cm H₂O) (With or Without Flow-By Option)

1. Explain purpose and procedure of CPAP trials to patient and family, and switch patient from resting settings to CPAP level. Instruct the patient to breathe normally, and monitor for signs and symptoms of intolerance (described earlier). If using protocol, refer to specific criteria.
(Level V: Clinical studies in more than one patient population and situation)

As with the T-piece, this method employs high-pressure, low-volume work. Prompt return to ventilator is necessary if excessive work and fatigue are to be prevented.[11–14]

2. After predetermined time interval on CPAP or with signs or symptoms of intolerance, place patient back on resting ventilator settings.
(Level V: Clinical studies in more than one patient population and situation)

Do not exceed predetermined wean trial duration. Adequate rest between trials and at night offsets fatigue and encourages effective respiratory muscle conditioning. The patient is placed back on the ventilator to rest until all data regarding weaning response can be assessed.[11–14]

3. Notify physician, nurse practitioner, or team of results of trials. If last step of wean plan or protocol has been attained, extubation should be considered. (If protocol is used, this step may be automatic.)

Intermittent Mandatory Ventilation and Synchronized Intermittent Mandatory Ventilation Weaning Method

1. Gradually and progressively decrease IMV/synchronized intermittent mandatory ventilation (SIMV) breaths.
(Level V: Clinical studies in more than one patient population and situation)

This method of weaning provides gradual decrements or full PPV support by permitting spontaneous breathing between periodic preset ventilator breaths. The preset breaths are progressively decreased as the patient assumes a greater proportion of the minute volume with spontaneous breathing.[17–20]

IMV/SIMV demand valves offer high resistance to breathing and produce a lag between the patient's initiation of a breath and delivery of the inspired gas during spontaneous breathing. These factors may increase the work of breathing and result in subsequent fatigue.[21] To avoid this, some use PSV between IMV breaths to offset the work associated with small tube sizes, circuit resistance, and high breathing rates. This method of weaning has been associated with prolonged weaning trial duration in at least one study.[22] It is therefore essential that a plan be in place for progressive weaning and that a clinical end point be predetermined (eg, IMV of 4). Another method used to decrease work between IMV breaths is the use of flow-by (see Procedure 31).[19, 23]

Procedure continued on following page

Procedure **for Weaning** *Continued*

Steps	Rationale	Special Considerations
2. Assess the patient for signs and symptoms of fatigue, inadequate gas exchange, and impaired breathing pattern with each decrement in IMV/SIMV support. *(Level IV: Limited clinical studies to support recommendations)*	Determines patient response to weaning.[17–20] A plan that clearly describes the end point of this method is essential. The multidisciplinary team may then more readily determine when extubation is appropriate. *(Level V: Clinical studies in more than one patient population and situation)*[8, 9]	Lower levels of IMV (ie, 4 or less), when not used with PSV or flow-by, are similar to strength conditioning trials.[16, 24] Adequate rest times should be ensured between trials and especially at night.

Pressure Support Weaning Method

Steps	Rationale	Special Considerations
1. Start at pressure support maximum (PSVmax) and decrease level according to the protocol or as clinically indicated (ie, no signs of intolerance). *(Level IV: Limited clinical studies to support recommendations)*	This weaning method provides for endurance conditioning. To that end, the level is gradually decreased as patient's endurance increases. PSVmax is the level that attains a spontaneous respiratory rate (RR) of 20 or less, absence of accessory muscle use, and a Vt of 8 to 12 mL/kg. Higher RRs and smaller Vts are generally acceptable during trials. Because the mode employs low-pressure, high-volume work, weaning intervals may be longer than with strengthening modes. Regardless, full support should be ensured at night and for rest, especially early in the weaning.[24–26]	With PSV, the selected level should not be arbitrarily determined. The pressure level should be increased if any sustained signs of intolerance occur. Work is gradually increased by lowering the level of PSV in increments.
2. Monitor patient responses to weaning. Return to full ventilatory support if signs of intolerance occur and when intended duration of trial has been reached. *(Level V: Clinical studies in more than one patient population and situation)*	PSV, despite requiring spontaneous effort, reduces the work of breathing associated with circuits, endotracheal tubes, and high breathing rates.[21] Fatigue, however, is posssible if the level is not high enough.[25, 26] PSVmax is used as a respiratory muscle rest level.	An incompletely inflated artificial airway cuff can create a leak that prevents the PSV cycle-off mechanism from activating (ie, the ventilator senses that flow is one fourth the original flow and cycles off).
3. When the clinical goal for PSV wean is accomplished (ie, 12 hours at lowest level) extubation or an additional step is discussed with the team. *(Level V: Clinical studies in more than one patient population and situation)*	If protocol is used, the next step may be automatic.[13, 14]	

Expected Outcomes

- Timely and successful discontinuance of PPV
- Comfortable and adequate breathing pattern during the weaning process

Unexpected Outcomes

- Tracheal injury
- Pulmonary barotrauma
- Cardiovascular depression
- Fatigue
- Hypoxemia
- Hypercapnia
- Dyspnea
- Unsuccessful, demoralizing weaning trials

Patient Monitoring and Care

Patient Monitoring and Care	Rationale	Reportable Conditions
		These conditions should be reported if they persist despite nursing interventions.
1. Evaluate overall patient stability (ie, physiologic, psychologic, and mechanical) in a systematic manner. Frequency of evaluation may vary depending on whether the patient requires STMV or LTMV. A multidisciplinary approach is encouraged.	Patient stability and overall condition must be considered before initiating active weaning trials. Premature attempts may be a harmful and frustrating for all involved. A multidisciplinary team approach ensures active attention to the diverse factors that affect weaning readiness. Refer to Tables 33–1, 33–2, and 33–3 for pulmonary-specific and comprehensive weaning assessment tools.	• Changes in weaning indices (pulmonary-specific and integrated) along with general factors that affect weaning
2. During weaning trials, pay attention to signs and symptoms of intolerance and respiratory muscle fatigue. If signs of intolerance occur, prompt return to PPV is required.	Trials continued despite emergence of signs of intolerance lead to fatigue and failure. Cardiopulmonary failure and collapse are potential outcomes.	• Signs of weaning trial intolerance (tachypnea, dyspnea, chest and abdominal asynchrony) • Agitation • Mental status changes • Significant decrease in SaO_2 (SaO_2 <90% or 10% decrease) • Changes in pulse rate or rhythm • Blood pressure increase or decrease
3. If no signs of intolerance occur during trials, continue until the patient achieves the trial criteria and report to team so that additional planning can occur (eg, extubation) or follow protocol steps to extubation.		

Documentation

Documentation should include the following:

- Patient and family education
- Individualized goals for weaning
- Procedure used for weaning (eg, T-piece, decreasing IMV/SIMV support, pressure support, flow-by positive end-expiratory pressure, or CPAP);
- Parameters used to assess patient readiness to wean and weaning trial tolerance such as ABGs, oximetry readings, BWAP score, negative inspiratory pressure, positive expiratory pressure, spontaneous Vt, vital capacity, MV, dynamic characteristics, static compliance measurements, airway resistance measurement, breathing pattern, and accessory muscle use

- Patient response to decrements in MV support
- Mode or method of weaning
- Duration of trial
- Level of support (if appropriate, as in PSV, flow-by, or CPAP)
- Unexpected outcomes
- Nursing interventions

References

1. Hanneman SK, Ingersoll GL, Knebel AR, Shekleton ME, Burns SM, Clochesy JM. Weaning from short-term mechanical ventilation: a review. *Am J Crit Care.* 1994;3:421–443.
2. Burns SM, Clochesy JM, Hanneman SK, Ingersoll GL, Knebel AR, Shekleton ME. Weaning from long-term mechanical ventilation. *Am J Crit Care.* 1995;4:4–22.
3. Knebel AR, Shekleton ME, Burns SM, Clochesy JM, Hanneman SK. Weaning from mechanical ventilatory support: refinement of a model. *Am J Crit Care.* 1998;7:149–152.
4. Hanneman SKG. Multidimensional predictors of success or failure with early weaning from mechanical ventilation after cardiac surgery. *Nurs Res.* 1994;43:4–10.
5. Morganroth ML, Morganroth JL, Nett LM, Petty TL. Criteria for weaning from prolonged mechanical ventilation. *Am J Crit Care.* 1984;144:1012–1016.
6. Burns SM, Burns JE, Truwit JD. Comparison of five clinical weaning indices. *Am J Crit Care.* 1994;3:342–352.
7. Yang KL, Tobin JM. A prospective study of indexes predicting the outcome of trials of weaning from mechanical ventilation. *N Engl J Med.* 1994;324:1445–1450.
8. Cohen IL, Bari N, Strosberg MA, et al. Reduction of duration and cost of mechanical ventilation in an intensive care unit by use of a ventilatory management team. *Crit Care Med.* 1991;19:1278–1284.
9. Burns SM, Marshall M, Burns JE, et al. Design, testing and results of an outcomes-managed approach to patients requiring prolonged ventilation. *Am J Crit Care.* 1998;7:45–47.
10. Scheinhorn DJ, Artinian BM, Catlin JL. Weaning from prolonged, mechanical ventilation: the experience at a regional weaning center. *Chest.* 1994;105:534–539.
11. Brochard L, Rauss A, Benito S, et al. Comparison of three methods of gradual withdrawal from ventilatory support during weaning from mechanical ventilation. *Am J Respir Crit Care.* 1994;150:896–903.
12. Esteban A, Frutos F, Tobin M, et al. A comparison of four methods of weaning patients from mechanical ventilation. *N Engl J Med.* 1995;332:345–350.
13. Ely EW, Baker AM, Dunagan DP, et al. Effect on the duration of mechanical ventilation of identifying patients capable of breathing spontaneously. *N Engl J Med.* 1998;335:1864–1869.
14. Kollef MH, Shapiro SD, Silver P, et al. A randomized, controlled trial of protocol-directed vesus physician-directed weaning from mechanical ventilation. *Crit Care Med.* 1997;25:557–574.
15. MacIntyre NR. Respiratory function during pressure support ventilation. *Chest.* 1986;89:677–683.
16. MacIntyre NR. Ventilatory modes and mechanical ventilatory support. *Crit Care Med.* 1997;25:1106–1107.
17. Banner MJ, Blanch PB, Kirby RR. Imposed work of breathing and methods of triggering a demand-flow continuous positive airway system. *Crit Care Med.* 1993;21:183–190.
18. Beydon L, Chasse M, Harf A, Lemaire F. Inspiratory work of breathing during spontaneous ventilation using demand values and continuous flow systems. *Am Rev Respir Dis.* 1988;138:300–304.
19. Gurevitch MJ, Gelmont D. Importance of trigger sensitivity in ventilator response delay in advanced chronic obstructive pulmonary disease with respiratory failure. *Crit Care Med.* 1989;17:354–359.
20. Gibney NRT, Wilson RS, Pontoppidan H. Comparison of work of breathing on high gas flow and demand valve continuous positive airway pressure systems. *Chest.* 1982;82:692–695.
21. Fiastro JF, Habib MP, Quan SF, Campbell SC. Comparison of standard weaning parameters and the work of breathing in mechanically ventilated patients. *Chest.* 1988;93:499–505.
22. Esteban A, Alia I, Ibanez J, Benito S, Tobin MJ and the Spanish Lung Failure Collaborative Group. Modes of mechanical ventilation and weaning: A national survey of Spanish hospitals. *Chest.* 1994;106:1188–1193.
23. Sassoon CSH, Lodia R, Rheeman CH, Kuei LL, Light RW, Mahutte CE. Inspiratory muscle work of breathing during flow-by, demand-flow, and continuous-flow systems in patients with chronic obstructive pulmonary disease. *Am Rev Respir Dis.* 1992;145:1219–1222.
24. MacIntyre NR. Weaning from mechanical ventilatory support: volume-assisting intermittent breaths versus pressure assisting every breath. *Respir Care.* 1988;33:121–125.
25. Brochard L, Harf A, Lorino H, Lemarie F. Inspiratory pressure support prevents diaphragmatic fatigue during weaning from mechanical ventilation. *Am Rev Respir Dis.* 1989;139:513–521.
26. Brochard L, Pluskwa F, Lemaire F. Improved efficacy of spontaneous breathing with inspiratory pressure support. *Am Rev Respir Dis.* 1987;136:411–415.

Additional Readings

Burns SM. Weaning from long-term mechanical ventilation. In: Chulay M, exec ed; Burns SM, series ed. *Protocols for Practice.* Aliso Viejo, Ca: American Association of Critical-Care Nurses; 1998.

Burns SM. Mechanical ventilation and weaning. In: Kinney MR, Dunbar SB, Brooks-Brunn J, Molter N, Vitello-Cicciu JM, eds. *AACN's Clinical Reference for Critical Care Nursing.* 4th ed. St. Louis, Mo: C.V. Mosby; 1998:607–633.

MacIntyre NR. Weaning mechanical ventilatory support. In: Dantzker DR, MacIntyre NR, Bakow ED, eds. *Comprehensive Respiratory Care.* Philadelphia, Pa: W.B. Saunders; 1995:735–742.

Tobin MJ, Alex CG. Discontinuation of mechanical ventilation. In: Tobin MJ, ed. *Principles and Practice of Mechanical Ventilation.* New York, NY: McGraw-Hill; 1994:1177–1206.

34

Automated External Defibrillation

P U R P O S E: An automated external defibrillator (AED) is a defibrillator that, by use of a computerized detection system, analyzes cardiac rhythms, distinguishes between those that require defibrillation and those that do not, and delivers a series of preprogrammed electric shocks. The AED is designed to allow early defibrillation by providers who have minimal or no training in rhythm recognition or manual defibrillation.

Charlotte A. Green
Karen K. Carlson

PREREQUISITE NURSING KNOWLEDGE

- Defibrillation is the therapeutic use of an electric shock that temporarily stops or stuns an irregularly beating heart and allows more coordinated electrical activity to resume. Physiologically, it is thought that the shock depolarizes the myocardium, terminates ventricular fibrillation (VF) or ventricular tachycardia (VT), and allows normal electric activity to occur. VF and pulseless VT are the only two rhythms amenable to conversion by an AED.
- Time is the major determining factor in the success of the defibrillation. For every minute defibrillation is delayed, the chance of success decreases by 7% to 10%.[1-4]
- The AED (Fig. 34–1) is attached to the patient using adhesive electrode pads. Through these pads, the rhythm is analyzed and shock delivered, if indicated. If the AED recognizes VF or VT, visual and verbal prompts will guide the operator to deliver a shock to the patient. The AED, not the operator, makes the decision about whether the rhythm is appropriate for defibrillation.
- The chance of the AED shocking inappropriately is very low. The AED should be applied only to unresponsive, nonbreathing, and pulseless patients. To keep artifact interference to a minimum, the patient should not be touched or moved during the analysis time.[3-6]
- Although defibrillation is the definitive treatment for pulseless VT and VF, the use of the AED is not a stand-alone skill but is used in conjunction with cardiopulmonary resuscitation (CPR).
- At this time, the AED is indicated for use only in adults. It should not be used in children under the age of 8 years or weighing less than 25 to 30 kg.[4]

- The use of AEDs in prehospital settings has increased the success of defibrillation. It is recommended that AEDs be placed on any nonmonitored unit where the response time of the resuscitation (ie, code) team is greater than 1 minute.[3, 7] It is also recommended that AEDs be placed in freestanding health care settings where health care providers are not familiar with rhythm recognition or defibrillation.
- Many manual defibrillators can be purchased that have AED capability allowing a tiered response (ie, those with different skill levels can use the same defibrillator).
- Most AEDs in use in the emergency medical system (EMS) or in the hospital have a method of recording the event. These can be in the form of rhythm strip printouts, audio and event recording devices, data cards, or computer chips that can print an event summary.[3]
- AEDs can be purchased with and without monitor screens. AEDs with screens may allow the provider with rhythm recognition skills to override the AED's analysis and recommendations.
- The most important safety issue that an AED operator must address is the possibility of inadvertently shocking a bystander or other provider at the scene. It is imperative that the operator clear the patient verbally and visibly, by looking from the patient's head to toe, before discharging energy to the patient.
- All defibrillation programs need to include training for the potential operators. Training should include psychomotor skills, troubleshooting, equipment maintenance, and how to interface with the advanced cardiac life support (ACLS) providers.[7]

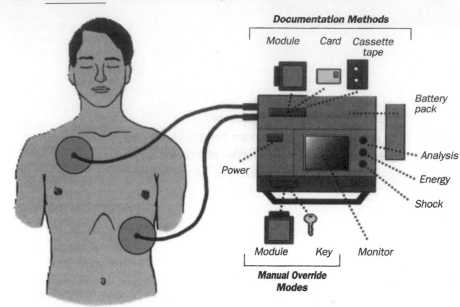

Documentation Methods

Module   Card   Cassette tape

Battery pack

Power

Analysis

Energy

Shock

Module   Key   Monitor

Manual Override Modes

■ ● **FIGURE 34–1.** Generic AED control panel. (From Cummins RO, Graves J. *ACLS Scenarios: Core Concepts for Case-Based Learning.* St. Louis, Mo: Mosby-Lifeline; 1996:52.)

- Specific information regarding the use of an institution's AED, including monitoring, recording, overriding, troubleshooting, and safety features, is available from the manufacturer. It is each provider's responsibility to be familiar with this information before using the AED.
- Once a resuscitation team (eg, 911 responders, code team, ACLS providers) arrives, they will assume responsibility for monitoring and treating the patient. Ideally, they should continue to use the AED to monitor and shock, if at all possible, allowing the AED provider to operate the AED according to ACLS instructions.[3] There are two reasons to change to a standard monitor and defibrillator: if the AED does not have a monitoring screen and if transport would interfere with the AED's ability to analyze. Some manufacturers have AEDs and manual defibrillators with compatible cables allowing a quick, smooth transition from one device to the other.

EQUIPMENT

- AED
- Disposable gloves
- Barrier device or airway management equipment
- Spare sets of gauze pads in sealed packages
- Hand towel
- Scissors
- Razor

Additional equipment, which will vary based on the model and abilities of the device, includes the following:

- Monitoring electrodes

- Spare charged battery
- Adequate electrocardiogram (ECG) paper
- Spare data card

PATIENT AND FAMILY EDUCATION

Most often, AEDs are used in emergency situations. Therefore, there is limited or no time to educate the family about the equipment and its uses. Occasionally after a sudden cardiac event, a patient may be discharged from an institution with an AED. In those situations, patient and family education would be vital.[4, 8]

PATIENT PREPARATION AND ASSESSMENT

Patient Assessment

- Establish that patient is unresponsive, nonbreathing, and pulseless. ➥**Rationale:** Patient must be unresponsive, pulseless, and nonbreathing to be a candidate for use of an AED.

Patient Preparation

- Ensure that skin is dry where electrodes or pads will be placed.[3, 4, 9] ➥**Rationale:** Good contact must be ensured to analyze the rhythm and to defibrillate most effectively. If excessive hair interferes with good contact, either shave the area before applying the pad or apply the pad and then immediately remove the pad and hair and apply a new pad in the same area.

Procedure **for Automated External Defibrillation**

Steps	Rationale	Special Considerations
1. Establish that patient is unresponsive, not breathing, and pulseless.	Patient must be unresponsive, pulseless, and nonbreathing to be a candidate for use of an AED.	
2. Call for AED; activate emergency response procedures for your settings.	Defibrillation is the definitive treatment for VF. Time is critical.	Knowing how to activate the emergency response team in your setting is vital.

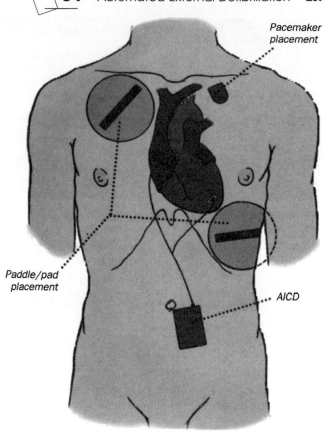

Pacemaker
placement

Paddle/pad
placement

AICD

■ ● **FIGURE 34-2.** AED pad placement. (From Cummins RO, Graves J. *ACLS Scenarios: Core Concepts for Case-Based Learning.* St. Louis, Mo: Mosby-Lifeline; 1996:52.)

Procedure	for **Automated External Defibrillation** *Continued*		

Steps	Rationale	Special Considerations
3. Perform CPR until the AED arrives.	Patient must be nonbreathing and pulseless to be a candidate for use of the AED. CPR will help keep the patient in a rhythm able to be defibrillated for a longer time, increasing the chance that defibrillation will be effective.	Personal protective equipment is used in all settings, including gloves and a mask-valve device or a barrier device.
4. Press the on button.	Most AEDs require a short period for a self-check of their circuitry. Simply opening the lid will turn on some AEDs.	
5. Attach the pads to the patient (Fig. 34-2): one pad below the right clavicle to the right of the sternum and the other below the left nipple on the mid-axillary line.		
6. Place pads firmly to eliminate air pockets and to form a complete seal. A. Do not place the pads over any medication or monitoring patches. B. Do not place an AED pad directly over an implanted device as this may interfere with the effectiveness of defibrillation (see Fig. 34-2). Try to stay at least 1 inch to the side of the power source of the pacemaker or internal cardiac defibrillator.	The AED uses the electrode pads to monitor and to shock. Good contact must be ensured to defibrillate most effectively.	Some models require attaching cables to the pads before placing them on the patient. Polarity of the pads is interchangeable for defibrillation purposes.[10] If ECG monitoring is being done, the QRS complex will be inverted if the positive and negative pads are reversed.

Procedure continued on following page

Procedure **for Automated External Defibrillation** *Continued*

Steps	Rationale	Special Considerations
7. Press the analyze button to analyze the patient's rhythm.	The machine needs to analyze the rhythm to determine the need for defibrillation.	Avoid CPR, transport, or any contact with the patient during the analyze mode.
8. If a shock is advised, clear the patient visually and verbally.	The AED has determined that the rhythm is either VF or VT; defibrillation is needed. Maintain safety for all of those around the patient. If people are touching the patient when the energy is discharged, they may also receive that shock.	Use a mnemonic such as "I'm clear, you're clear, we are all clear," and look at the patient head-to-toe while talking to ensure that no one is touching the patient. Another mnemonic is, "Shocking on three. One, I am clear. Two, you are clear. Three, we are all clear. Shocking now."
9. Push the shock button or buttons, as needed.	Delivering the shock quickly is the best way to reverse the pulseless rhythm.	The manufacturer presets the number of shocks and the energy level for each shock. The AED will give the operator a visual and verbal cue to push the shock button.
10. Reanalyze the rhythm.	The rhythm must be analyzed to determine if an additional shock is advised. Shocks are delivered in sets of three only if the AED determines that another shock is indicated.	Remember to clear the patient for analysis.
11. If a shock is advised, clear the patient and push the shock button.	The AED will now deliver shocks according to preprogrammed energy settings, typically based on the American Heart Association (AHA) AED algorithm (a series of three shocks at 200, 300, and 360 joules [J]).[3, 4]	
12. Repeat steps 10 and 11, as needed.	The AED will increase to 360 J for the third and subsequent shocks. No pulse check is needed between shocks.	Be sure to clear the patient for both analysis and shocking.
13. After the third shock, or if a no shock advised message occurs, check the pulse.	Checking the pulse determines whether the last shock restored a rhythm with a pulse and determines the need for continued CPR.	
14. If no pulse, do CPR for 1 minute or as standard.	Provides oxygen and circulation.	Most AEDs will have a CPR timer that will count down and alert you when the time for CPR is complete. Time interval is usually 1 minute based on AHA guidelines[3, 4] but can be configured to meet local protocols.
15. Repeat steps 7 to 14 if so advised until ACLS team arrives.	Algorithm is series of three shocks followed by 1 minute of CPR with the series repeated until resuscitation units arrive.	
16. If at any time a no shock advised message is given, check the pulse.	If the no shock advised message is given, the patient is not in a rhythm appropriate for defibrillation. A pulse must always be checked after a no shock advised message.	A no shock advised message does not imply that the patient has been resuscitated.
17. If a no shock advised message is received and there is no pulse, begin CPR.	CPR is the only option available at this time until advanced support arrives.	
18. If a no shock advised message is received and the patient has a pulse, check for breathing. If the patient is not breathing, begin rescue breathing 12 to 15 breaths per minute.	Defibrillation has been successful in restoring the patient's rhythm, but spontaneous respirations are not present.	

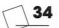

Procedure for Automated External Defibrillation *Continued*

Steps	Rationale	Special Considerations
19. Check blood pressure (BP) and treat as needed.	A perfusing rhythm has been restored. The patient needs to be evaluated and monitored until resuscitation team arrives.	Be aware that patients could return to their original, pulseless rhythm. Patients need to be monitored closely. If at any time patients lose their pulse, begin again at step 7.

Expected Outcomes

- Restoration of perfusing rhythm
- Restoration of spontaneous respirations

Unexpected Outcomes

- Operator or bystander shocked
- Skin burns

Patient Monitoring and Care

Patient Monitoring and Care	Rationale	Reportable Conditions
		These conditions should be reported if they persist despite nursing interventions.
1. Monitor vital signs and rhythm following resuscitation.	A patient experiencing VF or VT is at risk for the development of further cardiac instability and arrhythmias, including the recurrence of VF or VT.	• Change in vital signs from baseline • Arrhythmias
2. Administer appropriate antiarrhythmic agents as indicated.	Antiarrhythmic agents will decrease the risk of the development of further arrhythmias.	• Arrhythmias
3. Transport patient into appropriate follow-up care.	Hospitalized patients are transferred to a critical care unit; nonhospitalized patients should be transferred to an emergency department for follow-up care.	

Documentation

Documentation should include the following:

- Patient and family education
- Type of arrest (witnessed or unwitnessed)
- Preshock and postshock rhythms
- Baseline assessment
- CPR information (including start and stop times)
- Application of AED
- Time from AED activation to first shock
- Number of times patient was defibrillated
- Any complications
- Assessment following resuscitation (if applicable)
- Unexpected outcomes
- Nursing interventions

References

1. Weaver WD, Copass MK, Bufi D, Ray R, Hallstrom AP, Cobb LA. Improved neurologic recovery and survival after early defibrillation. *Circulation.* 1984;69:943–948.
2. Weaver WD, Cobb LA, Hallstrom AP, Fahrenbrunch C, Copass MK, Ray R. Factors influencing survival after out-of-hospital cardiac arrest. *J Am Coll Cardiol.* 1986;7:179–186.
3. Cummins RO, ed. *Textbook of Advanced Cardiac Life Support.* Dallas, Tx: American Heart Association; 1997:4.1–4.22.
4. Aufderheide TP, Stapleton ER, Hazinski MF. *Heartsaver AED for the Lay Rescuer and First Responder.* Dallas, Tx: American Heart Association; 1998.
5. Cummins RO, Eisenberg MS, Bergner L, Hallstrom A, Hearne T, Murray JA. Automatic external defibrillation: evaluation of its role in the home and in emergency medical services. *Ann Emerg Med.* 1984;13(9 pt 2):798–801.
6. Cummins RO, Eisenberg MS, Litwin PE, Graves JR, Hearne TR, Hallstrom AP. Automatic external defibrillators used by

emergency medical technicians: a controlled clinical trial. *JAMA.* 1987;257:1605–1610.

7. Mancini M, Kaye W. In-hospital first-responder automated external defibrillation: what critical care practitioners need to know. *Am J Crit Care.* 1998;7:314–319.

8. Cummins RO. From concept to standard-of-care? Review of the clinical experience with automated external defibrillators. *Ann Emerg Med.* 1989;18:1269–1275.

9. Physio-Control Corporation. *Defibrillation: What You Should Know.* Redmond, Wa: Physio-Control; 1998.

10. Weaver D, Martin JS, Wirkus MJ, et al. Influence of external defibrillator electrode polarity on cardiac resuscitation. *Pace.* 1993;16:285–289.

Additional Reading

Cummins RO, Grave J. *ACLS Scenarios: Core Concepts for Case-Based Learning.* St. Louis, Mo: Mosby-Lifeline; 1996:51–52.

35

Cardioversion

PURPOSE: Cardioversion is the therapy of choice for termination of hemodynamically unstable tachydysrhythmias. It may also be used to convert hemodynamically stable atrial fibrillation or atrial flutter into normal sinus rhythm.

Cynthia Hambach

PREREQUISITE NURSING KNOWLEDGE

- Understanding of the anatomy and physiology of the cardiovascular system, principles of cardiac conduction, basic dysrhythmia interpretation, and electrical safety is required.
- Advanced cardiac life support (ACLS) knowledge and skills are necessary.
- Synchronized cardioversion is recommended for termination of unstable paroxysmal supraventricular tachycardia, atrial fibrillation, atrial flutter, and unstable ventricular tachycardia with a pulse.[1-3] Because ventricular tachycardia is often a precursor to ventricular fibrillation, cardioversion has the potential to prevent this life-threatening dysrhythmia.[1]
- The electric current delivered with cardioversion depolarizes the myocardium in an attempt to restore the heart's coordinated impulse conduction as a single source of impulse generation. A countershock synchronized to the QRS complex allows for the electric current to be delivered outside the heart's vulnerable period.[1, 4, 7] This synchronization occurs a few milliseconds after the highest part of the R wave but before the vulnerable period associated with the T wave.[1, 4, 7]
- Cardioversion may be implemented in the patient with an emergent condition. The aforementioned dysrhythmias are converted by synchronized cardioversion when the patient develops symptoms from the rapid ventricular response.[7] Symptoms may include the following: hypotension, chest pressure, shortness of breath, decreased level of consciousness, pulmonary congestion, shock, congestive heart failure, and myocardial infarction.[1]
- Elective cardioversion may be used to convert hemodynamically stable atrial fibrillation or atrial flutter into normal sinus rhythm.[5, 7, 8] It may be initiated if antidysrhythmic medications have been unsuccessful.[4] Conversion to a regular rhythm is beneficial in patients with mitral stenosis, left ventricular hypertrophy, congestive heart failure, and myocardial ischemia.[7] When used to convert atrial fibrillation, anticoagulation is considered for a period of 3 weeks prior to cardioversion to decrease the risk of thromboembolism.[7-9] It may not be necessary if atrial fibrillation has been present for less than 48 hours.[9] Anticoagulation should be continued for 4 weeks

after cardioversion because of the possibility of delayed embolism.[7-9] Thromboembolism is less likely to occur in the patient with atrial flutter.[7, 9]
- If time and clinical condition permit, the patient should be given a combination of analgesia and sedation to minimize discomfort.[1-3, 5-7, 10]

EQUIPMENT

- Defibrillator/cardioverter monitor with electrocardiogram (ECG) oscilloscope/recorder capable of delivering a synchronized shock
- ECG cable
- Conductive gel or paste or prepackaged gelled conduction pads
- Intravenous sedative or analgesic pharmacologic agents as prescribed
- Bag-valve-mask device
- Flowmeter for oxygen administration
- Emergency suction and intubation equipment
- Emergency medications
- Emergency pacing equipment

PATIENT AND FAMILY EDUCATION

- Assess patient and family understanding of etiology of dysrhythmia. ➤**Rationale:** Assesses the patient and family understanding of condition and additional educational needs.
- Explain the procedure to the patient and family. ➤**Rationale:** Decreases anxiety and promotes patient compliance.[4]
- Explain the signs and symptoms of hemodynamic compromise associated with preexisting cardiac dysrhythmias to both patient and family. ➤**Rationale:** Enables the patient and family to recognize when the patient needs to notify the nurse or physician.
- Evaluate and discuss with the patient the need for long-term pharmacologic support. ➤**Rationale:** Allows the nurse to anticipate educational needs of the patient and family regarding specific discharge medications.
- Assess and discuss with the patient the need for lifestyle changes. ➤**Rationale:** Underlying pathophysiology may

necessitate alterations in the patient's current lifestyle and require a plan for behavioral changes.

PATIENT ASSESSMENT AND PREPARATION
Patient Assessment

- Assess ECG for tachydysrhythmias, including paroxysmal supraventricular tachycardia, atrial fibrillation, atrial flutter, and ventricular tachycardia, which could require synchronized cardioversion.   ➤➤*Rationale:* Tachydysrhythmias may precipitate deterioration of hemodynamic stability.[1]

- Assess vital signs and any associated symptoms of hemodynamic compromise with each significant change in ECG rate and rhythm.   ➤➤*Rationale:* Deterioration of vital signs or presence of associated symptoms indicates hemodynamic compromise that could become life threatening.[1]

- Assess presence or absence of peripheral pulses and level of consciousness.   ➤➤*Rationale:* This baseline determination assists in the detection of cardioversion induced peripheral embolization.[8]

- Obtain serum potassium, magnesium, and digitalis levels; arterial blood gases.   ➤➤*Rationale:* Electrolyte imbalances, acid-base disturbances, and digitalis toxicity significantly contribute to electrical instability and may potentiate postconversion dysrhythmias.[2] Hypokalemia should be corrected to prevent postconversion dysrhythmias. Although cardioversion is considered safe practice in patients taking digitalis glycosides, they are generally held on the day of cardioversion.[8]

Patient Preparation

- Ensure that patient and family understands preprocedural teaching. Answer questions as they arise and reinforce information as needed.   ➤➤*Rationale:* Evaluates and reinforces understanding of previously taught information.

- Validate that an informed consent has been obtained according to institutional policy.   ➤➤*Rationale:* Informed consent is advised prior to performing cardioversion unless the patient presents in a life-threatening state.[5]

- Establish patent intravenous access.   ➤➤*Rationale:* Medication administration may be required.[1, 5]

- Assist the patient to a supine position.   ➤➤*Rationale:* Supine positioning provides the best access for procedure initiation, intervention, and management of adverse effects.

- Remove all metallic objects from the patient.   ➤➤*Rationale:* Metallic objects are excellent conductors of electric current and could result in burns.

- Remove nitroglycerin patch from patient's chest or make sure the defibrillator pad or paddle does not touch the patch. (Level IV: Limited clinical studies to support recommendations).   ➤➤*Rationale:* The patch may impede transmission of the current. Older transdermal patches may have an aluminum backing that could cause an arcing of current when the paddle is placed over it. This may produce visual arcing, smoke, or chest burns.[1, 11–14]

- Give the patient nothing by mouth (NPO).   ➤➤*Rationale:* Decreases the risk of aspiration.

- Remove loose-fitting dentures, partial plates, or other mouth prostheses.   ➤➤*Rationale:* Decreases the risk of airway obstruction during the procedure. Evaluate individual situation (eg, dentures may facilitate a tighter seal for airway management).

- Preoxygenate the patient as appropriate to the condition.   ➤➤*Rationale:* Adequate oxygenation of cardiac tissue diminishes the risk of cerebral and cardiac complications.[1] Hypoxia can enhance electric instability after cardioversion.[2]

- Maintain a patent airway with oxygenation throughout the procedure.   ➤➤*Rationale:* Respiratory depression and hypoventilation can occur after administration of sedatives and analgesics.[2]

- If time allows, consider administering sedation and analgesia.   ➤➤*Rationale:* These medications will provide amnesia and decrease pain during procedure.[1–3, 5–7, 10]

Procedure	for Cardioversion

Steps	Rationale	Special Considerations
1. Wash hands.	Reduces transmissions of microorganisms; standard precautions.	
2. Connect patient to lead wires.	R wave must be sensed by the defibrillator to achieve synchronization for cardioversion.[1, 5–7]	
3. Select monitor lead displaying an R wave of sufficient amplitude to activate the synchronization mode of the defibrillator. In most models, synchronization is achieved when the monitoring lead produces a *tall* R wave. *(Level VI: Clinical studies in a variety of patient populations and situations to support recommendations)*	Synchronized cardioversion must sense the R wave to deliver the current outside the heart's vulnerable period.[1, 2, 5–7]	If a combination defibrillator/monitor is not being used, a converter cable must connect the monitor to the defibrillator to achieve synchronization.

| Procedure | **for Cardioversion** *Continued* |

Steps	Rationale	Special Considerations
4. Place the defibrillator in synchronization mode. Ensure that the patient's QRS complexes appear with a marker to signify correct synchronization of the defibrillator with the patient's ECG rhythm (Fig. 35–1). To confirm that the synchronization has been achieved, observe for visual flashing on the screen or listen for auditory beeps. If necessary, adjust the R wave gain until the synchronization marker appears on each R wave. *(Level VI: Clinical studies in a variety of patient populations and situations to support recommendations)*	Synchronization prevents the random delivery of an electric charge, which may potentiate ventricular defibrillation.[1, 2, 5–7]	
5. If defibrillator is unable to distinguish between the peak of the QRS complex and the peak of the T wave, as in polymorphic ventricular tachycardia, proceed with unsynchronized cardioversion.	This will avoid a delay or failure of shock delivery in synchronized mode.[1]	
6. Prepare the patient or paddles or both with proper conductive agent. *(Level VI: Clinical studies in a variety of patient populations and situations to support recommendations)* Conductive gel should be evenly dispersed on the defibrillator paddles and should adequately cover the surface, but should not be excessive, which can cause slippage or arcing of the current.[1, 5–7, 10, 20] Excessive perspiration also can affect conduction, causing arcing of current.	Reduces transthoracic resistance, thus enhancing electric conduction through subcutaneous tissue.[1, 3, 5, 7, 10, 15–19] Minimizes erythema from the electric current.[7]	Prepackaged gelled conductive pads are available for placement in area of paddle.[3, 6, 16] Never use alcohol-soaked pads because they are combustible when in contact with electric current. Do not use inappropriate gel because it will increase the transthoracic resistance and decrease the current given to the patient.[7, 18, 19] It may also cause burns or sparks, which can increase the risk of fire.[1, 18] Self-adhesive defibrillation pads connected directly to the defibrillator have been found to be as effective as paddles.[5, 10, 16, 20, 21–23] Advantages are their safety and convenience of use in any of the appropriate locations.[1, 16, 20–22] When using these pads, ensure that good contact is maintained to reduce transthoracic resistance and improve current flow.[7] *Procedure continued on following page*

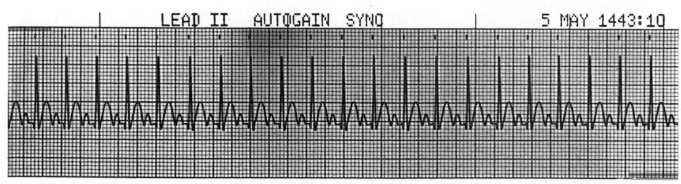

LEAD II   AUTOGAIN   SYNC   5 MAY 1443:10

■ ● **FIGURE 35–1.** R wave synchronization. Note the vertical synchronization marker above each R wave.

Procedure **for Cardioversion** *Continued*

Steps	Rationale	Special Considerations
7. Turn on ECG recorder for continuous printout.	Establishes a visual recording of the patient's current ECG status and response to intervention and provides a permanent record of the patient response to intervention.	
8. Follow these steps for paddle placement. A. Place one paddle at the heart's apex just to the left of the nipple at the midaxillary line. Place the other paddle just below the right clavicle to the right of the sternum (Fig. 35–2). *(Level VI: Clinical studies in a variety of patient populations and situations to support recommendations)* Avoid placing paddles over lead wires.[6]	Cardioversion is achieved by passing an electric current through the cardiac muscle mass to restore a single source of impulse generation. This pathway maximizes current flow through the myocardium.[1–3, 5–7, 10, 15, 16] Incorrect paddle placement may decrease current flow and fail to terminate the dysrhythmia.[7, 16]	A larger paddle size (12 to 13 cm) also decreases the transthoracic resistance and improves current flow.[1, 3, 7, 10, 15, 17, 23, 25, 26] If the paddle size is too large, it will result in inadequate contact with the skin, resulting in the current following an extracardiac pathway and missing the heart.[1, 7] Most paddles range from 8 to 12 cm in diameter and are effective.[10, 16, 24]
B. In women, the apex paddle is placed at the fifth to sixth intercostal space with the center of the paddle at midaxillary line.	Placement over a woman's breast should also be avoided to reduce transthoracic resistance.[9]	
C. Anterior-posterior placement may also be used. The anterior paddle is placed in the anterior left precordial area, and the posterior paddle is placed posteriorly behind the heart in the left infrascapular area. *(Level IV: Limited clinical studies to support recommendations)*	Both methods of paddle placement are effective.[1, 2, 3, 5–7, 10, 16, 24]	

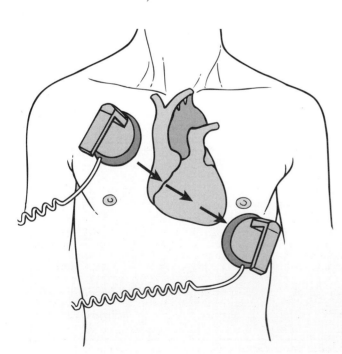

■ ● **FIGURE 35–2.** Paddle placement and current flow in cardioversion. (From Lewis S, Heitkemper M, Dirksen S. *Medical-Surgical Nursing: Assessment and Management of Clinical Problems.* 5th ed. St. Louis, Mo: Mosby; 2000: 935.)

Procedure **for Cardioversion** *Continued*

Steps	Rationale	Special Considerations
D. In the patient with a permanent pacemaker, do not place paddles directly over the pulse generator. *(Level IV: Limited clinical studies to support recommendations)*	Cardioversion over an implanted pacemaker may impair passage of current to the patient and cause the device to malfunction or become damaged.[1, 7, 8, 10, 15, 16, 27-32] Myocardial injury may also occur if the current flows down the lower resistance pathway of the lead wire.[7, 8, 28, 30]	Some authors recommend paddle placement at least 5 in (10 to 13 cm) from the pulse generator and lead wire.[6, 8, 15, 16, 27-29] Anterior-posterior placement is also suggested.[7, 27-30] The device should be assessed following any electric countershock.[1, 8, 10, 15, 27, 28, 30] Standby emergency pacing equipment should be available should pacemaker failure occur.[27-29, 31]
E. In the patient with a temporary pacemaker, turn off the pacemaker, disconnect the lead wires, and use standard paddle placement (Fig. 35–2).[16] The pacemaker wires should be insulated with a rubber glove.	This prevents the current from flowing to the pulse generator, avoiding the heart, and causing possible damage to the generator.[16]	
F. Paddle placement in the patient with an implantable cardioverter-defibrillator (ICD) is the same as standard paddle placement for cardioversion (see Fig. 35–2). Paddles should not be placed over the device.	Placement over the device could damage the unit or cause it to malfunction.[1]	The ICD should be checked after external countershock. ICD units with patch electrodes that cover part of the epicardium may decrease the current to the patient.
9. Charge defibrillator paddles as prescribed or in accordance with the recommendations of the American Heart Association. *(Level VI: Clinical studies in a variety of patient populations and situations to support recommendations)*	Defibrillator is charged with the lowest energy level required to convert the tachydsrhythmia (Table 35–1).[1, 33, 34]	
10. Disconnect oxygen source during actual cardioversion.[6]	Decreases the risk of combustion in the presence of electric current.[18]	Arcing of electric current in the presence of oxygen could precipitate an explosion and subsequent fire hazard.[18]
11. Apply 25 lb/in² pressure to each paddle against the chest wall.[2, 3, 6, 7, 16]	Firm paddle pressure will decrease transthoracic resistance, thus improving the flow of current across the axis of the heart.[3, 5, 7, 10, 15, 16, 19, 26] Tilting the paddles may cause skin burns.[5]	

Procedure continued on following page

Table 35–1 ● ■ ■ **American Heart Association Energy Level Recommendations for Treating Tachydysrhythmias**

Ventricular Tachycardia with Pulse	Polymorphic Ventricular Tachycardia with Pulse	Paroxysmal Supraventricular Tachycardia	Atrial Fibrillation	Atrial Flutter
First attempt: Cardiovert with 100 J	First attempt: Cardiovert with 200 J	First attempt: Cardiovert with 50 J	First attempt: Cardiovert with 100 J	First attempt: Cardiovert with 50 J
Second attempt: Cardiovert with 200 J	Second attempt: Cardiovert with 200–300 J	Second attempt: Cardiovert with 100 J	Second attempt: Cardiovert with 200 J	Second attempt: Cardiovert with 200 J
Subsequent attempts: Cardiovert with 300 J, then 360 J	Third attempt: Cardiovert with 360 J	Subsequent attempts: Cardiovert with 200 J, then 300 J, then 360 J	Subsequent attempts: Cardiovert with 300 J, then 360 J	Subsequent attempts: Cardiovert with 200 J, then 300 J, then 360 J

(Source: American Heart Association recommendations from Cummins RO. *Advanced Cardiac Life Support*. Dallas, Tex: American Heart Association; 1997.)

Procedure **for Cardioversion** *Continued*

Steps	Rationale	Special Considerations
12. State "all clear," and visually verify that everyone is clear of contact with patient, bed, and equipment.	Maintains safety to caregivers, because electric current can be conducted from the patient to another individual if contact occurs.[5]	
13. Verify that the defibrillator is in synchronization mode and that the patient's QRS complexes appear with a marker to signify correct synchronization of the defibrillator with the patient's ECG rhythm (see Fig. 35–1). *(Level VI: Clinical studies in a variety of patient populations and situations to support recommendations)*	Synchronization prevents the random delivery of an electric charge, which may potentiate ventricular fibrillation.[1, 2, 5–7]	
14. Depress both buttons on the paddles simultaneously and hold until defibrillator fires. In the synchronized mode, there will be a delay before the charge is released. This allows the sensing mechanism to detect the QRS complex.[2]	Depolarizes the cardiac muscle.	If self-adhesive defibrillation pads are used, charge will be delivered by depressing the discharge button on the defibrillator.
15. Observe monitor for conversion of the tachydysrhythmia and assess pulse. If pulse is noted, assess vital signs and level of consciousness.	Simultaneous depolarization of the myocardial muscle cells should reestablish a single source of impulse generation.[2, 5]	If unsuccessful in converting rhythm, proceed with repeated energy recommendations (see Table 35–1). Ensure that the defibrillator is still in synchronization mode. Many defibrillators will revert back to the unsynchronized mode after cardioversion.[1] Ventricular fibrillation may develop after cardioversion. If so, deactivate synchronizer and follow the procedure for defibrillation.[1, 5, 7] (See Procedure 36.)
16. Clean defibrillator, and remove any gel from paddles.	Conductive gel accumulated on the defibrillator paddles impedes surface contact and increases transthoracic resistance.	
17. Discard supplies in appropriate receptacle.	Standard precautions.	
18. Wash hands.	Reduces transmission of microorganisms; standard precautions.	

Expected Outcomes

- Reestablishment of a single source of impulse generation for the cardiac muscle
- Hemodynamic stability

Unexpected Outcomes

- Continued tachydysrhythmias
- Ventricular fibrillation progressing to cardiopulmonary arrest
- Bradycardia
- Asystole
- Pulmonary edema
- Systemic embolization
- Respiratory complications
- Hypotension
- Pacemaker or ICD dysfunction
- Skin burns

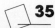

Patient Monitoring and Care

Patient Monitoring and Care	Rationale	Reportable Conditions
		These conditions should be reported if they persist despite nursing interventions.
1. Evaluate neurologic status before and after cardioversion. Reorient as needed to person, place, and time.	Temporary altered level of consciousness may occur following synchronized cardioversion. Cerebral emboli may develop as a postprocedure complication.[4,8]	• Change in level of consciousness
2. Monitor pulmonary status before and after cardioversion.	Respiratory centers of the brain may be depressed as a result of hypoxia or sedative or analgesic agents.[2]	• Slow, shallow respirations • Decrease in oxygen saturation as measured by pulse oximetry
3. Monitor cardiovascular status (blood pressure, heart rate, and rhythm) before and after cardioversion.	Dysrhythmias may develop after cardioversion.[4,5,7,8,35]	• Hypotension • Supraventricular dysrhythmias • Ventricular dysrhythmias • Bradycardia • Asystole
4. Continue to monitor ECG after procedure.	Dysrhythmias may develop after cardioversion.[4,5,7,8,35]	• Supraventricular dysrhythmias • Ventricular dysrhythmias • Bradycardia • Asystole
5. Prepare for possible intravenous antidysrhythmic medication.	Dysrhythmias may develop after conversion.[4,5,7,8,35] Antidysrhythmic medications may be used to prevent dysrhythmias from occurring after cardioversion.[1,7]	• Supraventricular dysrhythmias • Ventricular dysrhythmias • Bradycardia • Asystole
6. Evaluate for burns.	Erythema at electrode sites may be seen secondary to local hyperemia in the current pathway.[7] Skin burns may be caused by tilting of the paddles[5,7] or by an insufficient amount of conductive material.[7]	• Skin burns

Documentation

Documentation should include the following:

- Patient and family education
- Neurologic, pulmonary, and cardiovascular assessment before and after cardioversion
- Interventions to prepare the patient for cardioversion
- The joules (J) used and the number of cardioversion attempts made
- Printout ECG tracing depicting the cardiac rhythm before and after cardioversion
- Condition of skin of the chest wall
- Unexpected outcomes and nursing interventions

References

1. Cummins RO. *Advanced Cardiac Life Support.* Dallas, Tex: American Heart Association; 1997.
2. Correa LF. Electrical intervention in cardiac disease. In: Crawford MV, Spence MI, eds. *Commonsense Approach to Coronary Care.* 6th rev ed. St Louis, Mo: Mosby–Year Book; 1995:443–496.
3. Graber RF. Emergency defibrillation and cardioversion. *Patient Care.* 1989;23(1):193–196.
4. Dunn D, Corrubia N. Patient teaching: cardioversion. *RN.* 1993;56(1):45–48.
5. Dracup K. *Meltzer's Intensive Coronary Care: A Manual for Nurses.* 5th rev ed. Norwalk, Conn: Appleton & Lange; 1995.
6. Braun AE. What to do when a patient needs defibrillation or cardioversion. *Nursing.* 1991;21(7):50–54.
7. Tacker WA. *Defibrillation of the Heart: ICDs, AEDs, and Manual.* St Louis, Mo; Mosby–Year Book; 1994.
8. Lown B, deSilva RA. Cardioversion and defibrillation. In: Schlant RC, Alexander RW, eds. *Hurst's The Heart: Arteries*

and Veins. 8th rev ed. New York, NY: McGraw-Hill; 1994:843–846.

9. Kerber RE. Transthoracic cardioversion of atrial fibrillation and flutter: standard technique and new advances. *Am J Cardiol*. 1996;78(suppl 8):22–26.

10. Kerber RE. Electrical treatment of cardiac arrhythmias: defibrillation and cardioversion. *Ann Emerg Med*. 1993;22(pt 2):296–301.

11. Parke JD, Higgins SE. Hazards associated with chest application of nitroglycerin ointments. *JAMA*. 1982;248:427.

12. Babka JC. Does nitroglycerin explode? *N Engl J Med*. 1983;309:379.

13. Wrenn K. The hazards of defibrillation through nitroglycerin patches. *Ann Emer Med*. 1990;19:1327–1328.

14. Panacek EA, Munger MA, Rutherford WF, Gardner SF. Report of nitropatch explosions complicating defibrillation. *Am J Emerg Med*. 1992;10:128–129.

15. Ewy GA. Electrical therapy for cardiovascular emergencies. *Circulation*. 1986;74(suppl IV):IV-111–IV-116.

16. Woods SL, Sivarajan Froelicher ES, Halpenny CJ, Motzer SU. *Cardiac Nursing*. 3rd rev ed. Philadelphia, Pa: J.B. Lippincott; 1995.

17. Connell PN, Ewy GA, Dahl CF, Ewy MD. Transthoracic impedance to defibrillator discharge: effect of electrode size and electrode-chest wall interface. *J Electrocardiol*. 1973;6:313–317.

18. Hummel RS, Ornato JP, Weinberg SM, Clarke AM. Spark-generating properties of electrode gels used during defibrillation: a potential fire hazard. *JAMA*. 1988;260:3021–3024.

19. Sirna SJ, Ferguson DW, Charbonnier F, Kerber RE. Factors affecting transthoracic impedance during electrical cardioversion. *Am J Cardiol*. 1988;62:1048–1052.

20. Kerber RE, Martins JB, Kelly KJ, et al. Self-adhesive preapplied electrode pads for defibrillation and cardioversion. *J Am Coll Cardiol*. 1984;3:815–820.

21. Stults KR, Brown DD, Cooley F, Kerber RE. Self-adhesive monitor/defibrillation pads improve prehospital defibrillation success. *Ann Emerg Med*. 1987;16:872–877.

22. Wilson RF, Sirna S, White CW, Kerber RE. Defibrillation of high-risk patients during coronary angiography using self-adhesive, preapplied electrode pads. *Am J Cardiol*. 1987;60:380–382.

23. Dalzell GWN, Cunningham SR, Anderson J, Adgey AAJ. Electrode pad size, transthoracic impedance and success of external ventricular defibrillation. *Am J Cardiol*. 1989;64:741–744.

24. Kerber RE, Jensen SR, Grayzel J, Kennedy J, Hoyt R. Elective cardioversion: influence of paddle-electrode location and size on success rates and energy requirements. *N Engl J Med*. 1981;305:658–662.

25. Thomas ED, Ewy GA, Dahl CF, Ewy MD. Effectiveness of direct current defibrillation: role of paddle electrode size. *Am Heart J*. 1977;93:463–467.

26. Kerber RE, Grayzel J, Hoyt R, Marcus M, Kennedy J. Transthoracic resistance in human defibrillation: influence of body weight, chest size, serial shocks, paddle size and paddle contact pressure. *Circulation*. 1981;63:676–682.

27. Gould L, Patel S, Gomes GI, Chikshi AB. Pacemaker failure following external defibrillation. *PACE*. 1981;4:575–577.

28. Owen PM. The effects of external defibrillation on permanent pacemakers. *Heart Lung*. 1983;12:274–277.

29. Mathewson M, Dusek JL. DC countershock does not harm today's pacemakers . . . fact or myth? *Crit Care Nurse*. 1984;4(2):48.

30. Levine PA, Barold SS, Fletcher RD, Talbot P. Adverse acute and chronic effects of electrical defibrillation and cardioversion on implanted unipolar cardiac pacing systems. *J Am Coll Cardiol*. 1983;1:1413–1422.

31. Lau FYK, Bilitch M, Wintroub HJ. Protection of implanted pacemakers from excessive electrical energy of DC shock. *Am J Cardiol*. 1969;23:244–249.

32. Altamura G, Bianconi L, Lo Bianco F, et al. Transthoracic DC shock may represent a serious hazard in pacemaker dependent patients. *PACE*. 1995;18(part II):194–198.

33. Kerber RE, Martins JB, Kienzle MG, et al. Energy, current and success in defibrillation and cardioversion: clinical studies using an automated impedance-based method of energy adjustment. *Circulation*. 1988;77:1038–1046.

34. Kerber RE, Kienzle MG, Olshansky B, et al. Ventricular tachycardia rate and morphology determine energy and current requirments for transthoracic cardioversion. *Circulation*. 1992;85:158–163.

35. Eysmann SB, Marchlinski FE, Buxton AE, Josephson ME. Electrocardiographic changes after cardioversion of ventricular arrhythmias. *Circulation*. 1986;73:73–81.

Additional Readings

Correa LF. Electrical intervention in cardiac disease. In: Crawford MV, Spence MI, eds. *Commonsense Approach to Coronary Care*. 6th rev ed. St Louis, Mo: Mosby–Year Book; 1995:443–496.

Cummins RO, ed. *Advanced Cardiac Life Support*. Dallas, Tex: American Heart Association; 1997.

Kerber RE. Electrical treatment of cardiac arrhythmias: defibrillation and cardioversion. *Ann Emerg Med*. 1993;22(part 2):296–301.

Tacker WA. *Defibrillation of the Heart: ICDS, AEDs, and Manual*. St. Louis, Mo: Mosby–Year Book; 1994.

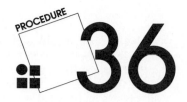

Defibrillation (External)

P U R P O S E: External defibrillation is performed to eradicate life-threatening ventricular fibrillation or pulseless ventricular tachycardia. The goal for defibrillation is to restore coordinated electric and mechanical pumping action, resulting in restored cardiac output, tissue perfusion, and oxygenation.

Virginia Wilson

PREREQUISITE NURSING KNOWLEDGE

- Understanding of the anatomy and physiology of the cardiovascular system, principles of cardiac conduction, basic dysrhythmia interpretation, and electric safety is required.
- External defibrillation is achieved by delivering a large random flow of electrons as a strong electric current through the heart over a brief period.[1] Defibrillator paddles placed over the patient's chest wall surface in the anterior-apex position maximize the current flow through the myocardium.[1, 2]
- Ventricular fibrillation is a lethal dysrhythmia. Early emergent defibrillation is the treatment of choice to restore normal electric activity and coordinated contractile activity.[1, 3]
- Advanced cardiac life support (ACLS) knowledge and skills are necessary.

EQUIPMENT

- Defibrillator with electrocardiogram (ECG) oscilloscope
- Defibrillator paddles of appropriate diameter (adult, 8.5 to 12 cm in diameter)
- Appropriate conductive materials (gel pads or conductive paste) or remote or hands-free adhesive defibrillation electrodes connected directly to the defibrillator
- Emergency pharmacologic agents
  - ❖ Epinephrine, 1 mg (10 mL of a 1:10,000 solution)
  - ❖ Lidocaine, 20 mg/mL
  - ❖ Lidocaine, 2 g in 500 mL D_5W
  - ❖ Bretylium, 500 mg/10 mL
  - ❖ Bretylium, 2 g in 500 mL D_5W
  - ❖ Procainamide, 20–30 mg/min up to 17 mg/kg total
  - ❖ Procainamide, 2 g in 500 mL D_5W
  - ❖ Sodium bicarbonate, 1 mEq/mL
  - ❖ Magnesium, 1 g, 2 mL of a 50% solution
- Flowmeter for oxygen administration
- Bag-valve-mask device capable of delivering 100% oxygen and large inflation volume
- Cardiac board
- Emergency suction and intubation equipment

- Emergency pacing equipment

PATIENT AND FAMILY EDUCATION

- Teaching may need to be performed after the procedure. **➤➤Rationale:** If the emergent defibrillation is performed in the face of hemodynamic collapse, education may be impossible until after the procedure has been performed.
- Assess patient and family understanding of the etiology of the dysrhythmia. **➤➤Rationale:** Assess the patient and family's knowledge level and additional educational needs.
- Explain the procedure to both the patient and the family. **➤➤Rationale:** Promotes understanding and encourages questions.
- Explain to both the patient and the family the signs and symptoms of hemodynamic compromise associated with preexisting cardiac dysrhythmias. **➤➤Rationale:** Enables the patient and the family to recognize when to contact the nurse or physician.
- Evaluate the patient's need for long-term pharmacologic support. **➤➤Rationale:** Anticipates educational needs of the patient and family regarding specific discharge medications.
- Assess and discuss with the patient the need for lifestyle changes. **➤➤Rationale:** Underlying pathology may necessitate alterations in patient's current lifestyle and require a plan for behavioral changes.
- Assess and discuss with the patient the need as applicable for an automatic implantable cardioverter-defibrillator. **➤➤Rationale:** Life-threatening dysrhythmias may persist after initial defibrillation and pharmacologic interventions. Recurrent ventricular dysrhythmias may represent a chronic condition for the patient.
- Assess and discuss with the patient the need as applicable for an emergency communication system. **➤➤Rationale:** People with recurrent life-threatening dysrhythmias are at risk for cardiac arrest.

PATIENT ASSESSMENT AND PREPARATION
Patient Assessment

- Determine current dysrhythmias, including paroxysmal tachycardia, atrial fibrillation, atrial flutter, atrial tachycardia, and ventricular tachycardia. ➤➤*Rationale:* Tachy-dysrhythmias often precede ventricular fibrillation, can be life threatening, and can precipitate deterioration of hemodynamic stability.

- Assess for current ventricular fibrillation. ➤➤*Rationale:* Ventricular fibrillation is life-threatening; if not terminated immediately, death will ensue.
- Assess vital signs. ➤➤*Rationale:* Blood pressure and pulse are absent in the presence of ventricular fibrillation because of the loss of cardiac output.

Patient Preparation

- Ensure that the patient and family understand preprocedural teaching (if time is available). Answer questions as they arise and reinforce information as needed. ➤➤*Rationale:* Evaluates and reinforces understanding of previously taught information.
- Place the patient on cardiac board in supine position. ➤➤*Rationale:* Supine positioning provides the best access

during the procedure and during intervention for and management of adverse effects. Cardiac board provides a hard surface for cardiopulmonary resuscitation.

- Place the patient in a safe environment, away from metallic objects and pooled water. ➤➤*Rationale:* Metallic objects and water are excellent conductors of electricity and may result in burns or arcing of current.
- Remove loose-fitting dentures, partial plates, or other prostheses. Evaluate individual situation; dentures may facilitate a tighter seal for airway management. ➤➤*Rationale:* Decreases risk of airway obstruction.
- Initiate basic life support (BLS) if immediate defibrillation is not available.[1, 3, 4] ➤➤*Rationale:* Maintains cardiac output to diminish irreversible organ and tissue damage.
- Oxygenate patient with bag-valve-mask device and 100% oxygen. ➤➤*Rationale:* Adequate oxygenation diminishes the risk of cerebral and cardiac complications.
- Place the defibrillator in the defibrillation mode. ➤➤*Rationale:* Defibrillation mode must be set to randomly disperse the electric charge because synchronization mode will not fire in the absence of a QRS complex.[1, 3]

Procedure for Defibrillation (External)

Steps	Rationale	Special Considerations
1. Wash hands.	Reduces transmission of microorganisms; standard precautions.	
2. Prepare the patient or paddles, or both with proper conductive agent. Conductive gel should be evenly dispersed on the defibrillator paddles. *(Level VI: Clinical studies in a variety of patient populations and situations to support recommendations)*	Conductive medium enhances electric conduction through subcutaneous tissue, decreases transthoracic resistance, and assists in minimizing burns from electric current.[5-7]	Pregelled conductive pads are available for placement in the area of the paddles. Never use alcohol-soaked pads because they are combustible when in contact with electric current. Hands-off defibrillator electrodes are an alternative method for defibrillation. Preliminary findings suggest (1) time reduction in actual defibrillation time, (2) reduced variability, (3) improved conversion rate, and (4) a reduction in loose lead artifact.[1, 8]
3. Ensure that the defibrillator cables are positioned to allow for adequate access to the patient.	Allows defibrillation to occur without excessive tension on cables.	
4. Turn on ECG recorder for continuous printout.	Establishes a visual recording of the patient's current ECG, verifies response to intervention, and provides a permanent record of the response to defibrillation.	
5. Place one paddle at the heart's apex, just to the left of the nipple in the midline axillary line. Place the other paddle just below the right clavicle to the right of the sternum. *(Level VI: Clinical studies in a variety of patient populations and situations to support recommendations) (see Fig. 35–2)*	Defibrillation is achieved by passing electric current through the cardiac muscle mass to restore a single source of impulse generation.[1]	Alternative placement locations include the following: anterior-left precordium/posterior behind the heart in the right infrascapular region, or anterior-left apex/posterior behind the heart in the right infrascapular region.[7] Avoid placing paddles over nitroglycerin patches, over the generators of permanent pacemakers, and over the generator of internal cardioverter-defibrillators.

Procedure	for Defibrillation (External) *Continued*

Steps	Rationale	Special Considerations
6. Charge defibrillator paddles as prescribed or in accordance with recommendations of the American Heart Association. *(Level VI: Clinical studies in a variety of patient populations and situations to support recommendations)*	Defibrillator is charged with the lowest energy level required to convert ventricular fibrillation or pulseless ventricular tachycardia.	Energy recommendations by the American Heart Association[1] for adults: first attempt: 200 joules (J), second attempt: 300 J, subsequent attempts: 360 J
7. Apply 25 lb/in² pressure to each paddle against the chest wall.	Decreases transthoracic resistance and improves the flow of the current across the axis of the heart.[2, 5, 6]	
8. State "all clear" or similar wording three times and visually verify that all personnel are clear of contact with patient, bed, and equipment.	Maximizes safety to self and caregivers because electric current can be conducted from the patient to another person if contact occurs.[1]	
9. Verify that the patient is still in ventricular fibrillation or pulseless ventricular tachycardia.	Ensures that defibrillation is necessary.	
10. Depress both buttons on the paddles simultaneously and hold until defibrillator fires. In the defibrillation mode, there will be an immediate release of the electric charge.[1, 3]	Depolarizes the cardiac muscle.	Charge may be delivered by depressing the discharge button on the defibrillator.
11. Assess for the presence of a carotid pulse, and observe the conversion of the dysrhythmia.	Assesses patient response to defibrillation.	
12. If unsuccessful, immediately charge the paddles to 300 J and repeat steps 5 to 11.	Immediate action increases the chance of successful depolarization of cardiac muscle.	Transthoracic resistance decreases with repeated shocks.[2]
13. If second attempt is unsuccessful, immediately charge the paddles to 360 J and repeat steps 5 to 11.	Immediate action increases the chance of successful depolarization of cardiac muscle.	
14. If third attempt is unsuccessful, initiate ACLS. *(Level VI: Clinical studies in a variety of patient populations and situations to support recommendations)*	Actions necessary to maintain the delivery of oxygenated blood to vital organs.	BLS must be continued throughout resuscitation.[1, 5]
15. If successful, obtain vital signs and assess patient.	Assesses patient response to defibrillation.	
16. Clean defibrillator and remove any gel. If hands-off defibrillation electrodes were used, evaluate the placement and integrity of electrodes.	Conductive gel accumulated on the defibrillator paddles impedes surface contact and increases transthoracic resistance. Hands-off defibrillation electrodes may crimp, crack, or fold with loss of adhesiveness.[8]	Loss of adhesive integrity in hands-off defibrillation electrodes occurs in restless or diaphoretic patients.
17. Discard used supplies and wash hands.	Reduces transmission of microorganisms; standard precautions.	

Expected Outcomes	Unexpected Outcomes
• Reestablishment of a single source of impulse generation for the cardiac muscle • Hemodynamic stability	• Cardiopulmonary arrest and death • Cerebral anoxia and brain death • Respiratory complications • Paddle burns • Asystole • Hypotension • Pacemaker or implantable cardioverter-defibrillator (ICD) dysfunction

Patient Monitoring and Care

Patient Monitoring and Care	Rationale	Reportable Conditions
		These conditions should be reported if they persist despite nursing interventions.
1. Evaluate neurologic status after defibrillation. Reorient as necessary to person, place, and time.	Temporary altered level of consciousness may occur following defibrillation.[1]	• Change in level of consciousness
2. Monitor pulmonary status after defibrillation.	Respiratory centers of the brain may be depressed as a result of hypoxia.[1]	• Change in respirations • Decreased oxygen saturation
3. Monitor cardiovascular status (blood pressure, heart rate, and rhythm) immediately after defibrillation and every 15 min until stable.	Dysrhythmias may develop after defibrillation.[1] Vital signs should stabilize after achieving a normal heart rate and rhythm.	• Dysrhythmias and abnormal vital signs
4. Continue to monitor the ECG after defibrillation.	Postdefibrillation dysrhythmias may occur.	• Dysrhythmias
5. Initiate intravenous antidysrhythmic pharmacologic therapy as prescribed.	Ventricular fibrillation is indicative of the myocardium's state of irritability. If antidysrhythmic therapy is not administered, recurrence of ventricular fibrillation is probable.	• Dysrhythmias despite antidysrhythmic therapy
6. Assess skin for burns.	Electric current in contact with subcutaneous tissue can cause loss of skin integrity.[1, 2]	• Skin burns
7. Monitor electrolytes.	Abnormal electrolytes may have contributed to the development of ventricular dysrhythmias. In addition, cellular and tissue perfusion returns with restoration of a pulse and blood pressure, but intracellular acidosis may remain after resuscitation.[1]	• Abnormal electrolyte results

Documentation

Documentation should include the following:

• Neurologic, respiratory, and cardiovascular assessments before and after defibrillation
• Nursing measures implemented to prepare patient for defibrillation, including joules used and the number of attempts made

• Printout ECG tracings depicting defibrillation and cardiac events
• Patient response to defibrillation
• Any unexpected outcomes and the interventions taken
• Patient and family education

References

1. Cummins RO. *Advanced Life Support.* Dallas, Tx: American Heart Association; 1997.
2. Kerber RE, Martins JB, Kelly KJ, Ferguson DW, Kouba C, Nensen SR, et al. Self-adhesive preapplied electrode pads for defibrillation and cardioversion. *J Am Coll Cardiol.* 1984;3:815–820.
3. Thomas ED, Ewy GA, Dahl CF, Ewy MD. Effectiveness of direct current defibrillation: role of paddle size. *Am Heart J.* 1977;93:463–467.
4. Cummins R, Sanders A, Mancici E, Hazinski MF. In-hospital resuscitation: a statement for healthcare professionals from the American Heart Association Cardiac Care Committee and the Advanced Cardiac Life Support, Basic Life Support, Pediatric Resuscitation and Program Administration Subcommittees. *Circulation.* 1997;95:2211–2212.
5. Emergency Cardiac Care Committees and Subcommittees, American Heart Association. Guidelines for cardiopulmonary resuscitation and emergency care. *JAMA.* 1992;268:2171–2298.
6. Gutgesell HP, Tacker HA, Geddes LA, Davis JS, Lie JT, McNamara DG. Energy dose for ventricular defibrillation of children. *Pediatrics.* 1976;58:898–901.
7. Kerber RE. Electrical treatment of cardiac arrhythmias: defibrillation and cardioversion. *Ann Emerg Med.* 1993;22:296–301.

8. Kloeck W, Cummins R, Chamberlain D, Bossaert L, Callanan V, Carli P, et al. Early defibrillation: an advisory statement from the Advanced Life Support Group of the International Liaison Committee on Resuscitation. *Circulation.* 1997;95: 2183–2184.

Additional Readings

Hearn P. Early defibrillation: lessons learned. *J Cardiovasc Nurs.* 1996;10:24–36.

Kloeck W, Cummins R, Chamberlain D, Bossaert L, Callanan V, Carli P, et al. The Universal Advanced Life Support Algorithm: an advisory statement from the Advanced Life Support Group of the International Liaison Committee on Resuscitation. *Circulation.* 1997;95:2180–2182.

Reiffel JA. Prolonging survival by reducing arrhythmia death: pharmacologic therapy of ventricular tachycardia and fibrillation. *Am J Cardiol.* 1997;96:2812–2829.

Tacker WA. *Defibrillation of the Heart: ICD's, AED's, and Manual.* St. Louis, Mo: Mosby–Year Book; 1994.

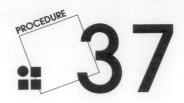

37

Defibrillation (Internal)

PURPOSE: Internal defibrillation is achieved by delivering an electric current directly to the myocardium's surface via an open thoracotomy approach or open sternotomy, as in the postoperative cardiovascular surgery patient. Internal defibrillation is used intraoperatively and in emergency thoracotomies.

Joan M. Vitello-Cicciu
Christine Moriarty
Kellie Smith

PREREQUISITE NURSING KNOWLEDGE

- Understanding of the anatomy and physiology of the cardiovascular system, principles of cardiac conduction, basic dysrhythmia interpretation, and safe use of electricity is required.
- Advanced cardiac life support (ACLS) knowledge and skills are necessary.
- Dosage calculations for emergency pharmacologic agents should be known.
- Clinical and technical competence related to use of the defibrillator is needed.
- Direct internal defibrillation eliminates transthoracic resistance; therefore, the recommended energy requirements are much lower than with external defibrillation.
- Internal paddle placement ensures that the axis of the heart is situated between the sources of current. Because the electric activity is chaotic, with no coordinated ventricular response, the electric current is randomly delivered to terminate ventricular fibrillation and restore cardiac output and reestablish tissue perfusion and oxygenation.
- Energy requirements for internal defibrillation range from 5 joules (J) to as high as 60 J. Ideal energy requirements that cause minimal damage to the myocardium and are effective for defibrillation have not been established.
- A study performed by Geddes et al[1] reported that an energy level of 5 J was sufficient in 50% of the human hearts internally defibrillated. Further conclusions of the study noted that energy levels between 10 J and 20 J were successful in terminating the dysrhythmias without myocardial necrosis developing in 90% of the patients studied.

EQUIPMENT

- Sterile gloves, goggles, gowns, and masks
- Open thoracotomy or sternotomy tray

- Sterile internal paddles (ensure their compatibility with defibrillator)
- Defibrillator with electrocardiogram (ECG) oscilloscope and recorder
- Flowmeter for oxygen administration
- Bag-valve-mask device capable of delivering 100% oxygen and large inflation volumes
- Emergency suction and intubation equipment
- Emergency pharmacologic agents per ACLS protocol
- Sterile suction system for chest suctioning
- Emergency pacemaker equipment

PATIENT AND FAMILY EDUCATION

- Teaching may need to be performed after the procedure. ➤*Rationale:* Because internal defibrillation is performed in the face of hemodynamic collapse, education is usually performed after the procedure.
- Explain to family the need for internal defibrillation of the patient with a life-threatening dysrhythmia. ➤*Rationale:* Clarification or reinforcement of information is an expressed family need to reduce anxiety.
- Assess and discuss, as applicable, with the patient and family the need for follow-up electrophysiologic studies (EPS). ➤*Rationale:* Enables patient and family to understand importance of EPS.
- Assess patient and family understanding of the underlying disease pathology. ➤*Rationale:* Prepares the patient and family for both expected and unexpected outcomes.
- Explain to patient and family the signs and symptoms of hemodynamic compromise associated with preexisting cardiac dysrhythmias. ➤*Rationale:* Enables the patient and family to recognize when the patient needs to contact health care providers.
- Evaluate the patient's need for long-term antidysrhythmic support. ➤*Rationale:* Allows the nurse to anticipate educational needs of the patient and family regarding specific discharge medications.

- Assess and discuss with the patient the need as applicable for lifestyle changes. ➨*Rationale:* Underlying pathophysiology may necessitate alterations in patient's current lifestyle and require a plan for behavioral changes.
- Assess and discuss with the patient the need as applicable for emergency communication plan. ➨*Rationale:* Patients with recurrent life-threatening ventricular dysrhythmias are at risk for cardiac arrest.

PATIENT ASSESSMENT AND PREPARATION
Patient Assessment

- Assess ECG for dysrhythmias, including ventricular ectopy and ventricular tachycardia. ➨*Rationale:* Ventricular dysrhythmias often precede ventricular fibrillation and precipitate deterioration of hemodynamic stability.
- Assess ECG for ventricular fibrillation. ➨*Rationale:* The development of ventricular fibrillation is life threatening, and if it is not terminated immediately, death will ensue.
- Assess vital signs with each significant change in ECG rate and rhythm. ➨*Rationale:* Blood pressure and pulse

are absent in the presence of ventricular fibrillation as a result of the loss of cardiac output.

Patient Preparation

- Place patient in supine position. ➨*Rationale:* Supine positioning provides the best access during the procedure and during intervention for management of adverse effects.
- Remove all metallic objects from the patient. ➨*Rationale:* Metallic objects are conductors of electric current and can cause burns.
- Prepare the patient's skin with antibacterial solution and drape the patient. ➨*Rationale:* Decreases the potential for nosocomial infection.
- Remove loose-fitting dentures, partial plates, or other mouth prostheses. Evaluate individual situation; dentures may facilitate a tighter seal for airway management. ➨*Rationale:* Decreases the risk of airway obstruction during the procedure.
- Have anesthesia present or readily available. ➨*Rationale:* Facilitates airway management or sedation.

Procedure **for Defibrillation (Internal)**

Steps	Rationale	Special Considerations
1. Initiate basic life support (BLS).	Decreases the risk of airway obstruction during the procedure; maintains oxygenation and perfusion.	External defibrillation should be attempted first whenever possible (see Procedure 36).
2. Don sterile gloves, mask, gown, and goggles. Assist physician or advanced practice nurse with opening the chest (see Procedure 39).	Maintains sterility; standard precautions.	Suctioning around the heart may be necessary before defibrillating if drainage or bleeding is present.
3. Insert debibrillator electric cord into a grounded electric wall outlet.	Prepares equipment.	
4. Place defibrillator in the defibrillation mode.	Defibrillation mode must be selected to deliver the electric charge immediately because the synchronization mode will not fire in the absence of a QRS complex.	
5. Turn on the ECG recorder for a continuous printout.	Establishes a visual recording of the patient's current ECG status and provides a permanent record of the patient's response to intervention.	
6. Once the physician or advanced practice nurse has positioned the internal paddles on the heart, connect the other end of the internal paddles to the defibrillator and charge the defibrillator paddles as prescribed (usually 5 to 20 J). *(Level IV: Limited clinical studies to support recommendations)*	Defibrillator is charged with the lowest energy level required to convert ventricular fibrillation and prevent any damage to the heart muscle.	One paddle is placed over the right atrium or right ventricle; the other paddle is placed over the apex (Fig. 37–1). Usually 5 to 20 J is sufficient to convert ventricular fibrillation.[2] Refer to defibrillator manufacturer's operation guidelines for specific recommendations.
7. State "all clear" three times and visually verify that all personnel are clear of contact with patient, bed, and equipment.	Electric current can be conducted from the patient to another person if contact occurs.	

Procedure continued on following page

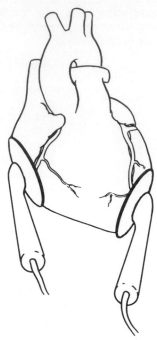

■ ● **FIGURE 37–1.** Paddle placement for internal defibrillation. (From Kinkade S, Lohrman JE. *Critical Care Nursing Procedures: A Team Approach.* Philadelphia, Pa: B.C. Decker; 1990.)

Procedure for **Defibrillation (Internal)** *Continued*

Steps	Rationale	Special Considerations
8. The physician or advanced practicie nurse depresses both buttons on the paddles simultaneously and holds until the defibrillator fires. In the defibrillation mode, there will be an immediate release of the electric charge.	Depolarizes cardiac muscle.	Charge may also be delivered by depressing the discharge button on the defibrillator until the charge is delivered.
9. Assess for the presence of a pulse, and observe for conversion of the dysrhythmia.	Simultaneous depolarization of the myocardial muscle cells may reestablish a single source of impulse generation.	
10. If first attempt is unsuccessful, immediately charge paddles and repeat steps 7 to 9.	Immediate action increases the chance for successful depolarization of cardiac muscle.	
11. If second attempt is unsuccessful, immediately charge paddles and repeat steps 7 to 9.	Immediate action increases the chance for successful depolarization of cardiac muscle.	
12. If third attempt is unsuccessful, initiate ACLS.	Actions are necessary to maintain the delivery of oxygenated blood to vital organs.	Recurrent ventricular fibrillation may necessitate surgical placement of an automatic implantable cardioverter-defibrillator. Open-chest compression must be resumed after third attempt, if not successful. Consider the need for pacing if rhythm converts to asystole.
13. If successful, obtain vital signs and assess the patient.	Assesses patient response to defibrillation.	

Procedure **for Defibrillation (Internal)** *Continued*

Steps	Rationale	Special Considerations
14. Prepare patient for transport to the operating room or prepare to assist with closing incision at bedside.	Surgical intervention is necessary when open-chest technique is used.	
15. Clean defibrillator, and remove blood or body fluids. Send used paddles for resterilization. Obtain sterile paddles to restock defibrillator cart.	Reduces transmission of microorganisms; sterile precautions; standard precautions.	
16. Discard used supplies and wash hands.	Reduces transmission of microorganisms; standard precautions.	

Expected Outcomes

- Reestablishment of a single source of impulse generation for the cardiac muscle
- Hemodynamic stability

Unexpected Outcomes

- Cardiopulmonary arrest and death
- Cerebral anoxia and brain death
- Respiratory complications
- Infection
- Myocardial damage caused by paddles

Patient Monitoring and Care

Patient Monitoring and Care	Rationale	Reportable Conditions
		These conditions should be reported if they persist despite nursing interventions.
1. Evaluate neurologic status after defibrillation. Reorient as necessary to person, place, and time.	Temporary altered level of consciousness may occur following defibrillation.[3]	• Change in level of consciousness
2. Monitor pulmonary status after defibrillation.	Respiratory centers of the brain may be depressed as a result of hypoxia.[3]	• Change in respirations • Decrease in oxygen saturation
3. Monitor cardiovascular status (blood pressure, heart rate, and rhythm) immediately after defibrillation and every 15 minutes until stable.	Dysrhythmias may develop after defibrillation.[3] Vital signs should stabilize after achieving a normal heart rate and rhythm.	• Dysrhythmias and abnormal vital signs
4. Continue to monitor the ECG after defibrillation.	Postdefibrillation dysrhythmias may occur.	• Dysrhythmias
5. Initiate intravenous antidysrhythmic pharmacologic therapy as prescribed.	Ventricular fibrillation is indicative of the myocardium's state of irritability. If antidysrhythmic therapy is not administered, recurrence of ventricular fibrillation is probable.	• Dysrhythmias despite antidysrhythmic therapy
6. Monitor electrolytes.	Abnormal electrolytes may have contributed to the development of ventricular dysrhythmias. In addition, cellular and tissue perfusion returns with restoration of a pulse and blood pressure, but intracellular acidosis may remain after resuscitation.[1]	• Abnormal electrolyte result
7. Monitor for signs of infection.	Disruption of skin integrity and introduction of foreign material into the thoracic cavity predisposes the patient to the risk of infection.	• Elevated white blood cell count, elevated temperature, pain at incisional site, erythema, or drainage from incisional site

▌Documentation

Documentation in the patient record should include the following:

- Neurologic, respiratory, and cardiovascular assessments before and after defibrillation
- Nursing measures implemented to prepare the patient for internal defibrillation, that is, joules used and number of attempts made
- Printout of ECG tracings depicting defibrillation and cardiac events

- Patient response to defibrillation
- Any unexpected outcomes and the interventions taken
- Time patient sent to the operating room
- Patient and family education

References

1. Geddes LA, Tacker WA, Rosborough J, et al. The electrical dose for ventricular defibrillation with electrodes applied directly to the heart. *J Thorac Cardiovasc Surg.* 1974;68:593–602.
2. Moore S. Jump-starting the heart A current review of defibrillation techniques and equipment. *JAMA* 1986;12:213–217.
3. Cummins RO. *Advanced Life Support.* Dallas, Tx: American Heart Association; 1997.

Additional Readings

Pugsley WB, Baldwin T, Treasure T, Sturridge MF. Low energy level internal defibrillation during cardiopulmonary bypass. *Eur J Cardiothorac Surg.* 1989;3:273–275.
Seifert PC. *Cardiac Surgery.* St. Louis, Mo: Mosby–Year Book; 1994:70–73, 151–152.

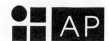

Emergent Open Sternotomy (Perform)

PURPOSE: The emergent open sternotomy in the postoperative patient after cardiac surgery is designed to identify and eliminate areas of persistent hemorrhage, relieve pericardial tamponade, and provide access for open cardiac massage.

Deborah G. LaMarr

PREREQUISITE NURSING KNOWLEDGE

- The anatomy and physiology of the cardiovascular system should be understood.
- Advanced cardiac life support (ACLS) knowledge and skills are necessary.
- Knowledge of suturing, sternal opening, sternal wiring, surgical instrumentation, and sternal exploration is necessary.
- This procedure is designed for postoperative patients after cardiac surgeries who have undergone the median sternotomy approach.
- Signs and symptoms of cardiac tamponade should be known.
- The emergent open sternotomy in the postoperative patient after cardiac surgery is indicated for exsanguinating hemorrhage or cardiac tamponade with imminent cardiac arrest.
- Early reexploration for persistent hemorrhage may reduce the requirement for homologous transfusions and may also lower the wound infection rate associated with an undrained mediastinal hematoma.
- Mediastinal reexploration for cardiac tamponade will decrease ventricular diastolic pressure. This decreased pressure will allow for increased ventricular filling and stroke volume, enhanced cardiac output, and globally improved systemic perfusion.
- Mechanical ventilation and sedation are prerequisites to sternal reexploration.
- Paralytic agents may be a necessary adjunct to sedation to improve oxygenation, diminish muscle activity, and enhance visualization in the operative field.
- Internal defibrillation may be necessary if life-threatening dysrhythmias occur (see Procedure 37).

EQUIPMENT

- Povidone-iodine solution
- Caps, masks, goggles, sterile gloves, and drapes
- Sterile dressing supplies
- Sterile open-chest set:
  - ❖ Rib spreader
  - ❖ Kelly clamps and skin snaps
  - ❖ Knife handle
  - ❖ Wire cutter
  - ❖ Scissors
- Prolene suture (cutting needle), other suture material according to preference
- Clip applicator and clips
- Syringes: 3 mL, 5 mL, 10 mL, 20 mL
- Electrocautery equipment: generator, cautery, grounding pad
- Knife blades: #10, #11, #15
- Sternal wires
- Large sterile suction catheter (eg, Yankeur)
- Suction container and tubing
- Sterile staple remover
- Sterile stapler and staples
- Emergency medication and resuscitation equipment

Additional equipment (to have available depending on patient status) includes the following:

- Analgesia or sedation as prescribed
- Blood products and intravenous IV solutions as prescribed
- Chest tubes and chest tube drainage system
- Epicardial wires
- Intra-aortic balloon pump or mechanical assist device

PATIENT AND FAMILY EDUCATION

- Teaching may be necessary after the procedure. ➤➤*Rationale:* If the emergent sternotomy is performed in the face of hemodynamic collapse, the education of the patient and family may be impossible until after the procedure has been performed.

- Explain the reason that the open sternotomy procedure was performed and its outcome or anticipated outcome. ➤*Rationale:* Clarifies information and encourages patient and family to ask questions and voice specific concerns about the procedure.

PATIENT ASSESSMENT AND PREPARATION

Patient Assessment

- Determine baseline hemodynamic and neurologic status. ➤*Rationale:* Identifies data that may indicate the need for emergent open sternotomy and provides comparison data.
- Assess medical history, specifically that related to coagulation disorders, renal disease with coexistent uremia, and functional status of the right and left ventricle. ➤*Rationale:* Provides essential data.
- Assess current laboratory data, specifically complete blood cell (CBC) count, platelet count, prothrombin time (PT), partial prothrombin time, (PTT) fibrinogen, and international normalized ratio (INR). ➤*Rationale:* Baseline coagulation studies need to be near normal to be eliminated as possible causes for ongoing hemorrhage.
- Signs and symptoms of cardiac tamponade requiring emergent sternotomy are as follows:

  ❖ Excessive chest tube drainage[1] as follows: 500 mL for 1 hour, 400 mL for 2 consecutive hours, or 300 mL for 3 consecutive hours
  ❖ Hypotension: mean arterial blood pressure less than 60 mm Hg
  ❖ Altered mental status
  ❖ Apical heart rate >110 beats per minute
  ❖ Narrowing of pulse pressure
  ❖ Distended neck veins

  ❖ Distant heart sounds
  ❖ Equilibrium of intracardiac pressures with right atrial, pulmonary capillary wedge, and (if measured) left atrial pressures being equal
  ❖ Decreased cardiac output and cardiac index
  ❖ Pulsus paradoxus
  ❖ Sudden decrease or cessation in chest tube drainage
  ❖ If time allows, obtain a chest radiograph to assess for evidence of widened mediastinum. ➤*Rationale:* Widening of the mediastinum on chest radiograph, especially the right heart border, could be indicative of mediastinal blood.
  ❖ If time allows, obtain a transthoracic echocardiogram in an attempt to identify a mediastinal clot. ➤*Rationale:* Aids the diagnosis and confirms the necessity for the open-sternotomy procedure.

Patient Preparation

- Ensure that the patient and family understand preprocedural teaching (if time available). Answer questions as they arise and reinforce information as needed. ➤*Rationale:* Evaluates and reinforces understanding of previously taught information.
- Obtain informed consent (this may not be possible if the procedure is an acute emergency). ➤*Rationale:* Protects rights of the patient and ensures a competent decision for the patient and the family.
- Ensure that patient's ventilation is maintained. ➤*Rationale:* Ensures that the patient's airway is protected and that oxygen needs are met.
- Position patient in supine position with head of bed flat. ➤*Rationale:* Ensures visualization of operative field.
- Prescribe analgesics or sedatives. ➤*Rationale:* Promotes comfort.

Procedure **for Emergent Open Sternotomy (Perform)**		
Steps	**Rationale**	**Special Considerations**
1. Call physician and operative team.	The physician can reassess the need for further surgical intervention. The operative team may be needed to assist at the bedside or to prepare the operating room if further exploration is needed.	Follow hospital standard.
2. Prepare electrocautery device for possible use: apply ground pad to patient's skin and attach grounding and cautery cables.	This device is used to terminate capillary oozing or bleeding.	
3. Ensure that a new sterile suction system is set up.	This will be used to suction the mediastinum during the procedure.	
4. Wash hands, and don gloves.	Reduces transmission of microorganisms; standard precautions.	
5. Remove old dressing and surgically prepare skin for incision: cleanse chest with antiseptic solution.	Inhibits microorganism transmission with surgical instrumentation.	Prepare skin from sternal notch to midabdomen and midclavicular line to midclavicular line.

Procedure for Emergent Open Sternotomy (Perform) *Continued*

Steps	Rationale	Special Considerations
6. Wash hands, and don caps, goggles, masks, sterile gowns, and gloves for all members of the health care team involved with the procedure.	Reduces transmission of microorganisms; sterile precautions; standard precautions.	All personnel in the room must don masks and caps.
7. Place four sterile towels and drape off each side around the sternotomy incision.	A large sterile field will supply room for placement of instruments.	Allows good view of the sternal notch.
8. Hand off the electrocautery and suction to assisting critical care nurse.	Assistance is needed if bleeding continues.	
9. With scalpel, open the wound down to the sternum, exposing the sternal wires.	Ensures visualization of sternal wires.	Staples can be removed with staple remover.
10. Cauterize oozing bleeding sites as needed.	Minimizes blood loss and enhances visualization of the surgical field.	
11. Cut sternal wires from top to bottom with wire cutter or untwist wires with heavy needle holder.	Wires will fatigue and break when untwisted with heavy needle holders.	
12. With hands, gently separate the sternum.	Caution must be taken to separate gently because heart, pacing wires, and grafts rest just under the sternal bone.	
13. Place the sternal retractor just under the sternal bone and crank open, exposing the heart; continuously palpate edges of retractor for potential caught grafts or wires.	Blades can trap and tear grafts and wires if caught and pulled apart when the retractor is cranked open.	
14. Place a finger over the bleeding site and suction the remainder of the chest, evacuating any clots.	Pressure on the bleeding site may minimize blood loss.	Resuscitate with IV fluids, inotropic medications, and blood products as necessary.
15. Assist the physician with control and ligation of major and minor bleeding sites, enhance sternal retraction, and provide suctioning and electrocautery as needed.	May eliminate the need for further reexploration and allows for full visualization of the surgical field.	The physician will determine if the patient needs to be transferred to the operating room for further surgical intervention.
16. Assist the physician with the placement of chest tubes or pacing wires as needed.	Pacing leads and chest tubes can be displaced during sternal retraction.	
17. Assist with placement of mechanical assist devices if needed.	Cardiac tamponade can conceal right or left ventricular dysfunction; mechanical assistance may be necessary to improve cardiac output.	
18. Assist patient transport to the operating room if necessary.	The patient may need surgical repair of coronary artery bypass grafts, cardiac valves, or the myocardium.	

Procedure continued on following page

AP This procedure should be performed only by physicians, advanced practice nurses, and other health care professionals (including critical care nurses) with additional knowledge, skills, and demonstrated competence per professional licensure or institutional standard.

Procedure	**for Emergent Open Sternotomy (Perform)** *Continued*

Steps	Rationale	Special Considerations
19. If the patient does not need to return to the operating room, assist the physician with reinsertion of the sternal wires as follows: grasp the sternal wire with the needle holder, then push through the sternum, anterior to posterior, on one side. Pull the wire through to the other sternal edge, pushing through the sternum posterior to anterior. Twist edges of wires together with the needle holder. Cut off excess wire.	Ensures sternal closure.	Caution must be taken not to penetrate the heart, pericostal vessels, lungs, or grafts with sternal wires. On occasion, if severe right or left ventricular dysfunction persists, the chest may need to be left open and covered with a sterile occlusive surgical dressing (eg, Gore-Tex patch).
20. Repeat a sternal wire reinsertion as described in step 19, placing each insertion 4 to 5 in apart until the sternum is closed.	Ensures sternal closure.	
21. Assist the physician with skin closure, according to preference.	Promotes wound healing.	The patient's chest may be left open and covered with a sterile, occlusive surgical dressing if severe ventricular dysfunction exists.
22. Apply dressing to the sternal incision, epicardial pacing wires, and chest tube sites.	Promotes aseptic management of the surgical incision and wound sites.	
23. Remove and discard personal protective equipment, discard used supplies, package instruments for sterilization, and wash hands.	Reduces transmission of microorganisms and body secretions; standard precautions.	

Expected Outcomes	Unexpected Outcomes
• Increased cardiac output • Increased tissue perfusion, including cerebral, renal, and peripheral perfusion • Standard chest tube drainage • Decreased need for homologous transfusion	• Severe right or left ventricular dysfunction • Continued bleeding or coagulation disorders • Myocardial or aortic perforation • Cardiac arrest • Pneumothorax • Myocardial infarction • Atrial and ventricular dysrhythmias • Pain

Patient Monitoring and Care

Patient Monitoring and Care	Rationale	Reportable Conditions
		These conditions should be reported if they persist despite nursing interventions.
1. Perform cardiovascular, peripheral vascular, and hemodynamic assessments every 15 to 30 minutes as patient status requires: assess level of consciousness; assess vital signs, cardiac index, and pulmonary artery pressures; and measure urine output.	Assess for adequacy of cerebral perfusion; hemodynamic instability can lead to cerebral anoxia. Demonstrates hemodynamic stability and volume status; recurrent tamponade or persistent myocardial arterial depression may develop during and after sternotomy. Validates adequate perfusion to the kidneys.	• Change in level of consciousness • Decrease in cardiac output and cardiac index, abnormal pulmonary artery pressures; equalizing pulmonary artery pressures; mean arterial blood pressure less than 60 mm Hg, changes in heart rate • Urine output <.5 mL/kg/hr
2. Assess heart and lung sounds every 2 hours and as needed.	Abnormal heart and lung sounds may indicate the need for additional treatment.	• Distant heart sounds or additional changes in heart and lung sounds.
3. Monitor coagulation and hematologic studies.	Coagulation and hematologic profiles will provide data that will indicate the risk of bleeding and indicate the need for additional treatment.	• Abnormal hemoglobin and hematocrit, PT, PTT, INR, platelets, fibrinogen
4. Monitor chest tube drainage.	Ensures adequate functioning of the chest tube drainage system.	• Cessation of chest tube drainage; increased chest tube drainage; clots in chest tube drainage system

Documentation

Documentation should include the following:

- Patient and family education
- Indications for the procedure and the procedure used
- Informed consent obtained
- Estimated blood loss
- Patient therapies and response; including hemodynamics, inotropic or vasopressor agents, ventilation, and neurologic status
- Unexpected outcomes
- Additional interventions

Reference

1. Lyerly H. *Handbook of Surgical Intensive Care.* Chicago, Ill: Year Book Medical Publishers; 1995:83–86.

Additional Readings

Bojar R, Mathisen D, Warner K. *Manual of Perioperative Care in Cardiac and Thoracic Surgery.* Boston, Mass: Blackwell Scientific Publications; 1994:989–999.

Borkon M, Schaff H, Gardner T, et al. Diagnosis and management of postoperative pericardial effusions and late cardiac tamponade following open-heart surgery. *Ann Thorac Surg.* 1981;31: 512–518.

Fairman R, Edmunds H. Emergency thoracotomy in the surgical care unit after open cardiac operation. *Ann Thorac Surg.* 1981;32:386–391.

Sabiston D, Spencer F. *Surgery of the Chest.* Philadelphia, Pa: W.B. Saunders; 1995:220–222.

39

Emergent Open Sternotomy (Assist)

P U R P O S E: The emergent open sternotomy in the postoperative patient after cardiac surgery is designed to identify and eliminate areas of persistent hemorrhage, relieve pericardial tamponade, and provide access for open cardiac massage.

Deborah G. LaMarr

PREREQUISITE NURSING KNOWLEDGE

- The anatomy and physiology of the cardiovascular system should be understood.
- Advanced cardiac life support (ACLS) knowledge and skills are necessary.
- This procedure is designed for postoperative patients after cardiac surgeries who have undergone the median sternotomy approach.
- Signs and symptoms of cardiac tamponade should be understood.
- The emergent open sternotomy in the postoperative patient after cardiac surgery is indicated for exsanguinating hemorrhage or cardiac tamponade with imminent cardiac arrest.
- Early reexploration for persistent hemorrhage may reduce the requirement for homologous transfusions and may also lower the wound infection rate associated with an undrained mediastinal hematoma.
- Mediastinal reexploration for cardiac tamponade will decrease ventricular diastolic pressure. This decreased pressure will allow for increased ventricular filling and stroke volume, enhanced cardiac output, and globally improved systemic perfusion.
- Mechanical ventilation and sedation are prerequisites to sternal reexploration.
- Paralytic agents may be a necessary adjunct to sedation to improve oxygenation, diminish muscle activity, and enhance visualization in the operative field.
- Internal defibrillation may be necessary if life-threatening dysrhythmias occur (see Procedure 37).

EQUIPMENT

- Povidone-iodine solution
- Caps, masks, goggles, sterile gloves, and drapes
- Sterile dressing supplies
- Sterile open-chest set:
  - ❖ Rib spreader
  - ❖ Kelly clamps and skin snaps
  - ❖ Knife handle
  - ❖ Wire cutter

- ❖ Scissors
- Prolene suture (cutting needle), other suture material according to preference
- Clip applicator and clips
- Syringes: 3 mL, 5 mL, 10 mL, 20 mL
- Electrocautery equipment: generator, cautery, grounding pad
- Knife blades: 10, 11, 15
- Sternal wires
- Large sterile suction catheter (eg, Yankeur)
- Suction container and tubing
- Sterile staple remover
- Sterile stapler and staples
- Emergency medication and resuscitation equipment

Additional equipment (to have available depending on patient status) includes the following:

- Analgesia or sedation as prescribed
- Blood products and intravenous (IV) solutions as prescribed
- Chest tubes and chest tube drainage system
- Epicardial pacing wires
- Intra-aortic balloon pump or mechanical assist device

PATIENT AND FAMILY EDUCATION

- Teaching may be necessary after the procedure. **➤➤Rationale:** If the emergent sternotomy is performed in the face of hemodynamic collapse, the education of the patient and family may be impossible until after the procedure has been performed.
- Explain the reason that the open sternotomy procedure was performed and its outcome or anticipated outcome. **➤➤Rationale:** Clarifies information and encourages patient and family to ask questions and voice specific concerns about the procedure.

PATIENT ASSESSMENT AND PREPARATION
Patient Assessment

- Determine baseline hemodynamic and neurologic status. **➤➤Rationale:** Identifies data that may indicate

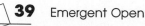

the need for emergent open sternotomy and provides comparison data.

- Assess medical history, specifically that related to coagulation disorders, renal disease with coexistent uremia, and functional status of the right and left ventricle. ➤*Rationale:* Provides essential data.
- Assess current laboratory data, specifically complete blood cell (CBC) count, platelet count, prothrombin time (PT), partial prothrombin time (PTT), fibrinogen, and international normalized ratio (INR). ➤*Rationale:* Baseline coagulation studies need to be near normal to be eliminated as possible causes for ongoing hemorrhage.
- Signs and symptoms of cardiac tamponade requiring emergent sternotomy:
  ❖ Excessive chest tube drainage[1] as follows: 500 mL for 1 hour, 400 mL for 2 consecutive hours, or 300 mL for 3 consecutive hours
  ❖ Hypotension: mean arterial blood pressure less than 60 mm Hg.
  ❖ Altered mental status
  ❖ Apical heart rate >110 beats per minute
  ❖ Narrowing of pulse pressure
  ❖ Distended neck veins
  ❖ Distant heart sounds
  ❖ Equilibrium of intracardiac pressures with right atrial, pulmonary capillary wedge, and (if measured) left atrial pressures being equal
  ❖ Decreased cardiac output and cardiac index
  ❖ Pulsus paradoxus
  ❖ Sudden decrease or cessation in chest tube drainage
- If time allows, obtain a chest radiograph as prescribed to assess for evidence of widened mediastinum. ➤*Rationale:* Widening of the mediastinum on chest radiograph, especially the right heart border, could be indicative of mediastinal blood.
- If time allows, obtain a transthoracic echocardiogram as prescribed in an attempt to identify a mediastinal clot. ➤*Rationale:* Aids the diagnosis and confirms the necessity for the open sternotomy procedure.

Patient Preparation

- Ensure that the patient and family understand preprocedural teaching (if time available). Answer questions as they arise and reinforce information as needed. ➤*Rationale:* Evaluates and reinforces understanding of previously taught information.
- Ensure that informed consent was obtained (this may not be possible if the procedure is an acute emergency). ➤*Rationale:* Protects rights of the patient and ensures a competent decision for the patient and the family.
- Ensure that patient's ventilation is maintained. ➤*Rationale:* Ensures that the patient's airway is protected and that oxygen needs are met.
- Position patient in supine position with head of bed flat. ➤*Rationale:* Ensures visualization of operative field.
- Administer analgesics or sedatives as prescribed. ➤*Rationale:* Promotes comfort.

Procedure for Emergent Open Sternotomy (Assist)

Steps	Rationale	Special Considerations
1. Call physician and operative team.	The physician can reassess the need for further surgical intervention. The operative team may be needed to assist at the bedside or to prepare the operating room if further exploration is needed.	Follow hospital standard.
2. Assist with preparation of the electrocautery device for possible use: apply ground pad to patient's skin and attach grounding and cautery cables.	This device is used to terminate capillary oozing or bleeding.	
3. Set up a new sterile suction system.	This will be used to suction the mediastinum during the procedure.	
4. Wash hands, and don gloves.	Reduces transmission of microorganisms; standard precautions.	
5. Assist with removing old dressing and surgically prepare skin for incision: cleanse chest with antiseptic solution.	Inhibits microorganism transmission with surgical instrumentation.	Prepare skin from sternal notch to midabdomen and midclavicular line to midclavicular line.
6. Wash hands, and don caps, masks, goggles, sterile gowns, and gloves for all members of the health care team involved with the procedure.	Reduces transmission of microorganisms; sterile precautions; standard precautions.	All personnel in the room must don masks and caps.
7. Assist with placement of sterile towels and drape off each side around the sternotomy incision.	A large sterile field will supply room for placement of instruments.	Allows good view of the sternal notch.

Procedure continued on following page

Procedure for Emergent Open Sternotomy (Assist) *Continued*

Steps	Rationale	Special Considerations
8. Assist with electrocautery and suction as needed.	Assistance is needed if bleeding continues.	
9. Assist as needed by supplying the wire cutters and aiding in the removal of cut wires from the surgical field.	Ensures that wires are adequately removed.	If staples are present, the staple remover will be needed.
10. Assist with cauterization of oozing bleeding sites as needed.	Minimizes blood loss and enhances visualization of the surgical field.	
11. Assist with control of bleeding, enhance sternal retraction, and suction as needed.	May eliminate the need for further exploration and allows for full visualization of the surgical field.	
12. Assist with the placement of chest tubes or pacing wires as needed.	Pacing leads and chest tubes can be displaced during sternal retraction.	
13. Assist with placement of mechanical assist devices if needed.	Cardiac tamponade can conceal right or left ventricular dysfunction; mechanical assistance may be necessary to improve cardiac output.	
14. Assist patient transport to the operating room if necessary.	The patient may need surgical repair of coronary artery bypass grafts, cardiac valves, or the myocardium.	
15. If the patient does not need to return to the operating room, assist the physician or advanced practice nurse with reinsertion of the sternal wires as needed.	Ensures sternal closure.	
16. Assist with skin closure.	Promotes wound healing.	
17. Apply dressing to the sternal incision, epicardial pacing wires, and chest tube sites.	Promotes aseptic management of the surgical incision and wound sites.	The patient's chest may be left open and covered with a sterile, occlusive surgical dressing if severe ventricular dysfunction exists.
18. Remove and discard personal protective equipment, discard used supplies, package instruments for sterilization, and wash hands.	Reduces transmission of microorganisms and body secretions; standard precautions.	

Expected Outcomes

- Increased cardiac output
- Increased tissue perfusion, including cerebral, renal, and peripheral perfusion
- Standard chest tube drainage
- Decreased need for homologous transfusion

Unexpected Outcomes

- Severe right or left ventricular dysfunction
- Continued bleeding or coagulation disorders
- Myocardial or aortic perforation
- Cardiac arrest
- Pneumothorax
- Myocardial infarction
- Atrial and ventricular dysrhythmias
- Pain

Patient Monitoring and Care

Patient Monitoring and Care	Rationale	Reportable Conditions
		These conditions should be reported if they persist despite nursing interventions.
1. Perform cardiovascular, peripheral vascular, and hemodynamic assessments every 15 to 30 minutes as patient status requires.		
A. Assess level of consciousness.	Assess for adequacy of cerebral perfusion; hemodynamic instability can lead to cerebral anoxia.	• Change in level of consciousness
B. Assess vital signs, cardiac index, and pulmonary artery pressures.	Demonstrates hemodynamic stability and volume status; recurrent tamponade or persistent myocardial arterial depression may develop during and after sternotomy.	• Decrease in cardiac output and cardiac index, abnormal pulmonary artery pressures; equalizing pulmonary artery pressures; mean arterial blood pressure less than 60 mm Hg, changes in heart rate
C. Measure urine output.	Validates adequate perfusion to the kidneys.	• Urine output <.5 mL/kg/hr
2. Assess heart and lung sounds every 2 hours and as needed.	Abnormal heart and lung sounds may indicate the need for additional treatment.	• Distant heart sounds or additional changes in heart and lung sounds
3. Monitor coagulation and hematologic studies.	Coagulation and hematologic profiles will provide data that will indicate the risk of bleeding and indicate the need for additional treatment.	• Abnormal hemoglobin and hematocrit, PT, PTT, INR, platelets, fibrinogen
4. Monitor chest tube drainage.	Ensures adequate functioning of the chest tube drainage system.	• Cessation of chest tube drainage; increased chest tube drainage; clots in chest tube drainage system

Documentation

Documentation should include the following:

- Patient and family education
- Indications for the procedure and the procedure used
- Informed consent obtained
- Estimated blood loss
- Patient therapies and response; including hemodynamics, inotropic or vasopressor agents, ventilation, and neurologic status
- Unexpected outcomes
- Additional interventions

Reference

1. Lyerly H. *Handbook of Surgical Intensive Care.* Chicago, Ill: Year Book Medical Publishers; 1995:83–86.

Additional Readings

Bojar R, Mathisen D, Warner K. *Manual of Perioperative Care in Cardiac and Thoracic Surgery.* Boston, Mass: Blackwell Scientific Publications; 1994:98–99.

Borkon M, Schaff H, Gardner T, et al. Diagnosis and management of postoperative pericardial effusions and late cardiac tamponade following open-heart surgery. *Ann Thorac Surg.* 1981; 31:512–518.

Fairman R, Edmunds H. Emergency thoracotomy in the surgical care unit after open cardiac operation. *Ann Thorac Surg.* 1981; 32:386–391.

Sabiston D, Spencer F. *Surgery of the Chest.* Philadelphia, Pa: W.B. Saunders, 1995:220–222.

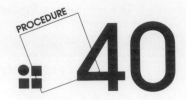

40 Pericardiocentesis (Assist)

PURPOSE: Pericardiocentesis is performed to remove fluid from the pericardial sac, to obtain a specimen for the differential diagnosis of pericardial effusion, and to prevent or treat cardiac tamponade. Cardiac output is usually improved after pericardiocentesis.

Ann Louise Jones

PREREQUISITE NURSING KNOWLEDGE

- Cardiovascular anatomy and physiology should be understood.
- Pericardial effusion is the abnormal accumulation of more than 50 mL of fluid in the pericardial sac.
- A pericardial effusion can be noncompressive or compressive. With a compressive effusion, there is increased pressure within the pericardial sac, which results in cardiac tamponade and resistance to cardiac filling.
- The presentation of acute and chronic fluid accumulation varies. A rapid collection of fluid (over minutes to hours) may result in hemodynamic compromise with volumes of less than 250 mL. Chronically developing effusions (over days to weeks) allow for hypertrophy and distention of the fibrous parietal membrane.[1] Therefore, a patient may accumulate 2000 mL or more of fluid before exhibiting hemodynamic compromise symptoms.[2]
- Symptoms of cardiac tamponade are not specific. Patients may exhibit signs and symptoms of an associated disease. With a decrease in cardiac output, the patient often develops tachycardia, tachypnea, pallor, cyanosis, impaired cerebral and renal function, sweating, hypotension, neck vein distention, and pulsus paradoxus.[3]
- The presence and amount of fluid in the pericardium are evaluated through chest radiograph, two-dimensional echocardiogram, and clinical findings.
- Once cardiac tamponade is verified, a pericardiocentesis is performed to remove fluid from the pericardial sac. An acute tamponade resulting in hemodynamic instability necessitates an emergency procedure.
- A critical care nurse assists with the pericardiocentesis and continuously monitors the patient's response to the procedure.
- Pericardiocentesis is commonly performed using a subxiphoid approach.
- Two-dimensional echocardiography is an option to guide the pericardiocentesis.[4]
- Failed pericardial drainage, reaccumulation of pericardial fluid, or cardiac injury may progress into cardiac tamponade requiring urgent or emergent chest exploration.

EQUIPMENT

- Pericardiocentesis tray (or thoracentesis tray)
- 16- or 18-G 3-in cardiac needle or catheter over the needle
- J-Guide wire, 0.035 diameter
- Vessel dilator, #7 Fr
- Pigtail catheter, #7 Fr
- Tubing and drainage bag or bottle (for continuous drainage setup)
- 30 mL povidone-iodine
- Two packs of 4 × 4 gauze sponges
- #11 knife blade with handle
- Sterile 50-mL, 10-mL, 5-mL, and 3-mL syringes
- Sterile drapes and towels
- Mask, surgical cap, sterile gown, and gloves for all personnel
- Sterile alligator clip cable
- Two three-way stopcocks
- 1% lidocaine (topical)
- Emergency cart (defibrillator, emergency respiratory equipment, emergency cardiac drugs, and temporary pacemaker)
- 12-lead electrocardiogram (ECG) machine
- 2-dimensional echography equipment (optional)
- Culture bottles and specimen tubes for fluid analysis
- 2- and 3-in tape

PATIENT AND FAMILY EDUCATION

- Instruct the patient and family regarding the reason pericardiocentesis is needed, give a description of the procedure, and explain expected outcomes and possible complications. **➤Rationale:** Information about the procedure decreases anxiety and apprehension.
- Instruct patient and family on potential signs and symptoms of recurrent pericardial effusion (ie, dyspnea, dull ache or pressure within the chest, dysphagia, cough, tachypnea, hoarseness, hiccups, or nausea).[5] **➤Rationale:** Early detection of pericardial effusion may prevent complications from heart compression.
- Instruct patient and family about patient's risk for recurrent pericardial effusion. **➤Rationale:** Predicting pericardial effusion may allow early detection of a life-threatening problem.

PATIENT ASSESSMENT AND PREPARATION

Patient Assessment

- Determine history of present illness as well as mechanism of injury (if applicable), past medical history, and current medical therapies. ➨*Rationale:* Needed to determine patient's present health, to identify potential risk factors, and to provide an opportunity for the nurse to establish a relationship with the patient.
- Determine baseline heart rate, cardiac rhythm, heart sounds (S1, S2, rubs), venous pressure, blood pressure, pulse pressure, SpO₂, respiratory status, and neurologic status.
- ➨*Rationale:* Need to compare baseline heart rate, cardiac rhythm, heart sounds (S1, S2, rubs), venous pressure, blood pressure, breath sounds, respiratory status and neurologic status to assess changes during or after procedure.
- Assess current laboratory values including complete blood cell (CBC) count, electrolytes, and coagulation profile. ➨*Rationale:* Needed to identify potential for cardiac dysrhythmias or abnormal bleeding.

Patient Preparation

- Ensure that the patient and family understand preprocedural teaching. Answer questions as they arise and reinforce information as needed. ➨*Rationale:* Evaluates and reinforces understanding of previously taught information.
- Validate that the informed consent has been signed. ➨*Rationale:* Protects rights of patient and makes competent decision possible for patient; however, under emergency circumstances, time may not allow form to be signed.
- Position patient comfortably in supine position with head of bed elevated 30 to 60 degrees. ➨*Rationale:* Facilitates aspiration of pericardial fluids and ease of breathing.
- Administer sedatives as prescribed. ➨*Rationale:* Reduces anxiety, promotes comfort, and decreases myocardial workload.
- Apply limb leads and connect to cardiac bedside monitoring system or to 12-lead ECG machine. ➨*Rationale:* ECG changes may indicate cardiac injury.

Procedure **for Pericardiocentesis (Assist)**

Steps	Rationale	Special Considerations
1. Wash hands, and apply personal protective gear.	Reduces transmission of microorganisms; standard precautions.	
2. Open pericardiocentesis tray and appropriate supplies using aseptic technique (other supplies are opened as needed).	Minimizes potential for infection.	
3. Ensure that patient is positioned comfortably in supine position (or with head of bed elevated up to 60 degrees).	Facilitates aspiration of fluids (elevated head of bed facilitates ease of breathing).	
4. Prepare skin by applying antibacterial solution.	Minimizes potential for infection.	Shaving the area may be necessary before applying antibacterial solution.
5. Assist personnel with donning mask, surgical cap, sterile gown, and gloves.	Maintains aseptic technique.	
6. Prepare syringe of topical 1% lidocaine.	Reduces patient's discomfort.	
7. Attach three-way stopcock, 3-in cardiac needle, and 50-mL syringe.	Provides mechanism to aspirate fluid.	
8. Assist physician in connecting one end of alligator clip to the metal portion of the needle and the other end to the V₁ lead of the ECG. Use bedside monitor or ECG machine (see Fig. 40–1).	Provides mechanism to identify myocardial injury. If the needle contacts the ventricle, ST depression should be seen. With atrial contact, PR segment elevation will occur. Maintains aseptic technique.	
9. Observe physician slowly insert needle into pericardial sac until fluid is aspirated.	Minimizes risk of cardiac injury.	The movement of the heart usually defibrinates blood in the pericardial space. Clotting indicates penetration of the heart.[6] *Procedure continued on following page*

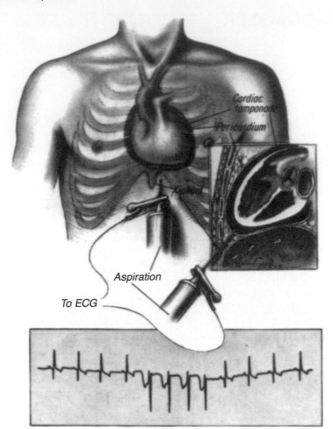

■ ● FIGURE 40–1. Illustration of subxiphoid pericardiocentesis with electrocardiographic monitoring. Note negative QRS deflection indicating myocardial contact. (From Sabiston DC Jr, Spencer FC. *Surgery of the Chest.* 6th ed. Philadelphia: W.B. Saunders; 1995.)

Procedure	for Pericardiocentesis (Assist) *Continued*

Steps	Rationale	Special Considerations
10. Continuously monitor bedside ECG or 12-lead ECG, vital signs, SpO₂, and venous pressure during needle aspiration, fluid withdrawal, and withdrawal of needle.	Detects myocardial injury; monitors results of procedure.	Emergent chest exploration may be necessary if aspiration is unsuccessful, pericardial fluid repeatedly accumulates, or complications develop.[7]
11. If indwelling catheter is placed to continuously drain large pericardial effusion, attach to sterile bag or bottle using aseptic technique (see Procedure 71).	Facilitates fluid drainage; minimizes potential for infection.	
12. Once needle has been withdrawn, cleanse antiseptic solution from skin and apply sterile dressing.	Minimizes skin breakdown and minimizes infection.	
13. Send pericardial fluid samples to laboratory for evaluation.	Provides diagnosis of organism involved in pericardial effusion.	Usual tests include body fluid cytology, cell count, electrolytes, routine aerobic and anaerobic cultures, acid-fast bacilli cultures, and other tests as indicated.
14. Continue bedside ECG monitoring and discontinue 12-lead ECG (if used).	Change in cardiac rhythm may indicate cardiac tamponade or injury.	

Procedure **for Pericardiocentesis (Assist)** *Continued*

Steps	Rationale	Special Considerations
15. Provide emotional support to the patient throughout the procedure.	Minimizes apprehension and anxiety.	
16. Dispose of used supplies.	Standard precautions.	
17. Wash hands.	Reduces transmission of microorganisms; standard precautions.	

Expected Outcomes

- Fluid removed from pericardial sac
- Relief of pain and discomfort
- Improved cardiac output
- Patient's blood pressure, venous pressure, heart sounds, pulse pressure, and cardiac rhythm within normal limits

Unexpected Outcomes

- Patient has drop in blood pressure, rise in venous pressure, cardiac dysrhythmias, or excessive bleeding.
- Patient has cardiac dysrhythmias.
- Patient has ST depression.
- Patient has PR segment elevation.

Patient Monitoring and Care

Patient Monitoring and Care	Rationale	Reportable Conditions
		These conditions should be reported if they persist despite nursing interventions.
1. Continuously monitor ECG; evaluate venous pressure, systemic blood pressure, heart sounds, SpO₂, and neurologic status before, during, and every 15 minutes immediately postprocedure until stable (if available, continuously monitor cardiac index and systemic vascular resistance [SVR]).	A change in these signs may indicate cardiac tamponade, cardiac injury, or hemodynamic instability.	• Rising venous pressure, falling arterial pressure, decrease in intensity of heart sounds, change in level of consciousness, or pulsus paradoxus; if applicable, abnormal cardiac index or SVR
2. Treat dysrhythmias as prescribed.	Dysrhythmias may lead to cardiac decompensation or arrest or both.	• Persistent dysrhythmias despite appropriate intervention
3. Auscultate heart and lung sounds immediately after procedure.	Evaluates potential fluid reaccumulation or puncture of lung.	• Asymmetric breath sounds, dyspnea, tachypnea, abrupt change in SpO₂, or decrease in heart sound intensity
4. Obtain portable chest radiograph immediately postprocedure.	Assesses for pneumothorax or hemothorax.	• Pneumothorax or hemothorax
5. Obtain two-dimensional echocardiogram within several hours (as prescribed).	Demonstrates adequate pericardial drainage.	• Pericardial effusion
6. Monitor pericardiocentesis site for bleeding.	Assesses for puncture of heart, lungs, stomach, or liver.	• Bleeding or hematoma at site; decrease in hemoglobin or hematocrit; changes in coagulation studies
7. Assess pericardiocentesis site for signs of infection.	Potential catheter-related sepsis.	• Erythema, edema, purulent drainage, or foul odor of site. Temperature >100.5°F (38°C).
8. Change dressing daily and as needed.	Minimizes potential for infection.	
9. Reposition patient for safety and comfort (usually supine in position); may raise head of bed 30 to 60 degrees.	Protects patient from injury and facilitates ease of breathing.	
10. Be prepared for chest exploration because of deterioration in patient's condition.	Deterioration may indicate development of further cardiac tamponade.	• Decreased blood pressure, dysrhythmias, increased venous pressure, change in mental or respiratory status, perspiration, or distant heart sounds

Continued on following page

Patient Monitoring and Care	Rationale	Reportable Conditions
11. Keep patient and patient's family informed about patient's condition. Be available to answer family's questions and facilitate meeting their needs as appropriate.	The unknown increases the anxiety and apprehension of the patient and the patient's family.	

Documentation

Documentation should include the following:

- Preprocedure instruction and patient and family's response
- Preprocedure and postprocedure blood pressure, venous pressure, heart sounds, level of consciousness, respiratory status, cardiac rhythm
- Medications administered
- Amount and consistency of postprocedure drainage

- Assessment of pericardiocentesis site
- Occurrence of unexpected outcomes
- ECG rhythm strips
- Nursing interventions required
- Specimens sent to laboratory

References

1. Focht G, Becker RC. Pericardiocentesis. In: Rippe JM, Irwin RS, Fink MP, et al., eds. *Intensive Care Medicine.* Boston, Mass: Little, Brown & Co; 1996:111–116.
2. Shabetai R. Treatment of pericardial disease. In: Smith TW, ed. *Cardiovascular Therapeutics: A Companion to Braunwald's Heart Disease.* Philadelphia, Pa: W.B. Saunders, 1996:742–746.
3. Spodick D. Percarditis, pericardial effusion, cardiac tamponade, and constriction. *Crit Care Clin.* 1989;5:455–476.
4. Douglas JM. The pericardium. In: Sabiston JR, Spencer FC, eds. *Surgery of the Chest.* Philadelphia, Pa: W.B. Saunders, 1995:1379–1380.
5. Muirhead J. Pericardial disease. In: Underhill SL, Woods SL, SaVarajan Froelicher ES, et al, eds. *Cardiac Nursing.* Philadelphia, Pa: J.B. Lippincott; 1989:111–116.
6. Yeston N, Grotz R, Loiacono L. Pericardiocentesis. In: Civetta JM, Taylor JW, Kirby RR, eds. *Critical Care.* Philadelphia, Pa: Lippincott-Raven; 1997:577–578.
7. Suddarth DS. *Lippincott Manual of Nursing Practive.* Philadelphia, Pa: J.B. Lippincott; 1991:310–311.

Additional Readings

Loeb S, McCloskey PW, Tryniszewski C. *Critical Care Procedures.* Springhouse, Pa: Springhouse Corp; 1994:225–229.
Lorell B. Pericardial disease. In: Braunwald AB, ed. *Heart Disease: A Textbook of Cardiovascular Medicine.* Philadelphia, Pa: W.B. Saunders; 1997:1478–1524.
Mavroukakis S, Stine A. Nursing management of adults with disorders of the coronary arteries, myocardium, or pericardium. In: Beare PG, Myers JL, eds. *Adult Health Nursing.* St. Louis, Mo: C.V. Mosby; 1998:597–603.

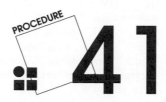

PROCEDURE

41

Atrial Electrogram

PURPOSE: An atrial electrogram (AEG) is obtained to determine the presence of atrial activity in a dysrhythmia or to identify the relationship between atrial and ventricular depolarizations.

Teresa Preuss
Debra J. Lynn-McHale

PREREQUISITE NURSING KNOWLEDGE

- The anatomy and physiology of the cardiovascular system, principles of cardiac conduction, and basic dysrhythmia interpretation should be understood.
- Principles of general electrical safety apply when using temporary invasive pacing. Gloves should always be worn when handling pacing electrodes to prevent microshock because even small amounts of electric current can cause serious dysrhythmias if transmitted to the heart.
- Advanced cardiac life support knowledge and skills are necessary.
- Indications for AEG are as follows:
  - ❖ When atrial activity is not clearly detected on electrocardiogram (ECG) monitoring
  - ❖ To determine the relationship between atrial and ventricular activity
  - ❖ To differentiate wide complex rhythms (ie, ventricular tachycardia and supraventricular tachycardia with aberrant ventricular conduction)
  - ❖ To differentiate narrow complex supraventricular tachycardias (ie, sinus tachycardia, atrial tachycardia, paroxysmal supraventricular tachycardia, atrial flutter, atrial fibrillation with relatively regular R-R intervals, or junctional tachycardia)
- Atrial electrograms can be performed by using a multichannel bedside ECG monitor that allows for simultaneous display of the AEG along with the surface ECG. A 12-lead ECG machine can also be used to obtain an AEG.
- An AEG is a method of recording electrical activity originating from the atria by using temporary atrial epicardial wires placed during cardiac surgery. Standard ECG monitoring records electrical events from the heart using electrodes located on the surface of the patient's body, which is a considerable distance from the myocardium. One limitation of ECG monitoring may be its inability to detect P waves effectively.
- Atrial electrograms detect electrical events directly from or in close proximity to the atria, providing a greatly

enhanced tracing of atrial activity. This enhanced tracing allows for comparison of atrial events with ventricular events and determination of the relationship between the two.
- It is important to accurately identify the epicardial atrial pacing wire or wires.
- The two types of AEGs that can be obtained from epicardial pacing wires are unipolar and bipolar.
- A *unipolar electrogram* measures electrical activity between one atrial epicardial wire and a surface ECG electrode. The *unipolar AEG* detects both atrial and ventricular activity.
- A *bipolar electrogram* detects electrical activity between the two atrial epicardial wires attached to the myocardium. The *bipolar AEG* predominantly detects atrial activity, because both electrodes are attached to the atria.

EQUIPMENT

- Clean gloves
- Temporary atrial epicardial pacing wires placed during cardiac surgery
- Alligator clips or AEG-modified patient lead wires
- Bedside multichannel ECG monitor and recorder or 12-lead ECG machine (ensure that biomedical safety standards are met and safe for use with epicardial wires)
- Sterile dressings and materials needed for site care

PATIENT AND FAMILY EDUCATION

- Assess the readiness to learn of patient and family and factors that affect learning. **➥Rationale:** Allows the nurse to individualize teaching.
- Provide information about the normal conduction system, normal and abnormal heart rhythms, and symptoms of abnormal heart rhythms. **➥Rationale:** Assists patient and family to understand the patient's condition and encourages the patient and family to ask questions.

- Provide information about the AEG, reason for the AEG, and explanation of the equipment. ➤➤*Rationale:* Decreases patient anxiety. Assists patient and family to understand the procedure, why it is needed, and how it will help the patient.
- Explain the patient's expected participation during the procedure. ➤➤*Rationale:* Encourages patient compliance.

PATIENT ASSESSMENT AND PREPARATION

Patient Assessment

- Assess cardiac rhythm for the presence of atrial activity. ➤➤*Rationale:* Determines the presence or absence of P waves and the potential need for an AEG.
- Assess cardiac rhythm for the relationship between atrial and ventricular activity. ➤➤*Rationale:* Determines the relationship between P waves and QRS complexes and the potential need for an AEG.

- Assess for dysrhythmias. ➤➤*Rationale:* Determines baseline cardiac rhythm.
- Assess for compromise of hemodynamic status (eg, systolic blood pressure less than 90 mm Hg; mean arterial pressure less than 60 mm Hg; altered level of consciousness (LOC); patient reports of dizziness, shortness of breath, nausea, vomiting, cool or clammy skin, or chest pain). ➤➤*Rationale:* Clinical parameters that reflect a decreased cardiac output indicate a need for immediate intervention.

Patient Preparation

- Ensure that the patient understands preprocedural teaching. Answer questions as they arise and reinforce information as needed. ➤➤*Rationale:* Evaluates and reinforces understanding of previously taught information.
- Expose patient's chest and identify epicardial pacing wires. ➤➤*Rationale:* Provides access to atrial pacing wires.

Procedure	for Atrial Electrogram

Steps	Rationale	Special Considerations
1. Wash hands, and don gloves.	Reduces transmission of microorganisms and body secretions; standard precautions.	Use of gloves prevents microshocks when handling epicardial wires.[1,2]
2. Expose and identify the atrial epicardial pacing wires.	It is important to differentiate the atrial from ventricular wires to ensure that the appropriate epicardial wires are used.	Typically, the atrial wires exit the chest to the right of the patient's sternum and the ventricular wires exit to the left of the patient's sternum (Fig. 41–1).

Obtaining a Unipolar AEG Using a Multichannel Bedside ECG Monitor—Lead I

1. Attach one atrial pacing wire to the alligator clip of the AEG-modified patient lead wire (Fig. 41–2).	One atrial pacing wire is used when obtaining a unipolar AEG.	

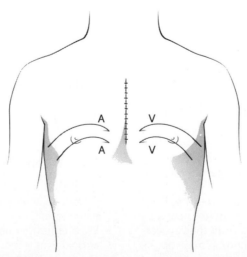

■ ● **FIGURE 41–1.** Atrial wires exit chest to the right of the patient's sternum. Ventricular wires exit chest to the left of the patient's sternum. (Drawing by Todd Sargood.)

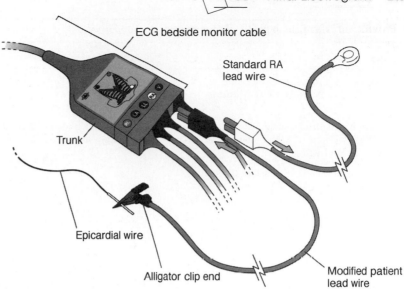

■ ● **FIGURE 41–2.** ECG bedside monitor cable with modified patient lead wire connected to epicardial wire. (Drawing by Todd Sargood.) ECG, electrocardiogram.

Labels: ECG bedside monitor cable; Standard RA lead wire; Trunk; Epicardial wire; Alligator clip end; Modified patient lead wire

Procedure for Atrial Electrogram *Continued*

Steps	Rationale	Special Considerations
2. Disconnect the surface ECG standard lead wire from the right arm (RA) port of the trunk of the ECG bedside monitor cable (see Fig. 41–2).		
3. Plug the AEG-modified patient lead wire into the RA port of the trunk of the ECG bedside monitor cable.	Connects the atrial pacing wire to the ECG bedside monitoring system.	Determine that ECG bedside monitoring system meets all safety requirements.
4. Select Lead I on the bedside ECG monitor.	Lead I detects electrical activity between the RA limb lead and the left arm (LA) limb lead. Because the atrial pacing wire is connected into the RA port, Lead I will detect the electrical activity between the atrial wire and the surface LA limb lead.	
5. Record a strip.	Displays AEG for analysis.	Dual-channel recorder permits the comparison of the surface ECG and the AEG.
6. Analyze AEG strip (Fig. 41–3).	Compares the surface ECG with the AEG. Identifies P waves and QRS complexes and determines the relationship between the P waves and the QRS complexes.	

Procedure continued on following page

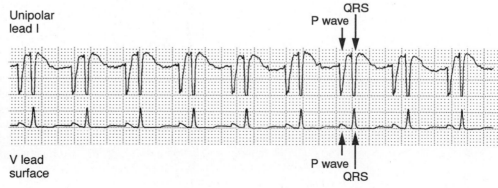

■ ● **FIGURE 41–3.** Unipolar AEG strip from Lead I. The surface ECG was obtained in the V lead. The unipolar AEG was obtained in lead I. Note that the atrial activity is magnified in lead I. AEG, atrial electrogram. ECG, electrocardiogram.

Unipolar lead I

V lead surface

P wave | QRS

Procedure **for Atrial Electrogram** *Continued*

Steps	Rationale	Special Considerations
Obtaining a Unipolar AEG Using a Multichannel Bedside ECG Monitor— V Lead		
1. Attach one atrial pacing wire to the alligator clip of the AEG-modified patient lead wire.	One atrial pacing wire is used when obtaining a unipolar AEG.	
2. Disconnect the surface ECG standard lead wire from the V lead port of the trunk of the ECG bedside monitor cable.		
3. Plug the AEG-modified patient lead wire into the V lead port of the trunk of the ECG bedside monitor cable.	Connects the atrial pacing wire to the ECG bedside monitoring system.	Determine that ECG bedside monitoring system meets all safety requirements.
4. Select V lead on the bedside ECG monitor.	Use of the precordial lead allows for detection of atrial electrical activity between the V lead and an indifferent limb lead in a unipolar configuration.	
5. Record a strip.	Displays AEG for analysis.	
6. Analyze AEG strip (Fig. 41–4).	Compares the surface ECG with the AEG. Identifies P waves and QRS complexes and determines the relationship between the P waves and the QRS complexes.	
Obtaining a Bipolar AEG Using a Multichannel Bedside ECG Monitor		
1. Attach both atrial pacing wires to alligators clips of two separate AEG-modified patient lead wires.	Two atrial pacing wires are used when obtaining a bipolar AEG.	
2. Disconnect the surface ECG standard lead wire from the RA and LA lead ports of the trunk of the ECG bedside monitor cable.		
3. Plug the AEG-modified patient lead wires into the RA and LA ports of the trunk of the ECG bedside monitor cable.	Connects the atrial pacing wires to the ECG bedside monitoring system.	Determine that ECG bedside monitoring system meets all safety requirements.
4. Select Lead I on the bedside ECG monitor.	Lead I detects electrical activity between the RA limb lead and the LA limb lead. Because the atrial pacing wires are connected into the RA and LA ports, Lead I will detect the electrical activity between the two atrial wires.	
5. Record a strip.	Displays AEG for analysis.	

Unipolar
V lead

QRS
P wave

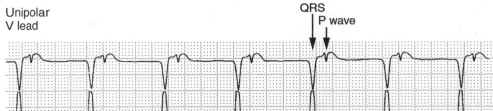

Lead II
surface

QRS

■ ● **FIGURE 41–4.** Unipolar AEG strip. The surface ECG was obtained in lead II. Based on the surface ECG, the rhythm appears to be junctional with no evidence of P waves or atrial activity. The unipolar AEG clearly demonstrates retrograde P waves that follow the QRS complex, thus confirming the junctional rhythm interpretation. AEG, atrial electrogram. ECG, electrocardiogram.

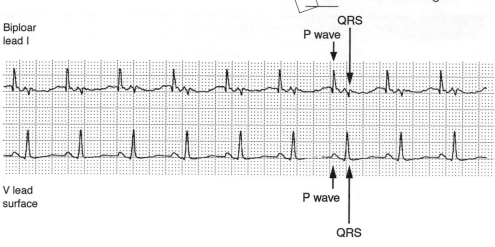

Bipolar
lead I

QRS

P wave

V lead
surface

P wave

QRS

■ ● **FIGURE 41–5.** Bipolar AEG strip of lead I. The surface ECG was obtained in the V lead. The bipolar AEG was obtained in lead I. Note that the atrial activity is magnified in lead I. Also note how small the ventricular activity is in lead I. AEG, atrial electrogram. ECG, electrocardiogram.

| Procedure | for Atrial Electrogram *Continued* |

Steps	Rationale	Special Considerations
6. Analyze AEG strip (Fig. 41–5).	Displays AEG for analysis. Compares the surface ECG with AEG. Identifies P waves and QRS complexes and determines the relationship between the P waves and the QRS complexes.	Dual-channel recorder permits the comparison of the surface ECG and the AEG. Bipolar tracings usually magnify atrial activity and minimize ventricular activity.
Obtaining a Unipolar AEG Using a 12-Lead ECG Machine		
1. Connect the patient to the 12-lead ECG machine (see Procedure 54).	Provides another method of obtaining an AEG.	Determine that the 12-lead ECG machine meets all safety requirements.
2. Attach one atrial epicardial pacing wire to the clip of the RA lead wire of the 12-lead ECG machine (Fig. 41–6).		
3. Run a 12-lead ECG.	Lead I measures the electrical activity between the RA and LA. Because the atrial pacing wire is connected to the RA lead, Lead I will detect the electrical activity between the atrial wire and the surface LA limb lead. Lead II measures the electrical activity between the RA and left leg (LL). Because the atrial pacing wire is connected to the RA lead, Lead II will detect the electrical activity between the atrial wire and the surface LL lead.	*Procedure continued on following page*

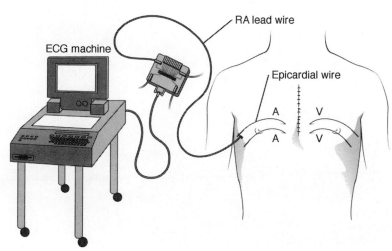

ECG machine

RA lead wire

Epicardial wire

A   V

A   V

■ ● **FIGURE 41–6.** Attach 12-lead ECG per procedure, except that the RA lead wire will connect to one of the atrial epicardial pacing wires. (Drawing by Todd Sargood.) ECG, electrocardiogram.

Procedure | **for Atrial Electrogram** *Continued*

Steps	Rationale	Special Considerations
4. Analyze Leads I and II.	Identifies P waves and QRS complexes and determines the relationship between the P waves and the QRS complexes.	

Obtaining a Bipolar AEG Using a 12-Lead ECG Machine

Steps	Rationale	Special Considerations
1. Connect the patient to the 12-lead ECG machine (see Procedure 54).	Provides another method of obtaining an AEG.	Determine that 12-lead ECG machine meets all safety requirements.
2. Attach one atrial epicardial pacing wire to the RA limb lead and the other atrial epicardial wire to the LA limb lead of the 12-lead ECG machine.	Connection to the limb leads of the ECG machine allows for the detection and recording of atrial electrical activity.	
3. Run a 12-lead ECG (Fig. 41–7).	Lead I measures the electrical activity between the RA and LA limb leads, which sense atrial activity from both epicardial wires, to provide a bipolar tracing.	
4. Analyze Lead I (see Fig. 41–7).	Displays bipolar AEG for analysis. Identifies P waves and QRS complexes and determines the relationship between the P waves and the QRS complexes.	Bipolar tracings usually magnify atrial activity and minimize ventricular activity. Using this method, unipolar AEGs are also obtained in Lead II and Lead III.

After AEG Is Obtained

Steps	Rationale	Special Considerations
1. Disconnect the atrial pacing wires from the alligator clip.	Removes equipment used for obtaining the AEG.	
2. Apply a dry sterile dressing to epicardial wire exit site(s).	Reduces the transmission of microorganisms; sterile precautions.	Follow institution guidelines for site care.
3. Place the uninsulated portion of the epicardial wires in an insulated material.	Prevents microshock.	
4. Discard disposable supplies, and wash hands.	Reduces the transmission of microorganisms; standard precautions.	

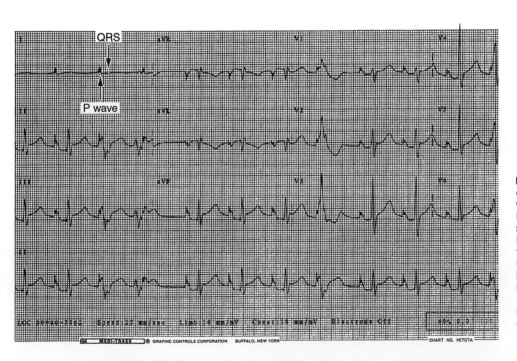

■ ● FIGURE 41–7. A 12-lead ECG obtained with two atrial pacing wires connected to the RA and LA lead wires. Lead I demonstrates a bipolar AEG. Note the P wave is greater in size than the QRS complex. Leads II and III demonstrate unipolar AEGs. In both leads II and III, atrial activity is enhanced. Throughout, the 12-lead ECG atrial activity is enhanced. AEG, atrial electrogram. ECG, electrocardiogram.

Expected Outcomes	Unexpected Outcomes
• Atrial activity is identified. • The relationship between atrial and ventricular activity is determined.	• Hemodynamically significant dysrhythmias • Dysrhythmias in which atrial activity is unclear or the relationship between atrial and ventricular activity is unclear • Microschocks causing dysrhythmias

Patient Monitoring and Care

Patient Monitoring and Care	Rationale	Reportable Conditions
		These conditions should be reported if they persist despite nursing interventions.
1. Evaluate the AEG for the presence of atrial activity and its relationship to ventricular activity. Compare with surface ECG for interpretation.	AEG will enhance atrial activity to allow for clarification of dysrhythmia origin.	• Inability to identify atrial activity
2. Monitor ECG rhythm for changes.	The underlying dysrhythmia may change during the AEG.	• Altered hemodynamic status caused by change in ECG rhythm
3. Monitor vital signs and LOC during the AEG and as needed.	Ensure adequate tissue perfusion.	• Hemodynamic instability or decrease in LOC
4. Evaluate and treat dysrhythmias.	Identification and treatment of dysrhythmias may improve patient outcome.	• Return of rhythm stability; change in cardiac rate or rhythm
5. Site care should be as follows:		
A. Cleanse the area surrounding the epicardial pacing wires with an antiseptic solution such as povidone-iodine.	Reduces infection. The Centers for Disease Control and Prevention (CDC) does not have a specific recommendation for care of epicardial pacing wires or site care.	• Any signs or symptoms of infection
B. Apply a dry sterile dressing with the date and time of the dressing change. Institution standard should be followed for frequency and type of dressing.	The CDC recommends that all patient dressings should be changed if the dressing becomes damp, loosened, or soiled.[3]	
C. Protect the exposed, uninsulated portion of the epicardial pacing wires in an insulated environment according to institution standards (eg, closed container, finger cots, insulated gloves).	Prevents microshocks and potentially lethal dysrhythmias.	

Documentation

Documentation should include the following:

- Patient and family education
- ECG tracings before, during, and after AEG
- AEG tracing with interpretation
- Hemodynamic status and LOC
- Patient toleration
- Occurrence of unexpected outcome
- Interventions taken

References

1. Finkelmeier BA, Salinger MH. The atrial electrogram: its diagnostic use following cardiac surgery. *Crit Care Nurse.* 1984;4:42–46.
2. Lynn-McHale DJ, Riggs KL, Thurman L. Epicardial pacing after cardiac surgery. *Crit Care Nurse.* 1991;11:62–77.
3. Pearson MD. Guidelines for prevention of intravascular device–related infections. *Am J Infect Control.* 1996;24:262–293.

Additional Readings

Bass LS, Schneider CL. Temporary epicardial electrodes. *Dimens Crit Care Nurs.* 1986;5:80–90.

Bumgarner LI. Diagnostic uses of epicardial electrodes after cardiac surgery. *Prog Cardiovasc Nurs.* 1992;7:21–24.

Sulzbach LM. The use of temporary atrial wire electrodes to record atrial electrograms in patients who had cardiac surgery. *Heart Lung.* 1985;14:540–548.

Sulzbach LM, Lansdowne LM. Temporary atrial pacing after cardiac surgery. *Focus Crit Care.* 1991;18:65–74.

Young LC. Atrial electrogram: an asset to ECG monitoring. *Crit Care Nurse.* 1981;1:14–18.

Overdrive Atrial Pacing *Continued*

	Rationale	Special Considerations
pacing wires, follow		
epicardial pacing	Atrial wires exit the chest to the right of the patient's sternum (see Fig. 41–1).	The atrial epicardial pacing wires can be verified by performing an atrial electrogram (see Procedure 41) or by atrial pacing (see Procedure 47).
negative terminal of ng cable to an atrial cing wire.	Pacing current is delivered through the negative terminal of the pulse generator; therefore, an epicardial pacing wire on the atrium must be connected to the negative terminal for the atrium to receive pacing impulses.	
positive terminal of ng cable to a second cing wire or to a	The pacing circuit is completed as energy reaches the positive electrode.	Additional options for a ground wire include a subcutaneous needle in the tissue on the chest or an ECG monitoring electrode on the chest near the epicardial wire exit site. The positive terminal of the connecting cable is then connected to the subcutaneous needle hub or to the metal nipple of the monitoring electrode with a double alligator clip.
the milliampere (mA/ on the pulse generator.	Settings are based on the characteristics of the patient's dysrhythmia and the threshold required for atrial capture.	The pacing rate is initially set at least 10 beats per minute higher than the intrinsic atrial rate (often 20% to 30% higher) for atrial tachycardia or atrial flutter. If the rhythm is atrial fibrillation, the pacing rate is usually set in the 300 to 350 pulses per minute range initially and may be increased to the maximum of 800 pulses per minute. An output of at least 10 mAs is recommended, and outputs up to 20 mAs are sometimes necessary.[1]
for a brief period r for several seconds), rminate pacing.	Short bursts of pacing stimuli at a rapid rate are intended to create refractory tissue in the atrium and interrupt the reentry circuit responsible for the tachyarrhythmia.[1, 3] These bursts can be repeated at faster rates and for longer intervals until the dysrhythmia terminates or changes.	Refer to the pulse generator's technical manual for instructions on how to initiate rapid atrial pacing. On termination of the dysrhythmia, the sinus node may be suppressed for a period, resulting in bradycardia, asystole, junctional or ventricular escape rhythms, or polymorphic ventricular tachycardia. It may be necessary to initiate temporary ventricular pacing or transcutaneous pacing for a period until normal sinus function returns.
connecting cable from pacing wires or from the cing electrode connector	Remove rapid atrial pacemaker.	Standard pacing can be resumed if necessary.

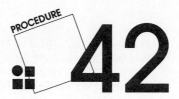
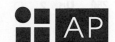

Overdrive Atrial Pacing

PURPOSE: Overdrive atrial pacing is used in an attempt to terminate reentrant atrial dysrhythmias, especially atrial flutter, and allow restoration of sinus rhythm. Sinus rhythm enhances cardiac output by allowing atrial contraction to contribute to ventricular filling.

Carol Jacobson

PREREQUISITE NURSING KNOWLEDGE

- Understanding of the anatomy and physiology of the cardiovascular system, principles of cardiac conduction, and basic and advanced dysrhythmia interpretation is necessary.
- Understanding of pacemakers is required to evaluate pacemaker function and the patient response to pacemaker therapy.
- Principles of general electrical safety apply when using temporary invasive pacing. Gloves should always be worn when handling pacing electrodes to prevent microshock, because even small amounts of electric current can cause serious dysrhythmias if they are transmitted to the heart.
- Clinical and technical competence related to use of an atrial pacing pulse generator or the rapid atrial pacing feature of a standard pulse generator is needed.
- Advanced cardiac life support (ACLS) knowledge and skills should be understood.
- Supraventricular dysrhythmias, such as atrial flutter, reentrant atrial tachycardia, atrioventricular (AV) nodal reentry tachycardia, and reentrant tachycardias that use an accessory pathway in Wolff-Parkinson-White (WPW) syndrome, can sometimes be terminated by overdrive atrial pacing.
- Atrial fibrillation occasionally terminates with overdrive atrial pacing, but this is not a reliable therapy for atrial fibrillation.
- Overdrive atrial pacing is most commonly performed using epicardial atrial pacing wires placed during cardiac surgery. A transvenous atrial pacing lead can also be used, especially now that temporary transvenous atrial leads with an active fixation (screw) tip are available to help keep the lead in the atrium.
- A pulse generator that is capable of overdrive atrial pacing should be selected. An atrial pacing pulse generator (Fig. 42–1) can be used to perform rapid atrial pacing. Some of the newer temporary pulse generators have a feature that can be used to perform rapid atrial pacing (Fig. 42–2).
- Overdrive atrial pacing involves the delivery of short bursts of rapid pacing stimuli through an epicardial atrial pacing wire or an atrial transvenous lead to the atrium. The physician or advanced practice nurse usually determines the duration and rate of the burst.
  - ❖ Typically, a 10- to 30-second burst at a rate 20% to 30% faster than the intrinsic atrial rate is initially used (eg, begin at a rate of 375 pulses per minute for atrial

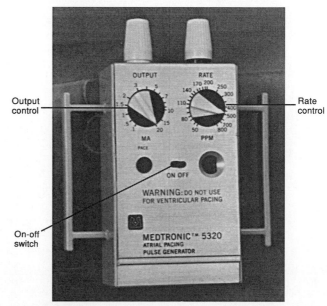

■ ● FIGURE 42–1. High-rate temporary atrial pulse generator for overdrive atrial pacing. (From Medtronic, Inc.)

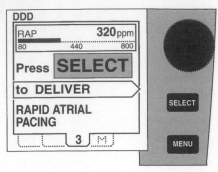

DDD

RAP   320 ppm
80   440   800

Press **SELECT**

to DELIVER

RAPID ATRIAL
PACING

3   M

SELECT

MENU

■ ● **FIGURE 42–2.** RAP (rapid atrial pacing). (From Medtronic,
Inc.)

flutter at a rate of 300).[1] An alternative approach is to
initiate atrial pacing at a rate 10 beats per minute
faster than the intrinsic atrial rate[1] (Fig. 42–3).

❖ Successive bursts are usually performed at gradually
increasing rates (maximum capability of pulse generator for overdrive atrial pacing is 800 pulses per
minute) and may be delivered for longer periods, up
to 1 minute.

• It is extremely important that the atrial pacing wire or
atrial pacing lead be correctly identified when initiating
overdrive pacing because pacing the ventricle at rapid
rates may result in ventricular tachycardia or ventricular
fibrillation.

• Rapid atrial pacing may result in degeneration of the
atrial rhythm to atrial fibrillation with a rapid ventricular
response.

• If an accessory pathway is present, rapid atrial pacing can
result in conduction to the ventricles over the accessory
pathway, leading to ventricular fibrillation.

• Overdrive suppression of the sinus node can result in
periods of bradycardia, asystole, junctional or ventricular
escape rhythms, or polymorphic ventricular tachycardia
on termination of the atrial tachyarrhythmia.

EQUIPMENT

• Clean gloves
• External pulse generator capable of rapid atrial pacing
• Connecting cable
• Cardiac monitor and recorder
• Materials for epicardial pacing wire site care
  ❖ Povidone-iodine pads or swabsticks
  ❖ Gauze
  ❖ Gauze pads
  ❖ Tape
• Insulating material for epicardial pacing wires or transve-
  nous pacing electrode connector pins (eg, finger cots,
  glove, needle caps)

Additional equipment (to have available depending on
patient status) includes the following:

• Defibrillator
• Emergency medications
• Airway management equipment
• Standard pulse generator or transcutaneous pacemaker

PATIENT AND FAMILY EDUCATION

• Explain procedure and its purpose to patient and family.
  ➻**Rationale:** Decreases patient and family anxiety and
  promotes cooperation with procedure.

• Reassure patient that the pacing will probably not be felt
  and that any sensation felt will most likely be a "flut-

tering" feeling in the chest.   ➻**Rationale:** Prepares patient and may decrease patient's anxiety.

PATIENT ASSESSMENT AND PREPARATION

Patient Assessment

• Assess electrocardiogram (ECG) rhythm and intervals,
  noting both atrial and ventricular rates.   ➻**Rationale:**
  Determines baseline cardiac conduction.

• Assess vital signs and hemodynamic or oxygenation parameters being monitored.   ➻**Rationale:** Determines
  baseline cardiovascular function.

• Assess signs and symptoms that might be caused by the
  dysrhythmia (eg, shortness of breath [SOB], dizziness,
  nausea, chest pain, signs of poor peripheral
  perfusion).   ➻**Rationale:** Determines patient response to
  dysrhythmia.

• Assess presence and patency of intravenous (IV) access.
  ➻**Rationale:** Ensures functional IV access.

• Note any medications that might have an effect on patient's rhythm or hemodynamic parameters (eg, beta
  blockers, calcium channel blockers, antidysrhythmics,
  digoxin).   ➻**Rationale:** Knowing the effects of drug
  therapy can alert the health care team to potential prob-

lems f
brady
blocke

Patien

• Ensure
  dural t
  force i
  and rei
  mation

• Initiate
  already
  visible
  capture
  tient's
  adverse
  to provi

• Place pa
  epicardi
  wire.
  care if n

• Place bl
  using an
  Aids in
  overdriv

Procedure for Overdrive Atrial Pacing	
Steps	**Rationale**
1. Wash hands.	Reduces transmission of micro standard precautions.
2. Don gloves.	Protects patient from microshoc pacing wires are being handled.[2]
3. Attach connecting cable to the external pulse generator, making sure that the positive (+) pole of the cable is connected to the (+) terminal of the pulse generator and the negative (−) pole of the cable is connected to the (−) terminal.	The connecting cable provides e length so the pulse generator doe have to be placed on the patient' or abdomen to reach pacing wire makes it easier to manipulate cor the pulse generator without havin bend over the patient to reach the
4. To use a transvenous atrial pacing lead, follow these steps:	The pacing stimulus travels from pulse generator to the negative te and energy will return to the pulse generator via the positive terminal
A. Identify the proximal and the distal electrode connector pins on the external portion of the atrial pacing lead.	
B. Connect the negative terminal of the connecting cable to the distal negative electrode connector pin.	Energy from the pulse generator is directed to the distal electrode in c with the atrium.
C. Connect the positive terminal of the connecting cable to the proximal positive electrode connecting pin.	The pacing circuit is completed as reaches the positive electrode.

Procedure for

Steps

5. To use epicardial
   these steps:
   A. Expose atria
      wires.

   B. Connect the
      the connecti
      epicardial pa

   C. Connect the
      the connecti
      epicardial p
      ground wire

6. Set the rate and
   output) controls

7. Pace the atrium
   (several beats
   then abruptly t

8. Disconnect the
   the epicardial
   transvenous p
   pins.

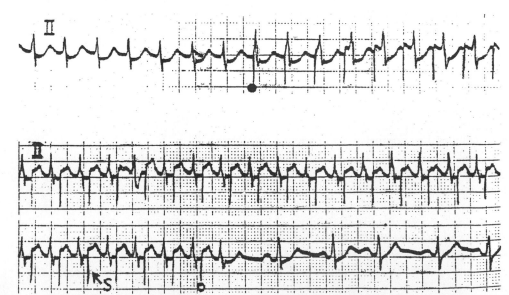

■ ● **FIGURE 42–3.** The top trace shows ECG lead II recorded during an episode of paroxysmal atrial tachycardia at a rate of 150
beats per minute. Beginning with the eighth beat in this trace (black dot), rapid atrial pacing at a rate of 165 beats per minute
was initiated. In the middle trace, which begins 12 seconds after the top trace, atrial capture is demonstrated clearly. In the
bottom trace, which is continuous with the middle trace, sinus rhythm appears when atrial pacing is terminated abruptly (open
circle). S, stimulus artifact. Paper recording speed 25 mm/s. (From Cooper TB, MacLean WAH, Waldo AL. Overdrive pacing for
supraventricular tachycardia: A review of theoretical implications and therapeutic techniques. *PACE.* 1978;1:200.)

■■ AP This procedure should be performed only by physicians,
advanced practice nurses, and other health care professionals (including critical care nurses) with additional knowledge, skills, and demonstrated competence per professional licensure or institutional standard.

Procedure **for Overdrive Atrial Pacing** *Continued*

Steps	Rationale	Special Considerations
9. Apply a sterile, occlusive dressing to pacing site.	Prevents transmission of microorganisms; standard precautions.	
10. Protect exposed pacing electrode connector pins or epicardial wires with insulating material (finger cots, needle covers, small glass test tubes). the insulated portion of the epicardial pacing wires can be neatly coiled on top of the gauze dressing, covered with another piece of gauze, and taped in place. Label each wire or dressing to identify atrial and ventricular pacing wires.	Prevents microshock, which can result in significant dysrhytmias.[2] Aids identification of pacing wires.	
11. Discard used supplies, and wash hands.	Reduces transmission of microorganisms; standard precautions.	

Expected Outcomes	Unexpected Outcomes
• Return to normal sinus rhythm • Stable or improved hemodynamic parameters	• Failure to capture atrium • Conversion to atrial fibrillation • Prolonged period of bradycardia or asystole following termination of tachyarrhythmia • Rapid conduction of atrial paced impulses to ventricle through an accessory pathway, resulting in ventricular tachycardia or ventricular fibrillation • Emergence of slow junctional or ventricular escape rhythm or polymorphic ventricular tachycardia following termination of tachyarrhythmia • Microshock resulting in ventricular tachycardia or fibrillation

Patient Monitoring and Care

Patient Monitoring and Care	Rationale	Reportable Conditions
		These conditions should be reported if they persist despite nursing interventions.
1. Monitor cardiac rhythm continuously at bedside during the procedure and after the procedure.	Allows for immediate recognition of rhythm changes or return of initial tachydysrhythmia.	• Rhythm changes • Return of initial tachydysrhythmia • Any significant or hemodynamically unstable dysrhythmia • Need for additional temporary pacing to maintain adequate heart rate following conversion of initial tachydysrhythmia

Continued on following page

AP This procedure should be performed only by physicians, advanced practice nurses, and other health care professionals (including critical care nurses) with additional knowledge, skills, and demonstrated competence per professional licensure or institutional standard.

Patient Monitoring and Care *Continued*

Patient Monitoring and Care	Rationale	Reportable Conditions
2. Monitor vital signs before initiating overdrive pacing, every 5 to 10 minutes during attempts to overdrive pace, with any significant rhythm change during procedure, and on termination of procedure. If patient is not hemodynamically stable following procedure, monitor vital signs every 5 to 10 minutes. Monitor vital signs per unit standards if patient is stable following procedure.	Changes in vital signs may indicate significant change in patient's condition. Blood pressure often improves with restoration of sinus rhythm and may deteriorate if ventricular rate accelerates because of overdrive pacing. If patient is on antidysrhythmic medications, changes in vital signs may indicate adverse drug reaction.	• Any significant change in vital signs, cardiac rhythm, or other monitored parameters
3. Site care to transvenous pacing lead site or epicardial wire exit site with povidone-iodine swabs, and apply sterile gauze dressing to exit site. Observe site for signs of infection or wire dislodgment.	Decreases incidence of infection.	• Redness or exudate around site, increased white blood cell count, or elevated temperature
4. Monitor patient's response to antidysrhythmic medications.	Antidysrhythmic medications may be necessary to prevent recurrence of initial tachydysrhythmia or to control ventricular rate.	• Prolongation of QT interval; rhythm changes

Documentation

Documentation should include the following:

- Patient and family education provided and an evaluation of their understanding of procedure
- Initial rhythm strip documenting cardiac rate and rhythm
- Initial vital signs and other pertinent physical assessment findings
- Pacemaker settings used
- Number of pacing attempts
- Rate and duration of successful pacing burst
- Postconversion rhythm

- Patient's response to procedure (eg, anxiety, pain)
- Postprocedure rhythm strip
- Postprocedure vital signs
- Any medications given during procedure
- Any unexpected outcomes
- Additional interventions

References

1. Waldo AL: Atrial flutter. In: Podrid PJ, Kowey PR: *Cardiac Arrhythmia: Mechanisms, Diagnosis, and Management.* Baltimore, Md: Williams & Wilkins; 1995.
2. Baas LS, Beery TA, Hickey CS: Care and safety of pacemaker electrodes in intensive care and telemetry nursing units. *Am J Crit Care.* 1997;6:302–311.

Additional Readings

Dreifus LS. *Pacemaker Therapy.* Philadelphia, Pa: F.A. Davis; 1983.
Roman-Smith P. Pacing for tachydysrhythmia. *AACN Clin Issues Crit Care Nurs.* 1991;2:132–139.

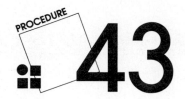

43

Implantable Cardioverter-Defibrillator

PURPOSE: The implantable cardioverter-defibrillator (ICD) is an implanted electronic device that is used to prevent sudden cardiac death (SCD) caused by malignant ventricular dysrhythmias. The ICD continuously monitors a patient's rhythm and attempts to convert ventricular tachycardia or ventricular fibrillation via antitachycardia pacing, cardioversion, defibrillation, or both.

Cathy M. Martin
Patricia Gonce Morton
Michael A. Nace

PREREQUISITE NURSING KNOWLEDGE

- The normal anatomy and physiology of the cardiovascular system, principles of cardiac conduction, and basic dysrhythmia interpretation should be understood.
- ICDs need to be understood to evaluate ICD function and the patient response to ICD therapy.
- Advanced cardiac life support knowledge and skills are necessary.
- Clinical and technical competence related to use of the external defibrillator is necessary.
- The ICD is used as a long-term therapy for patients at risk for SCD.
- Several studies support the efficacy of the ICD in prolonging the overall survival of patients as well as preventing SCD.[1-4]
- The American College of Cardiology/American Heart Association Task Force (ACC/AHA) revised the guidelines for the use of ICDs in 1998.[5] ICDs are most effective in patients who have had a cardiac arrest caused by ventricular fibrillation (VF) or ventricular tachycardia (VT) not caused by a transient or reversible cause.[5]
- The ICD system is composed of a pulse generator and a lead system (Fig. 43–1). The ICD system monitors the heart rate and cardiac rhythm and provides the energy for antitachycardia pacing, cardioversion, and defibrillation. The pulse generator contains antitachycardia pacing, cardioversion, and defibrillation. The pulse generator contains capacitors, circuits, and a lithium battery that will last approximately 3 to 5 years before requiring replacement.[6] Battery life depends on the number of times the device defibrillates.
- The first- and second-generation ICDs were implanted surgically using the sternotomy, thoracotomy, or subxiphoid approach.
- Early ICD models used two sets of leads. The first lead was placed in the superior vena cava. The second lead

was a ventricular patch, which was made of titanium mesh and rubber insulation and was sewn onto the epicardial surface of the ventricle. A two-patch system could be used as an alternative and the patches would typically be placed on the anterior right ventricle and the posterior left ventricle. The patch leads can be identified on chest radiograph by their mesh perimeter as well as the manufacturer's model number.[7] For early-model ICDs, the generator was implanted in the abdominal area.

- The newest ICD generators are implanted subcutaneously in the pectoral region. The lead system is in contact with the endocardial surface and consists of single, double, or triple leads. Current systems use a single tripolar endocardial lead that is capable of sensing the patient's heart rate and rhythm and also delivering the shock.[8] These lead

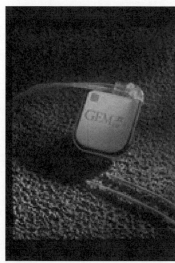

■ ● **FIGURE 43–1.** Photo of an ICD, the generator with lead wire. ICD, implantable cardioverter-defibrillator. (From Medtronic Inc.)

systems are inserted transvenously through the subclavian or cephalic vein and are positioned at the apex of the right ventricle and the superior vena cava.[9] This placement technique has decreased recovery time, perioperative complications, length of stay, and mortality.[7] Complications of the endocardial technique include lead dislodgment, lead fracture, and venous thrombosis.[7, 12]

- Current ICDs offer increased capabilities and are known as third-generation devices. On recognition of ventricular tachycardia or ventricular fibrillation, the third-generation ICDs provide tiered therapy, a type of multilevel therapy, to terminate the dysrhythmia. The first tier is usually antitachycardia pacing, and if it is ineffective, the second tier of therapy involves a low-energy cardioversion. The third tier is defibrillation and is used if the second tier fails to convert the rhythm. The fourth tier of therapy is ventricular demand pacing, and it is used if the previous tiers convert the rhythm to asystole or to a slow rate.
- Third-generation devices have various programmable features including antitachycardia pacing, low-energy cardioversion, defibrillation, antibradycardia pacing, set time to therapy, stored data, noninvasive electrophysiologic stimulation, variable energy outputs, and redetection algorithms. These features allow therapy to be individualized for each patient.[9]
- Defibrillator codes were developed in 1993 by the North American Society of Pacing and Electrophysiology (NASPE) and the British Pacing and Electrophysiology Group (BPEG) to describe the capabilities and operation of ICDs.[11] The defibrillator code is patterned after the pacemaker code; however, it has some important differences (Table 43–1).[12] The defibrillator code offers less information about the ICD's antibradycardia pacing function, but it offers more specific information about the shock functions.
- Magnet mode is an ICD feature that varies between manufacturers. If available on individual models, the magnet mode allows for suppression of therapy in an emergency. All health care providers caring for patients with an ICD must be trained in the proper use of this mode.[9] The magnet mode will deactivate the defibrillator capability of the ICD; however, the magnet mode will not interfere with the back-up pacing mode.
- Emotional adjustments vary with each patient and family. Patients may exhibit depression, anxiety, fear, and anger. Some patients view the device as an activity restriction and others see it as a life-saving device that will allow them to resume a normal life. Phantom shock[3] is a condition in which a patient's anxiety and concern about the delivery of a shock is so great that it affects the patient's daily activity. Support groups should be encouraged for patients receiving ICD therapy.

EQUIPMENT

- ECG monitor and recorder
- ECG electrodes

Additional equipment (to have available depending on need) includes the following:

- ICD interrogator (commonly obtained from the electrophysiology department)
- Magnet (doughnut or bar type)
- 12-lead ECG machine
- Analgesics as prescribed
- Emergency medications and resuscitation equipment
- Antidysrhythmics as prescribed

PATIENT AND FAMILY EDUCATION

- Assess learning needs, readiness to learn, and factors that will influence learning.   ➽*Rationale:* Allows the nurse to individualize teaching in a meaningful manner.
- Assess the patient and family understanding of ICD therapy and the reason for its use.   ➽*Rationale:* Provides information regarding knowledge level and necessity of additional teaching.
- Provide information about the normal conduction system, such as structure of the conduction system, source of heart beat, normal and abnormal heart rhythms, and symptoms of abnormal heart rhythms.   ➽*Rationale:* Understanding of the normal conduction system will assist the patient and family in recognizing the seriousness of the patient's condition and the need for ICD therapy.
- Provide information about ICD therapy including the reason for ICD, explanation of the equipment, what to expect during activation of the ICD, precautions and restrictions in activities of daily living, signs and symptoms of complications, and instructions on when to call the physician, and information on expected follow-up.   ➽*Rationale:* Understanding of ICD functioning and expectations after discharge assists the patient and family in developing realistic perceptions of ICD therapy. Information may improve compliance with restrictions and promote effective lifestyle management after discharge.
- Provide patient registration and identification (ID) card. Encourage patient to wear Medic Alert information and to carry ID card at all times.   ➽*Rationale:* Reinforces

---

Table 43–1 ▪■■   **NASPE/BPEG Defibrillator Code**

Position I	Position II	Position III	Position IV
Shock Chamber	Antitachycardia Pacing Chamber	Tachycardia Detection	Antibradycardia Pacing Chamber
O = None	O = None	E = Electrogram	O = None
A = Atrium	A = Atrium	H = Hemodynamic	A = Atrium
V = Ventricle	V = Ventricle		V = Ventricle
D = Dual (A + V)	D = Dual (A + V)		D = Dual (A + V)

BPEG, British Pacing and Electrophysiology Group; NASPE, North American Society of Pacing and Electrophysiology.
(From Bernstein AD, Camm AJ, Fletcher RD, et al. The NASPE/BPEG defibrillator code (NBD Code). *PACE.* 1993;16:1776; with permission.)

seriousness of patient condition and ensures that appropriate identifying information will be available to other health care providers if needed.

- Discuss the need for family members to learn cardiopulmonary resuscitation (CPR). ➠*Rationale:* Family should be prepared for an emergency situation (eg, if ICD does not convert life-threatening rhythm or ICD malfunctions.)
- Inform patients to activate the emergency medical services (EMS) system if they are alone or are having any symptoms such as dizziness, extreme fatigue, heart palpitations, and lightheadedness.[13] ➠*Rationale:* Activation of the EMS system will provide trained personnel to initiate advanced cardiac life support (ACLS).
- Teach the patient and family members to remain calm in the event of a shock. Instruct them to move to a safe place and sit down. Have someone stay with the patient if they can throughout the event. In the event of multiple shocks, or if the patient becomes unresponsive, someone should activate the EMS system or call 911. ➠*Rationale:* Activation of the EMS system will provide trained personnel to initiate ACLS.
- Instruct the patient to keep a log of all the events surrounding a shock (time of day, number of shocks, any symptoms felt before or after the shock, activity before the shock, any action taken by the patient or bystanders).[13–14] ➠*Rationale:* This information will help to evaluate the functioning of the ICD and the patient's response to the therapy.
- Inform the patients about their specific ICD and reason for the tones that may be emitted from the device. An audible tone may indicate battery depletion. Electromagnetic interference (EMI) may deactivate the ICD. If this occurs, the patient may hear an audible tone from the device indicating deactivation. The patient should move away from the source of EMI and notify the physician immediately if they hear a tone from the ICD.[14] ➠*Rationale:* The patient will need to be seen and have the ICD interrogated to determine if the ICD is activated or not.
- Inform the patient and partner that they will not be harmed if a shock is delivered when they are together. ➠*Rationale:* Prepares patient and family, encourages verbalization of feelings, and may decrease anxiety.
- Driving restrictions vary from state to state as well as among physicians. Patients should discuss plans for long trips and driving restrictions with their physician.[13–14] ➠*Rationale:* These restrictions may help to prevent lead fracture, generator migration, and motor vehicle accidents.
- Inform the patient and family of potential sources of EMI to the ICD. In the hospital these include the following:

magnetic resonance imaging (MRI),[14–15] diathermy, computed tomography (CT) scan, lithotripsy, electrocautery, radiation therapy, and nerve stimulator. Outside of the hospital these include the following: hand-held wands used by airport security, arc welders,[14] large transformers or motors, antitheft devices at stores or libraries,[7] cellular phones less than 6 inches away from the pulse generator,[14] the antenna of an operating citizens' band or ham radio,[7, 13–14] improperly grounded electric equipment,[7, 14] and hand-held tools less than 12 inches away from the pulse generator.[7] ➠*Rationale:* EMI can deactivate, deplete, or inhibit the pulse generator of the ICD.

PATIENT ASSESSMENT AND PREPARATION

Patient Assessment

- Assess ECG for cardiac rate and rhythm. ➠*Rationale:* Establishes baseline data.
- Assess intravenous (IV) access. ➠*Rationale:* IV access should be ensured in case emergency medications are needed.
- Identify whether the ICD is activated or deactivated. ➠*Rationale:* Provides essential data regarding the functioning of the ICD and treatment of ventricular tachycardia and ventricular fibrillation.
- Identify the type of ICD, the mode of function, and how it is programmed. ➠*Rationale:* Aids in assessment of what rate and rhythm will activate the device; whether antitachycardia pacing, cardioversion, defibrillation, and back-up pacing capabilities are present; and how they are set.
- Determine patient's ICD history: date of insertion, last battery change, most recent ICD check, how often the device is used, if the patient has experienced any problems with the ICD or ICD site, and any unexpected symptoms. ➠*Rationale:* The ICD history provides baseline information and may aid in determining any problems that might be occurring.
- Explore issues such as body image, lifestyle changes, and sexual concerns. ➠*Rationale:* Patients with ICDs may develop emotional, physical, and social changes. Referral for counseling may be necessary.

Patient Preparation

- Ensure that the patient and family understand teaching. Answer questions as they arise and reinforce information as needed. ➠*Rationale:* Evaluates and reinforces understanding of previously taught information.
- Provide analgesics or sedatives as prescribed and needed. ➠*Rationale:* Decreases discomfort or anxiety related to ICD therapy.

Procedure **for Implantable Cardioverter-Defibrillator**

Steps	Rationale	Special Considerations
1. Wash hands.	Reduces transmission of microorganisms; standard precautions.	
2. Prepare skin for application of ECG electrodes by washing with soap and water.	Proper skin preparation is essential to maintain appropriate skin-to-electrode contact.	It may be necessary to clip chest hair to ensure good skin contact with the electrodes.

Procedure continued on following page

Procedure for Implantable Cardioverter-Defibrillator *Continued*

Steps	Rationale	Special Considerations
3. Attach ECG leads to electrodes, place electrodes on patient's chest, record ECG.	Necessary to assess cardiac rhythm.	
4. If patient experiences ventricular tachycardia or ventricular fibrillation:		Run a continuous ECG strip of the dysrhythmia from the bedside monitor if possible.
A. Assess and stay with the patient.	Ensures patient safety, provides opportunity to assess patient's response to dysrhythmia.	
B. Wait for the device to function: antitachycardia pace, cardiovert, defibrillate.	The ICD will require a brief period (20–30 seconds) to assess the ventricular tachycardia or ventricular fibrillation and to initiate therapy.	
C. If the dysrhythmia continues, wait for the ICD to recharge and defibrillate again if indicated.	The ICD will reassess the cardiac rhythm, recharge, and defibrillate again as preprogrammed.	Time needs to be allotted for the ICD to defibrillate as it is preprogrammed.
D. If the ICD has been functioning as preprogrammed and still does not convert the dysrhythmia, initiate ACLS.	Provides emergency care.	Assess the patient's response to ventricular tachycardia; patient may be hemodynamically stable or unstable. Follow ACLS standards. Remain with the patient. Notify the physician or advanced practice nurse immediately, and prepare emergency equipment. Gloves should be worn to minimize the transmission of electric current to the health care providers when providing chest compressions.
E. Apply defibrillation paddles in one of the two following ways: Place at the heart's apex just to the left of the nipple in the midline axillary line and place the other paddle just below the right clavicle to the right of the sternum; or apply anterior-posterior defibrillation electrodes or paddles. The anterior paddle is placed in the anterior left precordial area and the posterior paddle is placed posteriorly behind the heart in the left infrascapular area.	The electric current will pass through the cardiac muscle.	Defibrillator paddles and defibrillation patches should not be placed over nitroglycerin patches or the ICD generator. The paddles and patches should be a minimum of 2 inches away from the generator when delivering external shocks.
F. If indicated, externally defibrillate the patient according to ACLS[16] (see Procedure 36).	Provides efficacious emergency care.	Some of the ICDs have preprogrammed pacing capability; thus, cardiac pacing may be initiated by the ICD if the result of defibrillation is asystole.
5. Deactivation of the ICD	The ICD may need to be deactivated if it is defibrillating a cardiac rhythm that is not ventricular tachycardia or ventricular fibrillation. If the device is functioning inappropriately, deactivation may be required to prevent harm to the patient.	Follow hospital standards to ensure that a nurse can deactivate an ICD. Inform physician of ICD deactivation. The following circumstances may require ICD deactivation: lead dislodgement, lead migration, lead fracture, inappropriate identification of the rhythm, inappropriate defibrillation threshold.[12, 21, 22]
A. Place a bar or doughnut magnet over the right upper corner of the pulse generator.	The magnet activates and deactivates the ICD.	A programmer may also be used to deactivate the ICD.
B. Listen for a synchronous tone that should occur simultaneously with each R wave (the tone will last for approximately 30 seconds).	A synchronous tone indicates that the ICD is activated.	

Procedure	**for Implantable Cardioverter-Defibrillator** *Continued*	

Steps	Rationale	Special Considerations
C. Listen for a constant tone.	A constant tone indicates that the ICD is deactivated.	
D. Remove the magnet after the constant tone is heard.		
6. Reactivation of an ICD	Turns the ICD on.	Follow hospital standards to ensure that a nurse can reactivate an ICD. An ICD can be inadvertently deactivated when the pulse generator is exposed to EMI. Some ICDs have audible tones that will be emitted if the ICD becomes deactivated. Interrogation will be required to determine if the ICD is activated or not.[9, 16, 19]
A. Place a bar or doughnut magnet over the right upper corner of the pulse generator.	The magnet activates and deactivates the ICD.	A programmer may also be used to activate the ICD.
B. Listen for a constant tone.	A constant tone indicates that the ICD is deactivated.	
C. Listen for a synchronous tone that should occur simultaneously with each R wave.	A synchronous tone indicates that the ICD is activated.	
D. Remove the magnet.		

Expected Outcomes	Unexpected Outcomes
• ICD detects life-threatening ventricular tachycardia or ventricular fibrillation. • ICD delivers appropriate therapy, including defibrillation as necessary. • Cardiac rhythm is converted to a hemodynamically stable rhythm. • Hemodynamic stability is achieved.	• Failure of the ICD to detect ventricular tachycardia or ventricular fibrillation • Failure of the ICD to convert life-threatening dysrhythmia despite appropriate therapy and defibrillation attempts • Failure of the back-up pacing system to pace if asystole is the result of defibrillation • Inappropriate defibrillation • Infection at generator site, tunneled region, or myocardium • Lead fracture or migration • Pulse generator migration • Pulse generator pocket hematoma • Venous thrombosis • Skin erosion

Patient Monitoring and Care		

Patient Monitoring and Care	Rationale	Reportable Conditions
		These conditions should be reported if they persist despite nursing interventions.
1. Monitor the ECG continuously.	Detects dysrhythmias.	• Dysrhythmias
2. Monitor the ICD for antitachycardia pacing, cardioversion, and defibrillation.	Detects functioning of the ICD.	• Ventricular dysrhythmias, ICD therapy and defibrillation, ICD malfunction

Continued on following page

Patient Monitoring and Care *Continued*

Patient Monitoring and Care	Rationale	Reportable Conditions
3. Assess the patient's response to ICD defibrillation, including cardiac rate and rhythm, level of consciousness, and vital signs.	Determines patient status and necessity for additional treatment.	• Cardiac rate and rhythm before and after defibrillation, level of consciousness, and vital signs
4. Evaluate and treat the patient for pain and anxiety.	ICD defibrillation may cause pain and may also increase patient anxiety.	• Pain and anxiety that are not relieved by prescribed analgesic or sedative
5. Assess ICD pulse generator site for evidence of manipulation.	Patient manipulation at the site may affect ICD therapy.	• Evidence of ICD pulse generator manipulation
6. Monitor for signs and symptoms of infection.	Placement of an invasive device may result in infection.	• Signs or symptoms of infection

▌Documentation

Documentation should include the following:

- ICD history
- Preprogrammed ICD parameters
- The status of the device, that is, if it is on or off
- Patient and family education
- Dysrhythmias
- ICD functioning
- Patient response to ICD therapy
- Occurrence of any unexpected outcomes
- Additional interventions

References

1. Saksena S. Survival of implantable cardioverter-defibrillator recipients: can the iceberg remain submerged. *Circulation.* 1992;85:1616–1618.
2. Fogoros RN: The effect of the implantable cardioverter defibrillator on sudden death and on total survival. *PACE.* 1993;16:506–508.
3. Sarter B, Callans D, Gottlieb C, et al. Implantable defibrillator diagnostic storage capabilities: evolution, current status, and future utilization. *PACE.* 1998;21:1287–1298.
4. Gottlieb C, Callans D, Marchlinski F. Implantable cardioverter defibrillators in the United States: understanding the benefits and the limitations of implantable cardioverter defibrillator therapy based on clinical trial results. *PACE.* 1998;21:2016–2020.
5. Gregoratos G, Chitlin MD, Epstein AE, et al. ACC/AHA guidelines for implantation of cardiac pacemakers and antiarrhythmia devices: a report of the ACC/AHA Task Force on Practice Guidelines (Committee on Pacemaker Implantation). *J Am Coll Cardiol.* 1998;31:1175–1206.
6. Harper P, VanRiper S. Implantable cardioverter defibrillator: a patient education model for the illiterate patient. *Crit Care Nurs.* April 1993;13(2):55–59.
7. McMahon-Busch M, Haskin JB. Pacemakers and implantable defibrillators. In: Woods SL, Froelicher ESS, Halpenny CJ, Motzer SA, eds. *Cardiac Nursing.* 3rd ed. Philadelphia, Pa: J.B. Lippincott; 1995;647–653.
8. Gonce Morton P. Patient management: cardiovascular system. In: Hudak C, Gallo BM, Gonce Morton P, eds: *Critical Care Nursing; A Holistic Approach.* 7th ed. Philadelphia, Pa: Lippincott-Raven Publishers, 1998;327–330.
9. Knight L, Livingston N, Gawlinski N, et al: Caring for patients with third generation implantable cardioverter defibrillators: from decision to implant to patient's return home. *Crit Care Nurs.* 1997;17:47–60.
10. Naccarelli GM. Implantable cardioverter/defibrillators. In: Willerson JT, Cohn JN, eds: *Cardiovascular Medicine.* New York, NY: Churchill Livingstone, 1995:1441–1452.
11. Gonce Morton P. The pacemaker and defibrillator codes: implications for critical care nursing. *Crit Care Nurs.* 1997;17:52–58.
12. Berstein AD, Camm AJ, Fletcher RD, et al. The NASPE/BPEG defibrillator code (NBD Code). *PACE.* 1993;16:1776.
13. Kruse L, Demarco M, Moyer P, et al. Keeping pace with implanted defibrillators. *RN.* August 1998;61(8):30–35.
14. Moser S, Crawford D, Thomas A. Updated care guidelines for patients with automatic implantable cardioverter defibrillators. *Crit Care Nurs.* April 1993;13(2):62–71.
15. Stemper C. Advanced life support. In: Sheehy S, ed. *Emergency Nursing Principles and Practice.* 3rd ed. St. Louis, MO: C.V. Mosby, 1992;160.
16. Howland-Gradman J, Kitt S. Cardiac emergencies. In: Kitt S, Selfridge-Thomas J, Proehl J, Kaiser J, eds. *Emergency Nursing: A Physiologic and Clinical Perspective.* 2nd ed. Philadelphia, Pa: W.B. Saunders; 1994;175–179.
17. Craney J, Gorman L. Conscious sedation and implantable devices: safe and effective sedation during pacemaker and implantable cardioverter defibrillator placement. *Crit Care Clin North Am.* 1997;9:325–334.
18. Brooks R, Ruskin J. The implantable cardioverter-defibrillator. In: Schlant R, Alexander R, eds. *The Heart, Arteries and Veins.* 8th ed. New York, NY: McGraw-Hill, 1994:847–857.
19. Betz M, Wood M, Ellenbogen K. Pacemakers and implantable cardioverter defibrillators in the intensive care unit setting. In: Ayers S, Grenvik P, Holbrook P, Shoemaker W, eds. *Textbook of Critical Care.* 3rd ed. Philadelphia, Pa: W.B. Saunders; 1995:513–521.

Additional Readings

Harper P, VanRiper S. Implantable cardioverter defibrillator: a patient education model for the illiterate patient. *Crit Care Nurs.* April 1993;13(2):55–59.

Moser S, Crawford D, Thomas A. Updated care guidelines for patients with automatic implantable cardioverter defibrillators. *Crit Care Nurs.* April 1993;13(2):62–71.

Schleicher CA. Implantable cardioverter defibrillator. In: Dressler DK, Gettrust KV, eds. *Plans of Care for Speciality Practice: Cardiovascular Citical Care Nursing.* Albany, NY: Delmar Publishers; 1994:257–267.

Web Sites

http://www.medtronic.com
http://www.guidant.com
http://www.biotronic.com
http://www.duff.net/zapper/zap1.htm

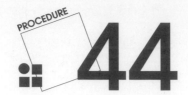

44

Permanent Pacemaker (Assessing Function)

PURPOSE: The purpose of permanent pacing is to establish an adequate heart rate and cardiac output when a chronic, recurrent conduction or impulse formation disturbance exists in the cardiac conduction system that is not secondary to a transient cause.

Francine E. Paschall
Ellen Strauss McErlean

PREREQUISITE NURSING KNOWLEDGE

- Understanding of normal anatomy and physiology of the cardiovascular system, principles of cardiac conduction, and basic dysrhythmia interpretation is needed.
- Understanding of pacemakers to evaluate pacemaker function and patient response to pacemaker therapy is necessary.
- Advanced cardiac life support knowledge and skills are necessary.
- Permanent pacing is indicated for clinical conditions that necessitate supplemental bradycardia support:
  ❖ Acquired atrioventricular (AV) block in adults
  ❖ Chronic bifascicular and trifascicular block
  ❖ AV block associated with acute myocardial infarction (MI)
  ❖ Sinus node dysfunction
  ❖ Hypersensitive carotid sinus syndrome and neurally mediated syndromes
  ❖ Interventricular conduction defects
  ❖ Symptomatic bradycardias
  ❖ Specific indications for dilated cardiomyopathy and hypertrophic cardiomyopathy[1]
- Permanent pacing also may be used to terminate or prevent tachydysrhythmias.
- Relative contraindications are as follows:
  ❖ Active infection (endocarditis, positive blood cultures)
  ❖ Bleeding (evidenced by increased blood coagulation studies)
- The pulse generator is implanted subcutaneously within the chest (pectoral placement), is typically made of stainless steel or titanium, and contains the electronic components as well as the battery necessary to sustain pacing (Fig. 44–1).
- A transvenous pacing lead is another component of the permanent pacing system and may be positioned in the right atrium, the right ventricle, or both chambers, depending on the type of pacing needed.

- Unipolar pacing involves placing a single lead in the heart. The distal tip is the negative electrode and is in contact with the myocardium. The positive electrode encompasses the metallic pacer case, located in the soft tissue. Energy is delivered from the negative electrode to the positive electrode causing myocardial depolarization. The electrocardiogram (ECG) tracing will show a large, easily visible spike.
- Bipolar pacing uses a single lead, where the distal tip is the negative electrode in contact with the myocardium. The positive electrode is located within 1 cm of the negative electrode. Energy is delivered from the negative electrode to the positive electrode, causing myocardial depolarization. The ECG tracing may show small spikes or the spikes may be invisible.
- Basic principles of cardiac pacing include sensing, pacing, and capture.
  ❖ Sensing refers to the ability of the pacemaker to detect intrinsic myocardial electrical activity. The pacemaker will either be inhibited from delivering a stimulus or will initiate an electrical impulse, based on the sensed

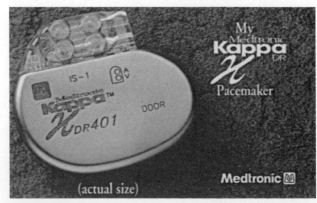

■ ● FIGURE 44–1. Permanent pulse generator. (From Medtronic USA, Inc.)

Spike   Ventricular paced beat

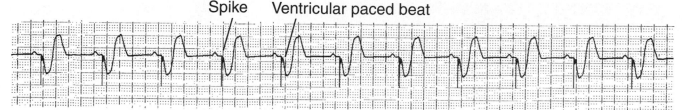

■ ● **FIGURE 44–2.** Single-chamber VVI pacing, normal operation.

activity. The action of the pacemaker will depend on the programmed response.

❖ Pacing occurs once the permanent pacemaker is activated and the requisite level of energy travels from the pacemaker through the transvenous lead wires to the myocardium. This is known as pacer "firing" and will be represented as a line or spike on the ECG recording (pacemaker spikes are shown in Figure 44–2).

❖ "Capture" refers to the successful stimulation of the myocardium by the pacemaker impulse that results in depolarization. It is evidenced on the ECG by a pacemaker spike/stimulus followed by either an atrial or ventricular complex, depending on the chamber being paced.

• Depending on the type of pacemaker, the pacemaker may be able to function in a single chamber, pacing either the atrium or the ventricle, or in both chambers. Pacemakers also may be programmed to include upper and lower rate limits, the amount of time the device waits between atrial and ventricular activity, the time period during which the pacemaker is unable to detect intrinsic activity, and the amount of energy delivered to the myocardium with each paced event. An international pacemaker code was developed to provide the clinician with a standard way to interpret pacemaker programming (Table 44–1). The nurse must be able to determine the programmed mode using the pacemaker code and to determine whether the device is functioning appropriately (Figs. 44–2 and 44–3).

• Recognition of inappropriate pacemaker function includes failure to pace, failure to sense; and failure to capture.

❖ Failure to pace: the pacemaker does not discharge a pacing stimulus at its programmed time to the myocardium, as evidenced by the absence of pacemaker spike on the ECG where expected.

❖ Failure to sense: the pacemaker has either detected

signals that mimic intrinsic cardiac activity or did not accurately identify intrinsic activity (undersensing). Oversensing is recognized on the ECG by pauses where paced beats were expected and prolongation of the interval between paced beats (Fig. 44–4). Undersensing is recognized on the ECG by inappropriate pacemaker spikes relative to the intrinsic electrical activity (pacemaker spikes occurring within the P wave, QRS complex, or T wave) and shortened distances between paced beats (Fig. 44–5).

❖ Failure to capture: the pacemaker has delivered a pacing stimulus that was unable to initiate depolarization of the myocardium and subsequent myocardial contraction. This is evidenced on the ECG by pacemaker spikes that are not followed by a P wave for atrial pacing or spikes not followed by a QRS complex for ventricular pacing (Fig. 44–6).

• Dual-chamber or DDD pacemakers contain pacing leads that are located in both the atrium and the ventricle. Pacing and sensing occur in both chambers. Pacing is inhibited by sensed atrial or ventricular activity. Sensed atrial activity will trigger a ventricular paced response in the absence of intrinsic ventricular activity within a programmed AV interval.

• The concept of rate-responsive pacing applies to those pacemaker implants that include a sensor and are designed to mimic normal changes in heart rate based on physiologic needs. Most commonly, the sensor reacts to motion and vibration or respirations and initiates an appropriate change in pacing rate, depending on the metabolic activity. These patients will have a pacemaker rate range.

• Electromagnetic interference (EMI) may interfere with pacemaker function. Electrocautery, cardiac electroversion, magnetic resonance imaging (MRI), radiation, diathermy, and extracorporeal shock wave lithotripsy are examples of sources of EMI that may disrupt the pacemaker-initiated electrical circuit.

Table 44–1 ●■■ **Generic Pacemaker Code**

I Chamber Paced	II Chamber Sensed	III Response to Sensing	IV Programmability, Rate Modulation	V Antitachycardia Function
O = None	O = None	O = None	O = None	O = None
A = Atrium	A = Atrium	T = Triggered	P = Simple programmable	P = Pacing
V = Ventricle	V = Ventricle	I = Inhibited	M = Multiprogrammable	S = Shock
D = Dual chamber (A and V)	D = Dual chamber (A and V)	D = Dual (T and I)	R = Rate modulation	D = Dual (P and S)

Adapted from NASPE/BPEG Generic Pacemaker Code, 1987.

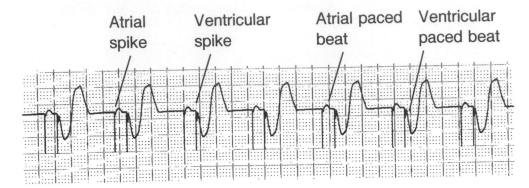

Atrial spike   Ventricular spike   Atrial paced beat   Ventricular paced beat

■ ● **FIGURE 44–3.** Dual-chamber DDD pacing, normal operation.

Atrial paced beat   Expected ventricular paced beat

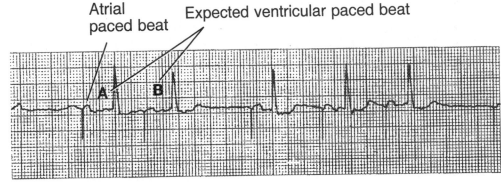

■ ● **FIGURE 44–4.** Ventricular oversensing. Ventricular spike expected at 150 ms. Ventricular spike and corresponding ventricular depolarization did not occur at points *A* and *B*.

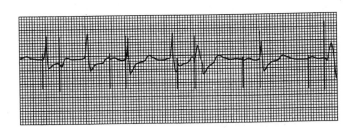

■ ● **FIGURE 44–5.** Ventricular undersensing. Pacer appears to be firing asynchronously. The third and sixth ventricular complexes represent concurrent intrinsic ventricular depolarization overlaid by inappropriate pacemaker fire.

Ventricular spike

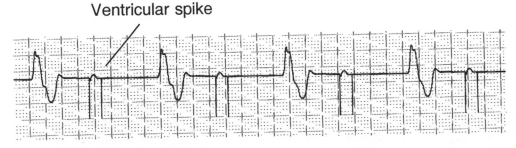

■ ● **FIGURE 44–6.** Failure to capture. All ventricular spikes show absence of corresponding ventricular depolarization.

EQUIPMENT

- ECG monitor and recorder
- ECG electrodes

Additional equipment as needed includes the following:

- Pacemaker magnet
- Pacemaker programmer

PATIENT AND FAMILY EDUCATION

- Assess learning needs, readiness to learn, and factors that will influence learning. ➤*Rationale:* Allows the nurse to individualize teaching in a meaningful manner.
- Provide information about the normal conduction system, such as structure of the conduction system, source of heart beat, normal and abnormal heart rhythms, and symptoms of abnormal heart rhythms. ➤*Rationale:* Understanding of the normal conduction system will assist the patient and family in recognizing the seriousness of the patient's condition and the need for permanent pacemaker therapy.
- Provide information about permanent pacing, including reason for pacing, explanation of the equipment, what to expect during permanent pacing, precautions and restrictions in activities of daily living, signs and symptoms of complications and instructions on when to call the physician, advanced practice nurse, or pacemaker clinic, and information on expected follow-up. ➤*Rationale:* Understanding of pacemaker functioning and expectations after discharge assists the patient and family in developing realistic perceptions of permanent pacing therapy. Information may improve compliance with restrictions and promote effective lifestyle management after discharge.
- Provide information about transtelephonic monitoring. ➤*Rationale:* Periodic pacemaker checks over the telephone may be required for routine monitoring or if there is a change in patient condition to evaluate pacemaker function.
- Provide patient registration and identification (ID) card. Encourage patient to wear "Medic Alert" information and to carry ID card at all times, especially if patient is admitted to the hospital. ➤*Rationale:* Reinforces seriousness of patient condition and ensures that appropriate identifying information will be available to other health care providers, if needed.

PATIENT ASSESSMENT AND PREPARATION
Patient Assessment

- Identify the programmed mode of the pacemaker. ➤*Rationale:* Knowledge of how the pacemaker is intended to respond is necessary to detect appropriate and inappropriate function.
- Identify the reason for permanent pacemaker support. ➤*Rationale:* Knowledge of the clinical indication will provide the nurse with baseline data when evaluating pacemaker function and patient response.
- Determine patient's pacemaker history: date of insertion, last battery change, most recent pacemaker check, whether the patient has experienced any problems with the pacemaker or pacemaker site, and any unexpected symptoms such as dizziness, chest pain, shortness of breath, or palpitations. ➤*Rationale:* The pacemaker history provides information useful in determining any problems that might be occurring.
- Assess ECG for appropriate pacemaker function. ➤*Rationale:* Evidence of inappropriate function will determine need for further testing.
- Assess patient's hemodynamic response to the paced rhythm. ➤*Rationale:* The patient's hemodynamic response will indicate how effective the pacemaker is in maintaining adequate cardiac output in response to the patient's physiologic needs. Evidence of adequate cardiac output is supported by systolic blood pressure greater than 90 mm Hg, mean arterial blood pressure greater than 60 mm Hg, no decrease in level of consciousness, and no complaints of fatigue, dizziness, shortness of breath, pallor, diaphoresis, or chest pain.

Patient Preparation

- Ensure that the patient and family understand teaching. Answer questions as they arise and reinforce information as needed. ➤*Rationale:* Evaluates and reinforces understanding of previously taught information.
- Assist patient to comfortable position. ➤*Rationale:* Promotes patient comfort.

Procedure **for Assessing Function of Permanent Pacemaker**

Steps	Rationale	Special Considerations
1. Wash hands.	Reduces transmission of microorganisms; standard precautions.	
2. Prepare skin for application of ECG electrodes by washing with soap and water.	Proper skin preparation is essential to maintain appropriate skin-to-electrode contact.	It may be necessary to clip chest hair to ensure good skin contact with the electrode.
3. Attach ECG leads to electrodes, place electrodes on patient's chest, and record ECG.	Necessary to assess cardiac rhythm.	A single-lead rhythm strip demonstrating visible P waves is adequate.[2] Lead II or MCL_6 generally provides the best P wave morphology if ECG lead availability is limited.

Procedure continued on following page

Procedure	for Assessing Function of Permanent Pacemaker *Continued*

Steps	Rationale	Special Considerations
4. Assess cardiac rhythm for the presence of pacemaker activity.	Allows for determination of pacemaker function. Troubleshoots programming of the pacemaker as well as the electrical response of the atria and ventricles.	Prerequisite knowledge of pacemaker programmed settings is necessary to adequately evaluate pacer function.
A. Identify atrial activity. Is the pacemaker programmed to detect atrial activity? Was the atrial activity sensed? What is the pacemaker programmed to do once atrial activity is sensed? If the pacemaker is programmed to trigger ventricular pacing with sensed atrial activity, is there a ventricular paced complex at the programmed AV interval? If not, is there an intrinsic QRS complex that occurred before the programmed AV interval?		
B. If there is no intrinsic atrial activity present, determine whether the pacemaker is programmed to pace the atrium. If atrial pacing should be occurring, determine the lower rate limit that the pacemaker will stimulate atrial activity (a paced atrial event should occur at the end of a ventricular-atrial interval). Evaluate whether the pacemaker is firing at this rate.	Troubleshoots programming of the pacemaker and atrial response.	If pacemaker spike is present but evidence of atrial capture is not present, attempt to assess the presence of atrial contraction by looking for the a wave in the central venous pressure (CVP) waveform (if available).
C. Look for ventricular activity. Is the pacemaker programmed to detect intrinsic activity? Is it sensed appropriately? What is the pacemaker programmed to do once ventricular activity is sensed? Does inhibition of ventricular pacing occur?	Determines the presence of ventricular activity and response to pacemaker actions.	
D. If there is no intrinsic ventricular activity, determine whether the pacemaker is programmed to pace the ventricles. If pacing should occur, identify the lower rate limit and determine whether ventricular pacing spikes are occurring at this rate. If ventricular pacing spikes are occurring at intervals that are longer than the lower rate limit, evaluate for oversensing of unwanted signals. If ventricular pacing spikes are occurring at intervals that are shorter than the lower rate limit, determine whether there is hidden atrial activity that is triggering a ventricular output (if appropriate for the programmed mode) or suspect undersensing. Determine whether each ventricular pacing spike is followed by a QRS complex. If the pacemaker has an upper rate limit, determine whether the patient is being paced appropriately once that limit has been reached.	Troubleshoots the relationship between pacemaker programming and ventricular response.	Look for the presence of P waves in the T wave.
E. If antitachycardia pacing is programmed, determine whether the tachycardia detection criterion has been met and if the pacemaker intervened appropriately.	Determines appropriate pacemaker function.	
5. Assess the patient's hemodynamic response.	It is possible for the patient to have the electrical activity of pacing occurring without the associated mechanical activity of cardiac contraction (pulseless electrical activity—PEA).	
6. If inappropriate pacemaker function is detected, notify the physician immediately.	Inappropriate pacemaker function may compromise the cardiac output and require immediate adjustment of settings or replacement of malfunctioning components.	

Expected Outcomes

- Adequate systemic tissue perfusion and cardiac output as evidenced by systolic blood pressure greater than 90 mm Hg, mean arterial blood pressure greater than 60 mm Hg, patient being alert and oriented, and no complaints of dizziness, shortness of breath, nausea, or vomiting because of hypotension or ischemic chest pain
- Absence of hemodynamically significant dysrhythmias
- Appropriate heart rate, proper sensing, and capture demonstrated on the ECG

Unexpected Outcomes

- Failure to sense with possibility of R on T phenomenon (initiation of ventricular tachycardia/fibrillation as a result of an improperly timed pacer spike)
- Failure to capture
- Failure to pace
- Pacemaker-mediated tachycardia: caused when a ventricular paced beat results in retrograde AV nodal conduction and produces a premature P wave. If the premature P wave is sensed, a ventricular output would follow, setting up an endless-loop tachycardia.[2]
- Pacemaker syndrome results from loss of AV synchrony with VVI and DVI pacing modes. Symptoms the patient may experience include chest pain, fatigue, and dyspnea.
- Pacing at an inappropriate rate
- Infection at the site
- Battery end of life

Patient Monitoring and Care

Patient Monitoring and Care	Rationale	Reportable Conditions
		These conditions should be reported if they persist despite nursing interventions.
1. Monitor the ECG continuously for the presence of a cardiac rate and rhythm that is consistent with the programmed parameters.	Indicates ongoing functioning of the permanent pacemaker.	• Failure of the pacemaker to perform as programmed; undersensing, oversensing
2. Evaluate the hemodynamic response to pacemaker therapy.	Provides ongoing assessment of patient's physiologic response to pacing.	• Deterioration of the patient's condition as evidenced by change in vital signs/hemodynamic parameters
3. Assess insertion site for evidence of manipulation.	Patient manipulation at the site may affect pacemaker therapy. "Twiddler's" syndrome has been noted to cause lead dislodgment and loss of pacemaker function.[1]	• Evidence of pacemaker manipulation
4. Monitor for signs and symptoms of infection.	Placement of an invasive device may result in infection.	• Signs or symptoms of infection

Documentation

Documentation should include the following:

- Pacemaker history
- Patient education and evaluation of patient and family understanding
- Programmed parameters
- ECG rhythm strip recording
- Evaluation of pacemaker function
- Vital signs and hemodynamic response
- Physical assessment parameters
- Unexpected outcomes
- Interventions required and evaluation of the interventions

References

1. American College of Cardiology and American Heart Association. Guidelines for implantation of cardiac pacemakers and antiarrhythmia devices. *JACC*. 1998;31:1175–1209.
2. Moses HW, Moulton KP, Miller BD, Schneider JA. *A Practical Guide to Cardiac Pacing*. Boston, Ma: Little, Brown; 1995:171–197.
3. Furman S, Hayes DL, Holmes DR. *A Practice of Cardiac Pacing*. Mount Kisco, NY: Futura Publishing; 1993:559–563.
4. Moses HW, Moulton KP, Miller BD, Schneider JA. *A Practical Guide to Cardiac Pacing*. Boston, Ma: Little, Brown; 1995:96, 114.

Additional Readings

Barbiere CC, Liberatore K. From emergent transvenous pacemaker to permanent implant. *Crit Care Nurse*. 1993;13:39–44.

Busch MM, Haskin JB. Pacemakers and implantable defibrillators. In: Woods SL, Froelicher ES, Halpenny CJ, Motzer SU, eds. *Cardiac Nursing*. 3rd ed. Philadelphia, Pa: J.B. Lippincott; 1995:618–661.

Morton PG. The pacemaker and defibrillator codes: implications for critical care nursing. *Crit Care Nurse*. 1997;17:50–59.

Platt S, Furman S, Gross JN, Andrews C, Benedek M. Transtelephone monitoring for pacemaker follow-up 1981–1994. *PACE*. 1996;19(12 part 1):2089–2098.

Van Orden Wallace CJ. Dual-chamber pacemakers in the management of severe heart failure. *Crit Care Nurse*. 1998;18:57–67.

Vardas PE. *Cardiac Arrhythmias, Pacing and Electrophysiology*. Boston, Ma: Kluwer Academic; 1998.

Witherall CL. Cardiac rhythm control devices. *Crit Care Nurs Clin North Am*. 1994;6:85–101.

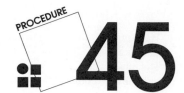

Temporary Transcutaneous (External) Pacing

P U R P O S E: Transcutaneous or external pacing is used to stimulate myocardial depolarization through the chest wall. External pacing is initiated as a temporary measure when there has been a failure of the normal conduction system of the heart to produce an electric impulse resulting in hemodynamic compromise or other debilitating symptoms in the patient.

Francine E. Paschall
Ellen Strauss McErlean

PREREQUISITE NURSING KNOWLEDGE

- The normal anatomy and physiology of the cardiovascular system, principles of cardiac conduction, and basic dysrhythmia interpretation should be understood.
- Transcutaneous pacemakers should be understood so that pacemaker function and the patient response to pacemaker therapy can be evaluated.
- Clinical and technical competence related to use of the transcutaneous pacemaker is necessary.
- Advanced cardiac life support knowledge and skills are necessary.
- Transcutaneous pacing is most commonly used to stimulate the myocardium to depolarize in the absence of an intrinsic rhythm, establish an adequate cardiac output and blood pressure to ensure tissue perfusion to vital organs, and reduce the possibility of ventricular dysrhythmias in the presence of bradycardia.
- Indications for transcutaneous pacing include the following:
  - ❖ Asystolic cardiac arrest (American Heart Association asystole treatment algorithm)[1]
  - ❖ Symptomatic bradycardia
  - ❖ Temporary bridge in the presence of long-term pacemaker failure, revision, or replacement before placement of temporary transvenous pacemaker
  - ❖ Temporary bridge in the presence of Type II second-degree atrioventricular (AV) heart block or third-degree AV heart block before placement of temporary transvenous pacemaker
  - ❖ Cardioactive drug toxicity
  - ❖ Anesthesia-induced bradycardia
  - ❖ Patients for whom temporary pacing is necessary yet for whom invasive techniques are contraindicated: those with immunosuppression, severe vascular disease, high-bleeding risk, and sepsis; pretransplant candidates; and posttransplant patients
  - ❖ Emergent overdrive suppression or termination of supraventricular and ventricular tachydysrhythmias before placement of temporary transvenous pacemaker
- External cardiac pacing is a method of stimulating myocardial depolarization through the chest wall via two large pacing electrodes. The electrodes are placed on the anterior and posterior chest wall and are attached by a cable to an external pulse generator that houses the pacemaker controls (Fig. 45–1).
- Basic principles of cardiac pacing include sensing, pacing, and capture:
  - ❖ *Sensing* refers to the ability of the pacemaker to detect intrinsic myocardial electrical activity. Sensing occurs if the pacemaker is in the synchronous or demand

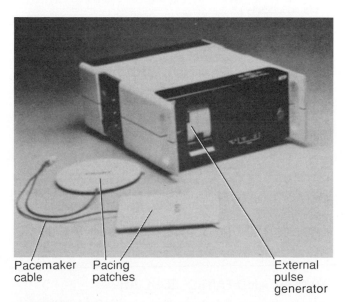

■ ● FIGURE 45–1. Temporary transcutaneous (external) pacemaker. (From Zoll Medical Corporation, Burlington, MA.)

mode. The pacemaker either will be inhibited from delivering a stimulus or will initiate an electrical impulse.

❖ *Pacing* occurs once the external pulse generator is activated and the specified level of energy travels from the external pulse generator through the pacing patches, through the patient's chest, to the myocardium. This is known as pacer *firing* and is represented as a *spike* on the electrocardiogram (ECG) tracing.

❖ *Capture* refers to the successful stimulation of the myocardium by the pacemaker impulse, resulting in depolarization. It is evidenced on the ECG by a pacemaker spike followed by either an atrial or a ventricular complex, depending on the chamber paced. External pacing provides only single-chamber ventricular pacing.

• An understanding of the various pacing modes is necessary:

❖ Temporary external pacing is capable of delivering ventricular asynchronous or ventricular synchronous pacing.

❖ Asynchronous pacing is initiated only in an emergency to establish an immediate rhythm.

❖ Synchronous pacing is the recommended mode of transcutaneous pacing. When the pacing rate is set above the patient's intrinsic heart rate, the patient will be paced continuously unless the pacemaker senses an intrinsic complex. If the pacemaker senses an intrinsic complex, the pacemaker will be inhibited from initiating a pacing impulse. When the pacing rate is set below the patient's intrinsic rate, the pacemaker will initiate pacing when the heart rate falls below the desired set rate.

• The efficacy of external pacing is influenced by a number of variables: the position and adherence of the pacing electrodes, the level of energy delivered to the myocardium, the presence of acidosis or electrolyte imbalances, concomitant drug therapy (especially antidysrhythmic therapy), and anatomic features of the patient (eg, barrel chest, obesity).

• Principles of general electric safety apply when using external pacing. Biomedical engineering or other medical safety personnel should be familiar with the manufacturer's specific recommendations with reference to safety.

EQUIPMENT

• External pacing generator and monitor unit (see Fig. 45–1)
• Pacing cable and pacing patches (see Fig. 45–1)

• Pacemaker electrodes
• ECG electrode patches
• ECG monitor and cable

Additional equipment (to have available depending on patient need) includes the following:

• Scissors to remove body hair
• Emergency medications and resuscitation equipment

PATIENT AND FAMILY EDUCATION

• Assess learning needs, readiness to learn, and factors that will influence learning. ➤*Rationale:* Individualizes

teaching so that it will be meaningful to the patient and family.

• Discuss basic facts about the normal conduction system, such as structure of the conduction system, source of heart rate, normal and abnormal heart rhythms, and symptoms of abnormal heart rhythms. ➤*Rationale:* Understanding of the normal conduction system will assist the patient and family in recognizing the seriousness of the patient's condition and the need for external pacing.

• Discuss basic facts about the external pacemaker, such as the reason for the pacemaker, explanation of the equipment, what to expect during the procedure, what to expect after the procedure, and adjuncts to pacing therapy (ie, medications). ➤*Rationale:* Understanding of pacemaker functioning and expectations of the procedure will assist the patient and family in developing a realistic perception of the procedure and how it will help the patient.

• Describe the potential sensations the patient may experience, such as involuntary muscular contraction. ➤*Rationale:* Prepares patient and family for what may be expected normally.

• Discuss possible interventions to alleviate discomfort experienced. ➤*Rationale:* Provides patient with an opportunity to validate perceptions. Gives the patient and family knowledge that interventions will be used to minimize the level of discomfort.

• If indicated, inform patient and family of the possibility of the need for transvenous or permanent pacing support. ➤*Rationale:* Prepares patient and family for additional therapy. If permanent pacing is required, the patient and family will need further instruction about possible lifestyle modifications and follow-up visits and information about the pacemaker to be implanted.

PATIENT ASSESSMENT AND PREPARATION

Patient Assessment

• Assess cardiac rhythm for the presence of bradydysrhythmias (including AV block), bradydysrhythmias associated with premature ventricular contractions, tachydysrhythmias, or asystole. ➤*Rationale:* The presence of these dysrhythmias may warrant the need for transcutaneous pacing.

• Determine hemodynamic response to the dysrhythmia, such as a systolic blood pressure of less than 90 mm Hg; altered level of consciousness; complaints of dizziness, shortness of breath, or nausea and vomiting; cool, clammy, diaphoretic skin; or the development of chest pain. ➤*Rationale:* The decision to intervene once specific cardiac dysrhythmias are noted depends on the effect of the dysrhythmia on the patient's cardiac output. Assessment of clinical parameters that reflect a decreased cardiac output will allow the health care team to determine whether pacing is indicated.

• Review of current medications. ➤*Rationale:* Medications such as digoxin, calcium channel blockers, and beta blockers alter AV nodal conduction and may be implicated as a cause for the dysrhythmia or reevaluated for concomitant effect on the conduction system. Other medications, especially antidysrhythmics, may alter the pacing threshold.

- Review current laboratory studies, including chemistry or electrolyte profile and digoxin or other cardioactive drug levels. ➛*Rationale:* Assists in determining if the need for external pacing was precipitated by metabolic disturbances or drug toxicity.

- Determine whether there is a physically large anterior-posterior diameter, a history of pericardial effusion, dilated cardiomyopathy, or pulmonary emphysema. ➛*Rationale:* These conditions may result in ineffective external pacing because of transthoracic impedance.

Patient Preparation

- Ensure that the patient and family understand preprocedural teaching. Answer questions as they arise and reinforce information as needed. ➛*Rationale:* Evaluates and reinforces understanding of previously taught information.

- Select chest and back placement sites and prepare the chest and back skin for placement of electrodes. Avoid contact with ECG electrodes, wires, and nitroglycerin patches and paste. ➛*Rationale:* Adequately preparing the skin, avoiding placement over bony structures and external wires, clipping body hairs, and avoiding open skin areas will reduce discomfort associated with external pacing. Placement over nitroglycerin patches and paste prevents conduction of electric current. Do not use benzoin for adherence because it increases the potential for skin burns.

- Consider administering sedation before initiating pacing. ➛*Rationale:* Transcutaneous pacing can be uncomfortable for the patient.

Procedure for Temporary Transcutaneous (External) Pacing

Steps	Rationale	Special Considerations
1. Wash hands.	Reduces transmission of microorganisms; standard precautions.	
2. Turn on pulse generator and monitor.	Ensures that equipment is functional.	Many devices work on battery or alternating current (AC) power.
3. Prepare the skin on the chest and back by washing with soap and water and trimming body hair with scissors, if necessary.	Removal of skin oils, lotion, and moisture will improve patch adherence and maximize delivery of pacing energy through the chest wall.	Optional step in an emergency. Skin preparation is an important consideration if high levels of energy are required for capture. Avoid use of flammable liquids to prepare skin (alcohol, benzoin) because of increased potential for burns. Avoid shaving chest hair because the presence of nicks in the skin under the pacing patches greatly increases patient discomfort.
4. Apply ECG electrodes of conventional three-lead, single-channel monitoring system. Connect ECG cable to monitor inlet of pulse generator.	Checks intrinsic rhythm and pacer sensing function.	Attachment of the ECG cable is optional in an emergency if asynchronous pacing is initiated (ie, asystole).
5. Adjust ECG lead and size to maximum R wave size.	Detection of intrinsic rhythm is necessary for proper demand pacing.	Lead II usually provides the most prominent R wave. (This step is unnecessary with asystole or asynchronous pacing.)
6. Apply the back (posterior, +) pacing electrode between the spine and left scapula at the level of the heart (Fig. 45–2).	Placement of pacing patches in the recommended anatomic location will enhance the potential for successful pacing.	Avoid placement over bone, because this increases the levels of energy required to pace, causing greater discomfort and the possibility of noncapture.
7. Apply the front (anterior, −) pacing electrode at the left, fourth intercostal space, midclavicular line (Fig. 45–3).	Placement of the pacing patches in the recommended anatomic location will enhance the potential for successful pacing.	Adjust position of electrode below and lateral to breast tissue to ensure optimal patch adherence. Avoid placement of electrodes over permanently placed devices such as implantable cardioverter-defibrillators (ICDs) or permanent pacemakers.

Procedure continued on following page

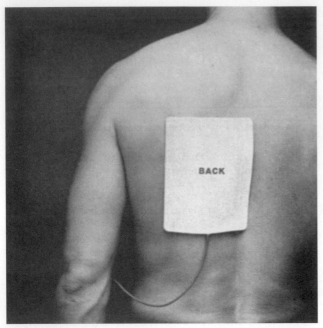

■ ● FIGURE 45–2. Location of the posterior (back) pacing electrode. (From Zoll Medical Corporation, Burlington, MA.)

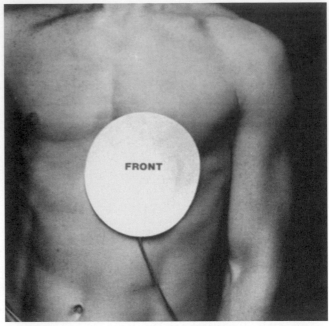

■ ● FIGURE 45–3. Location of the anterior (front) pacing electrode. (From Zoll Medical Corporation, Burlington, MA.)

Procedure	for Temporary Transcutaneous (External) Pacing *Continued*

Steps	Rationale	Special Considerations
8. When the patient is too unstable to allow posterior placement, the back electrode may be placed over the patient's right sternal area at the second or third intercostal space. The front electrode will be maintained at the apex (fourth or fifth intercostal space, midclavicular line; ie, standard anterior-anterior defibrillation paddle placement).	Facilitates ease of electrode placement for emergent pacing.	Pacing may be less effective with this method of electrode placement. Avoid placement of electrodes over bone, because this increases the levels of energy required to pace, causing greater discomfort and the possibility of noncapture.
9. Connect pacing electrodes to cable and connect to external pulse generator.	Necessary for the delivery of electric energy.	
10. Consider administering sedation before initiating pacing.	Transcutaneous pacing can be uncomfortable for the patient.	Evaluate the patient's hemodynamic status before administering sedation because of the potential for hypotension.
11. Set pacemaker settings as prescribed by the physician or advanced practice nurse, including rate, level of energy (output, mA), and mode, if available (demand/synchronous, nondemand/asynchronous) (Fig. 45–4).	Each patient may require different pacemaker settings to provide safe and effective external pacing. Pacing should be maintained at a rate that maintains adequate cardiac output but does not induce ischemia.	Follow hospital standards to ensure that a nurse can initiate transcutaneous pacing. Attempt to use the lowest level of energy necessary to pace consistently. The average adult can usually be paced with a current of 40 to 70 mA.[2] Use demand mode if available and nondemand mode only in the absence of an intrinsic rhythm.
12. Initiate pacing by slowly increasing the energy level (mA) delivered until consistent capture occurs at the prescribed rate. This is the threshold.	Use the lowest amount of energy that consistently results in myocardial capture and contraction to minimize discomfort.	Follow the manufacturer's specific recommendations for setting the energy level (mA) above threshold to maintain assurance of consistent capture and to maximize patient comfort.

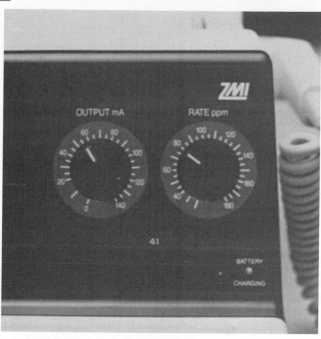

■ ● **FIGURE 45–4.** Pacemaker settings for external pacing. (From Zoll Medical Corporation, Burlington, MA.)

Procedure **for Temporary Transcutaneous (External) Pacing** *Continued*

Steps	Rationale	Special Considerations
13. Monitor ECG tracing pacer artifact and associated capture or sensing (Fig. 45–5).	Ensures adequate functioning of the pacer.	It is possible to see pacer artifact without consistent myocardial depolarization. Reevaluate threshold and increase energy levels as appropriate. Evaluate the ability of the pacer to recognize or sense an early native QRS complex.
14. Palpate patient's carotid or femoral pulse.	Ensures adequate blood flow with paced complexes.	It is possible to have electrical activity without associated mechanical contraction.
15. Evaluate patient comfort.	Pacing may be tolerated or uncomfortable for the patient.	Adjustments in threshold, changes in pacer patch location, or medication for sedation may be required.[3]
16. Discard used supplies, and wash hands.	Reduces transmission of microorganisms; standard precautions.	

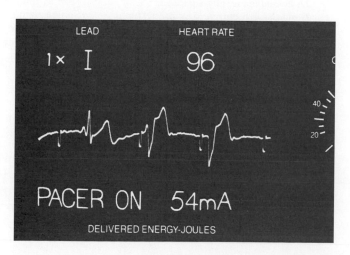

■ ● **FIGURE 45–5.** ECG tracing of external pacing. ECG, electrocardiogram. (From Zoll Medical Corporation, Burlington, MA.)

- Adequate systemic tissue perfusion and cardiac output as evidenced by blood pressure greater than 90 mm Hg systolic, alert and oriented patient, absence of dizziness or syncope, absence of shortness of breath, absence of nausea and vomiting caused by hypotension, and absence of ischemic chest pain
- Stable cardiac rhythm
- Adequate pacer function

- Failure of the pacemaker to sense patient's underlying rhythm with the possibility of R-on-T phenomenon (initiation of ventricular tachydysrhythmias as a result of an improperly timed spike on the T wave)
- Failure of the pacemaker to capture the myocardium
- Failure of the pacemaker to pace
- Discomfort, including skin burns from the delivery of high levels of energy through the chest wall, painful sensations, and skeletal muscle twitching

Patient Monitoring and Care

Patient Monitoring and Care	Rationale	Reportable Conditions
		These conditions should be reported if they persist despite nursing interventions.
1. Monitor vital signs hourly and as needed.	Ensures adequate tissue perfusion with paced beats. Adjustments in pacing rate may need to be made based on vital signs.	• Change in vital signs associated with signs and symptoms of significant hemodynamic deterioration
2. Monitor level of comfort: ○ Assess level of comfort. ○ Administer analgesic or sedative as needed. ○ Adjust level of energy to lowest level. ○ Evaluate patient response to interventions.	External delivery of energy through the chest wall may cause varying degrees of discomfort.	• Pain unrelieved by prescribed medications or interventions; patient intolerant of the prescribed medications (ie, severe nausea, hypotension, decreased respirations)
3. Obtain ECG recording to document pacing function every 4 hours and as needed.	Documentation of pacemaker efficacy is necessary for the patient record.	
4. Evaluate pacemaker function (capturing and sensing) with any changes in patient condition or vital signs.	Ensures continued functioning of pacemaker. Introduction of other variables such as electrolyte imbalance or metabolic changes may alter the level of energy required to pace effectively.	• Inability to maintain appropriate sensing and capture • Changes in patient condition that may affect appropriate pacer function and require physician intervention
5. Monitor heart rhythm for resolution of the hemodynamically significant dysrhythmia requiring treatment. This may require turning the pacemaker off to assess the underlying rhythm.	Indicates whether external pacing has been an effective method of treatment. Some manufacturers have the 4:1 feature (ie, Zoll allows assessment of baseline rhythm without turning the pacer off).	• Worsening of the baseline cardiac rhythm (eg, change from symptomatic second-degree heart block to complete heart block)
6. Evaluate the hemodynamic response to pacing by comparison to the baseline.	Evaluates the patient's physiologic response to pacing and ensures that it is optimal.	• Significant hemodynamic deterioration
7. Monitor skin integrity under the electrodes. ○ Assess skin integrity with routine physical assessment, minimally once every 24 hours but more frequently if pacing or defibrillation recurs through multifunction electrodes. ○ Change electrodes at least every 24 hours.	Change in skin integrity caused by burns or skin breaks will significantly alter patient's level of comfort and expose the patient to possible infection.	• Changes in skin integrity

Documentation

• Patient and family education	• Any medications administered during the initial procedure
• Patient preparation	• Pacing rate
• Date and time transcutaneous pacing is initiated	• Threshold level
• Description of events warranting intervention	• Milliamperage setting (mA)
• Vital signs and physical assessment before and after transcutaneous pacing	• Mode of pacing
	• Percentage of time paced if in demand mode
• ECG recordings before and after pacing	• Status of skin integrity when pacing electrodes are changed
• Patient tolerance and comfort level and related interventions	• Unexpected outcomes
	• Additional interventions

References

1. American Heart Association, Emergency Cardiac Care Committee and Subcommittees. Guidelines for cardiopulmonary resuscitation and emergency cardiac care. *JAMA.* 1992;268: 2213–2214.
2. Moses HW, Moulton KP, Miller BD, Schneider JA. *A Practical Guide to Cardiac Pacing.* Boston, Mass: Little, Brown, and Co; 1995:105–108.
3. Atlee JL. *Arrhythmias and Pacemakers.* Philadelphia, Pa: W.B. Saunders; 1996:270–274.

Additional Readings

American Heart Association, Emergency Cardiac Care Committee and Subcommittees. Guidelines for cardiopulmonary resuscitation and emergency cardiac care. *JAMA.* 1992;268:2213–2214.

Appel-Hardin S. The role of the critical care nurse in noninvasive temporary pacing. *Crit Care Nurse.* 1992;12:9–10.

Beeler L. Noninvasive temporary cardiac pacing in the emergency department: a review and update. *J Emerg Nurs.* 1993;19:202–205.

Braun AE. Emergency cardiac care: a quick response to life-threatening arrhythmias. *RN.* 1994;57:54–63.

Paraskos JA, Watts S. Emergency cardiac pacing. *Hosp Med.* 1996;32:35–41.

Pezzella DA. External pacing. *Prog Cardiovasc Nurs.* 1989;4:18–22.

Teplitz L. External pacemakers. *J Cardiovasc Nurs.* 1991;5:44–57.

Waggoner PC. External cardiac pacing. *AACN Clin Issues Crit Care Nurs.* 1991;2:118–125.

Wertz EM. External cardiac pacing. *Emergency.* 1994;26:53–56.

Winslow EH. Research for practice. External pacing in the field: poor results. *Am J Nurs.* 1994;94:24.

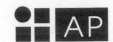

Temporary Transvenous Pacemaker Insertion (Perform)

P U R P O S E: The purpose of temporary cardiac pacing is to ensure or restore adequate heart rate and rhythm. A transvenous pacemaker is inserted as a temporary measure when the normal conduction system of the heart fails to produce an electrical impulse, resulting in hemodynamic compromise or other debilitating symptoms in the patient.

Deborah E. Becker

PREREQUISITE NURSING KNOWLEDGE

- Understanding of normal anatomy and physiology of the cardiovascular system, principles of cardiac conduction, and basic and advanced dysrhythmia interpretation is necessary.
- Understanding of temporary pacemakers is needed to evaluate pacemaker function and patient response to pacemaker therapy.
- Clinical and technical competence in central line insertion, temporary transvenous pacemaker insertion, and suturing is necessary.
- Clinical and technical competence is needed related to use of temporary pacemakers.
- Competence in chest x-ray interpretation should exist.
- Advanced cardiac life support knowledge and skills are necessary.
- Principles of general electrical safety apply when using temporary invasive pacing methods. Gloves should always be worn when handling electrodes to prevent microshock.
- The insertion of a temporary pacemaker is performed in both emergency and elective clinical situations. Temporary pacing may be used to stimulate the myocardium to contract in the absence of an intrinsic rhythm, to establish adequate cardiac output and blood pressure to ensure tissue perfusion to vital organs, to reduce the possibility of ventricular dysrhythmias in the presence of bradycardia, to supplement an inadequate rhythm with transient decreases in heart rate (ie, chronotropic incompetence in shock), or to allow the administration of medications (ie, beta blockers) to treat ischemia or tachydysrhythmias

in the presence of conduction system dysfunction or bradycardia.
- Temporary transvenous pacing is indicated for the following:
  ❖ Third-degree atrioventricular (AV) block (symptomatic congenital complete heart block, symptomatic acquired complete heart block)
  ❖ Type II AV block
  ❖ Dysrhythmias complicating acute myocardial infarction (symptomatic bradycardia, complete heart block, new bundle branch block with transient complete heart block, alternating bundle branch block)
  ❖ Sinus node dysfunction (symptomatic bradydysrhythmias, treatment of tachy-brady syndromes [sick sinus syndromes])
  ❖ Ventricular standstill or cardiac arrest
  ❖ Long QT syndrome with ventricular dysrhythmias
  ❖ Drug toxicity
  ❖ Postoperative cardiac surgery
  ❖ Prophylaxis with cardiac diagnostic or interventional procedures
  ❖ Chronotropic incompetence in the setting of cardiogenic shock
- When temporary transvenous pacing is used, the pulse generator is externally attached to a pacing lead wire that is inserted through a vein into the right atrium or ventricle.
- Veins used for the insertion of a transvenous pacing lead wire are subclavian, femoral, brachial, internal jugular, or external jugular.
- Single-chamber ventricular pacing is usually the most appropriate method in an emergency because the goal is to establish a heart rate as quickly as possible.
- The pacing lead is an insulated wire with two electrodes at the tip of the wire (Fig. 46–1).
- The pacing lead can be a hard-tipped or a balloon-tipped pacing catheter that is placed in direct contact with the myocardium. Most temporary leads are bipolar with the

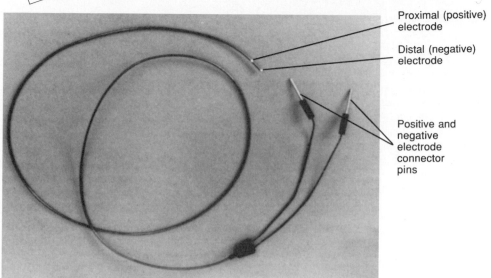

Proximal (positive) electrode

Distal (negative) electrode

Positive and negative electrode connector pins

■● **FIGURE 46–1.** Bipolar lead wire.

distal tip electrode separated from the proximal ring by 1 to 2 cm (see Fig. 46–1).

- Basic principles of cardiac pacing include sensing, pacing, and capture.
  - ❖ *Sensing* refers to the ability of the pacemaker device to detect intrinsic myocardial electrical activity. Sensing occurs if the pulse generator is in the synchronous or demand mode. The pacemaker either will be inhibited from delivering a stimulus or will initiate an electrical impulse.
  - ❖ *Pacing* occurs once the temporary pulse generator is activated and the requisite level of energy travels from the pulse generator through the temporary pacing lead wire to the myocardium. This is known as pacemaker "firing" and is represented as a "line" or "spike" on the electrocardiogram (ECG) recording.
  - ❖ *Capture* refers to the successful stimulation of the myocardium by the pacemaker, resulting in depolarization. It is evidenced on the ECG by a pacemaker spike followed by either an atrial or a ventricular complex, depending on the chamber being paced.
- Temporary pulse generator features include the following:
  - ❖ The temporary pulse generator houses the controls and the energy source for pacing.
  - ❖ There are pulse generators that can be used for single-chamber pacing with one set of terminals at the top of the pulse generator, into which the pacing wires are inserted (via connecting cable).
  - ❖ A dual-chamber pacemaker requires two sets of terminals for atrial and ventricular wires.
  - ❖ Different models of pacemakers use either dials or touch pads to change settings.
  - ❖ Pacing rate is determined by the rate dial or pad.
  - ❖ The AV interval dial or pad on a dual-chamber pacemaker controls the amount of time between atrial and ventricular stimulation (electronic P-R interval).
  - ❖ The energy delivered to the myocardium is determined by setting the output (mA or milliamperage) dial or pad on the pulse generator.
  - ❖ Dual-chamber pacing requires that mAs be set for both the atria and the ventricle.
- The ability of the pacemaker to detect the patient's intrinsic rhythm is determined by the pacing mode. In the asynchronous mode, the pacemaker functions as a fixed-rate pacemaker and is not able to sense any of the patient's inherent cardiac activity. In the synchronous mode, the pacemaker is able to sense the patient's inherent cardiac activity.
- The ability of the pacemaker to depolarize the myocardium is dependent on a number of variables: position of the electrode and degree of contact with viable myocardial tissue; level of energy delivered through the pacing wire; presence of hypoxia, acidosis, or electrolyte imbalances; fibrosis around the tip of the catheter; and concomitant drug therapy.[1]

EQUIPMENT

- Antiseptic skin preparation solution (povidone-iodine)
- Local anesthetic
- Sterile drapes, towels, masks, gowns, gloves, and dressings
- Balloon-tipped pacing catheter and insertion tray
- Pacing lead wire
- Pulse generator
- 9-volt battery for pulse generator
- Connecting cable
- Percutaneous introducer needle or 14-G needle
- Introducer sheath with dilator
- Guidewire (per physician or advanced practice nurse)
- Alligator clips
- Suture with needle, syringes, needles
- ECG monitor and recorder
- Supplies for dressing at insertion site

Additional equipment (to have available depending on patient need) includes the following:

- Emergency equipment
- Fluoroscopy
- 12-lead ECG machine

PATIENT AND FAMILY EDUCATION

- Assess learning needs, readiness to learn, and factors that will influence learning. ➣*Rationale:* Individualizes teaching in a manner that will be meaningful to the patient and the family.
- Discuss basic facts about the normal conduction system, such as structure of the conduction system, source of heart rate, normal and abnormal heart rhythms, and symptoms and significance of abnormal heart rhythms. ➣*Rationale:* Patient and family should understand why the procedure is necessary and what potential risks and benefits will be derived from undergoing this invasive procedure.
- Provide a basic description of the temporary pacemaker insertion procedure. ➣*Rationale:* Patient and family should be informed of the invasive nature of the procedure and any risks associated with the procedure. An understanding of the procedure may reduce anxiety associated with the procedure.
- Describe the precautions and restrictions required while the temporary pacemaker is in place, such as limitation of movement, avoiding handling the pacemaker or touching exposed portions of the electrode, and situations in which the nurse should be notified (eg, if the dressing becomes damp, if the patient experiences dizziness). ➣*Rationale:* Understanding potential limitations may improve patient compliance with restrictions and precautions.

PATIENT ASSESSMENT AND PREPARATION

Patient Assessment

- Assess cardiac rhythm for the presence of the dysrhythmia that necessitates placement of temporary cardiac pacing. ➣*Rationale:* Determines the need for invasive cardiac pacing.
- Assess the hemodynamic response to the dysrhythmia. Rhythm disturbances may significantly reduce cardiac output, with detrimental effects on perfusion to vital organs. ➣*Rationale:* Determines the urgency of the procedure. May indicate the need for temporing measures (such as vasopressors or transcutaneous pacing).
- Review current medications. ➣*Rationale:* Medications may be implicated as a cause for the dysrhythmia that led to the need for pacemaker therapy, or medications may need to be held as a result of concomitant effect. Other medications, such as antidysrhythmics, may alter the pacing threshold.
- Review current laboratory studies, including chemistry or electrolyte profile, arterial blood gases, and cardioactive drug levels. ➣*Rationale:* Assists in determining if the need for pacing was precipitated by metabolic disturbances or drug toxicity and establishes the pacing milieu.
- Presence and position of central venous access (if present). ➣*Rationale:* The temporary transvenous pacing catheter is advanced through the central venous circulation. If access is already established, it is necessary to ensure proper placement before the pacing catheter can be advanced through the circulatory system.

Patient Preparation

- Ensure that the patient and the family understand preprocedural teaching. Answer questions as they arise, and reinforce information as needed. ➣*Rationale:* Evaluates and reinforces understanding of previously taught information.
- Obtain informed consent. ➣*Rationale:* Protects rights of patient and makes competent decision possible for patient; however, under emergency circumstances, time may not allow consent form to be signed.
- Connect the patient to a five-lead monitoring system or to a 12-lead ECG machine. ➣*Rationale:* Facilitates the placement of the balloon-tipped catheter by indicating the position of the catheter during its placement. Also, allows for monitoring of the patient's cardiac rhythm during the procedure.
- Administer pain medication or sedation as prescribed. ➣*Rationale:* May be indicated depending on patient level of anxiety and pain. Sedation or pain medication may not be possible if patient is hypotensive.

Procedure for Insertion of a Temporary Transvenous Pacemaker

Steps	Rationale	Special Considerations
1. Wash hands.	Reduces transmissions of microorganisms; standard precautions.	
2. Connect patient to bedside monitoring system, and monitor ECG continuously.	Monitors intrinsic rhythm as well as rhythm during and after the procedure to evaluate for adequate rate and pacemaker function.	If the monitoring system is not a five-lead system, also connect the patient to the 12-lead ECG machine (see Procedure 54).
3. Assess pacemaker functioning, and insert a new battery into the pulse generator if needed.	Ensures functional pacemaker pulse generator.	There are different ways to assess battery function depending on model and manufacturer. Check manufacturer recommendations for specific instructions.
4. Attach the connecting cable to the pulse generator, connecting the "positive" on the cable to the "positive" on the pulse generator and the "negative" on the cable to the "negative" on the pulse generator.	Prepares the pacing system. The pacing stimulus will travel from the pulse generator to the negative terminal, and energy will return to the pulse generator via the positive terminal.	

Procedure for Insertion of a Temporary Transvenous Pacemaker *Continued*

Steps	Rationale	Special Considerations
5. Check the placement of the central venous access by chest x-ray before starting the procedure. If central venous access is needed, refer to Procedure 73.	Central venous access is needed for transvenous pacing.	
6. Prepare insertion site by clipping hair close to the skin in the area surrounding the insertion site.	Essential to prevent infection.	Shaving should be avoided because nicks in the skin may predispose patient to infection.
7. All personnel performing and assisting with the procedure should don masks, gowns, gloves, and caps.	Prevents infection and maintains standard precautions.	Gloves should be worn whenever the pacing electrodes are handled, to prevent microshock.
8. Cleanse site with antiseptic solution such as povidone-iodine solution.	Prevents infection.	
9. Drape the site with the sterile drapes.	Provides a sterile field and reduces the transmission of microorganisms.	
10. Administer local anesthetic to numb the insertion site.	A large-gauge introducer is used, which may cause discomfort during the insertion procedure.	Not necessary if central venous access is already in place.
11. Make a percutaneous puncture through the vein selected for the procedure (eg, jugular, subclavian, antecubital, or femoral vein). Refer to Procedure 73.	Allows for direct placement of the introducer.	
12. Insert the balloon-tipped catheter through the introducer, and advance the pacing lead.		
13. Inflate the balloon when the tip of the pacing lead is in the vena cava.	The air-filled balloon allows the blood flow to carry the catheter tip into the desired position in the right ventricle.	
14. Verify transvenous pacing lead placement by A. Using the V lead of the bedside monitoring system or the 12-lead ECG machine. B. Connect the patient to the limb leads. C. An alligator clip may be needed (Fig. 46–2). D. Attach the V lead of the ECG monitoring system or the 12-lead ECG machine to the negative electrode connector pin (distal pin) of the pacing electrode. E. Set the monitoring system to continuously record the V lead. F. Observe the ECG for ST segment elevation in the V lead recording (Fig. 46–3). G. Observe for left bundle branch block pattern and left axis deviation that can usually be identified.	The negative pacing electrode is positioned in the apex of the right ventricle. The ECG is then derived directly from the pacing electrode, and the position of the catheter tip is verified by the internal electrical recording that demonstrates ST segment elevation indicating contact with the myocardium.	Fluoroscopy may be needed to permit direct visualization of the pacing electrode. If fluoroscopy is used, all personnel must be shielded from the radiation with lead aprons or be positioned behind lead shields.

Procedure continued on following page

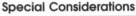

■ ● FIGURE 46–2. Alligator clips. ECG, electrocardiogram.

Procedure	**for Insertion of a Temporary Transvenous Pacemaker** *Continued*

Steps	Rationale	Special Considerations
15. After the electrodes are properly positioned, deflate the balloon and connect the external electrode pins to the pulse generator via the connecting cable. Ensure that the positive and negative electrodes are connected to the respective positive and negative terminals on the pulse generator via the connecting cable.	Energy from the pulse generator is directed to the negative electrode in contact with the ventricle. The pacing circuit is completed as energy reaches the positive electrode. The lead wires must be connected securely to the pacemaker to ensure appropriate sensing and capture and to prevent inadvertent disconnection.	It is recommended that a bridging connecting cable be used between the pacing wires and the pulse generator. Some lead wires may not have "negative" and "positive" marked on them. Polarity is established when the wires are placed in the connecting cable.
16. Refer to Procedure 47 for setting pacemaker settings and initiating pacing.		
17. Suture the pacing lead in place.	Prevents dislodgment.	
18. Apply a sterile, occlusive dressing over the site.	Prevents infection.	
19. Secure necessary equipment to provide some stability for the pacemaker, such as hanging pulse generator on an intravenous (IV) pole, strapping pulse generator to patient's torso, or hanging pulse generator from a carrying device.	The pulse generator should be protected from falling or becoming inadvertently detached by patient movement. Disconnection or tension on the pacing electrodes may lead to pacemaker malfunction.	
20. Discard used supplies, and wash hands.	Reduces transmission of microorganisms; standard precautions.	

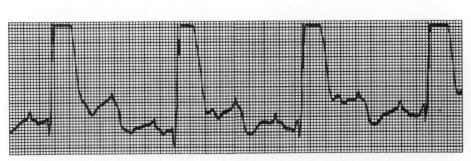

■ ● FIGURE 46–3. ECG rhythm recorded in the right ventricle: elevated ST segments when pacing electrode is wedged against the endocardial wall of the right ventricle. ECG, electrocardiogram. (From Meltzer LE, Pinneo R, Kitchell JR. *Intensive Coronary Care.* 4th ed. Bowie, Md: Robert J. Brady Co.; 1983: 233.)

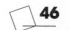

| Procedure | **Insertion of a Temporary Transvenous Pacemaker** *Continued* |

Steps	Rationale	Special Considerations
21. Obtain chest x-ray.	In the absence of fluoroscopy, an x-ray is essential to detect potential complications associated with insertion as well as to visualize lead position.	

Expected Outcomes

- ECG will show paced rhythm consistent with parameters set on pacemaker, as evidenced by appropriate heart rate, proper sensing, and proper capture.
- Patient will exhibit hemodynamic stability, as evidenced by systolic blood pressure greater than 90 mm Hg, mean arterial blood pressure greater than 60 mm Hg, alertness and orientation, and no syncope or ischemia.
- Pacemaker leads will be isolated from other electrical equipment by maintaining secure connections into pulse generator.

Unexpected Outcomes

- Inability to achieve proper placement of the pacing catheter
- Failure of the pacemaker to sense, causing competition between the pacemaker-initiated impulses and the patient's intrinsic cardiac rhythm
- Failure of the pacemaker to capture the myocardium
- Pacemaker oversensing causing the pacemaker to be inappropriately inhibited
- Stimulation of diaphragm causing hiccuping, possibly related to pacing the phrenic nerve, perforation, wire dislodgment, or excessively high pacemaker mA setting
- Development of phlebitis, thrombosis, embolism, or bacteremia
- Ventricular dysrhythmias from manipulation within the cardiac chamber
- Pneumothorax or hemothorax from the insertion procedure
- Myocardial perforation and cardiac tamponade from the insertion procedure and electrode placement
- Air embolism
- Lead dislodgment

Patient Monitoring and Care

Patient Monitoring and Care	Rationale	Reportable Conditions
		These conditions should be reported if they persist despite nursing interventions.
1. Monitor vital signs and hemodynamic response to pacing as often as patient condition warrants.	The goal of cardiac pacing is to improve cardiac output by increasing heart rate or by overriding life-threatening dysrhythmias.	• Change in vital signs associated with signs and symptoms of hemodynamic deterioration
2. Evaluate ECG for presence of paced rhythm or resolution of initiating dysrhythmia.	Proper pacemaker functioning is assessed by observing the ECG for pacemaker activity consistent with the parameters set.	• Inability to obtain a paced rhythm • Oversensing • Undersensing

3. Monitor patient's level of comfort.
  ○ Assess level of comfort.
  ○ Administer analgesic or sedative as needed.
  ○ Evaluate patient response to interventions.
	Discomfort may increase patient's anxiety and decrease tolerance of the procedure, causing hemodynamic compromise.	• Continual hiccups (may indicate wire perforation)
		• Unrelieved discomfort

Continued on following page

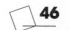 This procedure should be performed only by physicians, advanced practice nurses, and other health care professionals (including critical care nurses) with additional knowledge, skills, and demonstrated competence per professional licensure or institutional standard.

Patient Monitoring and Care *Continued*

Patient Monitoring and Care	Rationale	Reportable Conditions
4. Check and document sensitivity and threshold at least every 24 hours. Threshold may be checked by physicians in high-risk patients.	Prevents unnecessarily high levels of energy delivery to the myocardium. Threshold may be checked more frequently if the patient condition changes or pacer function is questioned.	• Problems with sensitivity or threshold
5. Change dressing as determined by institutional policy depending on the type of dressing used. ○ Cleanse surrounding area with antiseptic solution such as povidone-iodine. ○ Apply dry, sterile dressing and tape. ○ Record date of dressing change.	Decreases potential for infection.	• Signs of infection such as increased temperature, increased white blood cells, purulent drainage at the insertion site, or warmth or pain at the site
6. Monitor for other complications.	Early recognition leads to prompt treatment.	• Any signs of complications such as embolus, thrombosis, perforation of the myocardium, pneumothorax, hemothorax, or phlebitis
7. Monitor electrolytes.	Electrolyte imbalances may precipitate dysrhythmias.	• Abnormal electrolyte values
8. Ensure that all connections are secure at least daily.	Maintenance of tight connections is necessary to ensure proper pacer functioning.	• Inability to maintain tight connections with available equipment, jeopardizing pacing therapy

Documentation

Documentation should include the following:

- Patient and family education and response to education
- Date and time of insertion
- Date and time of initiation of pacing
- Description of events warranting intervention
- Vital signs and hemodynamic parameters before, during, and after procedure
- ECG monitoring strip recording before and after pacemaker insertion

- Type of wire inserted and location of insertion
- Pacemaker settings—mode, rate, output, sensitivity setting, threshold measurements, and whether pacemaker is on or off
- Patient response to procedure
- Complications and interventions
- Medications administered and patient response to medication
- Date and time pacing was discontinued

Reference

1. Morhadd MG, Dahlberg ST. Temporary cardiac pacing. In Rippe JM, Irwin RS, Fink MP, Cerra FB, Curley F, Herd SO, eds. *Procedure and Techniques in Intensive Care Medicine.* Philadelphia, Pa: Lippincott Williams & Wilkins; 1994:73–80.

Additional Readings

Atlee JL. *Arrhythmias and Pacemakers.* Philadelphia, Pa: W.B. Saunders; 1996:247–329.

Medtronic, Inc. *Cardiac Pacing and Patient Care.* Minneapolis, Mn: Author; 1997:1–40.

Moses HW, Moulton KP, Miller BD, Schneider JA. *A Practical Guide to Cardiac Pacing.* Boston, Ma: Little, Brown; 1995:89–112.

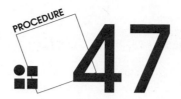

47

Temporary Transvenous and Epicardial Pacing

P U R P O S E: The purpose of temporary cardiac pacing is to ensure or restore an adequate heart rate and rhythm. Transvenous and epicardial pacing are initiated as temporary measures when there has been a failure of the normal conduction system of the heart to produce an electrical impulse, resulting in hemodynamic compromise or other debilitating symptoms in the patient.

Francine E. Paschall
Ellen Strauss McErlean

PREREQUISITE NURSING KNOWLEDGE

- Understanding of the normal anatomy and physiology of the cardiovascular system, principles of cardiac conduction, and basic dysrhythmia interpretation is needed.
- Understanding of temporary pacemakers in order to evaluate pacemaker function and the patient response to pacemaker therapy is necessary.
- Clinical and technical competence related to use of temporary pacemakers is essential.
- Advanced cardiac life support knowledge and skills are needed.
- Basic principles of hemodynamic monitoring are essential when assessing the efficacy of temporary pacing therapy. A working knowledge of the pulmonary artery (PA) catheter function and use relative to hemodynamic monitoring is a necessity when using a PA catheter with pacing function (see Procedure 66). Knowledge of the care of the patient with central venous catheter insertion and access is also necessary (see Procedure 74).
- Principles of general electrical safety apply when using temporary invasive pacing methods. Gloves should always be worn when handling electrodes to prevent microshock. In addition, the exposed proximal ends of pacing wires should be insulated when not in use to prevent microshock.[1]
- The insertion of a temporary pacemaker is performed in both emergency and elective clinical situations. Temporary pacing may be used to stimulate the myocardium to contract in the absence of an intrinsic rhythm, establish an adequate cardiac output and blood pressure to ensure tissue perfusion to vital organs, reduce the possibility of ventricular dysrhythmias in the presence of bradycardia, supplement an inadequate rhythm with transient decreases in heart rate (eg, chronotropic incompetence in shock), or allow the administration of medications (eg, beta blockers) to treat ischemia or tachydysrhythmias

in the presence of conduction system dysfunction or bradycardia.

- Temporary invasive pacing is indicated for the following:
  - ❖ Third degree atrioventricular (AV) block
    Symptomatic congenital complete heart block
    Symptomatic acquired complete heart block
  - ❖ Symptomatic second degree heart block
  - ❖ Dysrhythmias complicating acute myocardial infarction
    Symptomatic bradycardia
    Complete heart block
    New bundle branch block with transient complete heart block
    Alternating bundle branch block
  - ❖ Sinus node dysfunction
    Symptomatic bradydysrhythmias
    Treatment of bradycardia-tachycardia syndrome (sick sinus syndromes)
  - ❖ Ventricular standstill or cardiac arrest
  - ❖ Long QT syndrome with ventricular dysrhythmias
  - ❖ Drug toxicity
  - ❖ Postoperative cardiac surgery
    Symptomatic bradydysrhythmias
    Low cardiac output states
  - ❖ Prophylaxis with cardiac diagnostic or interventional procedures
  - ❖ Chronotropic incompetence in the setting of cardiogenic shock
- There are three primary methods of invasive temporary pacing: transvenous endocardial pacing, pulmonary artery catheter pacing, and epicardial pacing.
- Transvenous pacing
  - ❖ In temporary transvenous pacing, the pulse generator is externally attached to a pacing lead that is inserted through a vein into the right atrium or ventricle.

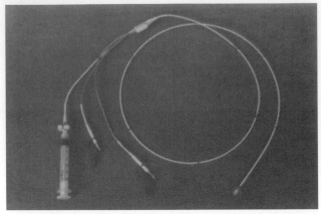

■ ● FIGURE 47–1. Balloon-tipped bipolar lead wire for transvenous pacing.

❖ Veins used for insertion of the pacing lead are the subclavian, femoral, brachial, internal jugular, or external jugular.

❖ Single chamber ventricular pacing is usually the most appropriate method in an emergency because the goal is to establish a heart rate as quickly as possible.

❖ Temporary atrial or dual chamber pacing can be initiated if the patient requires atrial contraction for improvement in hemodynamics.

❖ The pacing lead is an insulated wire with one or two electrodes at the tip of the wire.

❖ The pacing lead can be a hard-tipped or balloon-tipped pacing catheter that is placed in direct contact with the myocardium (see Fig. 47–1). Most temporary leads are bipolar, with the distal tip electrode separated from the proximal ring by 1 to 2 cm (see Fig. 46–1).

• Pacing via a PA catheter
  ❖ The use of a thermodilution PA catheter for temporary atrial or ventricular pacing can be done with combination catheters that are specifically designed for temporary pacing.
  ❖ The newest pacing PA catheter features atrial and ventricular ports for introduction of pacing wires (Fig. 47–2).
  ❖ Use of a PA catheter combines the capabilities of

PA pressure monitoring, thermodilution cardiac output measurement, fluid infusion, mixed venous oxygen sampling, and temporary pacing.

❖ One limitation of these multifunction catheters is that the simultaneous measurement of pulmonary artery wedge pressure (PAWP) and pacing is usually not possible. Balloon inflation can cause repositioning of the pacing electrode with catheter movement and measurement of PAWP may cause pacing to become intermittent.

• Temporary epicardial pacing
  ❖ Temporary epicardial pacing is a method of stimulating the myocardium through the use of Teflon-coated unipolar stainless steel wires that are sutured loosely to the epicardium after cardiac surgery.
  ❖ The epicardial wires may be attached to the right atrium for atrial pacing, the right ventricle for ventricular pacing, or both for AV pacing (Fig. 47–3).
  ❖ Once implanted on the epicardial surface, each pacing wire is brought through the chest wall before the chest is closed.
  ❖ Typically, the atrial wires are located on the right of the sternum and the ventricular wires exit to the left of the sternum (see Fig. 41–1).
  ❖ An external temporary pulse generator is then connected to the epicardial pacing wires via a bridging or connecting cable (Figs. 47–4, 47–5, and 47–6).

• Basic principles of cardiac pacing include sensing, pacing, and capture.
  ❖ *Sensing* refers to the ability of the pacemaker device to detect intrinsic myocardial electrical activity. Sensing occurs if the pulse generator is in the synchronous or demand mode. The pacemaker will either be inhibited from delivering a stimulus or will initiate an electrical impulse.

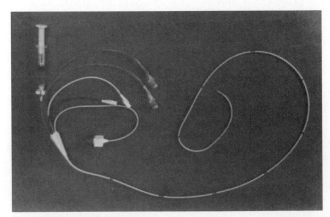

■ ● FIGURE 47–2. Pulmonary artery catheter with atrial and ventricular pacing lumens.

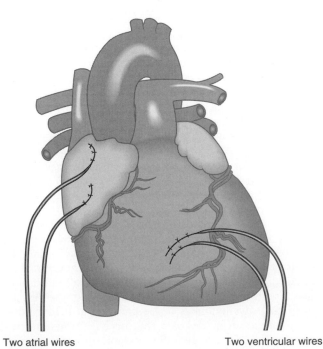

Two atrial wires   Two ventricular wires

■ ● FIGURE 47–3. Location of atrial and ventricular epicardial lead wires.

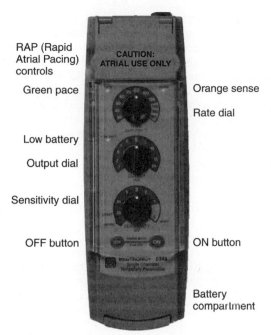

RAP (Rapid Atrial Pacing) controls

Green pace

Low battery

Output dial

Sensitivity dial

OFF button

CAUTION: ATRIAL USE ONLY

Orange sense

Rate dial

ON button

Battery compartment

■ ● **FIGURE 47–4.** Single-chamber temporary pulse generator. (From Medtronic USA, Inc.)

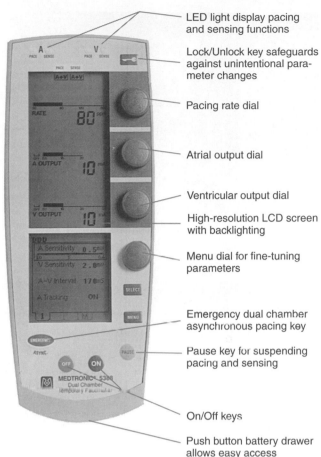

LED light display pacing and sensing functions

Lock/Unlock key safeguards against unintentional parameter changes

Pacing rate dial

Atrial output dial

Ventricular output dial

High-resolution LCD screen with backlighting

Menu dial for fine-tuning parameters

Emergency dual chamber asynchronous pacing key

Pause key for suspending pacing and sensing

On/Off keys

Push button battery drawer allows easy access

■ ● **FIGURE 47–6.** Dual-chamber temporary pulse generator. (From Medtronic USA, Inc.)

❖ *Pacing* occurs once the temporary pulse generator is activated and the requisite level of energy travels from the pulse generator through the temporary wires to the myocardium. This is known as pacemaker *firing* and is represented as a line or spike on the electrocardiogram (ECG) recording.

❖ *Capture* refers to the successful stimulation of the myocardium by the pacemaker, resulting in depolarization. It is evidenced on the ECG by a pacemaker spike, followed by either an atrial or ventricular complex, depending on the chamber being paced.

• Temporary pulse generator
  ❖ The temporary pulse generator houses the controls and energy source for pacing.
  ❖ There are pulse generators that can be used for single-chamber pacing that have one set of terminals at the top of the pulse generator into which the pacing wires are inserted (via connecting cable). See Figure 47–4.
  ❖ A dual-chamber pacemaker requires two sets of termi-

nals for the atrial and ventricular wires (see Figs. 47–6 and 47–7).
  ❖ Different models of pacemakers use either dials or touch pads to change settings.
  ❖ Pacing rate is determined by the rate dial or touch pad.
  ❖ The AV interval dial or pad on a dual-chamber pacemaker controls the amount of time between atrial and ventricular stimulation (electronic PR interval).
  ❖ The energy delivered to the myocardium is determined by setting the output (milliampere) dial or pad on the pulse generator.
  ❖ Dual chamber pacing requires that milliamperes be set for both the atria and the ventricle.

• The ability of the pacemaker to detect the patient's intrinsic rhythm is determined by the pacing mode. In the asynchronous mode, the pacemaker functions as a fixed-rate pacemaker and is not able to sense any of the patient's inherent cardiac activity. In the synchronous mode, the pacemaker is able to sense the patient's inherent cardiac activity.

• Reference to the pacemaker code aids in the assessment of pacing terminology (see Table 44–1).

• The ability of the pacemaker to depolarize the myocardium is dependent on a number of variables: the position of the electrode and degree of contact with viable myo-

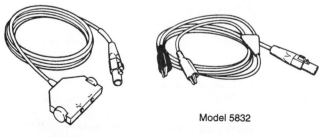

Model 5832

Model 5433A/ 5433V

■ ● **FIGURE 47–5.** Connecting cables. (From Medtronic USA, Inc.)

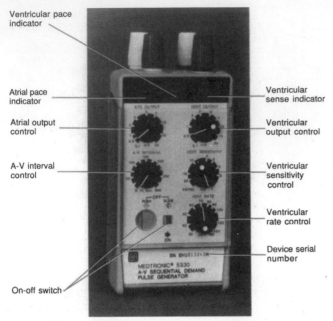

Ventricular pace indicator
Atrial pace indicator
Atrial output control
A-V interval control
A-V interval control
On-off switch
Ventricular sense indicator
Ventricular output control
Ventricular sensitivity control
Ventricular rate control
Device serial number

■ ● **FIGURE 47–7.** Dual-chamber temporary pulse generator. (From Medtronic USA, Inc.)

cardial tissue; the level of energy delivered through the pacing wire; the presence of hypoxia, acidosis, or electrolyte imbalances; fibrosis around the tip of the catheter; and concomitant drug therapy.[2]

EQUIPMENT

- Antiseptic skin preparation solution (povidone-iodine)
- Local anesthetic
- Sterile drapes, towels, masks, goggles, gowns, gloves, caps, and dressings
- Pacing lead wires
- Pulse generator
- 9-V battery for pulse generator
- Connecting cables
- Percutaneous introducer needle or 14-G needle
- Introducer sheath with dilator

- Guidewire (chosen by the physician or advanced practice nurse)
- Alligator clips (if necessary)
- Suture with needle, needles, syringes
- ECG monitor and recorder
- Supplies for dressing at insertion site

Additional equipment to have available, depending on need, includes the following:

- Emergency equipment
- Fluoroscopy
- Flush solution and pressure line set-up, if using PA catheter (see Procedure 69)

- 12-lead ECG machine

PATIENT AND FAMILY EDUCATION

- Assess learning needs, readiness to learn, and factors that will influence learning. ➤*Rationale:* Individualizes teaching in a manner that will be meaningful to the patient and family.

- Discuss basic facts about the normal conduction system, such as structure of the conduction system, source of heart rate, normal and abnormal heart rhythms, and symptoms or significance of abnormal heart rhythms. ➤*Rationale:* Patient and family should understand why the procedure is necessary and what potential risks and benefits will be derived from undergoing this invasive procedure.
- Provide a basic description of the temporary pacemaker insertion procedure. ➤*Rationale:* Patient and family should be informed of the invasive nature of the procedure and any risks associated with it. An understanding of the procedure may reduce anxiety.
- Describe the precautions and restrictions required while the temporary pacemaker is in place, such as limitation of movement, avoidance of handling the pacemaker or touching exposed portions of the electrode, and when to notify the nurse (eg, if the dressing becomes wet, if the patient is experiencing dizziness). ➤*Rationale:* Understanding potential limitations may improve patient compliance with restrictions and precautions.

PATIENT ASSESSMENT AND PREPARATION

Patient Assessment

- Assess cardiac rhythm for the presence of the dysrhythmia that necessitates placement of temporary cardiac pacing. ➤*Rationale:* Determines the need for invasive cardiac pacing.
- Assess the hemodynamic response to the dysrhythmia. Rhythm disturbances may significantly reduce cardiac output with detrimental effects on perfusion to vital organs. ➤*Rationale:* Determines the urgency of the procedure. May indicate the need for temporing measures, such as vasopressors or transcutaneous pacing.
- Review current medications. ➤*Rationale:* Medications may be a cause of the dysrhythmia that led to the need for pacemaker therapy, or medications may need to be held due to concomitant effect. Other medications, such as antidysrhythmics, may alter the pacing threshold.
- Review current laboratory studies including chemistry or electrolyte profile, arterial blood gases, or cardioactive drug levels. ➤*Rationale:* Assists in determining if the need for pacing was precipitated by metabolic disturbances or drug toxicity, and establishes the pacing milieu.

Patient Preparation

- Ensure that the patient and family understand preprocedural teaching. Answer questions as they arise, and reinforce information as needed. ➤*Rationale:* Evaluates and reinforces understanding of previously taught information.
- Validate that informed consent has been obtained. ➤*Rationale:* Protects rights of the patient and makes competent decision possible for the patient; however, under emergency circumstances, time may not allow the form to be signed.
- Administer pain medication or sedation as prescribed. ➤*Rationale:* May be indicated, depending on the patient's level of anxiety and pain. Sedation or pain medication may not be possible if the patient is hypotensive.

Procedure for Temporary Transvenous and Epicardial Pacing		
Steps	**Rationale**	**Special Considerations**

Initiating Temporary Pacing

Steps	Rationale	Special Considerations
1. Wash hands.	Reduces transmission of microorganisms; standard precautions.	
2. Connect patient to bedside monitoring system and monitor ECG continuously.	Monitor intrinsic rhythm as well as rhythm during and after the procedure to evaluate for adequate rate and pacemaker function.	
3. Assess pacemaker functioning and insert a new battery into the pulse generator, if needed (Figs. 47–8 and 47–9).	Ensures functional pacemaker pulse generator.	There are different ways to assess battery function, depending on the model and manufacturer. Check manufacturer recommendations for specific instructions.
4. Attach the connecting cable to the pulse generator, connecting the *positive* on the cable to the *positive* on the pulse generator, and the *negative* on the cable to the *negative* on the pulse generator.	Prepares the pacing system. The pacing stimulus will travel from the pulse generator to the negative terminal, and energy will return to the pulse generator via the positive terminal.	

Assisting with Insertion of Temporary Transvenous Pacing (Ventricular)

Steps	Rationale	Special Considerations
1. Follow steps 1 through 4 as listed earlier for Initiating Temporary Pacing.		
2. Prepare insertion site by clipping hair close to the skin in the area surrounding the insertion site.	Essential to prevent infection.	Shaving should be avoided because nicks in the skin may predispose patient to infection.
3. All personnel performing and assisting with the procedure should don masks, goggles, gowns, gloves, and caps.	Prevents infection and maintains standard precautions.	Gloves should be worn whenever handling the pacing electrodes to prevent microshock.[3]
4. Cleanse site with antiseptic solution such as povidone-iodine.	Prevents infection.	
5. Assist with administration of local anesthetic to numb the insertion site.	A large gauge introducer is used, which may cause discomfort during the insertion procedure.	

Procedure continued on following page

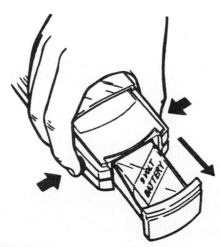

■ ● **FIGURE 47–8.** Replacing the battery. Press both battery drawer buttons to open the battery compartment and re-move the old battery. (From Medtronic USA, Inc.)

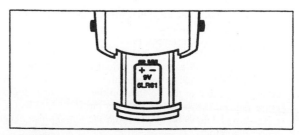

■ ● **FIGURE 47–9.** Placement of the new battery. Insert new battery, close the compartment, and press the "on" button. (From Medtronic USA, Inc.)

Procedure **for Temporary Transvenous and Epicardial Pacing** *Continued*

Steps	Rationale	Special Considerations
6. Assist the physician or advanced practice nurse as a percutaneous puncture is performed through the jugular, subclavian, antecubital, or femoral site.	Allows for direct placement of the introducer.	May be unnecessary if central venous access is already in place.
7. Assist as needed as the pacing lead is passed through the introducer.	Facilitates the insertion process.	If a balloon-tipped pacing lead is used, balloon inflation occurs when the tip of the pacing lead is in the vena cava. The air-filled balloon allows the blood flow to carry the catheter tip into the desired position in the right ventricle.
8. Verify transvenous pacing lead wire placement via one of the following: A. Fluoroscopy B. Bedside monitoring system or 12-lead ECG machine. If an ECG monitoring system or a 12-lead ECG machine is used ○ Connect the patient to the limb leads. ○ An alligator clip may be needed (see Fig. 46–2). ○ Attach the V lead of the ECG monitoring system or the 12-lead ECG machine to the negative electrode connector pin (distal pin) of the pacing lead wire (an alligator clip may be needed). ○ Set the monitoring system to continuously record the V lead. ○ Observe the ECG for ST segment elevation in the V lead recording (see Fig. 46–3). ○ In addition, a left bundle branch block pattern and left axis deviation usually can also be identified.	The pacing electrode is positioned in the apex of the right ventricle. Fluoroscopy allows direct visualization of the pacing electrode. The ECG is then derived directly from the pacing electrode, and the position of the catheter tip is verified by the internal electrical recording, which demonstrates ST segment elevation in contact with the myocardium.	If fluoroscopy is used, all personnel must be shielded from the radiation with lead aprons or be positioned behind lead shields.
9. After the pacing lead wire is properly positioned, connect the external electrode pins to the pulse generator via the connecting cable. Ensure that the positive and negative electrode connector pins are connected to the respective positive and negative terminals on the pulse generator via the connecting cable (Figs. 47–10 and 47–11).	Energy from the pulse generator is directed to the negative electrode. The pacing circuit is completed as energy reaches the positive electrode. The lead wires must be connected securely to the pacemaker to ensure appropriate sensing and capture and to prevent inadvertent disconnection.	It is recommended that a connecting cable be used between the pacing wires and the pulse generator. Some lead wires may not have *negative* and *positive* marked on them. Polarity is established when the wires are placed in the connecting cable.
10. **For AV demand pacing when atrial wires are placed in addition to ventricular wires,** connect atrial electrodes to atrial terminals and ventricular electrodes to the ventricular terminals. Attach the *positive* on the connecting cable to the *positive* on the pulse generator and the *negative* on the connecting cable to the *negative* on the pulse generator.	Ensures that atrial electrodes and ventricular electrodes are connected correctly to the pulse generator. Secure connections are essential for proper sensing and conduction of pacemaker energy. The pacing stimulus will travel from the pulse generator to the negative terminal and energy will return to the pulse generator via the positive terminal.	

| Procedure | **for Temporary Transvenous and Epicardial Pacing** *Continued* |

| Steps | Rationale | Special Considerations |

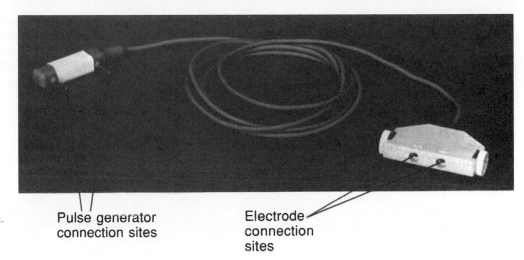

■ ● **FIGURE 47–10.** Connecting cable.

Pulse generator connection sites   **Electrode connection sites**

11. **For atrial pacing when atrial wires are placed,** connect atrial electrodes to atrial terminals. Attach the *positive* on the connecting cable to the *positive* on the pulse generator, and the *negative* on the connecting cable to the *negative* on the pulse generator. | Secure connections are essential for proper sensing and conduction of pacemaker energy. The pacing stimulus will travel from the pulse generator to the negative terminal and energy will return to the pulse generator via the positive terminal. |

Assisting with Insertion of a Temporary Pacemaker via a Pulmonary Artery Catheter

1. Follow steps 1 through 4 as listed earlier for Initiating Temporary Pacing.

2. Assist the physician or advanced practice nurse with insertion of the PA catheter (see Procedure 66). | | Pacing electrodes may be inserted at the time of PA catheter insertion, or they may be inserted at a later time, when temporary pacing is required because of a change in patient condition.

3. Obtain the appropriate pacing lead for insertion. | Only probes specifically manufactured for use with the PA catheter should be used. Check specific manufacturer's recommendations. | Continuous monitoring of the right ventricular pressure waveform via the pacing lumen is recommended before insertion of the electrode to ensure correct placement of the right ventricular port 1 to 2 cm distal to the tricuspid valve.
Procedure continued on following page

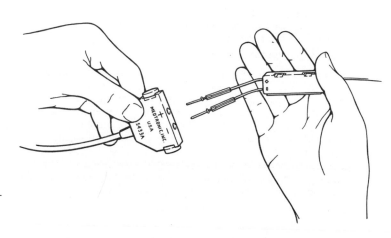

■ ● **FIGURE 47–11.** Inserting the lead wires into the connecting-bridging cable. (From Medtronic USA, Inc.)

Procedure **for Temporary Transvenous and Epicardial Pacing** *Continued*		
Steps	**Rationale**	**Special Considerations**
4. Assist the physician or advanced practice nurse with insertion of the pacing lead.	Close monitoring of the ECG during insertion of the pacing lead is necessary to detect potentially lethal dysrhythmias.	Follow specific manufacturer's instructions regarding pacing lead insertion and securing the pacing lead in place within the catheter lumen.
5. After the electrodes are properly positioned, connect the positive and negative electrode connector pins to the pulse generator via the connecting cable. Ensure that the positive and negative electrodes are connected to the respective positive and negative terminals on the pulse generator via the connecting cable.	Energy from the pulse generator is directed to the negative electrode. The pacing circuit is completed as energy reaches the positive electrode. The electrodes must be securely connected to the pulse generator to ensure appropriate sensing and capture as well as to prevent inadvertent disconnection.	Gloves should be worn whenever handling the pacing electrodes to prevent microshock.
Epicardial Pacing		
1. Follow steps 1 through 4 as listed earlier for Initiating Temporary Pacing.		
2. Don gloves.	Examination gloves should be worn whenever handling the epicardial wires to prevent microshock.	
3. Expose the epicardial pacing wires and identify the chamber of origin. Wires exiting to the right of the sternum are atrial in origin. Wires exiting to the left of the sternum are ventricular in origin (see Fig. 41–1).	Identifies correct chamber for pacing.	
4. Connect the epicardial wires to the pulse generator via the connecting cable. Ensure that the positive and negative electrodes are connected to the respective positive and negative terminals on the pulse generator via the connecting cable.	The epicardial wires must be securely connected to the pulse generator to ensure appropriate sensing and capture as well as to prevent inadvertent disconnection. Use of unipolar or bipolar configuration needs to be established. This is dependent on where the physician placed the epicardial wires. In a unipolar pacing system, there is only one electrode in contact with the chamber being paced (the negative electrode). The positive, or indifferent, electrode is commonly sewn to the subcutaneous tissue of the chest wall. With bipolar pacing, both electrodes are in direct contact with the myocardial tissue of the chamber being paced.	The wire connected to the negative terminal determines where the energy will be delivered. The wire connected to the positive terminal determines how the energy will return to the pulse generator. With AV demand pacing, be sure to place both atrial wires in the terminal labeled *atrium* (via cable) and ventricular wires in the terminal labeled *ventricle* (via cable). With bipolar pacing, either wire can be the negative electrode. With unipolar pacing (one electrode in contact with the heart), the epicardial wire must be the negative electrode and the skin wire must be the positive electrode.
All Methods of Temporary Pacing		
1. Determine the mode of pacing desired.	The pacing mode chosen should be the one that will best achieve the goal of pacing therapy. Possibilities include atrial or ventricular asynchronous, ventricular or atrial demand, or dual chamber demand pacing.	Asynchronous pacing in the presence of an intrinsic rhythm may result in "R on T," leading to a lethal dysrhythmia, and should only be used in the absence of an intrinsic rhythm.

Procedure	for Temporary Transvenous and Epicardial Pacing *Continued*	

Steps	Rationale	Special Considerations
2. Set the pacemaker mode, pacemaker rate, and level of energy (output or milliampere) as prescribed or as determined by sensitivity and stimulation threshold testing (see steps 3, 4, and 5).	Determination of pacemaker settings is based on patient response and the capture threshold measured after the wires are connected.	The demand mode is recommended to avoid competition between the pacemaker-initiated beats and the patient's intrinsic rhythm. Output is set to ensure capture of the myocardium. In AV demand pacing, separate output settings are used to ensure capture of the atrium and the ventricle.
3. Turn all settings to the lowest level and then turn on the pacemaker.	Establishes power source and ensures that the device does not start pacing until all settings have been determined.	
4. Determine sensitivity threshold (for each chamber as appropriate). A. Gradually turn the sensitivity dial counterclockwise (or to a higher numerical setting), and observe the pace indicator light for flashing. B. Slowly turn sensitivity dial clockwise (or to a lower numerical setting) until sense indicator light flashes and pace indicator light stops. This value is the *sensing threshold.* C. Set sensitivity dial to the number that was half the sensing threshold to provide 2:1 safety margin.	*Sensitivity threshold* is the level at which intrinsic myocardial activity is recognized by the sensing electrodes. For demand pacing, the sensitivity must be measured and set.	After sensitivity threshold is determined, some physicians prefer to set sensitivity settings all the way to the demand mode (most sensitive) or all the way to the asynchronous mode (least sensitive), regardless of sensitivity threshold. If sensitivity is set to the most sensitive, the pacemaker may be inappropriately inhibited because it may detect and interpret extramyocardial activity (eg, muscle movement, artifact) as actual myocardial activity. When determining sensitivity threshold, the milliamperes should be turned down to avoid the possibility of a pacemaker stimulus falling on the T wave (R on T phenomenon) and inducing a potentially lethal dysrhythmia.
5. Determine stimulation threshold (for each chamber as necessary): A. Set pacing rate approximately 10 beats above the patient's intrinsic rate. B. Gradually decrease output from 20 mA until capture is lost. C. Gradually increase mA until 1:1 capture is established. This is the stimulation threshold. D. Set the milliamperes at least two times higher than the stimulation threshold.[4] This output setting is sometimes referred to as the *maintenance threshold.*	The output dial regulates the amount of electrical current (milliamperes) that is delivered to the myocardium to initiate depolarization. The maintenance threshold is set at least two times above the stimulation threshold to allow for increases in the stimulation threshold without loss of capture.[4]	Individual institutional policies govern when threshold determination should be done and whether a nurse may test the stimulation threshold. Thresholds may not be determined if sensitivity is poor or if the patient's inherent heart rate is greater than 90 beats per minute. Threshold may increase or decrease within hours of electrode placement due to fibrosis at the tip of the catheter, medication administration (eg, some antidysrhythmics), alteration of position, or underlying pathology. In the case of dual chamber pacing, the threshold for each chamber must be assessed. This step should only be performed by a physician in a patient who is pacemaker-dependent for bradyarrhythmia.

Procedure continued on following page

Procedure	for **Temporary Transvenous and Epicardial Pacing** *Continued*

Steps	Rationale	Special Considerations
6. Assess rhythm for appropriate pacemaker function (Fig. 47–12): A. *Capture:* Is there a QRS complex for every ventricular pacing stimulus? Is there also a P wave for every atrial pacing stimulus? (see Fig. 47–12) B. *Rate:* Is the rate at or above the pacemaker rate if in the demand mode? C. *Sensing:* Does the sensitivity light indicate that every QRS complex is sensed?	ECG tracing should reflect appropriate response to pacemaker settings if functioning properly. Sometimes, P-wave activity may not be visible due to low voltage amplitude. If the patient is solely atrially paced, ventricular tracking and response should follow the atrial rate setting.	
7. After settings are adjusted for optimal patient response, place protective plastic cover over pacemaker controls, if available.	Pacemaker settings may be inadvertently altered by patient movement or handling if controls are not covered.	Patient may need reinforcement of educational content regarding touching the pacemaker.
8. Check institutional policy or obtain specific physician prescription regarding the purposeful wedging of the pulmonary artery (PA) pacing catheter that is being used actively for pacing therapy.	Intermittent capture has been noted during the wedging procedure as a result of movement of the electrode with catheter migration into the wedge position.[1]	Usually, the PA catheter is not wedged during pacing.
9. Assess patient response to pacing including blood pressure, level of consciousness, heart rhythm, and other hemodynamic parameters, if available.	Pacemaker settings are determined by patient response.	When single chamber ventricular pacing is used, a higher rate may be necessary to compensate for the loss of atrial contribution to cardiac output. Evaluate recurrence of ischemia with increased paced heart rate.
10. After the pacing lead is sutured into place, apply a sterile, occlusive dressing over the insertion site.	Prevents infection.	The epicardial electrodes and the insertion sites may be covered by a 4-in × 4-in dressing and taped to the chest. The wires may be placed over the dressing and covered with gauze. Finger cots may also be used to cover the wires.
11. Throughout the procedure, assess the patient's need for sedative or analgesic medication and administer as necessary.	The procedure may be anxiety producing as well as uncomfortable for the patient.	Close monitoring of blood pressure, heart rate, respiratory rate, and level of consciousness should be performed with the administration of medication.

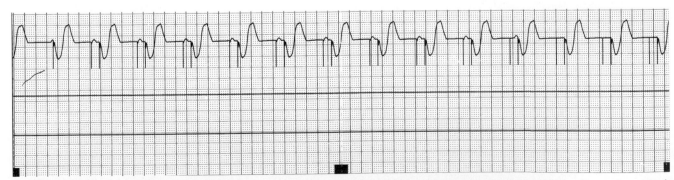

■ ● **FIGURE 47–12.** Pacemaker electrocardiogram strip of AV pacing. Note atrial pacing spike before each P wave and ventricular pacing spike before each QRS complex.

Steps	Rationale	Special Considerations
12. Secure necessary equipment to provide some stability for the pacemaker, such as hanging pulse generator on IV pole, strapping pulse generator to patient's torso, or hanging pulse generator around patient's neck (if ambulatory). ·	The pulse generator should be protected from falling or becoming inadvertently detached by patient movement. Disconnection or tension on the pacing electrodes may lead to pacemaker malfunction.	
13. Wash hands and discard used supplies.	Reduces transmission of microorganisms; standard precautions.	
14. Obtain chest radiograph as prescribed.	In the absence of fluoroscopy, a radiograph is essential to detect potential complications associated with insertion as well as to visualize lead position.	Not necessary for epicardial pacing.
15. Selectively restrict patient mobility depending on insertion site.	Prevents electrode dislodgment.	Check institutional policy regarding ambulation for the patient with a temporary pacemaker insertion.

Expected Outcomes

- ECG will show paced rhythm consistent with parameters set on pacemaker, as evidenced by appropriate heart rate, proper sensing, and proper capture.
- Patient will exhibit hemodynamic stability, as evidenced by a systolic blood pressure greater than 90 mm Hg, a mean arterial blood pressure greater than 60 mm Hg, being alert and oriented, and no syncope or ischemia.
- Pacemaker leads and wires will be isolated from other electrical equipment by maintaining secure connections into pulse generator. If disconnected from the pulse generator, the leads and wires should be insulated by a rubber glove finger (or other insulating material).[2]
- When pacing with a PA catheter, proper pacemaker function will be maintained during hemodynamic monitoring procedures.

Unexpected Outcomes

- Failure of the pacemaker to sense, causing competition between the pacemaker initiated impulses and the patient's intrinsic cardiac rhythm
- Failure of the pacemaker to capture the myocardium
- Pacemaker oversensing causing the pacemaker to be inappropriately inhibited
- Stimulation of the diaphragm causing hiccuping may be related to pacing the phrenic nerve, perforation, wire dislodgment, or excessively high pacemaker milliampere setting
- Development of phlebitis, thrombosis, embolism, or bacteremia
- Ventricular dysrhythmias from manipulation within the cardiac chamber
- Pneumothorax or hemothorax from the insertion procedure
- Myocardial perforation and cardiac tamponade from the insertion procedure and electrode placement
- Air embolism
- Lead dislodgment
- Pacemaker syndrome as a result of loss of AV synchrony with ventricular demand pacing
- Intermittent pacing function with PA catheter when obtaining wedge reading

Patient Monitoring and Care

Patient Monitoring and Care	Rationale	Reportable Conditions
		These conditions should be reported if they persist despite nursing interventions.
1. Monitor vital signs and hemodynamic response to pacing as often as patient condition warrants.	The goal of cardiac pacing is to improve cardiac output by increasing heart rate or by overriding life-threatening dysrhythmias.	• Change in vital signs associated with signs and symptoms of hemodynamic deterioration
2. Evaluate ECG for presence of paced rhythm or resolution of initiating dysrhythmia.	Proper pacemaker functioning is assessed by observing the ECG for pacemaker activity consistent with the parameters set.	• Inability to obtain a paced rhythm • Oversensing • Undersensing
3. Monitor patient's level of comfort: ○ Assess level of comfort. ○ Administer analgesic or sedative, as needed. ○ Evaluate patient response to interventions.	Discomfort may increase patient's anxiety and decrease tolerance of the procedure, causing hemodynamic compromise.	• Continual hiccups (may indicate wire perforation) • Unrelieved discomfort
4. Check and document sensitivity and stimulation threshold at least every 24 hours.	Ensures proper pacemaker functioning and prevents unnecessarily high levels of energy delivery to the myocardium. Threshold may be checked by physicians in high risk patients.	• Sensitivity and stimulation threshold may be checked more frequently if the patient condition changes or pacer function is questioned
5. Assess pacer functioning after the wedge procedure.	Intermittent pacing may occur during or after the wedge procedure, due to movement of the pacing electrode during wedging.	• Loss of capture after performing the wedge procedure
6. Change dressing as determined by institutional policy, depending on the type of dressing used. ○ Cleanse surrounding area with antiseptic solution, such as povidone-iodine. ○ Apply dry, sterile dressing and tape. ○ Record date of dressing change.	Decreases potential for infection.	• Signs of infection include increased temperature, increased white blood cell count, drainage at the insertion site, and warmth or pain at the insertion site
7. Monitor for other complications.	Early recognition leads to prompt treatment.	• Any signs of these complications, such as embolus, thrombosis, perforation of the myocardium, pneumothorax, hemothorax, or phlebitis
8. Monitor electrolytes.	Electrolyte imbalances may precipitate dysrhythmias.	• Abnormal electrolyte values
9. Ensure, at least daily, that all connections are secure.	Maintenance of tight connections is necessary to ensure proper pacer functioning.	• Inability to maintain tight connections with available equipment jeopardizes pacing therapy

Documentation

Documentation should include the following:

- Patient and family education
- Date and time of initiation
- Description of events warranting intervention
- Vital signs and hemodynamic parameters before, during, and after the procedure
- ECG monitoring strip recording before and after pacemaker insertion
- Type of wire inserted and location
- Pacemaker settings: mode, rate, output, sensitivity setting, threshold measurements, and whether the pacemaker is *on* or *off*

- Patient response to the procedure
- Complications and interventions
- Medications administered and patient response to the medication
- Date and time pacing was discontinued

References

1. Atlee JL. *Arrhythmius and Pacemakers*. Philadelphia, Pa: W.B. Saunders; 1996:247–329.
2. Busch MM, Haskin JB. Pacemakers and implantable defibrillators In: Woods SL, Sivarajan Froelicher ES, Halpenny CJ, Motzer SU, eds. *Cardiac Nursing*. 3rd ed. Philadelphia, Pa: J.B. Lippincott; 1995:618–661.
3. Baas LS, Beery TA, Hickey CS. Care and safety of pacemaker electrodes in intensive care and telemetry nursing units. *Am J Crit Care*. 1997;6:302–311.
4. Moses HW, Moulton KP, Miller BD, Schneider JA. *A Practical Guide to Cardiac Pacing*. Boston, MA: Little, Brown; 1995:89–112.

Additional Readings

Fitzpatrick A, Sutton R. A guide to temporary pacing. *BMJ* 1992;304:365–369.

Furman S, Hayes DL, Holmes DR. *A Practice of Cardiac Pacing*. Mount Kisco, NY: Futura Publishing; 1993:231–260.

Futterman LG, Lemberg L. Pacemaker update—part II: atrioventricular synchronous and rate-modulated pacemakers. *Am J Crit Care*. 1993;2:96–98.

Hickey CS, Baas LS. Temporary cardiac pacing. *AACN Clin Issues Crit Care Nurs*. 1991;2:107–117.

Lynn-McHale DJ, Riggs KL, Thurman L. Epicardial pacing after cardiac surgery. *Crit Care Nurse*. 1991;11(8):62–74.

Manion PA. Temporary epicardial pacing in the postoperative cardiac surgical patient. *Crit Care Nurse*. 1993;13(2):30–38.

Morton PG. The pacemaker and defibrillator codes: implications for critical care nursing. *Crit Care Nurse*. 1997;17(1):50–59.

Schurig L, Gura M, Taibi B, eds, for the *NASPE/CAP: Council of Associated Professionals. Educational Guidelines: Pacing and Electrophysiology*. 2nd ed. Armonk, NY: Futura Publishing; 1997.

Witherell CL. Cardiac rhythm control devices. *Crit Care Nurs Clin North Am*. 1994;6(1):85–101.

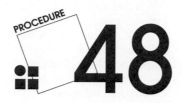

Intra-aortic Balloon Pump Management

PURPOSE: Intra-aortic balloon pump (IABP) therapy is designed to increase coronary artery perfusion, increase systemic perfusion, decrease myocardial workload, and decrease afterload.

Debra J. Lynn-McHale

PREREQUISITE NURSING KNOWLEDGE

- Understanding of the normal anatomy and physiology of the cardiovascular and peripheral vascular systems is needed.
- Principles of hemodynamic monitoring, electrophysiology and dysrhythmias, and coagulation should be understood.
- Clinical and technical competence related to use of IABPs is necessary.
- Advanced cardiac life support knowledge and skills are necessary.
- Indications for IABP therapy are as follows:
  - ❖ Cardiogenic shock
  - ❖ Refractory unstable angina
  - ❖ Recurrent ventricular dysrhythmias as a result of ischemia
  - ❖ Prophylaxis before cardiac surgery
  - ❖ Failure to wean successfully from cardiopulmonary bypass
  - ❖ Left ventricular failure after cardiopulmonary bypass
  - ❖ High-risk patients undergoing coronary artery angioplasty or additional interventional cardiology procedures
- Contraindications to IABP therapy are as follows:
  - ❖ Moderate to severe aortic insufficiency
  - ❖ Thoracic and abdominal aortic aneurysms
  - ❖ The relative value of IABP therapy in the presence of severe aortoiliac disease, major coagulopathies, and terminal disease should be evaluated individually.
- IABP therapy is an acute, short-term therapy for patients with reversible left ventricular failure or is an adjunct to other therapies for irreversible heart failure. Cardiac assistance with the IABP is performed to improve myocardial oxygen supply and reduce cardiac workload. Intra-aortic balloon (IAB) pumping is based on the principles of counterpulsation (Fig. 48–1).

- ❖ The events of the cardiac cycle provide the stimulus for balloon function, and the movement of helium gas between the balloon and the control console gas source produces inflation and deflation of the balloon.
- ❖ Recognition of the R wave or the QRS complex on the electrocardiogram (ECG) is the most commonly used trigger source.
- ❖ Inflation occurs during ventricular diastole, causing an increase in aortic pressure. This increased pressure displaces blood proximally to the coronary arteries and distally to the rest of the body. The result is an increase in myocardial oxygen supply and subsequent improvement in cardiac output.
- ❖ Deflation should occur just before ventricular systole

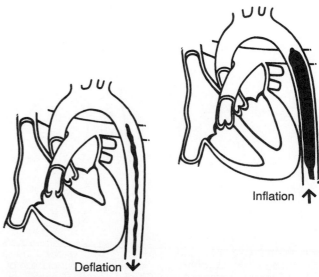

Inflation ↑

Deflation ▼

■ ● FIGURE 48–1. Counterpulsation. (From Datascope Corp., Montvale, New Jersey.)

or ejection. This decreases the pressure within the aortic root, reducing afterload and cardiac workload.

- Insertion and placement verification proceed as follows:
  ❖ The IAB catheter is commonly placed in the femoral artery via percutaneous puncture or arteriotomy.
  ❖ Surgical placement via the transthoracic approach also may be used.
  ❖ The IAB catheter should lie approximately 2 cm inferior to the subclavian artery and superior to the renal arteries. This position allows for maximum balloon effect without occlusion of other arterial supply (Fig. 48–2).
  ❖ The IAB should not fully occlude the aorta during inflation. It should be 85% to 90% occlusive.
  ❖ Fluoroscopy may be used to aid in proper IAB catheter positioning, especially for patients with a tortuous aorta.
  ❖ Correct catheter position is verified via radiography if fluoroscopy is not used during catheter insertion.
- The central lumen of many IAB catheters provides a means for monitoring aortic pressure.

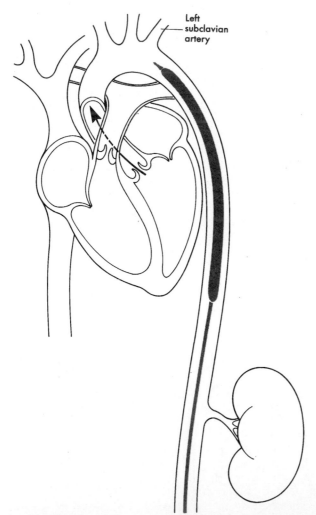

■ ● **FIGURE 48–2.** Intra-aortic balloon (IAB) positioned in the descending thoracic aorta, just below the left subclavian artery but above the renal artery. (From Quaal SJ. *Comprehensive Intraaortic Balloon Counterpulsation*, 2nd ed. St. Louis: Mosby–Year Book; 1993.)

- The mechanics of the control console vary from manufacturer to manufacturer.
- Timing methods of IABP therapy vary slightly from manufacturer to manufacturer. Using the traditional or conventional method, the IAB deflates before isovolumetric contraction. Using the real-time method, the inflation of the IAB extends throughout diastole.[1]
- Specific information concerning controls, alarms, troubleshooting, and safety features is available from each manufacturer and should be read thoroughly by the nurse before use of the equipment.

EQUIPMENT

- IABP, gas supply
- ECG and arterial pressure monitoring supplies
- IAB catheter (size range 8 to 10 Fr for adults; balloon catheters vary in balloon volumes)
- IAB catheter insertion kit
- Povidone-iodine solution
- Caps, goggles, masks, sterile gowns, gloves, and drapes
- Sterile dressing supplies
- O-silk suture on a cutting needle, used to suture catheter to skin
- Number 11 scalpel, used for skin entry
- 1% lidocaine without epinephrine, one 30-mL vial
- Stopcocks, one 2-way and one 3-way

- One Luer-Lok plug
- 500 mL normal saline with 1000 units of heparin or the flush solution recommended according to institution standards
- Hemodynamic monitoring tubing with transducer
- Analgesics and sedatives as prescribed
- Lead apron (needed if procedure is performed using fluoroscopy)
- Prescribed intravenous (IV) solutions
- Emergency medications and resuscitation equipment

Additional equipment to have available depending on patient status includes the following:

- Vasopressors as prescribed
- Antibiotics as prescribed

- Heparin infusion or dextran if prescribed

PATIENT AND FAMILY EDUCATION

- Assess patient and family understanding of IABP therapy and the reason for its use. ➔*Rationale:* Clarification or reinforcement of information is an expressed family need during times of stress and anxiety.
- Explain standard care to patient and family, including insertion procedure, IABP sounds, frequency of assessment, alarms, dressings, need for immobility of affected extremity, expected length of therapy, and parameters for discontinuation of therapy. ➔*Rationale:* Encourages patient and family to ask questions and voice specific concerns about the procedure.
- After catheter removal, instruct patient to report any warm or wet feeling on the leg and any dizziness or lightheadedness. ➔*Rationale:* Indicative of bleeding at the insertion site.

PATIENT ASSESSMENT AND PREPARATION

Patient Assessment

- Take past medical history, specifically related to competency of the aortic valve, aortic disease, or peripheral vascular disease. ➤*Rationale:* Provides baseline data regarding cardiac functioning and identifies contraindications to IABP therapy.
- Assess cardiovascular, hemodynamic, peripheral vascular, and neurovascular assessment. ➤*Rationale:* Provides baseline data.
- Assess the extremity for intended IABP catheter placement for quality and strength of femoral, popliteal, dorsalis pedal, and posterior tibial pulses. ➤*Rationale:* The IAB catheter will be inserted into the vasculature of the extremity exhibiting the best perfusion. Provides baseline data related to peripheral blood flow, which may be compromised by the IAB.
- Assess the current laboratory profile, including complete blood count (CBC), platelet count, prothrombin time (PT), partial thromboplastin time (PTT), bleeding time, and International Normalized Ratio (INR). ➤*Rationale:* Baseline coagulation studies are helpful in determining risk for bleeding. Platelet function may be affected by the mechanical trauma from balloon inflation and deflation.
- Assess signs and symptoms of cardiac failure requiring IABP therapy, including the following:
  - ❖ Unstable angina
  - ❖ Altered mental status
  - ❖ Heart rate greater than 110 beats per minute
  - ❖ Dysrhythmias
  - ❖ Systolic blood pressure less than 90 mm Hg

- ❖ Mean arterial pressure (MAP) less than 70 mm Hg with vasopressor support
- ❖ Cardiac index less than 2.4
- ❖ Pulmonary artery wedge pressure (PAWP) greater than 18 mm Hg
- ❖ Decreased mixed venous oxygen saturation (SvO_2)
- ❖ Inadequate peripheral perfusion
- ❖ Urine output less than 0.5 mL/kg per hour

➤*Rationale:* Physical signs and symptoms result from the heart's inability to adequately contract and from inadequate coronary or systemic perfusion.

Patient Preparation

- Ensure that the patient and family understand preprocedural teaching. Answer questions as they arise, and reinforce information as needed. ➤*Rationale:* Evaluates and reinforces understanding of previously taught information.
- Validate that the informed consent form has been signed. ➤*Rationale:* Protects rights of patient and makes competent decision possible for patient; however, under emergency circumstances, time may not allow form to be signed.
- Validate patency of central and peripheral venous intravenous access. ➤*Rationale:* Central access may be needed for vasopressor administration; peripheral access is needed for fluid administration.
- Place patient in a supine position and prepare the intended insertion site with antiseptic solution. ➤*Rationale:* Prepares site access and positioning for IAB insertion.

Procedure for Assisting with IAB Catheter Insertion

Steps	Rationale	Special Considerations
1. Wash hands, and don caps, goggles, masks, sterile gowns, and gloves for all health care personnel involved in the procedure.	Reduces transmission of microorganisms and body secretions; standard precautions.	
2. Turn on gas supply.	Activates the gas driving the balloon pump.	Check manufacturer's recommendations.
3. Sedate the patient as needed; the affected extremity may need to be restrained.	Movement of the lower extremity may inhibit insertion of the catheter or contribute to catheter kinking once the IAB is in place.	A sheet placed over the affected leg and tucked in or a knee immobilizer may minimize movement of the affected leg.
4. Establish ECG input to IABP console and obtain ECG configuration with optimal R wave amplitude and absence of artifact. Indirect ECG input can be obtained via "slave" of bedside ECG to IABP console.	The R wave, QRS complex, or arterial pressure waveform may be the trigger for balloon inflation and deflation. Patient cable from console establishes ECG.	A secondary ECG source is desirable in the event of lead disconnection or loss of trigger. Review manufacturer's instructions for selecting the appropriate trigger control. If the patient has a pacemaker, the trigger should be set to reject the pacemaker artifact.
5. Assist with placement of hemodynamic monitoring lines if they are not already present.	Hemodynamic monitoring is necessary for assessment and management of the patient requiring IABP therapy.	A radial arterial line is commonly inserted. The arterial line tracing is used to assess and optimize timing and also may be used as a trigger source.

Procedure continued on following page

Procedure for **Assisting with IAB Catheter Insertion** *Continued*

Steps	Rationale	Special Considerations
6. Complete IABP console preparation. Refer to instruction manual.	Ensures adequate functioning of the IABP device.	Models of the pump console vary. Review of manufacturer's instructions is recommended.
7. Remove IAB catheter from sterile packing and place the catheter and insertion tray on the sterile field.	Makes supplies available while maintaining sterility. Select the most appropriate size of balloon catheter. Most adult balloons are 40 mL in size. However, smaller balloon volumes (30 to 34 mL) are commonly placed in adults 5 ft 4 in and under, whereas larger balloon volumes (50 mL) are commonly placed in adults 6 ft and taller.	Catheters vary in volume of the balloon. An adequate volume is necessary to achieve optimal hemodynamic effects from IABP therapy.
8. Administer heparin bolus before arterial puncture, if prescribed.	Anticoagulation may decrease the incidence of thromboemboli related to the indwelling IAB catheter.	Systemic anticoagulation may not be used in all patients.
9. Attach the supplied one-way valve to the Luer tip of the distal end of the balloon lumen.	Creates a device for air removal from the balloon catheter.	Maintains wrap of balloon for insertion.
10. Pull back slowly on the syringe until all air is aspirated.	Removes air from the balloon, creating a vacuum.	
11. Disconnect the syringe only.	Prevents air entry back into the balloon.	Leave the one-way valve in place.
12. Lubricate the IAB catheter with sterile saline.	Decreases "drag" on the catheter during insertion.	
13. The central lumen of the IAB catheter should be flushed with heparinized saline before insertion.	Removes air from the central lumen.	If the catheter is not flushed before insertion, allow backflow of arterial blood before connection to the flush system.
14. Assist with introducer sheath or dilator assembly and insertion.	Prepares for balloon catheter entry.	Some IABs are inserted without a sheath. If the IAB is inserted via the sheathless method, only the dilator will be used.
15. Assist with balloon catheter insertion.	Catheter placement is a necessary part of IAB setup.	
16. Assist with removal of the one-way valve according to manufacturer's recommendations.	Releases the vacuum and readies the balloon for counterpulsation.	
17. If the central lumen of a double-lumen catheter is used to monitor arterial pressure, attach a three-way stopcock with continuous heparinized flush and transducer to the monitor. Set the alarms.	Monitors arterial pressure.	The central lumen, if used, must be attached to an alarm system because undetected disconnection could result in life-threatening hemorrhage.
18. Avoid fast flush and blood sampling from the central aortic lumen.	Air may enter the system during fast flush and also during blood sampling, resulting in air emboli.	Some manufacturers and institutions recommend hourly manual flush of central lumen lines. If fast flush is required, ensure that the IABP is "on standby" (not pumping) during the flush. However, the risk of air embolus entry or dislodging a thrombus at the lumen tip is a major concern. Refer to your institution's policy in regard to fast flush or manual flushing of central lumen catheters.

Procedure **for Assisting with IAB Catheter Insertion** *Continued*

Steps	Rationale	Special Considerations
19. Attach the balloon-lumen tubing to the pump console.	Attachment is necessary because the console programs and operates balloon counterpulsation.	
20. Follow steps for timing, troubleshooting, and patient monitoring.	Provides for appropriate operation of counterpulsation.	Many IABP consoles have features for automatic timing. Refer to specific manufacturer instructions.
21. Zero the pressure transducer.	Ensures accurate arterial pressure measurement, timing, maintenance, and functioning of the IABP.	Refer to specific manufacturer instructions.
22. Obtain a portable chest x-ray as soon as possible.	Correct IAB catheter position must be confirmed to prevent complications associated with interference of the arterial blood supply.	If fluoroscopy is used for insertion of the catheter, an x-ray immediately after placement is not necessary.
23. Apply a sterile dressing to the catheter insertion site.	Allows for aseptic management.	
24. Remove and discard personal protective equipment, and wash hands.	Reduces the transmission of microorganisms; standard precautions.	

Procedure **for Timing of the IABP**

Steps	Rationale	Special Considerations
1. Select an ECG lead that optimizes the R wave and decreases artifact.	The R wave is usually used to trigger the balloon.	An alternate trigger can also be used if necessary.
2. Time the IABP using the arterial waveform.	The arterial waveform assists in identifying accurate IAB inflation and deflation.	Refer to specific manufacturer instructions for automatic timing.
3. Set the IABP frequency to the every-other-beat setting (1:2 or 50%) (Fig. 48–3).	Comparison can be made between the assisted and unassisted arterial waveforms.	
4. Inflation		
A. Identify the dicrotic notch of the assisted systolic waveform (see Fig. 48–3).	The dicrotic notch represents closure of the aortic valve.	
B. Adjust inflation later to expose the dicrotic notch of the unassisted systolic waveform.	Identifies landmark for accurate inflation.	
C. Slowly adjust inflation earlier until the dicrotic notch disappears and a sharp V wave forms (see Fig. 48–3).	Balloon augmentation should occur after the aortic valve closes.	A sharp V wave may not be seen in patients with low systemic vascular resistance.
D. Compare the augmented pressure with the patient's unassisted systolic pressure.	Balloon augmentation should be equal to or greater than the patient's unassisted systolic blood pressure.	If balloon augmentation is less than the patient's systolic pressure, consider that the balloon is positioned too low, the patient is hypovolemic or tachycardic, or the balloon volume is set too low.

Procedure continued on following page

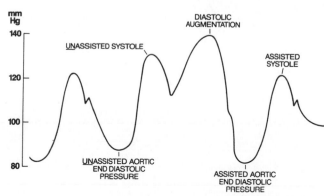

■ ● **FIGURE 48–3.** 1:2 intra-aortic balloon pump frequency. (From Datascope Corp., Montvale, New Jersey.)

Procedure for Timing of the IABP *Continued*

Steps	Rationale	Special Considerations
E. Adjust inflation if needed.	Necessary to achieve optimal diastolic augmentation.	Timing of inflation will vary slightly depending on the location of the arterial line.
		Aortic root: Inflate after exposing the dicrotic notch. Radial: Inflate 40 to 50 ms before the dicrotic notch. Femoral: Inflate 120 ms before the dicrotic notch (Fig. 48–4).
		Because of the distance of the radial and femoral arteries from the actual closure of the aortic valve, the arterial waveforms are delayed.

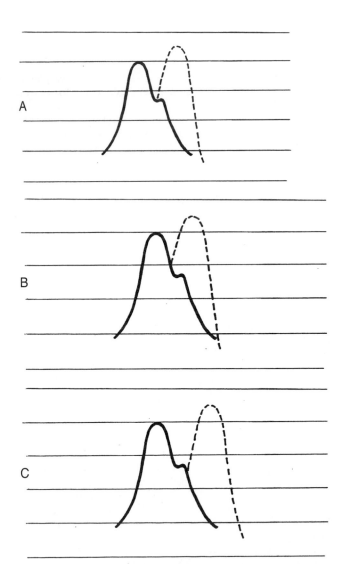

A

B

C

■ ● **FIGURE 48–4.** IABP inflation. *A,* Radial. *B,* Femoral. *C,* Central aortic. IABP, intra-aortic balloon pump.

Procedure for Timing of the IABP *Continued*		
Steps	**Rationale**	**Special Considerations**

5. Deflation

    A. Identify the assisted and unassisted aortic end-diastolic pressures and the assisted and unassisted systolic pressures. Ratio is 1:2 (50%) (see Fig. 48–3).

These landmarks are important in determining accurate IAB deflation.

    B. Set the balloon to deflate so that the balloon-assisted aortic end-diastolic pressure is as low as possible (lower than the patient's unassisted diastolic pressure) while still maintaining optimal diastolic augmentation and not impeding on the next systole (the assisted systole).

The assisted systolic pressure will be less than the unassisted systolic pressure as a result of a decrease in afterload, thus reducing the myocardial workload.

Reduction of afterload will decrease the energy required by the heart during systole. It is important to achieve afterload reduction without diminishing diastolic augmentation.

6. Set the IABP frequency to 1:1 (100%) (Fig. 48–5).

Ensures that each heartbeat is assisted.

7. Assess timing every hour and whenever the heart rate changes by more than 10 beats per minute or the rhythm changes.

Inappropriate timing prevents effective IABP therapy.

The computerized IABPs vary in the degree of adjustment to changes in heart rate and rhythm. Refer to specific manufacturer's guidelines for automatic timing adjustment.

8. Assess and intervene to correct inappropriate timing.

Ensures accurate timing and optimal functioning of the IABP.

    A. Problem: **Early inflation** (Fig. 48–6). Intervention: **Move inflation later.**

Inflation occurs before closure of the aortic valve, leading to premature aortic valve closure, increased left ventricular volume, and decreased stroke volume.

Procedure continued on following page

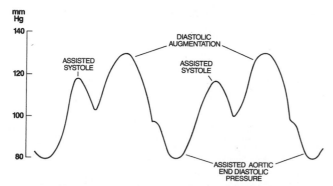

■ ● FIGURE 48–5. Correct intra-aortic balloon pump timing (1:1). (From Datascope Corp., Montvale, New Jersey.)

Timing Errors
Early Inflation

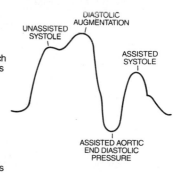

Inflation of the IAB prior to aortic valve closure

Waveform Characteristics:
- Inflation of IAB prior to dicrotic notch
- Diastolic augmentation encroaches onto systole (may be unable to distinguish)

Physiologic Effects:
- Potential premature closure of aortic valve
- Potential increased in LVEDV and LVEDP or PCWP
- Increased left ventricular wall stress or afterload
- Aortic regurgitation
- Increased MVO_2 demand

■ ● FIGURE 48–6. Early inflation. (From Datascope Corp., Montvale, New Jersey.)

Procedure	for Timing of the IABP *Continued*	
Steps	**Rationale**	**Special Considerations**
B. Problem: **Late inflation** (Fig. 48–7). Intervention: **Adjust inflation earlier.**	A delay in inflation leads to a decrease in coronary artery perfusion.	
C. Problem: **Early deflation** (Fig. 48–8). Intervention: **Adjust deflation later.**	Deflation occurs before the aortic valve opening, leading to low balloon augmentation and less or no afterload reduction; coronary artery perfusion may also be decreased.	Note the sharp diastolic wave after augmentation and the increase in the assisted systolic pressure.
D. Problem: **Late deflation** (Fig. 48–9). Intervention: **Adjust deflation earlier.**	Deflation occurs after the aortic valve has opened, leading to an increase in the aortic end-diastolic pressure and an increase in afterload.	Note the delayed diastolic wave after augmentation and the diminished assisted systole. If using the real-time method of timing, late deflation is not identified by changes in the aortic end-diastolic pressure but is identified by diminished assisted systolic pressure, increase in heart rate, increase in filling pressures, and decrease in cardiac output and cardiac index.

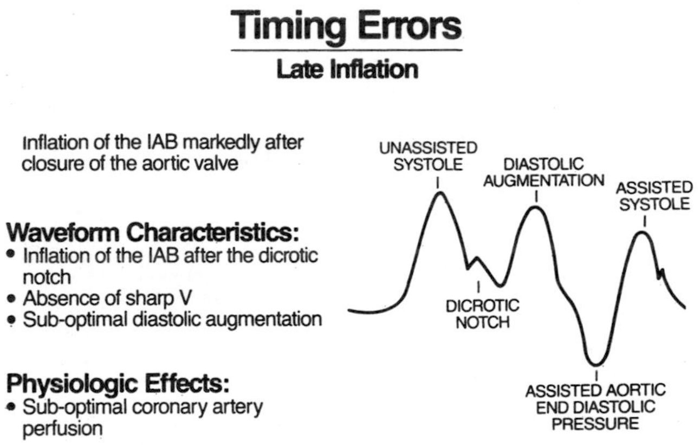

Timing Errors
Early Deflation

Premature deflation of the IAB during the diastolic phase

Waveform Characteristics:
- Deflation of IAB is seen as a sharp drop following diastolic augmentation
- Sub-optimal diastolic augmentation
- Assisted aortic end diastolic pressure may be equal to or less than the unassisted aortic end diastolic pressure
- Assisted systolic pressure may rise

Physiologic Effects:
- Sub-optimal coronary perfusion
- Potential for retrograde coronary and carotid blood flow
- Angina may occur as a result of retrograde coronary blood flow
- Sub-optimal afterload reduction
- Increased MVO_2 demand

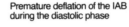

Timing Errors
Late Inflation

Inflation of the IAB markedly after closure of the aortic valve

Waveform Characteristics:
- Inflation of the IAB after the dicrotic notch
- Absence of sharp V
- Sub-optimal diastolic augmentation

Physiologic Effects:
- Sub-optimal coronary artery perfusion

■ ● **FIGURE 48–7.** Late inflation. (From Datascope Corp., Montvale, New Jersey.)

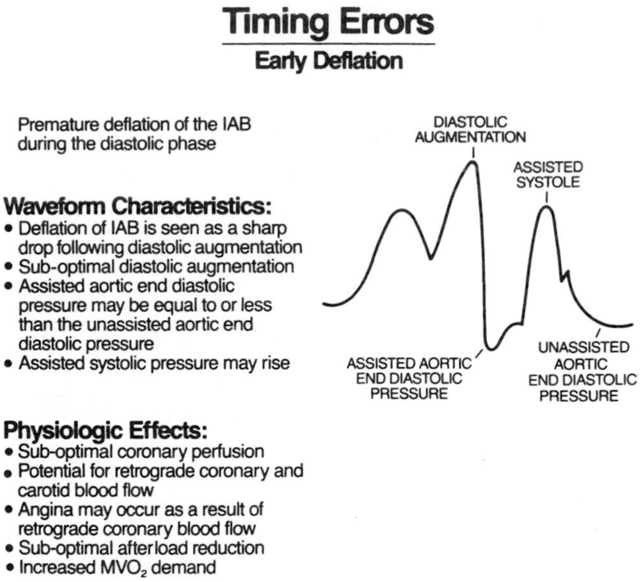

■ ● **FIGURE 48–8.** Early deflation. (From Datascope Corp., Montvale, New Jersey.)

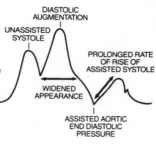

Timing Errors
Late Deflation

Deflation of the IAB late in diastolic phase as aortic valve is beginning to open

Waveform Characteristics:
- Assisted aortic end-diastolic pressure may be equal to or greater than the unassisted aortic end diastolic pressure
- Rate of rise of assisted systole is prolonged
- Diastolic augmentation may appear widened

Physiologic Effects:
- Afterload reduction is essentially absent
- Increased MVO$_2$ consumption due to the left ventricle ejecting against a greater resistance and a prolonged isovolumetric contraction phase
- IAB may impede left ventricular ejection and increase the afterload

■ ● **FIGURE 48–9.** Late deflation. (From Datascope Corp., Montvale, New Jersey.)

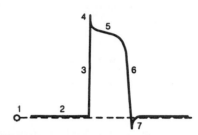

■ ● **FIGURE 48–10.** Normal balloon gas waveform. 1, zero baseline; 2, fill pressure; 3, rapid inflation; 4, peak inflation artifact; 5, plateau pressure or inflation plateau pressure; 6, rapid deflation; 7, peak deflation pressure and return to fill pressure. (From Arrow International.)

Procedure | **for Balloon Pressure Waveform**

Steps	Rationale	Special Considerations
1. Determine if the IABP console has a balloon pressure waveform.	Helium is shuttled in and out of the IAB catheter, and the balloon pressure waveform represents this movement.	Refer to specific manufacturer instructions regarding the balloon pressure waveform.
2. Assess the balloon pressure waveform.	Reflects pressure that is in the IAB.	
3. Determine if the balloon pressure waveform is normal (Fig. 48–10). A normal balloon pressure waveform	A normal balloon pressure waveform reflects that the IAB is inflating and deflating properly.	
A. Has a fill pressure (baseline pressure) slightly above zero.	Reflects pressure in the tubing between the IAB and the IABP driving mechanism.	
B. Has a sharp upstroke.	Occurs as gas inflates the IAB catheter.	
C. Has peak inflation artifact.	This overshoot pressure artifact is caused by gas pressure in the pneumatic line.[2]	
D. Has a pressure plateau.	This plateau is created as the IAB remains inflated during diastole.	The plateau indicates the length of time of inflation as well as whether full inflation (volume) has been delivered to the IAB. If there is no plateau pressure, the IAB may not be fully inflated.
E. Has a rapid deflation.	Gas is quickly shuttled from the IAB.	
F. Has a negative deflection below baseline, then returns to baseline.	Gas returns to the IABP console, then stabilizes within the system.	
4. Compare the balloon pressure waveform with the arterial pressure waveform (Fig. 48–11). Note the similarity in the width of the balloon pressure waveform and the augmented arterial waveform.	Demonstrates the relationship between the balloon pressure waveform and the arterial waveform. Reflects the effect of the balloon on the augmented arterial pressure.	
5. Determine if the balloon pressure waveform does not meet the description above.	Abnormal balloon pressure waveforms may indicate problems with the IAB or the IABP console.	Refer to specific manufacturer instructions regarding troubleshooting abnormal balloon pressure waveforms.

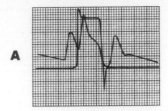

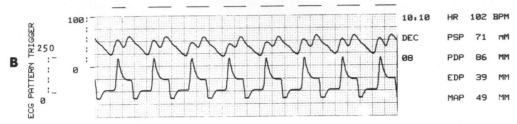

■ ● **FIGURE 48–11.** *A,* Balloon pressure waveform superimposed on the arterial pressure waveform. *B,* Actual recording of an arterial pressure waveform *(top)* and balloon gas waveform *(bottom)* from a balloon-pumped patient. (From Arrow International.)

Procedure **for Troubleshooting**

Steps	Rationale	Special Considerations
1. **Atrial fibrillation:** Set the IABP to inflate and deflate the majority of the patient's beats.	IABP therapy will not be 100% effective during atrial fibrillation (AF) because of the irregular rhythm.	The underlying cause of the AF should be treated. IABPs will automatically deflate the balloon on the R wave. Use the atrial fibrillation trigger mode or the R wave deflation mode. The real-time method of timing may track dysrhythmias better than traditional or conventional IABP timing.
2. **Tachycardia:** Change IABP frequency to 1:2.	Because diastole is shortened during tachycardia, the balloon augmentation time is shortened. Pumping every other beat may improve MAP.	The underlying cause of the tachycardia should be treated.
3. **Asystole**		
A. Switch trigger to arterial pressure.	This trigger can be used if there is at least a 15–mm Hg rise in arterial pressure.	Refer to the manufacturer's manual for this information because the minimum mm Hg needed to use this feature varies.
B. Set inflation to provide diastolic augmentation, and set deflation to occur before upstroke of the next systole.	Programs the machine for appropriate preset timing.	Preliminary research suggests that when used during cardiopulmonary resuscitation, IAB counterpulsation increases cerebral and coronary perfusion.[3]
(Level IV: Limited clinical studies to support recommendations)		
C. If chest compressions do not provide an adequate trigger ○ Turn to internal trigger ○ Set the rate at 60 to 80 beats per minute ○ Set the IABP frequency to 1:2 ○ Turn the balloon augmentation down to 50%	The internal trigger will keep the catheter moving so clot formation is minimized. Maintains consistent movement of IAB catheter. 1:2 frequency is adequate to prevent thrombus formation on the IAB catheter. Slight inflation and deflation of the IAB catheter will prevent clot formation.	

Procedure **for Troubleshooting** *Continued*

Steps	Rationale	Special Considerations
4. **Ventricular tachycardia or ventricular fibrillation**		
A. Ensure that personnel are cleared from the patient and equipment before cardioverting or defibrillating.	Prevents spread of energy to health care personnel. Maintains electrical safety.	
B. Cardiovert or defibrillate as necessary.	Converts rhythm.	The IABP console is electrically isolated.
5. **Loss of vacuum or IABP failure**		
A. Check and tighten connections on pneumatic tubing.	A loose connection may have contributed to loss of vacuum.	
B. Check the compressor power source.	Ensures that power is available to drive helium.	
C. Hand inflate and deflate the balloon every 5 minutes with half the total balloon volume if necessary.	Prevents clot formation along the dormant balloon.	
D. Change the IAB console.	Establishes power source and effective IABP therapy.	
6. **Suspected balloon perforation**		
A. Observe for loss of augmentation.	Gas may be gradually leaking from the balloon catheter.	Always set the alarms so the alarm will sound if there is a 10–mm Hg drop in diastolic augmentation.
B. Check for blood in the catheter tubing.	Blood in the tubing indicates that the balloon has perforated and that arterial blood is present.	It is possible for a balloon leak to be self-sealing as a result of the surface tension between the inside and the outside of the IAB membrane. This may be evidenced by the presence of dried blood in the catheter tubing. The dried blood may appear as a brownish, coffee-ground–like substance.
C. Assess for changes or lack of normal balloon pressure waveform.	The balloon pressure waveform may be absent if the balloon is unable to retain gas, or the pressure plateau may gradually decrease if the IAB is leaking gas.	
7. **Balloon perforation**		
A. Place the IABP on standby.	Prevents further IAB pumping and continued gas exchange.	Some IABP consoles will automatically shut off if a leak is detected. The IAB catheter should be removed within 15 to 30 minutes.
B. Clamp the IAB catheter.	Prevents arterial blood back-up.	
C. Disconnect the IAB catheter from the IABP console.	Prevents blood from backing up into the IABP console.	
D. Notify the physician.	The IAB catheter will need to be removed or replaced immediately.	If the IAB leak has sealed itself off, this may result in entrapment of the IAB in the vasculature. Surgical removal may be required.
E. Prepare for IAB catheter removal or replacement.	The IAB catheter should not lie dormant for longer than 30 minutes.	
F. Discontinue anticoagulation therapy.	Clotting will occur more readily if anticoagulation is stopped (necessary if removing the catheter).	

Procedure for Weaning and IAB Catheter Removal

Steps	Rationale	Special Considerations
1. Assess clinical readiness for weaning.	Optimal clinical and hemodynamic parameters validate readiness for weaning.	Patient hemodynamic status should be optimal before weaning of IABP therapy. Signs of clinical readiness include the following: no angina, heart rate less than 110 beats per minute, absence of lethal or unstable dysrhythmias, MAP greater than 70 mm Hg with minimal or no vasopressor support, PAWP less than 18 mm Hg, cardiac index greater than 2.4, mixed venous oxygen saturation between 60% and 80%, capillary refill less than 2 seconds, and urine output greater than 0.5 mL/kg per hour.
2. Change assist ratio to 1:2, and monitor patient response for 1 to 6 hours or as noted per institution's protocol.	Length of time required to wean from IABP therapy depends on hemodynamic response of patient and length of time patient has been receiving IABP therapy.	
3. If hemodynamic parameters remain satisfactory, further change ratio from 1:3 to 1:8 (depending on patient and balloon console assist frequencies, or as prescribed).	IABP consoles vary in assist ratios.	Refer to the institution's policy on weaning procedures.
4. Discontinue heparin or dextran 4 to 6 hours before IAB catheter removal, or reverse heparin with protamine (as prescribed) just before catheter removal.	This will decrease the likelihood of bleeding after balloon removal.	
5. Turn the IABP to standby or off.	Ensures deflation of IAB catheter.	
6. Assist the physician or advanced practice nurse with removal of the percutaneous balloon.	Facilitates removal.	
7. Ensure that pressure is held on the insertion site for 30 to 45 minutes after the IAB catheter is withdrawn. Ensure that hemostasis is obtained.	Decreases the incidence of bleeding and hematoma formation.	
8. Assess insertion site for signs of bleeding or hematoma formation before application of a sterile pressure dressing.	Assists in the detection of bleeding.	
9. Apply pressure dressing to the insertion site for 2 to 4 hours.	Minimizes bleeding from the insertion site.	
10. Monitor vital signs and hemodynamic parameters every 15 minutes × 4, every 30 minutes × 2, then every hour as the patient's condition warrants.	Validates patient stability or identifies hemodynamic compromise.	
11. Assess the quality of perfusion to the decannulated extremity immediately after removal and every 1 hour × 2, then every 2 hours.	Removal of the IAB catheter may dislodge thrombi on the catheter and lead to arterial occlusion.	
12. Maintain immobility of decannulation extremity and bedrest with the head of the bed no greater than 30 degrees for 8 hours.	Promotes healing and decreases stress at the insertion site.	

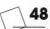

Expected Outcomes	Unexpected Outcomes
• Increased myocardial oxygen supply • Decreased myocardial oxygen demands • Increased cardiac output • Increased tissue perfusion, including cerebral, renal, and peripheral circulation	• Impaired perfusion to the extremity with the IAB catheter in place • Balloon perforation • Inappropriate IAB placement • Pain • Bleeding or coagulation disorders • Aortic dissection • Infection

Patient Monitoring and Care

Patient Monitoring and Care	Rationale	Reportable Conditions
		These conditions should be reported if they persist despite nursing interventions.
1. Perform systematic cardiovascular, peripheral vascular, and hemodynamic assessments every 15 to 60 minutes as patient status requires.		
• Level of consciousness	Assesses for adequate cerebral perfusion; thrombi may develop and dislodge during IABP therapy; the IAB may migrate, decreasing blood flow to the carotid arteries.	• Change in level of consciousness
• Vital signs and pulmonary artery pressures	Demonstrates effectiveness of IABP therapy.	• Unstable vital signs and significant changes in hemodynamic pressures, lack of response to IABP therapy
• Arterial line and IAB waveforms	Ensures effectiveness of IABP timing and therapy.	• Difficulty achieving effective IABP therapy
• Cardiac output, cardiac index, and systemic vascular resistance determinations	Demonstrates effectiveness of IABP therapy.	• Abnormal cardiac output, cardiac index, and systemic vascular resistance values
• Circulation to extremities	Validates adequate peripheral perfusion. If reportable conditions are found, they may indicate catheter or embolus obstruction of perfusion to extremity. Specifically, decreased perfusion to the left arm may indicate misplacement of the IAB catheter.	• Capillary refill greater than 2 seconds • Diminished or absent pulses (eg, antecubital, radial, popliteal, tibial, pedal) • Color pale, mottled, or cyanotic • Diminished or absent sensation • Pain • Diminished or absent movement • Cool or cold to touch
• Urine output	Validates adequate perfusion to the kidneys.	• Urine output <0.5 mL/kg per hour
2. Assess heart and lung sounds every 4 hours and as needed.	Abnormal heart and lung sounds may indicate the need for additional treatment. *Special Note:* When patient's condition permits, place the IABP on standby to accurately auscultate heart and lung sounds, because IABP therapy creates extraneous sounds and impairs heart and lung sound assessment.	• Abnormal heart and lung sounds

Continued on following page

Patient Monitoring and Care *Continued*

Patient Monitoring and Care	Rationale	Reportable Conditions
3. Maintain head of bed at less than 45 degrees.	Prevents kinking of the IAB catheter and migration of the catheter.	
4. Monitor for signs of inappropriate IAB placement.	The IAB catheter may be positioned too high or too low, thus occluding at the left subclavian, celiac, inferior or superior mesenteric, or renal arteries.	• Diminished or absent antecubital or radial pulse • Color of left arm pale, mottled, cyanotic • Diminished or absent sensation to left arm • Dampened radial arterial pressure waveform • Diminished or absent movement of left arm • Diminished or absent bowel sounds • Increased abdominal girth • Abdomen firm to touch • Tympany • Abdominal pain • Decreased urine output, less than 0.5 mL/kg per hour • Increased urine osmolality • Increased blood urea nitrogen or creatinine • Reduced IABP augmentation
5. Monitor for signs of balloon perforation.	In the event of balloon perforation, a very small amount of helium will be released into the aorta, potentially causing an embolic event.	• Blood or brown flecks in tubing • Loss of IABP augmentation • Control console alarm activation (eg, gas loss)
6. Maintain accurate IABP timing.	If timing is not accurate, cardiac output may decrease rather than increase.	
7. Log roll patient every 2 hours. Prop pillows to support patient and to maintain alignment. Consider use of pressure-relief devices. *(Level V: Clinical studies in more than one or two different patient populations and situations to support recommendations)*	Promotes comfort and skin integrity and prevents kinking of the IAB catheter. ***Special Note:*** Log rolling may not be tolerated in severely hemodynamically compromised patients; low-pressure beds are necessary for these patients. Low-pressure beds can decrease the occurrence of pressure ulcers in patients requiring IABP therapy.[4, 5]	
8. Immobilize the cannulated extremity with a draw sheet tucked under the mattress or by using a soft ankle restraint or a knee immobilizer.	Prevents dislogment and migration of the IAB catheter. ***Special Note:*** Assess skin integrity and perfusion distal to the restraint every hour.	
9. Initiate passive and active range-of-motion exercises every 2 hours to extremities that can be mobilized.	Prevents venous stasis and muscle atrophy.	
10. Assess the area around the IAB catheter insertion site every 2 hours and as needed for evidence of hematoma or bleeding.	IAB catheter inflation and deflation traumatize red blood cells and platelets. Anticoagulation therapy may alter hemoglobin and hematocrit and coagulation values.	• Bleeding at insertion site • Hematoma at insertion site

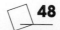

Patient Monitoring and Care	Rationale	Reportable Conditions
11. Maintain anticoagulation as prescribed, and monitor coagulation studies.	Prophylactic anticoagulation may be used to prevent thrombi and emboli development.	• Abnormal coagulation studies
12. Monitor patient for systemic evidence of bleeding or coagulation disorders.	Hematologic and coagulation profiles may be altered as a result of blood loss during balloon insertion, anticoagulation, and platelet dysfunction as a result of mechanical trauma by balloon inflation and deflation.	• Bleeding from IAB insertion site • Bleeding from incisions or mucous membranes • Petechiae or ecchymoses • Guaiac-positive nasogastric aspirate or stool • Hematuria • Decreased hemoglobin or hematocrit • Decreased filling pressures • Increased heart rate • Retroperitoneal hematoma • Pain in the lower abdomen, flank, thigh, or lower extremity
13. Change the IAB catheter site dressing every 24 hours • Cleanse site with normal saline. • Cleanse site with povidone-iodine solution for 1 minute. • Apply a sterile dressing; label with date, time, and nurse's initials.	Decreases incidence of infection and allows an opportunity for site assessment.	• Signs or symptoms of infection
14. Monitor for signs and symptoms of aortic dissection.	Aortic dissection may occur as a result of IAB placement into a false lumen in the aorta.	• Acute back, flank, testicular, or chest pain • Decreased pulses • Variation in blood pressure between left and right arms • Decreased cardiac output • Increased heart rate • Decreased hemoglobin and hematocrit • Decreased filling pressures
15. Assess and manage patient's pain.	The patient may experience pain from angina, IAB placement, or limited mobility.	• Unrelieved pain
16. Identify parameters that demonstrate clinical readiness to wean from IABP therapy.	Close observation of the patient's tolerance to weaning procedures is necessary to ensure that the body's oxygen demands can be met. The presence of these reportable conditions indicates that consideration should be given to weaning the patient from the IABP.	• No angina • Heart rate less than 110 beats per minute • Absence of lethal or unstable dysrhythmias • MAP greater than 70 mm Hg with little or no vasopressor support • PAWP less than 18 mm Hg • Cardiac index greater than 2.4 • Svo_2 between 60% and 80% • Capillary refill less than 3 seconds • Urine output greater than 0.5 mL/kg per hour

Documentation

Documentation should include the following:

- Patient and family education
- Insertion of IAB catheter (including size of catheter used and balloon volume)
- Peripheral pulses and neurovascular assessment of affected extremity
- Any difficulties in insertion
- IABP frequency
- Patient toleration
- Confirmation of placement (eg, chest x-ray)
- Insertion site assessment
- Hemodynamic status
- IABP pressures (unassisted end-diastolic pressure, unassisted systolic pressure, balloon augmented pressure, assisted systolic pressure, assisted end-diastolic pressure, and MAP)
- Occurrence of unexpected outcomes
- Additional nursing interventions taken

References

1. Cadwell CA, Tyson G. Real timing. In Quaal S, ed. *Comprehensive Intraaortic Balloon Counterpulsation.* 2nd edition. St. Louis, Mo: Mosby–Year Book; 1993.
2. Kalina J. Use of the balloon pressure waveform in conjunction with the augmented arterial pressure waveform. In: Quaal S, ed. *Comprehensive Intraaortic Balloon Counterpulsation.* 2nd ed. St. Louis, Mo: Mosby–Year Book; 1993.
3. Miller LW. Emerging trends in the treatment of acute myocardial infarction and the role of intra-aortic balloon pumping. *Card Assists.* 1986;3:1–3.
4. Jesurum J, Joseph K, Davis JM, Suki R. Balloons, beds, and breakdown. *Crit Care Nurs Clin N Am.* 1996;8:423–440.
5. Inman K, Sibbald W, Rutledge F, Clark BJ. Clinical utility and cost-effectiveness of an air suspension bed in the prevention of pressure ulcers. *JAMA.* 1993;269:1139–1142.

Additional Readings

Beaver K. Correlation of balloon pressure waveforms to troubleshooting gas leakage and restriction alarms. *Crit Care Nurs Clin N Am.* 1996;8:383–388.
Cadwell CA, Hobson KS, Pettis S, Blackburn A. Clinical observations with real timing. *Crit Care Nurs Clin N Am.* 1996;8:357–370.
Cadwell CA, Quaal SJ. Intra-aortic balloon counterpulsation timing. *Am J Crit Care.* 1996;5:254–261.
Goran SF. Understanding advanced hemodynamic concepts. *Crit Care Nurs Clin N Am.* 1996;8:371–381.

Gould KA, Kroha KL. Current intra-aortic balloon pump practice issues. *Crit Care Nurs Clin N Am.* 1996;8:477–490.
Hanlon-Pena PM, Ziegler JC, Stewart R. Management of the intra-aortic balloon pump patient. *Crit Care Nurs Clin N Am.* 1996;8:389–408.
Joseph DL, Spadoni SM. Timing waveform analysis. *Crit Care Nurs Clin N Am.* 1996;8:349–356.
Molnar HM. Intra-aortic balloon pump: nursing implications for patients with an iliac artery approach. *Am J Crit Care.* 1998;7:300–307.
Osborn C, Quaal SJ. Maximizing cardiopulmonary resuscitation in patients with intra-aortic balloon pumps. *Crit Care Nurse.* 1998;18:25–27.
Quaal SJ. *Comprehensive Intraaortic Balloon Counterpulsation.* 2nd ed. St. Louis, Mo: Mosby–Year Book; 1993.
Quaal SJ. Maintaining competence and competency in the care of the intra-aortic balloon pump patient. *Crit Care Nurs Clin N Am.* 1996;8:441–450.
Quaal SJ. Caring for the intra-aortic balloon pump patient: most frequently asked nursing questions. *Crit Care Nurs Clin N Am.* 1996;8:471–476.
Shin AE, Joseph D. Concepts of intraaortic ballon counterpulsation. *J Cardiovasc Nurs.* 1994;8:45–60.
Sitzer VA, Atkins PJ. Developing and implementing a standard of care for intra-aortic balloon counterpulsation. *Crit Care Nurs Clin N Am.* 1996;8:451–457.
Stavarski DH. Complications of IABP: preventable or not preventable? *Crit Care Nurs Clin N Am.* 1996;8:409–421.
Wojner AW. Assessing the five points of the intra-aortic balloon pump waveform. *Crit Care Nurse.* 1994;14:48–52.

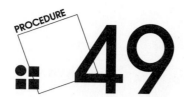

PROCEDURE

49

External Counterpressure with Pneumatic Antishock Garments

PURPOSE: External counterpressure accomplished with a pneumatic anti-shock garment (PASG) is designed as a short-term therapy to increase blood pressure, stabilize bleeding, and function as an effective splint for lower extremity or pelvic fractures.

Denise M. Lawrence

PREREQUISITE NURSING KNOWLEDGE

- The anatomy and physiology of the cardiovascular and peripheral vascular systems should be understood.
- Advanced cardiac life support (ACLS) knowledge and skills are necessary.
- Clinical and technical competence related to use of the pneumatic antishock garment is necessary.
- PASG is a short-term intervention used for patients experiencing acute trauma. PASG is used to control hemorrhage, increase blood pressure, and improve perfusion to the vital organs. PASG also functions as an effective splinting device for preventing blood loss, particularly when transport to definitive care is delayed.
- PASG may be used for patients with the following conditions:
  - ❖ Hypotension caused by blood loss or loss of vascular tone
  - ❖ Systolic blood pressure of less than 90 mm Hg
  - ❖ Penetrating injuries of the lower abdomen and lower extremities when transport time will exceed 20 minutes
  - ❖ For compression and splinting of fractures or external wounds of the lower abdomen, pelvis, or lower extremities when transport time will exceed 20 minutes
- Contraindications for PASG include the following:
  - ❖ Pulmonary edema
  - ❖ Congestive heart failure
  - ❖ Impaled foreign body of the lower torso
  - ❖ Pregnant patients
  - ❖ Abdominal wounds with evisceration
  - ❖ Tension pneumothorax
  - ❖ Cardiac tamponade
  - ❖ Head injuries with increased intracranial pressure
  - ❖ Diaphragmatic rupture
- Application of pneumatic counterpressure to the abdomen and legs causes pneumatic compression to the vessels.

This increases the pressure outside the vessel wall, increasing the peripheral vascular resistance. In addition, decreasing perfusion of the capillary beds of the lower extremities with pneumatic counterpressure will increase the blood pressure.
- PASG has three independently controlled compartments, each with its own high-pressure tubing and pressure control valve. The garment is made of heavy-duty nylon or polyvinyl. The PASG is manufactured in sizes appropriate for adults and children over 6 years of age. Velcro fasteners are used to secure the PASG to the abdomen and legs.
- Each compartment is connected to a separate tubing for air flow and pressurization. Each individual compartment tubing is interconnected to a single connection that is attached to a foot pump. Each tube contains two valves: (1) an on/off flow valve, which allows independent pressurization of the compartment, and (2) a pressure-relief or pop-off valve, which is a safety device to prevent inflation pressure from exceeding 104 mm Hg (Fig. 49–1).
- The abdominal compartment extends from the costal margins to the pubis. Each leg compartment extends from the groin crease to the ankle.

EQUIPMENT

- PASG
- Foot pump
- Blood pressure monitoring unit

Additional equipment to have available as needed includes the following:

- Intravenous solutions as prescribed
- Emergency medications and resuscitative equipment

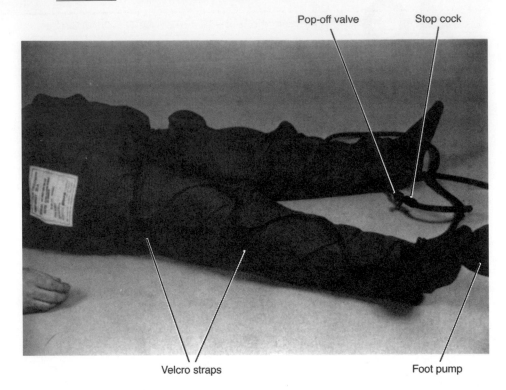

Pop-off valve   Stop cock

Velcro straps   Foot pump

■ ● **FIGURE 49–1.** Complete pneumatic antishock garment. (From Jastremski MS, Dumas M, Penalver L. *Emergency Procedures.* Philadelphia, Pa: WB Saunders; 1992: 363.)

PATIENT AND FAMILY EDUCATION

- Explain the purpose of the PASG and its anticipated benefits. ➤*Rationale:* Informs patient and family about the device. This information prepares the patient and family for what to expect and may decrease anxiety.
- Explain the procedure for PASG to the patient and family. ➤*Rationale:* Encourages patient and family cooperation and understanding of the procedure.

PATIENT ASSESSMENT AND PREPARATION

Patient Assessment

- Determine baseline cardiovascular, peripheral vascular, respiratory, and neurovascular status. ➤*Rationale:* Provides baseline information that may aid in determining the need for PASG.
- Assess for signs and symptoms of hemorrhagic shock. ➤*Rationale:* Physical signs and symptoms of shock may result from major blood volume loss and require immediate treatment.
- Assess skin, including possible sites of hemorrhage, be-

fore application of PASG. ➤*Rationale:* Once the trousers are applied, the area beneath the trousers will be difficult to assess.
- Assess baseline arterial blood gas and lactate levels. ➤*Rationale:* These levels can be used for comparison because metabolic acidosis can develop as a result of muscle necrosis and tissue ischemia.

Patient Preparation

- Ensure that the patient and family understand preprocedural teaching. Answer questions as they arise and reinforce information as needed. ➤*Rationale:* Evaluates and reinforces understanding of previously taught information.
- Ensure proper immobilization of spine. ➤*Rationale:* Spine alignment is maintained until spinal injury has been ruled out.
- Ensure that the patient has a decompressed bladder and stomach and patent airway. ➤*Rationale:* Increased abdominal and intrathoracic pressure can result in compromised airway, aspiration, and bladder rupture.

Procedure **for External Counterpressure with Pneumatic Antishock Garments**

Steps	Rationale	Special Considerations
Application of PASG		
1. Wash hands, and don gloves.	Reduces transmission of microorganisms; standard precautions.	
2. Search for and remove objects that are between the patient and the suit.	Removal of objects prevents patient injury.	Thorough assessment and documentation of skin integrity are essential before PASG application.

Procedure	for External Counterpressure with Pneumatic Antishock Garments *Continued*

Steps	Rationale	Special Considerations
3. Completely unfold PASG and lay it flat; smooth out wrinkles.	Prepares the device for use.	
4. Carefully logroll the patient, and place the PASG under the patient.	Maintains spine immobilization.	
5. Position the PASG so the abdominal section is positioned below the costal margin and the leg section ends at the ankle. *(Level VI: Clinical studies in a variety of patient populations and situations to support recommendations)*	Proper placement of trousers prevents respiratory compromise. Diaphragmatic compression interferes with thoracic movement.[1, 2, 4]	
6. Fold trousers around left leg and secure with Velcro. Repeat the procedure with right leg. Secure the PASG around the abdomen.	Prepares PASG.	Check dorsalis pedis and posterior tibial pulses before and after PASG application.
7. Attach foot pump and air tubes to the PASG. Ensure that all stopcocks are open.	Allows for trouser compartment inflation.	

Inflation of PASG

Steps	Rationale	Special Considerations
1. Open valves of the compartments to be inflated and close the valves of the compartments that will not be inflated.	Allows for proper inflation of device.	Leg-compartment inflation is contraindicated if there is an impaled object in the leg. Both extremity compartments must be inflated before inflation of the abdominal section.
2. Inflate the leg segment until the Velcro crackles or pressure gauge reads more than 100 mm Hg. *(Level V: Clinical studies in more than one or two different patient populations and situations to support recommendations)*	Inflation should increase the peripheral vascular resistance. This allows increased blood flow to the heart, brain, and kidneys.[1, 2, 4, 5]	
3. Inflate the abdominal segment if the patient's hemodynamic status does not improve. *(Level V: Clinical studies in more than one or two different patient populations and situations to support recommendations)*	Tamponade of intra-abdominal hemorrhage may be achieved by abdominal inflation.[1, 2, 4, 5]	Abdominal inflation is contraindicated in patients during pregnancy and in patients with impaled objects, evisceration, tension pneumothorax, penetrating chest trauma, or diaphragmatic rupture.
4. Monitor blood pressure for response during inflation.	Monitors hemodynamic status.	PASG is not a substitute for fluid volume replacement. Intravenous fluids should be administered as prescribed.
5. Continue inflation until desired blood pressure is achieved or maximal suit pressure is reached and the pop-off valve is activated. *(Level V: Clinical studies in more than one or two different patient populations and situations to support recommendations)*	Maintain PASG pressure at lowest level for which arterial pressure is stabilized.[1, 2, 4]	As a safety mechanism, release valves are activated when pressure in the suit exceeds 104 mm Hg or suit crackles.
6. When optimal blood pressure is reached, close all valves.	Prevents air leakage from valves.	

Procedure continued on following page

Procedure for External Counterpressure with Pneumatic Antishock Garments *Continued*

Steps	Rationale	Special Considerations
7. Do not suddenly remove PASG. *(Level V: Clinical studies in more than one or two different patient populations and situations to support recommendations)*	Sudden deflation without adequate fluid resuscitation may cause the patient's blood pressure to drop precipitously. Sequential release allows for a gradual return of blood flow. Intrasuit pressure is assessed to determine the amount of pressure exerted on the tissues.[1, 2, 4, 5]	
8. Assess the patient for clinical indicators that hemodynamic stability has been achieved.	Hemodynamic stability must be confirmed before safe deflation of PASG. Instability may occur before PASG deflation. Additional intravenous fluids may be required.	PASG should not be used for longer than 24 hours because of the potential for tissue damage.

Deflation of the PASG

Steps	Rationale	Special Considerations
1. Confirm hemodynamic stability before deflation.	PASG weaning should be considered when the patient's condition stabilizes, and before 24 hours of therapy.	Suggested parameters: systolic blood pressure greater than 90 mm Hg; heart rate, 60 to 120 beats/min; urine output, 0.5 mL/kg/hr; palpable peripheral pulses.
2. Prepare intravenous solutions as prescribed.	Blood pressure serves as a clinical parameter during the deflation process.	When blood pressure drops more than 5 to 10 mm Hg, prepare to administer intravenous fluid until blood pressure returns to baseline.
3. Initiate the deflation process with the abdominal wall compartment of the PASG.		
4. Deflate the PASG slowly by opening the stopcock.	Allows gradual release of the pressure.	
5. Monitor vital signs at time of deflation and every 5 to 10 minutes during deflation. *(Level V: Clinical studies in more than one or two different patient populations and situations to support recommendations)*	Compartment should be deflated sequentially to allow for gradual return of blood flow from the central circulation to prevent a sudden drop in circulatory blood volume.[1, 2, 4, 5]	
6. After the abdominal compartment is deflated and vital signs remain stable, deflate one leg at a time, continuing to assess vital signs.	Validates hemodynamic stability.	When blood pressure drops more than 5 to 10 mm Hg, stop deflation and prepare to administer intravenous fluid until blood pressure returns to baseline.
7. After deflation, continue to monitor the vital signs every 15 minutes for 1 hour, then every hour for 24 hours.		

Expected Outcomes	Unexpected Outcomes
• Control of hemorrhage • Hemodynamic stability • Proper placement of PASG	• Hemodynamic instability • Respiratory compromise • Continued hemorrhage • Compartment syndrome • Impaired skin integrity • Metabolic acidosis • Increased cerebral edema

Patient Monitoring and Care

Patient Monitoring and Care	Rationale	Reportable Conditions
		These conditions should be reported if they persist despite nursing interventions.
1. Perform ongoing assessment of cardiovascular system and document every 15 to 60 minutes as patient condition warrants.	Demonstrates effectiveness of PASG therapy; determines need for volume replacement.	• Significant changes in vital signs
2. Assess respiratory status and document every 15 to 60 minutes.	Abnormal respiratory status may indicate increased intrathoracic pressure and increased workload of heart.	• Tachypnea, cough, crackles, hypoxia, or distended neck veins
3. Assess circulation to the extremities every 15 to 60 minutes.	Validates adequate peripheral perfusion. Abnormal findings may indicate the development of compartment syndrome.	• Pain; pallor; diminished or absent movement, sensation, or pedal pulse; or capillary refill greater than 2 seconds
4. Monitor arterial blood gas and lactate levels.	May indicate development of muscle necrosis, tissue ischemia, and inadequate resuscitation.	• Abnormal arterial blood gas and lactate levels
5. Monitor intake and output.	Confirms adequate fluid resuscitation.	• Urine output of more than 0.5 mL/kg/hr
6. Monitor PASG pressures.	Pressure determines the amount of pressure exerted on the tissues beneath the garment.	• PASG pressure of more than 100 mm Hg
7. Monitor skin integrity before PASG inflation and after PASG deflation.	Skin integrity is difficult to assess once PASG is inflated. Once PASG is removed, vigilant skin assessment is necessary.	• Skin breakdown, redness, hematoma, and lacerations

Documentation

Documentation should include the following:

- Patient and family education
- Rationale for institution of PASG
- Vital signs
- Patient response to PASG therapy
- Laboratory studies
- Skin integrity assessment
- Time compartment was inflated and deflated
- Intake and output
- Unexpected outcomes
- Additional interventions

References

1. Maull K. Role of military antishock trousers. In: Ivatury RR, Cayten CG, ed. *The Textbook of Penetrating Trauma.* Media, Pa: Williams & Wilkins; 1996.
2. Cardona V, Hurn P, Bastnagel P, Scanlon E. *Trauma Nursing: From Resuscitation Through Rehabilitation.* 2nd ed. Philadelphia, Pa: W.B. Saunders; 1994.
3. Mattox KL, Bickell WH, Pepe PE, et al. Prospective randomized evaluation of antishock garment in penetrating cardiac wounds. *JAMA.* 1986;266:2398.
4. Chank AK, Dunford J, Hoyt DB, et al. MAST 96. *J Emerg Med.* 1996;4:419–424.
5. Chang FC, Harrison PB, Beech RR, et al. PASG: does it help in the management of traumatic shock? *J Trauma.* 1995;39:453–456.

Additional Reading

Lieberman JF, Maull KI. A critical review of the use of pneumatic antishock garment in trauma. *Contemp Surg.* 1989;34–37.

50

Ventricular Assist Devices

P U R P O S E: Ventricular assist devices (VADs) are used as mechanical bridges to heart transplantation and occasionally as bridges to recoverable myocardial events. VADs currently are being researched as a long-term alternative to heart transplantation.[1-4]

Lee Ann Ruess

PREREQUISITE NURSING KNOWLEDGE

- Understanding of the normal anatomy and physiology of the cardiovascular, peripheral vascular, and pulmonary systems is necessary.
- Principles of hemodynamic monitoring, cardiopulmonary bypass (CPB), electrophysiology and dysrhythmias, and coagulation should be understood.
- Clinical and technical competence related to use of VADs is essential.
- Advanced cardiac life support knowledge and skills are necessary.
- Indications for VAD therapy include the following:
  - ❖ Extension of CPB for postcardiotomy cardiogenic shock or for the inability to wean from CPB
  - ❖ Approved cardiac transplant candidate
  - ❖ Bridge to cardiac transplantation
  - ❖ Patients who meet the New York Heart Association (NYHA) classification IV and are failing to respond to medical therapy[2]
  - ❖ Bridge to recovery
- Relative contraindications of VAD therapy include the following:
  - ❖ Body surface area (BSA) <1.3 m²
  - ❖ Renal/liver failure unrelated to cardiac incident
  - ❖ Untreatable metastatic cancer
- Complications of VAD therapy may include hepatic dysfunction, the need for reoperation, bleeding, neurologic dysfunction, pulmonary dysfunction, renal dysfunction, infection, right ventricular failure, embolism, cardiac tamponade, and dysrhythmias.
- Effective cardiac assistance by the VAD is affected greatly by hypovolemia, hypertension, right ventricular failure (RVF), cardiac tamponade, and cardiac dysrhythmias; therefore, the interaction between the patient and the device requires close monitoring.
- The device is implanted surgically in the operating room. Correct device implantation is verified via radiography or fluoroscopy.

- Specific information concerning controls, alarms, trouble shooting, and safety features is available from each manufacturer and should be read thoroughly by the nurse before use of the equipment.
- Heartmate
  - ❖ ThermoCardiosystems (Woburn, MA) developed two implantable VADs used for left ventricular assistance.[5] The implantable pneumatic (IP) is powered pneumatically and serves as a predecessor to the electrically driven vented electric (VE) Heartmate[2] (Fig. 50–1).
  - ❖ The VAD (IP or VE) may be implanted into the peritoneum, anterior to the spleen and stomach, or in

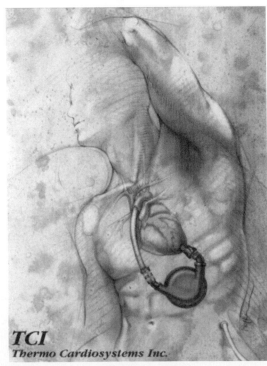

■ ● FIGURE 50–1. Heartmate implantable pneumatic (IP) ventricular assist device. (Thermocardiosystems, Woburn, MA.)

the preperitoneal pocket external to the abdominal viscera.[10]

❖ The blood chamber of the left ventricular assist device (LVAD) is supplied by cannulation from the left ventricle and is capable of holding 83 mL. It ejects blood through unidirectional valves into the ascending aorta.

❖ The blood chamber is divided by a flexible polyurethane diaphragm. An influx of pressurized air through the pneumatic tubing drives the flexible diaphragm and controls the duration of systole.

❖ The Heartmate operates by adjusting its ejection duration to maximize the patient's cardiac output. The systolic time of the blood pump cycle is identified as the ejection duration. This length of time is selected by the operator in any of the pump modes (fixed, automatic, and external) and is variable from 200 to 450 milliseconds. Increasing ejection duration may increase the ability to fully empty the blood pump, thereby increasing stroke volume.[9] However, a chosen ejection duration that is too long for the beat rate may limit the pumping rate per minute. In this case, stroke volume would increase, but the net effect may be a similar or decreased flow rate. Ejection duration should be long enough to fully empty the pump, but not too long to produce rate limitations.

• Thoratec
  ❖ The Thoratec VAD (Thoratec Laboratories Corp, Berkley, CA) is a pneumatically driven pump that can provide left, right, or biventricular support.[6]
  ❖ The device is positioned externally on the abdominal wall (Fig. 50–2).
  ❖ A pneumatically driven console controls pumping through a blood chamber. A diaphragm divides the air chamber from the blood sac. By alternating positive and negative pressure to the air chamber, the pump achieves ejection and filling of the blood sac. Although the blood sac is capable of holding 80 mL, full ejection is calculated using an average stroke volume of 65 mL.

  ❖ The Thoratec is driven by a dual-drive console, which contains two independent drive modules for left and right ventricular support. Patients with biventricular assist devices (BiVADs) require both modules, and patients with a right ventricular assist device (RVAD) or a LVAD require one module. When only one module is being used, the other module can serve as a back-up if pump failure should occur. The console supplies air pressure to eject blood from the pump into the arterial system and vacuum to assist pump filling. A full 65-mL stroke volume is possible from 20 to 110 beats per minute (bpm), providing cardiac outputs of 1.2 to 7.2 L/min. The console calculates VAD output automatically.

  ❖ The control modes for operation include fixed, automatic, and synchronous. A fixed rate allows the operator to choose a VAD rate that is asynchronous with the patient's intrinsic heart rate. The automatic mode is also asynchronous to the patient's intrinsic heart rate, but responds to changes in physiologic conditions. Synchronous is synchronized to the patient's intrinsic heart rate. It is triggered by the R wave of the electrocardiogram (ECG) and can be used to wean the patient following recovery of heart function.

• Abiomed
  ❖ The Abiomed 5000 BVS (Abiomed Cardiovascular Inc, Danvers, MA) is an extracorporeal, pneumatically driven pump capable of delivering left, right, or biventricular support.[7]
  ❖ The drive console controls systole by delivering air into the lower rigid plastic pumping chamber, displacing blood from the blood sac. Blood drains passively from the patient's atrium into the atrial chamber of the blood pump. When the atrial chamber of the blood pump is full and the pressure inside the atrial chamber exceeds the pressure inside the ventricular chamber, the tri-leaflet valve will open, allowing blood to flow into the ventricular chamber of the blood pump. Blood pump diastole is completed as soon as the ventricular chamber is filled with 100 mL. The diastolic filling time is adjusted automatically to changes in the patient's preload to ensure the ventricular chamber is completely filled to full capacity (100 mL). The system is programmed to consistently deliver a 70- to 80-mL stroke volume. It does so by keeping a running four beat average of previous stroke volumes and adjusting systolic duration to achieve the 70- to 80-mL goal.

  ❖ The vertically aligned pneumatic blood pumps are adjusted to optimize flow. The blood flow from the patient to the blood pump is passive and relies on gravity. The top of the blood pump should be between 0 and 10 inches below the level of the patient's atria (Fig. 50–3). Moving the pump above or below this level can affect flow. Preload can be adjusted by changing the height of the blood pump. Always allow 2 minutes for the system to adjust before making additional changes.

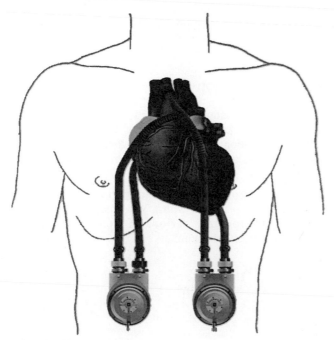

■ ● **FIGURE 50–2.** Thoratec biventricular assist device. (Thoratec Laboratories Corp., Berkeley, CA.)

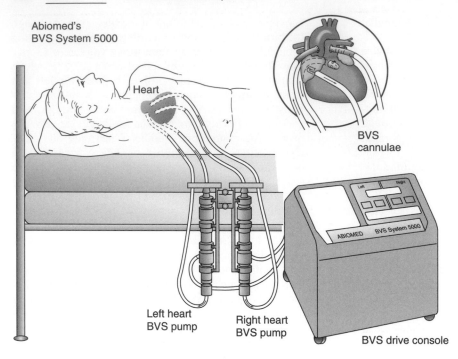

Abiomed's
BVS System 5000

Heart

BVS
cannulae

Left heart
BVS pump

Right heart
BVS pump

BVS drive console

■ ● **FIGURE 50–3.** ABIOMED's BVS 5000 System. (From Dixon JF, Farris CD. The ABIOMED BVS 5000 System. *AACN Clin Issues Crit Care.* 1991; 2(3):553.)

EQUIPMENT

- VAD drive console
- Connection cables (specific to device)
- Back-up drive console
- Emergency pump device (hand crank, foot pump, or bulb, depending on device)

  Additional equipment as needed includes the following:

- Emergency equipment

PATIENT AND FAMILY EDUCATION

- Assess patient and family understanding of VAD therapy and the reason for its use. **➠Rationale:** Clarification or reinforcement of information is an expressed patient and family need during times of stress and anxiety.
- Explain environment and care planned to the patient and family, including frequency of assessment, sounds and function of equipment, placement of device, explanation of alarms, dressings and therapy, decreased or assisted mobility, and parameters for discontinuation of therapy. **➠Rationale:** Provides information and encourages the patient and family to ask questions or voice concerns or fears related to the therapy.

PATIENT ASSESSMENT AND PREPARATION
Patient Assessment

- Assess past medical history, specifically related to competency of aortic/pulmonic valve, mitral/tricuspid valve,

primary pulmonary hypertension, right ventricular failure, left ventricular failure, and peripheral vascular disease. **➠Rationale:** Provides baseline data regarding cardiac functioning.

- Perform cardiovascular, hemodynamic, peripheral vascular, and neurovascular assessment. **➠Rationale:** Provides baseline data.
- Assess current laboratory profile, including complete blood count (CBC), platelet count, prothrombin time (PT), partial thromboplastin time (PTT), and international normalized ratio (INR). **➠Rationale:** Baseline coagulation studies are helpful in determining risk for bleeding. Platelet function may be affected by the mechanical trauma from the blood pump.

Patient Preparation

- Ensure that the patient and family understand preprocedural teaching. Answer questions as they arise and reinforce information as needed. **➠Rationale:** Evaluates and reinforces understanding of previously taught information.
- Provide emotional support to patient and family. **➠Rationale:** The patient with a VAD may be confined to the hospital for long periods of time, especially if awaiting a heart transplant.

Procedure **for Ventricular Assist Devices**

Steps	Rationale	Special Considerations
Re-initiating VAD Pumping after VAD Device Failure		
1. Check that the back-up VAD console is available.	Ensures continuation of therapy if the VAD device fails.	A back-up VAD device should be within 100 feet of the patient at all times.
2. Turn the power switch back on.	Reestablishes the power source to the VAD.	
3. Observe the control panel.	The control panel on the console continuously indicates the status of the system. The VAD system will go through a self-test after the system is turned on.	
4. Set the console to control volume or pressure and improve cardiac output.	Establishes VAD settings.	Set the device as prescribed by the physician. Each VAD functions differently. Refer to the manufacturer manual for specific information related to device settings.
5. Assess the VAD for complete filling and ejection.	Incomplete filling or ejecting will decrease the effectiveness of the VAD.	Incomplete filling may be due to hypovolemia, bleeding, right ventricular failure, ventricular recovery, tamponade, inadequate pharmacologic support, VAD cannula position, inflow cannula kinked, insufficient vacuum, or dysrhythmias.
Troubleshooting VAD Alarms		
1. Low flow		
A. Assess for obstruction of lines, and correct problem if present.	Obstructed blood lines will minimize flow.	
B. Check pump placement on chest x-ray.	Ensures correct VAD placement.	
C. Administer intravenous fluids as prescribed.	Adequate preload is necessary for effective cardiac output.	
D. Increase vasoactive support as prescribed.	May enhance hemodynamic functioning.	
2. High pressure		
A. Assess for obstruction of lines, and correct problem if present.	The VAD drive line or the blood pump lines may be kinked.	
B. Assess for adequate anticoagulation.	The blood pump lines may occlude due to thrombus formation.	
3. Low pressure		
A. Assess for disconnection, cracks, or leaks in the tubing, and correct problem if present.	Blood loss may occur if connections are loose.	
B. Administer intravenous fluids as prescribed.	Maintains adequate preload.	
4. Battery indicator		
A. Ensure that the VAD console is plugged in.	Establishes power source.	
B. Replace the VAD console, if necessary.	Establishes reliable power source.	

Procedure continued on following page

Procedure	**for Ventricular Assist Devices** *Continued*

Steps	Rationale	Special Considerations
5. Inadequate emptying		
A. Assess blood pump lines for kinks, and correct problem if present.	Kinks will inhibit emptying.	
B. Assess heart sounds.	Muffled heart sounds may indicate cardiac tamponade.	Assess for additional signs and symptoms of cardiac tamponade.
C. Assess anticoagulation status.	Thromboembolism may inhibit emptying.	
D. Consider decreasing volume.	Preload may be too high.	
E. Consider administration of vasodilators.	Afterload may be too high.	
6. Inadequate filling		
A. Assess intravascular volume.	Preload may be inadequate.	
B. Assess for active bleeding.	May contribute to hypovolemia.	
C. Assess for presence of dysrhythmias.	May contribute to inadequate myocardial filling.	
D. Assess for presence of jugular vein distention.	May indicate right ventricular failure.	
E. Assess heart sounds.	May indicate cardiac tamponade.	
F. If using Abiomed system, consider repositioning the blood pump.	May enhance preload.	

Expected Outcomes	Unexpected Outcomes
• Increased myocardial oxygen supply and decreased myocardial oxygen demand	• Device failure
• Increased cardiac output	• Device misplacement
• Increased tissue perfusion	• Pain
• Safe bridge to heart transplantation or recovery	• Bleeding and coagulation disorders
	• Multisystem organ failure

Patient Monitoring and Care

Patient Monitoring and Care	Rationale	Reportable Conditions
		These conditions should be reported if they persist despite nursing interventions.
1. Perform systematic cardiovascular, peripheral vascular, and hemodynamic assessment every 15 to 60 minutes as patient status requires.		
○ Level of consciousness	Assesses for adequacy of cerebral perfusion; thrombi may develop and dislodge during VAD therapy.	• Change in level of consciousness
○ Vital signs and pulmonary artery pressures	Demonstrates effectiveness of VAD therapy.	• Unstable vital signs and significant changes in hemodynamic pressures, lack of response to VAD therapy
○ Cardiac output (CO), cardiac index (CI), and systemic vascular resistance (SVR)	Demonstrates effectiveness of VAD therapy.	• Abnormal values

Patient Monitoring and Care *Continued*

Patient Monitoring and Care	Rationale	Reportable Conditions
○ Circulation to extremities	Validates adequate peripheral perfusion. If reportable conditions are found, they may indicate thrombotic or embolic obstruction of perfusion to an extremity.	• Capillary refill >2 seconds • Diminished or absent pulses (radial, popliteal, tibial, pedal) • Color pale, mottled, or cyanotic • Diminished or absent sensation • Pain • Diminished or absent movement • Cool or cold to touch
○ Urine output	Validates adequate perfusion to the kidneys.	• Urine output <0.5 mL/kg/hr
2. Assess heart and lung sounds every 4 hours and as needed.	Abnormal heart and lung sounds may indicate the need for additional treatment.	• New murmur • New S_3 or S_4 • Crackles or rhonchi • Muffled heart sounds
3. Monitor for signs of inadequate filling/emptying.	Adequate VAD function is dependent on appropriate volume status. Heartmate: more than 4 dashes (seen consistently) on console represents inadequate filling or emptying. Thoratec: inadequate emptying is noted by absence of a "flash" or incomplete squeezing together of the chambers in the pump. Abiomed: atrial and ventricular chambers will expand completely and collapse together completely when adequate filling/emptying occurs.	• Inadequate filling or emptying
4. Log roll patient every 2 hours. Prop pillows to support patient and to maintain alignment.	Promotes comfort and skin integrity and prevents kinking of the VAD drive lines. *Note:* This step is only for hemodynamically stable patients.	• Disruption of skin integrity
5. Initiate passive and active range-of-motion exercises every 2 hours.	Prevents venous stasis and muscle atrophy.	
6. Assess the area around the VAD insertion site every 2 hours and as needed for evidence of hematoma and bleeding.	Anticoagulation therapy increases the risk of bleeding.	• Bleeding at insertion site • Hematoma at insertion site
7. Assess coagulation studies: ○ Monitor CBC, platelet, and PT/PTT and INR as prescribed. ○ Activated clotting time (ACT) should be assessed every 3 to 4 hours.[3] This usually begins after the first 24 hours. Special note: Patients in atrial fibrillation may require higher ACT values.	The VAD will require prophylactic anticoagulation to prevent thrombi and emboli development.	• Abnormal values
8. Monitor patient for systemic evidence of bleeding or coagulation disorders.	Hematologic and coagulation profiles may be altered as a result of blood loss during VAD insertion, anticoagulation, and platelet dysfunction due to mechanical trauma by the VAD pumping blood.	• Bleeding from VAD insertion site • Bleeding from incisions or mucous membranes • Petechiae/ecchymosis • Guaiac-positive nasogastric aspirate or stool • Hematuria • Decreased hemoglobin/hematocrit • Decreased filling volumes • Increased heart rate

Continued on following page

Patient Monitoring and Care	Rationale	Reportable Conditions
9. Change the VAD site dressing every 24 hours and as needed.	Decreases incidence of infection and allows an opportunity for site assessment. *Special note*: Most manufacturers do not recommend using povidone-iodine because of degradation of the drive lines. Patients with open chest sites often require a physician at the bedside during dressing changes.	• Signs and symptoms of infection
10. Assess and manage patient's pain.	The patient may experience pain from VAD placement or limited mobility.	• Unrelieved pain
11. Identify parameters/signs that demonstrate adequate filling/emptying of blood pump.	Each device has its own specific parameters for adequate pumping: Heartmate: fixed rate assures a minimum heart rate; ejection duration changes to accommodate rate changes. Thoratec: fixed rate is asynchronous with the patient's intrinsic rate; set % systole is half the set heart rate and ensures an ejection time of 300 LVAD ms; drive pressure should be 100 mm Hg above systolic blood pressure and RVAD should be 100 mm Hg above systolic pulmonary pressure. Abiomed: height of the blood pumps should be 0 to 10 inches below the level of the atria. Movement of the pumps will affect preload or filling.	• High or low pressure alarms. • Urine output <0.5 mL/kg/hr • Systolic blood pressure (SBP) below limits • Cardiac output (CO) and cardiac index (CI) below limits • Additional guidelines as per hospital policy
12. Identify parameters that demonstrate clinical readiness to wean from VAD therapy.	Close observation of the patient's tolerance to weaning procedures is necessary to ensure that the body's cardiac output demands can be met without pump assistance. The presence of these reportable conditions indicate that consideration should be given to weaning the patient from the VAD. Slowly reducing the outflow from the VAD allows the native ventricle to eject enough stroke volume to maintain an adequate cardiac output. Special note: Most patients placed on a VAD are awaiting heart transplantation; therefore, weaning is not a consideration.	• No angina • Heart rate less than 110 beats per minute • Absence of lethal or unstable dysrhythmia • Mean arterial pressure (MAP) greater than 70 mm Hg with little or no vasopressor support • Pulmonary artery wedge pressure (PAWP) <18 mm Hg • CI >2.5 L/min • Svo_2 = 60% to 80% • Capillary refill <3 sec • Urine output >0.5 mL/kg/hr

Documentation

Documentation should include the following:

- Patient and family education
- Patient tolerance
- Confirmation of placement
- Hemodynamic status
- Pain
- Activity level
- Unexpected outcomes
- Additional interventions
- Heartmate: mode, ejection duration, alarm volume, drive line sites, rates, complete filling and emptying, flow

- Thoratec: mode, set rate, set % systole, LVAD and RVAD drive pressures, drive line sites, complete filling and emptying
- Abiomed: level of pump, complete filling and emptying, drive line sites, flow
- Backup drive console and emergency pump device

References

1. Arabia F, Paramesh V, Toporoff B, et al. Biventricular cannulation for the Thoratec ventricular assist device. *Ann Thoracic Surg.* 1998;66:2119–2120.
2. Chillocott S, Atkins P, Adamson R. Left ventricular assist as a viable alternative for cardiac transplantation. *Crit Care Nurs Q.* 1998;20:64–69.
3. DeRose J, Umana J, Argenziano M, et al. Implantable left ventricular assist devices provide an excellent outpatient bridge to transplantation and recovery. *J Am Coll Cardiol.* 1997;30:1773–1777.
4. Schmid C, Deng M, Hammel D, et al. Emergency versus elective/urgent left ventricular assist device implantation. *J Heart Lung Transplant.* 1998;17:1024–1028.
5. Thermo Cardiosystems, Inc. *Heartmate Training Manual.* Woburn, Mass: Author; 1991.
6. Thoratec Laboratories Corporation. *Thoratec VAD System: Mechanical Support.* Pleasanton, Ca: Author; 1997.
7. ABIOMED Cardiovascular, Inc. *Abiomed BVS 5000: Guide to Patient Management.* Danvers, Ma. Author; 1994.
8. Livingston E, Fisher C, Bibidakis E, et al. Increased activation of the coagulation and fibrinolytic systems leads to hemorrhagic complications during left ventricular assist implantation. *Circulation.* 1996;94(suppl II):II227–II234.
9. McCarthy P, Smedira N, Vargo R, et al. One hundred patients with the Heartmate left ventricular assist device: evolving concepts and technology. *J Thoracic Cardiovasc Surg.* 1998;115:904–912.
10. Mussivand T, Masters R, Hendry P, et al. Critical anatomic dimensions for intrathoracic circulatory assist devices. *Artif Organs.* 1992;16:281–285.

Additional Readings

Dixon JF, Farris DD. The ABIOMED BVS 5000 System. *AACN Clin Issues Crit Care Nurs.* 1991;2:552–561.

Henker R. Cardiac assist devices as a bridge to cardiac transplant. *AACN Clin Issues Crit Care Nurs.* 1991;2:598–605.

Ley SJ. The Thoratec ventricular assist device: nursing guidelines. *AACN Clin Issues Crit Care Nurs.* 1991;2:529–544.

51

Electrophysiologic Monitoring: Hardwire and Telemetry

PURPOSE: Continuous electrophysiologic monitoring is routinely performed for the majority of critically ill patients. A key component of electrophysiologic monitoring is the electrocardiogram (ECG). The ECG provides a continuous graphic picture of cardiac electric activity. The ECG can be used for diagnostic, documentation, and treatment purposes.

Mary G. McKinley

PREREQUISITE NURSING KNOWLEDGE

- Understanding of the anatomy and physiology of the cardiovascular system, principles of cardiac conduction, ECG lead placement, basic dysrhythmia interpretation, and electrical safety is required.
- Advanced cardiac life support (ACLS) knowledge and skills are necessary.
- Electrophysiologic monitoring, both by hardwire and telemetry, is indicated for all patients in critical care units as well as for patients in postanesthesia areas, operating rooms, and emergency departments.
- Electrophysiologic monitoring is designed to give a graphic display of the electrical activity in the heart generated by cardiac depolarization and repolarization.
- Hardwire ECG monitors have electrodes and lead wires that are attached directly to the patient. Impulses are transmitted directly from the patient to the monitor (Fig. 51–1).
- Telemetry systems have electrodes and lead wires that are attached from the patient to a battery pack that transmits impulses to the monitor via radio wave transmission (Fig. 51–2).
- Telemetry is useful in progressive ambulation and evaluation of toleration of activity. A disadvantage to telemetry can include increased distortion of the ECG pattern.
- Specific areas of the chest are used for electrode placement to obtain a view of the electrical activity in a particular area of the heart (commonly called a lead).

- ECG monitors can use a three- or five-lead wire system to provide the different views (leads) of the heart's electrical activity.
- Standardized placement of leads is important so that the information that is obtained is assessed within a common frame of reference and so appropriate judgments can be made on the patient's cardiac status. Alterations of electrode position may significantly distort the appearance of

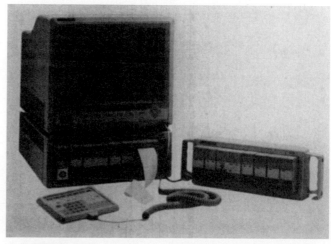

■ ● **FIGURE 51–1.** Bedside monitoring system. (From Hewlett-Packard.)

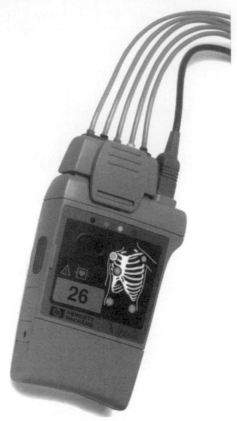

■ ● **FIGURE 51–2.** Telemetry monitoring system. (From Hewlett-Packard.)

the waveform and can lead to misdiagnosis or mistreatment.[1, 2]

- The two major factors that determine the views of the ECG deflection on the monitor are the location of the electrodes on the body and the direction of the cardiac impulse in relation to the position of the electrode.
- A basic rule of electrocardiography is the rule of electric flow. This rule notes that if electricity flows toward the positive electrode, the pattern produced on the monitor or graph paper will be upright. If the electricity flows away from the positive electrode (or toward the negative electrode), the pattern will be a downward deflection. Lead wires attached to the patient are coded (+, P, [positive] or −, N, [negative]; RA [right arm]; RL (right leg); LL [left leg] or LA [left arm]; V or C) in some way for ease in correct placement. Placement of the leads will give different views of the conduction through the heart.
- Information from the bedside via hardwire or telemetry can be transferred to a central monitor where it can be printed, stored, and analyzed (Fig. 51–3).
- Most monitoring systems provide a continuous readout of two or more leads simultaneously. This provides more information and a comparison of the ECG patterns. Optimal lead selection is based on the goals of monitoring for each patient's clinical situation.

EQUIPMENT

- ECG monitor (central and bedside monitor)
- Lead wires (no longer than 18 inches)
- Electrodes, pregelled and disposable
- Gauze pads or terry cloth washcloth
- Soap and water in basin
- Patient cable (should adapt to monitor and lead wires)
- ECG calipers
- Alcohol pads

Additional equipment to have available as needed includes the following:

- Skin preparation solution, such as skin barrier wipe or tincture of benzoin, if needed
- Battery pack (telemetry monitoring only)
- Pouch or pocket gown to hold telemetry unit (telemetry monitoring only)
- Scissors

PATIENT AND FAMILY EDUCATION

- Assess the readiness of the patient and family to learn. ➤*Rationale:* Anxiety and concerns the patient and family may have inhibit their ability to learn.
- Provide explanations of the equipment and alarms to both patient and family. ➤*Rationale:* Assists in making them feel more comfortable with monitoring and reduces anxiety.
- Reassure the patient and family that the monitor is constantly being reviewed and that any alterations or problems will be quickly treated. ➤*Rationale:* Reassures patient and family that immediate care is available.
- Emphasize that the patient should feel free to move about in bed. ➤*Rationale:* This will encourage movement on the part of the patient and allay fears about disruption of the monitoring system.

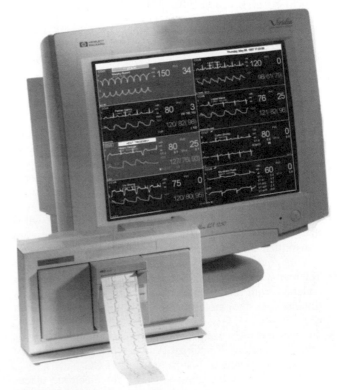

■ ● **FIGURE 51–3.** Central station system. (From Hewlett-Packard.)

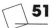

- Explain the importance of reporting any chest discomfort or pain. ➤➤*Rationale:* Ensures appropriate and timely interventions.

PATIENT ASSESSMENT AND PREPARATION
Patient Assessment

- Assess peripheral pulses, vital signs, heart sounds, level of consciousness, lung sounds, neck vein distention, presence of chest pain or palpitations, and peripheral circulatory disorders (ie, clubbing, cyanosis, and dependent edema). ➤➤*Rationale:* Physical signs and symptoms will result from alterations in the performance of the cardiovascular system.

- Assess history of cardiac dysrhythmias or cardiac problems. ➤➤*Rationale:* Provides baseline data and may guide selection of monitoring leads.

Patient Preparation

- Ensure that the patient and family understand preprocedural teaching. Answer questions as they arise and reinforce information as needed. ➤➤*Rationale:* Evaluates and reinforces understanding of previously taught information.
- Assist patient to supine position. ➤➤*Rationale:* Eases access to chest for electrode placement.

Procedure **for Electrophysiologic Monitoring**

Steps	Rationale	Special Considerations
1. Wash hands.	Reduces the transmission of microorganisms; standard precautions.	
2. Turn on computerized central monitoring system.	Once activated, the central monitoring system will sound alarm to notify nurse of problems with the ECG for interpretation and attention.	Nurse must verify patterns, evaluate computer interpretations, and assess the patient to confirm findings.
3. For telemetry monitoring, insert battery into telemetry unit, matching polarity markings on transmitter.	Batteries can fail if left sitting on the shelf or in the unit. Polarity must match for proper functioning of the unit.	Refer to manufacturer's recommendations about battery storage and replacement.
4. Ensure that the monitor is plugged into a grounded alternating current (AC) wall outlet.	Maintains electrical safety.	
5. Turn bedside monitor on.	Provides power source to monitor.	Equipment may require warm-up time.
6. Identify whether a three- or a five-lead wire system is available.	Assists in determining possible placement of electrodes and leads that can be viewed.	Optimal lead selection should be based on the goals of monitoring for each patient's clinical situation.
7. Check cable and lead wires for fraying, broken wires, or discoloration.	Detects conditions that may give inaccurate ECG trace.	Safety must be maintained. If equipment is damaged, obtain alternative equipment and notify biomedical engineer for repair.
8. Plug the patient cable into the monitoring system.	Hardware systems require a direct connection to the bedside monitoring system.	

9. Check that the lead wires are plugged into the patient cable correctly and securely.
  A. Three-lead system (Fig. 51–4):
   ○ The negative wire plugs into the opening marked *N*, −, or *RA*.
   ○ The positive wire plugs into the opening marked *P*, +, *LL*, or *LA*.
   ○ The ground wire plugs into the opening marked *G*, *Neutral*, or *RL*.
	Reduces chance of disconnection, distortion, or outside interference with ECG tracing.	Manufacturers code the lead connections so that correct attachments can be made. Often these are color coded, but they may be letter or symbol coded.

Procedure continued on following page

Procedure **for Electrophysiologic Monitoring** *Continued*

Steps	Rationale	Special Considerations
B. Five-lead system (Fig. 51–5): ○ The right arm wire plugs into the opening marked *RA*. ○ The left arm wire plugs into the opening marked *LA*. ○ The left leg wire plugs into the opening marked *LL*. ○ The right leg wire plugs into the opening marked *RL*. ○ The chest wire plugs into the opening marked *C* or *V*.		
10. Connect the electrodes to the lead wires before placing the electrodes on the patient.	Prepares monitoring system.	Placing electrodes on the chest and then attaching the lead wires can be uncomfortable for the patient and can contribute to the development of air bubbles in the electrode gel, which can decrease conduction.
11. Choose electrode placement. A. Three-lead system: ○ First choice: MCL_1 ○ Second choice: MCL_6 B. Five-lead system: ○ First choice: Single-lead monitoring: V_1, dual-lead monitoring: V_1, and the limb lead appropriate for clinical situation (see special considerations for tips). ○ Second choice: Substitute V_6 for V_1 when patient cannot have electrode at sternal border or when QRS complex amplitude is not adequate for optimized computerized monitoring.	Choice is based on constraints on chest wall space and type of information required or desired.	Tips for selection of limb lead appropriate for the clinical situation: 1. Atrial flutter: II, III, or AVF. 2. Inferior MI: II, III, or AVF—lead with maximum elevation of ST segment on 12-lead ECG. 3. Anterior MI: Select the lead with maximum elevation of ST segment on 12-lead ECG. 4. After angioplasty: Select III or AVF—whichever has tallest R wave. 5. If three channels are available, use V_1 + I + AVF.[3]
12. Identify the sternal notch or angle of Louis. A. Palpate the upper sternum to identify where the clavicles join the sternum (suprasternal notch).	The sternal notch identifies the second rib and thereby assists in locating the fourth intercostal space (ICS) so that accurate placement may be achieved.	

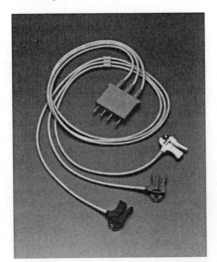

■ ● **FIGURE 51–4.** Three-lead cable. (From Hewlett-Packard.)

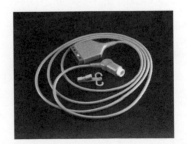

■ ● **FIGURE 51–5.** Five-lead cable. (From Hewlett-Packard.)

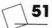

Procedure **for Electrophysiologic Monitoring** *Continued*

Steps	Rationale	Special Considerations
B. Slide fingers down the center of the sternum to the obvious bony prominence. This is the sternal notch, which identifies the second rib and provides the landmark for noting the fourth ICS. C. Locate the fourth ICS.		
13. Wash the skin with soap and water and dry it thoroughly, cleaning the area for the application of electrodes. *(Level IV: Limited clinical studies to support recommendations)*	Provides for adequate transmission of electrical impulses. Moist skin is not conducive to electrode adherence.[3–5]	It may be necessary to clip chest hair to ensure good skin contact with the electrode.
14. Clean the intended sites with alcohol pads. Consider using skin preparation solutions. *(Level IV: Limited clinical studies to support recommendations)*	Alcohol or skin preparations may be needed to remove oils, thus improving impulse transmission.[3–5]	Skin preparation solutions should not be applied to the area of the skin that will be in direct contact with the electrode gel because transmission of impulses may be decreased.
15. Abrade skin using a washcloth, scratch pad on electrode pack, or gauze pad.	Removes dead skin cells, promoting impulse transmission.	
16. Remove backing from the pregelled electrode and test the center of the pad for moistness.	Gel can dry out in storage; gel should be moist to allow for impulse transmission.	
17. Apply electrodes to sites, ensuring a seal. Avoid pushing on gel pad.	Electrodes must be placed tightly to prevent external influences from affecting the ECG. Pressing on the gel pad can cause gel to leak onto adhesive surface and may interfere with transmission.	

18. Place electrodes as follows:
 	
A. Three-lead stystem; MCL$_1$ and MCL$_6$ (Fig. 51–6):
  ○ Apply right arm (RA) electrode to the patient's left shoulder.
  ○ Apply left arm (LA) electrode at fourth ICS right sternal border.
  ○ Apply left leg (LL) electrode to the fifth ICS at midaxillary line.
  ○ Select lead I to obtain MCL$_1$ and lead II to obtain MCL$_6$.
	Proper positioning is essential to ensure correct view of leads.[1, 2]	Lead selection is based on chest wall constraints and clinical situation.

Procedure continued on following page

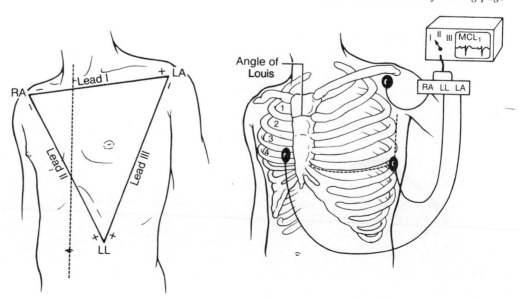

■ ● **FIGURE 51–6.** Three-lead application. (From Drew B. Bedside electrocardiographic monitoring. *AACN Clin Issues Crit Care.* 1993; 4(1):28.)

Angle of Louis

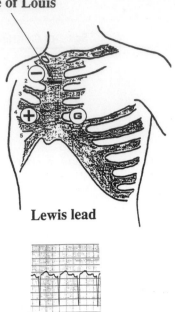

Lewis lead

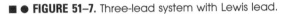

■ ● **FIGURE 51–7.** Three-lead system with Lewis lead.

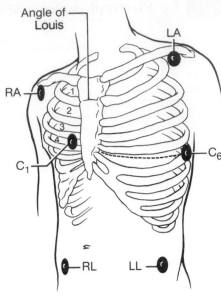

■ ● **FIGURE 51–8.** Five-lead application. (From Drew B. Bedside electrocardiographic monitoring. *AACN Clin Issues Crit Care.* 1993; 4(1):26.)

Procedure	for Electrophysiologic Monitoring *Continued*

Steps	Rationale	Special Considerations
B. Lewis lead (Fig. 51–7): ○ Apply right arm (RA) electrode at first ICS right sternal border. ○ Apply left arm (LA) electrode to fourth ICS right sternal border. ○ Apply left leg (LL) electrode to fourth ICS left sternal border.		Lewis lead offers the best visualization of P waves.
C. Five-lead system (Fig. 51–8): ○ Apply right arm (RA) to the right shoulder close to the junction of the right arm and torso. ○ Apply left arm (LA) to left shoulder close to the junction of the left arm torso. ○ Apply right leg (RL) electrode at the level of the lowest rib, on the right abdominal region or on the hip. ○ Apply left leg (LL) electrode at the level of the lowest rib on the left abdominal region or on the hip.	Arm electrodes that are placed under the clavicle or leg electrodes that are placed too high on the ribs can alter the point of view of the leads and results in inaccurate recording.[1,2]	
○ Apply the chest lead electrode on the selected site: V_1 fourth ICS right sternal border or V_6 fifth ICS midaxillary line. ○ Set lead selector or monitor to appropriate leads.	Only one precordial lead can be displayed—placement of the electrode identifies the lead used.	
19. For hardwire monitoring, fasten lead wire and patient cable to patient's gown, making a stress loop.	Decreases tension on lead wires to alleviate undue stress, causing interference or faulty recordings. Minimizes pulling on electrodes, which can be uncomfortable for the patient.	

Procedure	**for Electrophysiologic Monitoring** *Continued*

Steps	Rationale	Special Considerations
20. For telemetry monitoring, secure the transmitter in pouch or pocket in patient's gown.	Decreases tension on lead wires to alleviate undue stress, causing interference or faulty recordings. Minimizes pulling on electrodes, which can be uncomfortable for the patient. Transmitter must be secure so that it will not be dropped or damaged.	
21. Examine the ECG tracing on the monitor for the size of R and T waves.	The R wave should be approximately twice the height of the other components of the ECG to ensure proper detection by the heart rate counter in the equipment. Accuracy of the alarm system often depends on the R wave. If the T wave is nearly equal to the R wave, double counting can occur, resulting in false arms.	Manufacturers provide for calibration of the ECG to 1 mV, and monitors have size adjustments that can be used to increase or decrease the size of the ECG.
22. Obtain an ECG strip (Fig. 51–9) and interpret it for rhythm, rate, presence and configuration of P waves, length of PR interval, length of QRS complex, presence and configuration of T waves, length of QT interval, presence of extra waves (such as U waves), and presence of dysrhythmias.	Reviews the normal conduction sequence and identifies abnormalities that may require further evaluation or treatment.	
23. Set alarms. Upper and lower alarm limits are set on the basis of the patient's current clinical status and heart rate.	Activates the bedside or telemetry monitor alarm system.	Monitoring systems allow for setting alarms at beside or central console. Types of alarms may include rate (high or low), abnormal rhythms or complexes, pacemaker recognition, and others, depending on the manufacturer. *Caution:* turning off bedside alarms is not recommended. Alarms should be adjusted according to the known clinical status of the patient.
24. Discard used supplies and wash hands.	Reduces transmission of microorganisms; standard precautions.	

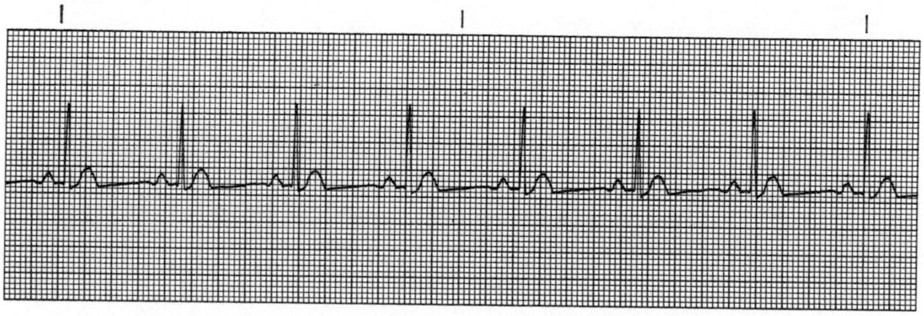

■ ● **FIGURE 51–9.** Monitor strip of clear pattern.

- Properly applied electrodes
- A clear monitor tracing displayed (see Fig. 51–9)
- Alarms set
- Prompt identification and treatment of dysrhythmias

- Altered skin integrity
- AC interference, also called 60-cycle interference (Fig. 51–10)
- Wandering baseline (Fig. 51–11)
- False alarms
- Artifact or waveform interference (Fig. 51–12)
- Microshock

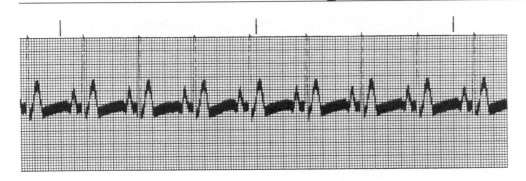

■ ● **FIGURE 51–10.** Monitor strip of 60-cycle interference.

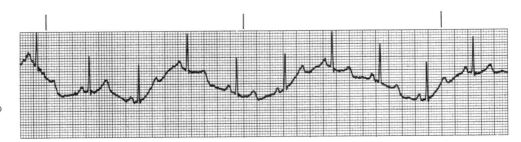

■ ● **FIGURE 51–11.** Monitor strip erratic baseline.

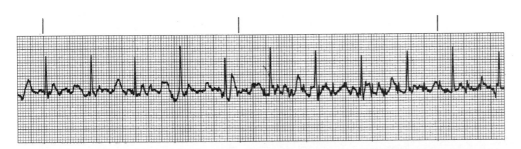

■ ● **FIGURE 51–12.** Monitor strip interference.

Patient Monitoring and Care

Patient Monitoring and Care	Rationale	Reportable Conditions
		These conditions should be reported if they persist despite nursing interventions.
1. Evaluate monitor pattern for the presence of P waves, QRS complex, a clear baseline, and absence of artifact or distortion. Obtain a rhythm strip on admission, every shift (as per institution protocol), and with rhythm changes.	A clear pattern is required to make accurate judgments about the patient's status and treatment.	• Changes in cardiac ECG complexes, rate, and rhythm
2. Evaluate the ECG pattern continually for dysrhythmias, assess patient tolerance of the change, and provide prompt nursing intervention.	Changes in the pattern may indicate significant problems for the patient and may require immediate intervention or additional diagnostic tests such as a twelve-lead ECG.	• Changes in cardiac rate and rhythm and hemodynamic instability.

Patient Monitoring and Care *Continued*

Patient Monitoring and Care	Rationale	Reportable Conditions
3. Evaluate skin integrity around the electrode on a daily basis, and change electrodes every 48 hours. Rotate sites when changing electrodes. Monitor skin for any allergic reaction to the adhesive or the gel. Change all electrodes if a problem occurs with one.	Skin integrity must be maintained to have a clear picture of the ECG. Replacing electrodes every 48 hours prevents drying of the gel. It may be necessary to change to different leads if sites become irritated. Electrode resistance changes as the gel dries, so changing all electrodes at once prevents differences in resistance between electrodes.[4, 6]	• Alteration in skin integrity
4. Check electrode placement every shift.	Accurate interpretation of many dysrhythmias depends on proper placement of electrodes and knowing which lead is being viewed.	

Documentation

Documentation should include the following:

• Patient and family education
• An initial or baseline strip, noting the lead, interprotation, any dysrhythmias, and treatments
• Routine strips according to institution protocol
• A monitor strip should be recorded whenever there is a change in the patient's rhythm, vital signs, or mental status; the patient experiences chest pain; there is a change in lead placement; and when evaluating the effect of antidysrhythmic agents
• Unexpected outcomes
• Additional nursing interventions

References

1. Drew B. Bedside electrocardiographic monitoring. *AACN Clin Issues.* 1993;4:25–32.
2. Drew B. Bedside electrocardiographic monitoring: state of the art for the 90's. *Heart Lung.* 1991;20:610–662.
3. Clochesy J, et al. Electrode site preparation: a follow-up. *Heart Lung.* 1991;20:27–30.
4. Drew B, Ide B, Sparacino P. Accuracy of bedside ECG monitoring: a report on current practices of critical care nurses. *Heart Lung.* 1991;20:597–609.
5. Medina V, Clochesy JM, Omery A. Comparison of electrode site preparation techniques. *Heart Lung.* 1989;18:456–460.
6. Jacobson C. Bedside cardiac monitoring. *AACN Research Based Practice Protocol, Technology Series.* Aliso Viejo, CA: American Association of Critical Care Publications; 1996:1–32.

Additional Readings

Alspach J. *Core Curriculum for Critical Care Nursing.* Philadelphia, Pa: W.B. Saunders; 1998.

Bucher L, Melander S. *Critical Care Nursing.* Philadelphia, Pa: W.B. Saunders; 1999.

Drew B, Tisdale L. ST segment monitoring for coronary artery reocclusion following thrombolytic therapy and coronary angioplasty: identification of optimal bedside monitoring leads. *Am J Crit Care.* 1993;2:280–292.

Drew B, Adams M, Pelter M, Wung S. ST segment monitoring with a derived 12-lead electrocardiogram is superior to routine cardiac care unit monitoring. *Am J Crit Care.* 1996;5:198–206.

Drew B, Pelter M, Adams M, Wung S, Chou T, Wolfe C. 12 lead ST-segment monitoring vs. single lead maximum ST-segment monitoring for detecting ongoing ischemia in patients with unstable coronary syndromes. *Am J Crit Care.* 1998;7:355–363.

Hartshorm J, Sole M, Lamborn M. *Introduction to Critical Care Nursing.* Philadelphia, Pa: W.B. Saunders; 1997:37–85.

Hebra J. The nurse's role in continuous dysrhythmia monitoring. *AACN Clin Issues.* 1994;5:178–185.

Thomason T, Riegel B, Carlson B, Gocka I. Monitoring electrocardiographic changes: results of a national survey. *J Cardiovasc Nurs.* 1995;9:1–9.

52

Extra Electrocardiographic Leads: Right Precordial and Left Posterior Leads

PURPOSE: Extra electrocardiographic (ECG) leads are used in conjunction with the standard 12-lead ECG to provide additional diagnostic information. Right precordial leads are useful in diagnosing right ventricular (RV) myocardial infarction (MI).[1-4] These right precordial leads are important because they enable clinicians to identify MI patients who are at high risk of developing atrioventricular (AV) conduction disturbances,[4] to predict the site of coronary artery occlusion,[5] and to guide appropriate hemodynamic monitoring and interventions.[6] Left posterior leads are used to aid in the detection of true posterior MI or left circumflex (LCX) coronary artery–related occlusion and to facilitate timely reperfusion treatment.[7-10] Recording left posterior leads can also help in the differential diagnosis of tall R waves in lead V_1 and V_2.[11]

Shu-Fen Wung
Barbara J. Drew

PREREQUISITE NURSING KNOWLEDGE

- Understanding of the anatomy and physiology of the cardiovascular system, basic rhythm interpretation, and electrical safety is required.
- Advanced cardiac life support (ACLS) knowledge and skills are necessary.
- Familiarity with principles of electrophysiology is necessary: The right precordial leads V_{1R} through V_{6R} and left posterior leads V_7 through V_9 are unipolar leads in which the chest electrode serves as the "exploring" electrode or positive pole of the lead. These precordial leads view the heart from the vantage point of their electrode positions on the chest, similar to the standard left precordial leads V_1 through V_6. To record right precordial or left posterior leads, the four limb electrodes (right arm [RA], left arm [LA], left leg [LL], and right leg [RL] are also required to create a central terminal (negative pole) and to stabilize the ECG recording.
- Accuracy in identifying anatomic landmarks to locate electrode sites and knowledge of importance of accurate electrode placement. It is essential for nurses to accurately locate the electrode positions for the standard 12-lead ECG because the same anatomic landmarks are used to locate the right precordial and left posterior leads. Accurate ECG interpretation is possible only when the recording electrodes are placed in the proper positions. Slight alterations of the electrode positions may significantly distort the appearance of the ECG waveforms and can lead to misdiagnosis.[12] Reliable comparison of serial (more than two ECGs recorded at different times) ECG recordings relies on accurate and consistent electrode placement. It is therefore recommended that an indelible marker be used to clearly identify the electrode locations to ensure that the same electrode locations are selected when serial ECGs are recorded.
- Nurses should be aware of body positional changes that can alter ECG recordings. Serial ECGs should be recorded with the patient in a supine position to ensure that all recordings are done in a consistent manner. Side-lying positions and elevation of the torso may change the position of the heart within the chest and can change the waveforms on the ECG recording.[13] If another position other than supine is clinically required, notation of the altered position should be made on the tracing.
- Nurses should be able to operate the 12-lead ECG machine used in the unit. Calibration of 1 millivolt (mV) = 10 mm and paper speed of 25 mm/s are standards used in clinical practice. For ST segment analysis, filter settings of 0.05 to 100 Hertz is recommended by the American Heart Association.[14] Any variation used for particular clinical purposes should be noted on the tracing. For

example, large QRS amplitudes require the use of a calibration of 5 mm/mV. Specific information regarding configuring the ECG machine, troubleshooting, and safety features is available from the manufacturer and should be read prior to use of the equipment.

- Nurses should be able to interpret recorded ECGs for the presence or absence of myocardial ischemia, infarction, and dysrhythmias so that patients can be treated appropriately. For example, acute inferior MI patients with RV involvement, determined by ST segment elevation in the right precordial leads, are at high risk for developing high-degree AV block. Nurses should monitor patients closely for conduction disturbances and anticipate the need for temporary pacing. Moreover, patients with RV infarction are prone to developing hypotension and shock that responds to treatment with intravenous (IV) fluids.

- Indications for recording a right precordial ECG are as follows:
  - ❖ Patients admitted for evaluation and treatment of suspected acute MI, especially those with inferior wall MI (ST segment elevation in leads II, III, and aVF)
  - ❖ To evaluate risk for developing AV node conduction disturbances and to anticipate treatment plans
  - ❖ To predict site of coronary artery occlusion (RV infarction occurs with proximal right coronary artery occlusion)
  - ❖ To determine risk of developing "volume-responsive" shock, in which case IV fluids are warranted and vasodilators (eg, IV nitroglycerin) are contraindicated

- Indications for recording a left posterior ECG are as follows:
  - ❖ Patients admitted for evaluation and treatment of acute or suspected MI, especially those with isolated ST segment depression in the left precordial ECG leads V_1 through V_3 or those with a nondiagnostic ECG
  - ❖ Presence of chest pain or "anginal equivalent" symptoms (eg, jaw, left shoulder or arm discomfort, or shortness of breath) or ST segment depression in the left precordial ECG leads V_1 through V_3 after catheter-based interventions of the LCX artery
  - ❖ Patients with any of these ECG characteristics indicative of posterior MI in lead V_1: R waves ≥6 mm in height, R wave ≥40 milliseconds (ms) in duration, R/S ratio ≥1, or S wave ≤3 mm. In lead V_2: R wave ≥15 mm in height, R wave ≥50 ms in duration, R/S ratio ≥1.5 or S wave ≤4 mm[15]
  - ❖ To differentiate true posterior infarction from other conditions that can cause tall R waves in lead V_1, such as RV hypertrophy, right bundle branch block, Wolff-Parkinson-White syndrome, and ventricular septal hypertrophy

EQUIPMENT

- Indelible marker
- 12-lead ECG machine with attached patient cable
- Lead wires (one end connects to the patient cable and one end connects to ECG electrodes on the patient)
- ECG electrodes

PATIENT AND FAMILY EDUCATION

- Describe the procedure and reasons for obtaining extra ECG leads. Reassure the patient that the procedure is painless. ➥*Rationale:* Clarifies information, reduces anxiety, and gains cooperation from the patient.

- Explain patient's role in assisting with the ECG recording and emphasize actions that improve the quality of the ECG tracing, such as relaxing, avoiding conversation and body movement, and breathing normally. ➥*Rationale:* Ensures patient's cooperation to improve the quality of the tracing and avoids unnecessarily repeating ECGs because of muscle artifact.

PATIENT ASSESSMENT AND PREPARATION

Patient Assessment

- Interpret previously recorded ECGs. ➥*Rationale:* Each patient has his or her own individual baseline ECG. Previous ECG recordings can help clinicians to determine whether a change is acute or chronic.

- Evaluate presence of anginal-type symptoms, such as these feelings in the chest: pain, pressure, tightness, heaviness, fullness, or squeezing sensation; radiated pain; or shortness of breath. ➥*Rationale:* Correlates ECG changes with patient's symptoms.

- Determine past medical history of cardiac disease, such as MI, and related interventions and medications. ➥*Rationale:* Knowledge about patient's prior cardiac history and medications can help in interpreting ECG recordings (Fig. 52–1). For example, digitalis therapy causes chronic ST segment depression that does not indicate ischemia. Therefore, a normal-looking isoelectric ST segment in a digitalized patient may indicate acute ischemia. Patients with prior posterior MI might have abnormal Q waves in the left posterior leads.

- Interpret standard 12-lead ECG for any signs of myocardial ischemia or infarction, as well as dysrhythmias. ➥*Rationale:* Nurses should be able to evaluate the standard 12-lead ECG for the location of ischemia or infarction and assess the possibility of RV and posterior involvement (Fig. 52–2).

Pre-PTCA

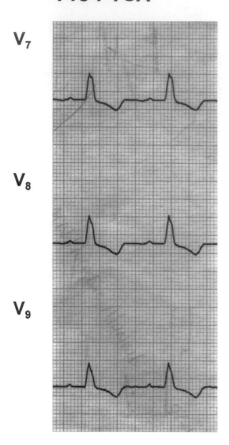

V₇

V₈

V₉

LCX Occlusion

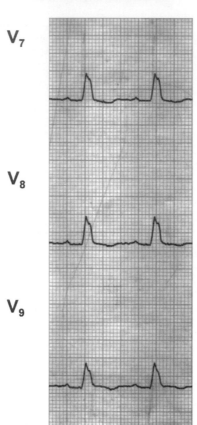

V₇

V₈

V₉

■ ● **FIGURE 52–1.** Baseline ST segment deviation as a result of left bundle branch block before percutaneous transluminal coronary angioplasty (pre-PTCA, left panel). During angioplasty balloon inflation of the proximal LCX coronary artery (LCX occlusion, right panel), the patient developed myocardial ischemia with chest pain radiating to the left arm. ST segments in the left posterior leads (V₇, ₈, and ₉) became elevated compared with the baseline pre-PTCA tracing, to produce a normal-looking, isoelectric ST segment. This ``pseudo-normalization'' of the ST segment during ischemia can be misinterpreted as normal without assessment of the baseline ECG.

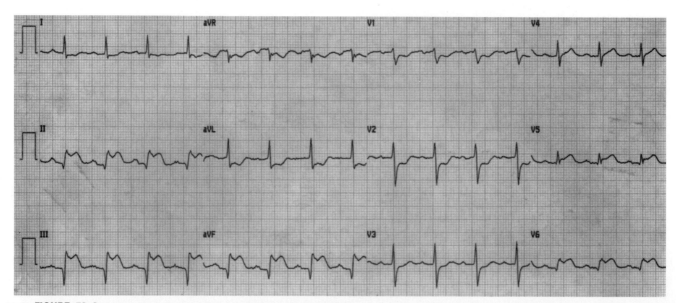

■ ● **FIGURE 52–2.** Initial ECG in a patient admitted to the emergency department with acute inferior myocardial infarction (elevated ST segments and Q waves in leads II, III, and aVF) with apical involvement (elevated ST segment in leads V₄, V₅, and V₆). ST segment depression in leads V₁, V₂, and V₃ is suggestive of posterior involvement. Left posterior and right precordial leads should be recorded to assess posterior and right ventricular involvement.

Procedure for Extra Electrocardiographic Leads

Steps	Rationale	Special Considerations
1. Wash hands.	Reduces transmission of microorganisms; standard precautions.	
2. Check patient cable and lead wires for fraying or broken wires.	Detects any condition that might cause the ECG recording to be incomplete or inaccurate.	If the equipment is damaged, obtain alternative equipment and notify biomedical engineer for repair.
3. Check the lead wires for accurate labels.	Obtains accurate ECG recordings.	
4. Plug ECG machine into a grounded wall outlet.	Maintains electrical safety.	Follow manufacturer's recommendation and institution's protocol on electrical safety per biomedical department.
5. Turn ECG machine on.	Activates the ECG machine.	Follow manufacturer's recommendation.
6. Program the ECG machine: paper speed of 25 mm/s; calibration of 10 mm/mV; filter settings of 0.05 to 100 Hertz. *(Level II: Theory based, no research data to support recommendations; recommendations from expert consensus group may exist)*	In accordance with clinical practice and recommendation for ST segment analysis by the American Heart Association (AHA).[14]	Follow manufacturer's recommendation in configuring ECG machine.
7. Place the patient in supine position. *(Level IV: Limited clinical studies to support recommendations)*	Body position changes can cause ST segment deviation as well as QRS waveform alteration.[13, 16]	If another position is clinically required, note the altered position on the ECG recording. ECGs should be recorded in the same body position to ensure ECG changes are not caused by a change in body position.
8. Expose the body parts for electrode placement.		Overexposing body parts may cause shivering and lack of privacy.
9. Identify electrode sites and mark with indelible marker.	When multiple ECG recordings are required, it is important to minimize ECG changes caused by altered electrode placement.[12]	After accurately identifying locations, an indelible marker should be used to mark the electrode sites.
Limbs leads		The limb leads are placed in the same way as when recording a standard 12-lead ECG (see Procedure 54).
○ Right arm (RA): inside right forearm ○ Left arm (LA): inside left forearm ○ Right leg (RL): anywhere on the body; by convention, usually on the right ankle or inner aspect of the calf ○ Left leg (LL): left ankle or inner aspect of the calf	RL electrode is a ground electrode that does not contribute to the ECG tracings.	

Procedure continued on following page

Procedure	**for Extra Electrocardiographic Leads** *Continued*	

Steps	Rationale	Special Considerations
Right precordial leads (see Fig. 52–3) ○ V_{1R}: fourth intecostal space (ICS) at left sternal border (same as V_2) ○ V_{2R}: fourth ICS at right sternal border (same as V_1) ○ V_{3R}: halfway between V_{2R} and V_{4R} ○ V_{4R}: right midclavicular line in the fifth ICS ○ V_{5R}: right anterior axillary line at the same horizontal level as V_{4R} ○ V_{6R}: right midaxillary line at the same horizontal level as V_{4R}	All patients with acute inferior wall MI should have right precordial leads recorded in addition to left precordial leads V_1 through V_6.[17] Accurate electrode placement is essential for obtaining valid and reliable data for ECG recordings. Slight alterations in the position of one precordial electrode may significantly distort the appearance of the cardiac waveforms and can have significant impact on the diagnosis.[12]	These right precordial leads are placed across the right precordium using the same landmarks that are used for the left precordial leads.[18] V_{1R} is at the same location as V_2, and V_{2R} is at the same location as V_1 in the standard 12-lead ECG (Fig. 52–4). The redundancy of V_1 (V_{2R}) and V_2 (V_{1R}) can be used to ensure that the ECGs are recorded accurately. Identify the sternal notch and move downward to locate the angle of Louis. The second ICS is located right below the angle of Louis.
Left posterior leads (see Fig. 52–5) ○ V_7: posterior axillary line at the same level as V_4 through V_6 ○ V_8: halfway between V_7 and V_9 ○ V_9: left paraspinal line at the same level as V_4 through V_6	Left posterior leads are placed to view the posterior wall of the heart. Left posterior leads should be recorded in patients admitted with the suspected posterior MI or known to have LCX artery disease.[7, 9, 10]	Help patient turn to the right side to expose the left side of the back. Make sure the patient is safely turned. V_{4-6} are located at the midclavicular line in the fifth ICS. Leads V_7 through V_9 are at the same horizontal level as V_4 through V_6.
10. Place the electrodes on the marked locations.	Secure the electrodes to obtain good quality of ECG recordings.	If limb plate electrodes are used, do not overtighten and cause discomfort. *Procedure continued on page 344*

Procedure continued on page 344

Right Precordial Leads

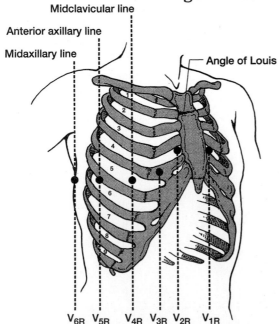

V_{1R}: 4th intercostal space (ICS) at left sternal border (same as V_2)

V_{2R}: 4th ICS at right sternal border (same as V_1)

V_{3R}: halfway between V_{2R} and V_{4R}

V_{4R}: right midclavicular line in the 5th ICS

V_{5R}: right anterior axillary line at the same horizontal level as V_{4R}

V_{6R}: right mid-axillary line at the same horizontal level as V_{4R}

Midclavicular line
Anterior axillary line
Midaxillary line
Angle of Louis
V_{6R} V_{5R} V_{4R} V_{3R} V_{2R} V_{1R}

■ ● **FIGURE 52–3.** Electrode locations for recording a right precordial ECG. (From Drew BJ, Ide B. Right ventricular infarction. *Progress Cardiovasc Nurs.* 1995; 10(2):46.)

Conventional 12–Lead ECG

Right Precordial Leads

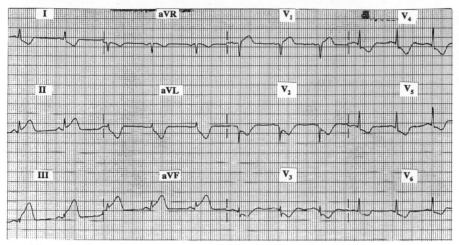

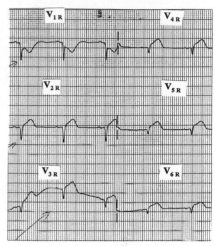

■ ● **FIGURE 52–4.** ST segment elevation in leads II, III, and aVF indicates acute inferior wall myocardial infarction. Three characteristics on the standard 12-lead ECG (left panel) are suggestive of a right ventricular infarction: A, diagnosis of inferior myocardial infarction, B, ST segment elevation in lead III exceeding that of lead II, and C, ST segment elevation is confined to V_1 without elevation in the remaining left precordial leads. Definitive diagnosis of right ventricular infarction is made by observing ST segment elevation ≥1 mm in one or more of the right precordial leads. In the right panel, ST elevation is seen in V_{2R} (V_1) through V_{6R}. (From Drew BJ, Ide B. Right ventricular infarction. *Progress Cardiovasc Nurs.* 1995; 10(2):46.)

Left Posterior Leads

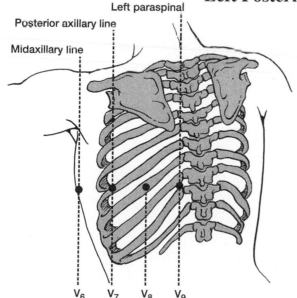

V_7: posterior axillary line at the same level as V_{4-6}

V_8: halfway between V_7 and V_9

V_9: left paraspinal line at the same level as V_{4-6}

■ ● **FIGURE 52–5.** Electrode locations for recording a left posterior ECG.

Procedure	**for Extra Electrocardiographic Leads** *Continued*	

Steps	Rationale	Special Considerations
11. Identify the number of available ECG channels for simultaneous recording in the ECG machine.	Newer multiple-channel machine can record up to 16 leads at a time that would allow simultaneous recording of a standard 12-lead ECG and 4 channels of right precordial leads V_{3R} through V_{6R} or 3 channels of left posterior leads V_7 through V_9.	If the ECG machine can record only 12 leads, record 3 separate ECGs: (1) standard 12-lead with left precordial leads, (2) right precordial leads, (3) left posterior leads. Some newer generation ECG machines may allow recording for more than 12 leads. For example, if the machine can record 16 leads, you could record 2 ECGs: (1) standard 12-lead plus right precordial leads (V_{3R}, V_{4R}, V_{5R}, and V_{6R}) and then (2) standard 12-lead plus left posterior leads (V_7, V_8, and V_9). However, an institutional protocol for recording these extra leads should be developed so that a consistent method is used to avoid confusion.

12. Connect the lead wires to the electrodes and record ECG. Correctly label the ECG tracings, noting the extra leads.
  A. Recording right precordial leads using a 12-lead ECG machine, connect as follows:
  ○ V_1 wire to electrode V_{1R},
  ○ V_2 wire to electrode V_{2R},
  ○ V_3 wire to electrode V_{3R},
  ○ V_4 wire to electrode V_{4R},
  ○ V_5 wire to electrode V_{5R}, and
  ○ V_6 wire to electrode V_{6R}.
  B. Recording left posterior leads using a 12-lead ECG machine, connect as follows:
  ○ V_4 wire to electrode V_7,
  ○ V_5 wire to electrode V_8, and
  ○ V_6 wire to electrode V_9.
	When the unipolar left precordial lead wires V_1 through V_6 are connected to the right precordial or left posterior electrodes, the ECG machine records signals from where the electrodes are placed.	Make notation on the ECG tracing that these are right precordial or RV leads. Change the labels on the ECG printouts. Change labels from V_1 to V_{1R}, V_2 to V_{2R}, V_3 to V_{3R}, V_4 to V_{4R}, V_5 to V_{5R} and V_6 to V_{6R}. Make a notation of "left posterior leads" and relabel appropriately on the ECG printouts. Change V_4 to V_7, V_5 to V_8, and V_6 to V_9. *(Note: Labels on the ECG printout depend on the connected lead wire and the location of the electrode.)*

13. Assess the quality of the tracing.	Ensures a clear tracing is obtained and no lead is off.	
14. Discard used supplies, and wash hands.	Reduces transmission of microorganisms; standard precautions.	

Expected Outcomes	Unexpected Outcomes
• Clean and accurate recording of ECG tracings allows clinicians to diagnose dysrhythmias and ischemia.	• Inaccurate lead placement: Electrode misplacement or incorrect lead connection. An accurate ECG interpretation is possible only when the recording electrodes are placed in the accurate positions on the body surface.
• Institutional protocol should be developed for recording the extra posterior and RV ECG leads according to the availability and type of the ECG machine so that the recording method is consistent.	• Failure to identify the recordings as either right precordial or left posterior ECGs and to change the ECG leads to their correct labels. This could lead to misdiagnosis.
	• Poor ECG tracing caused by electrical artifact either from external or internal sources. External artifact introduced by line current (60-cycle interference) may be minimized by disconnecting nearby electrical devices, unplugging the ECG machine and operating on battery, improving grounding, or replacing lead wires. Internal artifact may result from body movement, shivering, muscle tremors, and hiccups.

Patient Monitoring and Care

Patient Monitoring and Care	Rationale	Reportable Conditions
		These conditions should be reported if they persist despite nursing interventions.
1. Evaluate the ECG recordings for acute RV or posterior myocardial ischemia or infarction (Fig. 52–6). Record whether patient has chest pain on the ECG tracing. Use 0 to 10 score to quantify pain severity (eg, "8/10 chest pain").	To promptly initiate appropriate interventions, such as reperfusion treatment or vasodilators.	• Any abnormal ST segment deviation (elevation or depression) indicative of acute myocardial ischemia or infarction
2. Assess presence of chest pain or anginal equivalent symptoms (eg, jaw, left shoulder or arm discomfort, or shortness of breath).	Ischemia caused by decreased coronary blood flow or increased myocardial oxygen demand may produce anginal symptoms.	• Anginal symptoms, but do not ignore acute ST segment changes in an asymptomatic patient because 80% to 90% of ischemic episodes are clinically "silent"

Continued on following page

Standard 12-Lead ECG   **Left Posterior Leads**

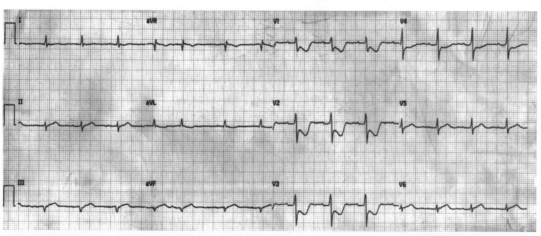 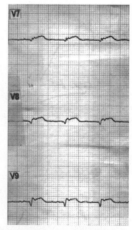

■ ● **FIGURE 52–6.** An ECG recorded in a 76-year-old diabetic patient during occlusion of the left circumflex artery. ST segment depression is observed in left precordial leads V$_{1-4}$, which suggests posterior MI (left panel). Left posterior leads V$_{7-9}$ are helpful in recording ST segment elevation that confirms posterior myocardial ischemia (right panel). Observing ST segment elevation in the contiguous posterior leads allows patients with acute MI to benefit from thrombolytic therapy that they would be denied from analysis of the standard 12-lead ECG alone.

Patient Monitoring and Care *Continued*

Patient Monitoring and Care	Rationale	Reportable Conditions
3. Check ECG for signs of AV node conduction disturbances in patients with RV infarction (eg, second or third degree AV block).	Right coronary artery (RCA) supplies blood to the AV node in 90% of patients. Occlusion of the RCA proximal to the RV branch decreases blood supply to the AV nodal artery. Incidence of high-degree AV block in inferior MI patients with RV involvement is significantly higher (48%) than in patients without RV MI (13%).[4]	• Acute MI patients with RV involvement, as evidenced by a QS pattern or ST segment elevation ≥ 1 mm in the right precordial leads[17]
Administration of atropine or isoproterenol could be used to maintain an adequate ventricular rate. Temporary external or transvenous pacing may be indicated.		
4. Assess hemodynamic status: Elevated mean atrial pressure, reduced cardiac output, hypotension, and prominent venous engorgement.	Hypotension and reduced cardiac output in patients with RV infarction could be attributed to inadequate left ventricular filling.[6]	• Cardiovascular and hemodynamic changes associated with RV infarction
In patients with RV infarction who exhibit shock, volume expansion is used to provide adequate left ventricular filling. Positive inotropic agents may also be indicated. Avoid use of vasodilators, such as nitroglycerin. Also avoid the use of diuretics such as furosemide (Lasix).	Volume expansion increases both the right and left ventricular filling pressures and restores arterial pressure and peripheral blood flow. Positive inotropic agents augment the contractile force of the residual functioning fibers in the damaged RV and increase right atrial contractile force. Vasodilators cause venous dilation and reduced preload. Diuretics reduce preload and left ventricular filling.[6]	• Changes in cardiovascular and hemodynamic status after intervention

Documentation

Documentation should include the following:

- Patient and family education
- The reason the extra leads are recorded (eg, suspected RV infarction, posterior MI
- Description of associated symptoms
- Interpretation of the ECGs recorded
- Interventions as indicated from the recorded ECG
- Occurrence of unexpected outcomes
- Additional interventions

References

1. Correale E, Battista R, Martone A, et al. Electrocardiographic patterns in acute inferior myocardial infarction with and without right ventricle involvement: classification, diagnostic and prognostic value, masking effect. *Clin Cardio.* 1999;22:37–44.
2. Madias J, Mahjoub M, Wijetilaka R. Standard 12-lead ECG versus special chest leads in the diagnosis of right ventricular myocardial infarction. *Am J Emerg Med.* 1997;15:89–90.
3. Croft C, Nicod P, Corbett J, et al. Detection of acute right ventricular infarction by right precordial electrocardiography. *Am J Cardiol.* 1982;50:421–427.
4. Bratt SH, de Zwaan C, Brugada P, et al. Right ventricular involvement with acute inferior wall myocardial infarction identifies high risk of developing atrioventricular nodal conduction disturbances. *Am Heart J.* 1984;107:1183–1187.
5. Bratt SH, Gorgels APM, Bar FW, et al. Value of the ST-T segment in lead V_{4R} in inferior wall acute myocardial infarction to predict the site of coronary arterial occlusion. *Am J Cardiol.* 1988;62:140–142.
6. Cohn JN, Guiha NH, Broder MI, et al. Right ventricular infarction: clinical and hemodynamic features. *Am J Cardiol.* 1974;33:209–214.
7. Brady W. Acute posterior wall myocardial infarction: electro-

cardiographic manifestations. *Am J Emerg Med.* 1998; 16:409–413.

8. Zalenski RJ, Rydman RJ, Sloan EP, et al. Value of posterior and right ventricular leads in comparison to the standard 12-lead electrocardiogram in evaluation of ST segment elevation in suspected acute myocardial infarction. *Am J Cardiol.* 1997;79:1579–1585.

9. Wung SF, Drew BJ. 18 lead ECG in the diagnosis of myocardial ischemia and its correlation to the culprit coronary artery. *Circulation.* 1998;(suppl)98: I-380.

10. Agarwal J, Khaw K, Aurignac F, et al. Importance of posterior chest leads in patients with suspected myocardial infarction, but nondiagnostic, routine 12-lead electrocaridogram. *Am J Cardiol.* 1999;83:323–326.

11. Casas RE, Marriott HJL, Glancy L. Value of leads V$_7$–V$_9$ in diagnosing posterior wall acute myocardial infarction and other causes of tall R waves in V$_1$–V$_2$. *Am J Cardiol.* 1997;80(4):508–509.

12. Drew BJ, Ide B. Importance of accurate lead placement. *Progress Cardiovasc Nurs.* 1994;Spring:44.

13. Adams MG, Drew BJ. Body positional effects on the ECG: implication for ischemia monitoring. *J Electrocardiol.* 1997;30:285–291.

14. Mirvis DM, Berson AS, Goldberger AL, et al. Instrumentation and practice standards for electrocardiographic monitoring in special care units. *Circulation.* 1989;79:464–471.

15. Haisty WK, Pahlm O, Wagner NB, et al. Performance of the automated complete Selvester QRS scoring system in normal subjects and patients with single and multiple myocardial infarction. *J Am Coll Cardiol.* 1992;19:341–346.

16. Drew BJ, Wung SF, Adams MG, et al. Bedside diagnosis of myocardial ischemia with ST segment monitoring technology: measurement issues for real-time clinical decision-making and trial designs. *J Electrocardiol.* 1998;30(suppl):157–165.

17. Funk M. Diagnosis of right ventricular infarction with right precordial ECG leads. *Heart Lung.* 1986;15:563–570.

18. Drew BJ, Ide B. Right ventricular infarction. *Progress Cardiovasc Nurs.* 1995;10:45–46.

19. Chow TC, Bel-Kahn JVD, Allen J, et al. Electrocardiographic diagnosis of right ventricular infarction. *Am J Med.* 1981;70:1175–1180.

20. Anderson HR, Nielsen DN, Hansen LG. The normal right chest electrocardiogram. *J Electrocardiol.* 1987;20:27–32.

Additional Readings

Kulkarni AU, Brown R, Ayoubi M, et al. Clinical use of posterior electrocardiographic leads: a prospective electrocardiographic analysis during coronary occlusion. *Am Heart J.* 1996;131:736–741.

Lopez-Sedon J, Coma-Canella I, Alcaswna S, et al. Electrocardiographic findings in acute right ventricular infarction: sensitivity and specificity of electrocardiographic alterations in right precordial leads V$_{4R}$, V$_{3R}$, V$_1$, V$_2$ and V$_3$. *J Am Coll Cardiol.* 1985;6:1273–1279.

Melendez LJ, Jones DT, Salcedo JR. Usefulness of three additional electrocardiographic chest leads (V$_7$, V$_8$, and V$_9$) in the diagnosis of acute myocardial infarction. *Can Med Assoc J.* 1978;119:745–748.

Perloff JK. The recognition of strictly posterior myocardial infarction by conventional scalar electrocardiography. *Circulation.* 1964;706–718.

Zalenski RJ, Cooke D, Rydman R, et al. Assessing the diagnostic value of an ECG containing leads V$_{4R}$, V$_8$, and V$_9$: the 15-lead ECG. *Ann Emerg Med.* 1993;22:786–793.

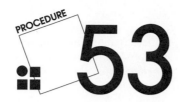

53

ST Segment Monitoring

P U R P O S E: Bedside ST segment monitoring is used to detect myocardial ischemia. This technology can be applied to patients who are diagnosed with acute coronary syndromes, including acute myocardial infarction (MI) and angina. For these patients, ST segment monitoring is valuable in determining the success of thrombolytic therapy or in detecting transient ischemia with unstable angina. This technology can also be used to detect abrupt reocclusion following transcatheter procedures (eg, angioplasty or stent).[1-6]

Michele M. Pelter
Mary G. Adams

PREREQUISITE NURSING KNOWLEDGE

- Understanding of the anatomy and physiology of the cardiovascular system, principles of cardiac conduction, ECG lead placement, basic dysrhythmia interpretation, and electrical safety is required.
- Advanced cardiac life support (ACLS) knowledge and skills are necessary.
- Myocardial ischemia has the following characteristics:[2-5]
  - ❖ It is associated with poor outcomes (ie, myocardial infarction and death).
  - ❖ It is a precursor to ventricular tachycardia.
  - ❖ It is transient or it can progress to infarction.
  - ❖ It is often not accompanied by chest pain (silent ischemia).
- ST segment monitoring may aid in the following:
  - ❖ Differentiation between the diagnosis of cardiac versus noncardiac chest pain
  - ❖ Detecton of silent myocardial ischemia.
  - ❖ Continuous evaluation of the patient's ECG, which is a more thorough method than periodic 12-lead ECGs because ischemia can be transient.
- Patients with left bundle branch block or pacemaker patterns may not be suitable for bedside ST segment monitoring. Left bundle branch block and pacemaker tracings may contribute to false positive alarms because of their distorted ST segments.
- A variety of bedside monitoring lead systems currently exist; however, not all bedside monitors are equipped with ST segment software.
- Lead-specific ST segment monitoring can be applied. The two most sensitive leads for detecting ischemia are leads V_3 and III.

EQUIPMENT

- Disposable electrodes
- Lead wires
- Bedside monitor with ST segment monitoring software capability
- Gauze pads or terry cloth washcloth
- Soap and water in basin
- Patient cable (should adapt to monitor and lead wires)
- ECG calipers
- Alcohol pads

Additional equipment to have available as needed includes the following:

- Skin preparation solution, such as skin barrier wipe, or tincture of benzoin, if needed
- Scissors
- Indelible marker

PATIENT AND FAMILY EDUCATION

- Explain the purpose of ST segment monitoring. ➥*Rationale:* Decreases patient and family anxiety.
- Encourage patient to report any symptoms of chest pain or anginal equivalent (eg, arm pain, jaw pain, shortness of breath, or nausea). ➥*Rationale:* Heightens patient's awareness of cardiac sensation and encourages communication of anginal pain.

PATIENT ASSESSMENT AND PREPARATION

Patient Assessment

- Identify medical history of cardiac risk factors, cardiac disease, and cardiac procedures. ➥*Rationale:* Identifies patients at risk for myocardial ischemia.
- Assess baseline cardiac rate and rhythm. ➥*Rationale:* Provides baseline data.
- Identify baseline ST segment levels before initiating ST segment monitoring. ➥*Rationale:* Identifies the patient's baseline ST segment level for comparison to subsequent changes.

349

Patient Preparation

• Ensure that the patient and family understand preprocedural teaching. Answer questions as they arise and reinforce information as needed.   ➡*Rationale:* Evaluates and reinforces understanding of previously taught information.

• Place patient in a resting supine position in bed and expose patient's torso while maintaining modesty.
  ➡*Rationale:* Eases access to chest for electrode placement.

Procedure **for ST Segment Monitoring**

Steps	Rationale	Special Considerations
1. Wash hands.	Reduces transmission of microorganisms; standard precautions.	
2. Identify accurate electrode placement (Fig. 53–1; see Procedures 51 and 54).	Ensures accurate ECG data.[7]	
3. Wash the skin with soap and water and dry it thoroughly, cleaning the area for the application of electrodes. (*Level IV: Limited clinical studies to support recommendations*)	Provides for adequate transmission of electrical impulses. Moist skin is not conducive to electrode adherence.[7-9]	It may be necessary to clip chest hair to ensure good skin contact with the electrode.
4. Clean the intended sites with alcohol pads. Consider using skin preparation solutions. (*Level IV: Limited clinical studies to support recommendations*)	Alcohol or skin preparations may be needed to remove oils, thus improving impulse transmission.[7-9]	
5. Abrade skin using a washcloth, scratch pad on electrode pack, or gauze pad.	Removes dead skin cells, promoting impulse transmission.	
6. If possible, mark any precordial location with a black indelible marker.	Prevents inaccurate electrode placement after bathing or inadvertent removal of the electrode.	Continuous ST segment monitoring trends depend on stable electrode placement. Sudden changes in ST segment trends often indicate electrode movement.
7. Connect ECG leads to electrodes before placing electrodes on the patient (see Procedure 51).	Prepares monitoring system.	

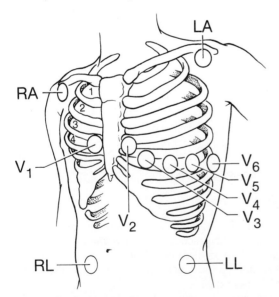

■ ● **FIGURE 53–1.** Correct lead placement for ST segment monitoring using continuous 12-lead monitoring. Limb electrodes must be located as close as possible to the junction to the limb and the torso. To diminish the impact of respirations on the tracing, it is especially important that the LL electrode be placed well below the level of the umbilicus. For V_1, the electrode is located at the fourth intercostal space to the right of the sternum. V_2 is in the same fourth intercostal space just to the left of the sternum, and V_4 in the fifth intercostal space on the midclavicular line. Placement of lead V_3 is halfway on a straight line between leads V_2 and V_4. Leads V_5 and V_6 are positioned on a straight line from V_4, with V_5 in the anterior axillary line and V_6 in the midaxillary line.

Procedure for ST Segment Monitoring

Steps	Rationale	Special Considerations
8. Select monitoring leads.	Any ECG lead can be used for ST segment monitoring.[10]	If continuous 12-lead ECG monitoring is unavailable, then lead-specific ischemia monitoring is encouraged. For example, lead III is sensitive to inferior ischemia and V_3 is sensitive to anterior or posterior ischemia.
9. If required by the bedside monitor manufacturer, identify the ECG complex landmarks.	Prepares monitoring system.	Refer to manufacturer's recommendations.
10. Set ST segment alarm threshold according to hospital policy.	Maximizes the sensitivity and specificity of ST segment monitoring and may reduce unnecessary false alarms.	The criteria for ischemia detection will vary from 1 mm of ST segment deviation (elevation or depression) in one ECG lead to 2 mm of ST segment deviation in two ECG leads (Fig. 53–2).
11. Print baseline ECG tracing to evaluate the quality of the signal and secure for future reference.	Ensures a quality baseline ECG for comparing subsequent changes because ST segment monitoring is based on continuous trending.	
12. If possible, obtain an ECG with the patient in both right and left side-lying positions and secure these for future reference.	Comparison of side-lying ECGs to ECGs from subsequent alarms may prevent false positive ST segment deviations caused by changes in body position from being interpreted as genuine ischemia.[11]	
13. Discard used supplies, and wash hands.	Reduces transmission of microorganisms; standard precautions.	

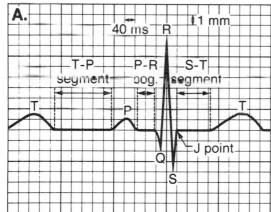
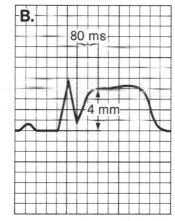
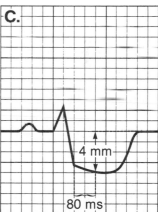

■ ● **FIGURE 53–2.** *A,* Normal electrocardiographic complex. Measurement points used in ST segment analysis are indicated. The PR segment is used to identify the isoelectric line. The ST segment begins at the J point, which is the end of the QRS complex. The ST segment measurement point can be measured at 60 or 80 ms past the J point. *B,* ST segment elevation. The ST segment shown measures +4 mm. The measurement point used is 80 ms past the J point. *C,* ST segment depression. The ST segment shown measures −4 mm. The measurement point used is 80 ms past the J point. (From Tisdale LA, Drew BJ. ST segment monitoring for myocardial ischemia. *AACN Clin Issues Crit Care Nurs.* 1993:4(1):36.)

- Accurate ECG monitoring that allows clinicians to interpret ST segment changes
- Detection and treatment of myocardial ischemia
- An increase in the number of bedside alarms when ST segment software is initiated. These may be caused by the following: (1) actual ischemia, (2) body position changes, (3) transient dysrhythmias, (4) heart rate changes, (5) noisy signal, or (6) lead misplacement.[12]

- Skin sensitivity to electrodes
- Undetected ST segment changes

Patient Monitoring and Care

Patient Monitoring and Care	Rationale	Reportable Conditions
		These conditions should be reported if they persist despite nursing interventions.
1. Confirm adequate electrode and lead wire placement every shift.	Enhances quality bedside ST segment monitoring.	
2. Evaluate ST segment trends routinely while obtaining vital signs.	Ensures that there are no significant deviations in the ST segment.	• Change in ST segment trends
3. Interpret all ST segment alarms and determine the cause (eg, ischemia, change in rhythm, dysrhythmia, noisy signal, lead misplacement, body position change).	Ensures accurate interpretation.	• ST segment elevation or depression

Documentation

Documentation should include the following:

- Patient and family education
- Initiation of ST segment bedside monitoring
- ECG leads selected for ST segment monitoring
- Alarm settings
- ST segment trending summary, ie, "no ST segment deviation seen in leads II or III"
- Presence and intensity of chest pain or anginal equivalent
- Unexpected outcomes
- Additional interventions taken

References

1. Dellborg M, Topol EJ, Swedberg K. Dynamic QRS complex and ST segment vector cardiographic monitoring can identify vessel patency in patients with acute myocardial infarction treated with reperfusion therapy. *Am Heart J.* 1991;122:943–948.
2. Drew BJ, Adams MG, Pelter MM, Wung SF: ST segment monitoring with a derived 12-lead electrocardiogram is superior to routine cardiac care unit monitoring. *Am J Crit Care.* 1996;5:198–206.
3. Gottlieb SO, Weisfeldt ML, Ouyang P, Mellitis ED, Gerstenblith G. Silent ischemia as a marker for early unfavorable outcomes in patients with unstable angina. *N Engl J Med.* 1986;314:1214–1218.
4. Krucoff MW, Parente AR, Bottner RK, et al. Stability of multi-lead ST-segment "fingerprints" over time after percutaneous transluminal coronary angioplasty and its usefulness in detecting reocclusion. *Am J Cardiol.* 1988;61:1232–1237.
5. Langer A, Freeman MR, Armstrong PW. ST segment shift in unstable angina: pathophysiology and association with coronary anatomy and hospital outcome. *J Am Coll Cardiol.* 1989;13:1495–1502.
6. Klootwijk P, Meij S, Greem C, Veldkamp RF, Ross AM, Armstrong PW. Non-invasive prediction of reperfusion and coronary artery patency by continuous ST segment monitoring in the GUSTO-I trial. *Eur Heart J.* 1996;17:689–698.
7. Drew BJ, Ide B, Sparacino P. Accuracy of bedside ECG monitoring: a report on the current practices of critical care nurses. *Heart Lung.* 1991;20:597–607.
8. Clochesy JM, Cifani L, Howe K. Electrode site preparation: A follow-up. *Heart Lung.* 1991;20:27–30.
9. Medina V, Clochesy JM, Omery A. Comparison of electrode site preparation techniques. *Heart Lung.* 1989;18:456–460.
10. Drew BJ, Tisdale LA. ST segment monitoring for coronary artery reocclusion following thrombolytic therapy and coronary angioplasty: identification of optimal bedside monitoring leads. *Am J Crit Care.* 1993;2:280–292.
11. Adams MG, Drew BJ. Body position effects on the ECG: implication for ischemia monitoring. *J Electrocardiol.* 1997;30:285–291.

12. Drew BJ, Wung SF, Adams MG, Pelter MM. Bedside diagnosis of myocardial ischemia with ST-segment monitoring technology: Measurement issues for real-time clinical decision making and trial design. *J Electrocardiol.* 1998; 30(suppl):157–165.

Additional Readings

Adams MG, Pelter MM, Wung SF, Taylor CA, Drew BJ. Frequency of silent myocardial ischemia with 12-lead ST segment monitoring in the coronary care unit: are there sex-related differences? *Heart Lung* 1999;28:81–86.

Amanullah AM, Lindvall K: Prevalence and significance of transient predominantly asymptomatic myocardial ischemia on Holter monitoring in unstable angina pectoris, and correlation with exercise test and thallium-201 myocardial perfusion imaging. *Am J Cardiol.* 1993;72:144–148.

Bush HS, Ferguson JJ, Angelini P, Willerson JT. Twelve-lead electrocardiographic evaluation of ischemia during percutaneous transluminal coronary angioplasty and its correlation with acute reocclusion. *Am Heart J.* 1990;121:1591–1599.

Currie P, Ashby D, Saltissi S. Prognostic significance of transient myocardial ischemia on ambulatory monitoring after acute myocardial infarction. *Am J Cardiol.* 1993;71:773–777.

Dellborg M, Gustafsson G, Riha M, Swedberg K. Dynamic changes of the QRS complex in unstable angina pectoris. *Int J Cardiol.* 1992;36:151–162.

Doevendans PA, Gorgels AP, van der Zee R, Partouns J, Bar FW, Wellens HJJ. Electrocardiographic diagnosis of reperfusion during thrombolytic therapy in acute myocardial infarction *Am J Cardiol.* 1995;75:1206–1210.

Drew BJ, Pelter MM, Adams MG, Wung SF, Chou TM, Wolfe CL. 12-lead ST segment monitoring vs single-lead maximum ST-segment monitoring for detecting ongoing ischemia in patients with unstable coronary syndromes. *Am J Crit Care.* 1998;7:355–363.

Drew BJ. Bedside ECG monitoring: state of the art for the 1990's. *Heart Lung.* 1991;20:610–623.

Drew BJ, Krucoff MW. Multilead ST-segment monitoring in patients with acute coronary syndromes: a consensus statement for healthcare professionals. ST-Segment Monitoring Practice Guideline International Working Group [Review]. *Am J Crit Care.* 1999;8:372–386.

Gottlieb SO, Weisfeldt ML, Ouyang P, Mellitis ED, Gerstenblith G. Silent ischemia predicts infarction and death during 2 year follow-up of unstable angina. *J Am Coll Cardiol.* 1987;10:756–760.

Krucoff MW, Croll MA, Pope JE, Granger CB, O'Connor CM, Sigmon KN. Continuous 12-lead ST-segment recovery analysis in the TAMI 7 study: performance of a non-invasive method for real-time detection of failed myocardial reperfusion. *Circulation.* 1993;88:437–446.

Larsson H, Jonasson T, Rinqvist I, Fellenius C, Wallentin L. Diagnostic and prognostic importance of ST recording after an episode of unstable angina or non-Q-wave myocardial infarction. *Eur Heart J.* 1992;13:207–212.

Mizutani M, Freedman SB, Barns E, Ogasawara S, Bailey BP, Bernstein L. ST monitoring for myocardial ischemia during and after coronary angioplasty. *Am J Cardiol.* 1990;66:389–393.

Wagner GS. Marriott's Practical Electrocardiology. Baltimore, MD: Williams & Wilkins; 1994.

54

Twelve-Lead Electrocardiogram

PURPOSE: A 12-lead electrocardiogram (ECG) provides information about the electrical system of the heart from 12 different views or leads. Common uses of a 12-lead ECG include diagnosis of acute coronary syndromes, identification of dysrhythmias, and determination of effects of medications or electrolytes on the heart's electrical system.

Mary G. McKinley

PREREQUISITE NURSING KNOWLEDGE

- Understanding of the anatomy and physiology of the cardiovascular system, principles of cardiac conduction, ECG lead placement, basic dysrhythmia interpretation, and electrical safety is required.
- Advanced cardiac life support (ACLS) knowledge and skills are necessary.
- Clinical and technical competence in the use of the 12-lead ECG machine and recorder is necessary.
- A 12-lead ECG provides different views or leads of the electrical activity of the heart. The leads are the standard limb leads (I, II, III), and the augmented limb leads (aVR, aVF, and aVL), and the six chest leads (V_1 to V_6).
- The standard and augmented leads view the heart from the vertical or frontal plane (Fig. 54–1), and the chest leads view the heart from the horizontal plane (Fig. 54–2).
- The graphic display consists of the P, Q, R, S, and T waves, which represent the electrical activity within the heart.
- Serial 12-lead ECGs (more that two ECGs recorded at

different times) may be obtained. The accuracy of interpretation relies on consistent electrode placement. Indelible markers may be used to identify the electrode locations to ensure that the same placement is used when serial ECGs are recorded.

EQUIPMENT

- 12-lead ECG machine and recorder
- Electrodes
- Gauze pads or terry cloth washcloth
- Soap and water in basin
- Patient cable and lead wires

Additional equipment to have available as needed includes the following:

- Alcohol pads
- Skin preparation solution such as skin barrier wipe or tincture of benzoin
- Indelible marker

PATIENT AND FAMILY EDUCATION

- Assess the readiness of the patient to learn. ➤*Rationale:* Anxiety and concerns of the patient and family may inhibit their ability to learn.

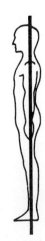

■ ● **FIGURE 54–1.** Vertical plane leads—I, II, III, aV$_R$, aV$_L$, aV$_F$.

■ ● **FIGURE 54–2.** Horizontal plane leads—V$_1$ to V$_6$.

- Provide explanations of the equipment and the procedure to both patient and family. ➤➤*Rationale:* Information may decrease anxiety.
- Emphasize that the patient should not talk but should relax, lie still, and breathe normally. ➤➤*Rationale:* Chest movement can distort the ECG picture.
- Reassure the patient and family that the 12-lead ECG will be reviewed and that any alterations or problems will be addressed. ➤➤*Rationale:* Patients and families need to be reassured that immediate care is available if it is needed.

PATIENT ASSESSMENT AND PREPARATION
Patient Assessment

- Assess peripheral pulses, vital signs, heart sounds, level of consciousness, lung sounds, neck vein distention, presence of chest pain or palpitations, and peripheral circulatory disorders (ie, clubbing, cyanosis, and dependent edema). ➤➤*Rationale:* Physical signs and symptoms will result from alterations in performance of the cardiovascular system.
- Assess history of cardiac dysrhythmias or cardiac problems. ➤➤*Rationale:* Provides baseline data.
- Assess previous 12-lead ECGs. ➤➤*Rationale:* Provides baseline data.

Patient Preparation

- Ensure that the patient and family understand preprocedural teaching. Answer questions as they arise and reinforce information as needed. ➤➤*Rationale:* Evaluates and reinforces understanding of previously taught information.
- Assist the patient to a supine position. ➤➤*Rationale:* Eases access to chest for electrode placement; changes in body position may affect the accuracy of the ECG recording.

Procedure for Twelve-Lead Electrocardiogram

Steps	Rationale	Special Considerations
1. Wash hands.	Reduces transmission of microorganisms; standard precautions.	
2. Check cable and lead wires for fraying, broken wires, or discoloration.	Detects conditions that will give an inaccurate ECG trace.	If equipment is damaged, obtain alternative equipment and notify biomedical engineer for repair.
3. Plug ECG machine into grounded alternating current (AC) wall outlet.	Maintains electrical safety.	
4. Turn ECG machine on.	Equipment may require warm-up time.	Follow manufacturer's recommendations.
5. Ensure that the patient is in the supine position, not touching the bedrails or foot board.	Provides adequate support for limbs so that muscle activity will be minimal. Touching the bedrails or foot board may increase the chance of distortion of the trace. Body position changes can cause alterations in the ECG trace.	The supine position is best, but Fowler or others may be used for comfort. If another position is clinically required, note the position on the tracing. ECGs should be recorded in the same position to ensure that changes are not caused by changes in body position.
6. Expose only the necessary parts of the patient's legs, arms, and chest.	Provides warmth, which reduces shivering.	Shivering may interfere with the recording.
7. Identify lead sites:	Ensures accuracy of lead placement.	Mark the sites with an indelible marker if serial ECGs are anticipated.
A. Limb leads (Fig. 54–3)	Promotes correct positioning of limb leads. Ensures an accurate tracing of the heart from a view in the vertical and frontal plane.	Limb leads should be placed in fleshy areas, and bony prominences should be avoided. The limb leads need to be placed equidistant from the heart and should be positioned in approximately the same place on each limb.

Procedure continued on following page

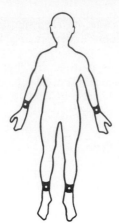

■ ● FIGURE 54–3. Limb lead placement in 12-lead electrocardiogram.

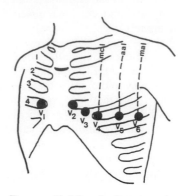

Precordial lead placement

■ ● FIGURE 54–4. Precordial lead placement.

Procedure	**for Twelve-Lead Electrocardiogram** *Continued*

Steps	Rationale	Special Considerations
B. Chest leads (Fig. 54–4), as follows: Identify the angle of Louis or the sternal notch; V_1 at the fourth intercostal space right sternal border; V_2 at the fourth intercostal space left sternal border; V_3 equidistant between V_2 and V_4; V_4 fifth intercostal space at the midclavicular line; V_5 horizontal level to V_4 at the anterior axillary line; V_6 horizontal level to V_4 at the midaxillary line.	Angle of Louis or sternal notch will assist with identifying the second rib for correct placement of precordial leads in appropriate intercostal space. Accurate placement ensures correct electrical tracing of the heart from the horizontal plane. Slight alterations in the position of any of the precordial leads may significantly alter the ECG and can have impact on diagnosis and treatment.[1]	
8. For pregelled electrodes, remove backing and test for moistness. For adhesive electrodes, remove backing and check the sticky, adhesive pad—it should be sticky.	Allows for appropriate conduction of impulses.	Gel must be moist. If pregelled electrodes are not moist or adhesive electrodes are not sticky, replace the electrode.
9. Apply electrodes securely.	Electrode must be secure to prevent external influences from affecting the ECG.	
10. Fasten lead wires to limb electrodes, avoiding bending or strain on wires, and use correct lead-to-electrode connection.	Provides for correct lead-to-limb connection.	
11. Identify multiple-channel machine recording setting (Fig. 54–5).	Multiple-channel machines will run three or more leads simultaneously and can be set to run leads in different configurations.	Obtain the tracing that is needed for the clinical situation.
12. Check the settings on the ECG machine: paper speed, 25 mm/s; sensitivity, 1 or 10 mm/s; baseline at center.	Ensures an accurate trace within standard limits for proper interpretation.	Manufacturers provide a calibration check in the machine to identify the sensitivity setting. Most machines have automatic settings that do this.

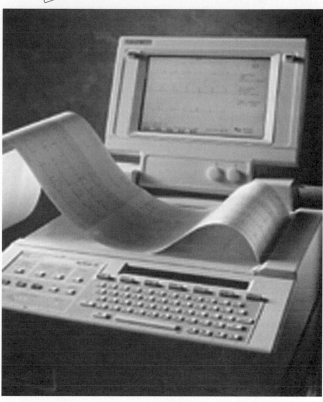

■ ● **FIGURE 54–5.** Multiple channel machine. (From Hewlett-Packard.)

Procedure for **Twelve-Lead Electrocardiogram** *Continued*

Steps	Rationale	Special Considerations
13. Turn on the recorder. Most systems record each lead for 3 to 6 seconds and automatically mark the correct lead.	The ECG must be accurately marked and have a clear baseline without artifact for correct interpretation. Three to six seconds is all that is needed for permanent record; more may be obtained on a rhythm strip. A rhythm strip is a long recording of a lead. Lead II is commonly used.	
14. Record the chest leads as above. *Note:* A multiple-channel machine may run the limb and chest leads simultaneously.	The chest leads may be set up and done automatically by the machine. Tracing should be free of respiratory artifact.	Respiratory artifact can be common in doing the chest leads and may require position changes to ensure a good baseline. If sequential ECGs are to be obtained, chest lead sites should be marked to ensure that the same lead sites will be used in subsequent ECGs.
15. Examine the tracing to see if it is clear, and repeat the ECG if it is not.	While the patient is still connected to the machine, the nurse should examine the ECG to see if any leads of the entire ECG need to be repeated.	
16. Interpret the recording for rhythm, rate, presence and configuration of P waves, length of PR interval, length of QRS complex, configuration and deviation of the ST segment, presence and configuration of T waves, length of QT interval, presence of extra waves (such as U waves), and identification of dysrhythmias.	Reviews the normal conduction sequence and identifies abnormalities that may require further evaluation or treatment.	

Procedure continued on following page

| Procedure | **for Twelve-Lead Electrocardiogram** *Continued* |

Steps	Rationale	Special Considerations
17. Evaluate ECG for any signs of ischemia, injury, or infarct as well as other significant myocardial alterations.	Identifies pathophysiologic processes that may require further evaluation or treatment.	
18. Disconnect the equipment, and clean the gel off the patient (if necessary) and prepare the equipment for future use.	Increases patient comfort.	
19. Discard used equipment, and wash hands.	Reduces transmission of microorganisms; standard precautions.	

Expected Outcomes	Unexpected Outcomes
• A clear 12-lead recording obtained (Fig. 54–6) • Prompt identification of abnormalities	• Altered skin integrity • Inaccurate lead placement or limb lead reversal (Fig. 54–7) • AC interference, also called 60-cycle interference (see Fig. 51–10) • Wandering baseline (see Fig. 51–11) • Artifact or waveform interference (see Fig. 51–12)

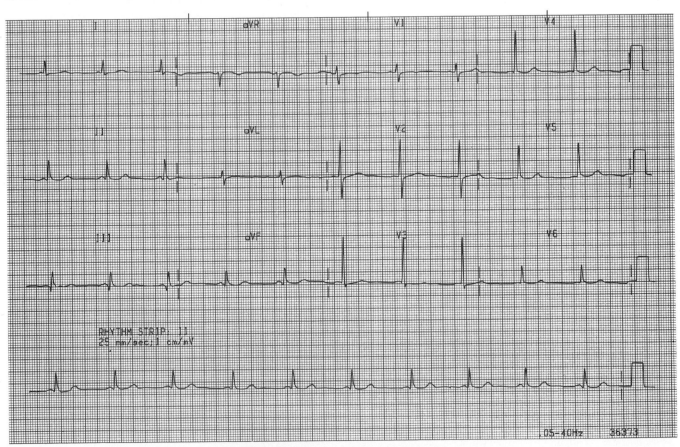

■ ● **FIGURE 54–6.** Clear 12-lead ECG recording.

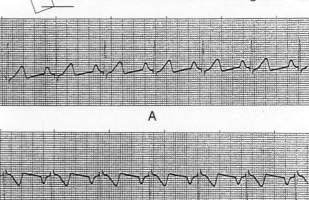

A

B

■ ● **FIGURE 54–7.** Limb lead reversal on 12-lead electrocardiogram in lead I. *A,* With correct placement. *B,* With incorrect placement.

Patient Monitoring and Care

Patient Monitoring and Care	Rationale	Reportable Conditions
		These conditions should be reported if they persist despite nursing interventions.
1. Obtain an ECG as prescribed and as needed (eg, for angina or dysrhythmias).	Provides determination of myocardial ischemia, injury, and infarction. Aids in diagnosis of dysrhythmias.	• Angina, dysrhythmias, or abnormal 12-lead ECG
2. Compare 12-lead ECG to previous ECGs.	Determines normal and abnormal findings.	• Any changes in the 12-lead ECG

Documentation

Documentation should include the following:

- Patient and family education
- The fact that a 12-lead ECG was obtained
- Reason for the 12-lead ECG
- Symptoms that the patient experienced, such as chest pain or palpitations
- Follow-up to the ECG, as indicated
- Unexpected outcomes
- Additional nursing interventions

Reference

1. Drew B. Bedside electrocardiographic monitoring. *AACN Clin Issues.* 1993;4:25–32.

Additional Readings

Abedin Z, Conner R. *12-Lead ECG Interpretation: The Self Assessment Approach.* Philadelphia, Pa: W.B. Saunders; 1989.

Alspach J. *Core Curriculum for Critical Care Nursing.* Philadelphia, Pa: W.B. Saunders; 1998.

Bucher L, Melander S. *Critical Care Nursing.* Philadelphia, Pa: W.B. Saunders; 1999.

Drew B, Adams M, Pelter M, Wung S. Bedside diagnosis of myocardial ischemia with ST segment monitoring technology: measurement for real time clinical decision making and trial designs. *J Electrocardiol.* 1998;30(suppl):157–165.

Drew B, Pelter M, Adams M, Wung S, Chou T, Wolfe C. 12 lead ST-segment monitoring vs. single lead maximum ST-segment monitoring for detecting ongoing ischemia in patients with unstable coronary syndromes. *Am J Crit Care.* 1998;7:355–363.

Drew B, Pelter M, Adams M, Wung S, Caldwell M. Comparison of standard and derived 12 lead electrocardiogram for diagnosis of coronary angioplasty induced myocardial ischemia. *Am J Cardiol.* 1997;79:639–644.

Drew B, Tisdale L. ST segment monitoring for coronary artery reocclusion following thrombolytic therapy and coronary angioplasty: identification of optimal bedside monitoring leads. *Am J Crit Care.* 1993;2:280–292.

Drew B, Adams M, Pelter M, Wung S. ST segment monitoring with a derived 12-lead electrocardiogram is superior to routine cardiac care unit monitoring. *Am J Crit Care.* 1996; 5:198–206.

Drew B. Bedside electrocardiographic monitoring: state of the art for the 90's. *Heart Lung.* 1991;20:610–662.

Drew B, Ide B, Sparacino P. Accuracy of bedside ECG monitoring: a report on current practices of critical care nurses. *Heart Lung.* 1991;20:597–609.

Finefrock S. Continuous 12 lead ST segment monitoring. *J Emerg Nurs.* 1995;21:413–416.

Hartshorn J, Sole M, Lamborn M. *Introduction to Critical Care Nursing.* Philadelphia, Pa: W.B. Saunders; 1997:37–85.

Morton P. Using 12 lead to detect ischemia, injury or infarct. *Crit Care Nurse.* 1996;16:85–94.

Thomason T, Riegel B, Carlson B, Gocka I. Monitoring electrocardiographic changes: results of a national survey. *J Cardiovasc Nurs.* 1995;9:1–9.

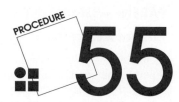

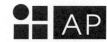

55

Arterial Catheter Insertion (Perform)

P U R P O S E: Arterial lines are used to continuously monitor blood pressure. They may be used to monitor the effects of vasoactive medications, for arterial administration of medications, for hemodynamic monitoring, and for frequent arterial blood gas and laboratory sampling.

Deborah E. Becker

PREREQUISITE NURSING KNOWLEDGE

- Knowledge of the anatomy and physiology of the vasculature and adjacent structures is important.
- Nurses must be adequately prepared to insert arterial catheters. This preparation should include specific educational content about arterial catheter insertion and opportunities to demonstrate clinical competency.
- Principles of hemodynamic monitoring should be understood.
- Clinical competence in suturing is necessary.
- Conditions that warrant the use of arterial pressure monitoring include patients with the following:
  - Acute hypotension or hypertension (hypertensive crisis)
  - Hemodynamic instability or circulatory collapse
  - Cardiac arrest
  - Hemorrhage
  - Shock from any cause
  - Continuous infusion of vasoactive medications
  - Frequent arterial blood gas measurements
  - Nonpulsatile blood flow (ie, those using nonpulsatile ventricular assist devices or receiving extracorporeal membrane oxygenation)
  - Intra-aortic balloon pump therapy
  - Neurologic injury
  - Coronary interventional procedures
  - Major surgical procedures
  - Multiple trauma
  - Respiratory failure
  - Sepsis
  - Obstetric emergencies

- Noninvasive, indirect blood pressure measurements determined by auscultation of Korotkoff sounds distal to an occluding cuff consistently average 10 to 20 mm Hg lower than simultaneous direct measurement.[1]
- Arterial waveform inspection can help rapidly diagnose the presence of valvular disorders, the effects of dysrhythmias on perfusion, the effects of the respiratory cycle on blood pressure, and the effects of intra-aortic balloon pumping or ventricular assist devices on blood pressure.
- The preferred artery for arterial catheter insertion is the radial artery (see Fig. 72–1). Though this artery is smaller than the ulnar artery, it is more superficial and can be more easily stabilized during the procedure.[2] Some research has found that the brachial artery is a safe and reliable alternative site for arterial puncture and line placement.[3]
- At times, the femoral artery may be used for arterial catheter insertion. The use of this artery can be technically difficult because of the proximity of the femoral artery to the femoral vein (see Fig. 72–2).
- The most common complications associated with arterial puncture include pain, vasospasm, hematoma formation, infection, hemorrhage, and neurovascular compromise.[3, 4, 5]
- Site selection is as follows:
  - Use the radial artery as first choice. Perform modified Allen test to determine patency of radial and ulnar arteries before performing arterial puncture (see Fig. 72–3). Normal palmar blushing is complete before 7 seconds, indicating a positive result; 8 to 14 seconds is considered equivocal; and 15 or more seconds indicates a negative test. Doppler flow studies or plethys-

---

AP This procedure should be performed only by physicians, advanced practice nurses, and other health care professionals (including critical care nurses) with additional knowledge, skills, and demonstrated competence per professional licensure or institutional standard.

mography can also be performed to ensure the presence of collateral flow. Research shows these studies to be more reliable than the Allen test.[6] Thrombosis of the arterial cannula is a common complication. Ensuring collateral flow distal to the puncture site is important for preventing ischemia.

❖ Use the brachial artery as the second choice, except in the presence of poor pulsation caused by shock, obesity, or a sclerotic vessel (eg, because of previous cardiac catheterization). The brachial artery is larger than the radial artery. Hemostasis after arterial cannulation is enhanced by its proximity to the bone if the entry point is approximately 1.5 inches above the antecubital fossa.

❖ Use the femoral artery in the case of cardiopulmonary arrest or altered perfusion to the upper extremities. The femoral artery is a large superficial artery located in the groin. It is easily palpated and punctured. Complications related to femoral artery puncture include hemorrhage and hematomas because bleeding can be difficult to control, inadvertent puncture of the femoral vein because of its close proximity to the artery, infection because aseptic technique is difficult to maintain in the groin area, and limb ischemia if the femoral artery is damaged.

EQUIPMENT

- 2-in, 20-G, nontapered Teflon cannula-over-needle or prepackaged kit with a 6-in, 18-G Teflon catheter with appropriate introducer and guide wire
- Hemodynamic monitoring system (see Procedure 69)
- Monitoring equipment consisting of a connecting cable, monitor, oscilloscope display screen, and recorder
- Nonsterile gloves and goggles

- Sterile gloves
- Alcohol pads on swabsticks
- Povidone-iodine pads or swabsticks
- Sterile 4 × 4 gauze pads
- Suture material
- 1% lidocaine without epinephrine, 1 mL to 2 mL
- 3-mL syringe with 25-G needle
- Chux
- Sterile towels
- 2-in tape

Additional supplies to have available as needed include the following:

- Bath towel
- Small wrist board

PATIENT AND FAMILY EDUCATION

- Explain the procedure and reason for arterial line insertion. ➥*Rationale:* Decreases patient and family anxiety.
- Explain to the patient that the procedure may be uncomfortable but that a local anesthetic will be used first to alleviate most of the discomfort. ➥*Rationale:* Elicits patient cooperation and facilitates insertion.
- Explain patient's role in assisting with insertion. ➥*Rationale:* Elicits patient cooperation and facilitates insertion.
- Tell patient about potential complications and how they

can be prevented. ➥*Rationale:* Fully informs patient of complications as well as alleviates anxiety.

PATIENT ASSESSMENT AND INTERVENTION
Patient Assessment

- Obtain medical history including history of diabetes, hypertension, peripheral vascular disease, vascular grafts, arterial vasospasm, thrombosis, or embolism. Obtain history of prior coronary artery bypass graft surgery in which radial arteries were removed for use as conduits. ➥*Rationale:* Extremities with any of the above problems should be avoided as sites for cannulation because of their potential for complications. Patients with diabetes mellitus or hypertension are at higher risk of arterial or venous insufficiency. Previously removed radial arteries are a contraindication for ulnar artery cannulation.
- Assess medical history of coagulopathies, use of anticoagulants, vascular abnormalities, or peripheral neuropathies. ➥*Rationale:* Assists in determining safety of procedure and aids in site selection.
- Assess allergy history (eg, allergy to lidocaine, EMLA cream, antiseptic solutions, or tape). ➥*Rationale:* Decreases the risk of allergic reactions.
- Presence of collateral flow to the area distal to the arterial catheter should be evaluated before cannulating the artery. For radial or ulnar arterial lines, a modified Allen test should be performed. ➥*Rationale:* Ensures presence of collateral flow to the hand to reduce complications.
- Assess the intended insertion site for the presence of a strong pulse. ➥*Rationale:* Identification and localization of the pulse increases the chance of a successful arterial cannulation.

Patient Preparation

- Ensure that the patient and family understand preprocedural teaching. Answer questions as they arise and reinforce information as needed. ➥*Rationale:* Evaluates and reinforces understanding of previously taught information.
- Obtain informed consent. ➥*Rationale:* Protects the rights of the patient and makes competent decision possible for the patient; however, under emergency circumstances, time may not allow form to be signed.
- Place patient supine in the bed with the limb that the arterial catheter will be inserted into resting comfortably on the bed. ➥*Rationale:* Provides patient comfort and facilitates insertion.
- Place a towel under the back of the wrist to hyperextend the wrist and tape it in place (if the radial artery is being used). ➥*Rationale:* Positions arm and brings the artery closer to the surface.
- Elevate and hyperextend the patient's arm. Support the arm with a pillow (when using the brachial artery). ➥*Rationale:* Increases accessibility of artery.
- When using the femoral artery, position patient supine with the leg straight. ➥*Rationale:* Provides best position for localizing the femoral artery pulse.

Procedure for Performing Arterial Catheter Insertion

Steps	Rationale	Special Considerations
1. Wash hands.	Reduces transmission of microorganisms; standard precautions.	
2. If the radial artery is to be used, perform the modified Allen test before arterial catheter insertion (see Fig. 72–3). *(Level II: Theory based, no research data to support recommendations; recommendations from expert consensus group may exist)*	The modified Allen test is recommended before a radial artery puncture to assess the patency of the ulnar artery and to assess for an intact superficial palmar arch.[2, 4, 7, 8]	
A. With the patient's hand held overhead, instruct the patient to open and close his or her hand several times.	Forces the blood from the hand.	If the patient is unconscious or unable to perform the procedure, clench the fist passively for the patient.
B. With the patient's fist clenched, apply direct pressure on the radial and ulnar arteries.	Obstructs the flow of blood to the hand.	
C. Instruct the patient to lower and open his or her hand.	Observe for pallor.	Performed passively if the patient is unconscious or unable to assist.
D. Release the pressure over the ulnar artery and observe the hand for the return of color.[4, 8]	Return of color within 7 seconds indicates patency of the ulnar artery and an intact superficial palmar arch and is interpreted as a positive Allen test. If color returns between 8 and 14 seconds, the test is considered equivocal. If it takes 15 or more seconds for color to return, the test is considered a negative test.	If the test is negative, the modified Allen test should be performed on the opposite hand.
3. Wash hands, and don goggles and gloves.	Reduces transmission of microorganisms; minimizes splash; standard precautions.	
4. Prepare site, beginning with the alcohol. Starting at the insertion site, cleanse outward, using a circular motion while applying friction. Repeat. Continue cleansing in a similar fashion using povidone-iodine.	Limits the introduction of potentially infectious skin flora into the vessel during the puncture. Combination of cleansing solutions enhances the antibacterial and antifungal actions of the agents.	The povidone-iodine solution should not be removed. Drying is not necessary. Application time is the chemical kill.
5. Change to sterile gloves.	Reduces the transmission of microorganisms; standard precautions.	
6. Drape area around the site with sterile towels.	Provides a sterile field and minimizes transmission of organisms.	
7. Locally anesthetize the puncture site. *(Level IV: Limited clinical studies to support recommendations)*	Provides local anesthesia for arterial puncture.	It has been reported that most patients experience pain during arterial puncture.[8]
A. Use a 1-mL syringe with a 25-G needle to draw up 0.5 mL 1% lidocaine without epinephrine.	Minimizes vessel trauma. Absence of epinephrine decreases the risk of peripheral vasoconstriction.	Recent research, exploring the efficacy of lidocaine ointment and EMLA cream as alternatives to intradermal lidocaine, shows promising results.[9–11] If used, the manufacturer's recommendations should be followed. *Procedure continued on following page*

Steps	Rationale	Special Considerations
B. Aspirate before injecting the local anesthetic.	Determines whether or not a blood vessel has been inadvertently entered.	
C. Inject intradermally and then with full infiltration around the intended arterial insertion site. Use approximately 0.2 to 0.3 mL for an adult.	Decreases the incidence of localized pain while injecting all skin layers. Most patients reported a reduction in pain when a local, intradermal anesthetic agent was used before arterial puncture.[8]	
8. Perform percutaneous puncture of the selected artery.		
A. Palpate and stabilize the artery with the index and middle fingers of the nondominant hand.	Increases the likelihood of correctly locating the artery and decreases the chance of the vessel rolling.	
B. With the needle bevel up and the syringe at a 30- to 60-degree angle to the radial or brachial artery, puncture the skin slowly. Adjust the angle to a 60- to 90-degree angle to the femoral artery.	A slow, gradual thrust promotes entry into the artery without inadvertently passing through the posterior wall.	
9. Advance the needle and the cannula until blood return is noted in the hub, then slowly advance the catheter about ¼ to ½ in farther to ensure that the cannula is in the artery.	Advancing the cannula further ensures that the entire cannula is in the artery and not just the tip of the stylet.	
10. Level the catheter to the skin, then continue to advance the cannula to its hub with a firm, steady, rotary action.	The rotary action helps to advance the catheter through the skin.	
11. Correct postioning is confirmed by the presence of pulsatile blood return on removal of the stylet.	Arterial blood is pulsatile, which confirms intra-arterial placement.	
12. Once positioning is confirmed, remove the stylet and connect the catheter to the hemodynamic monitoring system.	Maintains catheter patency and monitors arterial blood pressure.	
13. Zero the monitoring system and activate the alarm system (see Procedure 56).	Prepares monitoring system; provides notification of abnormal blood pressure parameters and system disconnections.	
14. Suture the arterial catheter in place.	Maintains arterial line positioning; reduces chance of accidental dislodgment.	
15. Apply dry sterile dressing and label insertion information.	Provides sterile environment; reduces infection.	
16. Discard used supplies; dispose of needles and other sharp objects in appropriate containers; wash hands.	Safely removes sharp objects; reduces the transmission of microorganisms; standard precautions.	

Expected Outcomes	Unexpected Outcomes
• Successful cannulation of the artery	• Pain or severe discomfort during insertion procedure
• Ability to obtain blood samples from the arterial line	• Complications of puncture or vasospasm
• Neurovascular system intact	• Complications after puncture, such as the following: change in color, temperature, or sensation of extremity used for insertion; or hematoma, hemorrhage, infection, or clot at insertion site
• Alterations in hemodynamic stability identified and treated accordingly	• Inability to cannulate the artery

Patient Monitoring and Care

Patient Monitoring and Care	Rationale	Reportable Conditions
		These conditions should be reported if they persist despite nursing interventions.
1. Observe insertion site for signs of hemostasis after procedure.	Postinsertion bleeding can occur in any patient but is more likely to occur in patients with coagulopathies or patients receiving anticoagulation therapy.	• Excessive bleeding, hematoma • Changes in vital signs
2. Assess the arterial catheter insertion site and involved extremity for signs of postinsertion complications.	Arterial catheter insertion can result in neurovascular compromsie of the extremity distal to the puncture site.	• Changes in color, size, temperature, sensation, or movement in the extremity used for arterial catheter insertion
3. Monitor arterial catheter insertion site for signs of local infection.	Infection related to the procedure may result from failure to maintain asepsis during insertion. Use of the femoral site for arterial line insertion may be related to an increased incidence of local infection.	• Erythema, warmth, hardness, tenderness, or pain at arterial line insertion site • Presence of purulent drainage from arterial line insertion site

Documentation

Documentation should include the following:

- Patient and family education
- Performance of the Allen test before insertion and its results (when using radial artery)
- Arterial site used
- Insertion of arterial line (date, time, and initials should go on the dressing itself)
- Size of cannula-over-needle catheter used
- Any difficulties in insertion
- Patient tolerance
- Appearance of site
- Appearance of limb, capillary refill time, and temperature of extremity after insertion is complete
- Occurrence of unexpected outcomes
- Nursing interventions taken

References

1. Venus B, Mathru M, Smith R. Direct versus indirect blood pressure measurements in the critically ill patients. *Heart Lung.* 1985;14:228–231.
2. Hadaway LC. Anatomy and physiology related to intravenous therapy. In: Terry J, Baranowski L, Lonsway RA, Hedric C, eds. *Intravenous Therapy: Clinical Principles and Practice.* Philadelphia, Pa: W.B. Saunders; 1995:97.
3. Okeson GC, Wulbrecht PH. The safety of brachial artery puncture for arterial blood sampling. *Chest.* 1998;114:748–751.
4. Buffington S. Specimen collection and testing. In: *Nursing Procedures.* 2nd ed. Springhouse, Pa: Springhouse Corp; 1996:145–147.
5. Giner J, Casan P, Belda J, Gonzalez M, Miralda R, Sanchis J. Pain during arterial puncture. *Chest.* 1996;110:1443–1445.

▪▪ AP   This procedure should be performed only by physicians, advanced practice nurses, and other health care professionals (including critical care nurses) with additional knowledge, skills, and demonstrated competence per professional licensure or institutional standard.

6. Qvist J, Peterfreund R, Perlmutter G. Transient compartment syndrome of the forearm after attempted radial artery cannulation. *Anesth Analogs.* 1996;83:183–185.

7. Perucca R. Obtaining vascular access. In: Terry J, Baranowski L, Lonsway RA, Hedric C, eds. *Intravenous Therapy: Clinical Principles and Practice.* Philadelphia, Pa: W.B. Saunders; 1995:386.

8. Cummins RO, ed. *Advanced Cardiac Life Support.* Dallas, Tex: American Heart Association; 1997:13.9–13.10.

9. Hussey VM, Poulin MV, Fain JA. Effectiveness of lidocaine hydrochloride on venipuncture sites. *AORN J.* 1997;66:472–475.

10. Lander J, Nazarali S, Hodgins M, Friesen E, McTavish J, Ouellette J, et al: Evaluation of a new topical anesthetic agent: a pilot study. *Nurs Res.* 1996;45:50–52.

11. Nott M, Peacock J. Relief of injection pain in adults: EMLA cream for 5 minutes before venipuncture. *Anaesthesia.* 1990;45:772–774.

Additional Readings

Imperial-Perez F, McRae M. *Protocols for Practice: Hemodynamic Monitoring Series—Arterial Pressure Monitoring.* Aliso Viejo, Calif: American Association of Critical-Care Nurses; 1998.

Riker J. Vascular complications after femoral artery catheterization in burn patients. *J Trauma.* 1996;41:904–905.

Seneff M. Arterial line placement and care. In: Irwin RS, Rippe JM, Cerra FB, Curley FJ, Heard SO. *Procedures and Techniques in Intensive Care Medicine.* 2nd ed. Philadelphia: Lippincott Williams & Wilkins; 1999:36–46

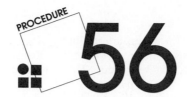

56

Arterial Catheter Insertion (Assist), Care, and Removal

P U R P O S E: Arterial pressure lines are used to continuously monitor blood pressure, to titrate vasoactive agents, and to obtain serial blood gases or other laboratory specimens in critically ill patients.

Rose B. Shaffer

PREREQUISITE NURSING KNOWLEDGE

- Knowledge of the anatomy and physiology of the vasculature and adjacent structures is important.
- Principles of hemodynamic monitoring should be understood.
- Conditions that warrant the use of arterial pressure monitoring include patients with the following:
  ❖ Acute hypotension or hypertension (hypertensive crisis)
  ❖ Hemodynamic instability or circulatory collapse
  ❖ Cardiac arrest
  ❖ Hemorrhage
  ❖ Shock from any cause
  ❖ Continuous infusion of vasoactive medications
  ❖ Frequent arterial blood gas measurements
  ❖ Nonpulsatile blood flow (ie, those using ventricular assist devices or receiving extracorporeal membrane oxygenation)
  ❖ Intra-aortic balloon pump therapy
  ❖ Neurologic injury
  ❖ Coronary interventional procedures
  ❖ Major surgical procedures
  ❖ Multiple trauma
  ❖ Respiratory failure
  ❖ Sepsis
  ❖ Obstetric emergencies
- Arterial pressure represents the forcible ejection of blood from the left ventricle into the aorta and out into the arterial system. During ventricular systole, blood is ejected into the aorta, generating a pressure wave. Because of the intermittent pumping action of the heart, this arterial pressure wave is generated in a pulsatile manner (Fig. 56–1). The ascending limb of the aortic pressure wave (anacrotic limb) represents an increase in pressure because of left ventricular ejection. The peak of this ejection is the peak systolic pressure, which is normally 100 to 140 mm Hg in adults. After reaching this peak, the ventricular pressure declines to a level below aortic pressure, and the aortic valve closes, marking the end of

ventricular systole. The closure of the aortic valve produces a small rebound wave that creates a notch known as the *dicrotic notch*. The descending limb of the curve (diastolic downslope) represents diastole and is characterized by a long declining pressure wave, during which the aortic wall recoils and propels blood into the arterial network. The diastolic pressure is measured as the lowest point of the diastolic downslope and is normally 60 to 80 mm Hg.

- The difference between the systolic and diastolic pressures is called the *pulse pressure*, with a normal value of 40 mm Hg.
- Arterial pressure is determined by the relationship between blood flow through the vessels (*cardiac output*) and the resistance of the vessel walls (*systemic vascular resistance*). The arterial pressure is therefore affected by

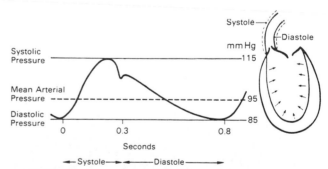

■ ● FIGURE 56–1. The generation of a pulsatile waveform. This is an aortic pressure curve. During systole, the ejected volume distends the aorta and aortic pressure rises. The peak pressure is known as the *aortic systolic pressure*. After the peak ejection, the ventricular pressure falls, and when it drops below the aortic pressure, the aortic valve closes, which is marked by the dicrotic notch, the end of the systole. During diastole, the pressure continues to decline and the aortic wall recoils, pushing the blood toward the periphery. The trough of the pressure wave is the *diastolic pressure*. The difference between systolic and diastolic pressure is the *pulse pressure*. (From Smith JJ, Kampine JP. *Circulatory Physiology*. Baltimore, Md: Williams & Wilkins; 1980:55.)

any factors that change either cardiac output or systemic vascular resistance.

- The average arterial pressure during a cardiac cycle is called the *mean arterial pressure* (MAP). It is not the average of the systolic plus the diastolic pressures because during the cardiac cycle, the pressure remains closer to diastole for a longer period than to systole (at normal heart rates). The MAP is calculated automatically by most patient monitoring systems; however, it can be calculated roughly by using the following formula:

$$MAP = \frac{(systolic\ pressure) + (diastolic\ pressure \times 2)}{3}$$

- MAP represents the driving force (perfusion pressure) for blood flow through the cardiovascular system. MAP is at its highest point in the aorta. As blood travels through the circulatory system, systolic pressure increases and diastolic pressure decreases, with an overall decline in the MAP (Fig. 56–2).
- The location of the arterial catheter depends on the patient's age, the condition of the arterial vessels, and the presence of other catheters (ie, the presence of a dialysis shunt is a contraindication for placing an arterial catheter in the same extremity). Once inserted, the arterial catheter causes little or no discomfort to the patient and allows continuous blood pressure assessment and intermittent blood sampling. If intra-aortic balloon pump therapy is required, arterial pressure may be directly monitored from the tip of the balloon in the aorta.

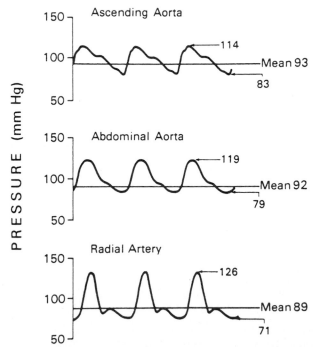

■ ● FIGURE 56–2. Arterial pressure from different sites in arterial tree. The arterial pressure waveform will vary in configuration depending on the location of the catheter. With transmission of the pressure wave into the distal aorta and large arteries, the systolic pressure increases and the diastolic pressure decreases; with a resulting heightening of the pulse, pressure declines steadily. (From Smith JJ, Kampine JP. *Circulatory Physiology*. Baltimore, Md: Williams & Wilkins; 1980: 57.)

- When arterial pulse waveforms are recorded from sites distal to the aorta, changes in the arterial waveforms often occur. The anacrotic limb becomes more peaked and narrowed, with increased amplitude; therefore, the systolic pressure in distal sites is higher than the systolic pressure recorded from a more central site (see Fig. 56–2). The diastolic downslope may demonstrate a secondary wave, and the dicrotic notch becomes less prominent from distal sites.
- There are several potential complications associated with arterial pressure monitoring. Infection at the insertion site can develop and cause sepsis. Clot formation in the catheter can lead to arterial embolization. The catheter can cause vessel perforation with extravasation of blood and flush solution into the tissues. Lastly, the distal extremity can develop circulatory or neurologic impairment.

EQUIPMENT

- 10% povidone-iodine solution
- Alcohol pads or swab-sticks
- 1% lidocaine solution without epinephrine
- 10-mL syringe with an 18-G and a 22-G needle
- 3-mL syringe with a 25-G needle
- Chux
- Sterile towels
- 1- to 2-in (2.5- to 5-cm) over-the-needle catheter (14- 18-G for adults)
- Sterile 4 × 4 gauze pads
- Tape
- Hemodynamic monitoring system: pressure device, flush bag, pressurized tubing, transducer, monitor cable, and monitor (see Procedure 69)
- Nonsterile gloves, sterile gloves, and goggles
- Suture materials

Additional equipment to have available as needed includes the following:

- Arm board
- Transparent dressing
- Bath towel

PATIENT AND FAMILY EDUCATION

- Assess patient and family understanding of the reason for arterial line insertion, including how the arterial pressure is displayed on the bedside monitor.   ➤*Rationale:* Decreases patient and family anxiety.
- Explain the standard of care to the patient and family, including insertion procedure, alarms, dressings, potential need for immobility of affected extremity, and length of time catheter is expected to be in place.   ➤*Rationale:* Encourages patient and family to ask questions and voice concerns about the procedure.
- Explain the patient's expected participation during the procedure.   ➤*Rationale:* Encourages patient cooperation during insertion.
- Explain the importance of keeping the affected extremity immobile.   ➤*Rationale:* Encourages patient compliance to prevent catheter dislodgment and ensures more accurate waveform.
- Instruct the patient to report any warmth, redness, pain, or wet feeling at the insertion site at any time, including

after catheter removal.   ➡*Rationale:* May indicate infection, bleeding, or disconnection of the tubing.

PATIENT ASSESSMENT AND PREPARATION
Patient Assessment

- Obtain medical history, including diabetes, hypertension, peripheral vascular disease, vascular grafts, arterial vasospasm, thrombosis, or embolism. Obtain history of prior coronary artery bypass graft surgery in which radial arteries were removed for use as conduits.   ➡*Rationale:* Extremities with any of these problems should be avoided as sites for cannulation because of their potential for complications. Patients with diabetes mellitus or hypertension are at higher risk of arterial or venous insufficiency. Previously removed radial arteries arc a contraindication for ulnar artery cannulation.
- Obtain specific neurovascular and peripheral vascular assessment of the extremity to be used for arterial cannulation, including assessment of color, temperature, presence and fullness of pulses, capillary refill, and motor and sensory function (as compared with opposite extremity). *Note*: A modified Allen test is performed before cannulation of a radial or ulnar artery (see Fig. 72–3).   ➡*Rationale:* Identifies any circulatory or neurologic impairment before cannulation to avoid potential complications.

Patient Preparation

- Ensure that the patient and family understand preprocedural teaching. Answer questions as they arise and reinforce information as needed.   ➡*Rationale:* Evaluates and reinforces understanding of previously taught information.
- Ensure that informed consent was obtained.   ➡*Rationale:* Protects rights of patient and makes competent decision possible for the patient; however, under emergency circumstances, time may not allow form to be signed.
- Place the patient's extremity in the appropriate position with adequate lighting of insertion site.   ➡*Rationale:* Prepares site for cannulation and facilitates accurate insertion.

Procedure **for Assisting with Insertion, Care and Removal of Arterial Pressure Lines**

Steps	Rationale	Special Considerations
1. Wash hands.	Reduces transmission of microorganisms; standard precautions.	
2. If catheter is to be inserted in the radial or ulnar artery, perform a modified Allen's test (see Fig. 72–3). *(Level II: Theory based, no research data to support recommendations; recommendations from expert consensus group may exist)*	Ensures adequacy of collateral blood flow of upper extremity to be cannulated.[1-5]	

Procedure continued on page 371

When the fast flush of the continuous flush system is activated and quickly released, a sharp upstroke terminates in a flat line at the maximal indicator on the monitor and hard copy. This is then followed by an immediate rapid downstroke extending below baseline with just 1 or 2 oscillations within 0.12 seconds (minimal ringing) and a quick return to baseline. The patient's pressure waveform is also clearly defined with all components of the waveform, such as the dicrotic notch on an arterial waveform, clearly visible.

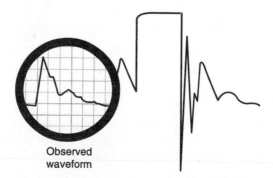

Square wave test configuration

Observed waveform

■ ● **FIGURE 56–3A.** Optimally damped system. Dynamic response test (square wave test) using the fast flush system normal response. (Fig. 56–3 from Darovic GO, Vanriper S, Vanriper J. Fluid-filled monitoring systems. In: Darovic GO. *Hemodynamic Monitoring.* 2nd ed. Philadelphia, Pa: WB Saunders; 1995:161–162.)

Intervention

There is no adjustment in the monitoring system required.

The upstroke of the square wave appears somewhat slurred, the waveform does not extend below the baseline after the fast flush and there is no ringing after the flush. The patient's waveform displays a falsely decreased systolic pressure and false high diastolic pressure as well as poorly defined components of the pressure tracing such as a diminished or absent dicrotic notch on arterial waveforms.

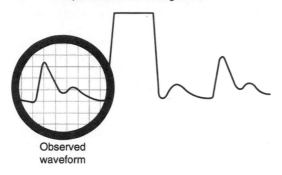

Square wave test configuration

Observed
waveform

Intervention

To correct for the problem:
1. Check for the presence of blood clots, blood left in the catheter following blood sampling, or air bubbles at any point from the catheter tip to the transducer diaphragm and eliminate these as necessary.
2. Use low compliance (rigid), short (less than 3 to 4 feet) monitoring tubing.
3. Connect all line components securely.
4. Check for kinks in the line.

■ ● **FIGURE 56–3B.** Overdamped system. Dynamic response test (square wave test) using the fast flush system damped response.

The waveform is characterized by numerous amplified oscillations above and below the baseline following the fast flush. The monitored pressure wave displays false high systolic pressures (overshoot), possibly false low diastolic pressures, and "ringing" artifacts on the waveform.

Square wave test configuration

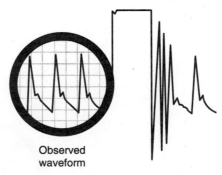

Observed
waveform

■ ● **FIGURE 56–3C.** Underdamped system. Dynamic response test (square wave test) using the fast flush system underdamped response.

Intervention

To correct the problem, remove all air bubbles (particularly pinpoint air bubbles) in the fluid system, use large-bore, shorter tubing, or use a damping device.

Procedure **for Assisting with Insertion, Care, and Removal of Arterial Pressure Lines**
Continued

Steps	Rationale	Special Considerations
3. When preparing flush bag, mix solution of heparinized saline if heparin use is not contraindicated. *(Level V: Clinical studies in more than one or two different patient populations and situations to support recommendations)* *Note:* Do not use heparinized dextrose solutions. *(Level VI: Clinical studies in a variety of patient populations and situations to support recommendations)*	Catheters flushed with heparinized saline are more likely than those flushed with nonheparinized saline to remain patent up to 72 hours.[6, 7] Use of heparin is contraindicated in patients with heparin-induced thrombocytopenia or heparin allergy. Dextrose supports the growth of microorganisms. These solutions have been associated with infection.[8, 9]	Follow institutional protocol for amount of heparin per milliliter of flush solution, usually 1 to 4 U/mL. Other factors that promote patency of the arterial line besides heparinized saline include the following: male sex, longer catheters, larger vessels, and short-term use of the catheter.[6]
4. Use a closed tubing system if possible. *(Level IV: Limited clinical studies to support recommendations)*	May reduce the risk of nosocomial infection.[9, 10]	
5. Consider using tubing with an in-line blood discard reservoir. *(Level IV: Limited clinical studies to support recommendations)*	May reduce the risk of nosocomial anemia.[11, 12]	

Assisting with Insertion

Steps	Rationale	Special Considerations
1. Wash hands, and don gloves and goggles.	Reduces transmission of microorganisms; standard precautions.	
2. Prepare hemodynamic monitoring system (see Procedure 69).	Prepares monitoring system.	
3. Immobilize site during catheter insertion.	Facilitates insertion; may prevent needle from lacerating vessel wall during insertion.	Sedation may be necessary if the patient is restless.
4. Assist with catheter insertion.	Allows for smooth, cooperative effort.	
5. Once catheter is positioned, connect tubing with Luer-Lok adapter to arterial catheter.	Provides secure attachment and allows signal to be transmitted to monitor via transducer.	Catheter must be held in place while connections are made.
6. Observe waveform and perform a dynamic response test (square wave test; Fig. 56–3).	Results indicate whether or not the system is damped.	
7. Assist with securing or suturing catheter in place.	Catheter is at risk of becoming dislodged until secured.	
8. Once the catheter is secured in place, apply a sterile, occlusive dressing.	Provides sterile environment; reduces infection.	Refer to institutional policy. Studies of the efficacy of using antimicrobial ointments at the catheter site to prevent infection are contradictory. The Centers for Disease Control and Prevention do not recommend the routine application of topical antimicrobial ointment to the insertion site of peripheral venous catheters but do not make a specific recommendation for peripheral arterial catheters.[9] Additionally, studies reveal controversy about which dressing to use over arterial insertion sites to prevent infection—transparent or gauze dressings. More research is needed, specifically with respect to peripheral arterial catheters.

Procedure continued on following page

Procedure for Assisting with Insertion, Care and Removal of Arterial Pressure Lines *Continued*

Steps	Rationale	Special Considerations
9. Apply armboard if necessary.	Ensures correct position of extremity for optimal waveform.	
10. Level and zero the transducer (see Procedure 69).	Prepares monitoring system.	
11. Set alarm parameters according to patient's current blood pressure.	Alarms should always be on to detect pulseless electrical activity, hypotension, hypertension, accidental disconnection, accidental removal of catheter, or overdamping of waveform.	
12. Discard used supplies and wash hands.	Reduces transmission of microorganisms; standard precautions.	
13. Run a waveform strip and record baseline pressures.	Obtains baseline data.	Never rely on digital values because the values are averaged calculations.

Procedure for Troubleshooting an Overdamped Waveform

Steps	Rationale	Special Considerations
1. Identify the overdamped waveform (Fig. 56–4).	Identifies problem.	
2. Check the patient.	A sudden hypotensive episode can look like an overdamped waveform (Fig. 56–5).	
3. Check that the pressure bag is inflated to 300 mm Hg.	Underinflation or overinflation can distort the waveform.	
4. Perform a dynamic response test if the arterial waveform seems to be overdamped (see Fig. 56–3).	Overdamping should be assessed immediately to ensure waveform accuracy and to prevent clotting of the catheter.	
5. If the waveform is overdamped, follow these steps:		
A. Check the arterial line insertion site for catheter positioning.	In the radial site, wrist movement—or in the femoral site, leg flexion—can cause catheter kinking or dislodgment and result in an ovedamped waveform.	
B. Check the system for air bubbles and eliminate them if they are found.	Air bubbles can be a cause of an overdamped system; air bubbles can also cause emboli.	
C. Check the tubing system for leaks or disconnections and correct the problem if it is found.	Ensure that all connections are tight.	

Procedure continued on page 374

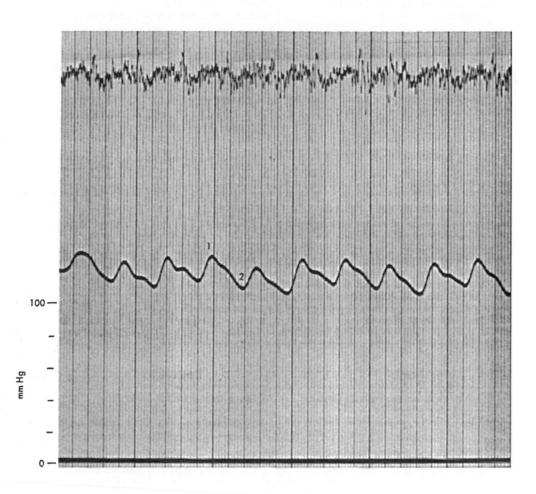

■ ● **FIGURE 56–4.** Over-damped arterial waveform (*1* = systole; *2* = diastole). (From Daily EK, Schroeder JS. *Hemodynamic Waveforms.* St. Louis, Mo: Mosby-Year Book; 1990: 110.)

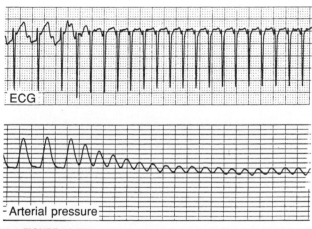

■ ● **FIGURE 56–5.** Patient developed a superventricular tachycardia (SVT) with a fall in arterial pressure. Note how the arterial line appears overdamped but is in fact reflecting a severe hypotensive episode associated with the tachycardia.

Procedure **for Troubleshooting an Overdamped Waveform** *Continued*

Steps	Rationale	Special Considerations
D. Attempt to aspirate and flush catheter as follows:	Assists with the withdrawal of air in tubing or clots that may be at catheter tip.	
Note: A catheter with an overdamped waveform should always be aspirated before flushing.	Using the fast-flush device or flushing with a syringe first may force a clot at the catheter tip into the arterial circulation.	
○ Wash hands, and don gloves.	Reduces transmission of microorganisms; standard precautions.	
○ Attach a 10-mL syringe to the blood sampling port of the stopcock closest to the patient.	A 10-mL syringe generates less pressure.	
○ Turn stopcock off to flush bag.	Opens the system from the patient to the syringe.	
○ Gently attempt to aspirate; if resistance is felt, reposition the extremity and reattempt aspiration. If resistance is still felt, stop and notify the physician or advanced practice nurse.	Allows check on catheter patency. Normally, blood should be aspirated into the syringe without difficulty.	
○ If blood is aspirated, remove 3 mL, turn stopcock off to patient, and discard the 3-mL sample.	Removes any clotted material within the catheter.	All blood wastes should be disposed of following standard precautions.
○ Hold a 4 × 4 gauze pad over the blood sampling port of stopcock. Activate fast-flush device to clear stopcock of blood.	Removes blood residue from stopcock, where it could be a reservoir for bacterial growth.	
○ Turn stopcock off to blood sampling port and replace it with a sterile occlusive cap.	Maintains sterility and closed system.	
○ Use fast-flush device to clear line of blood.	Prevents arterial line from clotting.	
6. Discard used supplies, and wash hands.	Reduces transmission of microorganisms; standard precautions.	

Procedure **for Troubleshooting an Underdamped Waveform**

Steps	Rationale	Special Considerations
1. Identify the underdamped waveform (see Fig. 56–3C).	Identifies problem.	
2. Wash hands.	Reduces transmission of microorganisms; standard precautions.	
3. Check the system for air bubbles and eliminate them if they are found.	Air bubbles can contibute to underdamping; air bubbles can also cause emboli.	
4. Check the length of the pressurized tubing system.	Ensure that the tubing length is minimized.	
5. Consider use of a damping device.	These devices mechanically alter damping.	Follow institution standard regarding use of damping devices.
6. Wash hands.	Reduces transmission of micoorganisms; standard precautions.	

Procedure for Arterial Line Dressing Change

Steps	Rationale	Special Considerations
1. Frequency of dressing change is determined by type of dressing material used and unit policy.	Prevents infection at insertion site.	The Centers for Disease Control and Prevention recommend replacing the dressing when the catheter is replaced (at least every 96 hours); when the dressing becomes damp, loosened, or soiled; or if inspection of the site is required.[9]
A. Wash hands, and don gloves.	Reduces transmission of microorganisms; standard precautions.	
B. Gently remove old dressings, being careful not to place tension on arterial catheter.	Prevents inadvertent dislodgment of catheter.	If excessive tape is used, use extreme care to secure the catheter while removing the tape. A second health care provider may be needed to assist with dressing removal to prevent accidental dislodgment or removal of the arterial catheter.
C. Observe for signs of infection.	Early detection may prevent bacteremia.	An infected catheter is removed, and the tip is sent for culture.
D. Cleanse insertion site with 10% povidone-iodine solution and allow to dry.	Iodine solutions need to air dry for maximum effectiveness and to help prevent the growth of bacteria at the insertion site.	
E. Replace dressing using aseptic technique.	Decreases risk of infection.	
F. Discard used supplies and wash hands.	Reduces transmission of microorganisms; standard precautions.	

Procedure for Removal of Arterial Catheter

Steps	Rationale	Special Considerations
1. Wash hands, and don gloves and goggles.	Reduces transmission of microorganisms; standard precautions.	Refer to institutional policy regarding removal of arterial catheters from sites other than radial or ulnar arteries.
2. Turn off continuous infusion, and turn off monitoring alarms.	Prevents flush solution from leaking and prevents false alarms.	
3. Attach syringe to blood sampling port, turn stopcock off to flush bag, and draw blood back through the tubing.	Ensures there is no clot in the catheter.	If unable to draw blood back, notify physician or advanced practice nurse.
4. Apply pressure distal to the insertion site.	Prepares for removal.	
5. Pull out catheter using a sterile 4 ×4 gauze pad to cover site as catheter is pulled out.	Prevents splashing of blood.	
6. Immediately apply firm pressure with a sterile 4 × 4 gauze pad proximal to the insertion site.	Prevents bleeding.	
7. Continue to apply pressure for a minimum of 5 minutes for radial or ulnar artery site.	Achieves hemostasis.	Longer periods of direct pressure may be needed to achieve hemostasis in patients receiving systemic heparin or thrombolytics or those with catheters in larger arteries (ie, in the femoral artery). With large catheters used for angiography or intra-aortic balloon pump therapy, direct pressure may be held for 30 to 60 minutes followed by bedrest for 6 to 8 hours after catheter removal.
8. Apply a pressure dressing to the insertion site.	A pressure dressing will help prevent rebleeding.	Dressing should not encircle extemity to prevent ischemia of extremity.
9. Discard supplies and wash hands.	Reduces transmison of microorganisms; standard precautions.	

Expected Outcomes	Unexpected Outcomes
• Minimal discomfort from arterial catheter	• Pain or discomfort from arterial catheter insertion site
• Maintenance of baseline hemoglobin and hematocrit levels	• Redness, warmth, edema, or drainage at or from the insertion site
• Adequate circulation to the involved extremity	• Elevated temperature or elevated white blood cell count
• Adequate sensory and motor function of the extremity	• Decreased hemoglobin and hematocrit
• Remaining euvolemic	• Impaired peripheral tissue perfusion (ie, edema, coolness, pain, paleness, or slow capillary refill of fingers or toes of cannulated extremity)
	• Impaired sensory or motor function of the extremity
	• Catheter disconnection with significant blood loss
	• Fluid volume overload

Patient Monitoring and Care

Patient Monitoring and Care	Rationale	Reportable Conditions
		These conditions should be reported if they persist despite nursing interventions.
1. Monitor neurovascular and peripheral vascular assessments of the cannulated extremity immediately after catheter insertion and every 4 hours, or more often if warranted, or according to unit policy.	Validates adequate peripheral circulation and neurovascular integrity. Changes in pulses, color, temperature, or capillary refill may indicate ischemia, arterial spasm, or neurovascular compromise.	• Diminished or absent pulses • Pale, mottled, or cyanotic appearance of extremity • Extremity that is cool or cold to the touch • Capillary refill time of more than 2 seconds • Diminished or absent sensation • Diminished or absent motor function • Pallor or cyanosis

2. Check arterial line flush system every 1 to 4 hours to ensure the following:
  ○ Pressure bag is inflated to 300 mm Hg.
  ○ Fluid is present in flush bag.
  ○ Flush system is delivering 1 to 3 mL/h.
	Ensures accuracy of pressure waveform and functioning of system.
	Necessary for proper function of flush device and to prevent backflow of blood into catheter and tubing.
	Catheter will clot off if fluid is not continuously infusing.
	Maintains catheter patency and prevents fluid overload.	

3. Monitor for overdamped or underdamped waveform.
 	
  ○ An overdamped waveform is characterized by a flattened waveform, a diminished or absent dicrotic notch, or a waveform that does not fall to baseline (see Fig. 56–4).
 	
  ○ An underdamped waveform is characterized by catheter fling.
	An optimally damped system provides an adequate waveform with appropriate blood pressure readings.
	With an overdamped waveform, systolic pressure may be read inaccurately low. Common causes of overdamped waveform include the following: air bubbles in system, use of compliant tubing, loose connections in system, too many stopcocks in system, cracked stopcock, arterial cannula occlusion, catheter tip against arterial wall, and insufficient pressure in pressure bag.
	With an underdamped waveform, systolic pressures may be read inaccurately high. Common causes of an underdamped waveform include the following: excessive tubing length, movement of the catheter in the artery, patient movement, and air bubbles in the system.
		• Overdamped or underdamped waveform that cannot be corrected with troubleshooting procedures

Patient Monitoring and Care	Rationale	Reportable Conditions
4. Perform a dynamic response test every 8 to 12 hours or when the system is opened to air or when the accuracy of readings is in question (see Fig. 56–3).	An optimally damped system provides an accurate waveform.	• Overdamped or underdamped waveform that cannot be corrected with troubleshooting procedures
5. Zero the transducer during initial setup and before insertion, if the transducer and the monitoring cable are disconnected, if the monitoring cable and the monitor are disconnected, and when the values obtained do not fit the clinical picture. Follow manufacturer's recommendations for both disposable and reusable systems.	Ensures accuracy of the hemodynamic monitoring system; minimizes risk of contamination of the system.	
6. Observe insertion site for signs of infection.	Infected catheters must be removed as soon as possible to prevent bacteremia. The tip should be sent for culture.	• Purulent drainage • Tenderness or pain at insertion site • Elevated temperature • Elevated white blood cells
7. Change the catheter site, pressure tubing, flush bag, and transducer every 96 hours or with each change of the catheter if it is changed more frequently. The flush bag may need to be changed more frequently if it is empty of solution. *(Level IV: Limited clinical studies to support recommendations)*	Changing the flush bag and system more often than every 96 hours may cause contamination and increase the risk of infection.[9, 13, 14]	
8. Run an arterial pressure strip and obtain measurement of the arterial pressures during end-expiration.	Eliminates the effect of the respiratory cycle on arterial pressure.	
9. Obtain an arterial waveform strip to place on the patient's chart at the start of each shift or whenever there is a change in the waveform.	The printed waveform allows assessment of the adequacy of the waveform, damping, or respiratory variation.	
10. Monitor hemoglobin or hematocrit daily or whenever a significant amount of blood is lost through the catheter (eg, through accidental disconnection).	Allows assessment of nosocomial anemia.	• Changes in hemoglobin and hematocrit

Documentation

Documentation should include the following:

- Patient and family education
- Peripheral vascular and neurovascular assessment before and after the procedure
- Date and time of insertion with size of catheter placed
- Condition of insertion site
- Patient response to insertion procedure

- Type of flush solution used
- Intake of flush solution (eg, 3 mL/h)
- Initial insertion recorded and waveform labeled with the date, time, and systolic and diastolic pressures
- Unexpected outcomes
- Additional nursing interventions

References

1. Buffington S. Specimen collection and testing. In: *Nursing Procedures*. 2nd ed. Springhouse, Pa: Springhouse Corp; 1996:145–147.
2. Hadaway LC. Anatomy and physiology related to intravenous therapy. In: Terry J, Baranowski L, Lonsway RA, Hedric C, eds. *Intravenous Therapy: Clinical Principles and Practice*. Philadelphia, Pa: W.B. Saunders; 1995:97.
3. Perucca R. Obtaining vascular access. In: Terry J, Baranowski L, Lonsway RA, Hedric C, eds. *Intravenous Therapy: Clinical Principles and Practice*. Philadelphia, Pa: W.B. Saunders; 1995:386.
4. Cummins RO, ed. *Advanced Cardiac Life Support*. Dallas, Tex: American Heart Association; 1997:13.10.
5. DeGroot KD, Damato G. Monitoring intra-arterial pressure. *Crit Care Nurse*. 1986;6:74–78.
6. American Association of Critical-Care Nurses. Evaluation of the effects of heparinized and nonheparinized flush solutions on the patency of arterial pressure monitoring lines: the AACN Thunder Project. *Am J Crit Care*. 1993;2:3–15.
7. Kulkarni M, Elsner C, Ouellet D, Zeldin R. Heparinized saline versus normal saline in maintaining patency of the radial artery catheter. *Can J Surg*. 1994;27:37–42.
8. Mermel LA, Maki DG. Epidemic bloodstream infections from hemodynamic pressure monitoring: signs of the times. *Infect Control Hosp Epidemiol*. 1989;10:47–53.
9. Pearson ML. Guideline for prevention of intravascular device-related infections. *Infect Control Hosp Epidemiol*. 1996;17:438–473.
10. Crow S, Conrad SA, Chaney-Rowell C, King JW. Microbial contamination of arterial infusions used for hemodynamic monitoring: a randomized trial of contamination with sampling through conventional stopcocks versus a novel closed system. *Infect Control Hosp Epidemiol*. 1989;10:557–561.
11. Peruzzi WT, Parker MA, Lichtenthal PR, Cochran-Zull C, Toth B, Blake M. A clinical evaluation of a blood conservation device in medical intensive care unit patients. *Crit Care Med*. 1993;21:501–506.
12. Silver MJ, Jubran H, Stein S, McSweeney T, Jubran F. Evaluation of a new blood-conserving arterial line system for patients in intensive care units. *Crit Care Med*. 1993;21:507–511.
13. Luskin RL, Weinstein RA, Nathan C, Chamberlin WH, Kabins SA. Extended use of disposable pressure transducers. *JAMA*. 1986;255:916–920.
14. O'Malley MK, Rhaume FS, Cerra FB, McComb RC. Value of routine pressure monitoring system changes after 72 hours. *Crit Care Med*. 1994;22:1424–1430.

Additional Readings

Aherns TS, Taylor LA. *Hemodynamic Waveform Analysis*. Philadelphia, Pa: W.B. Saunders; 1992.
Clark CA. Harmon EM. Hemodynamic monitoring: arterial catheters. In: Taylor RW, Civetta JM, Kirby RR. *Techniques and Procedures in Critical Care*. Philadelphia, Pa: J.B. Lippincott; 1990:218–231.
Clark VL, Kruse JA. Arterial catheterization. *Crit Care Clin*. 1992;8:687–697.
Daily EK, Schroeder JS. *Techniques in Bedside Hemodynamic Monitoring*. 5th ed. St Louis, Mo: C.V. Mosby; 1994.
Darovic GO. *Hemodynamic Monitoring: Invasive and Noninvasive Clinical Application*. 2nd ed. Philadelphia, Pa: W.B. Saunders; 1995.
Dech ZF. Blood conservation in the critically ill. *AACN Clin Issues Crit Care Nurs*. 1994;5:169–177.
Gleason E, Grossman S, Campbell C. Minimizing diagnostic blood loss in critically ill patients. *Am J Crit Care*. 1992;1:85–90.
Gorny DA. Arterial blood pressure measurement technique. *AACN Clin Issues Crit Care Nurs*. 1993;4:66–80.
Hoffman KK, Weber DJ, Samsa GP, Rutala WA. Transparent polyurethane film as an intravenous catheter dressing: a meta-analysis of the infection risks. *JAMA*. 1992;267:2072–2076.
Imperial-Perez F, McRae M. *Protocols for Practice: Hemodynamic Monitoring Series—Arterial Pressure Monitoring*. Aliso Viejo, Calif: American Association of Critical-Care Nurses; 1998.
Pizov R, Cohen M, Weiss Y, Segal E, Cotev S, Perel A. Positive end-expiratory pressure-induced hemodynamic changes are reflected in the arterial pressure waveform. *Crit Care Med*. 1996;24:1381–1387.

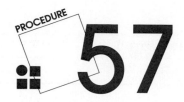

57

Blood Sampling from Arterial Pressure Lines

PURPOSE: Blood sampling from arterial pressure lines is performed to obtain blood specimens for arterial blood gas analysis or for other laboratory testing.

Rose B. Shaffer

PREREQUISITE NURSING KNOWLEDGE

- Understanding of sterile technique is necessary.
- Understanding of vascular anatomy and physiology is needed.
- Understanding of gas exchange and acid-base balance is necessary.
- Technique for specimen collection and labeling should be understood.
- Principles of hemodynamic monitoring should be understood.
- Knowledge regarding care of patients with arterial lines and stopcock manipulation is essential in order to draw blood from arterial pressure lines (see Procedure 56).

EQUIPMENT

- Nonsterile gloves
- Sterile 4 × 4 gauze pad
- Appropriate blood specimen tubes (or arterial blood gas [ABG] kit)
- Labels with patient's name and appropriate identifying data
- Laboratory forms

Additional equipment as needed includes the following:

- Alcohol pads or swabsticks
- Vacutainer®
- "Needleless" Vacutainer Luer-Lok adapter needle
- Bag of ice
- Extra blood specimen tube (for discard)
- Syringes, 5 mL and 10 mL
- Sterile dead-end cap

PATIENT AND FAMILY EDUCATION

- Assess patient and family understanding of the reason for blood sampling from the arterial line. **➤➤Rationale:** Alleviates anxiety and promotes understanding.

- Explain procedure to patient and family. **➤➤Rationale:** Alleviates anxiety and encourages questions.
- Explain that pressure waveform and digital display of blood pressure will be absent during blood sampling procedure. **➤➤Rationale:** Alleviates anxiety.
- Explain the importance of keeping the affected extremity immobile. **➤➤Rationale:** Encourages patient compliance during blood withdrawal.

PATIENT ASSESSMENT AND PREPARATION

Patient Assessment

- Assess patency of arterial line. **➤➤Rationale:** If arterial line is clotted, blood sampling will not be able to be performed.
- Assess previous laboratory results. **➤➤Rationale:** Provides data for comparison.

Patient Preparation

- Ensure that the patient and family understand preprocedural teaching. Answer questions as they arise and reinforce information as needed. **➤➤Rationale:** Evaluates and reinforces understanding of previously taught information.
- Expose the stopcock to be used for blood sampling and position the patient's extremity so that the site can easily be accessed. **➤➤Rationale:** Prepares site for blood withdrawal.

Procedure	for Blood Sampling from Arterial Pressure Lines

Steps	Rationale	Special Considerations

"NEEDLELESS" VACUTAINER

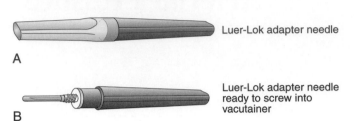

Luer-Lok adapter needle

A

Luer-Lok adapter needle
ready to screw into
vacutainer

B

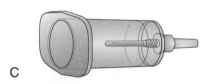

Luer-Lok adapter needle
screwed into vacutainer
with cap off

C

■ ● **FIGURE 57–1.** ''Needleless'' Vacutainer Luer-Lok adapter needle.

Steps	Rationale	Special Considerations
1. Wash hands, and don gloves.	Reduces transmission of microorganisms; standard precautions.	
2. If drawing an ABG, open ABG kit and use plunger to rid excess heparin from syringe.	An excess amount of heparin may alter ABG results.	
3. Attach needleless Vacutainer Luer-Lok adapter needle to Vacutainer (Fig. 57–1).	Prepares for blood sampling.	If possible, use needleless system for obtaining blood samples to prevent needlestick injury.
4. Suspend arterial line alarms.	Prevents alarm from sounding as waveform is lost during blood draw.	
5. Turn stopcock off to patient (Fig. 57–2).	Prevents backflow of blood from arterial line when three-way stopcock blood sampling port is opened.	There will be loss of arterial waveform and digital display.

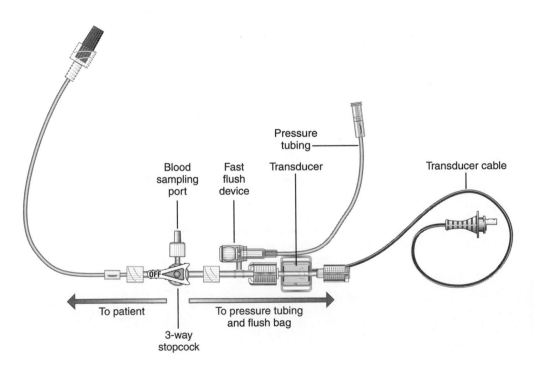

Pressure
tubing

Blood
sampling
port

Fast
flush
device

Transducer

Transducer cable

OFF

To patient

To pressure tubing
and flush bag

3-way
stopcock

■ ● **FIGURE 57–2.** Disposable transducer with continuous flush device. In this picture, the stopcock is turned ''off'' to the patient.

| Procedure | for Blood Sampling from Arterial Pressure Lines *Continued* |

Steps	Rationale	Special Considerations
6. Remove sterile occlusive cap from blood sampling port of three-way stopcock closest to patient.	Prepares for blood sampling.	If using a system where blood samples are obtained through a rubber diaphragm, swab the area with alcohol before entering the system.
7. Place Vacutainer with "needleless" Luer-Lok adapter needle into blood sampling port of three-way stopcock (Fig. 57–3).	Prepares for blood sampling.	
8. Attach one blood specimen tube (for discard) into Vacutainer without engaging it.		
A. When obtaining blood for ABGs, use a discard volume of two times the dead-space volume of the catheter and tubing to the sampling site. *(Level IV: Limited clinical studies to support recommendations)*	Use of this discard volume prevents dilution of the ABG sample by saline and excess heparin.[1]	
B. When obtaining blood for coagulation studies from a heparinized arterial line, use a discard volume of six times the dead-space volume of the catheter and tubing to the sampling site. *(Level VI: Clinical studies in a variety of patient populations and situations to support recommendations)*	Use of this discard volume prevents contamination of specimen with heparin, preventing inaccurate coagulation results.[2, 3]	This recommendation does not apply to patients receiving systemic heparin therapy or thrombolytics. More research is needed with these populations.
9. Turn the stopcock off to the flush bag.	Opens arterial line to vacutainer.	
10. Completely engage blood specimen tube into the Vacutainer.	Engages vacuum to withdraw blood from the line.	
11. Remove the minimal volume of blood needed for discard (see step 8).	Clears line of any flush solution that may affect laboratory results.	If possible, use blood-conserving closed system to avoid nosocomial anemia (Fig. 57–4).

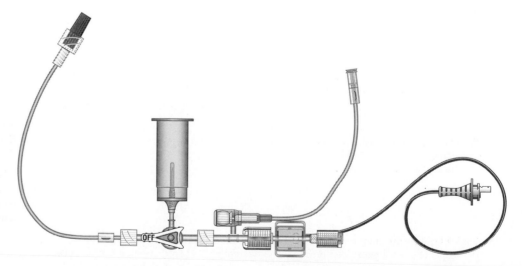

■ ● **FIGURE 57–3.** Vacutainer with "needleless" Luer-Lok needle attached to blood sampling port of three-way stopcock. The stopcock is "off" to the patient.

Procedure continued on following page

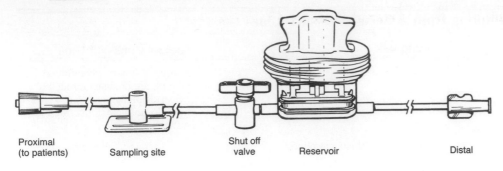

Proximal
(to patients)   Sampling site   Shut off
                                                          valve   Reservoir   Distal

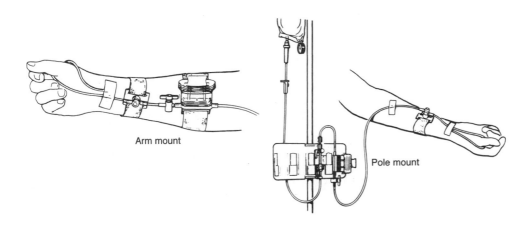

Arm mount

Pole mount

■ ● **FIGURE 57–4.** VAMP system for needleless blood withdrawal from hemodynamic lines. (Courtesy of Baxter-Edwards Laboratories.)

Procedure	**for Blood Sampling from Arterial Pressure Lines** *Continued*

Steps	Rationale	Special Considerations
12. Remove discard specimen.	Discards blood that also contains flush solution.	Place the discard specimen away from the field so as not to mistake it with the actual blood specimens for laboratory analysis.
13. Attach blood specimen tubes into Vacutainer, and engage each one, obtaining the appropriate blood specimens.		If drawing laboratory specimens (including coagulation studies and ABG), draw the routine laboratory studies first, then draw the ABG and coagulation studies.
A. If drawing an ABG with other laboratory studies, turn stopcock off to patient, remove Vacutainer, and attach ABG syringe to blood sampling port.	Prepares for connection of ABG syringe.	
B. Turn stopcock off to flush bag.	Opens arterial line to ABG syringe.	
C. Gently aspirate the ABG sample.	Obtains ABG sample while minimizing vessel trauma.	
14. Remove last blood specimen tube from Vacutainer (or remove ABG syringe) and turn stopcock off to patient.	Detaches the specimen.	Expel any air bubbles from the ABG syringe. Follow institution standard regarding use of ice. Commonly, the ABG specimen is placed on ice if any anticipated delay in sending the specimen to laboratory is anticipated.
15. Fast flush the remaining blood from the stopcock onto a gauze pad or into a discard syringe or blood specimen tube.	Prevents clotting of blood in blood sampling port so that blood can be drawn at later time. Also removes blood residue from stopcock, where it could be a reservoir for bacterial growth.	Follow institution standard.

Procedure	for Blood Sampling from Arterial Pressure Lines *Continued*

Steps	Rationale	Special Considerations
16. Place a new, sterile occlusive cap on blood sampling port.	Maintains sterility of system.	
17. Turn stopcock on to the patient and flush bag (off to blood sampling port) and use fast-flush device to clear line of blood.	Prevents arterial line from clotting.	Some monitoring systems may include an option to reinfuse the blood to the patient after the laboratory sample is obtained.
18. Turn alarms back on and ensure waveform returns.	Provides accurate waveform and blood pressure monitoring.	
19. Discard used supplies, and wash hands.	Prevents transmission of microorganisms; standard precautions.	
20. Label specimen and complete laboratory form per institutional protocol.	Helps the laboratory to perform the analysis accurately.	For ABGs, note the percent of oxygen therapy, respiratory rate, and ventilator settings, if appropriate, as well as the patient's temperature and time the specimen was drawn. Expedite the delivery of samples to laboratory.

Expected Outcomes

- Adequate blood sample with minimal blood loss
- No hemolysis of specimens
- No arterial spasm
- Arterial line patency maintained

Unexpected Outcomes

- Inadequate blood sample
- Hemolysis of specimens
- Dilution of specimens, causing inaccurate laboratory results
- Arterial spasm

Patient Monitoring and Care

Patient Monitoring and Care	Rationale	Reportable Conditions
		These conditions should be reported if they persist despite nursing interventions.
1. Use minimal volume of blood discard.	Helps prevent nosocomial anemia.	
2. Monitor hemoglobin or hematocrit daily or if a significant amount of blood loss occurs.	Allows early detection of nosocomial anemia.	• Changes in hemoglobin or hematocrit levels
3. Attempt to group blood draws together whenever possible.	Diminishes number of times the system is entered to help minimize the risk of infection.	
4. Before and after the blood withdrawal, assess and evaluate the arterial waveform.	Ensures accurate arterial pressure monitoring.	
5. Obtain laboratory specimen results.	Monitors test results.	• Abnormal specimen results

Documentation

Documentation should include the following:

- Patient and family education
- Time and type of specimen drawn
- Results of blood tests, when available
- Unexpected outcomes
- Additional nursing interventions

References

1. Preusser BA, Lash J, Stone KS, Winningham ML, Gonyon D, Nickel JT. Quantifying the minimum discard sample required for accurate arterial blood gases. *Nurs Res.* 1989;38:276–279.
2. Harper J. Use of intraarterial lines to obtain coagulation samples. *Focus Crit Care.* 1988;15:51–55.
3. Laxson CJ, Titler MG. Drawing coagulation studies from arterial lines: an integrative literature review. *Am J Crit Care.* 1994;3:16–22.

Additional Readings

Dirks JL. Innovations in technology: continuous intra-arterial blood gas monitoring. *Crit Care Nurs.* 1995;15:19–27.

Imperial-Perez F, McRae M. *Protocols for Practice: Hemodynamic Monitoring Series—Arterial Pressure Monitoring.* Aliso Viejo, Ca: American Association of Critical-Care Nurses; 1998.

58

Blood Sampling from Pulmonary Artery Line

P U R P O S E : Blood is removed from the pulmonary artery (PA) catheter to determine mixed venous oxygen saturation or to obtain a blood sample for laboratory analysis.

Teresa Preuss
Debra J. Lynn-McHale

PREREQUISITE NURSING KNOWLEDGE

- An understanding of sterile technique is needed.
- An understanding of cardiovascular and pulmonary anatomy and physiology is necessary.
- An understanding of gas exchange and acid-base balance is important.
- An understanding of technique for specimen collection and labeling is necessary.
- Principles of hemodynamic monitoring should be understood.
- Knowledge about the care of patients with pulmonary artery lines and stopcock manipulation is essential to draw blood from the pulmonary artery line (see Procedure 66).
- The most frequent blood specimen obtained from the pulmonary artery is one for mixed venous oxygen analysis.
- Routine blood sampling from the pulmonary artery catheter is not recommended because entry into the sterile system may increase the incidence of catheter-related infection.

EQUIPMENT

- Nonsterile gloves
- Goggles or fluid shield face mask
- Syringes, 5 mL and 10 mL
- Sterile 4 × 4 gauze pad
- Blood specimen tubes
- Blood gas sampling syringe
- Sterile dead-end cap
- Laboratory slips and specimen labels

Additional equipment to have available as needed includes the following:

- Alcohol swabs
- Vacutainer® (Becton Dickinson, Marlton, NJ)
- Needleless Vacutainer Luer-Lok adapter
- Bag of ice
- Extra blood specimen tube (for discard)

PATIENT AND FAMILY EDUCATION

- Explain purpose for blood sampling. ➤**Rationale:** Teaching provides information and may reduce anxiety and fear.
- Explain the patient's expected participation during the procedure. ➤**Rationale:** Encourages patient assistance.

PATIENT ASSESSMENT AND PREPARATION

Patient Assessment

- Assess cardiopulmonary and hemodynamic status, including abnormal lung sounds, respiratory distress, dysrhythmias, diminished pulses, decreased mentation, agitation, skin color changes, peripheral edema, jugular vein distention, chest pain, cough, and fever. ➤**Rationale:** These signs and symptoms could necessitate blood sampling for venous oxygenation.
- Assess for a decrease in cardiac output related to changes in preload, afterload, or contractility. ➤**Rationale:** Mixed venous blood samples are used to evaluate changes in cardiopulmonary function that affect cardiac output.

Patient Preparation

- Ensure that the patient understands preprocedural teaching. Answer questions as they arise and reinforce information as needed. ➤**Rationale:** Evaluates and reinforces understanding of previously taught information.
- Position patient so that stopcock for blood sampling is exposed. ➤**Rationale:** Improves ease of obtaining blood sample and minimizes the contamination of the stopcock.

Procedure   for Blood Sampling from Pulmonary Artery Line

Steps	Rationale	Special Considerations
1. Wash hands, and don gloves and goggles or fluid shield face mask.	Reduces transmission of microorganisms and body fluids; standard precautions.	
2. If drawing an arterial blood gas (ABG), sample, open ABG kit and use plunger to rid excess heparin from syringe.	Prepares ABG syringe.	
3. If using a Vacutainer, attach needleless Vacutainer Luer-Lok adapter to Vacutainer.	Prepares for blood sampling.	If possible, use a needleless system for obtaining blood samples to prevent needlestick injury.
4. Suspend pulmonary artery (PA) alarms.	Prevents alarm from sounding because the PA waveform is lost during blood draw.	
5. Remove the dead-end cap from the stopcock of the distal lumen of the PA catheter.	Prepares the line for blood sampling.	If using a system where blood samples are obtained through a rubber diaphragm, swab the area with an alcohol wipe before entering the system.
6. Place a sterile syringe or Vacutainer with needleless Luer-Lok adapter needle into the top port of the stopcock.	Prepares for blood sampling.	
7. Turn the stopcock off to the monitoring system.	The syringe or Vacutainer will then be in direct contact with the PA.	
8. Slowly and gently aspirate and observe as blood enters the syringe, and withdraw approximately 2.5 times the dead space of the catheter or engage the blood specimen tube into the Vacutainer and remove the discard volume.[1]	Clears the catheter of flush solution.	If using a blood specimen tube for discard, use one large enough for the appropriate dead space volume. If possible, use a blood-conserving closed system to avoid nosocomial anemia.
9. Turn the stopcock off to the syringe or Vacutainer.	Stops blood flow and closes all ports of the stopcock.	
10. Remove the syringe or the discard specimen and discard in appropriate receptacle.	Removes discard.	
11. Insert an ABG syringe into the stopcock or attach the ABG syringe to the Vacutainer system.	Prepares for removal of a blood sample.	
12. Turn the stopcock off to the hemodynamic flush system.	Prepares for blood sampling.	
13. Slowly aspirate the ABG sample.	Slow aspiration is important to prevent contamination of the mixed venous sample with arterial blood from the pulmonary capillaries.	
14. Turn the stopcock off to the patient.	Prevents bleeding.	
15. Remove the ABG syringe.	Detaches the specimen.	
16. Expel any air bubbles from the ABG syringe and cap the syringe.	Ensures accuracy of ABG results.	
17. Fast flush the remaining blood from the stopcock onto a gauze pad or into a discard syringe or blood specimen tube.	Clears blood from the system.	Some monitoring systems may include an option to reinfuse the blood to the patient after the laboratory sample is obtained.

	Procedure	**for Blood Sampling from Pulmonary Artery Line** *Continued*	

Steps	Rationale	Special Considerations
18. Turn the stopcock off to the top port of the stopcock.	This opens the system up for continuous PA pressure monitoring.	
19. If the system was open, attach a new, sterile dead-end cap to the top port of the stopcock.	Maintains a closed, sterile system.	
20. Flush the remaining blood in the PA catheter back into the patient.	Promotes patency of the PA catheter.	
21. Turn the alarms back on.	Activates the alarm system.	
22. Observe the monitor for return of the PA waveform.	Ensures continuous monitoring of the PA waveform.	
23. Label the specimen and laboratory form.	Properly identifies the patient and laboratory tests to be performed.	
24. Send the specimen for analysis.		Label the blood-gas laboratory slip as a mixed venous sample. Follow the hospital policy about using ice for ABG samples.
25. Discard used supplies, and wash hands.	Reduces transmission of microorganisms; standard precautions.	

Expected Outcomes	Unexpected Outcomes
• Adequate blood sample with minimal blood loss • PA catheter line patency maintained	• Inability to obtain laboratory sample • Dilution of specimen causing inaccurate laboratory results • Arterial sample obtained instead of mixed venous oxygen sample for blood-gas analysis

Patient Monitoring and Care

Patient Monitoring and Care	Rationale	Reportable Conditions
		These conditions should be reported if they persist despite nursing interventions.
1. Before and after the blood withdrawal, assess and evaluate PA waveform.	Ensures that the PA catheter is properly positioned.	
2. Correlate venous oxygen saturation results with measured cardiac output.	Svo_2 is usually decreased when the cardiac output is decreased.	• Abnormal mixed venous oxygen saturation, cardiac output, cardiac index, and afterload

Documentation

Documentation should include the following:

- Patient and family education
- Time and date the blood sample was taken
- Blood tests performed
- Any difficulties with PA catheter blood sampling
- Nursing interventions performed
- Unexpected outcomes

Reference

1. Preusser BA, Lash J, Stone KS, Winningham ML, Gonyon D, Nickel JT. Quantifying the minimum discard sample required for accurate arterial blood gases. *Nurs Res.* 1989;38:276–279.

Additional Readings

Ahrens TS, Taylor LA. *Hemodynamic Waveform Analysis.* Philadelphia, Pa: W.B. Saunders; 1992.

Darovic GO. *Hemodynamic Monitoring: Invasive and Noninvasive Clinical Application.* 2nd ed. Philadelphia, Pa: W.B. Saunders; 1995.

Schactman M, Scott C, Silva VM, Wolff CA. *Hemodynamic Monitoring.* El Paso, Tex: Skidmore-Roth Publishing; 1995.

59

Cardiac Output Measurement Techniques (Invasive)

PURPOSE: Cardiac output (CO) measurements are performed to monitor cardiovascular status. CO measurements are used to evaluate patient response to clinical interventions, mechanical assist devices, and vasoactive medications. CO measurements are essential in caring for critically ill patients with hemodynamic instability.

Kathleen Ahern Gould
Colette Hartigan
Suzanne Farley Keane

PREREQUISITE NURSING KNOWLEDGE

- Understanding of the normal anatomy and physiology of the cardiovascular system and pulmonary system is necessary.
- Understanding of basic dysrhythmia recognition and treatment of life-threatening dysrhythmias is necessary.
- The principles of aseptic technique and infection control should be understood.
- Understanding of the pulmonary artery (PA) catheter (see Fig. 66–1) and the location of the PA catheter in the heart and PA (see Fig. 66–2) is necessary.
- Understanding of the setup of the hemodynamic monitoring system (see Procedure 69) is necessary.
- Competence in the use and clinical application of hemodynamic waveforms and values obtained with a pulmonary artery catheter is necessary. Hemodynamic waveform interpretation of right atrial pressure (RAP), pulmonary artery pressure (PAP), and pulmonary artery wedge pressure (PAWP) provide confirmation of proper catheter placement.
- Knowledge of vasoactive medication therapy and its effect on cardiac tissue, coronary vessels, and vascular smooth muscles is needed.
- *Cardiac output* is defined as the amount of blood ejected by the left ventricle in 1 minute and is the product of stroke volume (SV) and heart rate (HR).

$$CO = SV \times HR$$

- *Stroke volume*, the amount of blood ejected by the left ventricle (LV) with each contraction, is the difference between left ventricular end-diastolic volume and left ventricular end-systolic volume. Normal SV is calculated to be between 60 and 100 mL per contraction.
- The normal CO is 4 to 8 L/min. The four physiologic factors that affect CO are preload, afterload, contractility, and heart rate.

- ❖ *Preload* of the left side of the heart refers to the amount of blood in the LV at the end of diastole and is measured by the PAWP. When preload or end-diastolic volume increases, the muscle fibers are stretched. The increased tension or force of cardiac contractions that accompanies an increase in diastolic filling is called the Frank-Starling law. The Frank-Starling law allows the heart to adjust its pumping ability to accommodate various levels of venous return.[1]
- ❖ *Afterload* of the left side of the heart refers to the amount of pressure or force the LV must generate to eject blood into the systemic circulation. Changes in vascular resistance (the force opposing blood flow within the vessels) has a direct effect on afterload. The cardiac muscle exerts effort to maintain SV in conditions such as aortic stenosis, hypertension, or other vasoconstrictive states. The systolic force of the heart is decreased in conditions that cause vasodilation. Vascular resistance is affected by several factors including length and radius of the blood vessel, arterial blood pressure, and venous constriction or dilation.[1]
- ❖ *Contractility* is defined as change in the strength of cardiac muscle contraction caused by factors other than preload stretch. Contractility is stimulated by the sympathetic nervous system and is increased by the release of calcium and norepinephrine and is decreased by parasympathetic neural stimulation, acidosis, and hyperkalemia. Contractility and HR are inherent to the cardiac tissues but can be influenced by neural, humoral, and pharmacologic factors.
- ❖ The last physiologic factor that affects CO is *heart rate*. Although the sinus atrial node dictates HR, many factors may affect changes in cardiac rate and rhythm. A decrease in HR can be the result of increased parasympathetic neural stimulation, decreased sympathetic

neural stimulation, or decreased body temperature. An increase in HR can be triggered by exercise, catecholamine release, or hypotension. At HRs greater than 180 beats per minute, there may be inadequate time for diastolic filling, resulting in decreased CO. A systematic assessment of all determinants of CO is essential for defining factors affecting CO for each patient (Fig. 59–1).

- Cardiac index is a more precise measurement of cardiac function than is cardiac output because calculation of cardiac index incorporates the patient's body surface area.
- Refer to Table 59–1 for normal hemodynamic values and calculations.
- At the bedside, cardiac measurements are obtained via the intermittent bolus thermodilution CO method (TDCO) or the continuous CO (CCO) method.
- The TDCO method proceeds as follows:
  ❖ An injectate (5% dextrose in water) of a known volume (10 mL) and temperature (room temperature) is injected into the right atrium (RA) or proximal port of the PA catheter. This injectate exits in the RA where it mixes with blood and flows through the right ventricle to the PA.
  ❖ A thermistor, near the distal tip of the catheter, detects the temperature change and sends a signal to the CO computer. The change in temperature over time is plotted as a curve. CO is mathematically calculated from the area under the curve and is displayed digitally and graphically on the oscilloscope (Fig. 59–2). The area under the curve is inversely proportional to the flow rate of blood. Thus a high CO is associated with a small area under the curve, whereas a low CO is associated with a large area under the curve (Fig. 59–3).

Table 59–1 ■■■ Hemodynamic Parameters

Parameters	Calculations	Normal Value
CO		
SV	$\dfrac{CO \times 1000}{HR}$	60–100 mL/per beat
SVI	$\dfrac{SV}{BSA}$	35–75 mL/m² per beat
CI	$\dfrac{CO}{BSA}$	2.8–4.2 L/min/m²
HR		60–100 BPM
Preload		
CVP		2–6 mm Hg
RAP		4–6 mm Hg
LAP		4–12 mm Hg
PAD		5–15 mm Hg
PAWP		4–12 mm Hg
RVEDP		0–8 mm Hg
LVEDP		4–10 mm Hg
Afterload		
SVR	$\dfrac{MAP - CVP/RAP \times 80}{CO}$	900–1600 dynes/sec/cm^{-5}
SVRI	$\dfrac{MAP - CVP/RAP \times 80}{CI}$	1970–2390 dynes/sec/cm^{-5}
PVR	$\dfrac{PAM - PAWP \times 80}{CO}$	155–255 dynes/sec/cm^{-5}
PVRI	$\dfrac{PAM - PAWP \times 80}{CI}$	255–285 dynes/sec/cm^{-5}
Contractility		
EF	$\dfrac{LVEDV \times 100}{SV}$	60%–75%
	$\dfrac{RVEDV \times 100}{SV}$	45%–50%
Pressures		
BP		$\dfrac{100\text{--}140}{60\text{--}90}$
MAP	DBP + ⅓ (SBP − DBP)	70–105 mm Hg

From Whalen DA, Keller R. Cardiovascular patient assessment. In: Kinney MR, Brooks-Brunn J, Molter N, Dunbar SB, eds. *AACN Clinical Reference for Critical Care Nursing.* 4th ed. St. Louis, Mo: Mosby–Year Book; 1998:299.

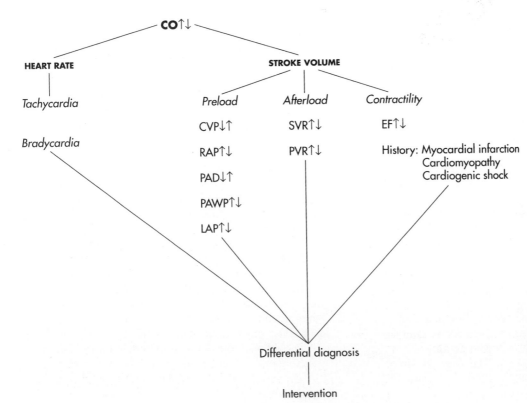

FIGURE 59–1. Systematic assessment of the determinants of cardiac output may assist the clinician in defining the etiologic factors of cardiac output alteration more precisely. (From Whalen DA, Keller R. Cardiovascular patient assessment. In: Kinney MR, Brooks-Brunn J, Molter N, Dunbar SB, Vitello-Cicciu JM, eds. *AACN Clinical Reference for Critical Care Nursing.* 4th ed. St. Louis, Mo: Mosby-Year Book; 1998: 300.)

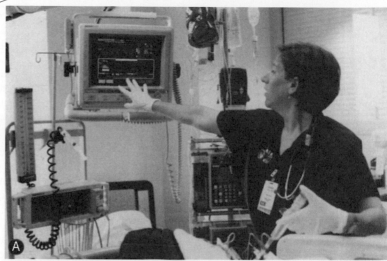

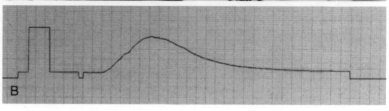

■ ● FIGURE 59–2. *A,* Examining cardiac output curves to establish reliability of values. *B,* Normal cardiac output curve with rapid upstroke and smooth progressive decrease in temperature sensing. (From Ahrens T. Hemodynamic monitoring. *Crit Care Nurs Clin N Am.* 1999;11(1):28.)

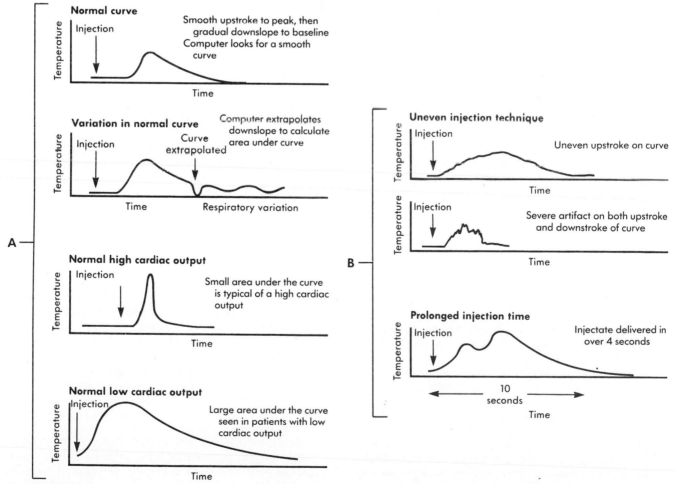

■ ● FIGURE 59–3. *A,* Variations in the normal cardiac output curve seen in certain clinical conditions. *B,* Abnormal cardiac output curves that will produce an erroneous cardiac output value. (From Thelan LA, Davie JK, Urden LD. *Textbook of Critical Care Nursing: Diagnosis and Management.* St. Louis, Mo: C. V. Mosby; 1998: 470.)

❖ There are limitations to the use of the TDCO method. For accuracy to be maintained, specific assumptions must be met. These assumptions include adequate mixing of blood and injectate, forward blood flow, steady baseline temperature in the PA, and appropriate technique.[2]

- Commercially available closed system delivery sets (CO sets) can be used with both room temperature and ice temperature injectate (Fig. 59–4).
- The CCO method proceeds as follows:
  ❖ CCO can be obtained using a heat-exchange CO catheter. This catheter has a membrane that allows for heat exchange with blood in the right atria. Continuous measurement of CO can be performed without the need for injected fluid.
  ❖ The PA catheter with CCO capability contains a thermal filament situated in the right ventricle. This filament emits a pulsed signal in a 30- to 60-second sequence,[2] allowing for adequate mixing of blood with heat as it passes through the ventricle. A bedside computer displays digital readings updated every 30 to 60 seconds, reflecting the average CO of the preceding 3 to 6 minutes. The CCO eliminates the need for fluid boluses, reduces contamination risk, and provides a continuous CO trend.[3, 6, 7]
  ❖ Because the CCO monitor constantly displays and frequently updates the CCO, treatment decisions may be expedited. Derived hemodynamic calculations (eg, cardiac index [CI] systemic vascular resistance) could be obtained with greater frequency, providing information when assessing response to therapies that affect hemodynamics. However, technology assessment, patient selection criteria, and patient outcomes using the CCO method are ongoing.[7–11]
  ❖ Adequate mixing of blood and indicator (heat) is required for accurate CCO measurements. Conditions that prevent appropriate mixing or directional flow of the indicator (heat) or blood include intracardiac shunts or tricuspid regurgitation.
  ❖ The CCO method is based on the same physiologic principle as the TDCO method: the indicator-dilution technique. The TDCO method uses a bolus of injectate as the indicator for measurement of CO. The CCO method uses the heat signals produced by the thermal filament as the indicator. This device provides a time-averaged rather than an instantaneous CO reading.[15] CCO values are influenced by the same principles as TDCO.
  ❖ Body temperatures greater than 40°C to 43°C may not be appreciated by CCO catheters. The heated thermal filament has a temperature limit to a maximum of 44°C (111.2°F). CCO computers are calibrated by the manufacturer to produce reliable calculations within a temperature range of 30°C to 40°C (86°F to 104°F) or 31°C to 43°C (87.8°F to 109.4°F). An error message will appear if the temperature in the PA is out of range.
  ❖ Infusions through proximal lumens should be limited to maintaining patency of lumen. Concomitant infusions through the proximal lumen can theoretically affect CCO measurements. Studies have shown that such infusions can cause variations in TDCO measurements. To date, no published data describing the effect of concurrent central line infusions on the accuracy of CCO measurements are available.[15]

❖ Because bolus injections are not required with the CCO method, the prevalence of user error is theoretically reduced.[21, 22]
❖ The CCO catheter can be used to obtain both CCO and TDCO measurements. Comparison results using both methods may be obtained. Comparison of TDCO and CCO methods support the use of CCO as a reliable method.[8, 9, 12, 23]

EQUIPMENT

- Nonsterile gloves
- Cardiac monitor
- Bedside hemodynamic monitoring system
- PA catheter (in place)
- CO computer or module
- Connecting cables
- Injectate temperature probe
- Injectate solution

Additional equipment as needed includes the following:

- Four 10-mL syringes (prefilled or empty)
- Injectate solution bag with intravenous (IV) tubing and three-way Luer-Lok stopcock
- Ice
- Setup for CCO
- Printer

PATIENT AND FAMILY EDUCATION

- Explain the procedure for CO and the reason for its measurement. ➺*Rationale:* Decreases patient and family anxiety.
- Explain the monitoring equipment involved, the frequency of measurements, and the goals of therapy. ➺*Rationale:* Encourages patient and family to ask questions and voice specific concerns about the procedure.
- Explain any potential variations in temperature the patient may or may not experience when iced injectate is used. ➺*Rationale:* Acknowledges patients' varying physical responses to injectate and possible perception of cold solution.

PATIENT ASSESSMENT AND PREPARATION

Patient Assessment

- Assess the patient's vital signs, fluid balance, heart and breath sounds, skin color, temperature, mentation, peripheral pulses, cardiac rate and rhythm, and hemodynamic variables. ➺*Rationale:* Clinical information provides data regarding blood flow and tissue perfusion.
- Assess history of medication therapy, including medication allergies and current pharmacologic regime. ➺*Rationale:* Current information may provide insights into CO results related to existing medical condition or medication regime.
- Assess past medical history for presence of coronary artery disease, presence of valvular heart disease, intracardiac pressures, ejection fraction, and overall ventricular function. ➺*Rationale:* Provides baseline information regarding cardiovascular status.
- Assess PAP, RAP, and PAWP waveforms. ➺*Rationale:* Ensures PA catheter is positioned properly.

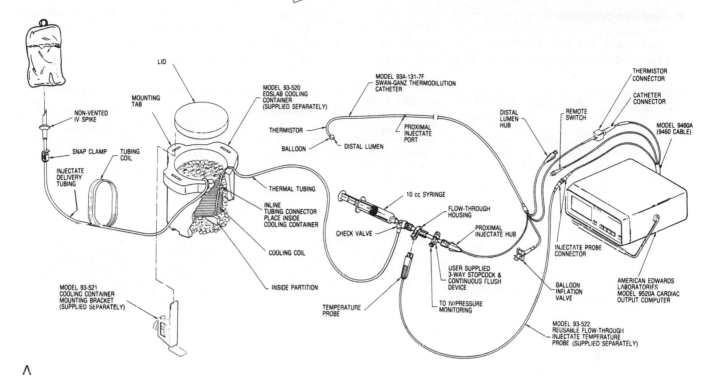

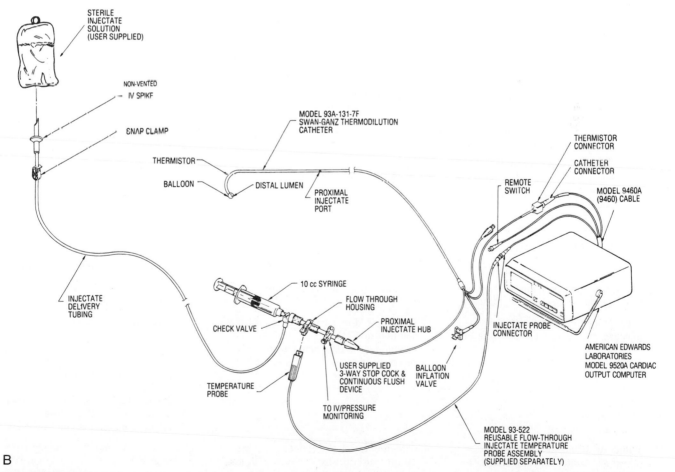

■ ● **FIGURE 59–4.** CO set preparations for cardiac output measurement. *A*, Iced temperature injectate preparation. *B*, Room temperature injectate preparation. (From Baxter Edwards Corporation.)

Patient Preparation

• Ensure that patient and family understand preprocedural teaching. Answer questions as they arise and reinforce information as needed. ➤➤*Rationale:* Evaluates and reinforces understanding of previously taught information.

• Assist patient to supine position. ➤➤*Rationale:* CO measurements are most accurate in the supine position.

Procedure **for Measurement of Cardiac Output**

Steps	Rationale	Special Considerations
1. Select the injectate delivery system—open or closed method. *(Level IV: Limited clinical studies to support recommendation)*	Closed system has infection control benefits by reducing multiple entries into the system.[14]	Closed system may eliminate cost and time expenditures of individual syringe preparation.
2. Select room temperature (19°C to 25°C) or iced temperature (0°C to 12°C) injectate. *(Level VI: Clinical studies in a variety of different patient populations and situations to support recommendation)*	Room temperature injectate may be used for most patients. Iced injectate may improve accuracy of CO measurement for patients with low or high COs.	Research on room temperature versus iced temperature injectates supports the accuracy of either method when 10-mL injectate volume is used.[13–16, 18, 20] However, additional research is needed in patients with low and high COs.

Procedure **for Closed Method of Syringe Preparation**

Steps	Rationale	Special Considerations
1. Wash hands, and don gloves.	Reduces transmission of microorganisms; standard precautions.	
2. Use 5% dextrose in water (D₅W).	The specific gravity of D_5W is a component in the formula used to derive CO by the TDCO method. The use of saline can result in a 2% decrease in TDCO measurement.[13]	Normal saline may be used if the patient's medical condition requires.
3. Aseptically connect the IV tubing to the injectate solution.	Prepares system.	
4. Hang the IV injectate solution on an IV pole, and prime the tubing.	Eliminates air from the tubing.	
5. Connect injectate tubing to the proximal lumen of the PA catheter via a three-way Luer-Lok stopcock (see Fig. 59–4).	Connects the injectate solution to the PA catheter.	
6. Connect the injectate syringe to the three-way stopcock (see Fig. 59–4).	The syringe will be used for solution injection.	Connect the system so that the CO syringe will be in a straight line with the PA catheter to decrease resistance when injecting solution.
7. Connect the in-line temperature probe (see Fig. 59–4).	Measures injectate temperature.	
8. If using iced injectate, set up the iced injectate system (eg, CO set) (see Fig. 59–4A).	If using iced injectate, cool the injectate solution to 0°C to 12°C (32°F to 53°F), depending on the manufacturer recommendation of the system in use.	Coiled tubing systems that are immersed in an ice bath are commercially available. Follow manufacturer guidelines for current equipment used. Cool injectate may be prearrhythmic in some patients.[16] CO set may also be used without ice to deliver closed system room temperature injectate.
9. Withdraw 10 mL of injectate. *(Level IV: Limited clinical studies to support recommendations)*	Common injectate volumes are 5 mL or 10 mL for critically ill adults with low, normal, and high CO.[14, 17]	10 mL is the most commonly used volume. When fluid restriction is important, the 5-mL bolus may be used.

Procedure **for Closed Method of Syringe Preparation** *Continued*

Steps	Rationale	Special Considerations
10. Select the computation constant consistent with injectate *volume* and injectate *temperature*. Also, confirm the type and size of PA catheter and confirm injectate delivery system.	The computation constant is set on the CO computer. Tables to facilitate the computation constant determination are provided by the manufacturer. The computation constant needs to be accurate for valid and reliable CO measurements.	Carefully select the correct computation constant for iced temperature or room temperature injection. Confirm setting on CO computer.
11. Connect CO cable to PA catheter.	Prepares system.	
12. Turn on CO computer or module.	Provides energy.	
13. Note the injectate temperature.	The injectate temperature should be at least 10° less than the patient's temperature.[18]	
14. Position the patient supine, with the head of the bed elevated up to 20 degrees or as patient's clinical condition warrants. (*Level V: Clinical studies in more than one or two different patient populations and situations to support recommendations*)	Studies of patients in supine position with head of bed flat or elevated 20 degrees have shown no significant differences in TDCO measurements.[3-5] Consistency in patient position may increase reliability in consecutive CO readings.	Patient's medical condition may determine positioning. Consistent positioning with CO readings and documentation of positioning should be noted on patient's record. Some patients may be more susceptible to position change. Comparison to CO in flat position may be warranted.
15. Verify the position of the PA catheter. Note the RA waveform from the proximal port and the PA waveform from the distal port.	Proper positioning of PA catheter ensures that the distal thermistor is located in the pulmonary artery. The distal thermistor wire calculates the time-temperature data. Excessive coiling of the catheter in the RA or right ventricle can result in poor positioning of the distal thermistor in relation to the injectate port.[19]	Improper positioning of PA catheters may result in false values.[8, 13, 14] Fluoroscopy and chest x-ray can be used to verify position. Catheter coiling may occur in patients with large dilated right ventricles.[19]
16. Observe the patient's cardiac rhythm.	Dysrhythmias or frequent ectopy may affect CO measurement.	
17. If possible, consider restricting infusions delivered through the introducer or other central lines. (*Level IV: Limited clinical studies to support recommendations*)	TDCO measurements obtained while receiving other infusions can vary CO measurements (by as much as 40% higher) obtained when no other infusions were being concomitantly infused.[13]	
18. Confirm computation constant.	Recheck computation constant before each series of CO measurements.	
19. Withdraw injectate into syringe.	Prepares for injection.	
20. Support stopcock with palm of nondominant hand.	Minimal handling (less than 30 seconds) of the syringe is recommended to avoid variations in injectate temperature that may introduce error into the CO calculation.	Syringe holders or automatic injector devices are available and can be used to aid in injectate administration.
21. Observe patient's respiratory pattern. Prepare to administer injectate at the end-expiratory phase in the respiratory cycle.	Significant variations in transthoracic pressure during respiration can affect CO.	
22. Activate CO computer, and wait for ready message.	The CO or module needs to be ready before injecting solution.	Manufacturer recommendations may vary.
23. Administer the injectate bolus rapidly and smoothly in 4 seconds or less. (*Level IV: Limited clinical studies to support recommendations*)	Prolonged injection time may result in false low CO. Rates of 2 to 4 seconds for injection of 5 to 10 mL of injectate yield accurate results.[2, 13, 14, 16]	Prolonged injection time interferes with time and temperature calculations.

Procedure continued on following page

Procedure for Closed Method of Syringe Preparation *Continued*

Steps	Rationale	Special Considerations
24. Determine the CO by observing the digital display and the CO curve (see Fig. 59–3).	The CO curve needs to be a normal curve. A normal curve starts at baseline and has a smooth upstroke and a gradual downstroke. If the CO curve is not normal, the CO measurement obtained from the injection should be discarded. Abnormal contours of the curve may indicate improper catheter position. Abnormal CO curve may represent technical error.	Normal CO is 4 to 8 L/min. Abnormal CO curves may also provide information about the patient's abnormal clinical condition, such as tricuspid valve regurgitation.
25. Repeat steps 18 to 24.	Discard CO measurements that do not have normal CO curves. Also discard values that are beyond the 10% range in the cycle of three injections.[2, 13]	Subsequent injections should be performed approximately 1 to 2 minutes apart. Consistent volumes and temperatures are necessary for accuracy.
26. Obtain the CO measurement by calculating the average of three measurements within 10% of a middle (median) value. *(Level IV: Limited clinical studies to support recommendations)*	Determines CO value.	
27. Return proximal stopcock at RA lumen to original position.	Initiates continued hemodynamic monitoring.	
28. Resume flow of infusions.	Continues therapy.	
29. Observe PA and RA waveforms on the monitor.	Continues hemodynamic monitoring.	
30. Discard used supplies, and wash hands.	Reduces transmission of microorganisms; standard precautions.	
31. Determine hemodynamic calculations.	Assesses hemodynamic status.	

Procedure for Open Method of Syringe Preparation

Steps	Rationale	Special Considerations
1. Wash hands, and don gloves.	Reduces transmission of microorganisms; standard precautions.	
2. Prepare syringes or obtain manufactured prefilled syringes for CO determination.	Prepares injectate for CO determination.	
3. Clean injectate port of D_5W IV bag with an alcohol wipe, or apply a dispensing port to the bag's injectate port.	Reduces surface contamination. Dispensing port negates the use of needles or needleless drawing system and reduces the incidence of accidental needlesticks.	Not necessary if using manufactured, prefilled, sterile syringes.
4. Aseptically withdraw injectate solution from the IV bag into three 10-mL syringes and cap securely.	Prepares injectate for at least three CO measurements.	Additional syringes may be necessary because syringes may be inadvertently dropped or contaminated.
5. If not using immediately, label container or syringes with the date and time that they were prepared.	Prefilled syringes at bedside or in refrigerator must be labeled (eg, "for CO injection only").	

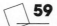

Procedure	**for Open Method of Syringe Preparation** *Continued*	

Steps	Rationale	Special Considerations
6. If using iced injectate, cool the syringes by filling the syringe container with sterile water and ice.	Iced slush is used to cool syringes.	Not necessary if using room temperature syringes. Handling of iced syringe may cause warming inconsistent with selected temperature. Cool injectate may be prearrhythmic in some patients.[16]
7. Select the computation constant consistent with injectate volume and injectate temperature. Also confirm the type and size of the PA catheter and confirm the injectate delivery system.	The computation constant is set on the CO computer. Tables to facilitate the computation constant determination are provided by the manufacturer. The computation constant needs to be accurate for valid and reliable CO measurements.	Carefully select the correct computation constant for iced temperature or room temperature injection. Confirm setting on CO computer.
8. Follow steps 11 to 17 of the closed method.		
9. Remove cap from the right atrial stopcock.	Prepares stopcock.	
10. Aseptically connect one of the sterile CO injectate syringes onto the right atrial stopcock.	Reduces risk of introducing microorganisms into the system.	
11. Turn the stopcock so that it is closed to the flush solution and open between injectate syringe and the patient.	Prepares system for injectate administration.	
12. Follow steps 20 to 26 of the closed method.	Obtains CO measurements.	Asepsis is essential as the stopcock is turned appropriately and syringes are changed between injectates.
13. After the last injectate is completed, return the stopcock so that the system is open between the patient and the transducer; aseptically remove the last injectate syringe; and place a new, sterile, dead-end cap on the stopcock port.	Closes the system; maintains sterility of the system.	
14. Observe PA and RA waveforms on the monitor.	Continues hemodynamic monitoring.	
15. Discard used supplies, and wash hands.	Reduces transmission of microorganisms; standard precautions.	

Procedure	**for Measurement of Cardiac Output Using Continuous Cardiac Output Method**

Steps	Rationale	Special Considerations
1. Connect the CO cable to the PA catheter.	Prepares system.	
2. Turn on the CO computer.	Provides energy.	
3. Observe the right atrial waveform. The proximal lumen of the PA catheter should be located in the RA.	A right atrial waveform indicates that the thermal filament is properly placed. The thermal filament should be located in the right ventricle between the infusion port and the distal tip of the catheter. Advancement of the thermal filament into the PA will result in erroneous measurements.	The thermal filament should float free in the right ventricle to prevent loss of indicator (heat) into the cardiac tissue. If loss of indicator occurs, CO will be overestimated, giving erroneous readings. The position of the catheter can also be confirmed by chest radiographs.

Procedure continued on following page

Procedure **for Measurement of Cardiac Output Using Continuous Cardiac Output Method**
Continued

Steps	Rationale	Special Considerations
4. Position patient supine with the head of the bed elevated up to 20 degrees. *(Level II: Theory based, no research data to support recommendations; recommendations from expert consenus group may exist)*	Position for CCO consistent with TDCO measurements.	Studies are needed to describe the effect of patients' body position on CCO measurements.
5. Check heat signal indicator on the CO computer.	CCO systems relate the quality of the heat signal by assessing the quality of the measured thermal signal. Relationships are in response to thermal noise or signal-to-noise ratio.	CCO monitors provide messages for troubleshooting signal-to-noise ratio interferences. Refer to manufacturer recommendations. Technologic advances provide success in suppressing the effects of blood thermal noise.[14]
6. Note that the CCO readings occur at different times and are measured with different phases of the respiratory cycle.	Continuous data collection reflects phasic changes in the respiratory cycle.	
7. Document CCO in conjunction with other hemodynamic findings.	CCO provides measurements that are averaged over the preceding 3 to 6 minutes.	CCO is calculated by a bedside computer displaying graphic trends and by a continuous graphic reading that is updated every 30 to 60 seconds.
8. Validate CCO with patient's clinical status and concurrent hemodynamic findings.	CCO is a global assessment parameter and must be appreciated as part of the patient's total hemodynamic profile at a given time.	CCO method eliminates many of the potential user and technique-related errors associated with intermittent bolus CO. Research demonstrates clinically acceptable correlation between the TDCO technique and the CCO method in the steady state.[7, 9, 11] Studies need to continue in patients during periods of acute hemodynamic instability and in specific patient populations in which there is structural or functional heart damage.

Expected Outcomes

- An accurate measurement of CO is obtained.
- Hemodynamic profile and derived parameters available continuously or intermittently are accurately assessed.
- Sterile integrity of PA lines is maintained.

Unexpected Outcomes

- Inability to accurately measure CO
- Erroneous readings because of technical error
- Erroneous readings because of equipment error
- Occlusion of proximal PA line
- Contamination of system

Patient Monitoring and Care

Patient Monitoring and Care	Rationale	Reportable Conditions
		These conditions should be reported if they persist despite nursing interventions.
1. Maintain patency of PA lines (see Procedure 69).	Line patency is essential for accurate readings.	- Inability to establish patency
2. Monitor PA waveform for confirmation of hemodynamic waveforms.	Proper placement determines accurate hemodynamics and CO measurement.	- Difficulty providing manual flush - Abnormal PA waveforms consistent with PA line malposition

Patient Monitoring and Care *Continued*

Patient Monitoring and Care	Rationale	Reportable Conditions
3. Maintain sterility of PA line and ports.	Reduces the risk of catheter-related infections.	• Fever, site redness, drainage, or symptoms consistent with infection
4. Calculate cardiac index, system vascular resistance, and other parameters as prescribed or indicated.	Determines hemodynamic function.	• Abnormal cardiac index, systemic vascular resistance, or other hemodynamic values
5. Monitor vital signs and respiratory status hourly and as required.	Change in vital signs or respiratory status may indicate hemodynamic compromise.	• Sudden or significant change in patient's clinical status
6. Calculate additional fluid volume for bolus method or continuous infusion into patient's total fluid volume.	Additional volume added intermittently should be included in total intake for accurate fluid volume assessment.	• Signs or symptoms of fluid overload (eg, respiratory distress, crackles, increased PA pressures, systemic edema)
7. Assess patient's response to therapy instituted based on hemodynamic parameters.	Hemodynamic monitoring may expedite treatment decisions and provide direction for positive patient outcomes.	• Significant change in CO or hemodynamic status

Documentation

Documentation should include the following:

- Patient and family education
- CO, cardiac index, systemic vascular resistance
- Characteristics and reliability of CO curve
- Continuous or Intermittent bolus method
- Volume and temperature of injectate
- Concurrent vital signs and hemodynamic measurements
- Titration or administration of pharmacologic agents affecting CO
- Significant medical or nursing interventions affecting CO (eg, intra-aortic balloon pump therapy, volume expanders, position changes, other clinical factors)
- Unexpected outcomes
- Additional interventions

References

1. Stewart S, Vitello-Cicciu JM. Cardiovascular clinical physiology. In: Kinney MR, Brooks-Brunn J, Molter N, Dunbar SB, Vitello-Cicciu JM, eds. *AACN Clinical Reference for Critical Care Nurse.* 4th ed. St. Louis: Mosby–Year Book; 1998:249–276.
2. Headley JM. Invasive hemodynamic monitoring: applying advanced technologies. *Crit Care Nurs.* 1998 Nov;21(3):73–84.
3. Grap MJ, Cantley M, Munro CL, Corley MC. Use of backrest elevation in critical care: a pilot study. *Am J Crit Care.* 1999;8(1):495–496.
4. Evans D. The use of position during critical illness: current practice and review of the literature. *Aust Crit Care.* 1994;7:16–21.
5. Driscoll A, Shanahan A, Crommy L, Foong S, Gleason A. The effect of patient positioning on reproducibility of cardiac output measurements. *Heart Lung.* 1995;24:38–44.
6. Albert N, Spear B, Hammell J. Agreement and clinical utility of 2 techniques for measuring cardiac output in patients with low cardiac ouptput. *Am J Crit Care.* 1998;8(1):464–467.
7. Medin DL, Brown DT, Wesley R, Cunnion RE, Gnibene FP. Validation of continuous thermodilution cardiac output in critically ill patients with analysis of systematic errors. *J Crit Care.* 1998;13(4):184–189.
8. Kalassian KG, Raffin TA. The technique of thermodilution cardiac output measurements. *J Crit Illness.* 1996;11:249–256.
9. Boldt J, Menges T, Wollbruck M, Hammerman H, Hempelmann G. Is continuous cardiac output measurement using theramodilution reliable in the critically ill patient? *Crit Care Med.* 1994;22:1913–1918.
10. Ditmyer CE, Shively M, Burns CB. Comparison of continuous with intermittent bolus thermodilution cardiac output measurement. *Am J Crit Care.* 1995;4:460–465.
11. Mihaljevic T, Von Segesser LK, Tonz, M, Leskosek B, Seifert B, Jenni R, Turina M. Continuous versus bolus thermodilution cardiac output measurement: a comparative study. *Crit Care Med.* 1995;23:944–949.

12. Rading G, Keyl C, Liebold A. Interoperative evaluation of a continuous versus intermittent bolus thermodilution technique of cardiac surgical patients. *Eur J Anesthesiology.* 1998;15(2): 196–201.

13. Gawlinski A. *Protocols for Practice: Hemodynamic Monitoring Series—Cardiac Output Monitoring.* Aliso Viejo, CA: American Association of Critical-Care Nurses; 1998.

14. Woods S, Oshuthorpe S. Cardiac output determination. AACN CL issue. *Crit Care Nurs.* 1993;4(1):81–97.

15. Kiely M, Byers LA, Greewood R. Thermodilution measurement of cardiac output in patients with low output: room temperature versus iced injectate. *Am J Crit Care.* 1998;7(6):436–438.

16. Zellinger M. *Advanced Concepts in Hemodynamics; Current Issues in Critical Care Nursing.* New York, NY: Medical Information Services; 1995.

17. McCloy K, Leung S, Beldon J. Effects of injectate volume on thermodilution measurements of cardiac output in patients with low ventricular ejection fraction. *Am J Crit Care.* 1999;8(2):86–92.

18. Gardner PE, Bridges EJ. Hemodynamic monitoring. In Woods SL, Sivarajan-Froelicher ES, Halpenny CJ, Motzer SV, eds. *Cardiac Nursing.* 3rd ed. Philadelphia: JB Lippincott; 1995:424–458.

19. Kerns M. Hemodynamic data. In: *The Cardiac Catheterization Handbook.* 1999. St. Louis, Mo: Mosby–Year Book; 1999:123–223.

20. Elkayam U, Berkley R, Azen S, et al. Cardiac output by thermodilution technique: effect of injectate's volume and temperature on accuracy and reproducibility in the critically ill patient. *Chest.* 1983;84:418–422.

21. Goede DS, Ackerman MA. We've come a long way: from fick to continuous cardiac output monitoring. *Am J Nurs.* 1994;94(suppl):24–29.

22. Gardner P, Woods S. Hemodynamic monitoring. In: Woods SL, ed. *Cardiac Nursing.* 3rd ed. Philadelphia, Pa: JB Lippincott; 1995:424–458.

23. Marcum J, Liberatone K, Willard G. A comparison of varying injectate volumes in determining thermodilution cardiac output in critically ill post-surgical patients. *Am J Crit Care.* 1995;2:262.

Additional Readings

Ahrens T. Hemodynamic monitoring. *Crit Care Nurs Clin N Am.* 1999;11(1):19–31.

Brandsteller RD, Grant GR, Estillo M, Rahim F, Singh K, Gitlier B. Swan-Ganz catheter: misconceptions, pitfalls, and incomplete user knowledge—an identified trilogy in need of correction. *Heart Lung: J Acute Crit Care.* 1998;27(4):218–222.

Burchell SA, Yu M, Takiguchi SA, Ohta RM, Meyers SE. Evaluation of a continuous cardiac output and mixed venous oxygen saturation catheter in critically ill surgical patients. *Crit Care Med.* 1997;25(3):388–391.

Cason CL, Lambert W. Positioning during hemodynamic monitoring. *DCCN.* 1993;12:226–233.

Daily EK, Schroeder JF. *Techniques in Bedside Hemodynamic Monitoring.* 5th ed. St. Louis, Mo: Mosby–Year Book; 1994.

Doering L, Dracupk K. Comparisons of cardiac output in supine and lateral positions. *Nurs Res.* 1988;37:114–118.

Headley JM. Strategies to optimize the cardiorespiratory status of the critically ill. *AACN Clin Issues Crit Care Nurs.* 1995;6:121–134.

Headley J. *Invasive Hemodynamic Monitoring: Physiological Principles and Clinical Application.* Irvine, Ca: Baxter Health Care Corp; 1996.

Munro HM, Wood CE, Taylor BL, Smith GB. Continuous invasive cardiac output monitoring: the Baxter/Edwards Critical Care Swan-Ganz Intelli Cath and Vigilance system. *Clin Intensive Care.* 1994;5:52–55.

Pesola GR, Rostata HP, Carlon GC. Room temperature thermodilution cardiac: central venous vs. right ventricular port. *Am J Crit Care.* 1992;1:76–80.

Pulmonary artery catheter consensus conference: consensus statement. *Crit Care Med.* 1997;25:910–925.

Taylor RW. Controversies in pulmonary artery catheterization. *New Horiz.* 1997;5:1–296.

Whalen DA, Keller R. Cardiovascular patient assessment. In: Kinney MR, Brooks-Brunn J, Molter N, Dunbar SB, Vitello-Cicciu JM, eds. *AACN Clinical Reference for Critical Care Nurse.* 4th ed. St. Louis, Mo: Mosby–Year Book; 1998:227–319.

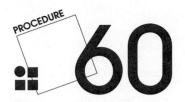

60

Central Venous/ Right Atrial Pressure Line Removal

PURPOSE: Central venous catheters are removed when therapy is completed, a mechanical malfunction has occurred, the catheter has become occluded or malpositioned, or the patient has developed a catheter-related infection.

Marie Arnone

PREREQUISITE NURSING KNOWLEDGE

- The normal anatomy and physiology of the cardiovascular system should be understood.
- Clinical and technical competence in central line removal is necessary.
- The anatomy and physiology of the vasculature and adjacent structures of the neck should be known.
- The nurse will need to validate that the catheter has been removed intact. Knowing the catheter design and length will assist the nurse in determining if the catheter is removed completely.[1]
- Migration of bacteria from the skin surface along the subcutaneous tract to the bloodstream has been designated as the primary mechanism in the pathogenesis of catheter-related septicemia. Disinfecting the skin before removing the catheter will decrease recolonization of the skin and catheter insertion site.[2, 3]
- Air embolism can occur during the removal of the catheter. Air embolism after the removal of the catheter is a result of air drawn in along the subcutaneous tract and into the vein. During inspiration, negative intrathoracic pressure is transmitted to the central veins. Any opening external to the body to one of these veins may result in aspiration of air into the central venous system. The pathologic effects depend on the volume and rate of air aspirated. The risk of air embolism is decreased if the nurse has the patient supine with the head of the bed flat or in the Trendelenburg position and if the patient is able to exhale and not breathe while the catheter is being removed.[1]

EQUIPMENT

- Goggles, mask, and gloves
- Alcohol pads or swabsticks
- Povidone-iodine pads or swabsticks
- Suture removal kit or sterile scissors
- 4 × 4 gauze pads
- 2 × 2 gauze pads
- One roll of 2-inch tape

Additional equipment to have available if needed includes the following:

- Culture tube to culture tip of catheter

PATIENT AND FAMILY EDUCATION

- Explain the procedure for catheter removal to patient and family. **➤➤Rationale:** Enhances patient and family understanding, increases patient cooperation, and reduces anxiety.
- Instruct the patient to report any signs and symptoms of shortness of breath, chest pain, or other changes. **➤➤Rationale:** May aid in early recognition of complications.

PATIENT ASSESSMENT AND PREPARATION

Patient Assessment

- Review laboratory data for platelet count, prothrombin time (PT), partial prothromboplastin time (PTT), and international normalized ratio (INR). **➤➤Rationale:** Pressure on the catheter site may be required for a longer period if coagulation studies are abnormal.
- Determine if patient is receiving anticoagulant therapy. **➤➤Rationale:** Pressure on the catheter site may be required for a longer period.
- Assess vital signs. **➤➤Rationale:** Provides baseline data.
- Observe the catheter site for signs and symptoms of infection (eg, redness, warmth at site, tenderness, or presence of drainage). **➤➤Rationale:** Culturing of the catheter site and catheter tip is indicated for diagnosis and treatment of catheter-related infection.

Patient Preparation

- Ensure that the patient and family understand preprocedural teaching. Answer questions as they arise and reinforce information as needed. **➤➤Rationale:** Evaluates and reinforces understanding of previously taught information.

- Position the patient supine with the head of the bed flat or in a slight Trendelenburg position. **➤Rationale:** A normal pressure gradient exists between atmospheric air and the central venous compartment that promotes air entry if the compartment is open. The lower the site of entry below the heart, the lower the pressure gradient, thus minimizing the risk of venous air embolism.

- Start a new peripheral intravenous (IV) line or ensure that an existing peripheral IV is patent. **➤Rationale:** Establishes IV access for fluids or medications.

Procedure for Central Venous/Right Atrial Pressure Line Removal

Steps	Rationale	Special Considerations
1. Wash hands.	Reduces transmission of microorganisms; standard precautions.	
2. Open sterile packages—suture removal kit or sterile scissors and sterile gauze pads.	Prepares supplies for use.	
3. Turn off IV infusion.	Prevents saturating the bed, patient, or work area with IV solution on catheter removal.	
4. Put on personal protective equipment (goggles, mask, and gloves).	Reduces transmission of microorganisms; standard precautions.	
5. Remove the catheter dressing and discard.	Exposes the catheter site.	
6. Remove examination gloves and don a clean pair of gloves.	Reduces the transmission of microorganisms; standard precautions.	
7. Starting with the insertion site, using concentric circles, cleanse the skin with alcohol or povidone-iodine or both.	Prevents contamination of the wound by skin microorganisms.[2, 3]	Cleanse an area approximately 2 in in diameter. Allow to dry.
8. Ensure that the head of the bed is flat. Remove the pillow and have the patient turn his or her head away from the catheter.	Positions the patient for central line removal and reduces the transmission of microorganisms.	
9. Carefully cut the suture, and pull the suture through the skin.	Allows for removal of the catheter.	Be sure that the entire suture is removed. Retained sutures can form epithelialized tracts that can lead to infection.
10. Instruct the patient to take a deep breath in and hold it.	This will minimize air being accidentally drawn into the systemic venous circulation.	
11. Remove the catheter, following these steps: A. Grasp the catheter with the dominant hand and slowly withdraw the catheter in one continuous motion. B. With the nondominant hand, quickly apply pressure over the puncture site with a sterile 4 × 4 gauze pad.	Withdrawing the catheter with a continuous motion decreases trauma to the vein. The distal end of a multilumen catheter should be removed quickly because the exposed proximal and medial openings could permit the entry of air.	If there are signs of infection, send the catheter tip to the laboratory for culture and sensitivity testing.

Procedure	for Central Venous/Right Atrial Pressure Line Removal *Continued*	

Steps	Rationale	Special Considerations
12. Maintain pressure for 2 to 5 minutes until hemostasis has been achieved.	Prevents bleeding and hematoma formation.	Pressure may be needed for longer if the patient has been receiving anticoagulant therapy or if coagulation studies are abnormal.
13. Once hemostasis has been achieved, apply an occlusive, sterile dressing over the site.	Minimizes infection at the site.	
14. Inspect the catheter after it is removed.	Ensures that the entire catheter has been removed.	
15. Discard used supplies and wash hands.	Reduces transmission of microorganisms; standard precautions.	

Expected Outcomes	Unexpected Outcomes
• Catheter will be removed intact. • Hemostasis will occur at catheter site.	• Inability to remove catheter • Catheter not removed intact • Air embolism • Pulmonary embolism • Catheter site infection • Difficulty attaining hemostasis at puncture site

Patient Monitoring and Care

Patient Monitoring and Care	Rationale	Reportable Conditions
		These conditions should be reported if they persist despite nursing interventions.
1. Obtain vital signs before and after the central venous catheter is removed.	Changes in heart rate, blood pressure, and respiratory rate may indicate pulmonary air embolism. If an embolus is suspected, position patient on his or her left side.	• Changes in vital signs; suspicion of pulmonary embolism
2. Assess the dressing for the first 15 minutes, then every 15 minutes for the next hour, for bleeding.	Assesses for hemostasis and early evidence of bleeding.	• Bleeding or hematoma development
3. Observe the catheter site daily for signs of infection.	Infection of the skin site may occur after the removal of the catheter.	• Redness, tenderness, or drainage at the catheter site • Elevated temperature or white blood cell counts
4. Remove the dressing and assess for site closure 24 hours after removal.[3]	Verifies healing and closure of the site.	• Abnormal healing

Documentation

Documentation should include the following:

- Patient and family education
- Date and time of catheter removal
- Site assessment
- Culture specimen sent (if appropriate)
- Ease of catheter removal
- Evaluation of the catheter

- Length of time pressure applied to obtain hemostasis
- Application of occlusive dressing
- Patient tolerance of the procedure
- Unexpected outcomes and interventions

References

1. Andris DA, Krzywda EA. Central venous access: clinical practice issues. *Nurs Clin North Am.* 1997;32:719–740.
2. Pearson ML. Special communication guideline for prevention of intravascular device-related infections. Part I. Intravascular device-related infections: an overview. *Am J Infect Control.* 1996;24:262–293.
3. Treston-Aurand J, Olmsted RN, Allen-Bridson K, Craig CP. Impact of dressing materials on central venous catheter infection rates. *J Intravenous Nurs.* 1997;20:201–206.

Additional Readings

Darovic G. *Hemodynamic Monitoring: Invasive and Noninvasive Clinical Application.* 2nd ed. Philadelphia, Pa: W.B. Saunders; 1995.

Lau CE. Transparent and gauze dressing and their effect on infection rates of central venous catheters: a review of past and current literature. *J Intravenous Nurs.* 1996;19:240–245.

61

Central Venous/ Right Atrial Pressure Line Site Care

PURPOSE: Site care of the central venous pressure line allows for assessment of the catheter insertion site for signs of infection or catheter dislodgment, skin integrity, and the integrity of the suture. Site care involves cleansing the area around the catheter to minimize the growth of microorganisms.

Marie Arnone

PREREQUISITE NURSING KNOWLEDGE

- The normal anatomy and physiology of the cardiovascular system should be understood.
- The principles of aseptic technique and infection control should be understood.
- Infection has been identified as a potentially life-threatening complication of central venous catheterization. Appropriate care of the catheter site is considered to have primary importance in decreasing the risk for catheter-related sepsis.
- Migration of bacteria from the skin surface along the subcutaneous tract to the bloodstream has been designated as the primary mechanism in the pathogenesis of catheter-related septicemia.
- Signs and symptoms of catheter infection and septicemia should be known.
- The dressing should be examined for evidence of moisture and evaluated for its ability to provide a protective barrier. Moisture is more likely to be seen in the critical care patient who is receiving frequent suctioning and when high humidification is used during ventilatory support and oxygen therapy. The thorax has a greater density of cutaneous flora and a higher skin temperature than other areas. These factors play a major role in the risk of infection with central venous catheters placed in the chest or neck.
- The differences between transparent dressings and gauze dressings should be understood. The nurse needs to be aware of the advantages and disadvantages of each type of dressing. The advantages of transparent dressings are that they allow visualization of the site and improved patient comfort. Transparent dressings are semipermeable and may require fewer dressing changes. The disadvantages are that they are more expensive than gauze, they may allow for the accumulation of moisture, they are difficult to apply to diaphoretic patients, and they may increase the opportunity of microorganism transmission. Gauze dressings absorb moisture and are less expensive.

The major disadvantage of a gauze dressing is the lack of visualization of the insertion site.

EQUIPMENT

- Nonsterile gloves
- Sterile gloves
- Alcohol pads or swabsticks
- Povidone-iodine pads or swabsticks
- Transparent dressing or sterile 2 × 2 gauze
- Skin protectant pad or swabstick
- Roll of 2-in tape

PATIENT AND FAMILY EDUCATION

- Explain dressing change procedure. ➤*Rationale:* Decreases patient anxiety.
- Explain the importance of patient positioning during dressing change. ➤*Rationale:* Increases patient cooperation and decreases potential for contamination.

PATIENT ASSESSMENT AND PREPARATION

Patient Assessment

- Assess the patient's arm, shoulder, neck, and chest on the same side as the catheter insertion site for signs of pain, swelling, or tenderness. ➤*Rationale:* Assessment is made to evaluate for thrombophlebitis or venous thrombosis.
- Evaluate the patient's clinical status for signs and symptoms of infection or sepsis, that is, fever, chills, change in mental status, hypotension, leukocytosis with left shift, respiratory alkalosis, metabolic acidosis, or glucose intolerance. ➤*Rationale:* Careful assessment of clinical status and the catheter site is performed to evaluate for catheter sepsis.
- Assess the patient's history for sensitivity to antiseptic solutions. ➤*Rationale:* Decreases risk of allergic reactions.

Patient Preparation

- Ensure that the patient and family understand preprocedural teaching. Answer questions as they arise and reinforce information as needed. **➤Rationale:** Evaluates and reinforces understanding of previously taught information.
- If the patient is on ventilatory support, assess the patient's need for suctioning before beginning the procedure. **➤Rationale:** Minimizes the risk of catheter site contamination by secretions and avoids disruption during the procedure.
- Instruct the patient to turn his or her head, or turn the patient's head, away from the insertion site. **➤Rationale:** Minimizes contamination of the site with microorganisms from the patient's respiratory tract.

Procedure **for Central Venous/Right Atrial Pressure Line Site Care**

Steps	Rationale	Special Considerations
1. Wash hands, and don gloves.	Reduces transmission of microorganisms; standard precautions.	
2. Remove the central venous line dressing.	Exposes the catheter site for inspection and site care.	
3. Inspect the catheter, insertion site, suture, and surrounding skin.	Assesses for signs of infection, catheter dislodgment, leakage, or loose sutures.	
4. Remove and discard gloves, and put on a sterile pair of gloves.	Maintains aseptic technique.	
5. Beginning at the insertion site, using concentric circles, cleanse the catheter and the skin around the insertion site with alcohol pads or swabsticks.	Débrides the skin and removes moisture.	Friction is important to débride the skin.
6. Cleanse the catheter and skin with the povidone-iodine pads or swabsticks as described in the previous step and allow them to dry.	Reduces the rate of recolonization of skin microflora.	To be effective, povidone-iodine needs to be in contact with the skin for 2 minutes.[4]
7. Apply skin protectant to the skin.	Protects the skin from injury on tape removal.	Do not apply within 1 in (2.5 cm) around the insertion site.
8. Apply transparent dressing or cover site with 2 × 2 gauze dressing.	Provides a sterile environment.	
9. Cover the gauze with tape, leaving the catheter hub and tubing connection exposed.	Provides occlusive seal to prevent site contamination.	
10. Split a piece of tape in a Y configuration.	Prepares for application around catheter hub and tubing.	
11. Slip the tape under the catheter hub and tubing connection until the end of the split is tight against the tape covering of the gauze or the transparent dressing.	Secures the catheter and may prevent dislodgment.	Use prepackaged catheter protecting tapes if available.
12. Chevron cross the wings of the tape over the dressing.	Secures the tape to prevent dislodgment.	
13. Apply a second piece of tape, covering the tape wings and catheter hub and tubing connection.	Secures connections and prevents inadvertent dislodgment.	
14. Tape the tubing to the arm, or loop the tubing and tape to the chest or neck dressing.	Reduces tension on catheter caused by patient movement.	
15. Discard used supplies and wash hands.	Reduces the transmission of microorganisms; standard precautions.	

Expected Outcomes

- Dressing remains dry, sterile, and intact.
- The catheter site remains free from infection.
- Catheter remains in place without dislodgment.

Unexpected Outcomes

- Catheter-related infection
- Acccidental removal of the catheter or malpositioning of the tip
- Impaired integrity of the skin under the dressing

Patient Monitoring and Care

Patient Monitoring and Care	Rationale	Reportable Conditions
		These conditions should be reported if they persist despite nursing interventions.
1. Assess dressing every 2 to 4 hours and as necessary.	Ensures occlusive, dry sterile dressing.	
2. Follow institution standard for frequency and type of dressing change.	The Centers for Disease Control and Prevention (CDC) have made no recommendation for the frequency of routine central venous line dressing changes but recommend replacing the dressing when the dressing becomes damp, loosened, or soiled or when inspection of the site is necessary.[4]	• Signs or symptoms of infection
3. Assess for signs and symptoms of infection.	Catheter should be removed if signs of infection are present.	• Redness, pain, or drainage at the insertion site; elevated temperature; elevated white blood cell count

Documentation

Documentation should include the following:

- Patient and family education
- Date and time of the procedure
- Condition of catheter site
- Type of dressing applied
- Documentation on the dressing should include date and time of dressing change and initials of person changing the dressing
- Unexpected outcomes
- Additional interventions

References

1. Andris DA, Krzywda EA. Central venous access: clinical practice issues. *Nurs Clin North Am.* 1997;32:719–740.
2. Lau CE. Transparent and gauze dressings and their effect on infection rates of central venous catheters: a review of past and current literature. *J Intravenous Nurs.* 1996;19:240–245.
3. Managram AJ, Horan TC, Person ML, et al. Guideline for prevention of surgical site infection. *Infect Control Hosp Epidemiol.* 1999;24:247–278.
4. Pearson ML. Special communication guideline for prevention of intravascular device-related infections. Part I. Intravascular device-related infections: an overview. *Am J Infect Control.* 1996;24:272–293.
5. Treston-Aurand J, Olmsted RN, Allen-Bridson K, Craig CP. Impact of dressing materials on central venous catheter infection rates. *J Intravenous Nurs.* 1997;20:201–206.

Additional Reading

Darovic G. *Hemodynamic Monitoring: Invasive and Noninvasive Clinical Application.* 2nd ed. Philadelphia, Pa: W.B. Saunders; 1995.

62

Central Venous/ Right Atrial Pressure Monitoring

P U R P O S E: The central venous pressure (CVP) or the right atrial pressure (RAP) is the pressure measured at the tip of a catheter placed within a central vein or the right atrium (RA). Measurements provide information about the patient's fluid volume status and right ventricular (RV) function. The CVP or RAP allows for evaluation of right-sided heart hemodynamics and evaluation of patient response to therapy. For the purpose of this skill, CVP and RAP are used interchangeably, and the water manometer and mercury transducer methods of pressure measurement are described.

Marie Arnone

PREREQUISITE NURSING KNOWLEDGE

- Understanding of the normal anatomy and physiology of the cardiovascular system is necessary.
- Understanding of the principles of aseptic technique and infection control is necessary.
- Principles of hemodynamic monitoring should be understood.
- Invasive lines increase susceptibility to infection. Adherence to aseptic technique when handling these lines can decrease the potential for infection.[8]
- CVP influences and is influenced by venous return and cardiac function. Although the CVP is used as a measure of changes in the right ventricle, the relationship is not linear. Because the right ventricle has the ability to expand and alter its compliance, changes in volume can occur with little change in pressure.
- A single reading of a CVP is not significant. Monitoring trends in CVP readings is more meaningful.
- Normal CVP is 2 to 7 mm Hg.
- The CVP represents right-sided heart preload or the volume of blood found in the right ventricle at the end of diastole.
- CVP values can be obtained by using a hemodynamic monitoring system or a fluid manometer system.
- Understanding of a, c, and v waves is necessary. The *a wave* reflects right atrial contraction. The *c wave* reflects closure of the tricuspid valve. The *v wave* reflects the right atrial filling during ventricular systole.
- The nurse needs to be technically and clinically competent in using the monitoring system chosen for obtaining CVP measurements. Hemodynamic monitoring systems allow for analysis of the waveform and measurement of the pressure. Water manometers provide only a numerical value.[4] If changing from one system to the other, it is important to know that the values will be different. Water

manometers measure centimeters of water pressure, whereas transducers measure mm Hg. Water manometer values will be higher than mercury readings. The formula for conversion is as follows: cm $H_2O \div 1.36 =$ mm Hg.[1-4]
- CVP readings can be affected by location of the air-fluid interface of the monitoring system (see Procedure 69).
- CVP values are useful in determining hypervolemia, hypovolemia, effect of medication therapy (especially medication that decreases preload), and cardiac function (Table 62–1).[7]

EQUIPMENT

- Hemodynamic monitoring system (see Procedure 69)
- Bedside monitor
- Analog recorder
- Carpenter's level

Table 62–1 ●■■ **Central Venous Pressure**

Conditions Causing Increased CVP

Elevated vascular volume
Increased cardiac output (hyperdynamic cardiac function)
Depressed cardiac function (RV infarct, RV failure)
Cardiac tamponade
Constrictive pericarditis
Pulmonary hypertension
Chronic left ventricular failure

Conditions Causing Decreased CVP

Reduced vascular volume*
Decreased mean systemic pressures (eg, as in late shock states)
Venodilation (drug induced)

---

*Be aware that although the measured CVP is low, cardiac function may be depressed, normal, or hyperdynamic when there is reduced vascular volume.

Additional equipment to have available as needed includes the following:

- Water manometer and intravenous (IV) fluid

PATIENT AND FAMILY EDUCATION

- Discuss the purpose of the CVP catheter with both patient and family. ➤➤*Rationale:* Reduces anxiety and includes patient and family in plan of care.
- Discuss the purpose of CVP monitoring with patient and family. ➤➤*Rationale:* Keeps the patient and the family informed and may reduce anxiety.

PATIENT ASSESSMENT AND PREPARATION

Patient Assessment

- Assess for signs and symptoms of fluid volume deficit, including weakness, thirst, decreased urine output, increased urine specific gravity, output that is greater than intake, sudden weight loss or gain, decreased pulmonary wedge pressure, hemoconcentration, hypernatremia, postural hypotension, tachycardia, decreased skin turgor, dry mucous membranes, decreased pulse pressure, weak and thready pulse, abnormal paradoxical pulse on arterial line waveform, and altered mental status.[1] ➤➤*Rationale:* The patient's clinical picture should correlate with CVP value. Fluid volume deficit will usually result in a decreased CVP.
- Assess for signs and symptoms of fluid volume excess, including dyspnea, orthopnea, anxiety, sudden weight gain, intake greater than output, pulmonary congestion, abnormal breath sounds (e.g., crackles), S_3 heart sound, dependent edema, pleural effusion, anasarca, tachypnea, dilutional decrease in hemoglobin and hematocrit, tachycardia, dysrhythmias, blood pressure change, increased pulmonary artery pressures or pulmonary wedge pressure,

jugular vein distention, oliguria, urine specific gravity changes, altered electrolytes, and altered mental status.[1] ➤➤*Rationale:* The patient's clinical picture should correlate with CVP values. Fluid volume overload will usually result in an elevated CVP.
- Assess for signs and symptoms of air embolus, including a sucking sound on inspiration, dyspnea, tachypnea, hypoxia, hypercapnia, wheezing, a bell-shaped air bubble in the pulmonary outflow tract on the chest x-ray film, increased pulmonary artery pressures, tachycardia, cyanosis, jugular vein distention, hypotension, increased systemic vascular resistance, substernal chest pain, ST segment changes on electrocardiogram (ECG), cor pulmonale, cardiac arrest, lightheadedness, confusion, anxiety, fear of dying, aphasia, localized neurologic deficits, hemiplegia, unresponsiveness, and seizures. ➤➤*Rationale:* Air embolus is a rare but potentially fatal complication of CVP catheterization. This may develop during insertion, with an accidental disconnection of the catheter, or during catheter removal.
- Assess for signs and symptoms of infection. Potential for infection can occur with improper catheter care or contamination. Contamination may occur during insertion or any time while the catheter is in place.[8, 9] ➤➤*Rationale:* Infection is a complication of any invasive line.

Patient Preparation

- Ensure that the patient and family understand preprocedural teaching. Answer questions as they arise and reinforce information as needed. ➤➤*Rationale:* Evaluates and reinforces understanding of previously taught information.
- Place patient in supine position with the head of the bed flat or elevated 45 degrees.[3, 7] ➤➤*Rationale:* Allows for accurate leveling of the air-fluid interface of the monitoring system with the atria.

Procedure for Central Venous/Right Atrial Pressure Monitoring

Steps	Rationale	Special Considerations
CVP Measurement Using Water Manometer Method		
1. Wash hands.	Reduces transmission of microorganisms; standard precautions.	
2. Locate the phlebostatic axis (see Procedure 69).	Ensures accuracy of measurement.	Once the phlebostatic axis has been identified, the nurse should mark the patient's skin with an indelible marker at the level. This will ensure that future readings are taken at the same location.
3. Place the zero level of the water manometer at the level of the phlebostatic axis (Figs. 62–1 and 62–2).	Levels the water manometer for accurate measurements.	If the water manometer is attached to an IV pole, use a carpenter's level to ensure that the zero level of the manometer is level with the phlebostatic axis.
4. Turn the water manometer stopcock open to the flush bag (Fig. 62–3, system A).	Permits fluid to fill the water manometer.	

Procedure continued on page 411

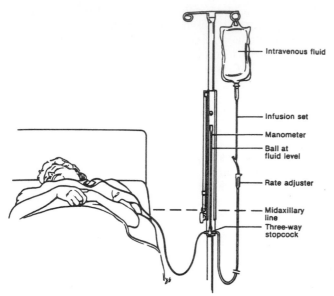

■ ● **FIGURE 62–1.** Central venus pressure water manometer flush system. This manometer is attached to the IV pole, and the height is adjusted to the phlebostatic axis using a carpenter's level. (From Hudack C. *Critical Care Nursing: A Holistic Approach.* Philadelphia: J.B. Lippincott; 1989:123.)

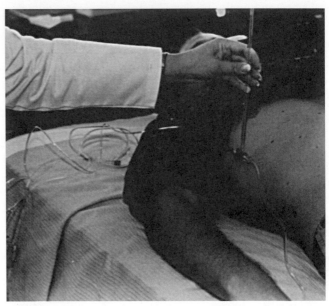

■ ● **FIGURE 62–2.** Water manometer placed at phlebostatic axis on patient.

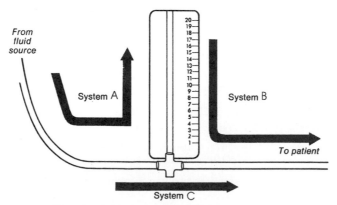

■ ● **FIGURE 62–3.** Central venous pressure measurement. *A,* Stopcock closed to patient for filling of manometer. *B,* Stopcock closed to fluid source and open to patient. *C,* Stopcock closed to manometer with fluid system opened to patient. (From Hudak C. *Critical Care Nursing: A Holistic Approach.* Philadelphia: J.B. Lippincott; 1989:122.)

Procedure	for Central Venous/Right Atrial Pressure Monitoring *Continued*	
Steps	**Rationale**	**Special Considerations**
5. Open the IV tubing roller clamp so that fluid flows from the IV fluid bag into the water manometer.	Prepares the water manometer for pressure measurement. If fluid is allowed to overflow the top of the manometer, contamination can result.	
A. Fill the manometer two-thirds full or above the level of the expected CVP measurement.	Underfilling the water manometer will result in an inaccurate measurement.	
B. Ensure that there are no air bubbles in the manometer.		
C. Close the roller clamp on the IV tubing.		
6. Turn the water manometer stopcock open to the patient and closed to the IV solution (see Fig. 62–3, system B).	Allows fluid to flow into the patient until the fluid column equalizes with the pressure in the right atrium.	
7. Observe the fluid column closely.	If the manometer is allowed to empty, air may enter the patient.	The fluid column may fall rapidly. Care should be taken not to allow all of the fluid to flow out of the manometer.
8. The fluid column should fall quickly and then fluctuate gently at the point where the fluid column equalizes with the right atrial pressure. Measure the CVP reading.	The pressure within the manometer equalizes with the pressure in the right atrium. The height of the fluid column reflects the right atrial pressure.	Fluid level will fluctuate with the patient's respiratory cycle once the fluid has equalized. The CVP measurement should be recorded at end-expiration.
9. Turn the water manometer stopcock open to the flush solution and the patient (see Fig. 62–3, system C), and regulate the roller clamp for the prescribed rate.	Prevents clotting of catheter and reestablishes IV flow.	
10. Wash hands.	Reduces transmission of microorganisms; standard precautions.	

CVP Measurement Using a Hemodynamic Monitoring System

1. Wash hands.	Reduces the transmission of microorganisms; standard precautions.	
2. Validate waveform as CVP on bedside monitor.	Ensures that catheter is in proper location.	
3. Level the air-fluid interface of the monitoring system to the phlebostatic axis (see Procedure 69).	Ensures accuracy in measurement.	
4. Run a dual-channel strip of the ECG and right atrial waveform.	Right atrial pressures should be determined from the graphic strip, as the effect of ventilation can be identified.	
5. Measure CVP or RAP at end-expiration.	Measurement is most accurate as the effects of pulmonary pressures are minimized.	
6. Using the dual-channel recorded strip, draw a vertical line from the beginning of the P wave of one of the ECG complexes down to the RA waveform. Repeat this with the next ECG complex.	Compares electric activity with mechanical activity. Usually three waves will be present on the RA waveform.	
7. Align the PR interval with the RA waveform (Fig. 62–4).	The a wave correlates with this interval.	

Procedure continued on page 413

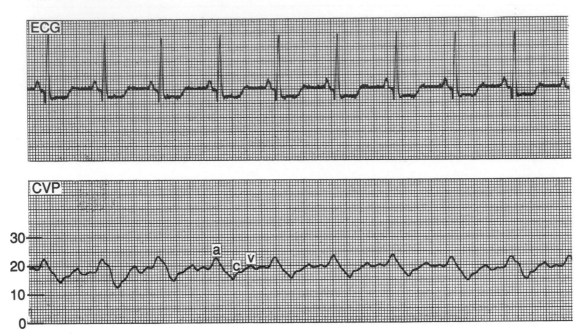

■ ● **FIGURE 62–4.** CVP waveform with a, c, v waves present. The a wave is usually seen just after the P wave of the ECG. The c wave appears at the time of the RST junction on the ECG. The v wave is seen in the TP interval. CVP, central venous pressure; ECG, electrocardiogram.

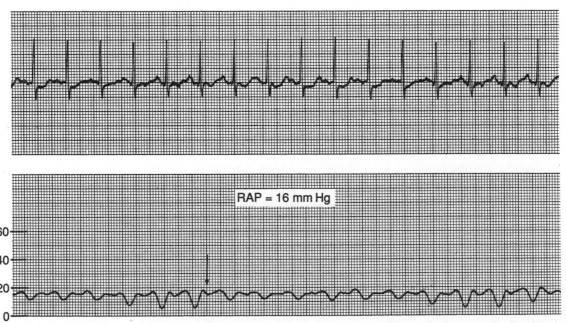

■ ● **FIGURE 62–5.** Reading RAP from paper printout at end-expiration in a spontaneously breathing patient. While observing the patient, identify inspiration. The point just before inspiration is end-expiration. Arrow indicates points of end-expiration. Reading is taken as a mean value. The RAP value for this patient is 16 mm Hg. RAP, right atrial pressure.

Steps	Rationale	Special Considerations
8. Identify the a wave (see Fig. 62–4).	The a wave is seen approximately 80 to 100 ms after the P wave. The c wave follows the a wave, and the v wave follows the c wave.	The a wave reflects atrial contraction. The c wave reflects closure of the tricuspid valve. The v wave reflects filling of the right atrium during ventricular systole.
9. Identify the scale of the RA tracing.	Aids in determining pressure measurement.	
10. Measure the mean of the a wave to obtain the pressure (Fig. 62–5).	The a wave represents atrial contraction and reflects right ventricular filling at end-diastole.	
11. Wash hands.	Reduces transmission of microorganisms; standard precautions.	

Expected Outcomes

- Accurate CVP measurments
- CVP readings that correlate with physical findings

Unexpected Outcomes

- Air embolus or other complication
- Inaccurate readings
- CVP readings that do not correlate with physical findings
- Redness, drainage, edema at insertion site, pain, fever, or elevated white blood cell count

Patient Monitoring and Care

Patient Monitoring and Care	Rationale	Reportable Conditions
		These conditions should be reported if they persist despite nursing interventions.
1. Monitor the patient's vital signs every 2 hours or more frequently if the patient's condition indicates.	Monitoring vital signs will alert the nurse to the beginning signs and symptoms of complications or infections.	• Changes in vital signs
2. Continuous monitoring of CVP waveform if using the hemodynamic monitoring system.	Changes in waveform may indicate change in catheter position or change in patient condition.	• Abnormal CVP values or waveforms
3. Measure CVP every 2 hours and as needed if using the water manometer method.	Indicate changes in patient condition.	• Abnormal CVP values

Documentation

Documentation should include the following:

- Patient and family education
- Cardiopulmonary assessment
- Assessment and labeled CVP waveform if appropriate
- IV intake, including amount of flush solution
- Assessment of fluid balance
- Unexpected outcomes
- Additional interventions

References

1. American Association of Critical Care Nurses. *Outcome Standards for Nursing Care of the Critically Ill.* Laguna Nigel, Calif: American Association of Critical-Care Nurses; 1990.
2. Andris DA, Krzywda EA. Central venous access: clinical practice issues. *Nurs Clin North Am.* 1997;32:719–740.
3. Clochesy JM. Hemodynamic monitoring. In: *Critical Care Nursing.* Philadelphia, Pa: W.B. Saunders; 1993.
4. Darovic G. Monitoring central venous pressure: hemodynamic monitoring. In: *Invasive and Noninvasive Clinical Applications.* 2nd ed. Philadelphia, Pa: W.B. Saunders; 1995.
5. Krzywda EA. Central venous access—catheters, technology, and physiology. *MEDSURG Nurs.* 1998;7:132–139.
6. Levins TT. Central intravenous lines: your role. *Nursing.* 1996;26:48–49.
7. Gardner PE, Bridges EJ. Hemodynamic monitoring. In: Woods SL, Sivarajan ES, Halpenny CJ, Underhill-Motzer S, eds. *Cardiac Nursing.* 3rd ed. Philadelphia, Pa: J.B. Lippincott; 1995:424.
8. Pearson ML. Special communication guideline for prevention of intravascular device-related infections. Part I. Intravascular device-related infections: an overview. *Am J Infect Control.* 1996;24:262–293.

Additional Readings

Keckeisen M. *Protocols for Practice: Hemodynamic Monitoring Series—Pulmonary Artery Pressure Monitoring.* Aliso Viejo, Calif: American Association of Critical-Care Nurses; 1997.
Mangram AJ. Guideline for prevention of surgical site infection. *Infect Control Hosp Epidemiol.* 1999;20:247–278.

63

Left Atrial Pressure Line, Care and Assisting with Removal

P U R P O S E: The left atrial catheter measures pressure from the left atrium to assess left ventricular function in the postoperative cardiac surgical patient. The left atrial catheter provides information about left-sided intracardiac pressure. Hemodynamic information obtained with the left atrial catheter is used to guide therapeutic intervention, including administration of fluids and diuretics and titration of vasoactive and inotropic medications.

Joan M. Vitello-Cicciu
Donna M. Rosborough

PREREQUISITE NURSING KNOWLEDGE

- Cardiovascular anatomy and physiology should be understood.
- Understanding of basic dysrhythmia recognition and treatment of life-threatening dysrhythmias is necessary.
- Advanced cardiac life support knowledge and skills are necessary.
- Understanding of the setup of the hemodynamic monitoring system is necessary (see Procedure 69).
- Understanding of hemodynamic monitoring (see Procedure 66) is necessary.
- Principles of aseptic techniques should be understood.
- The left atrial pressure (LAP) waveform is configured similarly to that of a pulmonary artery wedge pressure waveform (Fig. 63–1).
- Understanding of a, c, and v waves is necessary. The *a wave* reflects left atrial contraction. The *c wave* reflects closure of the mitral valve. The *v wave* reflects passive filling of the left atrium during left ventricular systole.
- The LAP is measured with a polyvinyl catheter placed in the left atrium during cardiac surgery. The left atrial catheter can be inserted via a needle puncture of the right superior pulmonary vein, with subsequent threading into the left atrium, or it can be inserted via a direct cannulation of the left atrium through a needle puncture at the intra-atrial groove.[1]
- LAP monitoring may be used[2] in the following situations:
  - ❖ For patients with prosthetic tricuspid or pulmonic valves, where a pulmonary artery catheter is contraindicated
  - ❖ For patients with abnormal heart anatomy (eg, those with a single ventricle or tricuspid atresia)
  - ❖ For patients with high pulmonary artery pressures (PAPs), which interfere with the accuracy of the pulmonary artery wedge pressure (PAWP)

  - ❖ To provide accurate information when vasoconstricting medications are infused in conjunction with pulmonary vasodilator medications
- The normal LAP is 6 to 12 mm Hg.
- One danger of using this catheter is the potential for air or blood clot emboli to enter the left atrium and be carried to the brain or other body organs. Close attention to the hemodynamic monitoring system and assessment of the waveform is imperative.

EQUIPMENT

- Left atrial catheter (inserted in operating room)
- Hemodynamic monitoring system (see Procedure 69)

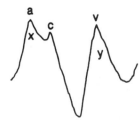

■ ● FIGURE 63–1. LAP waveform and its components: *a* wave—the presystolic wave resulting from atrial contraction; *x* descent—the down slope of the *a* wave caused by atrial relaxation; *c* wave—a sharp inflection caused by mitral valve closure; *v* wave—an atrial pressure wave rising to a peak during late ventricular systole caused by filling of the atrium while the mitral valve is closed; *y* descent—the down slope of the *v* wave caused by early diastolic runoff through the mitral valve. Changes in the waveform configuration may indicate valve or myocardial disease. For example, an elevated *a* wave is seen in mitral stenosis and an elevated *v* wave in mitral insufficiency. Both the *a* and *v* waves are Q-elevated in cardiac tamponade. LAP, left atrial pressure.

• Sterile dressing supplies

Additional equipment to have available if needed includes the following:

• Air filter (institution specific) between left atrial (LA) catheter and hemodynamic monitoring pressure tubing

PATIENT AND FAMILY EDUCATION

• Assess patient and family understanding of LAP monitoring.   ➤*Rationale:* Provides information about patient and family knowledge.
• Discuss purpose of the catheter.   ➤*Rationale:* Informs patient and family and may decrease anxiety.
• Discuss the location of the catheter and the importance of not touching this line or putting tension on this line with both patient and family.   ➤*Rationale:* Prevents line contamination and inadvertent line removal.

PATIENT ASSESSMENT AND PREPARATION
Patient Assessment

• Determine baseline hemodynamic, cardiovascular, peripheral vascular, and neurovascular status.   ➤*Rationale:* Provides data that can be used to compare with LAP.
• Assess current laboratory values profile, including coagulation studies.   ➤*Rationale:* Identifies laboratory value abnormalities. Baseline coagulation studies are helpful in determining the risk for bleeding.

Patient Preparation

• Ensure that the patient and family understand teaching. Answer questions as they arise and reinforce information as needed.   ➤*Rationale:* Evaluates and reinforces understanding of previously taught information.
• Sedate the patient as necessary.   ➤*Rationale:* An agitated or restless patient could accidentally pull the LA line out.

Procedure   for Care of the Left Atrial Pressure Line

Steps	Rationale	Special Considerations
1. Wash hands.	Reduces transmission of microorganisms; standard precautions.	
2. Check the hemodynamic monitoring system (see Procedure 69) for the following: A. Flush bag has solution. B. Flush bag is under pressure. C. Connections are tight. D. The entire system is air free.	Ensures that the hemodynamic monitoring system is set up appropriately.	The LA hemodynamic monitoring system is set up in the operating room.
3. Connect the pressure cable from the left atrial transducer to the bedside monitor.	Connects the LA catheter to the bedside monitoring system.	
4. Set the scale on the bedside monitor for LAP monitoring.	Permits waveform analysis.	The scale for LAP is commonly set at 20 mm Hg.
5. Level the left atrial air-fluid interface (zeroing stopcock) to the phlebostatic axis (see Procedure 69).	The phlebostatic axis approximates the level of the atria and should be used as the reference point for patients in the supine position.	The reference point for the atria changes when a patient is in the lateral position (see Procedure 69).
6. Secure the system to the patient's chest or arm.	Ensures that the air-fluid interface (zeroing stopcock) is maintained at the level of the phlebostatic axis. If the air-fluid interface is above the phlebostatic axis, the LAP will be falsely low. If the air-fluid interface is below the phlebostatic axis, the LAP will be falsely high.	The point of the phlebostatic axis should be marked with an indelible marker.
7. Zero the left atrial hemodynamic monitoring system (see Procedure 69).	Zeroing negates the effects of atmospheric pressure.	
8. Position the patient in the supine position with the head of the bed from 0 to 45 degrees.	Ensures the accuracy of LAP.	
9. Run a dual-channel strip of the ECG and the left atrial waveform (Fig. 63–2).	LAPs should be determined from the graphic strip as the effect of ventilation can be identified.	

Procedure	**for Care of the Left Atrial Pressure Line** *Continued*

Steps	Rationale	Special Considerations
10. Measure LAP at end-expiration.	Measurement is most accurate as the effects of pulmonary pressures are minimized.	
11. Using the dual-channel recorded strip, draw a vertical line from the beginning of the P wave of one of the ECG complexes down to the LAP waveform. Repeat this with the next ECG complex.	Compares electrical activity with mechanical activity. Three waveforms will be present between the two lines drawn.	
12. Align the end of a QRS complex of the ECG strip with the LAP waveform.	Compares electrical activity with mechanical activity.	
13. Identify the a wave.	The a wave correlates with the end of the QRS complex. The c wave follows the a wave, and the v wave follows the c wave.	

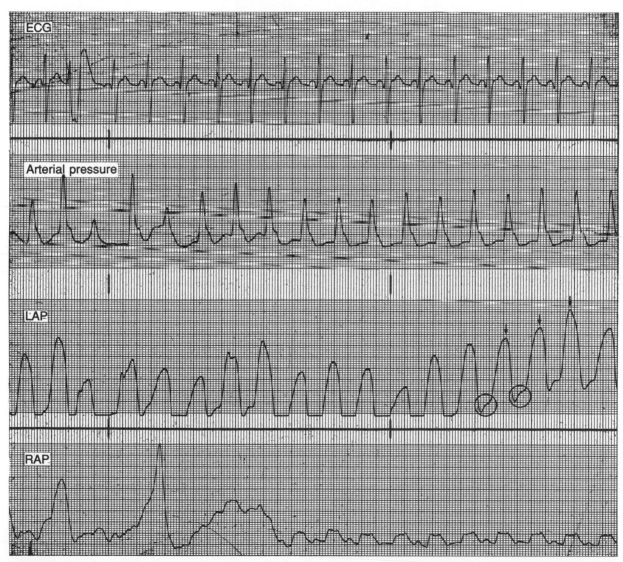

■ ● **FIGURE 63–2.** LAP catheter that has slipped into the LV. Note anacrotic notch on upstroke of LV waveform *(circled)*. Note also that paper was not calibrated in this example. LAP, left atrial pressure; LV, left ventricle.

Procedure continued on following page

Procedure	for Care of the Left Atrial Pressure Line *Continued*

Steps	Rationale	Special Considerations
14. Measure the mean of the a wave to obtain the LAP.	The a wave represents left atrial contraction as the left ventricle is filled during disastole.	If the patient's positive end-expiratory pressure (PEEP) is more than 10 mL H_2O, adjustments in determining the pressure may be necessary.
15. Set alarms. Upper and lower alarm limits are set on the basis of the patient's current clinical status and LAP values.	Activates the bedside and central alarm system.	
16. Continuously monitor waveform for any changes (overdamping, left ventricular waveform, or absence of waveform) and correlate with changes in physical findings.	Indicates problems with the LA catheter that require troubleshooting.	Overdamping may be caused by a hypovolemic state, air in the system, or a clot in the catheter. The presence of a left ventricular waveform (see Fig. 63–2) indicates that the catheter has migrated into the left ventricle. An absent waveform may be caused by cardiac arrest, clotted catheter, perforated left ventricle, or a problem within the hemodynamic monitoring system. It is important in all of these situations *not* to irrigate the catheter.[3]
17. Do not use the LA catheter for blood withdrawal, administration of medications, or for IV therapy. The catheter is for pressure monitoring purposes only.	Each time the line is entered, there is a significant risk of introducing air emboli or bacteria directly into the heart.	Bacterial contamination of this line is of great concern because it sits within the heart.
18. Wash hands.	Reduces transmission of microorganisms; standard precautions.	

Procedure	for Assisting with Removal of LA Line

Steps	Rationale	Special Considerations
1. Wash hands, and don gloves.	Reduces transmission of microorganisms; standard precautions.	
2. Position patient in the supine position.	Prepares patient and provides access to site.	
3. Turn the stopcock off to the patient, so that the catheter is shut off to the flush solution.	Turns off administration of flush solution and stops hemodynamic monitoring.	
4. Remove dressing.	Prepares for LA catheter removal.	
5. Clip sutures if present.	Frees LA catheter for removal.	
6. Assist the physician or advanced practice nurse as needed with catheter removal and hold firm pressure on the site.	Provides needed assistance.	
7. Apply a sterile, occlusive dressing to site.	Decreases the risk of infection until insertion site has healed.	
8. Dispose of used supplies and wash hands.	Reduces transmission of microorganisms; standard precautions.	

- Normal cerebral, myocardial, and peripheral perfusion
- LAP readings that correlate with physical findings
- Normal LAP value (6 to 12 mm Hg)
- LAP catheter removed when prescribed

- Infection
- Hemorrhage at removal site
- Air embolus
- Cardiac tamponade caused by LA line removal
- Retention, migration, or embolization of the catheter[4]

Patient Monitoring and Care	Rationale	Reportable Conditions
		These conditions should be reported if they persist despite nursing interventions.
1. Continuously monitor LA waveform and obtain pressure measurements every hour and as needed.	Identifies trends in monitoring.	• Abnormal LAP values
2. Monitor LAP hemodynamic monitoring system every 1 to 2 hours for integrity of the system and for presence of air bubbles in the system.	Could result in air embolism. If air is observed, it must be removed immediately.	• Air in the system that requires assistance with removal
3. Zero the system at the time of the patient's admission to the intensive care unit (ICU), if the transducer and the monitoring cable become disconnected, if the monitoring cable and the monitor become disconnected, and when the values obtained do not fit the clinical picture. Follow manufacturer's recommendations for disposable and reusable systems.	Ensures accuracy of the hemodynamic monitoring system; minimizes risk of contamination of the system.	
4. Change hemodynamic monitoring system (flush solution, pressure tubing, transducer and stopcock) every 72 hours. *(Level V: clinical studies in more than one or two different patient populations and situations to support recommendations)* Follow manufacturer's recommendations for reusable transducer systems.	The Centers for Disease Control and Prevention (CDC)[5] and research findings[6-8] recommend that the hemodynamic flush system can be used safely for 72 hours. This recommendation is based on research conducted with disposable pressure monitoring systems used for peripheral and central lines. No studies report this data specific to left atrial catheters.	
5. Follow institution standard for frequency and type of dressing change.	Decreases risk of infection at catheter site. The CDC[5] have made no recommendations for the frequency of routine left atrial catheter dressing changes. For central lines, the CDC recommend replacing dressings when the dressings become damp, loosened, or soiled or when inspection of the site is necessary.	
6. Follow institution standard for application of antimicrobial ointment to the LA catheter site.	Routine use of antimicrobial ointment at central venous catheter insertion sites is not recommended.[4] Specific data are not available related to LA catheter sites.	

Continued on following page

Patient Monitoring and Care	Rationale	Reportable Conditions
7. Before removal of the LA catheter, assess the prothrombin time (PT), partial thromboplastin time (PTT), international normalized ratio (INR), and platelets.	Ensures that the patient will not have any difficulty forming a clot at the LA insertion site after its removal. Failure to form a clot can lead to cardiac tamponade. PT, PTT, and INR values should be normal before the catheter is removed. Platelet count should be at least 60,000/mm³ before the catheter is removed.	• Abnormal coagulation results
8. After removal of the LA catheter, follow these steps: ○ Maintain bedrest for 2 hours. ○ Monitor vital signs and chest tube drainage every 15 minutes × 4, then every 30 minutes × 2, then again in 1 hour.	Changes in vital signs and bleeding from the chest tube (>100 mL/h) suggests that the insertion site had not clotted off and that the patient is hemorrhaging.	• Abnormal vital signs; excessive chest tube bleeding

Documentation

Documentation should include the following:

- Patient and family education
- Left atrial pressure waveform (label the a and v waves, inspiration and expiration, and the location where LAP was read)
- Amount of intake of flush solution
- Assessment of dressing or catheter insertion site or both
- Unexpected outcomes
- Additional interventions

References

1. Recker DH. Procedure for left atrial catheter insertion. *Crit Care Nurse.* 1985;5:36–41.
2. Bojar RM. *Manual of Perioperative Care in Cardiac and Thoracic Surgery.* Boston, Mass: Blackwell Scientific Publications; 1989:17, 233.
3. Tayor T. Monitoring left atrial pressures in the open-heart surgical patient. *Crit Care Nurse.* 1985;6:62–68.
4. Akl BF, Pett SB, Wernly JA, et al. Unusual complication of direct left atrial pressure monitoring line. *J Thorac Cardiovasc Surg.* 1984;88:1033–1035.
5. Pearson M. Hospital infection control practices advisory committee: guideline for prevention of intravascular device-related infections. *Infect Control Hosp Epidemiol.* 1996;17:438–473.
6. O'Mailley MK, Rhame FS, Cerra FB, McComb RC. Value of routine pressure monitoring system changes after 72 hours of use. *Crit Care Med.* 1994;22:1424–1430.
7. Ducharme FM, Gautier M, Lacroix J, Lafleur L. Incidence of infection related to arterial catheterization in children: a prospective study. *Crit Care Med.*1988;16:272–276.
8. Luskin RL, Weinstein RA, Nathan C, Chamberlin WH, Kabins SA. Extended use of disposable pressure transducers: a bacteriologic evaluation. *JAMA.* 1986;255:916–920.

Additional Readings

Leitman BS, Naidich DP, McGuinness G, McCauley DI. The left atrial catheter: its uses and complications. *Radiology.* 1992;185:611–612.

Rao PS, Sathyanarayana PV. Transseptal insertion of left atrial line: a simple and safe technique. *Ann Thorac Surg.* 1993;785–786.

Yeo TC, Miller FA Jr, Oh JK, Freeman WK. Retained left atrial catheter: an unusual cardiac source of embolism identified by transesophageal echocardiography. *J Am Soc Echocardiogr.* 1998;11:66–70.

64

Noninvasive Hemodynamic Monitoring: Impedance Cardiography

P U R P O S E : Impedance cardiography (ICG) is a continuous, noninvasive method to obtain hemodynamic data (cardiac output, left ventricular preload, afterload, and contractility) and assess thoracic fluid status.

Kathryn T. Von Rueden

PREREQUISITE NURSING KNOWLEDGE

- Understanding of cardiovascular anatomy and physiology is necessary.
- The principles of hemodynamic monitoring should be understood.
- Impedance (Z) is resistance to flow of electrical current. ICG measures electrical resistance changes in the thorax using four sets of external electrodes to input a high-frequency, low-amplitude current (similar to an apnea monitor). Fluids, such as blood and plasma, are good conductors of electricity and lower impedance.
- Blood volume and flow velocity increases and decreases in the ascending aorta during systole and diastole. Pulsatile flow generates electrical impedance changes. Impedance to electrical current decreases during systole due to increased blood volume, flow velocity, and alignment of red blood cells. Thus, the measurement of the magnitude and velocity of impedance changes directly reflect ascending aortic blood flow and left ventricular function.
- The dZ/dt (change in impedance/change in time) waveform depicts the change in impedance related to time and is similar to the aortic blood flow waveform (Fig. 64–1).
- Myocardial contractility is assessed by the dZ/dt and acceleration contractility index (ACI) values. Both are measured from the upslope of the dZ/dt curve during systole. Normal range of dZ/dt is 0.8 to 2.5 ohms/s; normal range of ACI is 2 to 5 ohm/s.[1] Higher values reflect enhanced left ventricular contractility.
- The dZ/dt value of >0.3 ohms/s indicates good impedance signal quality and is necessary to obtain reliable hemodynamic data. A dZ/dt of less than 0.3 ohms/s is occasionally observed when myocardial contractility is extremely poor or if the thorax is very fluid filled (eg, Zo <13 ohms).

- Zo is the measurement of the base or average thoracic impedance and reflects all of the fluid in the thorax. Greater amounts of fluid in the intravascular, interstitial, or intracellular spaces reduce thoracic electrical impedance and decrease the Zo. Because intravascular blood volume is relatively constant, a decrease in Zo usually reflects alveolar and interstitial edema; however, bleeding in the chest or pleural effusions also will decrease the Zo value. Normal Zo ranges from 20 to 30 ohms in most adults; women tend to have slightly higher values than men.

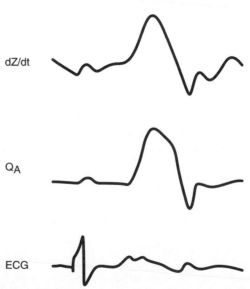

■ ● FIGURE 64–1. Relationship of dZ/dt impedance waveform, ascending aortic blood flow tracing, and ECG. (Courtesy of Renaissance Technology, Inc.)

Table 64–1 ●■■ **Impedance Cardiography Hemodynamic and Thoracic Fluid Parameters**

Parameter	Definition	Normal Values
Cardiac output (CO)	CO: liters of blood flow/min from left ventricle	4–8 L/min
Cardiac index (CI)	CI: CO/body surface area (m²)	2.5–4.5 L/min/m²
Stroke volume (SV)	SV: blood volume ejected/beat from left ventricle	60–100 mL/beat
SV index (SVI)	SVI: stroke volume/body surface area	33–47 mL/beat/m²
Systemic vascular resistance (SVR)	SVR: afterload, resistance to ejection of blood during left ventricular contraction	800–1200 dyne/s/cm⁻⁵
SVR index (SVRI)	SVRI: SVR/body surface area	1360–2200 dyne/s/cm⁻⁵/m²
Change in impedance/ time (dZ/dt)	Magnitude and rate of impedance change, direct reflection of force of left ventricular contraction; dZ/dt >0.3 required for optimal signal	0.8–2.5 ohms/s
Acceleration contractility index (ACI)	Direct reflection of myocardial contractility, calculated from rate of change in blood flow acceleration in the ascending aorta	2–5 ohms/s²
Preejection period (PEP)	Systolic time interval, measuring length of time for isovolumetric contraction, from ECG Q wave to opening of aortic valve	0.05–0.12 s
Ventricular ejection time (VET)	Systolic time interval, measuring the length of time for left ventricular ejection, from the opening to closing of aortic valve	0.25–0.35 s
Left cardiac work index (LCWI)	Reflection of myocardial oxygen demand	3–5 kg/min/m²
Thoracic fluid status (Zo)	Base thoracic impedance; reflects intravascular, interstitial, alveolar, and intracellular fluid	Men, 20–30 ohms Women, 25–35 ohms Infants, 30–45 ohms
	Zo <20 ohms: indicative of abnormal fluid accumulation in thorax	
	Zo <18 ohms: associated with interstitial pulmonary edema in acute heart failure exacerbation	
	Zo <15 ohms: associated with alveolar pulmonary edema in acute heart failure exacerbation	

ECG, electrocardiogram.

- Zo, dZ/dt, mean arterial pressure, central venous pressure (CVP) and the electrocardiogram (ECG) are used in the calculations of impedance-based hemodynamic parameters.

- Impedance-based cardiac output is calculated from stroke volume and heart rate. Precise determination of the aortic valve opening and closing (ventricular ejection time) and the maximum point of blood flow velocity (dZ/dt$_{max}$) are essential for accurate stroke volume measurement[1-4] (Fig. 64–2).

- Table 64–1 lists the ICG hemodynamic and thoracic fluid parameters, definitions, and normal values.

- Indications for hemodynamic monitoring using ICG are varied.[5, 6] Primary indications include the following:
  ❖ Potential for or signs and symptoms of pulmonary or cardiovascular dysfunction[7-10]
  ❖ Evaluation of a patient's thoracic fluid and hemodynamic status in locations outside of areas that can provide the close observation required for invasive hemodynamic monitoring[9, 11-14]
  ❖ Evaluation and differentiation of cardiac or pulmonary cause of shortness of breath[11, 12, 15]
  ❖ Evaluation of etiology and management of hypotension or hypoperfusion[7, 9, 11]
  ❖ Evaluation and titration of pharmacologic therapy[11, 16, 17]
  ❖ Evaluation of myocardial contractility and diagnosis of rejection following cardiac transplantation[18]
  ❖ Indication and justification for insertion of pulmonary artery catheter (dZ/dt <0.3)[4, 9]

  ❖ Hemodynamic monitoring following discontinuation of pulmonary artery catheter[4, 9]
  ❖ Pacemaker rate and atrioventricular delay timing to optimize stroke volume and cardiac output[19, 20]

- Contraindication to impedance cardiography monitoring: The ICG monitor should not be used for patients with impedance-driven pacemakers that calculate minute ventilation to regulate pulse generator pacing rate. The ICG impedance current interferes with the pacemaker imped-

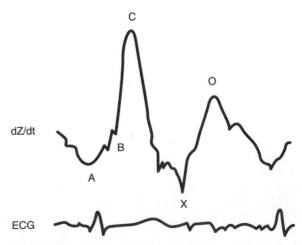

■ ● **FIGURE 64–2.** ECG and normal dZ/dt waveform. A, late ventricular diastole; B, opening of aortic valve; C, dZ/dt$_{max}$; X, closure of aortic valve; O, early ventricular diastolic filling. (Courtesy of Renaissance Technology, Inc.)

ance current and may cause pacemaker rate acceleration.[21]

EQUIPMENT

- Impedance cardiography monitor
- Impedance cardiography monitor cable
- Patient interface lead array
- ICG electrodes
- ECG electrodes
- Thoracic-length measurement calipers (manufacturer dependent)
- Blood pressure measuring device (to obtain systemic vascular resistance)

PATIENT AND FAMILY EDUCATION

- Explain the purpose of monitoring thoracic fluid and hemodynamic status. ➡*Rationale:* Enhances the understanding of the importance of physiologic assessment and monitoring and may reduce anxiety.
- Explain that four sets of impedance electrodes and three ECG electrodes are placed on the thorax and connected to leads. ➡*Rationale:* Decreases patient anxiety and elicits cooperation during electrode placement.
- Explain that impedance cardiography monitoring poses no risks or complications and causes little discomfort for the patient. Leads may limit mobility and electrodes may cause discomfort when removed from the skin. ➡*Rationale:* Decreases patient anxiety.

PATIENT ASSESSMENT AND PREPARATION
Patient Assessment

- Obtain the patient's vital signs and complete a cardiovascular assessment. ➡*Rationale:* Collects baseline data.
- Assess the patient's ability to be supine with the head of the bed less than 30 degrees for 3 to 5 minutes during placement of ICG electrodes. ➡*Rationale:* Patient may not tolerate supine position due to pain, discomfort, or difficulty breathing.

Patient Preparation

- Ensure that the patient understands preprocedural teaching. Answer questions as they arise and reinforce information as needed. ➡*Rationale:* Evaluates and reinforces understanding of previously taught information.
- Place the patient supine with head of the bed elevated no more than 30 degrees for electrode placement. ➡*Rationale:* Proper electrode placement (and, if necessary, accurate thoracic length measurement) is achieved with the patient in a supine, or nearly supine, position. Alternative positions are standing or sitting upright at 90 degrees.
- Prepare the skin for placement of electrodes by cleaning the skin with soap and water, cleaning with an alcohol pad, and using the abrasive pad provided with ICG electrodes. If necessary, clip body hair. ➡*Rationale:* Improves ICG electrode adherence and signal transmission.

Procedure for Noninvasive Hemodynamic Monitoring

Steps	Rationale	Special Considerations
1. Wash hands, and don gloves	Reduce transmission of microorganisms; standard precautions.	
2. Turn on ICG monitor, and enter patient data: A. Name B. Height and weight C. Adult D. Gender E. CVP (or use default CVP value) F. Blood pressure	Data are used to calculate hemodynamic parameters and indexed values, such as cardiac index and stroke volume index.	A noninvasive blood pressure device may be "slaved" into the ICG monitor for automatic blood pressure and systemic vascular resistance (SVR) updates, thus making manual entry of blood pressure unnecessary. Data entry requirements may vary by manufacturer.
3. Note the thoracic length calculated by the monitor.	A thoracic length is calculated based on patient height and will appear on the patient data screen. The thoracic length is important to ensure accurate electrode placement.	
4. Ensure that the patient is in the supine position with the head of the bed less than 30 degrees.	Flat position straightens torso and affords better exposure for accurate electrode placement.	Options for patients who do not tolerate the nearly supine position include sitting upright at 90 degrees or standing position.

Procedure continued on following page

| Procedure | **for Noninvasive Hemodynamic Monitoring** *Continued* |

Steps	Rationale	Special Considerations
5. Identify the landmarks for placement of the *upper thoracic ICG electrodes* (Fig. 64–3). Place the *dot,* or sensing portion of the electrode, in line with the ears, at the junction of the shoulders and the base of the neck. Place the upper thoracic dot electrodes directly opposite from each other.	Upper ICG electrode sets are placed to define the upper limit of the thorax. Dot portions should be placed 180 degrees opposite from each other to obtain the optimal signal and accurate measurements.	Proper placement of dot portion at the juncture of the shoulder and neck is critical to accurate data acquisition. The dot portion of the electrodes should not be placed on the sides of the neck. *Note*: The dot portions are placed below the ears in the location at the base of the neck, where a necklace would naturally rest.
6. Place the *strip,* or current-emitting portion of the upper electrode, at least 5 cm above the dot portion.	Signal strength is improved by placing the strip portion at a distance greater than 5 cm above the dot portion of the upper thoracic electrodes. Increasing the distance between the dot and strip portions improves signal strength; thus, placing the upper strips just below the ears or on the forehead will enhance the signal.	Separation of the sending (strip) and sensing (dot) portions of the electrode allows greater distance between the dot and strip and maintains the minimum 5 cm separation if the patient bends his or her head and neck toward the shoulder.
7. Note the proper thoracic length provided on the patient data screen of the monitor. Using the thoracic length caliper and keeping the ruled edge parallel to the spine, measure down from one of the upper thoracic dot electrodes to identify the position for the *lower thoracic dot electrode* (see Fig. 64–3). Place the *dot* (sensing) portion of electrode in the midaxillary line at the distance identified by the calipers with the *strip* (current-emitting) portion of the electrode below the dot port. Note: Thoracic length measurement is manufacturer dependent.	Lower ICG electrode sets are placed to define the lower limit of the thorax. The anatomic landmark for the lower thoracic dot electrodes is the point lateral to the junction of the sternum and xiphoid process. *Accurate thoracic length and electrode placement are critical for accurate stroke volume calculation.* Thoracic length that is too long due to placement of the lower thoracic electrode too low causes an overestimation of stroke volume and cardiac output, and vice versa, and all parameters can be affected by abdominal contents causing erroneous data.	Alternate method for placement of lower thoracic electrodes: identify the junction of the sternum and xiphoid process, and place the dot (sensing) portion of the ICG electrode *directly lateral* to that point. This method may be difficult in some patients due to their anatomy, obesity, or location of dressings; for example, over a sternotomy incision. Proper placement of the dot portion at the level of the sternal-xiphoid junction is critical to accurate data acquisition.
8. Repeat thoracic length measurement with the caliper on the opposite side of thorax and place the lower ICG electrode.	Dot portions should be placed 180 degrees opposite from each other to obtain the optimal signal and accurate measurements.	ICG electrodes are typically placed on opposite sides at the base of the neck and lateral from the sternal-xiphoid junction. Dressings or skin tears may necessitate rotating electrode placement to a more anterior to posterior position. If using an alternative electrode placement method, again locate the sternal-xiphoid junction and place the second set of lower thoracic electrodes *directly lateral to* that point, 180 degrees opposite the initially placed set.

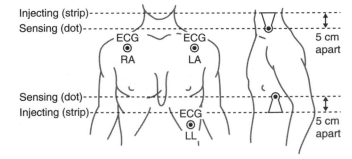

■ ● FIGURE 64–3. Placement sites of impedance cardiography electrodes defining the upper and lower limits of the thorax. The distance between the sensing (dot) electrodes is the thoracic length. (Courtesy of Renaissance Technology, Inc.)

Procedure **for Noninvasive Hemodynamic Monitoring** *Continued*

Steps	Rationale	Special Considerations
9. Ensure accurate thoracic length and correct electrode placement on opposite sides of the thorax. *(Level V: Clinical studies in more than one or two different patient populations and situations to support recommendations)*	Proper electrode placement is essential for acquisition of accurate hemodynamic and thoracic fluid status data.[22–25]	
10. If ECG electrodes are not integrated into the impedance electrodes, place the ECG electrodes in a lead that produces an upright R wave.	An upright R wave is necessary for signal processing.	The best leads for producing an upright R wave are leads II and V_6. Placing all three electrodes closer together on the chest may improve the amplitude of the R wave. If a pacemaker is in use, the R wave must be larger than the pacer spike. Be careful to not reverse the ECG polarity, which would produce a downward R wave and upright S wave. The ECG obtained from the ICG monitor is not for diagnostic use, but is important for hemodynamic calculations.
11. Attach the upper ICG electrodes to the short patient leads and the lower ICG electrodes to the longer patient leads (black to black, white to white). Connect the ECG leads and ICG lead array to the monitoring cable and monitor.		
12. Observe dZ/dt waveform and ECG displayed on monitor.	Hemodynamic calculations depend on artifact-free ICG and ECG signals. DZ/dt should be >0.3 ohms. R wave of ECG must be upright	

Troubleshooting

1. Display screen does not show ECG or ICG waveforms.
   A. Ensure power source is hospital-grade, grounded outlet.
   B. Ensure all "power" or "on" switches are activated.
   C. Ensure electrodes are in direct contact with skin.
   D. Ensure leads are properly connected to electrodes, monitoring cable, and ICG monitor.

2. There is excessive noise or 60-cycle interference on ECG or ICG waveforms.
   A. Ensure power source is hospital-grade, grounded outlet.
   B. Eliminate nonhospital-grade equipment plugged into same outlet.
   C. Ensure electrodes are in direct contact with skin.

Electrodes need to be in direct contact with skin that is free of hair and not placed over dressings or tape in order to allow ICG signal transmission via the electrode surface.

Skin preparation for ICG electrode placement is based on the same principles that apply to skin preparation for typical ECG monitoring (see Procedure 51).

Procedure continued on following page

Procedure for Noninvasive Hemodynamic Monitoring *Continued*

Steps	Rationale	Special Considerations
D. Ensure leads are properly connected to electrodes and monitoring cable.		
E. Ask patient to momentarily hold still to eliminate possible motion artifact as a cause of interference.		
3. There is a small, damped dZ/dt waveform, dZ/dt >0.3 ohms. Verify proper ICG electrode placement and skin contact. Assess Zo and dZ/dt for extremely low values. Options: A. Continue monitoring; dZ/dt will increase as thoracic fluid status improves and Zo increases with appropriate interventions. B. Consider invasive means to obtain hemodynamic data.	Extremely low Zo that occurs with a large volume of thoracic fluid may dampen the dZ/dt.[9]	Inability to obtain ICG hemodynamic data supports and may be considered an indication for invasive hemodynamic monitoring; for example, insertion of a pulmonary artery catheter.[5]
4. ICG data do not correspond to patient clinical presentation. A. Verify correct electrode placement.	Accurate electrode placement and thoracic length are critical to reliable hemodynamic data acquisition.	
B. Reassess thoracic length and placement of lower ICG electrodes.		
C. Ensure good electrode contact with skin.		
D. Ensure that leads are properly connected to all electrodes.		
E. Validate that correct patient height, weight, and other data have been entered.		
F. Update blood pressure or mean arterial pressure (MAP) to update the SVR calculation.	The cardiac output and SVR are updated continuously or recalculated by the ICG monitor. The displayed SVR may be erroneous if the blood pressure has changed and the current SVR is calculated based on a blood pressure or MAP that was entered several hours before.	Blood pressure should be routinely updated in the monitor if a noninvasive blood pressure monitoring device is not slaved into the ICG monitor.
G. Update the CVP pressure in the ICG monitor if large changes (eg, >10 mm Hg) have occurred in the CVP or the patient has become hypotensive.	Although the CVP has minimal impact on the SVR in most situations, if a patient is hypotensive with a low MAP (eg, <60 mm Hg) and has a high CVP >15 mm Hg), the SVR calculation will be affected and the CVP should be updated.	CVP entered into the monitor may be measured from a CVP catheter or from assessment of the height of the jugular vein pulsation. CVP entered into the ICG monitor must be in mm Hg.

Expected Outcomes

- Generation of reliable, continuous hemodynamic and thoracic fluid status parameters
- Hemodynamic and thoracic fluid data incorporated into patient evaluation and management

Unexpected Outcomes

- Hemodynamic parameters do not reflect clinical presentation.

Patient Monitoring and Care

Patient Monitoring and Care	Rationale	Reportable Conditions
		These conditions should be reported if they persist despite nursing interventions.
1. Assess baseline and trends in thoracic fluid status (Zo). Normal values: men: 20–30 ohms; women: 25–35 ohms.	Men tend to have slightly lower Zo than women due to anthropometric differences.[26] Zo less than 20 ohms, in most patients, is indicative of increased thoracic fluid. Rapid Zo decrease may be due to intrathoracic bleeding. Gradual decrease is associated with pulmonary edema. Rapid Zo rise may be due to pneumothorax. Gradual rise is an expected response to diuretic therapy and reduction of preload, or a reduction in afterload or improved left ventricular contractility, which facilitates forward flow through the pulmonary vasculature and reduce pulmonary congestion. A Zo decrease necessitates an evaluation of cardiac output, preload (using physiologic fluid challenge; see preload assessment), afterload, and contractility to establish cause of thoracic fluid accumulation, cardiac or noncardiac origin. Acute pulmonary edema and heart failure exacerbation are associated with Zo <18 ohms (reflects interstitial edema) and Zo <15 ohms (reflects alveolar edema).[11, 12] A normal Zo in the presence of respiratory distress typically indicates a pulmonary cause of shortness of breath, rather than cardiac origin.	• A Zo decrease of 2 ohms, indicating increased thoracic fluid accumulation; no change in Zo following therapy to relieve pulmonary vascular congestion
2. Assess baseline and trends in continuously displayed cardiac output (CO) or cardiac index (CI): ○ Normal: CO 4–8 L/min ○ Normal: CI 2.5–4.5 L/min/m² ○ Formula: $CO = SV^* \times HR$ *Use SVI for CI calculation.	Cardiac output and cardiac index are global reflections of cardiac function. Changes in or abnormal CO/CI are related to altered heart rate, preload, afterload, or contractility. Evaluate the determinants of CI to establish the cause of a change and institute appropriate interventions.	• Per institution's standard hemodynamic guidelines; for example, new or continued CO <3.5 L/min or CI <2.2 L/min/m² or sustained cardiac index decrease of 0.5 L/min/m² (unrelated to sedation, analgesia, or sleep)—assess and report or initiate management protocol; negligible or absent desired or expected response to therapy
3. Assess baseline and changes in preload by evaluating stroke volume (SV) response to physiologic fluid challenge: ○ Measure and note SV with head of bed elevated. ○ Place patient supine or lift legs for "physiologic fluid bolus." ○ Measure and note SV change. ○ Normal: SV 60–100 mL ○ Normal SV index: 33–47 mL/beat/m² ○ Formula: $SV = L^3/4.2 \times VET \times dZ/dt_{max}/Zo$	Preload is ventricular end-diastolic volume. Assessment of SV response to a physiologic fluid challenge reflects preload status.[16] (Fig. 64–4) Evaluate preload status with physiologic fluid bolus initially and when CI decreases by 0.5 L/min/m² or Zo decreases by 2 ohms. Interpretation of SV response to physiologic fluid bolus[16, 27-29]: normal: moderate (~30%) SV increase; hypovolemia: large (~50%) SV increase; left ventricular dysfunction or volume overload: no change in SV or a decrease in SV.	• Based on preload assessment, new-onset hypovolemia or left ventricular dysfunction, especially when associated with a reduction in CI or Zo, should be treated based on institution protocol or reported.

Continued on following page

Patient Monitoring and Care	Rationale	Reportable Conditions

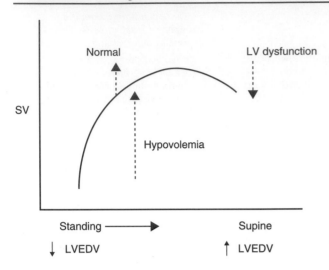

SV

Standing ———▶   Supine

↓ LVEDV   ↑ LVEDV

■ ● **FIGURE 64–4.** Stroke volume response to physiologic fluid bolus based on Frank-Starling curve in normal, hypovolemic, or hypervolemic–left ventricular dysfunction states. LV, left ventricle; LVEDV, left ventricular end-diastolic volume; SV, stroke volume.

4. Assess baseline and trends in afterload:
   - ○ Systemic vascular resistance (SVR). SVR normal: 800–1200 dyne/s/cm^{-5}
   - ○ SVR index normal: 1360–2200 dyne/s/cm^{-5}/m^2
   - ○ Formula: SVR =

$$\frac{MAP - CVP}{CO^*} \times 80$$

   *Use CI for SVR index calculation.

SVR is measure of resistance to left ventricular emptying. Afterload is inversely related to cardiac output and stroke volume.
Ensure SVR is based on current blood pressure or MAP (manually enter or verify that noninvasive blood pressure [NIBP] slaved into ICG monitor is functioning) and update default CVP based on measured CVP or jugular venous pressure estimation. Increased SVR often reflects compensatory mechanisms to maintain perfusion.
Vasodilation causes SVR to decrease.
Monitor SVR to establish response to therapies such as administration of vasodilators or vasoconstricting agents, or volume or thermoregulation interventions.

- • SVR that has risen above or fallen below normal range or target value
- • Negligible or absent desired or expected response to therapy

5. Assess baseline and trends in left ventricular contractility:
   - ○ Acceleration contractility index (ACI)
     Normal: 2–5 ohms/sec^2
     Formula: d^{2}Z/dt^2/Zo
   - ○ DZ/dt
     Normal: 0.8–2.5 ohms

ACI and dZ/dt measure blood flow acceleration in the ascending aorta and directly reflect left ventricular contractility. Impaired contractility is reflected by low ACI and dZ/dt.[18, 30, 31] Values increase with improved contractile force. Monitor ACI and dZ/dt for an increase to validate appropriate patient response to, for example, positive inotropic agent administration. DZ/dt reflects contractility, but may be diminished in patients with low Zo.[9]

- • Unexpected decrease in ACI or dZ/dt from baseline values
- • Negligible or absent desired/expected response to therapy

6. Assess hemodynamic parameters and Zo for trends every 1 to 2 hours, following interventions, and as needed.

Documentation

Documentation should include the following:

- Patient and family education
- Initiation of ICG hemodynamic monitoring
- Head-of-bed elevation for initial and subsequent documentation of hemodynamic and thoracic fluid status parameters
- Initial ICG parameters and stroke volume response to physiologic fluid challenge
- Routine every 1 to 2 hours, ICG parameters and trends
- Hemodynamic and Zo responses to therapeutic interventions
- Optional: printout of dZ/dt waveform
- Unexpected outcomes
- Additional interventions

References

1. Wang X, Sun H, VanDeWater J. Time frequency distribution technique in biological signal processing. *Biomed Instrument Technology.* 1995;29:203–212.
2. Wang X, VanDeWater J, Sun H, et al. Hemodynamic monitoring by impedance cardiography with an improved signal processing technique. *Proc IEEE Eng Med Biolog.* 1993;15:699–670.
3. Shoemaker W, Wo C, Bishop M, et al. Multicenter trial of a new thoracic bioimpedance device for cardiac output estimation. *Crit Care Med.* 1994;22:1907–1912.
4. VanDeWater J, Wang X. Development of a new impedance cardiograph. *J Clin Engineer.* 1995;20:218–223.
5. Von Rueden K, Turner M. Advances in continuous, noninvasive hemodynamic surveillance: impedance cardiography. *Crit Care Nurs Clin North Am.* 1999;11:63–75.
6. McFetridge J, Sherwood A. Impedance cardiography for noninvasive measurement of cardiac output. *Nurs Res.* 1999;48:109–113.
7. Bishop M, Shoemaker W, Wo C. Non-invasive cardiac index monitoring in gun shot wound victims. *Acad Emerg Med.* 1996;7:682–688.
8. Jonsson F, Madsen P, Jorgensen L, Lunding M, Secher N. Thoracic electrical impedance and fluid balance during aortic surgery. *Acta Anaesthesol Scand.* 1995;39:513–517.
9. Shoemaker W, Belzberg H, Wo C, et al. Multicenter study for noninvasive monitoring as alternatives to invasive monitoring in early management of acutely ill emergency patients. *Chest.* 1998;114:1643–1652.
10. Thangathurai D, Charbonnet C, Roessler P, et al. Continuous intraoperative noninvasive cardiac output monitoring using a new thoracic bioimpedance device. *J Cardiothorac Vasc Anesth.* 1997;11:440–444.
11. Milzman D, Moskowitz L, Samaddar R, Janchar T. Thoracic impedance monitoring of cardiac output in the ED improves heart failure resuscitation. *J Cardiac Failure.* 1998;4:31.
12. Milzman D, Hogan C, Han C, et al. Continuous, noninvasive cardiac output monitoring quantifies acute congestive heart failure in the ED. *Crit Care Med.* 1997;25:A47.
13. Frantz A. Home cardiac monitoring and technology. In: Gorski L, ed. *High Tech Home Care Manual.* Supplement #2. Rockville, Md: Aspen Publishing; 1996.
14. Frantz A, Lynn C. Cardiac technology in the home. *Home Health Care Management and Practice.* 1999;11:9–16.
15. Pickett B, Buell J. Usefulness of the impedance cardiogram to reflect left ventricular diastolic function. *Am J Cardiol.* 1993;71:1099–1103.
16. Hubbard W, Fish D, McBrien D. The use of impedance cardiography in heart failure. *Int J Cardiol.* 1986;12:71–79.

17. Scherhag A, Pfleger S, deMey C, et al. Continuous measurement of hemodynamic alterations during pharmacologic cardiovascular stress using automated impedance cardiography. *J Clin Pharmacol.* 1997;37:21S–28S.
18. Weinhold C, Reichenspurner H, Fulle P, Nollert G, Reichart B. Registration of thoracic electrical bioimpedance for early diagnosis of rejection after heart transplantation. *Heart Lung Transplant.* 1993;12:832–836.
19. Ovsyshcher I, Furman S. Impedance cardiography for cardiac output estimation in pacemaker patients: review of the literature. *PACE.* 1993;16:1412–1422.
20. Ovsyshcher I, Zimlichman R, Katz A, Bondy C, Furman S. Measurements of cardiac output by impedance cardiography in pacemaker patients at rest: effects of various atrioventricular delays. *J Am Coll Cardiol.* 1993;21:761–767.
21. Aldrete J, Brown C, Daily J, Buerke V. Pacemaker malfunction due to microcurrent injection from a bioimpedance noninvasive cardiac output monitor. *J Clinical Monitor.* 1995;11:131–133.
22. Jensen L, Yakimets J, Teo KK. A review of impedance cardiography. *Heart Lung.* 1995;24:183–193.
23. Fuller H. The validity of cardiac output measurement by thoracic impedance: a meta-analysis. *Clin Invest Med.* 1992;15:103–112.
24. Lamberts R, Visser K, Zijlstra W. *Impedance Cardiography.* Assen, The Netherlands: Van Gorcum; 1984.
25. O'Connell A, Tibballs J, Coulthard M. Improving agreement between thoracic bioimpedance and dye dilution cardiac output estimation in children. *Anaesth Intens Care.* 1991; 19:434–440.
26. Metry G, Wikstrom B, Linde T, Danielson B. Gender and age differences in transthoracic bioimpedance. *Acta Physiol Scand.* 1997;161:171–175.
27. Soubiran C, Harant I, Glisezinski I, et al. Cardio-respiratory changes during the onset of head-down tilt. *Aviat Space Environ Med.* 1996;67:648–653.
28. Kassis E. Cardiovascular response to orthostatic tilt in patients with severe congestive heart failure. *Cardiovasc Res.* 1987;21:362–368.
29. Larsen F, Mogensen L, Tedner B. Influence of furosemide and body posture on transthoracic electrical impedance in AMI. *Chest.* 1986;90:733–737.
30. Koerner K, Borzotta A, Wilson J. Screening for coronary artery disease will impedance cardiography. *Crit Care Med.* 1997;25:A47.
31. Feng S, Okuda N, Fujinami T, et al. Detection of impaired left ventricular function in coronary artery disease with acceleration index in the first derivative of the transthoracic impedance change. *Clin Cardiol.* 1988;11:843–847.

Additional Readings

DaMaria AN, Raisinghani A. Comparative overview of cardiac output measurement methods: has impedance cardiography come of age? *CHF.* 2000;6:60–73.

Greenberg B, Hermann D, Pranulis M, et al. Reproducibility of impedance cardiography hemodynamic measures in clinically stable heart failure patients. *CHF.* 2000;6:74–80.

Heethaar RM, van Oppen A, Ottenhoff FA, et al. Thoracic electrical bioimpedance: suitable for monitoring stroke volume during pregnancy? *Eur J Obstet Gynecol Reprod Biol.* 1995;58:183–190.

Miles DS, Gotshall R, Golden J, et al. Accuracy of electrical impedance cardiography for measuring cardiac output in children with congenital heart defects. *Am J Cardiol.* 1988;61:612–616.

Peacock WH, Albert N, Kies P, et al. Bioimpedance monitoring: better than chest x-ray for predicting abnormal pulmonary fluid? *CHF.* 2000;6:86–89.

Taler S, Augustine JE, Textor S. A hemodynamic approach to resistant hypertension. *CHF.* 2000;6:90–93.

Ventura H, Pranulis M, Young C, Smart F. Impedance cardiography: a bridge between research and clinical practice in the treatment of heart failure. *CHF.* 2000;6:94–102.

Von Rueden K, Turner M, Lynn C. Noninvasive, continuous hemodynamic and thoracic fluid status monitoring: impedance cardiography. *RN.* 1999;62:52–58.

Woltjer H, Bogaar H, Bronzwaer J, et al. Prediction of pulmonary capillary wedge pressure and assessment of stroke volume by noninvasive impedance cardiography. *Am Heart J.* 1997;134:450–455.

Wright R, Gilbert J. Clinical decision making in patients with congestive heart failure: the role of thoracic electrical bioimpedance. *CHF.* 2000;6:81–85.

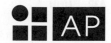

Pulmonary Artery Catheter Insertion (Perform)

P U R P O S E: Pulmonary artery (PA) catheters are used to determine hemodynamic status in critically ill patients. PA catheters provide information about right- and left-sided intracardiac pressures and cardiac output. Additional functions available are fiberoptic monitoring of mixed venous oxygen saturation, intracardiac pacing, and assessment of right ventricular volumes and ejection fraction. Hemodynamic information obtained with a PA catheter is routinely used to guide therapeutic intervention, including administration of fluids and diuretics and titration of vasoactive and inotropic medications.

Desiree A. Fleck

PREREQUISITE NURSING KNOWLEDGE

- The normal anatomy and physiology of the cardiovascular system should be understood.
- The anatomy and physiology of the vasculature and adjacent structures of the neck must be known.
- Principles of sterile technique should be understood.
- Clinical and technical competence in central line insertion and suturing is necessary.
- Clinical and technical competence in PA catheter insertion is essential.
- Competence in chest x-ray interpretation is necessary.
- Understanding of basic dysrhythmia recognition and treatment of life-threatening dysrhythmias is necessary.
- Advanced cardiac life support knowledge and skills are necessary.
- Understanding of basic pulmonary artery pressure monitoring (see Procedure 66) is needed.
- Understanding of a, c, and v waves is necessary. The *a wave* reflects atrial contraction. The *c wave* reflects closure of the atrioventricular valve. The *v wave* reflects passive filling of the atria during ventricular systole.
- Information can be gathered regarding cardiac output (CO), cardiac index (CI), systemic vascular resistance (SVR), pulmonary vascular resistance (PVR), stroke volume/stroke index (SV/SI), and right heart pressures—pulmonary artery pressure (PAP) and right atrial pressure (RAP), and a reflection of left ventricular end diastolic pressure (LVEDP) and volume (LVEDV).

- There are several types of PA catheters with different functions (eg, pacing, mixed venous oxygenation saturation monitoring, or right ventricular volume monitoring). Catheter selection is based on patient need.
- The PA catheter contains a proximal lumen port, a distal lumen port, a thermistor lumen port, and a balloon inflation lumen port (see Fig. 66–1). Some catheters also have an infusion port that can be used for the infusion of medications and intravenous fluids.
- The distal lumen port is used to monitor systolic, diastolic, and mean pressures in the PA. The proximal lumen (or injectate) port is used to monitor the right atrial pressure and to inject the solution used to obtain cardiac outputs. The balloon inflation lumen port is used to obtain pulmonary artery wedge pressure (PAWP).
- The standard PA catheter is 7.5 Fr and 110 cm long. The tip of the catheter should reach the PA after being advanced 45 to 55 cm from the internal jugular vein or 70 to 80 cm from a femoral or an antecubital vein. There are black marks every 10 cm to demonstrate where the catheter is positioned.
- Central venous access may be obtained in a variety of places (see Table 73–1).
- The right subclavian vein is a more direct route than the left subclavian vein for placing a PA catheter because the catheter does not cross the midline of the thorax.[1, 2]
- The risk of a pneumothorax is minimized by using an internal jugular vein. The preferred site for catheter insertion is the right internal jugular vein. The right internal jugular vein is a "straight shot" to the right atrium.
- Knowledge of West's lung zones helps attain proper placement of the PA catheter (Fig. 65–1). The PA catheter should lay in lung zone 3, below the level of the left atrium in the dependent portion of the lung.[3] In lung zone 3, both arterial and venous pressures exceed alveolar

431

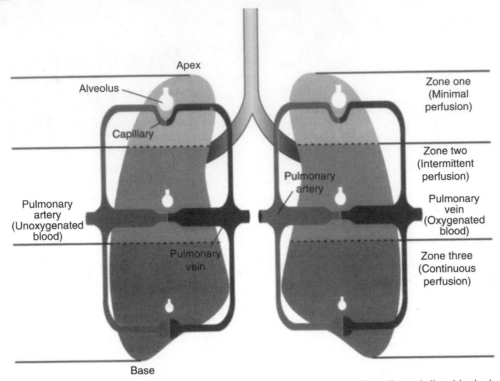

Apex

Alveolus

Capillary

Pulmonary
artery
(Unoxygenated
blood)

Pulmonary
vein

Pulmonary
artery

Zone one
(Minimal
perfusion)

Zone two
(Intermittent
perfusion)

Pulmonary
vein
(Oxygenated
blood)

Zone three
(Continuous
perfusion)

Base

■ ● **FIGURE 65–1.** West's lung zones. Schema of the heart and lungs demonstrating the relationship between the cardiac chambers and vessels and the physiologic zones of the lungs. Zone 1 (PA>Pa>Pv): absence of blood flow. Zone 2 (Pa>PA>Pv): intermittent blood flow. Zone 3 (Pa>Pv>PA): continous blood flow, resulting in an open channel between the pulmonary artery catheter and the left atrium. PA, pulmonary artery; Pa, pressure arterial; Pv, pressure venous. (From Copstead LC. *Perspectives on Pathophysiology*. Philadelphia: WB Saunders; 1995: 442.)

pressure, and PAWP reflects vascular pressures rather than alveolar pressures.[3]

- Common indications for insertion of a PA catheter include the following:
  - ❖ Myocardial infarction (MI) complicated by hemodynamic instability, heart failure, cardiogenic shock, mitral regurgitation, ventral septal rupture, subacute cardiac rupture with tamponade, and postinfarction ischemia
  - ❖ Hypotension:
    Hypotension unresponsive to fluid replacement
    Hypotension and congestive heart failure
    Tamponade, significant dysrhythmias, right ventricular infarct, acute pulmonary embolism, and tricuspid insufficiency
  - ❖ Anesthesia in cardiac surgery:
    Evidence of previous MI
    Resection of ventricular aneurysm
    Coronary artery bypass graft (reoperation)
    Coronary artery bypass graft (left main or complex coronary disease)
    Complex cardiac surgery (multivalvular surgery), high-risk surgery (pulmonary hypertension)
  - ❖ General surgery:
    Vascular procedures (abdominal aneurysm repair, aorto-bifemoral bypass)
    High-risk patients
    Hypotensive anesthesia

  - ❖ Cardiac disorders:
    Unstable angina requiring vasodilator therapy
    Congestive heart failure unresponsive to conventional therapy
    Pulmonary hypertension during acute drug therapy
    Distinguishing cardiogenic from noncardiogenic pulmonary edema
    Constrictive pericarditis or cardiac tamponade
    Evaluation of pulmonary hypertension for precardiac transplant work-up

  - ❖ Pulmonary disorders:
    Acute respiratory failure with chronic obstructive pulmonary diseases
    Cor pulmonale with pneumonia
    Optimization of positive end-expiratory pressure (PEEP) and volume therapy in patients with adult respiratory distress syndrome

  - ❖ Patients requiring intra-aortic balloon pump therapy
  - ❖ Critically ill pregnant patient (severe preeclampsia with unresponsive hypertension, pulmonary edema, persistent oliguria)
  - ❖ Extensive multisystem infection
  - ❖ Severe shock states
  - ❖ Drug overdose
  - ❖ Major trauma or burn
  - ❖ Azotemia

- Relative contraindications to PA catheter insertion include the following:

❖ Preexisting left bundle branch block
❖ Presence of fever (greater than 101°F or 38°C)
❖ Mechanical tricuspid valve
❖ Coagulopathic state

EQUIPMENT

• Percutaneous equipment tray or introducer kit
• PA catheter (non-heparin–coated catheters are available)
• Sheath introducer
• Sterile catheter sleeve
• Bedside hemodynamic monitoring system with pressure and cardiac output monitoring capability
• Pressure cables for interface with the monitor
• Cardiac output cable with a thermistor/injectate sensor
• Pressure transducer system, including flush solution recommended according to institution standard, a pressure bag or device, pressure tubing with flush device, and transducers (see Procedure 69)

• Sterile normal saline intravenous fluid for flushing catheter and introducer ports
• Povidone-iodine solution or alcohol if allergic
• Caps, masks, sterile gowns, sterile gloves, and sterile drapes
• 1% lidocaine without epinephrine
• Sterile basin or cup
• Sterile water or normal saline
• Sterile dressing supplies
• Stopcocks

Additional equipment to have available as needed includes the following:

• Fluoroscope
• Emergency equipment
• Indelible marker

PATIENT AND FAMILY EDUCATION

• Explain the procedure and reason for catheter insertion. ➼*Rationale:* Decreases patient and family anxiety.
• Explain the need for sterile technique and that the patient's face may be covered. ➼*Rationale:* Decreases patient anxiety and elicits cooperation.

PATIENT ASSESSMENT AND PREPARATION
Patient Assessment

• Determine medical history of cervical disk disease or difficulty obtaining vascular access. ➼*Rationale:* Increases risk of complications of insertion.

⊞ **AP** This procedure should be performed only by physicians, advanced practice nurses, and other health care professionals (including critical care nurses) with additional knowledge, skills, and demonstrated competence per professional licensure or institutional standard.

• Determine medical history of pneumothorax or emphysema. ➼*Rationale:* Patients with emphysematous lungs may be at higher risk for puncture and pneumothorax depending on approach.
• Determine medical history of anomalous veins. ➼*Rationale:* Patients may have history of dextrocardia or transposition of great vessels, leading to greater difficulty in placing catheter.
• Assess intended insertion site. ➼*Rationale:* Scar tissue may impede placement of catheter.
• Assess cardiac and pulmonary status. ➼*Rationale:* Some patients may not tolerate a supine or Trendelenburg position for extended periods.
• Assess vital signs and pulse oximetry. ➼*Rationale:* Provides baseline data.
• Assess for electrolyte imbalances (potassium, magnesium, and calcium). ➼*Rationale:* Electrolyte imbalances may increase cardiac irritability.
• Assess for left bundle branch block. ➼*Rationale:* There are reports of right bundle branch block associated with PA catheter insertion. Caution should be used because complete heart block may ensue.[5]
• Assess for heparin sensitivity or allergy. ➼*Rationale:* PA catheters are heparin bonded, although non-heparin–bonded catheters are available. If patient has a heparin allergy or has a history of heparin-induced thrombocytopenia, use a non-heparin–coated catheter.[7]
• Assess for coagulopathic state or recent anticoagulant or thrombolytic therapy. ➼*Rationale:* These patients are more likely to have complications related to bleeding.
• Assess for risks and benefits of PA catheter insertion. ➼*Rationale:* Complications do occur with PA catheter insertion and studies are controversial about the efficacy of PA catheter use.[2, 6, 8–11]

Patient Preparation

• Ensure that the patient understands preprocedural teaching. Answer questions as they arise and reinforce information as needed. ➼*Rationale:* Evaluates and reinforces understanding of previously taught information.
• Obtain informed consent or ensure it has been obtained. ➼*Rationale:* Protects rights of patient and makes competent decision possible for patient.
• Place patient in supine position and prepare area with povidone-iodine solution. ➼*Rationale:* Prepares site access for PA catheter insertion.
• If patient is obese or muscular and the preferred site is the internal jugular vein or subclavian vein, place towel posteriorly between shoulder blades. ➼*Rationale:* Will help extend the neck and provide better access to subclavian and internal jugular veins.
• If using arm vein, stabilize arm on padded arm board. ➼*Rationale:* Will aid visualization of arm veins.
• Drape sterile drapes over prepared area. ➼*Rationale:* Provides aseptic work area.

Procedure	for Pulmonary Artery Catheter Insertion (Perform)

Steps	Rationale	Special Considerations
1. Wash hands; all health care personnel involved in the procedure should don caps, masks, sterile gowns, and gloves.	Reduces transmission of microorganisms and body secretions; standard precautions.	
2. Obtain central venous access (see Procedure 73).	The PA catheter is inserted into a central vein.	
3. Open the PA catheter kit.		
4. Estimate the length of catheter needed by holding the catheter over the insertion site to the sternal notch.	Helps ensure proper placement. The catheter should reach the PA after being advanced 45 to 55 cm from the internal jugular vein or 70 to 80 cm from a femoral or an antecubital vein.	Before inserting catheter, attempt to curl catheter in direction it will float.
5. Hand off ports of the PA catheter to the critical care nurse for connection to the hemodynamic monitoring system.	Connects the ports to the flush system; connects the transducers to the bedside monitor.	
6. Flush all open lumens.	Removes air from the PA catheter.	
7. Insert the recommended amount of air into the balloon and immerse the inflated balloon in sterile water or normal saline.	Checks for integrity of the balloon.	If an air leak is present, air bubbles will be noted.
8. Ensure that the PA catheter thermistor is connected to the cardiac output monitor or module.	Allows the core or blood temperature to be monitored and is needed for cardiac output measurement.	
9. If a PA catheter with the ability to monitor mixed venous oxygenation is being inserted, the fiberoptics should be calibrated before removal from the package (see Procedure 13).	Calibrates the system.	Calibrate the catheter according to the manufacturer's guidelines.
10. Ensure that the critical care nurse has zeroed the hemodynamic monitoring system.	Prepares the monitoring system so that PA pressures can be obtained during catheter insertion.	
11. Insert the catheter through the sterile sheath.	Maintains sterility of the PA catheter to allow repositioning of the catheter.	
12. While observing the monitor and the markings on the PA catheter (Fig. 65–2), follow these steps: A. Advance the catheter through the introducer to the superior vena cava into the right atrium. B. Inflate the balloon with 1.5 mL of air. C. Advance the catheter through the tricuspid valve, into the right ventricle. D. Continue to advance the catheter from the right ventricle through the pulmonic valve into the PA. E. Advance the catheter to the PA wedge position. F. Deflate the balloon.	Waveforms and values change while moving from the superior vena cava to the right atrium to the right ventricle to the pulmonary artery and into the wedge position.	When inserting into the subclavian vein, have the patient bring his or her ear to the shoulder on the side of the insertion site. This creates a sharp angle between the jugular and subclavian veins and may help prevent misdirection of the catheter into the internal jugular vein. During insertion, monitor the ECG tracing for dysrhythmias.

Steps	Rationale	Special Considerations

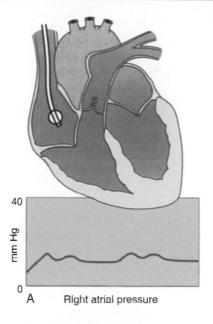

A Right atrial pressure

B Right ventricular pressure

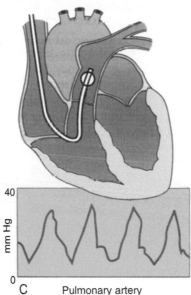

■ ● FIGURE 65–2. Catheter advancing through the heart with appropriate waveforms. (Adapted from Bucher L, Melander S. *Critical Care Nursing.* Philadelphia: WB Saunders; 1999: 123.)

C Pulmonary artery

D Pulmonary artery occlusive pressure

Steps	Rationale	Special Considerations
13. Ensure proper placement by rewedging the PA catheter, and confirm placement with paper tracing.	Ensures proper placement and accurate readings.	
14. Extend the sterile sheath over the catheter and secure in place.	Maintains catheter sterility for catheter repositioning.	Research has not yet determined how long the sheath remains sterile.
15. Apply an occlusive, sterile dressing.	Reduces incidence of infection.	
16. Obtain a chest x-ray.	Confirms catheter placement.	
17. Discard used supplies, and wash hands.	Reduces transmission of microorganisms; standard precautions.	

AP This procedure should be performed only by physicians, advanced practice nurses, and other health care professionals (including critical care nurses) with additional knowledge, skills, and demonstrated competence per professional licensure or institutional standard.

Expected Outcomes	Unexpected Outcomes
• Accurate placement of pulmonary artery catheter	• Pneumothorax or hemothorax
• Adequate and appropriate waveforms	• Infection
• Ability to obtain accurate information about cardiac pressures	• Ventricular dysrhythmias
• Evaluation of information to guide therapeutic interventions	• Misplacement (eg, carotid artery, subclavian artery)
	• Hemorrhage
	• Hematoma
	• Pericardial or ventricular rupture
	• Venous air embolism
	• Cardiac tamponade
	• Sepsis
	• Pulmonary artery infarction
	• Pulmonary artery rupture
	• Pulmonary artery catheter balloon rupture
	• Pulmonary artery catheter knotting
	• Heparin-induced thrombocytopenia or thrombosis

Patient Monitoring and Care

Patient Monitoring and Care	Rationale	Reportable Conditions
		These conditions should be reported if they persist despite nursing interventions.
1. Perform systematic cardiovascular, peripheral vascular, and hemodynamic assessments before and immediately following insertion:		
○ Assess level of consciousness.	Assesses for signs of adequate perfusion; air embolism may present with restlessness; patient may present with decreased level of consciousness if the catheter is advanced into the carotid artery.	• Change in level of consciousness
○ Assess vital signs.	Demonstrates response to procedure and effectiveness of therapies performed.	• Changes in vital signs
○ Assess postinsertion hemodynamic values: pulmonary artery systolic pressure (PASP), pulmonary artery diastolic pressure (PADP), RAP, pulmonary artery wedge pressure, CO, CI, SVR, and other parameters as needed.	Assesses patient status.	• Abnormal hemodynamic pressures or cardiac parameters
2. Monitor site for hematoma or hemorrhage.	If coagulopathies are present, may require pressure dressing.	• Hemorrhage that does not stop • Hematoma
3. Assess heart and lung sounds.	Abnormal heart or lung sounds may indicate cardiac tamponade, pneumothorax or hemothorax.	• Diminished or muffled heart sounds • Absent or diminished breath sounds unilaterally
4. Assess results of chest x-ray.	Ensures adequate placement in lung zone 3 below the level of the left atrium.	• Abnormal chest x-ray results
5. Monitor for signs of cardiac tamponade and air embolism.	Identifies complications.	• Signs or symptoms of cardiac tamponade or air embolism

Documentation

Documentation should include the following:

- Patient and family education
- Informed consent
- Insertion of PA catheter and sheath introducer
- Type and size of catheter placed
- Size of introducer sheath
- PA pressure values on insertion (RAP, right ventricular systolic and diastolic pressures, pulmonary artery systolic and diastolic pressures, PCWP)
- Graphic strip of insertion
- Insertion site of PA catheter
- Centimeter mark at edge of introducer

- Any difficulties encountered during placement (ventricular ectopy, new bundle branch blocks)
- Patient tolerance
- Confirmation of placement (eg, chest x-ray)
- Initial values after placement of catheter (PAPs, PCWP, RAP, CO, CI, systemic vascular resistance, pulmonary vascular resistance, SvO_2)
- Occurrence of unexpected outcomes
- Additional interventions

References

1. Amin DK, Shah PK, Swan HJC. Deciding when hemodynamic monitoring is appropriate. *J Crit Illness*, 1993;8:1053–1061.
2. Herbert KA, Glancy DL. Indications for Swan-Ganz catheterization. *Heart Dis Stroke*. 1994;3:196–200.
3. West JB, Dollery CT, Naimark A. Distribution of blood flow in isolated lung: relation to vascular and alveolar pressure. *J Appl Physiol*. 1964;19:713–724.
4. Bridges EJ, Woods SL. Pulmonary artery measurement: state of the art. *Heart Lung*. 1993;22:99–111.
5. Gardner PE, Bridges EJ. Hemodynamic monitoring. In: Woods SL, Sivarajan-Froelicher ES, Halpenny CJ, Motzei SU, eds. *Cardiac Nursing*. 3rd ed. Philadelphia, Pa: J.B. Lippincott; 1995:474–458.
6. Pulmonary Artery Consensus Conference Participants. Pulmonary Artery Catheter Consensus Conference: consensus statement. *Crit Care Med*. 1997;25:6,910–925.
7. Silver D, Kapsch DN, Tsoi EK. Heparin-induced thrombocytopenia, thrombosis, and hemorrhage. *Ann Surg*. 1983;198:301–306.
8. Iberti TJ, Fischer EP, Leibowitz AB, Panacek EA, Silverstein JH, Albertson TE. A multicenter study of physicians' knowledge of the pulmonary artery catheter. *JAMA*. 1990;22:2928–2933.
9. Iberti TJ, Daily EK, Leibowitz AB, Schecter CV, Fischer EP, Silverstein JH. Assessment of critical care nurses' knowledge of the pulmonary artery catheter. *Crit Care Med*. 1994;22:1674–1678.
10. Burns D, Burns D, Shively M. Critical care nurses' knowledge of pulmonary artery catheters. *Am J Crit Care*. 1996;5:49–54.
11. Morris AH, Chapman RH. Wedge pressure confirmation by aspiration of pulmonary capillary blood. *Crit Care Med*. 1985;13:756–759.

Additional Readings

Ahrens TS, Taylor LK. *Hemodynamic Waveform Analysis*. Philadelphia, Pa: W.B. Saunders; 1992.

American Association of Critical Care Nurses. Evaluation of the effects of heparinized and nonheparinized flush solutions on the patency of arterial pressure monitoring lines: The AAC Thunder Project. *Am J Crit Care*. 1993;2:3–15.

Amin DK, Shah PK, Swan HJC. The Swan-Ganz catheter: techniques for avoiding common errors. *J Crit Illness*. 1993;8:1263–1271.

Amin DK, Shah PK, Swan HJC. The technique of inserting a Swan-Ganz catheter. *J Crit Illness*. 1993;8:1147–1156.

Chernow B. Pulmonary artery flotation catheters: a statement by the American College of Chest Physicians and the American Thoracic Society. *Chest*. 1997;111:261.

Connors AF, Speroff T, Dawson NV, et al. The effectiveness of right heart catheterization in the initial care of critically ill patients. *JAMA*. 1996;276:11,889–897.

Daily EK, Schroeder JS. *Techniques in Bedside Hemodynamic Monitoring*. 5th ed. St Louis, Mo: C.V. Mosby; 1994.

Darovic GO. *Hemodynamic Monitoring: Invasive and Noninvasive Clinical Application*. Philadelphia, Pa: W.B. Saunders, 1995.

Friesinger GC, Williams SV, ACP/ACC/AHA Task Force on Clinical Privileges in Cardiology. Clinical competence in hemodynamic monitoring. *J Am Coll Cardiol*. 1990;15:1460.

Gardner PE. Pulmonary artery pressure monitoring. *AACN Clin Issues Crit Care Nurs*. 1993;4:98–119.

Ginosar Y, Pizov R, Sprung CL. Arterial and pulmonary artery catheters. In: *Critical Care Medicine*. St Louis, Mo: C.V. Mosby; 1995.

Keckeisen M. Protocols for practice: Hemodynamic monitoring series—pulmonary artery pressure monitoring. Aliso Viejo, CA: American Association of Critical-Care Nurses; 1997.

Marion PL. *The ICU Book*. Philadelphia, Pa: Lea & Febiger; 1991.

Pulmonary Artery Catheter Consensus Conference Participants. Pulmonary Artery Catheter Consensus Conference: consensus statement. *Crit Care Med*. 1997;25:910–925.

Putterman C. The Swan-Ganz catheter: a decade of hemodynamic monitoring. *J Crit Care*. 1989;4:127–146.

Quail SJ. Quality assurance in hemodynamic monitoring. *AACN Clin Issues Crit Care*. 1993;4:197–205.

■■ AP This procedure should be performed only by physicians, advanced practice nurses, and other health care professionals (including critical care nurses) with additional knowledge, skills, and demonstrated competence per professional licensure or institutional standard.

Staudinger T, Locker GJ, Laczika K, et al: Diagnostic validity of pulmonary artery catheterization for residents at an intensive care unit. *J Trauma.* 1998;44:902–906.

Steingrub JS, Celori G, Vickers-Lahti M. Therapeutic impact of pulmonary artery catheterization in a medical/surgical ICU. *Chest.* 1991;99:1451.

Swan JHC. What role today for hemodynamic monitoring. *J Crit Illness.* 1993;8:1043–1050.

Swan JHC, Ganz W, Forrester JS. Catheterization of the heart in a man with the use of a flow-directed balloon-tipped catheter. *N Engl J Med.* 1970;280:447.

The American Society of Anesthesiologists' Task Force on Pulmonary Artery Catheterization. Practice guidelines for pulmonary catheterization. *Anesthesiology.* 1993;78:380–394.

Urban N. Hemodynamic clinical profiles. *AACN Clin Issues Crit Care Nurs.* 1990;1:119–130.

Venus B, Mallory DL. Vascular cannulation. In: *Critical Care.* 2nd ed. Philadelphia, Pa: J.B. Lippincott; 1992.

66

Pulmonary Artery Catheter Insertion (Assist) and Pressure Monitoring

PURPOSE: Pulmonary artery (PA) catheters are used to determine hemodynamic status in critically ill patients. PA catheters provide information about right- and left-sided intracardiac pressures and cardiac output (CO). Additional functions available are fiberoptic monitoring of mixed venous oxygen saturation, intracardiac pacing, and assessment of right ventricular volumes and ejection fraction. Hemodynamic information obtained with a PA catheter is routinely used to guide therapeutic intervention, including administration of fluids and diuretics and titration of vasoactive and inotropic medications.

Debra J. Lynn-McHale
Teresa Preuss

PREREQUISITE NURSING KNOWLEDGE

- Understanding of cardiovascular anatomy and physiology is essential.
- Understanding of pulmonary anatomy and physiology is needed.
- Principles of aseptic technique should be understood.
- Understanding of basic dysrhythmia recognition and treatment of life-threatening dysrhythmias is necessary.
- Advanced cardiac life support knowledge and skills are necessary.
- Understanding of the anatomy of PA catheter (Fig. 66–1) and the location of PA catheter in heart and pulmonary artery (Fig. 66–2) is necessary.
- Understand the setup of the hemodynamic monitoring system (see Procedure 69).
- Be able to recognize the waveforms that occur during insertion, including right atrial (RA), right ventricular (RV), PA, and pulmonary artery wedge (PAW) (Fig. 66–3).
- Understand a, c, and v waves: the a wave reflects atrial contraction, the c wave reflects closure of the atrioventricular valve, and the v wave reflects passive filling of the atria during ventricular systole (Figs. 66–4 and 66–5).
- Indications for PA catheter therapy (see Procedure 65 for additional indications) are as follows
  - ❖ Aid in the diagnosis of complications after acute myocardial infarction (MI) that may include heart failure, cardiogenic shock, papillary muscle rupture, mitral regurgitation, ventricular septal rupture, or cardiac rupture with tamponade
  - ❖ Assessment of ventricular function in heart failure
  - ❖ Management of high-risk cardiac patients undergoing

surgical procedures during preoperative, intraoperative, or postoperative periods
  - ❖ Differentiation of hypotensive states, such as hypovolemia, sepsis, heart failure, and cardiac tamponade
  - ❖ Hemodynamic monitoring and evaluation of patients with major organ dysfunction who require fluid management and infusion of vasoactive medications, such as patients with burns, trauma, acute respiratory distress syndrome (ARDS), or gastrointestinal bleeding
- There are no absolute contraindications to hemodynamic monitoring with a PA catheter, but an assessment of risk versus benefit to the patient should be considered. Relative contraindications to pulmonary artery catheter insertion include preexisting left bundle branch block, presence of fever, mechanical tricuspid valve, and coagulopathic state.
- Understanding of normal hemodynamic values is necessary (see Table 59–1).
- The pulmonary artery catheter contains a proximal lumen port, a distal lumen port, a thermistor lumen port, and a balloon-inflation lumen port. Some catheters also have an infusion port that can be used for infusion of medications and intravenous fluids.
- The distal lumen port is used to monitor systolic, diastolic, and mean pressures in the pulmonary artery. The proximal lumen (or injectate) port is used to monitor the right atrial pressure and inject the solution used to obtain CO. The balloon-inflation lumen port is used to obtain PAW pressure (PAWP).
- The PA diastolic pressure and the PAWP are indirect measures of left ventricular end-diastolic pressure (LVEDP). Usually, the PAWP is approximately 1 to 4 mm Hg less than the pulmonary artery diastolic pressure (PADP). Because these two pressures are similar, the

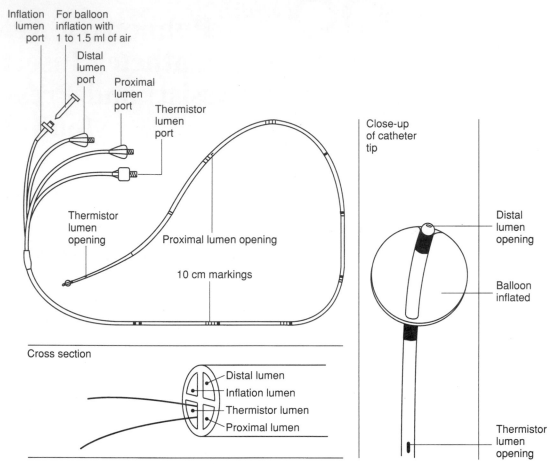

Inflation lumen port

For balloon inflation with 1 to 1.5 ml of air

Distal lumen port

Proximal lumen port

Thermistor lumen port

Thermistor lumen opening

Proximal lumen opening

10 cm markings

Cross section

Distal lumen
Inflation lumen
Thermistor lumen
Proximal lumen

Close-up of catheter tip

Distal lumen opening

Balloon inflated

Thermistor lumen opening

■ ● **FIGURE 66–1.** Anatomy of the pulmonary artery (PA) catheter. The standard no. 7.5-Fr thermodilution PA catheter is 110 cm in length and contains four lumens. It is constructed of radiopaque polyvinyl chloride. In 10-cm increments, there are black markings on the catheter beginning at the distal end. At the distal end of the catheter is a latex rubber balloon of 1.5-mL capacity, which, when inflated, extends slightly beyond the tip of the catheter without obstructing it. Balloon inflation cushions the tip of the catheter and prevents contact with the right ventricular wall during insertion. The balloon also acts to float the catheter into position and allows measurement of the pulmonary artery wedge pressure. Note black bands on catheter that indicate length of insertion. Narrow black bands represent 10-cm lengths and wide black bands indicate 50-cm lengths. (From Visalli F, Evans P. The Swan-Ganz catheter: a program for teaching safe, effective use. *Nursing 81.* 1981; 11 (1).)

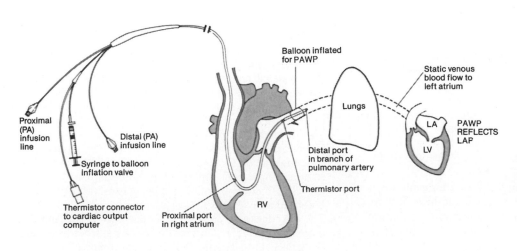

Balloon inflated for PAWP

Static venous blood flow to left atrium

Lungs

LA

LV

PAWP REFLECTS LAP

Proximal (PA) infusion line

Distal (PA) infusion line

Syringe to balloon inflation valve

Thermistor connector to cardiac output computer

Proximal port in right atrium

Distal port in branch of pulmonary artery

Thermistor port

RV

■ ● **FIGURE 66–2.** Pulmonary artery (PA) catheter location within heart. Pulmonary artery wedge pressure (PAWP) is an indirect measure of left atrial and left ventricular end-diastolic pressure. (From Kersten LD. *Comprehensive Respiratory Nursing.* Philadelphia, Pa: WB Saunders; 1989: 758.)

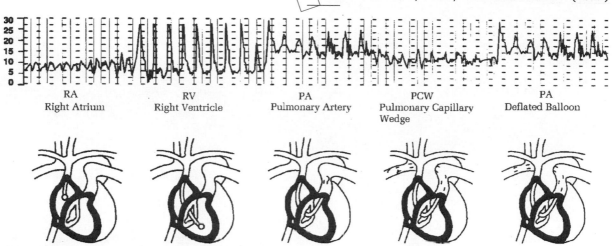

■ ● **FIGURE 66–3.** Schematic of waveform progression as a pulmonary artery catheter is inserted through the various cardiac chambers. (From Abbott Critical Care Systems, Mountain View, Ca.)

PADP commonly is followed. This minimizes the frequency of balloon inflation and thus decreases the potential of balloon rupture.

- Differences between the PADP and the PAWP may exist for patients with pulmonary hypertension, chronic obstructive lung disease, ARDS, pulmonary embolus, and tachycardia.
- Pulmonary artery pressures may be elevated due to pulmonary artery hypertension, pulmonary disease, mitral valve disease, left ventricular failure, atrial or ventricular left-to-right shunt, pulmonary emboli, or hypervolemia.
- Pulmonary artery pressures may be decreased due to hypovolemia or vasodilation.
- Elevated a and v waves may be evident in right atrial pressure (RAP)/CVP and in PAWP waveforms. These

elevations may occur in patients with cardiac tamponade, constrictive pericardial disease, and hypervolemia.
- Elevated a waves in the RAP/CVP waveform may occur in patients with pulmonic or tricuspid stenosis, right ventricular ischemia or infarction, right ventricular failure, pulmonary artery hypertension, and atrioventricular (AV) dissociation.
- Elevated a waves in the PAWP waveform may occur in patients with mitral stenosis, acute left ventricular ischemia or infarction, left ventricular failure, and AV dissociation.
- Elevated v waves in the RAP/CVP waveform may occur in patients with tricuspid insufficiency.
- Elevated v waves in the PAWP waveform may occur in patients with mitral insufficiency or ruptured papillary muscle.

■ ● **FIGURE 66–4.** Identification of a, c, and v waves in the waveform for right atrial and central venous pressure (RA/CVP). Atrial waveforms are characterized by three components: a, c, and v waves. The a wave reflects atrial contraction, the c wave reflects closure of the tricuspid valve, and the v wave reflects passive filling of the atria. (From Ahrens TS, Taylor LK. *Hemodynamic Waveform Analysis.* Philadelphia, Pa: WB Saunders; 1992.)

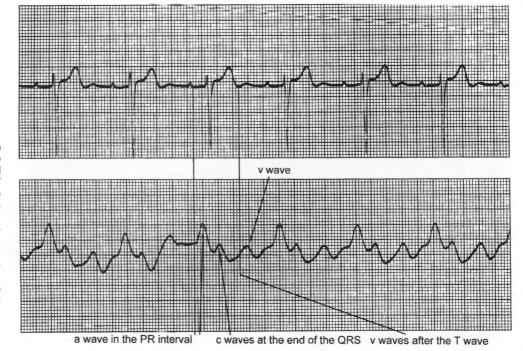

v wave

a wave in the PR interval   c waves at the end of the QRS   v waves after the T wave

ECG

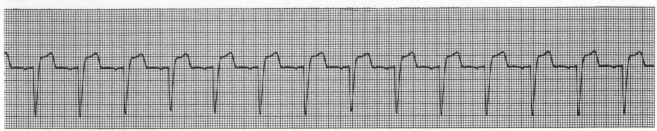

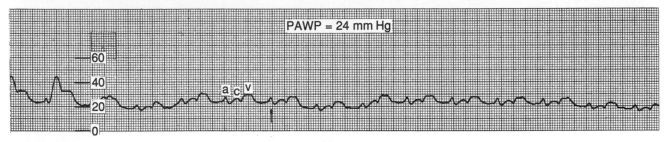

■ ● **FIGURE 66–5.** Normal pulmonary artery wedge pressure (PAWP) waveform and components. Note delay in *a, c,* and *v* waves because of the time it takes for the mechanical events to show a pressure change. This waveform is from a spontaneously breathing patient. The arrow indicates end-expiration, where the mean of *a* wave pressure is measured.

- Insertion and placement verification should occur as follows:
  ❖ The PA catheter may be inserted through the subclavian, internal jugular, femoral, external jugular, or antecubital veins.
  ❖ The standard 7.5-F PA catheter is 110 cm long and has black markings at 10-cm increments to facilitate insertion and positioning (Fig. 66–1). The catheter should reach the PA after being advanced 45 to 55 cm from the internal jugular vein or 70 to 80 cm from a femoral or an antecubital vein.
  ❖ Verification of PA catheter placement is validated by waveform analysis. Correct catheter placement demonstrates a PAW tracing when the balloon is inflated and a PA tracing when the balloon is deflated.
  ❖ Catheter placement is also verified by chest x-ray.

EQUIPMENT

- Percutaneous equipment tray/introducer kit
- PA catheter (non–heparin-coated PA catheters are available)
- Sheath introducer and sterile catheter sleeve
- Pressure cables for interface with the monitor
- Cardiac output cable with a thermistor/injectate sensor
- Pressure transducer system, including flush solution recommended according to institution standard, a pressure bag or device, pressure tubing with flush device, and transducers.

- Sterile normal saline intravenous fluid for flushing catheter and introducer ports
- Povidone-iodine solution
- Caps, masks, sterile growns, sterile gloves, and sterile drapes
- 1% lidocaine without epinephrine
- Sterile basin or cup
- Sterile water or normal saline
- Sterile dressing supplies
- Stopcocks
- Dead-end caps

Additional equipment as needed includes the following:

- Fluoroscope
- Emergency equipment
- Indelible marker

PATIENT AND FAMILY EDUCATION

- Assess patient and family readiness to learn and identify factors that affect learning. ➤*Rationale:* Allows the nurse to individualize teaching.
- Provide information about the PA catheter, reason for the PA catheter, and explanation of the equipment. ➤*Rationale:* Assists patient and family to understand the procedure, why it is needed, and how it will help the patient. Decreases patient and family anxiety.
- Explain the patient's expected participation during the procedure. ➤*Rationale:* Encourages patient involvement.

PATIENT ASSESSMENT AND PREPARATION
Patient Assessment

- Determine baseline hemodynamic, cardiovascular, peripheral vascular, and neurovascular status. ➤*Rationale:* Provides data that can be used for comparison with postinsertion assessment data and hemodynamic values.
- Determine baseline pulmonary status. If the patient is mechanically ventilated, note the type of support, ventilator mode, and presence or absence of positive end-expiratory pressure (PEEP) or continuous positive airway pressure (CPAP). ➤*Rationale:* The presence of mechanical ventilation alters hemodynamic waveforms.
- Assess past medical history specifically related to problems with venous access sites, cardiac anatomy, and pulmonary anatomy. ➤*Rationale:* Identification of obstructions or disease should be made prior to insertion attempt.

- Assess current laboratory profile, including electrolyte and coagulation studies. ➤➤*Rationale:* Identifies laboratory abnormalities. Baseline coagulation studies are helpful in determining risk for bleeding. Electrolyte imbalances may increase cardiac irritability.

Patient Preparation

- Ensure that the patient and family understands preprocedural teaching. Answer questions as they arise and reinforce information as needed. ➤➤*Rationale:* Evaluates and reinforces understanding of previously taught information.

- Ensure that informed consent has been obtained. ➤➤*Rationale:* Protects the rights of the patient and makes a competent decision possible for patient.
- Validate patency of peripheral IV line. ➤➤*Rationale:* Access may be needed for adminstration of emergency medications or fluids.
- Place patient in supine position. ➤➤*Rationale:* Prepares patient for skin preparation, catheter insertion, and setup of sterile field.
- Sedate the patient or provide prescribed analgesics as needed. ➤➤*Rationale:* Movement of patient may inhibit insertion of PA catheter.

Procedure **for Pulmonary Artery Catheter Insertion (Assist) and Pressure Monitoring**

Steps	Rationale	Special Considerations
Assisting with PA Catheter Insertion		
1. Wash hands.	Reduces possible transmission of microorganisms and body secretions; maintains standard precautions.	
2. Follow institutional standard for adding heparin to flush solution (see Procedure 69).	Heparinized flush solutions are commonly used to minimize thrombi and fibrin deposits on catheters that might lead to thrombosis or bacterial colonization of the catheter.	Although heparin may prevent thrombosis,[1] it has been associated with thrombocytopenia and other hematologic complications.[2] Research is needed regarding use of heparin versus normal saline to maintain PA line patency.
3. Prime or flush the entire pressure transducer system (see Procedure 69).	Removes air bubbles. Air bubbles introduced into the patient's circulation can cause air embolism. Air bubbles within the tubing will dampen the waveform.	Air is more easily removed from the hemodynamic tubing when the system is not under pressure.
4. Wash hands, and don caps, masks, sterile gowns, and gloves for all health care personnel involved in procedure.	Reduces possible transmission of microorganisms and body secretions; maintains standard precautions.	
5. Maintain pressure in the pressure bag or device at 300 mm Hg.	The flush device delivers 1 to 3 mL/hr to maintain patency of the hemodynamic system.	
6. Assist physician or advanced practice nurse with opening the PA catheter and introducer kits.	Aids in maintaining sterility.	
7. Connect hemodynamic flush system to appropriate distal and proximal ports of the PA catheter and flush all lumens.	Removes air from the pulmonary artery catheter.	
8. Connect the pressure cables from the RA and PA transducers to the bedside monitor.	Connects the pulmonary artery catheter to the bedside monitoring system.	
9. Connect the thermistor of the PA catheter to the CO monitor or module.	Allows the core temperature to be monitored and is needed for CO measurement.	
10. If a PA catheter with the ability to monitor mixed venous oxygenation is being inserted, the fiberoptics should be calibrated prior to removal from the package (see Procedure 13).	Calibrates the system.	Follow manufacturer guidelines for catheter calibration.

Procedure continued on following page

Procedure for Pulmonary Artery Catheter Insertion (Assist) and Pressure Monitoring
Continued

Steps	Rationale	Special Considerations
11. Set the scales for each pressure tracing.	Permits waveform analysis.	The scale for the RA/CVP pressure commonly is set at 20 mm Hg, and the PA scale commonly is set at 40 mm Hg. Scales are adjusted based on patient pressures.
12. Examine the PA catheter for defects in construction and check balloon integrity.	Faulty catheters should be replaced.	The inflated balloon can be placed in a container of sterile normal saline or water. No air bubbles should be seen. If air bubbles are seen, there is a defect in the balloon integrity.
13. Zero the system connected to the distal end of the PA catheter by turning the stopcock off to the patient, opening it to air, and zeroing the monitoring system (see Procedure 69).	Prepares the monitoring system so that PA pressures can be obtained during catheter insertion.	
14. The physician or advanced practice nurse may place a sterile plastic sleeve over the PA catheter, attaching it to the PA catheter before the catheter is inserted.	A sterile sleeve may prevent contamination of the PA catheter and allows repositioning of the catheter after the initial insertion.	Research has not yet determined how long the sleeve remains sterile.
15. As insertion begins, continuously run an ECG and PA distal waveform strip.	Provides documentation of insertion PA pressures and dysrhythmias.	A dual-channel recorder is preferred, because then the ECG and the PA waveform can be simultaneously recorded.
16. After the tip of the PA catheter is in the right atrium, inflate the balloon with no more than 1.25 to 1.5 mL of air and close the gate valve or the stopcock (Fig. 66–6).	The presence of the tip of the catheter in the right atrium is validated by waveform analysis (see Fig. 66–3). Closing the gate valve or the stopcock holds air in the balloon during insertion.	The inflated balloon advances the PA catheter through the right side of the heart and into the PA, minimizing the chance of endocardial damage.
17. Observe for RV, PA, and then PAW waveforms (see Fig. 66–3).	Placement in the PA is validated by waveform analysis.	Monitor the ECG tracing as the PA catheter is inserted, because ventricular dysrhythmias may occur because of right ventricular irritability. Right ventricular pressures can be obtained only during insertion.
18. Verify that the catheter is in the proper position. When the balloon is deflated, the monitor will show a PA tracing; when the balloon is inflated, the monitor will show a PAW tracing.	When the balloon is inflated, the catheter floats from the pulmonary artery to a smaller arteriole (Fig. 66–3).	The catheter should reach the PA after being advanced 45 to 55 cm from the internal jugular or subclavian vein or 70 to 80 cm from a femoral or antecubital vein. Placement may vary depending on patient size.

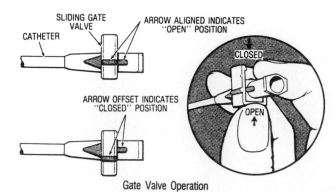

■ ● **FIGURE 66–6.** Gate valve in open position on pulmonary artery (PA) (distal) lumen of PA catheter. (From Baxter Edwards Corporation.)

Procedure **for Pulmonary Artery Catheter Insertion (Assist) and Pressure Monitoring**
Continued

Steps	Rationale	Special Considerations
19. Open the balloon inflation gate valve or stopcock after the pulmonary artery catheter is in place.	The gate valve and stopcock are closed during insertion to retain air in the balloon. The air is then released so that continuous monitoring of the PA waveform can be performed.	
20. Level the RA air-fluid interface (zeroing stopcock) and the PA air-fluid interface (zeroing stopcock) to the phlebostatic axis.	The phlebostatic axis approximates the level of the atria and should be used as the reference point for patients in the supine position.	The reference point for the atria changes when a patient is in the lateral position (see Procedure 69).
21. Secure the system to the patient's chest or arm or to a pole mount.	Ensures that the air-filled interface (zeroing stopcock) is maintained at the level of the phlebostatic axis. If the air-fluid interface is above the phlebostatic axis, PA pressures will be falsely low. If the air-fluid interface is below the phlebostatic axis, PA pressures will be falsely high.	The point of the phlebostatic axis should be marked with an indelible marker, especially if using a pole-mount setup.
22. Zero both the right atrial and pulmonary artery hemodynamic monitoring systems (see Procedure 69).	Ensures accuracy of the system with the established reference point.	
23. Observe the waveform and perform a dynamic response test (square wave test) (see Fig. 56–3A).	Results indicate whether the system is correctly damped.	
24. Place a sterile, occlusive dressing on the insertion site.	Reduces the risk of infection.	
25. Set alarms. Upper and lower alarm limits are set on the basis of the patient's current clinical status and hemodynamic values.	Activates the bedside and central alarm system.	
26. Discard used supplies, and wash hands.	Reduces the transmission of microorganisms; standard precautions.	

Obtaining PA Pressure Measurements

RA/CVP

1. Position patient in the supine position with the head of the bed from 0 to 45 degrees. *(Level VI: Clinical studies in a variety of patient populations and situations to support recommendations)*	Studies have determined that central venous and PA pressures are accurate in this position.[3–8]	Central venous and PA pressures may be accurate for patients in the supine position with the head of the bed elevated up to 60 degrees,[9] yet additional studies are needed to support this. Studies have not demonstrated the accuracy of hemodynamic values for patients in the lateral position.[6, 8, 10, 11]
2. Run a dual-channel strip of the ECG and RA waveform (Fig. 66–7).	RA pressures should be determined from the graphic strip, because the effect of ventilation can be identified.	Digital data can be used to determine RA pressure if ventilation does not affect the RA pressure waveform.
3. Measure RA pressure at end expiration.	Measurement is most accurate as the effects of pulmonary pressures are minimized.	

Procedure continued on following page

Procedure	**for Pulmonary Artery Catheter Insertion (Assist) and Pressure Monitoring**
	Continued

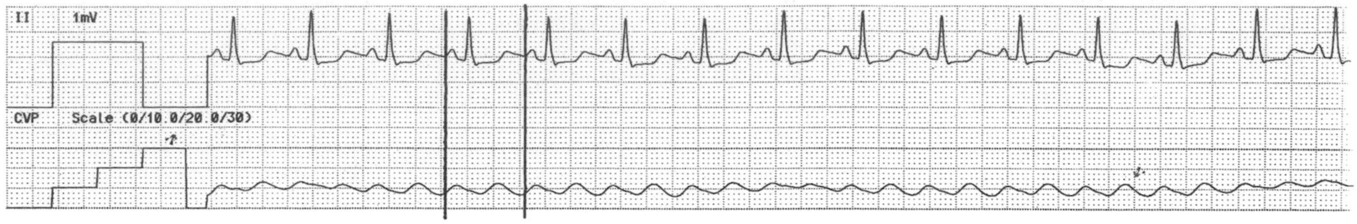

Steps	Rationale	Special Considerations

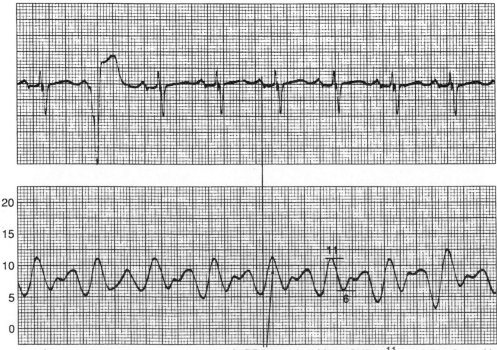

■ ● FIGURE 66–7. Note vertical lines drawn from the beginning of the P wave of two of the electrocardiogram (ECG) complexes down to the right atrial (RA) waveform. The first positive deflection of the RA waveform is the *a* wave, the second positive deflection is the *v* wave. The *c* wave, which would lie between the *a* wave and the *v* wave, is not evident in this strip.

Steps	Rationale	Special Considerations
4. Using the dual-channel recorded strip, draw a vertical line from the beginning of the P wave of one of the ECG complexes down to the RA waveform. Repeat this with the next ECG complex (see Fig. 66–7).	Compares electrical activity to mechanical activity. Usually three waves will be present on the RA waveform.	Rarely, the c wave will not be present.
5. Align the PR interval with the RA waveform.	The a wave correlates with this interval.	
6. Identify the a wave.	The a wave is seen approximately 80 to 100 milliseconds after the P wave. The c wave follows the a wave, and the v wave follows the c wave.	The a wave reflects atrial contraction. The c wave reflects closure of the tricuspid valve. The v wave reflects passive filling of the atria (Fig. 66–4).
7. Identify the scale of RA tracing (Fig. 66–8).	Aids in determining pressure measurement.	RA scale commonly is set at 20 mm Hg.
8. Measure the mean of the a wave to obtain the RA pressure (RAP) (see Fig. 66–8).	The a wave represents atrial contraction and reflects right ventricular filling at end diastole.	

a wave in PR interval   Mean CVP = $\frac{11}{6}$, or 8.5 or 9 mm Hg

■ ● FIGURE 66–8. Obtaining measurements of right atrial and central venous pressures (RA/CVP). Aligning the *a* wave on the RA/CVP waveform with the PR interval on the electrocardiogram facilitates accurate measurement of RA/CVP at end-diastole. (From Ahrens TS, Taylor LK. *Hemodynamic Waveform Analysis.* Philadelphia, Pa: WB Saunders; 1992.)

Procedure for **Pulmonary Artery Catheter Insertion (Assist) and Pressure Monitoring**
Continued

Steps	Rationale	Special Considerations
PA Systolic and Diastolic Pressures		
1. Position patient in the supine position with the head of the bed from 0 to 45 degrees. (*Level VI: Clinical studies in a variety of patient populations and situations to support recommendations*)	Studies have determined that central venous and PA pressures are accurate in this position.[3-8]	Central venous and PA pressures may be accurate for patients in the supine position with the head of the bed elevated up to 60 degrees,[9] yet additional studies are needed to support this. Studies have not demonstrated the accuracy of hemodynamic values for patients in the lateral position.[6, 8, 10, 11]
2. Run a dual-channel strip of the ECG and PA waveform (Fig. 66–9).	PA pressures should be determined from the graphic strip, because the effect of ventilation can be identified.	
3. Measure PA pressure at end expiration.	Measurement is most accurate as the effects of pulmonary pressures are minimized.	
4. Identify the QT interval on the ECG strip.	Demonstrates ventricular depolarization.	
5. Align the QT interval with the PA waveform.	Compares electrical activity to mechanical activity.	
6. Identify the scale of the PA tracing.	Aids in determining pressure measurement.	PA scale is commonly set at 40 mm Hg.
7. Measure the PA systolic pressure at the peak of the systolic waveform on the PA waveform (see Fig. 66–9).	This reflects the highest systolic pressure.	

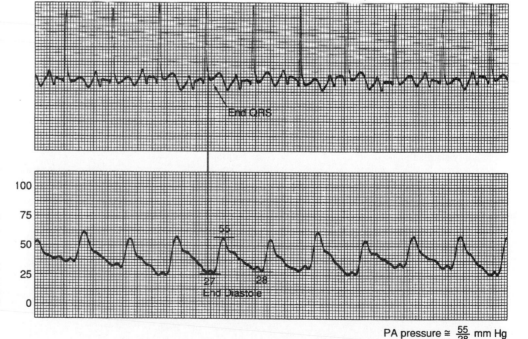

■ ● **FIGURE 66–9.** Obtaining measurements of pressure in the pulmonary artery (PA). For systolic pressure, align the peak of the systolic waveform with the QT interval on the electrocardiogram (ECG). For PA diastolic pressure, use the end of the QRS as a marker to detect the PA diastolic phase, and obtain the reading just before the upstroke of the systolic waveform. (From Ahrens TS, Taylor LK. *Hemodynamic Waveform Analysis.* Philadelphia, Pa: WB Saunders; 1992.)

PA pressure $\cong \frac{55}{28}$ mm Hg

Procedure continued on following page

Procedure **for Pulmonary Artery Catheter Insertion (Assist) and Pressure Monitoring**
Continued

Steps	Rationale	Special Considerations
8. Align the end of the QRS complex with the PA waveform (see Fig. 66–9).	The end of the QRS complex correlates with ventricular end-diastolic pressure.	
9. Measure the PA diastolic pressure at the point of the intersection of this line (Fig. 66–9).	This point occurs just before the upstroke of the systolic pressure.	
PAWP		
1. Position patient in the supine position with the head of the bed from 0 to 45 degrees. *(Level VI: Clinical studies in a variety of patient populations and situations to support recommendations)*	Studies have determined that central venous and PA pressures are accurate in this position.[3–8]	Central venous and PA pressures may be accurate for patients in the supine position with the head of the bed elevated up to 60 degrees,[9] yet additional studies are needed to support this. Studies have not demonstrated the accuracy of hemodynamic values for patients in the lateral position.[6, 8, 10, 11]
2. Fill the PA syringe with 1.5 mL of air.	More than 1.5 mL of air may rupture the PA balloon and the pulmonary arteriole.	
3. Connect the PA syringe to gate valve or stopcock of the balloon port of the PA catheter (see Fig. 66–6).	This port is designed for PA balloon air inflation.	
4. Run a dual-channel strip of the ECG and PA waveform.	The PAW pressures should be determined from the graphic strip, because the effect of ventilation can be identified.	
5. Slowly inflate the balloon with air until the PA waveform changes to a PAW waveform (Fig. 66–10).	A slight resistance is usually felt during inflation of the balloon. Overinflation of the balloon can cause pulmonary arteriole infarction or rupture, resulting in life-threatening hemorrhage.[12]	Only enough air is needed to convert the PA waveform to a PAW waveform. Thus, the entire amount of 1.5 mL of air is not necessarily needed.
6. Inflate the PA balloon for no more than 8 to 15 seconds (two to four respiratory cycles).	Prolonged inflation of the balloon can cause pulmonary arteriole infarction and rupture, with life-threatening hemorrhage.[12]	
7. Disconnect syringe from the balloon-inflation port.	Allows air to passively escape from the balloon.	Active withdrawal of air from the balloon can weaken the balloon, leading to balloon rupture.
8. Observe the monitor as the PAW waveform changes back to the PA waveform.	Ensures adequate balloon deflation.	
9. Expel air from the syringe.	The syringe should remain empty so that accidental balloon inflation does not occur.	
10. Reconnect the empty syringe to the end of the balloon-inflation port.	The syringe that is manufactured for the PA catheter should be connected to the PA line so that it is not lost. This syringe can only be filled with 1.5 mL of air, thus serving as a safety feature to minimize the chance of balloon overinflation.	
11. Close the gate valve or stopcock at the end of the balloon-inflation port.	Prevents accidental use of the balloon-inflation port.	

Procedure	for Pulmonary Artery Catheter Insertion (Assist) and Pressure Monitoring

Continued

Steps	Rationale	Special Considerations

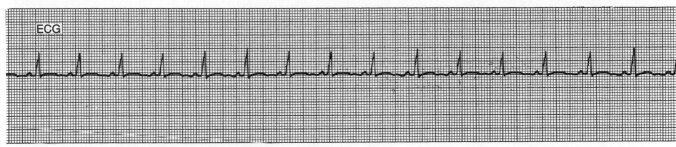

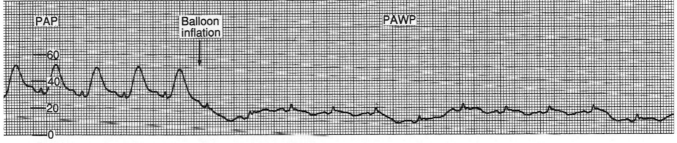

■ ● **FIGURE 66–10.** Change in pulmonary artery pressure (PAP) waveform to pulmonary artery wedge pressure (PAWP) waveform with balloon inflation. The balloon is inflated while observing the bedside monitor for change in the waveform. Balloon inflation *(arrow)* in patient with normal PAWP.

Steps	Rationale	Special Considerations
12. Using the dual-channel recorded strip, draw a vertical line from the beginning of the P wave of one of the ECG complexes down to the PAW waveform. Repeat this with the next ECG complex.	Compares electrical activity to mechanical activity. Two to three waves will be present on the PAW waveform.	C waves commonly are not present on PAW waveforms due to the distance the pressure needs to travel back to the transducer.
13. Align the end of a QRS complex of the ECG strip with the PAW waveform (Fig. 66–11).	Compares electrical activity to mechanical activity.	
14. Identify the a wave (see Fig. 66–11).	The a wave correlates with the end of the QRS complex. The c wave follows the a wave, and the v wave follows the c wave.	If only two waves are present, the first wave is the a wave and the second wave is the v wave.
15. Identify the scale of the PAW tracing.	Aids in determining pressure measurement.	PA scale commonly is set at 40 mm Hg.
16. Measure the mean of the a wave to obtain the PAWP (see Fig. 66–5).	The a wave represents atrial contraction and reflects left ventricular filling at end diastole.	If the PEEP is being used and the PEEP is more than 10 cm H_2O, adjustments in determining the pressures may be necessary. Follow institutional standard.
17. Compare the PADP with the PAWP.	The PAWP is commonly 1 to 4 mm Hg less than the PADP. Significant differences between PADP and PAWP may exist for patients with pulmonary hypertension, chronic obstructive lung disease, ARDS, pulmonary embolus, and tachycardia. PADPs that correlate with PAWPs represent left ventricular filling pressures.	

Procedure continued on following page

Steps	Rationale	Special Considerations

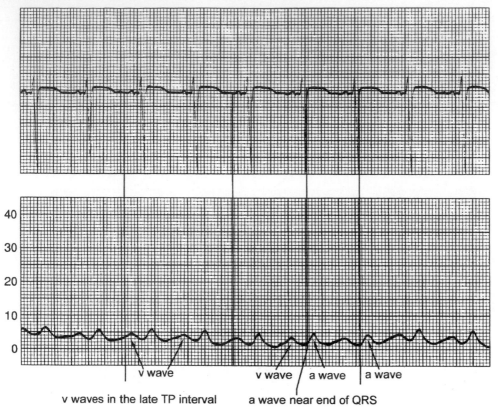

v waves in the late TP interval

a wave near end of QRS

■ ● **FIGURE 66–11.** Obtaining measurement of pulmonary artery wedge pressure (PAWP). For accurate readings, align the *a* wave from the PAWP waveform with the end of the QRS on the electrocardiogram (ECG) at end-diastole. (From Ahrens TS, Taylor LK. *Hemodynamic Waveform Analysis.* Philadelphia, Pa: WB Saunders; 1992.)

Steps	Rationale	Special Considerations
18. Follow PA diastolic pressures if there is a close correlation between PADP and PAWP.	Ensures accuracy of determination of left ventricular filling pressures.	Miminizes the number of times the PA balloon is inflated.
19. Follow the PAWP if there is greater than a 4 mm Hg difference between PAWP and PADP.	Ensures accuracy of measurements.	

Measurement of Hemodynamic Pressures at End Expiration

Steps	Rationale	Special Considerations
1. Measure all hemodynamic pressures at end expiration to ensure accuracy.	Atmospheric and alveolar pressures are approximately equal at end expiration. Intrathoracic pressure is closest to zero at end expiration. Measurement of hemodynamic pressures is most accurate at end expiration, because pulmonary pressures have minimal effect on intracardiac pressures.	
2. Determine end expiration by observing the rise and fall of the chest during breathing and use graphic hemodynamic, respiratory, or continuous airway pressures waveforms.	Aids in determining accuracy of end expiration.	

Determining End Expiration for the Patient Breathing Spontaneously

Steps	Rationale	Special Considerations
1. Record a strip of the PA waveform.	A labeled recording aids in determination of accurate hemodynamic pressure values.	In patients who are breathing spontaneously, the normal inspiratory:expiratory ratio is approximately 1:2.

Procedure	**for Pulmonary Artery Catheter Insertion (Assist) and Pressure Monitoring** *Continued*	

Steps	**Rationale**	**Special Considerations**
2. Note that the pressure waveform dips down during the inspiratory phase of breathing (Fig. 66–12).	Pleural pressure decreases during spontaneous inspiration, and this decrease is reflected by a fall in the cardiac pressures.	
3. Note that the pressure waveform elevates during the expiratory phase of breathing (see Fig. 66–12).	As pleural pressures equalize, the cardiac pressures reflect a more true normal.	
4. Measure the pressure at the end of the expiratory phase (see Fig. 66–12).	Ensures accurate determination of pressure values.	

Determining End Expiration for the Patient Receiving Mechanical Ventilation

1. Record a strip of the PA waveform.	A labeled recording aids in determination of accurate hemodynamic pressure values.	
2. Note that the pressure waveform elevates as a breath is delivered by the ventilator (Fig. 66–13).	As the ventilator delivers a breath to the lungs, an increase in pleural pressure results. This increase in pleural pressure causes an increase in intracardiac pressures.	
3. Note that the pressure waveform dips down as the breath is exhaled (see Fig. 66–13).	As the mechanical breath is exhaled, pulmonary pressures decrease and intracardiac pressures are more accurately reflected.	

Determining End Expiration for the Patient Receiving Intermittent Mandatory Mechanical Ventilation

1. If the patient is receiving intermittent mandatory ventilation, measure the pressure during the end expiration.	Ensures accurate determination of pressure values.	

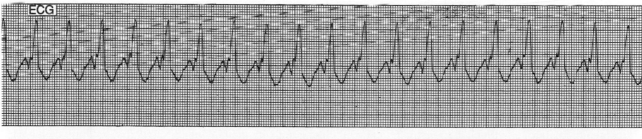
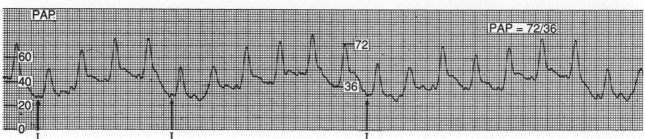

■ ● FIGURE 66–12. Respiratory fluctuations of pulmonary artery pressure (PAP) waveform in a spontaneously breathing patient. The location of inspiration (I) is marked on the waveform. The points just before inspiration are end-expiration, where readings will be taken.

Procedure continued on page 453

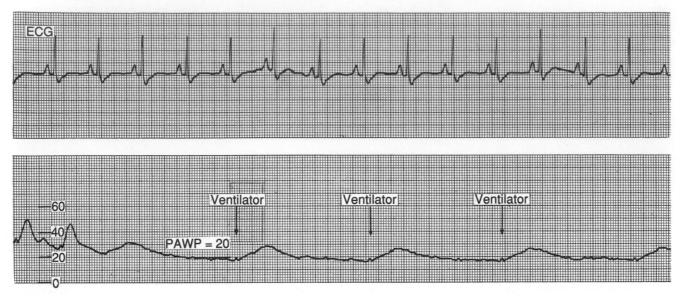

■ ● FIGURE 66–13. Mechanically ventilated patient (on pressure support–type ventilator) who had no spontaneous respiration because of neuromuscular blocking agent (vecuronium). The point of end-expiration is located just before the ventilator artifact.

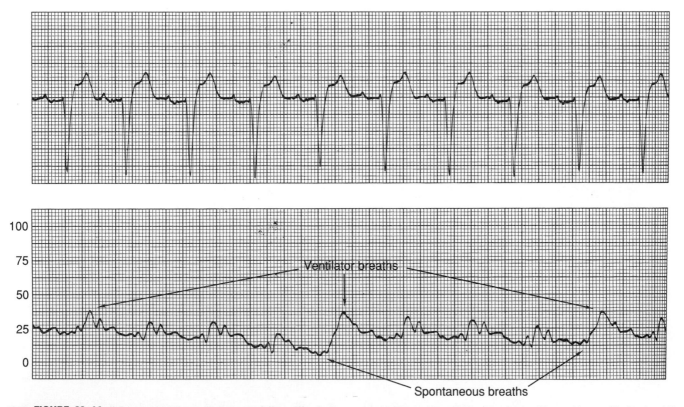

■ ● FIGURE 66–14. IMV mode of ventilation and the effect on a pulmonary artery (PA) waveform. (From Ahrens TS, Taylor LK. *Hemodynamic Waveform Analysis.* Philadelphia, Pa: WB Saunders; 1992:182.)

Procedure for Pulmonary Artery Catheter Insertion (Assist) and Pressure Monitoring
Continued

Steps	Rationale	Special Considerations
2. Note that the pressure waveform elevates as a breath is delivered by the ventilator (Fig. 66–14).	As the ventilator delivers a breath to the lungs, an increase in pleural pressure results. This increase in pleural pressure causes an increase in intracardiac pressures.	
3. Note that the pressure waveform dips down as the breath is exhaled (see Fig. 66–14).	As the mechanical breath is exhaled, pulmonary pressures decrease and intracardiac pressures are more accurately reflected.	
4. Identify the patient's spontaneous breath (see Fig. 66–14).	This breath may occur just prior to triggered ventilator breaths.	
5. Determine end expiration.	Ensures accuracy of measuremnts.	

Expected Outcomes

- Accurate placement of the pulmonary artery catheter
- Adequate and appropriate waveforms
- Ability to obtain accurate information about cardiac pressures
- Evaluation of information obtained to guide therapeutic interventions

Unexpected Outcomes

- Pneumothorax or hemothorax
- Infection
- Ventricular dysrhythmias
- Misplacement (eg, carotid artery, subclavian artery)
- Hemorrhage
- Hematoma
- Pericardial or ventricular rupture
- Venous air embolism
- Cardiac tamponade
- Sepsis
- Pulmonary artery infarction
- Pulmonary artery rupture
- Pulmonary artery catheter balloon rupture
- Pulmonary artery catheter knotting
- Heparin-induced thrombocytopenia or thrombosis

Patient Monitoring and Care

Steps	Rationale	Reportable Conditions
		These conditions should be reported if they persist despite nursing interventions.
1. Zero the transducer during intial setup or before insertion, if disconnection occurs between the transducer and the monitoring cable, if disconnection occurs between the monitoring cable and the monitor, and when the values obtained do not fit the clinical picture. Follow manufacturer recommendations for disposable and reusable systems.	Ensures accuracy of hemodynamic monitoring system; minimizes the risk of contamination of the system.	

Continued on following page

Steps	Rationale	Reportable Conditions
2. Place sterile dead-end caps on all stopcocks. Replace with new, sterile caps whenever the caps are removed.	Stopcocks can be a source of contamination. Stopcocks that are part of the initial setup are commonly vented. Vented caps need to be replaced with nonvented caps to maintain sterility.	
3. Monitor pressure transducer system (pressure tubing, transducer, stopcocks, etc.) for air and eliminate air from the system.	Air emboli are potentially fatal.	• Suspected air emboli
4. Obtain hemodynamic values (pulmonary artery systolic pressure [PASP], PADP, RAP) hourly and as necessary with condition changes.	Monitors patient status.	• Abnormal hemodynamic pressures or significant changes in hemodynamic pressures
5. Obtain CO, CI, and systemic vascular resistance and additional parameters immediately after catheter insertion and as necessary per patient condition.	Monitors patient status.	• Abnormal hemodynamic parameters or significant changes in hemodynamic parameters
6. Change hemodynamic monitoring system (flush solution, pressure tubing, transducers, and stopcocks) every 72 hours. *(Level V: Clinical studies in more than one or two different patient populations and situations to support recommendations)* Follow manufacturer recommendations for reusable transducer systems. The flush solution may need to be changed more frequently if empty.	The Centers for Disease Control and Prevention (CDC)[1] and research findings[13-15] recommend that the hemodynamic flush system can be used safely for 72 hours. This recommendation is based on research conducted with disposable pressure monitoring systems used for peripheral and central lines. This time frame may be extended,[13, 15] yet this is not currently recommended by the CDC.	
7. Perform a dynamic response test every 8 to 12 hours, when the system is opened to air, or when the accuracy of readings is in question (see Fig. 56-3A–C).	An optimally damped system provides an accurate waveform.	• Overdamped or underdamped waveform that cannot be corrected with troubleshooting procedures
8. Label tubing with date and time system was hung.	Identifies when system needs to be changed.	
9. Maintain pressure bag or device at 300 mm Hg.	At 300 mm Hg the flush device will deliver approximately 1 to 3 mL/hour to maintain patency of the system.	
10. Do not fast-flush catheter for longer than 2 seconds.[16]	Pulmonary artery rupture may occur with prolonged flushing of high-pressure fluid.	
11. Use aseptic technique when withdrawing from or flushing catheter.	Prevents bacterial contamination of system.	
12. Clear system of all traces of blood after blood withdrawal, including stopcocks.	Blood can become medium for bacterial growth. Clots also may be flushed into line if all blood is not eliminated.	
13. Maintain sterility and integrity of plastic sheath covering catheter.	Any tear in sheath will break sterile barrier, making catheter repositioning no longer possible.	• Defects in integrity of plastic sleeve
14. Do not infuse fluids such as whole blood or albumin via catheter lumens.	Viscous blood may occlude the catheter. Accuracy of the PA monitoring system may be adversely affected.	

Patient Monitoring and Care *Continued*

Steps	Rationale	Reportable Conditions
15. Follow institutional standard for frequency and type of dressing change.	Decreases risk of infection at catheter site. The CDC has made no recommendation for the frequency of routine PA catheter dressing change, but recommends replacing dressing when the dressing becomes damp, loosened, soiled, or when inspection of the site is necessary.[1]	• Signs or symptoms of infection
16. Date, time, and initial dressing change.	Ensures consistency of dressing change and indicates when next change will occur.	
17. Follow institutional standard for application of antimicrobial ointment to catheter sites.	Routine use of antimicrobial ointment at central venous catheter insertion sites is not recommended.[1]	
18. Obtain PA waveform strips to place on the patient's chart at the start of each shift or whenever there is a change in the waveform.	The printed waveform allows assessment of the adequacy of the waveform, damping, or respiratory variation.	

Documentation

Documentation should include the following:

- Patient and family education
- Insertion of the PA catheter
- External marking of PA catheter noted at exit site
- Patient tolerance
- Confirmation of PA catheter placement (eg, waveforms, chest x-ray)
- Site assessment
- Hemodynamic status
- PA pressures (RA/CVP, PA systolic and diastolic, PAWP)
- Waveforms (RA/CVP, PAP, PAWP)
- CO/CI and SVR
- Occurrence of unexpected outcomes and interventions

References

1. Pearson ML. Hospital infection control practices advisory committee: guideline for prevention of intravascular device-related infections. *Infect Control Hosp Epidemiol.* 1996;17:438–473.
2. Chong BH. Heparin-induced thrombocytopenia. *Br J Haematol.* 1995;89:431–439.
3. Wilson AE, Bermingham-Mitchell K, Wells N, Zachary K. Effect of backrest position on hemodynamic and right ventricular measurments in critically ill adults. *Am J Crit Care.* 1996;5:264–270.
4. Chulay M, Miller T. The effect of backrest elevation on pulmonary artery and pulmonary capillary wedge pressures in patients after cardiac surgery. *Heart Lung.* 1984;13:138–140.
5. Woods SL, Mansfield LW. Effect of body position upon pulmonary artery and pulmonary capillary wedge pressures in noncritically ill patients. *Heart Lung.* 1976;5:83–90.
6. Cason CL, Holland CL, Lambert CW, Huntsman KT. Effects of backrest elevation and position on pulmonary artery pressures. *Cardiovascular Nursing.* 1990;26:1–5.
7. Clochesy J, Hinshaw AD, Otto CW. Effects of change of position on pulmonary artery and pulmonary capillary wedge pressure in mechanically ventilated patients. *National Intravenous Therapy Association.* 1984;7:223–225.
8. Keating D, Bolyard K, Eichler E, Reed J III. Effect of sidelying positions on pulmonary artery pressures. *Heart Lung.* 1986;15:605–610.
9. Laulive JL. Pulmonary artery pressures and position changes in the critically ill adult. *Dimensions Crit Care Nurs.* 1982;1:28–34.
10. Groom L, Frisch SR, Elliot M. Reproducibility and accuracy of pulmonary artery pressure measurement in supine and lateral positions. *Heart Lung.* 1990;19:147–151.
11. Kennedy GT, Bryant A, Crawford MH. The effects of lateral body positioning on measurements of pulmonary artery and pulmonary wedge pressures. *Heart Lung.* 1984;13:155–158.
12. Hannan AT, Brown M, Bigman O. Pulmonary artery catheter induced hemorrhage. *Chest.* 1984;85:128–131.
13. O'Malley MK, Rhame FS, Cerra FB, McComb RC. Value of routine pressure monitoring system changes after 72 hours of use. *Crit Care Med.* 1994;22:1424–1430.
14. Ducharme FM, Gauthier M, Lacroix J, Lafleur L. Incidence of infection related to arterial catheterization in children: a prospective study. *Crit Care Med.* 1988;16:272–276.
15. Luskin RL, Weinstein RA, Nathan C, Chamberlin WH, Kab-

ins SA. Extended use of disposable pressure transducers: a bacteriologic evaluation. *JAMA*. 1986;255:916–920.

16. Daily EK, Schroeder JS. *Techniques in Bedside Hemodynamic Monitoring*. 5th ed. St. Louis, Mo: Mosby; 1994.

Additional Readings

Ahrens TS, Taylor LA. *Hemodynamic Waveform Analysis*. Philadelphia, Pa: W.B. Saunders; 1992.

Darovic GO. *Hemodynamic Monitoring: Invasive and Noninvasive Clinical Application*. 2nd ed. Philadelphia, Pa: W.B. Saunders; 1995.

Keckeisen M. *Protocols for Practice: Hemodynamic Monitoring Series—Pulmonary Artery Pressure Monitoring*. Aliso Viejo, Ca: American Association of Critical-Care Nurses; 1997.

Schactman M, Scott C, Silva VM, Wolff CA. *Hemodynamic Monitoring*. El Paso, Tx: Skidmore-Roth Publishing; 1995.

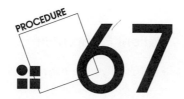

67

Pulmonary Artery Pressure Line, Removal

PURPOSE: The pulmonary artery (PA) catheter is removed when the patient's condition is improved sufficiently that hemodynamic monitoring is no longer necessary, when there is risk of complications from the presence of the catheter (eg, dysrhythmias, pulmonary infarction), or when there is risk of infection associated with the prolonged use of intravascular lines.

Teresa Preuss
Debra J. Lynn-McHale

PREREQUISITE NURSING KNOWLEDGE

- Cardiovascular anatomy and physiology should be understood.
- Normal values for intracardiac pressures should be known.
- Normal coagulation values should be known.
- Normal waveform configurations for right atrial pressure (RAP), right ventricular pressure (RVP), pulmonary artery pressure (PAP), and pulmonary artery wedge pressure (PAWP) should be understood.
- Venous access routes should be known.
- Principles of aseptic technique should be understood.
- Advanced cardiac life support knowledge and skills are necessary.
- Potential complications associated with removal of PA catheter should be known.
- In collaboration with the physician, determine when the PA catheter should be discontinued.
- Indications for the removal of the PA catheter include the following:
  ❖ The patient's condition no longer requires hemodynamic monitoring.
  ❖ Complications occured because of the presence of the PA catheter.
  ❖ PA catheter has been in use for more than 5 days.[1]
  ❖ Patient shows evidence of infection that may be associated with the PA catheter.
- Contraindications to percutaneous removal of PA catheter or introducer include the following:
  ❖ Patient's coagulation values are prolonged.
  ❖ The PA catheter is not in the proper position (eg, the PA catheter is knotted).
  ❖ A permanent or temporary transvenous pacemaker is present (this should be removed by a physician or with a physician present).

EQUIPMENT

- 1.5-mL syringe
- Gloves, clean gown, and face mask with shield
- 4 × 4 gauze pads
- Central line dressing kit
- Two moisture-proof absorbent pads

Additional equipment to have available as needed includes the following:

- Suture removal kit
- Sterile specimen container (needed if culture of catheter tip will be obtained)

PATIENT AND FAMILY EDUCATION

- Explain the procedure and the reason for catheter removal. ➥*Rationale:* Provides information and decreases anxiety.
- Explain the importance of lying still during the catheter removal. ➥*Rationale:* Ensures patient compliance and facilitates safe removal of the catheter.
- Instruct patient and family to report any bleeding or discomfort at the insertion site during or after catheter removal. ➥*Rationale:* Indentifies patient discomfort and assists with identification and prompt treatment of bleeding.

PATIENT ASSESSMENT AND PREPARATION

Patient Assessment

- Assess ECG, vital signs, and circulation to affected extremity. ➥*Rationale:* Serves as baseline data.
- Assess current coagulation values of patient. ➥*Rationale:* If patient has abnormal coagulation study results, hemostasis may be difficult to obtain after the PA catheter is removed.

- Verify catheter position by waveform analysis or chest x-ray.   ➤*Rationale:* Ensures accuracy of catheter position.
- Determine if patient has a permanent or temporary transvenous pacemaker.   ➤*Rationale:* PA catheter removal by a critical care nurse is usually contraindicated in the presence of a permanent or temporary transvenous pacemaker. Entanglement of the PA catheter and the pacemaker electrodes can occur.
- Assess integrity of the PA catheter.   ➤*Rationale:* The PA catheter should be removed by the physician if visible kinks or cracks are noted.

Patient Preparation

- Ensure that the patient understands preprocedural teaching. Answer questions as they arise and reinforce information as needed.   ➤*Rationale:* Evaluates and reinforces understanding of previously taught information.
- Place patient in supine position with the head of the bed flat or in a slight Trendelenburg position.   ➤*Rationale:* A normal pressure gradient exists between atmospheric air and the central venous compartment that promotes air entry if the compartment is open. The lower the site of entry below the heart, the lower the pressure gradient, thus minimizing the risk of venous air embolism.

| Procedure | **for Pulmonary Artery Pressure Line, Removal** |

Steps	Rationale	Special Considerations
1. Wash hands.	Reduces transmission of microorganisms; standard precautions.	
2. Place moisture-proof absorbent pad under the patient's upper torso and another under the PA catheter.	Contains any bloody drainage associated with removal and serves as a receptacle for the contaminated catheter.	
3. Ensure that the patient is positioned in the supine position so that the PA catheter and introducer are readily visible (eg, turn patient's head away from insertion site).	Decreases risk of infection.	If the PA catheter is in the femoral vein, extend the patient's leg and ensure that the groin area is adequately exposed.
4. Transfer or discontinue intravenous (IV) solution and flush solutions.	Ensures a closed system and prevents air from entering the system.	
5. Open supplies.	Prepares for removal.	
6. Wash hands.	Reduces transmission of microorganisms; standard precautions.	
7. Apply face mask with shield and clean gown, and don gloves.	Reduces transmission of microorganisms; standard precautions. Prevents splashing of body fluids to face during the procedure.	
8. Remove syringe from balloon inflation port, ensure that the gate valve or stopcock is in the open position, and observe PA waveform (see Fig. 66–9).	Allows air to passively escape from balloon and ensures adequate balloon deflation.	Myocardial or valvular tissues can be damaged if PA catheter is removed with the balloon inflated.
9. Turn stopcocks off to the patient.	Prepares for removal.	
10. Remove old dressing.	Signs of infection may determine the need to send a culture of the catheter tip.	
11. Clip sutures.	Frees PA catheter for removal.	
12. Unlock the sheath from the introducer.	Prepares for removal.	
13. Ask patient to take a deep breath in and hold it.	Minimizes risk of venous air embolus.[2]	
14. While securing introducer, gently withdraw PA catheter using a steady motion.	Ensures removal of an intact catheter.	Observe ECG tracing during removal. If resistance is met, do not continue to remove catheter and notify physician immediately. Resistance may be caused by catheter knotting, kinking, or wedging.
15. Place PA catheter on moisture-proof absorbent pad and check to be sure that the entire catheter was removed.	Allows for assessment of the catheter.	

Procedure **for Pulmonary Artery Pressure Line, Removal** *Continued*

Steps	Rationale	Special Considerations
16. Send tip of the PA catheter, if needed, to the laboratory for analysis.	Verifies the presence or absence of catheter-related infection.	
17. If the introducer remains in place, perform site care and apply a sterile dressing to the site.	Decreases risk of infection at insertion site.	Some introducers require a cap to be placed over the diaphragm site.[2]
18. If the introducer is to be removed, clip sutures securing the introducer.	Frees introducer for removal.	
19. Ask patient to take a deep breath in and hold it.	Minimizes risk of venous air embolus.	
20. Withdraw introducer using a steady motion with a 4 × 4 gauze pad held firmly over insertion site.	Minimizes risk of venous air embolus.	If resistance is met, do not continue to remove introducer and notify physician immediately. Resistance may be caused by kinks or cracks.
21. Lay introducer on moisture-proof absorbent pad. Check to be sure that all of the introducer was removed.	Allows for assessment of the introducer.	
22. Apply firm, direct pressure over insertion site with gauze pad until bleeding has stopped.	Ensures hemostasis.	Because a large vein was used for insertion, it may take up to 10 minutes for hemostasis to occur.
23. Apply sterile occlusive dressing to insertion site.	Decreases risk of infection at insertion site.	
24. Dispose of used supplies and wash hands.	Reduces transmission of microorganisms; standard precautions.	

Expected Outcomes

- PA catheter will be removed.
- Introducer may or may not be removed.

Unexpected Outcomes

- Dysrhythmias
- Myocardial valvular damage
- PA rupture
- Thrombosis
- Venous air emboli
- Uncontrolled bleeding
- Infection
- Unable to percutaneously remove PA catheter
- Hematoma

Patient Monitoring and Care

Patient Monitoring and Care	Rationale	Reportable Conditions
		These conditions should be reported if they persist despite nursing interventions.
1. PA catheters and introducer sheath should be changed at least every 5 days.	The CDC recommend replacement of PA catheters at least every 5 days and to replace introducer sheath every 5 days even if the catheter is removed.[1]	• Catheter in place longer than 5 days
2. Monitor cardiac rate and rhythm during catheter withdrawal.	Ventricular dysrhythmias may occur as the PA catheter passes through the right ventricle.	• Ventricular dysrhythmias occurring after the PA catheter is removed

Continued on following page

Patient Monitoring and Care	Rationale	Reportable Conditions
3. After removal of the PA catheter and introducer, assess the PA catheter site for signs of bleeding every 15 minutes × 2, every 30 minutes × 2, then 1 hour later.	Bleeding or a hematoma can develop if there is still bleeding from the vessel.	• Abnormal vital signs or signs of bleeding
4. Date, time, and initial the dressing.	Indicates when dressing was placed.	

Documentation

Documentation should include the following:

- Patient and family education
- Patient assessment before and after removal of the PA catheter
- Patient's response to procedure

- Date and time of removal
- Occurrence of unexpected outcomes
- Nursing interventions taken

References

1. Public Health Service, U.S. Department of Health and Human Services. *Guideline for Prevention of Intravascular Device-Related Infections.* Atlanta, Ga: Centers for Disease Control and Prevention; 1995.
2. Wadas TM. Pulmonary artery catheter removal. *Crit Care Nurse.* 1994;14:62–72.

Additional Readings

Ahrens TS, Taylor LA. *Hemodyanamic Waveform Analysis.* Philadelphia, Pa: W.B. Saunders; 1992.
Darovic GO. *Hemodynamic Monitoring: Invasive and Noninvasive Clinical Application.* 2nd ed. Philadelphia, Pa: W.B. Saunders; 1995.
Schactman M, Scott C, Silva VM, Wolff CA. *Hemodynamic Monitoring.* El Paso, Tex: Skidmore-Roth Publishing; 1995.

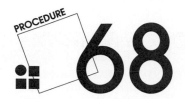

PROCEDURE 68

Pulmonary Artery Pressure Lines, Troubleshooting

PURPOSE: Troubleshooting of the pulmonary artery (PA) catheter is done to maintain catheter patency, to ensure that data from the PA catheter is accurate, and to prevent the development of catheter-related and patient-related complications.

Debra J. Lynn-McHale
Teresa Preuss

PREREQUISITE NURSING KNOWLEDGE

- Understanding of cardiovascular anatomy and physiology is necessary.
- Understanding of pulmonary anatomy and physiology is required.
- Understanding of basic dysrhythmia recognition and treatment of life-threatening dysrhythmias is necessary.
- Advanced cardiac life support knowledge and skills are necessary.
- Principles of aseptic technique should be understood.
- Understanding of the anatomy of PA catheters (see Fig. 66–1) and the location of the PA catheter in the heart and pulmonary artery (see Fig. 66–2) is important.
- The set-up of the hemodynamic monitoring system should be understood (see Procedure 69).
- The waveforms that occur during insertion should be recognized, including right atrial (RA), right ventricular (RV), pulmonary artery (PA), and pulmonary artery wedge (PAW) (see Fig. 66–3).
- Understanding of a, c, and v waves is necessary. The *a wave* reflects atrial contraction. The *c wave* reflects closure of the atrioventricular valve. The *v wave* reflects passive filling of the atria during ventricular systole (see Figs. 66–4 and 66–5).
- Normal hemodynamic values should be known (see Table 59–1).
- The pulmonary artery diastolic pressure (PADP) and the pulmonary artery wedge pressure (PAWP) are indirect measures of left ventricular end-diastolic pressure (LVEDP). Usually, the PAWP is approximately 1 to 4 mm Hg less than the PADP. Because these two pressures are similar, the PADP is commonly followed. This minimizes the frequency of balloon inflation, thus decreasing the potential of balloon rupture.
- Differences between the PADP and the PAWP may exist for patients with pulmonary hypertension, chronic obstructive lung disease, adult respiratory distress syndrome, pulmonary embolus, and tachycardia.
- Pulmonary artery pressures (PAPs) may be elevated because of pulmonary artery hypertension, pulmonary disease, mitral valve disease, left ventricular failure, atrial or ventricular left-to-right shunt, pulmonary emboli, or hypervolemia.
- PAPs may be decreased because of hypovolemia or vasodilation.
- Elevated a and v waves may be evident in RA or central venous pressure (CVP) and in PAW waveforms. These elevations may occur in patients with cardiac tamponade, constrictive pericardial disease, and hypervolemia.
- Elevated a waves in the RA or CVP waveform may occur in patients with pulmonic or tricuspid stenosis, right ventricular ischemia or infarction, right ventricular failure, pulmonary artery hypertension, and atrioventricular (AV) dissociation.
- Elevated a waves in the PAW waveform may occur in patients with mitral stenosis, acute left ventricular ischemia or infarction, left ventricular failure, and AV dissociation.
- Elevated v waves in the RA or CVP waveform may occur in patients with tricuspid insufficiency.
- Elevated v waves in the PAW waveform may occur in patients with mitral insufficiency or ruptured papillary muscle.

EQUIPMENT

- Syringes (3 mL or 10 mL)
- Sterile dead-end caps
- Stopcocks
- Pressure transducer system
- Connecting cable
- Sterile flush solution
- Pressure bag or device

Additional equipment to have available as needed includes the following:

- Available emergency equipment

PATIENT AND FAMILY EDUCATION

- Explain troubleshooting procedures. **➤Rationale:** Keeps patient and family informed and reduces anxiety.

- Explain the patient's expected participation during the procedure. ➤➤*Rationale:* Encourages patient compliance.
- Instruct patient and family of signs and symptoms to report to critical care nurse, including chest pain, palpitations, new cough, tenderness at insertion site, and chills. ➤➤*Rationale:* Encourages the patient to report signs of discomfort and potential PA catheter complications.

PATIENT ASSESSMENT AND PREPARATION

Patient Assessment

- Monitor PA waveforms continuously. ➤➤*Rationale:* The PA catheter may migrate forward into a wedged position or may loop around and fall into the right ventricle.
- Assess the configuration of the PA catheter waveforms.

➤➤*Rationale:* Thrombus formation at the catheter lumen may be evidenced by an overdamped waveform.
- Assess hemodynamic and cardiovascular status. ➤➤*Rationale:* The patient's clinical assessment should correlate with the PA catheter readings.
- Assess the patient and PA catheter site for signs of infection. ➤➤*Rationale:* Infection can develop because of the invasive nature of the PA catheter.

Patient Preparation

- Ensure that the patient understands preprocedural teaching. Answer questions as they arise and reinforce information as needed. ➤➤*Rationale:* Evaluates and reinforces understanding of previously taught information.
- Validate patency of intravenous lines. ➤➤*Rationale:* Access may be needed for administration of emergency medication or fluids.

Procedure	for Pulmonary Artery Pressure Lines, Troubleshooting

Steps	Rationale	Special Considerations
Troubleshooting an Overwedged Balloon		
1. Wash hands.	Reduces transmission of microorganisms; standard precautions.	
2. Identify overwedged waveform (Fig. 68–1).	Determines need for troubleshooting.	Overinflation of the balloon can cause pulmonary arteriole infarction or rupture resulting in life-threatening hemorrhage.[1]
3. Remove syringe from gate valve or stopcock of PA inflation port.	Passively removes air from the PA balloon.	
4. Note the change in PA waveform from the overinflated waveform to the PA waveform.	As the balloon deflates, the PA waveform returns.	
5. Fill the syringe with 1.5 mL of air.	More than 1.5 mL of air may rupture the PA balloon and the pulmonary arteriole.	

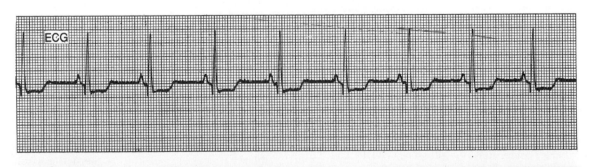

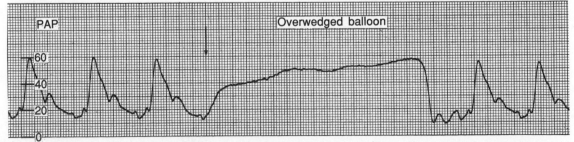

■ ● **FIGURE 68–1.** Balloon inflation *(arrow)* in patient with elevated wedge pressure. Overwedging of balloon (balloon has been overinflated). The danger of overinflating the balloon is that the PA vessel may rupture from the pressure of the balloon. PA, pulmonary artery.

Procedure	for Pulmonary Artery Pressure Lines, Troubleshooting *Continued*

Steps	Rationale	Special Considerations
6. Connect the PA syringe to the gate valve or stopcock of the balloon port of the PA catheter.	This port is designed for PA balloon air inflation.	
7. Slowly inflate the balloon with air until the PA waveform changes to a PAW waveform (see Fig. 66–10).	Only enough air is needed to convert the PA waveform to a PAW waveform.	
8. Inflate the PA balloon for no more than 8 to 15 seconds.	Avoids prolonged pressure on the pulmonary arteriole.	
9. Disconnect syringe from the balloon inflation port.	Allows air to passively escape from the balloon.	
10. Observe the monitor as the PAW waveform changes back to the PA waveform.	Ensures adequate balloon deflation.	
11. Expel air from the syringe.	Syringe should remain empty so that an accidental balloon inflation does not occur.	
12. Reconnect the empty syringe to the end of the balloon inflation port.	Retains safety syringe.	
13. Wash hands.	Reduces transmission of microorganisms; standard precautions.	

Troubleshooting an Absent Waveform

1. Wash hands, and don gloves.	Reduces transmission of microorganisms; standard precautions.	
2. Check to see if there is a kink in the pulmonary artery catheter.	Kinks may inhibit waveform transmission.	
3. Check pressure bag and ensure that all connections are tight.	Loose connections will allow air into the system and can overdamp or eliminate the waveform.	
4. Ensure stopcock is open to transducer (Fig. 68–2).	Stopcocks open to the system allow waveform transmission from the vascular system to the monitor; closed stopcocks will prevent waveform transmission to the monitor and oscilloscope.	
5. Ensure that the transducer cable is securely plugged into the monitor.	No waveform will be transmitted without proper electric connection.	
6. Ensure that correct monitor parameters are turned on.	Required for specific parameter monitoring.	
7. Ensure correct scale has been chosen for pressure being monitored; for example, 40 mm Hg scale is used for PA monitoring.	A larger scale (eg, 100 mm Hg) will cause the waveform to be smaller and possibly to not be visible on the oscilloscope.	
8. Zero the monitoring system (see Procedure 69).	Ensures accurate functioning of the monitoring system.	
9. Aspirate through the stopcock of the catheter to check for adequate blood return.	Ensures patency of the PA catheter.	A clotted catheter will have no waveform and no blood return when aspirated.

Procedure continued on following page

Procedure	**for Pulmonary Artery Pressure Lines, Troubleshooting** *Continued*	
Steps	**Rationale**	**Special Considerations**
10. Replace the monitoring cable.	A faulty cable can result in an absent waveform.	
11. Replace the transducer or pressure monitoring tubing.	A faulty transducer can result in an absent waveform.	
12. Notify the advanced practice nurse or the physician if troubleshooting is unsuccessful.	The catheter will need to be removed or replaced.	
13. Discard used supplies, and wash hands.	Reduces transmission of microorganisms; standard precautions.	

Troubleshooting an Overdamped Waveform

1. Wash hands, and don gloves.	Reduces transmission of microorganisms; standard precautions.	
2. Record overdamped waveform (Fig. 68–3).	Waveform can be compared with previous waveforms.	
3. Ensure that all connections are tight.	Loose connections will allow air into the system and can overdamp the waveform.	
4. Ensure that pressure bag or device is delivering 300 mm Hg.	Low counterpressure from bag will result in an overdamped waveform.	
5. Perform a dynamic response test (square wave test; see Fig. 56–3*B*).	Overdamped waveforms provide inaccurate pulmonary artery waveforms.	
6. Check all tubing for air bubbles. If air exists within the transducer, follow these steps: 　A. Turn the stopcock off to the patient. 　B. Remove the dead-end cap of the top port of the stopcock. 　C. Fast flush the air from the transducer and system. 　D. Place a new sterile dead-end cap on the top port of the stopcock. 　E. Turn the stopcock open to the patient (see Fig. 68–2). 　F. Monitor the waveform.	Removes air from the system, prevents the air from entering the patient, and ensures accurate monitoring of waveforms.	

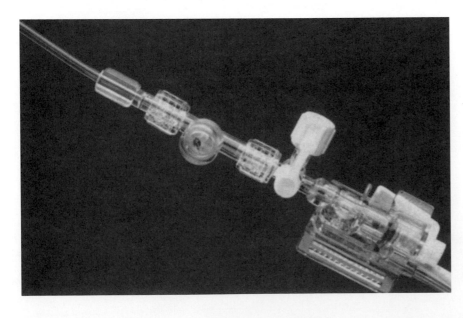

■ ● **FIGURE 68–2.** (From Ahrens T. *Hemodynamic Waveform Recognition.* Philadelphia: WB Saunders; 1993: 125.)

Procedure continued on page 466

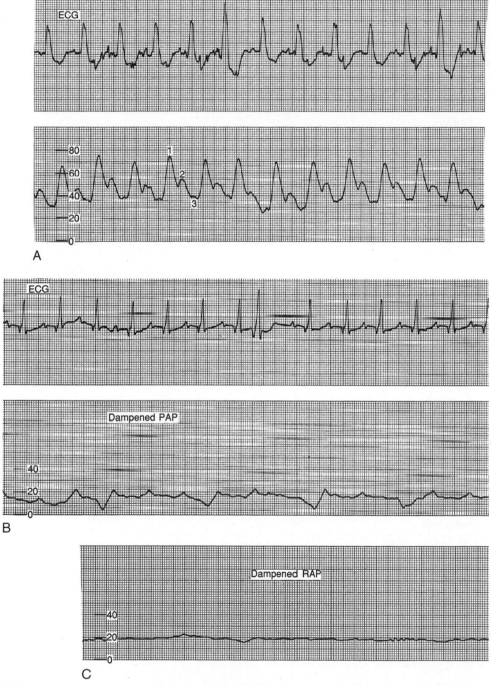

■ ● FIGURE 68–3. Effects of overdamping on PAP and RAP waveforms. *A,* Normal PAP waveform with elevated PA pressures. (*1* = PA systole; *2* = dicrotic notch; *3* = PA diastole). *B,* Overdamped PAP waveform. *C,* Overdamping of RAP waveform. Overdamping of the waveform may be due to clots at catheter tip, catheter against vessel or heart wall, air in lines, stopcock partially closed or deflated pressure bag. PA, pulmonary artery; PAP, pulmonary artery pressure; RAP, right atrial pressure.

Procedure	for Pulmonary Artery Pressure Lines, Troubleshooting *Continued*

Steps	Rationale	Special Considerations

Steps

If air exists between the pressure bag and a stopcock, follow these steps:

A. Turn the stopcock off to the patient.

B. Remove the dead-end cap from the top port of the stopcock.

C. Fast flush the air from the system.

D. Place a new sterile dead-end cap on the top port of the stopcock.

E. Open the stopcock to the monitoring system.

F. Observe the waveform.

If the air is between the patient and a stopcock, follow these steps:

A. Remove the dead-end cap from the top port of the stopcock.

B. Connect a 10-mL syringe to the stopcock.

C. Turn the stopcock off to the monitoring system.

D. Gently pull the air back into the syringe.

E. When all air is removed, turn the stopcock off to the patient.

F. Fast flush the blood from the top port of the stopcock.

G. Turn the stopcock off to the top port of the stopcock.

H. Remove the syringe.

I. Place a new sterile dead-end cap on the top of the stopcock.

J. Fast flush the system.

K. Monitor the waveform.

7. Aspirate through the stopcock of the catheter to check for adequate blood return.

A. Remove the dead-end cap from the top port of the stopcock.

B. Connect a 10-mL syringe to the stopcock.

C. Turn the stopcock off to the monitoring system.

D. Gently aspirate until blood enters the syringe.

E. Turn the stopcock open to the patient (see Fig. 68–2).

F. Fast flush the blood back into the patient.

G. Turn the stopcock off to the patient.

H. Fast flush the blood from the top port of the stopcock.

I. Remove the syringe from the top port of the stopcock.

J. Turn the stopcock open to the monitoring system (see Fig. 68–2).

K. Fast flush the system.

L. Monitor the waveform.

Rationale

Ensures that blood flows easily within the catheter and assesses for the presence of clots.

Procedure	for Pulmonary Artery Pressure Lines, Troubleshooting *Continued*

Steps	Rationale	Special Considerations
8. Notify the advanced practice nurse or physician if troubleshooting is unsuccessful.	The catheter will need to be removed or replaced.	
9. Discard used supplies, and wash hands.	Reduces transmission of microorganisms; standard precautions.	

Troubleshooting a Continuously Wedged Waveform

Steps	Rationale	Special Considerations
1. Wash hands.	Reduces transmission of microorganisms; standard precautions.	
2. Identify wedged waveform (see Fig. 66–5).	Confirms need for troubleshooting.	Continuous monitoring of the PA waveform is necessary to assess for the presence of the PA waveform. PA catheters should be wedged for only 10 to 15 seconds to obtain a PAWP measurement.
3. Remove the PA balloon syringe and ensure that the gate valve or stopcock is open and that the balloon is deflated.	Ensures that air is not trapped within the PA balloon.	
4. Assist the patient in changing position, or if possible, ask the patient to cough.	This may help to get the catheter to float out of the wedge position.	Monitor the PA waveform for a change from a PAW waveform to a PA waveform.
5. If troubleshooting is unsuccessful, notify the advanced practice nurse or physician.	Immediate repositioning of the catheter is necessary as prolonged wedging can lead to rupture or ischemia of the PA.	
6. Never flush a wedged PA catheter.	Flushing the catheter in the wedged position may lead to PA rupture and hemorrhage.	
7. Wash hands.	Reduces transmission of microorganisms; standard precautions.	

Troubleshooting a Catheter in the Right Ventricle (RV)

Steps	Rationale	Special Considerations
1. Wash hands.	Reduces transmission of microorganisms; standard precautions.	
2. Identify RV waveform (Fig. 68–4).	The RV waveform resembles the PA waveform. The RV waveform, however, does not have a dicrotic notch. In addition, the diastolic pressure of the RV waveform is lower than the PADP. The normal PADP is 8 to 15 mm Hg, the normal RV diastolic pressure is 0 to 8 mm Hg.	
3. Inflate PA balloon with 1.5 mL of air.	The inflated PA balloon may readily float into position in the PA.	
4. Observe for change in waveform from RV to PA to PAW (see Fig. 66–3).	Waveform analysis aids in identification of PA catheter position.	
5. Remove the syringe from the PA balloon port.	Air will be released passively from the PA balloon.	
6. Observe the waveform.	The waveform should change from the PAW waveform to a PA waveform.	
7. If RVP waveform is still present, inflate the PA balloon port with 1.5 mL of air.	An inflated PA balloon cushions the catheter tip and prevents endocardial irritation.	The PA catheter tip may cause ventricular dysrhythmias. If the PA balloon is inflated, the ventricular dysrhythmias may decrease as the inflated balloon may cause less irritation of the endocardium.

Procedure continued on following page

Procedure **for Pulmonary Artery Pressure Lines, Troubleshooting** *Continued*

Steps	Rationale	Special Considerations
8. Assist the patient with a change of position.	The inflated PA catheter may float into the PA after a position change.	
9. Observe for change in waveform from RV to PA to PAW (see Fig. 66–3).	Waveform analysis aids identification of PA catheter position.	
10. Remove the syringe from the PA balloon port.	Deflates the PA balloon.	
11. If troubleshooting is unsuccessful, notify the advanced practice nurse or physician.	The PA catheter cannot remain in the right ventricle because it may trigger life-threatening ventricular dysrhythmias. Immediate repositioning is necessary.	If ventricular dysrhythmias are present, consider temporarily leaving the balloon inflated until the catheter is repositioned in the PA.
12. Wash hands.	Reduces transmission of microorganisms; standard precautions.	

Troubleshooting an Inability to Wedge the PA Catheter

1. Wash hands.	Reduces transmission of microorganisms; standard precautions.	
2. Check positioning of the PA catheter.	Most PA catheters are in correct position if the external markings of the catheter are between 45 and 55 cm. The PA catheter tip may not be distal enough in the PA to float into the wedge position.	
3. Ensure that the PA balloon is inflated with a maximum 1.5 mL of air.	The full 1.5 mL of air may be necessary to wedge some PA catheters. An insufficient amount of air can prevent wedging.	Repositioning the patient may aid in changing the position of the catheter and may facilitate successful wedging of the PA catheter.

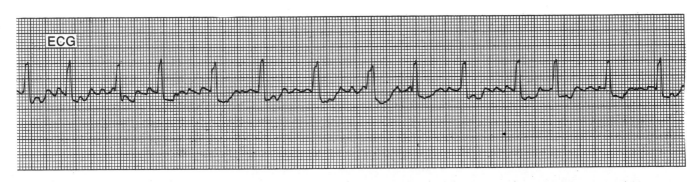

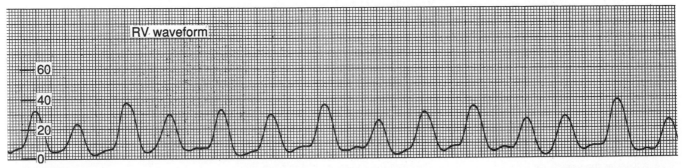

■ ● **FIGURE 68–4.** RVP waveform. This was seen coming from the PA (distal) lumen of a PA catheter. The catheter had become coiled in the RV. PA, pulmonary artery; RV, right ventricle; RVP, right ventricular pressure.

Procedure	for Pulmonary Artery Pressure Lines, Troubleshooting *Continued*

Steps	Rationale	Special Considerations
4. Resistance should be felt when inflating the PA balloon.	Resistance is present when the PA balloon is intact.	The balloon may rupture because of overinflation, frequent inflations, or repeated aspiration of air from the balloon rather than allowing it to passively deflate.
5. If no resistance is felt or if blood is aspirated from the balloon lumen, follow these steps: A. Immediately discontinue balloon inflation attempts. B. Tape the balloon inflation port closed. C. Label the tape that the balloon should not be used.	If the balloon is ruptured, no resistance will be felt during an inflation attempt. Blood may also come back through the balloon lumen.	
6. If the balloon is ruptured or troubleshooting is unsuccessful, notify the advanced practice nurse or physician.	A new PA catheter may be placed or PADP may be followed if the PADPs correlated with the PAWPs.	
7. Wash hands.	Reduces transmission of microorganisms; standard precautions.	

Troubleshooting Unexpected Changes in PAP

1. Wash hands.	Reduces transmission of microorganisms; standard precautions.	
2. Ensure patient is in supine position with head of bed less than or equal to 45°. *(Level VI: Clinical studies in a variety of patient populations and situations to support recommendations)*	Research has demonstrated that pressures are most accurate in this position.[2-7]	
3. Ensure that the air-fluid interface (zeroing stopcock) is level with phlebostatic axis (see Procedure 69).	Ensures accurate pressure values. If transducer is higher or lower than phlebostatic axis, pressures will be inaccurate.	
4. Zero the hemodynamic monitoring system (see Procedure 69).	Ensures accuracy of monitoring system.	
5. Check for air bubbles in pressure monitoring system and eliminate bubbles if present.	Air will overdamp waveform (see Fig. 68-3), resulting in lower readings.	
6. Obtain hemodynamic parameters and correlate with patient assessment data.	Hemodynamic and assessment data should correlate.	Faulty catheters may provide inaccurate data that may necessitate their removal or replacement.
7. If PAP changes are accurate, titrate fluids or vasoactive agents or notify advanced practice nurse or physician.	Hemodynamic data guide therapeutic intervention.	
8. Wash hands.	Reduces transmission of microorganisms; standard precautions.	

Troubleshooting Blood Backup into a PA Catheter or Pressure Transducer System

1. Wash hands, and don gloves.	Reduces transmission of microorganisms; standard precautions.	
2. Turn stopcock off to patient.	Prevents blood from going into transducer.	If blood reaches the transducer, it may have to be replaced.

Procedure continued on following page

| Procedure | for Pulmonary Artery Pressure Lines, Troubleshooting *Continued* |

Steps	Rationale	Special Considerations
3. Ensure that all connections are tight and that all stopcocks are closed to air and have dead-end caps.	Loose connections or open stopcocks will cause a decrease in pressure within the fluid-filled system and blood may exert a back pressure into the pressure tubing.	A crack in the system would necessitate replacing the entire monitoring system.
4. Ensure that the pressure bag is inflated to 300 mm Hg.	Low pressure from the bag will result in blood back-up.	
5. Once the source of the problem is located and corrected, flush the entire line to remove blood from the system.	Blood can become a medium for bacterial growth.[8] Prevents clot formation within monitoring system.	
6. Zero the hemodynamic monitoring system (see Procedure 69).	Ensures accuracy of monitoring system.	
7. Monitor PA waveform.	Ensures presence of the correct waveform and system functioning.	
8. Discard gloves, and wash hands.	Reduces transmission of microorganisms; standard precautions.	

Troubleshooting When Patient Coughs Up Blood or Develops Bloody Secretions from Endotracheal Tube During PA Catheter Monitoring

1. Wash hands, and don gloves.	Reduces transmission of microorganisms; standard precautions.	
2. Notify physician immediately.	PA perforation with hemorrhage is a lethal complication of a PA catheter.	
3. Maintain patency of airway.	Prevents hypoxemia and respiratory arrest.	Prepare for intubation as needed.
4. Remain with patient for monitoring and reassurance.	Reduces anxiety and fear; provides essential assessment.	

5. Be prepared to follow these steps:
  A. Send blood specimen for coagulation studies and type and crossmatch.
  B. Obtain chest x-ray.
  C. Prepare patient for the operating room.
	Blood loss from the PA can be fatal. Immediate surgical repair of the PA is necessary.	

Expected Outcomes	Unexpected Outcomes
• Normal pulmonary tissue perfusion	• PA balloon rupture
• Absence of PA catheter-related dysrhythmias	• Pulmonary infarction and rupture
• Absence of signs of PA catheter-related infection	• PA catheter-related infection resulting in sepsis
• Absence of discomfort associated with PA catheter	• Discomfort at PA catheter insertion site
• Accurate pulmonary artery waveforms and pressures	• Ventricular tachycardia unresponsive to antidysrhythmic medications

Patient Monitoring and Care

Patient Monitoring and Care	Rationale	Reportable Conditions
		These conditions should be reported if they persist despite nursing interventions.
1. The PA waveforms should be continuously monitored.	Provides assessment of proper placement of PA catheter and abnormal waveforms such as PAW or RV waveforms.	• Abnormal waveforms (eg, continued PAW tracing and RV tracings)
2. Pressure alarms should be set and turned on at all times.	Alerts critical care nurse to pressure changes and to disconnections in the pressure monitoring system.	• Abnormal hemodynamic values
3. Evaluate hemodynamic monitoring system and waveform configurations.	Ensures that the system is intact and functioning appropriately.	• Abnormal waveforms
4. Monitor hemodynamic status (PA, PAP or PAW, RA, cardiac output or cardiac index, systemic vascular resistance, etc.).	Guides appropriate therapy.	• Abnormal hemodynamic monitoring values
5. Monitor patient for catheter-related infections.	The PA catheter should be replaced at the first sign of site infection.	• Signs and symptoms of infection
6. Assess hemodynamic waveforms and pressure values before and after troubleshooting.	Identifies that troubleshooting has been successful.	• Unsuccessful troubleshooting attempts

Documentation

Documentation should include the following:

- Patient and family education
- Occurrence of unexpected outcomes and interventions
- Patient toleration
- Site assessment

References

1. Hannan AT, Brown M, Bigman O. Pulomonary artery catheter induced hemorrhage. *Chest.* 1984;85:128–131.
2. Wilson AE, Bermingham-Mitchell K, Wells N, Zachary K. Effect of backrest position on hemodynamic and right ventricular measurements in critically ill adults. *Am J Crit Care.* 1996;5:264–270.
3. Chulay M, Miler T. The effect of backrest elevation on pulmonary artery and pulmonary capillary wedge pressures in patients after cardiac surgery. *Heart Lung.* 1984;13:138–140.
4. Woods SL, Mansfield LW. Effect of body position upon pulmonary artery and pulmonary capillary wedge pressures in noncritically ill patients. *Heart Lung.* 1976;5:83–90.
5. Cason CL, Holland CL, Lambert CW, Huntsman KT. Effects of backrest elevation and position on pulmonary artery pressures. *Cardiovasc Nurs.* 1990;26:1–5.
6. Clochesy J, Hinshaw AD, Otto CW. Effects of change of position on pulmonary artery and pulmonary capillary wedge pressure in mechanically ventilated patients. *National Intraven Therapy Assoc.* 1984;7:223–225.
7. Keating D, Bolyard K, Crawford MH. The effects of lateral body positioning on measurements of pulmonary artery and pulmonary wedge pressures. *Heart Lung.* 1986;15:605–610.
8. Public Health Service, U.S. Department of Health and Human Services. *Guideline for Prevention of Intravascular Device-Related Infections.* Atlanta, Ga: Centers for Disease Control and Prevention; 1995.

Additional Readings

Ahrens TS, Taylor LA. *Hemodynamic Waveform Analysis.* Philadelphia, Pa: W.B. Saunders; 1992.

Darovic GO. *Hemodynamic Monitoring: Invasive and Noninvasive Clinical Application.* 2nd ed. Philadelphia, Pa: W.B. Saunders; 1995.

Keckeisen M. *Protocols for Practice: Hemodynamic Monitoring Series—Pulmonary Artery Pressure Monitoring.* Aliso Viejo, Calif: American Association of Critical-Care Nurses; 1997.

Laulive JL. Pulmonary artery pressures and position changes in the critically ill adult. *Dimens Crit Care Nurs.* 1982;1:28–34.

Schactman M, Scott C, Silva VM, Wolff CA. *Hemodynamic Monitoring.* El Paso, Tex: Skidmore-Roth Publishing; 1995.

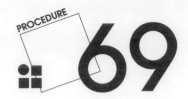

Single and Multiple Pressure Transducer Systems

PURPOSE: To provide a catheter-to-monitor interface so that intravascular and intracardiac pressures can be measured. The transducer detects a biophysical event and converts it to an electronic signal.

Marie Arnone

PREREQUISITE NURSING KNOWLEDGE

- Understanding of the normal anatomy and physiology of the cardiovascular system is needed.
- Principles of aseptic technique should be understood.
- Fluid-filled pressure monitoring systems used for bedside hemodynamic pressure monitoring are based on the principle that a change in pressure at any point in an unobstructed system results in similar pressure changes at all other points of the system.
- Pressure transducers, when attached to a monitoring system, sense a dynamic signal from the intravascular and intracardiac changes and transmit these changes to the bedside monitor. Waveform patterns reflect directly the flow and pressure sensed.
- Invasive measurement of intravascular (arterial) pressure requires insertion of a catheter into an artery.
- Invasive measurement of intracardiac (right atrial and pulmonary artery) pressures requires insertion of a catheter into the heart and pulmonary artery.
- Both reusable and disposable transducers are available. Disposable transducers are more commonly used because of their improved dynamic frequency response, reduced pressure drift, and potentially improved infection control.[1, 2]
- Usually, a hemodynamic monitoring system is set up to measure pulmonary artery systolic, diastolic, mean, and wedge pressures. Another hemodynamic monitoring system is usually set up to measure right atrial pressure.
- Arterial pressure monitoring requires a single transducer for continuous monitoring of blood pressure.
- To ensure accuracy of the hemodynamic values obtained from any transducer system, leveling and zeroing are essential.

EQUIPMENT

- Invasive catheter
- Noncompliant pressure tubing
- Pressure transducers
- Analog recorder
- 500-mL bag of normal saline intravenous (IV) solution
- Pressure bag or device
- Monitoring system (central and bedside monitors)
- Pressure monitoring cables
- Indelible marker
- Dead-end caps

Additional equipment as needed includes the following:

- Heparin
- 3-mL syringe
- Vial of sterile water
- Carpenter level
- Transducer connector for IV pole
- Stopcocks
- 4 × 4 gauze pads

PATIENT AND FAMILY EDUCATION

- Assess patient and family understanding of hemodynamic monitoring and the reason for its use. ➤**Rationale:** Clarification or reinforcement of information is an expressed patient and family need.
- Explain the procedure for hemodynamic monitoring. ➤**Rationale:** Prepares the patient and the family for what to expect; may decrease anxiety.
- Explain the waveforms on the bedside monitor, and explain how they assist the health care team in treatment decisions. ➤**Rationale:** Prepares the patient and the family for what to expect at the bedside; may decrease anxiety.

PATIENT ASSESSMENT AND PREPARATION
Patient Assessment

- Assess patient for conditions that may warrant the use of a hemodynamic monitoring system, including hypotension or hypertension, cardiac failure, cardiac arrest, hemorrhage, hypoxemia, metabolic acidosis or alkalosis, respiratory acidosis or alkalosis, positive fluid balance, oliguria, anuria, diminished mental status, and laboratory abnormalities. ➤**Rationale:** Provides data regarding signs and symptoms of hemodynamic instability.
- Obtain past medical history of coagulopathies, use of anticoagulants, vascular abnormalities, and peripheral

neuropathies. ➤*Rationale:* Assists in determining safety of procedure and aids in site selection.

Patient Preparation

• Ensure that the patient and the family understand preprocedural teaching. Answer questions as they arise, and reinforce information as needed. ➤*Rationale:* Evaluates and reinforces understanding of previously taught information.

• Position patient in the supine position with the head of bed flat or elevated up to 45 degrees. ➤*Rationale:* Prepares the patient for hemodynamic monitoring.

Procedure **for Single and Multiple Pressure Transducer Systems**

Steps	Rationale	Special Considerations
Transducer Setup		
1. Wash hands.	Reduces transmission of microorganisms; standard precautions.	
2. Determine the number of pressure cables required.	Prepares bedside monitoring system.	Some monitors necessitate a 5- to 15-minute time to warm up before monitoring.
3. Plug transducer cables into appropriate pressure modules on bedside monitor.	Allows for signal transmission to oscilloscope.	
4. Turn on monitor screen.	Prepares monitor.	Most monitor screen displays are programmed to show the waveforms in an order that corresponds to a particular jack for the cable (eg, the top cable position corresponds to the first waveform position on the screen).
5. Set the appropriate scale for the pressure being measured.	Necessary for visualization of the complete waveform and to obtain accurate readings. Waveforms vary in amplitude depending on the pressure within the system. The scale for right atrial pressure and central venous pressure is commonly set at 20 mm Hg, the scale for pulmonary artery pressure is commonly set at 40 mm Hg, and the scale for arterial blood pressure is commonly set at 180 mm Hg.	Some monitors are preprogrammed to display scales that correspond to the jack for cable insertion (eg, first position arterial, second pulmonary artery, third right atrial). Adjustments to the scale may be required.
6. Obtain premixed flush solution, or prepare flush solution.		Follow institutional protocol for amount of heparin per milliliter of flush solution, usually 1 to 4 U/mL.
A. Use a collapsible IV bag.	Collapsible IV bags allow fluid to be pressurized.	
B. Use a 500-mL IV bag of normal saline. *(Level VI: Clinical studies in a variety of patient populations and situations to support recommendations)*	Normal saline is preferred. Solutions containing dextrose increase the incidence of infection.[3, 4]	
C. When preparing flush bag, mix solution of heparinized saline if use of heparin is not contraindicated. *(Level V: Clinical studies in more than one or two different patient populations and situations to support recommendations)*	Heparinized flush solutions are commonly used to minimize thrombi and fibrin deposits on catheters that might lead to thrombosis or bacterial colonization of the catheter. Catheters flushed with heparinized saline are more likely than those flushed with nonheparinized saline to remain patent for up to 72 hours.[1, 5]	Use of heparin is contraindicated in patients with heparin-induced thrombocytopenia or heparin allergy. Research is needed regarding use of heparin versus normal saline to maintain pulmonary artery line patency.
D. Label IV bag indicating the dose of heparin (if used), the date and time of addition, and your initials.	Identifies contents of the IV flush bag and identifies when the IV bag needs to be changed.	

Procedure continued on following page

Procedure	for Single and Multiple Pressure Transducer Systems *Continued*

Steps	Rationale	Special Considerations
7. Spike outlet port of IV flush solution with tubing.	Allows access to IV flush solution.	Separate flush systems are needed if invasive catheters are inserted at different times.
A. One flush system is used if a triple line kit is used for pulmonary artery and arterial monitoring (Fig. 69–1).	Provides a system to monitor three pressures.	Use the minimal number of stopcocks needed.
B. One flush system can be used for arterial monitoring (Fig. 69–2).	Provides a system to monitor arterial pressure.	Use the minimal number of stopcocks needed.
C. One flush system is used if a bifurcated system is used for pulmonary artery and right atrial monitoring (Fig. 69–3).	Provides a system to monitor two pressures.	Use the minimal number of stopcocks needed.
D. Two flush systems may be used, or the second port of the IV flush solution can be used if two pressurized tubing systems are needed.	Provides a system to monitor two or three pressures.	
8. Open the IV roller clamp, and squeeze the drip chambers to fill the chamber half full.	Primes the drip chamber.	It is important to fill the drip chamber halfway to prevent air bubbles from entering the tubing. Filling halfway will allow the nurse to see that the solution is flowing when performing a manual flush of the invasive line.
9. Close the roller clamp, and insert the IV bag into the pressure bag or device on the IV pole. Do not inflate the pressure bag.	Priming the tubing under pressure increases turbulence and may cause air bubbles to enter the tubing.	Air should never be allowed to develop in a hemodynamic system. Micro or macro air emboli can migrate to major organs and present a life-threatening complication.

Single Reusable Transducer

1. Wash hands.	Reduces transmission of microorganisms; standard precautions.	
2. Remove the protective cover from the transducer.	Begins assembly of the hemodynamic monitoring system.	
3. With a sterile syringe, draw up 1 mL of sterile water, and drip the sterile water onto the transducer diaphragm. Do not overfill (Fig. 69–4).	Water on the diaphragm establishes an interface between the dome membrane and the diaphragm surface.	Maintain sterility of the internal dome and diaphragm. Manufacturer recommendations may vary as to the type and amount of solution.
4. Assemble the dome transducer system (Fig. 69–5).		Use the minimal number of stopcocks needed.
A. Attach the sterile transducer dome to the diaphragm.	Prepares the transducer.	
B. Assemble and connect the pressurized tubing.	Prepares the system.	
C. Flush all the air out of the system.	Eliminates air from the system.	
D. Replace any stopcocks with air vents with closed dead-end caps.	Vented caps are placed by the manufacturer and permit sterilization of the entire system. These vented caps need to be replaced with nonvented caps to prevent bacteria or air from entering the system.	
E. Inflate the pressure bag or device to 300 mm Hg.	Pressure bags inflated to 300 mm Hg will allow approximately 1 to 3 mL per hour of flush solution to be delivered through the catheter, thus maintaining catheter patency and minimizing clot formation.	

Procedure continued on page 479

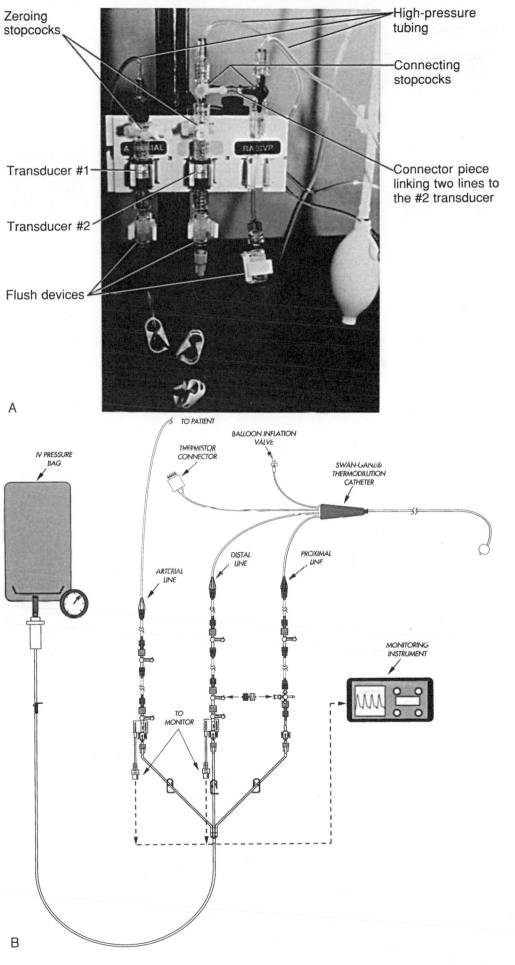

■ ● **FIGURE 69–1.** Monitoring three pressures from two transducers with a multiple pressure transducer system.

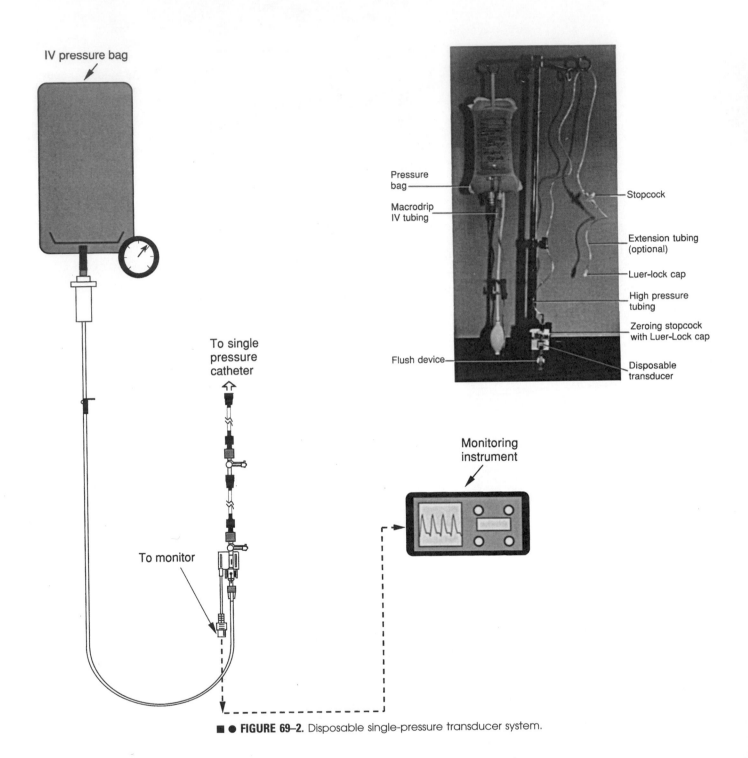

IV pressure bag

Pressure
bag

Macrodrip
IV tubing

Stopcock

Extension tubing
(optional)

Luer-lock cap

High pressure
tubing

Zeroing stopcock
with Luer-Lock cap

Flush device

Disposable
transducer

To single
pressure
catheter

Monitoring
instrument

To monitor

■ ● **FIGURE 69–2.** Disposable single-pressure transducer system.

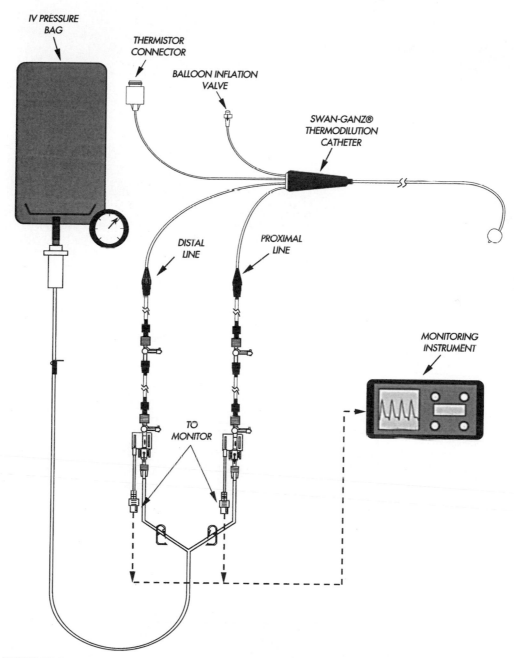

IV PRESSURE
BAG

THERMISTOR
CONNECTOR

BALLOON INFLATION
VALVE

SWAN-GANZ®
THERMODILUTION
CATHETER

DISTAL
LINE

PROXIMAL
LINE

MONITORING
INSTRUMENT

TO
MONITOR

■ ● **FIGURE 69–3.** Monitoring two pressures from two transducers with a multiple pressure transducer system.

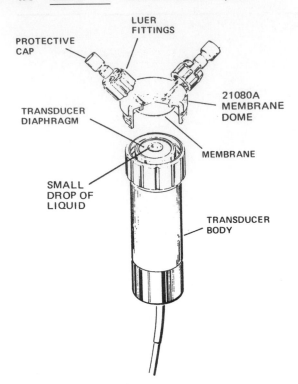

■ ● FIGURE 69–4. The components of a reusable pressure transducer. A drop of sterile water is placed on the diaphragm to establish a fluid interface between the dome chamber and the transducer diaphragm.

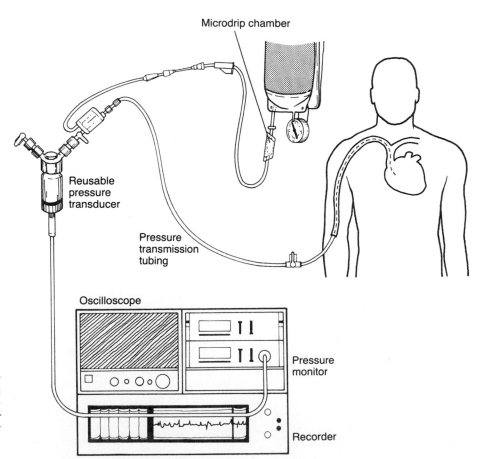

■ ● FIGURE 69–5. A fluid system for pulmonary artery pressure monitoring coupled with electronic instrumentation. (From Darovic Go, ed. *Hemodynamic Monitoring.* 2nd ed. Philadelphia: WB Saunders; 1995: 151.)

Procedure	**for Single and Multiple Pressure Transducer Systems** *Continued*

Steps	Rationale	Special Considerations
Single or Multiple Disposable Transducers		
1. Wash hands.	Reduces transmission of microorganisms; standard precautions.	
2. Open the prepackaged pressure transducer kit using aseptic technique.	Prepares the hemodynamic monitoring pressurized system.	Assemble the pressure transducers, pressure tubing, and stopcocks if not preassembled by the manufacturer.
3. Check all connections to be sure they are secure.	Ensures that the connections are tight; prepares the system.	
4. Flush the entire system, including transducers, all stopcocks, and pressure tubing, with the flush solution.	Eliminates air from the system.	
5. Replace any vented caps with Luer-Lok or dead-end caps, and tighten securely.	Vented caps are placed by the manufacturer and permit sterilization of the entire system. These vented caps need to be replaced with sterile nonvented caps to prevent bacteria and air from entering the system.	
6. Inflate the pressure bag or device to 300 mm Hg.	Pressure bags inflated to 300 mm Hg will allow approximately 1 to 3 mL per hour of flush solution to be delivered through the catheter, thus maintaining catheter patency and minimizing clot formation.	
Leveling the Transducer		
1. Wash hands.	Reduces transmission of microorganisms; standard precautions.	
2. Position the bed so that the patient is supine with the head of the bed flat or elevated no more than 45 degrees. *(Level VI: Clinical studies in a variety of patient populations and situations to support recommendations)*	Studies have demonstrated that central venous and PA pressures are accurate in this position.[6-11]	Central venous and pulmonary artery pressures may be accurate for patients in the supine position with the head of the bed elevated up to 60 degrees,[12] yet additional studies are needed to support this. Studies have not demonstrated the accuracy of hemodynamic values for patients in the lateral position.[8-10, 13, 14]
3. Locate the phlebostatic axis for the supine position (Fig. 69–6).	The phlebostatic axis is at approximately the level of the atria and should be used as the reference point for the air-fluid interface.	The reference point for the left lateral decubitus position is the fourth intercostal space at the left parasternal border (Fig. 69–7B).[15] The reference point for the right lateral decubitus position is the fourth intercostal space (ICS) at the midsternum (see Fig. 69–7A).[15]

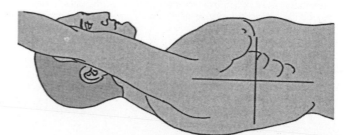

■ ● **FIGURE 69–6.** Phlebostatic axis in the supine patient.

Procedure continued on following page

Procedure	for Single and Multiple Pressure Transducer Systems *Continued*

Steps	Rationale	Special Considerations
A. Identify the fourth ICS on the edge of the sternum. B. Draw an imaginary line along the fourth ICS laterally, along the chest wall. C. Draw a second imaginary line from the axilla downward, midway between the anterior and posterior chest walls. D. Where these two lines cross is the level of the phlebostatic axis. E. Mark the point of the phlebostatic axis with an indelible marker.		
4. Place the carpenter's level with one end at the phlebostatic axis and the other end on the air-fluid interface (zeroing stopcock). Move the air-fluid interface up or down until the carpenter is level.	Ensures that the air-fluid interface is level with the phlebostatic axis.	If the transducers are patient mounted, place the pulmonary artery distal air-fluid interface at the phlebostatic axis and the pulmonary artery proximal air-fluid interface directly next to the phlebostatic axis. The arterial air-fluid interface is usually placed close to the insertion site. Secure systems in place with a 4 × 4 gauze pad between the transducers and the patient's skin for comfort.

Zeroing the Transducer

1. Wash hands.	Reduces transmission of microorganisms; standard precautions.	
2. Turn the stopcock off to the patient.	Prepares the system for the zeroing procedure.	
3. Remove the nonvented cap from the stopcock, opening the stopcock to air.	Allows the monitor to use atmospheric pressure as a reference for zero.	

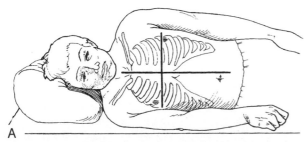 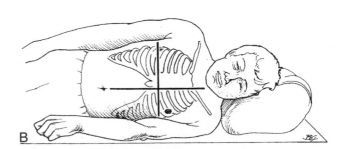

■ ● FIGURE 69–7. Reference points for the hemodynamic monitoring system for patients in lateral positions. *A,* For the right lateral position, the reference point is the intersection of the fourth intercostal space and midsternum. *B,* For the left lateral position, the reference point is the intersection of the fourth intercostal space and the left parasternal border. (From Keckeisen M. *Protocols for Practice: Hemodynamic Monitoring Series—Pulmonary Artery Monitoring.* Aliso Viejo, Ca: American Association of Critical-Care Nurses; 1997: 12.)

Steps	Rationale	Special Considerations
4. Push and release the zeroing button on the bedside monitor. Observe the digital reading until it displays a value of zero.	The monitor will automatically adjust itself to zero. Zeroing negates the effects of atmospheric pressure.	Some monitors require that the zero be turned and adjusted manually. Some systems also may require calibration. Refer to manufacturer guidelines for specific information.
5. Place a new, sterile cap on the stopcock.	Maintains sterility.	
6. Turn the stopcock so that it is open to the patient.	Permits pressure monitoring and maintains catheter patency.	
7. Discard used supplies, and wash hands.	Reduces transmission of microorganisms; standard precautions.	

Expected Outcomes

- Hemodynamic monitoring system is set up aseptically.
- Air-fluid interface of the transducer is leveled to the phlebostatic axis.
- Hemodynamic monitoring system is zeroed.

Unexpected Outcomes

- Loose connections within the hemodynamic monitoring system
- Stopcocks left open to air without dead-end caps
- Air bubbles within the system
- Pressure bag not inflated to 300 mm Hg

Patient Monitoring and Care

Patient Monitoring and Care	Rationale	Reportable Conditions
1. Check flush bag every 1 to 4 hours.	Ensures that flush bag contains solution to maintain catheter patency.	
2. Check that flush bag is maintained at 300 mm Hg every 1 to 4 hours and as needed.	Maintains catheter patency.	
3. **Arterial lines.** Change the flush bag and hemodynamic monitoring system (pressure tubing, transducer, and stopcocks) every 96 hours or with each change of the catheter if it is changed more frequently than every 96 hours. The flush bag may need to be changed more frequently if empty of solution. *(Level V: Clinical studies in more than one or two different patient populations and situations to support recommendations)* Follow manufacturer recommendations for reusable transducer systems.	Changing the system more often than every 96 hours may cause contamination and increase the risk of infection.[4, 16, 17]	

Continued on following page

Patient Monitoring and Care	Rationale	Reportable Conditions
4. **Pulmonary artery lines.** Change the flush bag and the hemodynamic monitoring system (pressure tubing, transducers, and stopcocks) every 72 hours. The flush bag may need to be changed more frequently if empty of solution. *(Level V: Clinical studies in more than one or two different patient populations and situations to support recommendations)* Follow manufacturer recommendations for reusable transducer systems.	The Centers for Disease Control and Prevention (CDC)[4] and research findings[16–18] recommend that the hemodynamic flush system can be used safely for 72 hours. This recommendation is based on research conducted with disposable pressure monitoring systems used for peripheral and central lines.	
5. Zero the hemodynamic monitoring system during initial setup or before insertion, after insertion, if disconnection occurs between the transducer and the monitoring cable, if disconnection occurs between the monitoring cable and the monitor, and when the values obtained do not fit the clinical picture. Follow manufacturer recommendations for both disposable and reusable systems.	Ensures accuracy of the hemodynamic monitoring system; minimizes risk of contamination of the system.	
6. Check hemodynamic monitoring system every 1 to 4 hours and as needed.	Ensure that all connections are tightly secured and that there are no cracks in the system. Ensure that the system is closed with dead-end caps on all stopcocks. Ensure that the system is free of air bubbles.	
7. Set hemodynamic monitoring system alarms.	Provides immediate alarm for high and low pressures.	

Documentation

Documentation should include the following:

- Patient and family education
- Date and time of hemodynamic monitoring system setup
- Hemodynamic monitoring system leveling and zeroing
- Type of flush solution
- Unexpected outcomes
- Additional nursing interventions

References

1. American Association of Critical Care Nurses. Evaluation of the effects of heparinized and nonheparinized flush solutions on the patency of arterial pressure monitoring lines: the AACN Thunder Project. *Am J Crit Care.* 1993;2:3–15.
2. Gardner RM, Hollingsworth KW. Technologic advances in invasive pressure monitoring. *J Cardiovasc Nurs.* 1988;2:52–55.
3. Mermel LA, Maki DG. Epidemic bloodstream infections from hemodynamic pressure monitoring: signs of the times. *Infect Control Hosp Epidemiol.* 1989;10:47–53.
4. Pearson ML. Guideline for prevention of intravascular device-related infections. *Infect Control Hosp Epidemiol.* 1996;17:438–473.
5. Kulkarni M, Elsner C, Ouellet D, Zeldin R. Heparinized saline versus normal saline in maintaining patency of the radial artery catheter. *Can J Surg.* 1994;27:37–42.
6. Chulay M, Miller T. The effect of backrest elevation on pulmonary artery and pulmonary capillary wedge pressures in patients after cardiac surgery. *Heart Lung.* 1984;13:138–140.
7. Wilson AE, Bermingham-Mitchell K, Wells N, Zachary K. Effect of backrest position on hemodynamic and right ventricular measurements in critically ill adults. *Am J Crit Care.* 1996;5:264–270.
8. Cason CL, Holland CL, Lambert CW, Huntsman KT. Effects of backrest elevation and position on pulmonary artery pressures. *Cardiovasc Nurs.* 1990;26:1–5.
9. Clochesy J, Hinshaw AD, Otto CW. Effects of change of

position on pulmonary artery and pulmonary capillary wedge pressure in mechanically ventilated patients. *National Intraven Therapy Assoc.* 1984;7:223–225.

10. Keating D, Bolyard K, Eichler E, Reed J III. Effect of sidelying positions on pulmonary artery pressures. *Heart Lung.* 1986;15:605–610.

11. Woods SL, Mansfield LW. Effect of body position upon pulmonary artery and pulmonary capillary wedge pressures in noncritically ill patients. *Heart Lung.* 1976;5:83–90.

12. Laulive JL. Pulmonary artery pressures and position changes in the critically ill adult. *Dimensions Crit Care Nurs.* 1982;1:28–34.

13. Groom L, Frisch SR, Elliot M. Reproducibility and accuracy of pulmonary artery pressure measurement in supine and lateral positions. *Heart Lung.* 1990;19:147–151.

14. Kennedy GT, Bryant A, Crawford MH. The effects of lateral body positioning on measurements of pulmonary artery and pulmonary wedge pressures. *Heart Lung.* 1984;13:155–158.

15. Keckeisen M. *Protocols for Practice: Hemodynamic Monitoring Series—Pulmonary Artery Pressure Monitoring.* Aliso Viejo, Ca: American Association of Critical-Care Nurses; 1997.

16. Luskin RL, Weinstein RA, Nathan C, Chamberlin WH, Kabins SA. Extended use of disposable pressure transducers. *JAMA.* 1986;255:916–920.

17. O'Malley MK, Rhaume FS, Cerra FB, McComb RC. Value of routine pressure monitoring system changes after 72 hours. *Crit Care Med.* 1994;22:1424–1430.

18. Ducharme FM, Gauthier M, Lacroix J, Lafleur L. Incidence of infection related to arterial catheterization in children: a prospective study. *Crit Care Med.* 1988;16:272–276.

Additional Readings

Bridges EJ, Woods SL. Pulmonary artery pressure measurements: state of the art. *Heart Lung.* 1993;22(2):101.

Cason CL, Lambert CW. Positioning during hemodynamic monitoring: evaluating the research. *Dimens Crit Care Nurs.* 1993;12:226–233.

Darovic G. Fluid-filled monitoring systems. In: Darovic GO, ed. *Hemodynamic Monitoring: Invasive and Noninvasive Clinical Application.* 2nd ed. Philadelphia; Pa: WB Saunders; 1995:149–175.

Gardner PE, Bridges EJ. Hemodynamic monitoring. In: Woods SI, Sivarajan ES, Halpenny CJ, Underhill-Motzer S, eds. *Cardiac Nursing.* 3rd ed. Philadelphia, Pa: JB Lippincott; 1995:424.

Imperial-Perez F, McRae M. *Protocols for Practice: Hemodynamic Monitoring Series—Arterial Pressure Monitoring.* Aliso Viejo, Ca: American Association of Critical-Care Nurses; 1998.

Lambert CW, Cason CL. Backrest elevation and pulmonary artery pressures: Research analysis. *Dimens Crit Care Nurs.* 1990;9:327–335.

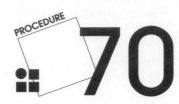

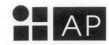

70

Arterial and Venous Sheath Removal

P U R P O S E: Arterial and venous sheaths are placed during cardiac catheterization and interventional cardiac procedures. Achieving and maintaining hemostasis after their removal is essential.

Amy L. Schueler
Rose B. Shaffer

PREREQUISITE NURSING KNOWLEDGE

- Knowledge of the anatomy of the femoral artery and vein and of the technique for the percutaneous approach to insertion of the arterial and venous sheaths is needed.
- Knowledge of the anticoagulation used after interventional procedures and of the appropriate tests used to determine timing of sheath removal is necessary.
- Technical and clinical competence in removing arterial and venous sheaths is needed.
- A variety of hemostasis options are available, including the following:
  - ❖ Manual compression
  - ❖ Mechanical compression devices (eg, C-clamp, Femostop) (Fig. 70–1)
  - ❖ Collagen plug devices (eg, VasoSeal, Angioseal)
  - ❖ Percutaneous suture closure devices (eg, Perclose).
- Manual compression, mechanical compression, and collagen plug devices may be applied by a variety of specially trained individuals (eg, physicians, registered nurses, technicians, advanced practice nurses, or physician assistants).
- Percutaneous suture closure devices are usually deployed by the physician at the end of the procedure.
- Regardless of the method used to achieve hemostasis, ongoing assessment and monitoring of the puncture site, as well as assessment of peripheral vascular and neurovascular status of the affected extremity, are the responsibility of the registered nurse.
- Sheath removal can be associated with many complications, including the following:

- ❖ External bleeding at the site
- ❖ Internal bleeding (eg, retroperitoneal bleeding)
- ❖ Vascular complications (eg, hematoma, pseudoaneurysm, arteriovenous [AV] fistula, thrombus, or embolus)
- ❖ Neurovascular complications (sensory or motor changes in affected extremity)
- ❖ Vasovagal complications
- Studies indicate that early removal of sheaths decreases complications.[1, 2]

EQUIPMENT

- Cardiac monitoring system
- Alcohol pad or swabsticks
- Povidone pad, swabsticks, or solution
- Nonsterile gloves

- Protective eyewear
- Dressing supplies
- Suture removal kit
- Indelible marker
- Syringe and needles

Additional equipment as needed includes the following:

- Readily available emergency medications and resuscitation equipment
- Selected hemostasis option (if using device other than manual compression)
- Activated clotting time (ACT) test tube or machine

- Noninvasive automatic blood pressure cuff
- 1% lidocaine (without epinephrine)

PATIENT AND FAMILY EDUCATION

- Explain the procedure to the patient and the family.
  ➤**Rationale:** Teaching provides information and may help

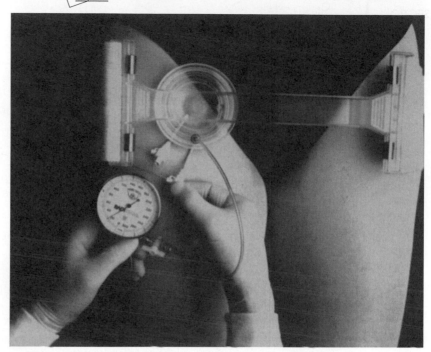

■ ● FIGURE 70–1. Femostop in correct position. (From Barbiere C. A new device for control of bleeding after transfemoral catheterization. *Crit Care Nurse.* 1995; 15(1):52.)

decrease anxiety and fear. It encourages patient to ask questions and voice concerns about the procedure.

- Explain the importance of bedrest, of head of bed no greater than 30 degrees, and of keeping affected extremity straight for a specified time to maintain hemostasis after the procedure. ➤➤*Rationale:* Elicits patient cooperation and decreases risk of bleeding, hematoma, or other vascular complications.

- Explain that the procedure may produce discomfort and that pressure will be felt at the site until hemostasis is achieved. Encourage the patient to report discomfort. ➤➤*Rationale:* Prepares the patient for what to expect.

- After sheath removal, instruct the patient to report any warm, wet feeling or pain at the puncture site. Also, instruct the patient to report any numbness or tingling or sensory or motor changes in the affected extremity. ➤➤*Rationale:* Aids in the early recognition of complications.

PATIENT ASSESSMENT AND PREPARATION

Patient Assessment

- Assess for medical history of bleeding disorders. ➤➤*Rationale:* May increase the risk of bleeding or vascular complications.

- Assess the complete blood count (CBC), platelet count, prothrombin time (PT) with international normalized ratio (INR), partial thromboplastin time (PTT), and ACT. ➤➤*Rationale:* Laboratory results should be within normal limits to decrease the risk of bleeding after sheath removal.

- Assess electrocardiogram (ECG) rhythm and vital signs. ➤➤*Rationale:* Establishes baseline data. In patients with systolic blood pressure >150 mm Hg, medications

should be considered to lower the blood pressure in order to achieve and maintain hemostasis.

- Assess extremity distal to the sheath for quality and strength of pulses, color, temperature, sensation, and movement. ➤➤*Rationale:* Establishes baseline assessment before sheath removal.

- Assess for patency of intravenous access. ➤➤*Rationale:* Allows for emergency medication or fluids to be administered if necessary.

Patient Preparation

- Ensure that the patient and the family understand preprocedural teaching. Answer questions as they arise, and reinforce information as needed. ➤➤*Rationale:* Evaluates and reinforces understanding of previously taught information.

- Administer analgesia before removal of sheaths. ➤➤*Rationale:* Facilitates pain management.

- Place the patient with the head of the bed flat or less than 15 degrees. ➤➤*Rationale:* Improves ability to achieve hemostasis.

- Mark the distal pulses with the indelible marker. ➤➤*Rationale:* Facilitates ability to locate pulses after procedure.

- If using a mechanical device to maintain pressure, position the belt of the device as indicated under the patient. ➤➤*Rationale:* The device will be positioned for use after sheath removal. Patient movement will be minimized after sheath removal.

⊞ AP This procedure should be performed only by physicians, advanced practice nurses, and other health care professionals (including critical care nurses) with additional knowledge, skills, and demonstrated competence per professional licensure or institutional standard.

Procedure for Arterial and Venous Sheath Removal

Steps	Rationale	Special Considerations
1. Wash hands, and don gloves and protective eyewear.	Reduces the risk of transmission of microorganisms; standard precautions.	
2. Turn off arterial line alarms.	Monitoring no longer needed; prevents alarm sounding.	
3. Remove arterial and venous sheath dressing.	Prepares for sheath removal.	
4. Turn the stopcock off to the patient and turn off the intravenous fluids.	Prevents back flow of blood and forward flow of fluids.	
5. Don sterile gloves.	Maintains asepsis.	
6. Clean the arterial and venous sites with antiseptic solution before removal.	May decrease the risk of infection.	Follow institutional standard.
7. Remove sutures.	Prepares for removal of sheath.	
8. Consider subcutaneously infiltrating the area around the catheter sites with 1% lidocaine.	May reduce the discomfort experienced during sheath removal.	
9. Palpate the femoral pulse.	Allows for more accurate positioning of hemostasis option (manual or mechanical).	
10. Position the hemostasis option (manual or mechanical) 0.5 to 1 cm above the site where the arterial sheath enters the skin. *(Level IV: Limited clinical studies to support recommendations)*	The arterial puncture site is superior and medial to the actual skin puncture site. The arterial sheath is inserted at a 45-degree angle to the artery.	Studies vary on the use of manual versus mechanical compression to achieve hemostasis of the femoral artery.[3, 4] If the patient is obese or has a large abdomen, a second person may be needed to assist with sheath removal and with accurate placement of the hemostasis option.
11. Simultaneously depress the hemostasis option (manual or mechanical) and gently remove the arterial sheath from the femoral artery during exhalation.	Prevents external bleeding. Pulling the arterial sheath during the exhalation phase of the respiratory cycle may prevent the patient from "bearing down" during arterial sheath removal.	Never withdraw the sheath if resistance is met. Notify the physician.
12. Continue to apply pressure. A. Maintain manual pressure, or B. Maintain mechanical device.	Pressure is needed to achieve hemostasis.	If using a mechanical device, set the pressure of the mechanical device according to the manufacturer's recommendation and institutional standard.
13. Assess the circulation to the extremity distal to the site of the sheath removal.	Verifies adequate circulation while achieving hemostasis.	The pulse may decrease during application of full pressure but should not be obliterated completely. If manual compression is being performed, another person is needed to assess distal perfusion.
14. Palpate the area around the arterial site.	Determines if any bleeding may have occurred or is occurring around the arterial site.	
15. Leave the hemostasis option (manual or mechanical) in place for 20 to 30 minutes.	Allows for adequate hemostasis to be achieved.	Follow institutional standard. Tissue damage may occur if prolonged pressure is maintained (eg, 2 to 3 hours).[5]

Procedure for Arterial and Venous Sheath Removal *Continued*

Steps	Rationale	Special Considerations
16. After hemostasis is achieved, remove the hemostasis option.	Once hemostasis is achieved, pressure is no longer necessary.	If using a mechanical device, follow the manufacturer's recommendations, institutional standard, or physician prescription regarding the gradual reduction of pressure from the device. Notify the physician if unable to achieve hemostasis.
17. Remove the venous sheath, and maintain manual pressure for approximately 5 minutes or until hemostasis is achieved.	Achieves hemostasis.	
18. Apply sterile dressing to both arterial and venous sites.	Minimizes infection at the sites.	
19. Discard used supplies, and wash hands.	Reduces the transmission of microorganisms; standard precautions.	

Expected Outcomes

- Arterial and venous sheaths are removed with hemostasis achieved.
- There is adequate circulation to the extremity distal to the site of sheath removal (positive sensation, movement, capillary refill, color, temperature, pulse).
- There is no evidence of hematoma or bruit.
- Cardiovascular and hemodynamic stability is achieved.

Unexpected Outcomes

- Inability to remove the arterial or venous sheaths
- Hematoma development
- Retroperitoneal bleed
- Pseudoaneurysm
- Vagal response during removal of arterial sheath
- Hemodynamic instability
- Impaired perfusion to the extremity distal to the site of sheath removal
- Angina

Patient Monitoring and Care

Patient Monitoring and Care	Rationale	Reportable Conditions
		These conditions should be reported if they persist despite nursing interventions.
1. Assess peripheral vascular and neurovascular status of the affected extremity after arterial sheath removal: Q 15 min × 4, Q 30 min × 2, Q 60 min × 4. Restart the peripheral vascular and neurovascular status after mechanical compression is removed.	A thrombus or embolus may precipitate changes in peripheral or neurovascular status, requiring early intervention.	• Decrease or change in strength of pulses in affected extremity (diminished or absent) • Cold or cool to touch • Paresthesia • Pallor, cyanosis • Pain • Inability to move extremity or toes

Continued on following page

⠿ AP This procedure should be performed only by physicians, advanced practice nurses, and other health care professionals (including critical care nurses) with additional knowledge, skills, and demonstrated competence per professional licensure or institutional standard.

Patient Monitoring and Care *Continued*

Patient Monitoring and Care	Rationale	Reportable Conditions
2. Obtain vital signs after removal of the arterial sheath: Q 15 min × 4, Q 30 min × 2, Q 60 min × 4. Restart vital-sign monitoring after mechanical compression is removed.	Changes in vital signs may occur because of vasovagal response or blood loss.	• Changes in vital signs
3. Monitor ECG.	Detects presence of dysrhythmias.	• Dysrhythmias
4. Assess puncture site: Q 15 min × 4, Q 30 min × 2, Q 60 min × 4. Restart puncture site assessment after mechanical compression is removed.	Detects presence of bleeding.	• Bleeding at arterial or venous sites • Hematoma development
5. After hemostasis is achieved, the patient's head of bed can be elevated up to 30 degrees. *(Level V: Clinical studies in more than one or two different patient populations and situations to support recommendations)*	Minimizes back discomfort and does not increase complications.[6, 7]	
6. Maintain bedrest for 6 to 8 hours after the sheath is removed. *(Level V: Clinical studies in more than one or two different populations and situations to support recommendations)*	Minimizes back discomfort and minimizes complications of bedrest.[7–9]	

Documentation

Documentation should include the following:

- Patient and family education
- Date and time of sheath removal
- Site of arterial and venous sheath removal
- Quality of arterial and venous sheath removed: (eg, intact, cracked)
- Any difficulties with removal
- Patient tolerance
- Any medications used
- Time to hemostasis
- Method of hemostasis
- Site assessment
- Vital signs—heart rate, blood pressure, respiratory rate, rhythm
- Neurovascular checks to affected extremity
- Occurrence of unexpected outcomes
- Nursing interventions required or actions taken
- Evaluation of any nursing intervention required

References

1. Bowden S, Matsco M, Worrey J. Time of removal of femoral sheaths after interventional procedures: comparison of hemoglobin and hematocrit values. *Am J Crit Care.* 1998;7:197–199.
2. Homes L, Holabaugh S. Using the continuous quality improvement process to improve the care of patients after angioplasty. *Crit Care Nurse.* 1997;17:56–65.
3. Bogart BA. Time to hemostasis: a comparison of manual versus mechanical compression of the femoral artery. *Am J Crit Care.* 1995;4:149–156.
4. Simon A, Bumgarner B, Clark K, Israel S. Manual versus mechanical compression for femoral artery hemostasis after cardiac catheterization. *Am J Crit Care.* 1998;7:308–313.
5. Barbiere C. A new device for control of bleeding after transfemoral catheterization. *Crit Care Nurse.* February 1995:51–53.
6. Sulzbach LM, Munro BH, Hirshfeld JW. A randomized clinical trial of the effect of bed position after PTCA. *Am J Crit Care.* 1995;4:221–226.
7. Coyne C, Baier W, Perra B, Sherer BK. Controlled trial of backrest elevation after coronary angiography. *Am J Crit Care.* 1994;3:282–288.
8. Keeling AW, Knight E, Taylor V, Nordt LA. Postcardiac catheterization time-in-bed study: enhancing patient comfort through nursing research. *Appl Nurs Res.* 1994;7:14–17.
9. Lau KW, Ran A, Koh TH, Koo CC, Quek S, Ng A, Johan A. Early ambulation following diagnostic 7 French cardiac catheterization: a prospective randomized trial. *Cath Cardiovasc Diag.* 1993;28:34–38.

Additional Readings

Bowden SM, Worrey JA. Assessing patient comfort: local infiltration of lidocaine during femoral sheath removal. *Am J Crit Care.* 1995;4:368–369.

Christensen BV, Manion RV, Iacarella CL, et al. Vascular complications after angiography with and without the use of sandbags. *Nurs Res.* 1998;11:51–53.

O'Brien C, Recker D. How to remove a femoral sheath. *Am J Nurs.* October 1992:34–37.

Rudisill P, Williams L, Craig S. Study of mechanical versus manual-mechanical compression following various interventional cardiology procedures. *J Cardiovasc Nurs.* 1997;11:15–22.

Schickel S, Nones Cronin S, Mize A, Voelker C. Removal of femoral sheaths by registered nurses: issues and outcomes. *Crit Care Nurse.* 1996;16:32–36.

Simon A, Bumgarner B, Clark K, Israel S. Manual versus mechanical compression for femoral artery hemostasis after cardiac catheterization. *Am J Crit Care.* 1998;7:308–313.

Tremko L, Understanding diagnostic cardiac catheterization. *Am J Nurs.* 1997;97:16K–16R.

71 Pericardial Catheter Management

P U R P O S E: An indwelling pericardial catheter allows for the slow and complete evacuation of a pericardial effusion. The catheter also allows for the infusion of medications such as antibiotics or chemotherapeutic agents into the pericardial space.

Kathy McCloy

PREREQUISITE NURSING KNOWLEDGE

- Understanding of the anatomy and physiology of the cardiovascular system, principles of cardiac conduction, electrocardiogram (ECG) lead placement, basic dysrhythmia interpretation, and electrical safety is required.
- Understanding of sterile technique is necessary.
- Advanced cardiac life support knowledge and skills are necessary.
- Collection of fluid in the pericardial space is termed pericardial effusion.
- The pericardial space normally contains 15 to 50 mL of fluid.[1] Injury of the pericardium causes increased production of pericardial fluid, formation of fibrin, and cellular proliferation.[2] Causes of pericardial effusion are numerous and include infection, malignant neoplasms, autoimmune disorders, kidney failure, heart failure, acute myocardial infarction, trauma, radiation exposure, inflammatory disorders, and myxedema.[1, 3] Pericardial effusion may also be medication induced, idiopathic, or a complication of invasive procedures.
- Pericardiocentesis is an effective treatment for pericardial effusion (see Procedure 40). An indwelling pericardial catheter may be left in place following pericardiocentesis to drain excess pericardial fluid.
- The pericardial catheter may be connected to a closed drainage system (Fig. 71–1).
- The pericardial catheter may also be left in place to allow installation of certain medications, (ie, nonabsorbable corticosteroid or antineoplastic agents) depending on the patient's underlying disease state.[1]
- The indwelling pericardial catheter should usually be removed within 24 to 48 hours after placement to avoid the risk of infection and iatrogenic pericarditis.[4] However, the indwelling pericardial catheter may be left in place for longer periods of time to ensure resolution of pericardial effusion and cardiac tamponade.[1, 2] Pericardial catheters are usually removed when the total amount of drainage has decreased to less than 25 to 30 mL over 24 hours.[5] To date, research-based evidence does not exist that defines the timing of pericardial catheter removal.

EQUIPMENT

- Pericardial catheter
- Sterile gloves
- Sterile isotonic normal saline for irrigation
- Syringes
- Alcohol pads or swabsticks
- Povidine-iodine pads or swabsticks
- Sterile 4 × 4 gauze
- Occlusive dressing
- Tape
- Three-way stopcock
- Drainage tubing
- Pericardial drainage bag

PATIENT AND FAMILY EDUCATION

- Explain the need for the indwelling pericardial catheter and the reason for insertion. **➤Rationale:** Teaching de-

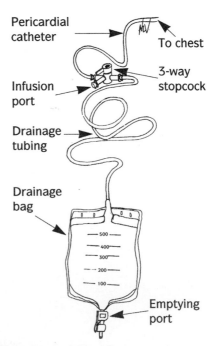

■● FIGURE 71–1. Indwelling pericardial catheter system. (From Hammel WJ. Care of patients with an indwelling pericardial catheter. *Crit Care Nurse.* 1998; 18(5):40–45.)

creases patient and family anxiety; meets patient and family needs for information.

- Explain the need for frequent monitoring in the intensive care unit while the pericardial catheter remains in place. ➺***Rationale:*** Decreases patient and family anxiety; meets patient and family needs for information.
- Explain that the catheter may be uncomfortable and cause some discomfort at the insertion site, possibly with inspiration, and that pain medication will be administered to promote comfort. ➺***Rationale:*** Facilitates effective pain management; decreases patient and family anxiety.

PATIENT ASSESSMENT AND PREPARATION

Patient Assessment

- Assess cardiovascular and hemodynamic status: heart rate, blood pressure (BP), respiratory rate, pulmonary artery pressure (PAP), pulmonary artery wedge pressure (PAWP), right atrial pressure (RAP), cardiac output (CO), cardiac idex (CI), heart sounds, and peripheral

pulses. ➺***Rationale:*** Establish patient's baseline for future comparison.
- Assess for dyspnea, tachypnea, tachycardia, muffled heart sounds, precordial dullness to percussion, impaired consciousness; hypotension (systolic BP less than 100 mm Hg or decreased from patient's baseline); increased jugular venous pressure; pulsus paradoxus (inspiratory fall in systolic BP) greater than 12 to 15 mm Hg; equalization of RAP, PAWP, and pulmonary artery diastolic pressure, low CO/CI.[3] ➺***Rationale:*** Assesses for signs and symptoms of cardiac tamponade.

Patient Preparation

- Ensure that the patient and family understand preprocedural teaching. Answer questions as they arise and reinforce information as needed. ➺***Rationale:*** Evaluates and reinforces understanding of previously taught information.
- Administer analgesia or anxiolytic before the pericardial catheter insertion. ➺***Rationale:*** Facilitates pain management and reduces anxiety.

Procedure for Pericardial Catheter Management

Steps	Rationale	Special Considerations
1. Wash hands.	Reduces transmission of microorganisms; standard precautions.	
2. Assist the physician with the pericardiocentesis (see Procedure 40).	The pericardial catheter is inserted by the physician during the pericardiocentesis.	The pericardial catheter may also be inserted in the operating room or in a special procedure environment (cardiac catheterization laboratory, interventional laboratory, etc.).
3. Determine that connections between the pericardial catheter, tubing, stopcock, and drainage bag are tight.	Ensures that the integrity of the system is intact.	
4. Observe the drainage of pericardial fluid.	Ensures pericardial catheter patency.	Pericardial fluid is commonly straw-colored, serous drainage. An echocardiogram is performed after the pericardiocentesis to assess for reaccumulation of pericardial fluid.
5. Place drainage tubing and drainage bag lower than the catheter insertion point.	Promotes drainage and prevents catheter blockage.	
6. Empty the pericardial drainage bag at least every 8 hours.		
A. Wash hands, and don gloves.		
B. Turn stopcock off to the patient.	Prevents pneumopericardium.	
C. Open the emptying port.		
D. Empty the pericardial drainage into a collection container.		
E. Measure the amount of drainage.		
7. If a drainage bag is not in use, aspirate the pericardial fluid every 4 to 6 hours or as clinically indicated through a three-way stopcock using sterile technique.[4]	Removes excess pericardial fluid; ensures catheter patency.	Follow institutional standards regarding personnel permitted to aspirate pericardial catheters (eg, registered nurse, physician).
A. Wash hands, and don sterile gloves.	Reduces the transmission of microorganisms; standard precautions. Prepares for aseptic technique.	

Procedure continued on following page

Procedure	for Pericardial Catheter Management *Continued*

Steps	Rationale	Special Considerations
B. Remove the cap from the three-way stopcock.		
C. Clean the infusion port of the three-way stopcock with an alcohol swab.	Decreases the risk of infection.	
D. Attach a sterile, 60-mL syringe to the three-way stopcock.	Connects to the port for pericardial fluid removal.	
E. Turn the stopcock on to the syringe and patient.	Permits removal of pericardial fluid.	
F. Gently aspirate pericardial fluid.	Gentle removal is necessary to avoid pericardial injury.	Pericardial fluid samples may be collected for selected diagnostic tests (eg, protein, glucose; hematocrit, white blood cell count; bacterial or fungal culture).
G. Measure the amount of drainage.	Needed for assessing and recording output.	
H. After each fluid withdrawal, flush the pericardial catheter with 2.0 to 5.0 mL of sterile normal saline.	Clears pericardial catheter and maintains catheter patency.	Monitor vital signs and ECG while flushing the pericardial catheter.
I. Return the three-way stopcock off to the infusion port.	Maintains closed system; prevents pneumopericardium.	
J. Place a new sterile cap on the infusion port.	Maintains asepsis.	
K. Discard drainage and used supplies, and wash hands.	Reduces transmission of microorganisms; standard precautions.	
Managing Pericardial Catheter Blockage		
1. Determine if the drainage system is lower than the insertion point and reposition if needed.	Facilitates drainage.	
2. Assess if there is an external mechanical cause of pericardial catheter blockage and, if present, correct. Consider:	Relieves mechanical obstruction to flow of pericardial fluid.	
A. Correct tubing kinks.		
B. Remove tubing that may be compressed under the patient.		
C. Turn the patient.		
3. Assess for tubing disconnection and, if loosened, reconnect.	Ensures intact pericardial drainage system.	
4. Determine if the stopcock is in the incorrect position and, if needed, correct the position.	Facilitates pericardial fluid collection.	
5. If the above steps do not relieve the catheter blockage, then:	Attempts to relieve blockage.	Follow institutional standards regarding personnel permitted to aspirate pericardial catheters (eg, registered nurse or physician).
A. Wash hands, and apply sterile gloves.	Reduces transmission of microorganisms; standard precautions. Prepares for aseptic technique.	
B. Turn the stopcock off to the drainage bag.	Decreases the risk of infection.	
C. Remove the cap from the stopcock.		
D. Clean the infusion port of the stopcock with an alcohol swab.		
E. Flush the pericardial catheter with 2.0 to 5.0 mL of heparinized normal saline, as prescribed (eg, 30 units of heparin per mL of normal saline).	Attempts to improve pericardial catheter patency. Heparinized saline may be used if the drainage is serous or fibrous in consistency.[5]	Monitor vital signs and ECG while flushing the pericardial catheter.

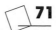

Procedure	for Pericardial Catheter Management *Continued*

Steps	Rationale	Special Considerations
F. Turn the stopcock off to the infusion port.	Allows drainage of flush solution and pericardial fluid.	Deduct flush solution from measurement of pericardial drainage.
G. Determine if pericardial fluid is draining.		
6. If the above measures do not remove the catheter blockage, consider changing the pericardial drainage tubing.		
7. If measures do not remove the catheter blockage, notify the physician.		

Care of the Pericardial Catheter Insertion Site

1. Wash hands, and don gloves.	Reduces transmission of microorganisms; standard precautions.	
2. Remove dressing.	Prepares for site care.	
3. Assess the catheter, insertion site, suture, and surrounding skin.	Assess for signs of infection, catheter dislodgment, leakage, or loose sutures.	
4. Remove and discard gloves and put on a sterile pair of gloves.	Maintains aseptic technique.	
5. Beginning at the insertion site, using concentric circles, cleanse the catheter and skin around the insertion site with alcohol pads or swabsticks.	Debrides the skin and removes moisture.	
6. Cleanse the catheter and skin with providone pads or swabsticks as described in the previous step and allow to dry.	Reduces the rate of recolonization of skin microflora.	
7. Apply sterile, occlusive dressing.	Provides a sterile environment.	
8. Label dressing with date, time, and initials.	Identifies last dressing change.	
9. Discard used supplies, and wash hands.	Reduces the transmission of microorganisms; standard precautions.	

Infusion of Medications Through Pericardial Catheters

1. Wash hands, and don sterile gloves.	Reduces the transmission of microorganisms; standard precautions. Prepares for aseptic technique.	
2. Review physician prescription for type and amount of medication, rate of infusion, and length of dwell time.	Ensures the accuracy of medication administration.	
3. Cleanse the infusion port of the stopcock with an alcohol pad or swabstick.	Decreases risk of infection.	
4. Connect the medication or solution (via tubing or syringe) to the infusion port of the stopcock.	Prepares for infusion.	Infusion of medication into the pericardial space may cause iatrogenic cardiac tamponade.
5. Turn the stopcock off to the pericardial drainage bag.	Prevents installation of medication into drainage bag.	
6. Infuse the medication or solution slowly as per physician prescription.	Provides treatment of underlying pathology.	Assess patient closely for pain as the medication or solution is administered into the pericardial space. Stop the infusion if chest pain similar to anginal pain develops or if the patient develops signs or symptoms of cardiac tamponade.

Procedure continued on following page

Procedure	for Pericardial Catheter Management *Continued*

Steps	Rationale	Special Considerations
7. If the medication is to dwell in the pericardial space before the reestablishment of pericardial drainage:		
A. Flush the pericardial catheter with 2.0 to 5.0 mL of sterile normal saline.	Ensures that the medication is instilled in the pericardial space and does not lie in the catheter.	
B. Turn the stopcock off to the patient.	Allows the medication or solution to dwell in the pericardial space.	
C. Follow dwell time as prescribed.	Maintains medication in the pericardial space.	
D. After the dwell time is complete, turn the stopcock off to the infusion port.	Allows pericardial drainage collection to resume.	
8. Measure the amount of the solution infused and the drainage collected.	Ensure that the volume of drainage collected is equal to or greater than the volume of solution instilled.	

Expected Outcomes	Unexpected Outcomes
• Patent pericardial drainage system	• Infection
• Resolution of pericardial effusion	• Pain
• Hemodynamic stability	• Catheter blockage
• Free of infection	• Reaccumulation of pericardial fluid
• Free of pain and discomfort	• Cardiac tamponade
• Medications administered as prescribed	• Dysrhythmias

Patient Monitoring and Care

Patient Monitoring and Care	Rationale	Reportable Conditions
		These conditions must be reported if they persist despite nursing interventions.
1. Perform systematic cardiovascular and hemodynamic assessments every 60 minutes and as patient status requires.	Monitors for cardiac tamponade and pericardial catheter-related problems.	• Signs of cardiac tamponade[3]; dyspnea, tachypnea, tachycardia, hypotension, increased jugular venous pressure, pulsus paradoxus, muffled heart sounds, precordial dullness to percussion, altered level of consciousness; equalization of RAP, PAP diastolic, PAWP; CI less than 2.5 L per minute; dysrhythmias
2. Assess patency of the pericardial catheter drainage system every hour and as needed.	Pericardial catheter blockage may predispose the patient to reaccumulation of pericardial fluid that may lead to cardiac tamponade.	• Cessation of pericardial drainage • Signs and symptoms of cardiac tamponade
3. Assess the amount and type of fluid draining from the pericardial catheter hourly and as needed.	Monitors type and amount of pericardial fluid drainage.	• Change in amount or color of pericardial drainage from patient's baseline
4. Change the pericardial dressing every 24 hours and when the dressing becomes damp, loosened, or soiled.	Provides an opportunity to assess for signs and symptoms of infection. Infective pericarditis is associated with high mortality and morbidity rates.[3, 4]	• Elevated WBCs • Elevated temperature, greater than 38.5°C • Signs and symptoms of infection at insertion site (pain, erythema, drainage)

Patient Monitoring and Care	Rationale	Reportable Conditions
5. Change the pericardial tubing and drainage bag every 72 hours.[2]	Reduces the incidence of infection.	
6. Assess and manage patient pain/discomfort.	The patient may experience chest pain or pleuritic type pain while the pericardial catheter is in place.	• Inadequate pain relief with analgesics
7. Identify parameters that demonstrate clinical readiness for removal of the indwelling pericardial catheter.	Facilitates early removal of the pericardial catheter; decreases infection risk.	• Pericardial drainage less than 25 to 30 mL over the previous 24 hours • Hemodynamic stability as evidenced by systolic BP greater than 100 mm Hg, CI greater than 2.5 L/min, no pulsus paradoxus, no equalization of RAP, PAP diastolic, PAWP • Absence of pericardial effusion demonstrated on two-dimensional (2-D) echo

Documentation

Documentation should include the following:

- Patient and family education
- Patient toleration of indwelling pericardial catheter
- Pericardial catheter insertion site assessment
- Dressing changes, tubing changes, drainage bag changes
- Amount of pericardial drainage each shift, including net volumes when catheter is flushed or medications infused
- Volumes of injectate or aspirate
- Characteristics of pericardial drainage: color, consistency, and any changes
- Hemodynamic status
- Pain associated with indwelling pericardial catheter
- Occurrence of unexpected outcomes
- Nursing interventions

References

1. Lorell BH. Pericardial disease. In: *Heart Disease: A Textbook of Cardiovascular Medicine*. 5th ed. Philadelphia, Pa: W.B. Saunders, 1997:1478–1534.
2. Hamel WJ. Care of patients with an indwelling pericardial catheter. *Crit Care Nurse*. October 1998; 18:40–45.
3. Freed M, Grines C. Pericardial disease: In: *Essentials of Cardiovascular Medicine*. Birmingham, Mi: Physician's Press; 1994:417–427.
4. Lorell BH, Grossman W. Restrictive cardiomyopathy and cardiac tamponade. In: *Cardiac Catheterization, Angiography, and Intervention*. 5th ed. Baltimore, Md: Williams & Wilkins; 1995:801–823.
5. Tsang TS, Freeman WK, Sinak LJ, Seward, JB. Echocardiographically guided pericardiocentesis: evolution and state-of-the-art technique. *Mayo Clin Proc*. July 1998; 73:647–652.

Additional Reading

Drummond JB, Seward JB, Tsang TS, Hayes SN, Miller FA. Outpatient two-dimensional echocardiography-guided pericardiocentesis. *J Am Soc Echocardiogr*. May 1998; 11:433–435.

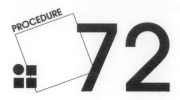

72

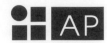

Arterial Puncture

> **P U R P O S E:** Arterial puncture is performed to obtain a sample of blood for arterial blood gas (ABG) analysis. This analysis measures blood pH and the partial pressure of oxygen (Pao_2) and carbon dioxide ($Paco_2$). ABG samples can also be analyzed for oxygen saturation (Sao_2) and for bicarbonate (Hco_3^-) values. These analyses are done primarily to evaluate a patient's oxygenation status, acid-base balance, and ventilation.[1] Additional laboratory tests (eg, ammonia and lactate levels) also may be performed on arterial blood samples.

Linda Bucher

PREREQUISITE NURSING KNOWLEDGE

- Nurses must be adequately prepared to perform an arterial puncture. This preparation should include specific educational content regarding arterial puncture and opportunities to demonstrate clinical competency.

- Principles of aseptic technique should be understood.

- Knowledge of the anatomy and physiology of the vasculature and adjacent structures is important.

- The brachial artery, a continuation of the axillary artery in the upper extremity, bifurcates just below the elbow (Fig. 72–1). From the bifurcation, the ulnar artery moves down the forearm on the medial side and the radial artery on the lateral side (see Fig. 72–1).[2]

- The preferred artery for arterial puncture is the radial artery. Although this artery is smaller than the ulnar artery, it is more superficial and can be more easily stabilized during the procedure.[2] Some research has found that the use of the brachial artery is a safe and reliable alternative site for arterial puncture.[3]

- At times, the femoral artery may be used for arterial puncture. The use of this artery can be technically difficult because of the proximity of the artery to the femoral vein (Fig. 72–2).

- Patient indications for ABGs will vary and can include patients with chronic obstructive pulmonary disease, acute respiratory distress syndrome (ARDS), and pneu-

monia. ABG analysis frequently is performed on patients experiencing shock, cardiopulmonary resuscitation (CPR), and changes in respiratory therapy or status.[1]

- Arterial cannulation should be considered for patients who require frequent arterial blood samples, continuous arterial pressure monitoring, or evaluation of vasoactive medication therapy (see Procedure 55).[4]

- The most common complications associated with arterial puncture include pain, vasospasm, hematoma formation, infection, hemorrhage, and neurovascular compromise.[1, 3, 5]

- Site selection proceeds as follows:
  - ❖ Use the radial artery as first choice. The radial artery

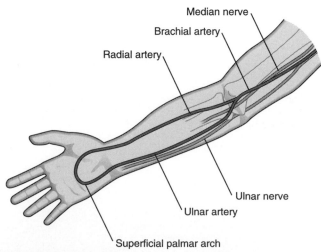

■ ● FIGURE 72–1. Anatomic landmarks for locating the radial and brachial arteries.

■■ AP This procedure should be performed only by physicians, advanced practice nurses, and other health care professionals (including critical care nurses) with additional knowledge, skills, and demonstrated competence per professional licensure or institutional standard.

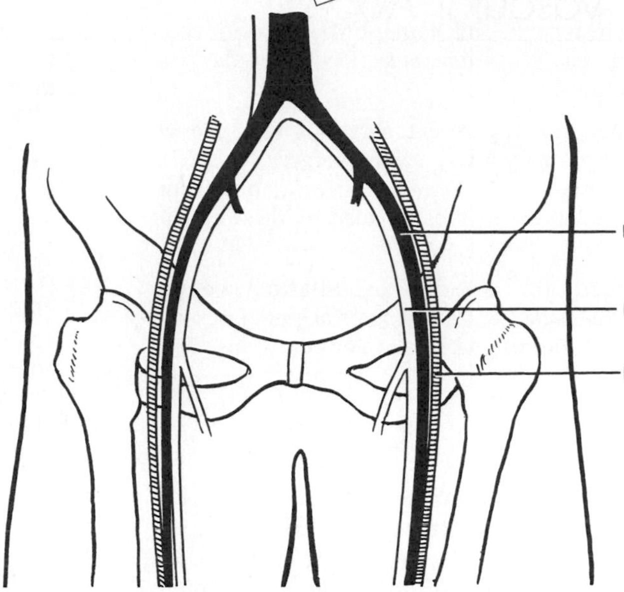

■ ● **FIGURE 72–2.** Anatomic landmarks for locating the femoral artery.

is small and easily stabilized as it passes over a bony groove located at the wrist (see Fig. 72–1).

❖ Use the brachial artery as second choice, except in the presence of poor pulsation due to shock, obesity, or sclerotic vessel (eg, because of previous cardiac catheterization). The brachial artery is larger than the radial artery. Hemostasis after arterial puncture is enhanced by its proximity to bone if the entry point is approximately 1½ inches above the antecubital fossa (see Fig. 72–1).

❖ Use the femoral artery in the case of cardiopulmonary arrest or altered perfusion to the upper extremities. The femoral artery is a large superficial artery located in the groin (see Fig. 72–2). It is easily palpated and punctured. Complications related to femoral artery puncture include hemorrhage and hematomas, because bleeding can be difficult to control; inadvertent puncture of the femoral vein, due to the close proximity of the vein to the artery; infection, because aseptic technique in the groin area is difficult to maintain; and limb ischemia if the femoral artery is damaged.

EQUIPMENT

• One prepackaged ABG kit that contains the following:
  ❖ One 20- to 25-G, 1- to 1½-in-long hypodermic needle; longer needles are required for brachial and femoral artery puncture
  ❖ One 1- to 5-mL glass or plastic syringe with a rubber stopper or cap
  ❖ One 1-mL ampule of sodium heparin, 1:1000 concentration
  ❖ Two 2-in × 2-in gauze pads
  ❖ Two povidone-iodine pads
  ❖ Two alcohol pads
  ❖ One plastic bag (for transport of sample to laboratory)
• One adhesive bandage
• Appropriate laboratory form, specimen label
• One pair of examination gloves and goggles

Additional supplies as needed include the following:

• Small rolled towel (to support patient's wrist)
• 1% lidocaine (without epinephrine), 1- to 2-mL, or eutectic mixture of local anesthetics (EMLA) cream
• Ice

PATIENT AND FAMILY EDUCATION

• Explain the reason for the arterial puncture to the patient and family. ➥*Rationale:* Clarification of information is an expressed patient and family need and helps to diminish anxiety, enhance acceptance, and encourage questions.

• Describe the overall steps of the procedure, including the patient's role in the procedure. ➥*Rationale:* Decreases patient anxiety, enhances cooperation, and provides an opportunity for the patient to voice concerns; prevents accidental movement during the procedure.

PATIENT ASSESSMENT AND PREPARATION

Patient Assessment

• Assess for factors that influence ABG measurements, including anxiety, endotracheal suctioning, nebulizer treatment, change in oxygen therapy, patient positioning, body temperature, metabolic rate, and respiratory rate. ➥*Rationale:* Stated conditions or therapies can alter blood gas analysis.

• Assess current anticoagulation therapy or known blood dyscrasia. ➥*Rationale:* Anticoagulation therapy or blood dyscrasias could prolong hemostasis at the puncture site and increase risk of hematoma formation or hemorrhage.

- Assess allergy history (eg, lidocaine, EMLA cream, antiseptic solutions, tape).   ➤➤*Rationale:* Decreases the risk of allergic reactions.

- Determine history of any recent surgeries (eg, use of radial artery for coronary artery bypass surgery [CABS]), fistulas, or shunts.   ➤➤*Rationale:* Arterial puncture should be avoided in extremities affected by these conditions.

- Determine need for arterial cannulation versus puncture.   ➤➤*Rationale:* Repeated arterial punctures increase patient discomfort and risk of complications.

Patient Preparation

- Ensure that the patient and family understand preprocedural teaching. Answer questions as they arise and reinforce information as needed.   ➤➤*Rationale:* Evaluates and reinforces understanding of previously taught information.

- If patient is receiving oxygen, check that therapy has been underway for at least 15 minutes before obtaining ABGs.[1]   ➤➤*Rationale:* Provides adequate time to realize the effect of oxygen therapy on ABG analysis.

- If patient has received a nebulizer treatment, wait 20 minutes after completion of treatment before obtaining ABGs.[1]   ➤➤*Rationale:* Provides adequate time to realize the effect of treatment on ABG analysis.

- Position the patient appropriately.   ➤➤*Rationale:* Enhances accessibility to the insertion site and promotes patient comfort.
  - ❖ Radial artery puncture: (1) Assist patient to a semirecumbent position.   ➤➤*Rationale:* Position of comfort decreases anxiety and may facilitate respiratory effort. (2) Elevate and hyperextend the wrist. A small, rolled towel may be placed under the wrist for support.   ➤➤*Rationale:* Moves the artery closer to the skin surface making the artery easier to palpate. (3) Palpate for the presence of a strong radial pulse.   ➤➤*Rationale:* Identification and localization of the pulse increase the chance of a successful arterial puncture.
  - ❖ Brachial artery puncture: (1) Assist patient to a semirecumbent position.   ➤➤*Rationale:* Position of comfort decreases anxiety and may facilitate respiratory effort. (2) Elevate and hyperextend the patient's arm. A small pillow may be placed under the arm for support.   ➤➤*Rationale:* Increases accessibility for puncture. (3) Rotate the patient's arm and palpate for the presence of a strong brachial pulse.   ➤➤*Rationale:* Identification and localization of the pulse increase the chance of a successful arterial puncture.
  - ❖ Femoral artery puncture: (1) Assist patient to a supine, straight-leg position.   ➤➤*Rationale:* Provides best position for localizing the femoral artery pulse. (2) Palpate for the presence of a strong femoral pulse.   ➤➤*Rationale:* Identification and localization of the pulse increase the chance of a successful arterial puncture.

Procedure **for Arterial Puncture**

Steps	Rationale	Special Considerations
1. Wash hands.	Reduces transmission of microorganisms; standard precautions.	Ensure that hospital policy permits RNs to perform radial, brachial, and femoral arterial punctures.
2. If the radial artery is to be used, perform the modified Allen test prior to puncture (Fig. 72–3). *(Level II: Theory based, no research data to support recommendations; recommendations from expert consensus group may exist)*	The modified Allen test is recommended before a radial artery puncture to assess the patency of the ulnar artery and an intact superficial palmar arch.[1, 2, 4, 6]	
A. With the patient's hand held overhead, instruct the patient to open and close his or her hand several times.	Forces the blood from the hand.	If the patient is unconscious or unable to perform procedure, clench the fist passively for the patient.
B. With the patient's fist clenched, apply direct pressure on the radial and ulnar arteries.	Obstructs the flow of blood to the hand.	
C. Instruct the patient to lower and open his or her hand.	Observe for pallor.	Performed passively if patient is unconscious or unable to assist.
D. Release the pressure over the ulnar artery and observe the hand for return of color.[1, 6]	Return of color within 7 seconds indicates patency of the ulnar artery and an intact superficial palmar arch and is interpreted as a *positive* Allen test. If color returns between 8 to 14 seconds, the test is considered equivocal. If it takes 15 or more seconds for color to return, the test is considered a negative test.	If the test is *negative,* the modified Allen test should be performed on the opposite hand.

Procedure **for Arterial Puncture** *Continued*

Steps	Rationale	Special Considerations

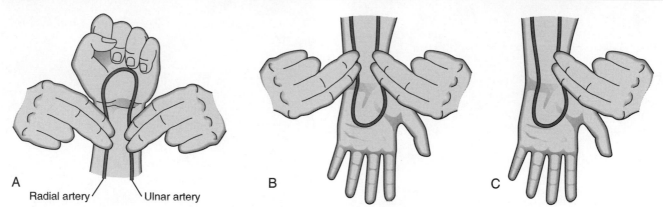

A   Radial artery   Ulnar artery   B   C

▪ ● **FIGURE 72–3.** Modified Allen test. Elevate patient's hand and instruct patient to open and close fist several times. *A,* With patient's fist clenched, simultaneously occlude the radial and ulnar arteries. *B,* Instruct patient to lower and open fist. Observe for pallor in the patient's hand. *C,* Release the pressure over the ulnar artery, and observe the hand for the return of color. (From Bucher L, Melander SD. *Critical Care Nursing.* Philadelphia: WB Saunders; 1999.)

3. Heparinize syringe and needle.

   A. Assemble a 22-G needle on syringe and prime the entire syringe barrel and needle with 1 mL of heparin. Once done, expel the heparin from the syringe.

        Prevents specimen coagulation.

        Excess heparin in the syringe can lower pH and $Paco_2$.

        A small-bore needle is less likely to cause vasospasm of the artery during the procedure.

   B. Eliminate any visible air bubbles from syringe.

        Maintains accuracy of ABG values.

4. Don goggles and gloves.

        Reduces transmission of microorganisms and body secretions; standard precautions.

5. Prepare site, beginning with the alcohol pads. Starting at the insertion site, cleanse outward, using a circular motion while applying friction. Repeat. Continue cleansing in a similar fashion using the two povidone-iodine pads.

        Limits the introduction of potentially infectious skin flora into the vessel during the puncture. Combination of cleansing solutions enhances the antibacterial and antifungal actions of the agents.

        The povidone-iodine solution should not be removed. Drying is not necessary. Application time (at least 30 seconds) is the chemical kill.

6. Locally anesthetize the puncture site. *(Level IV: Limited clinical studies to support recommendations)*

        Provides local anesthesia for arterial puncture.

        It has been reported that most patients experience pain during arterial puncture.[6]

   A. Use a 1-mL syringe with a 25-G needle to draw up 0.5 mL of 1% lidocaine without epinephrine.

        Minimizes vessel trauma. Absence of epinephrine decreases the risk of peripheral vasoconstriction.

        Research exploring the efficacy of lidocaine ointment and EMLA cream as alternatives to intradermal lidocaine shows promising results.[7–9] If used, the manufacturer's recommendations should be followed.

   B. Aspirate before injecting the local anesthetic.

        Determines whether or not a blood vessel has been inadvertently entered.

   C. Inject intradermally and then with full infiltration around artery puncture site. Use approximately 0.2 to 0.3 mL for an adult.

        Decreases the incidence of localized pain while injecting all skin layers. Most patients reported a *reduction* in pain when a local, intradermal anesthetic agent was used prior to arterial puncture.[6]

▪▪ AP This procedure should be performed only by physicians, advanced practice nurses, and other health care professionals (including critical care nurses) with additional knowledge, skills, and demonstrated competence per professional licensure or institutional standard.

Procedure continued on following page

Steps	Rationale	Special Considerations

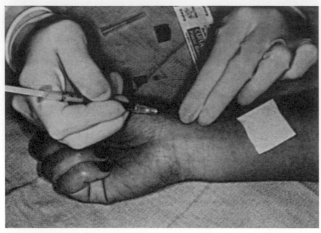

■ ● **FIGURE 72–4.** Radial artery puncture.

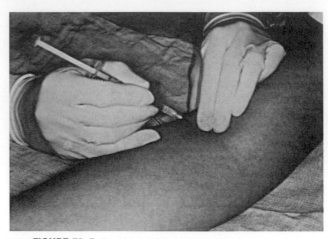

■ ● **FIGURE 72–5.** Brachial artery puncture.

7. Perform percutaneous puncture of the selected artery.

A. Palpate and stabilize the artery with the index and middle fingers of nondominant hand. | Increases the likelihood of correctly locating the artery and decreases chance of vessel rolling. | Use sterile gloves if site of artery puncture is palpated after it is antiseptically prepared.

B. With the needle bevel up and the syringe at a 30- to 60-degree angle to the radial or brachial artery, puncture skin slowly (Fig. 72–4 and 72–5). For a femoral artery puncture, a 60- to 90-degree angle is used (Fig. 72–6). | A slow, gradual thrust will promote entry into the artery without inadvertently passing through the posterior wall. | Enter at an angle that is comfortable for your hand. Certainty of position is more important than angle entry. If too much force is used, the needle may touch the periosteum of the bone and cause considerable pain.

C. Observe syringe for flashback of blood. | Pulsation of blood into the syringe verifies that the artery has been punctured. | Flashback occurs more easily with a glass syringe than a plastic syringe. Gentle aspiration may be necessary with a plastic syringe.

D. If puncture is unsuccessful, withdraw needle to skin level, angle slightly toward artery, and readvance. Do not withdraw needle. | Prevents necessity of a second puncture and changes needle angle to facilitate location of artery. | Excessive probing of the artery may cause injury to it, as well as to the nerve.

8. Obtain 1 to 5 mL of blood. | More than 1 mL of blood allows for rechecking and additional studies, if necessary. | Sample volumes will vary with equipment used. An accurate ABG can be done on as little as 1 mL of blood.

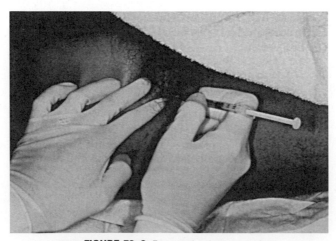

■ ● **FIGURE 72–6.** Femoral artery puncture.

Procedure **for Arterial Puncture** *Continued*

Steps	Rationale	Special Considerations
9. Withdraw needle while stabilizing barrel of syringe.	Prevents inadvertent aspiration of air during withdrawal.	Equipment may vary. Should a safety guard be available, it should be snapped onto the needle using a one-handed technique by gently pressing the device against a hard surface.
10. Press a gauze pad firmly over the puncture site for at least 5 minutes or until hemostasis is established.[1] Never ask the patient to assist in applying the pressure. Cover puncture site with adhesive bandage once hemostasis is achieved.[1, 10]	Hematomas and hemorrhage can occur if pressure is not applied and maintained correctly. Hematomas can cause circulatory impedance and pain and can predispose to infection. The patient's status can be unpredictable, and he or she should not be involved in this aspect of the procedure. If the patient fails to apply and maintain pressure, the risk of hematoma and hemorrhage increases.	If patient is receiving anticoagulation therapy or has a bleeding dyscrasia, pressure may need to be applied for as long as 15 minutes. If bleeding persists, an ice pack can be placed over the site while maintaining firm pressure.
11. Check syringe for air bubbles and express any air bubbles by slowly ejecting some of the blood onto a 2-in × 2-in gauze pad.	Air bubbles can alter the PaO_2 results.	If a safety guard is present, it should be removed and a blood/air filter should be placed on the syringe. Excess air should be evacuated through the blood/air filter.
12. Seal the needle or tip of syringe immediately using a rubber stopper or cap, respectively. Gently roll the syringe for 30 seconds.	Prevents leakage of blood and air from entering the sample. Mixes blood and heparin, thus preventing clot formation.	
13. Immerse sample into ice in plastic bag and prepare to transport to laboratory.[1, 10]	Ice decreases temperature of sample to 4°C. This slows oxygen metabolism and may enhance accuracy of results.	Follow hospital policy regarding necessity of the use of ice for ABG samples.
14. Label specimen and complete laboratory form per instutional protocol. Note the percent of oxygen therapy, respiratory rate, and ventilator settings, if appropriate, as well as the patient's temperature and time the specimen was drawn.	Helps the laboratory to perfom the analysis accurately.	Policies may vary regarding the type of patient information required for laboratory analysis.
15. Expedite delivery of sample to laboratory.	Ideally, blood gas analysis should be performed within 10 minutes of collection to ensure accuracy of results.[10]	
16. Dispose of used supplies properly, and wash hands.	Reduces transmission of microorganisms; standard precautions.	

Expected Outcomes	**Unexpected Outcomes**
• ABG sample is collected correctly such that accuracy of results is enhanced.	• Pain/severe discomfort during procedure
• Puncture site remains free of hematoma, hemorrhage, and infection.	• Complication during the puncture: vasospasm
• Neurovascular system remains intact (free of complications).	• Complications following the puncture: changes in the color, size, temperature, sensation, or pulse of extremity used for arterial puncture; hematoma, hemorrhage, or infection at puncture site
• Alterations in ABGs are identified and treated accordingly.	

██ AP This procedure should be performed only by physicians, advanced practice nurses, and other health care professionals (including critical care nurses) with additional knowledge, skills, and demonstrated competence per professional licensure or institutional standard.

Patient Monitoring and Care	Rationale	Reportable Conditions
		These conditions should be reported if they persist despite nursing interventions.
1. Observe puncture site for signs of hemostasis postprocedure.	Postpuncture bleeding can occur in any patient but is more likely to occur in patients with coagulopathies or patients who are receiving anticoagulation therapy.	• Excessive bleeding, hematoma • Changes in vital signs
2. Assess the puncture site and involved extremity for signs of postpuncture complications.	Arterial puncture can result in neurovascular compromise of the extremity distal to the puncture site.	• Changes in color, size, temperature, sensation, movement, or pulse in the extremity used for arterial puncture
3. Monitor puncture site for signs of local infection.	Infection related to the procedure may result from failure to maintain asepsis during puncture. Use of the femoral site for puncture may be related to increased incidence of local infection.	• Erythema, warmth, hardness, tenderness, or pain at puncture site • Presence of purulent drainage from puncture site

Documentation

Documentation should include the following:

- Patient and family education
- Results of the modified Allen test
- Arterial site used
- Local anesthetic used (if applicable)
- Patient's tolerance of procedure
- Patient's temperature and amount and type of oxygen therapy
- Postpuncture site assessment and care
- Disposition of sample, results, and analysis
- Unexpected outcomes
- Additional nursing interventions

References

1. Buffington S. Specimen collection and testing. In: *Nursing Procedures.* 2nd ed. Springhouse, Pa: Springhouse Corp; 1996:145–147.
2. Hadaway LC. Anatomy and physiology related to intravenous therapy. In: Terry J, Baranowski L, Lonsway RA, Hedric C, eds. *Intravenous Therapy: Clinical Principles and Practice.* Philadelphia, Pa: W.B. Saunders; 1995:97.
3. Okeson GC, Wulbrecht PH. The safety of brachial artery puncture for arterial blood sampling. *Chest.* 1998;14:748–751.
4. Perucca R. Obtaining vascular access. In: Terry J, Baranowski L, Lonsway RA, Hedric C, eds. *Intravenous Therapy: Clinical Principles and Practice.* Philadelphia, Pa: W.B. Saunders; 1995:386.
5. Giner J, Casan P, Belda J, et al. Pain during arterial puncture. *Chest.* 1996;110:1443–1445.
6. Cummins RO, ed. *Advanced Cardiac Life Support.* Dallas, Tx: American Heart Association; 1997:13.9–13.10.
7. Hussey VM, Poulin MV, Fain JA. Effectiveness of lidocaine hydrochloride on venipuncture sites. *AORN J.* 1997;66:472–475.
8. Lander J, Nazarali S, Hodgins M, et al. Evaluation of a new topical anesthetic agent: A pilot study. *Nurs Res.* 1996;45:50–52.
9. Nott M, Peacock J. Relief of injection pain in adults: EMLA cream for 5 minutes before venepuncture. *Anaesthesia.* 1990;45:772–774.
10. Flynn JC. Special collection procedures. In: Flynn JC, ed. *Procedures in Phlebotomy.* 2nd ed. Philadelphia, Pa: W.B. Saunders, 1999:124–125.

Additional Readings

Flynn JC. *Procedures in Phlebotomy.* 2nd ed. Philadelphia, Pa: W.B. Saunders; 1999.
Nursing Procedures. 2nd ed. Springhouse, Pa: Springhouse Corp; 1996.
Potter PA, Perry AG, eds. *Basic Nursing: A Critical Thinking Approach.* 4th ed. St. Louis, Mo: Mosby; 1999.
Terry J, Baranowski L, Lonsway RA, Hedrick C, eds. *Intravenous Therapy: Clinical Principles and Practice.* Philadelphia, Pa: W.B. Saunders; 1995.

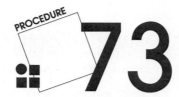
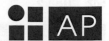
Central Venous Catheter Insertion (Perform)

P U R P O S E: Central venous catheters are inserted to measure and obtain right atrial pressure (RAP) and central venous pressure (CVP). Clinically useful information can be obtained about right ventricular function, cardiovascular status, and fluid balance in patients who do not require pulmonary artery pressure monitoring. Central venous catheters also are placed for infusion of vasoactive medications, total parenteral nutrition, and hemodialysis access.[1, 2] In addition, central venous catheters are used to administer medication and intravenous (IV) products to patients with limited peripheral IV access.

Desiree A. Fleck

PREREQUISITE NURSING KNOWLEDGE

- Understanding of the normal anatomy and physiology of the cardiovascular system is needed.
- Clinical and technical competence in central line insertion and suturing is necessary.
- Principles of sterile technique should be understood.
- Knowledge of the anatomy and physiology of the vasculature and adjacent structures of the neck is required.
- Competence in chest x-ray interpretation is needed.
- Advanced cardiac life support knowledge and skills are necessary.
- Indications for a CVP line include the following:
  - ❖ Blood loss
  - ❖ Hypotension following major surgery
  - ❖ Right ventricular ischemia or infarction
  - ❖ Hemodialysis access
  - ❖ Total parenteral nutrition
  - ❖ Lack of peripheral venous access
  - ❖ Assessment of hypovolemia or hypervolemia
- The CVP is particularly helpful after major surgery, during active bleeding.
- The CVP is helpful in differentiating right ventricular failure from left ventricular failure. The CVP is commonly elevated during or following right ventricular failure, ischemia, or infarction because of decreased compliance of the right ventricle while the pulmonary artery wedge pressure is normal.[1–3]
- The CVP can be helpful in determining hypovolemia. The CVP value is low if the patient is hypovolemic. Venodilation also decreases CVP.

- Relative contraindications of CVP line insertion include the following:
  - ❖ Fever
  - ❖ Coagulopathies
  - ❖ Presence of pacemakers
- The CVP provides information regarding right heart filling pressures and right ventricular function and volume.
- CVP can be measured using a water manometer system (see Procedure 62) or via a hemodynamic monitoring system (see Procedures 62 and 69).
- The CVP waveform is identical to the right atrial pressure (RAP) waveform.
- The normal CVP value is 2 to 6 mm Hg.
- ECG monitoring is essential in determining accurate interpretation of the CVP value.
- Understanding of a, c, and v waves: the a wave reflects right atrial contraction; the c wave reflects closure of tricuspid valve; and the v wave reflects right atrial filling during ventricular systole (see Fig. 74–1).
- Dysrhythmias may alter CVP or RA pressure waveforms.
- Central venous access may be obtained in a variety of sites (see Table 73–1).[6]
  - ❖ The risk of a pneumothorax is minimized by using an internal jugular vein. The preferred site for catheter insertion is the right internal jugular vein. The right internal jugular vein is a "straight shot" to the right atrium.
  - ❖ The right or left subclavian veins are also sites for central catheter placement. Placement of a central catheter through the right subclavian vein is a shorter and more direct route than the left subclavian vein, because it does not cross the midline of the thorax.[2]
  - ❖ Femoral veins may be accessed but have the strong disadvantage of forcing the patient to be on bedrest with immobilization of that leg.
- Presence of pacemakers may alter choices in placement of CVP lines, because there is a risk of dislodging pacemaker leads when inserting CVP lines.

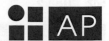

Table 73–1 ■■■ **Sites, Complications, and Success Rates**

Access Site	Complications	Success Rates (%)
Internal jugular vein	Carotid artery puncture Carotid artery cannulation	60–90
Right subclavian vein	Pneumothorax Tension pneumothorax Thoracic duct puncture Decreased success rate with inexperience	70–98
Left subclavian vein	Pneumothorax Tension pneumothorax Thoracic duct puncture Decreased success rate with inexperience	70–98

Femoral vein	Infection
	Arterial puncture
	Failure rate during
	  hypotension and shock
	Inability to thread central
	  catheters
		75–99

- Complications may occur during or after insertion of a central venous catheter (Tables 73–1 and 74–1).

EQUIPMENT

- Basic phlebotomy kit or CVP insertion kit
- Catheter of choice (single, dual, or triple lumen) usually supplied with insertion needle, syringe, and guidewire
- Sterile towels
- 1% lidocaine without epinephrine
- One 25-G 5/8 needle
- Large package of 4×4 gauze sponges
- Suture kit (hemostat, scissors, needle holder)
- 3-0 or 4-0 nylon suture with curved needle
- Three-way stopcock
- Syringes: one 10- to 12-mL syringe, two 3- to 5-mL syringes, two 22-G, 1½-in needles
- Masks, caps, goggles (shield and mask combination may be used), sterile gloves, and sterile gowns
- Number 11 scalpel
- Package of alcohol pads or swabsticks
- Package of povidone-iodine pads or swabsticks
- Skin protectant pad or swabstick
- Roll of 2-in tape
- Dressing supplies
- Moisture-proof underpad
- Antiseptic solution
- Nonsterile gloves
- 0.9% sodium chloride, 10–30 mL

Additional equipment as needed includes the following:

- Hemodynamic monitoring system (see Procedure 69)
- IV solution with Luer-Lok administration set for IV infusion
- Luer-Lok extension tubing
- Bedside monitor and oscilloscope

PATIENT AND FAMILY EDUCATION

- Assess patient and family understanding of CVP and explain need for CVP insertion. ➥*Rationale:* Clarification and understanding of information decreases patient and family anxiety levels.
- Explain procedure and time involved. ➥*Rationale:* Increases patient's cooperation and decreases patient and family anxiety levels.
- Explain the need for sterlie technique and that the patient's face may be covered. ➥*Rationale:* Decreases patient anxiety and elicits cooperation.

PATIENT ASSESSMENT AND PREPARATION
Patient Assessment

- Determine past medical history of pneumothorax/emphysema. ➥*Rationale:* Emphysematous lungs may be at increased risk for puncture and pneumothorax, depending on the approach.
- Determine past medical history of anomalous veins. ➥*Rationale:* Patients may have history of dextracardia or transposition of great vessels, leading to greater difficulty in placing the catheter.
- Assess intended insertion site. ➥*Rationale:* Scar tissue may impede placement of catheter. Previous surgery and previous placement of CVP may cause a thrombus to be present.
- Assess cardiac and pulmonary status. ➥*Rationale:* Some patients may not tolerate a supine or Trendelenburg position for extended periods.
- Assess vital signs and pulse oximetry. ➥*Rationale:* Provides baseline data.
- Assess electrolyte levels. ➥*Rationale:* Electrolyte abnormalities may increase cardiac irritability.
- Assess for heparin sensitivity or allergy.[5] ➥*Rationale:* Central venous catheters are heparin bonded, although non–heparin-bonded catheters are available. If patient has a heparin allergy or has a history of heparin-induced thrombocytopenia, use a non–heparin-coated catheter.
- Assess coagulopathic status or recent anticoagulant or thrombolytic therapy. ➥*Rationale:* These patients are more likely to have complications related to bleeding.

Patient Preparation

- Ensure that the patient and family understand preprocedural teaching. Answer questions as they arise and reinforce information as needed. ➥*Rationale:* Evaluates and reinforces understanding of previously taught information.
- Obtain informed consent. ➥*Rationale:* Protects the rights of the patient and makes a competent decision possible for the patient; however, under emergency circumstances, time may not allow for this form to be signed.
- Prescribe sedation if needed. ➥*Rationale:* Patient may need sedation to ensure adequate cooperation and appropriate placement. During the procedure, restlessness and altered level of consciousness may represent a pneumothorax, hypoxia, or placement in the carotid artery.
- Place patient in supine position and prep area with povidone-iodine solution or alcohol if the patient is allergic to iodine (see Fig. 74–2). ➥*Rationale:* Prepare access sites for central venous catheter insertion. Decreases risk of infection.
- If patient is obese or muscular and the preferred site is the internal jugular vein or subclavian vein, place towel posteriorly between shoulder blades. ➥*Rationale:* Helps extend the neck and provide better access to subclavian and internal jugular veins.
- Drape sterile drapes over prepped area. ➥*Rationale:* Provides aseptic work area.

Procedure for Central Venous Catheter Insertion (Perform)

Steps	Rationale	Special Considerations

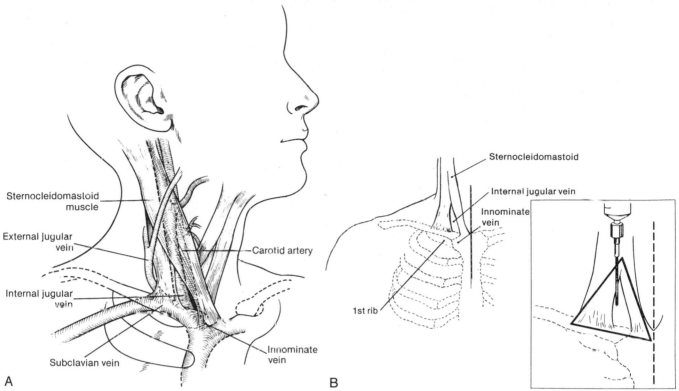

FIGURE 73–1. Anatomy of internal jugular vein. *A,* Anatomy of the internal jugular vein showing its lower location within the triangle formed by the sternocleidomastoid muscle and the clavicle. *B,* Relationship of external anatomic landmarks to underlying internal jugular vein. Triangle drawn over clavicle and sternal and clavicular portions of the sternocleidomastoid muscle is centered over internal jugular vein *(inset).* (From Dailey EK, Schroeder JS. *Techniques in Bedside Hemodynamic Monitoring.* St. Louis, Mo: C.V. Mosby; 1994. Daily PO, Griepp RB, Shumway NE. Percutaneous internal jugular vein cannulation. *Arch Surg.* 1970; 101:534–536. Copyright 1970 American Medical Association.)

Steps	Rationale	Special Considerations
1. Determine anatomy of access site.	Helps ensure proper placement of catheter.	
2. Wash hands, and don caps, masks, sterile gowns and gloves for all health care personnel involved with procedure.	Reduces transmission of microorganisms and body secretions; standard precautions.	
3. Check landmarks again for intended catheter insertion site.	Ensures proper placement of catheter.	
4. Estimate the length of catheter needed. This can be done by holding catheter from insertion site to sternal notch.	Helps ensure proper placement.	

Internal Jugular Vein (Fig. 73–1)

Steps	Rationale	Special Considerations
1. Locate the carotid artery by palpation.	Helps prevent placing the sheath in the carotid artery.	
2. Identify the jugular vein and mark it if necessary.	Identifies intended insertion site.	

AP This procedure should be performed only by physicians, advanced practice nurses, and other health care professionals (including critical care nurses) with additional knowledge, skills, and demonstrated competence per professional licensure or institutional standard.

Procedure continued on following page

Procedure **for Central Venous Catheter Insertion (Perform)** *Continued*

Steps	Rationale	Special Considerations
3. Turn the patient's head to the contralateral side.	Helps identify the landmarks.	
4. Place the patient in a 15- to 25-degree Trendelenburg position.	Helps to decrease risk of air embolism. Helps engorge the veins to help identify correct site.	
5. Identify the internal jugular vein from the triangle between the medial aspect of the clavicle, the medial aspect of the sternal head, and the lateral head of the sternocleidomastoid muscle (see Fig. 73–1).	A high entry can be made from a posterior approach, a lateral approach, an anterior approach, or a central approach.	
6. Administer a local anesthetic and locate the internal jugular vein with a small needle 3 to 4 cm above the medial clavicle and 1 to 2 cm within the lateral border of the sternocleido-mastoid muscle.	Provides patient comfort and aids in insertion.	
7. Attach a 3- or 5-mL syringe with 2 or 3 mL 1% lidocaine to the 18-G needle. Align the needle with the syringe parallel to the medial border of the clavicular head of the sternocleido-mastoid muscle. Aim at a 30-degree angle to the frontal plane over the internal jugular vein, toward the ipsilateral nipple.	Helps to anesthetize below the subcutaneous tissue. If the needle bevel is directed medially, the bevel aids in directing the guidewire medially.	
8. Use the Seldinger technique for placement of the catheter (Fig. 73–2).	This technique is the preferred method of central venous catheter placement. This technique uses a dilator and guidewire.	
9. Puncture the skin and advance the needle while maintaining slight negative pressure until free flow of blood is obtained.	Slight negative pressure helps to ensure placement into the vein and decreases the risk of air embolism and pneumothorax.	If free flow of blood is not obtained, remove and redirect the needle 5 to 10 degrees more laterally.
10. After free flow of blood is obtained, have the patient hold his or her breath or hum while the syringe is detached and insert the soft-tipped guidewire 10 to 15 cm through the needle. Remove the needle, wipe the guidewire with the sterile 4 × 4 gauze, and instruct the patient to breathe normally.	Free flow of blood indicates the needle is in the vessel. Holding the breath or humming decreases risk of air embolus.	
11. With a number 11 blade, make a small (2- to 3-mm) stab wound at insertion site.	Eases insertion of introducer through the skin.	
12. Insert the dilator through the skin, over the guidewire, until 10 to 15 cm of wire extends beyond the dilator. Remove the dilator.	Dilator enlarges the vessel and skin opening, easing the insertion of the introducer.	
13. Insert the catheter over the guidewire until 10 to 15 cm of wire extends beyond the catheter. Remove guidewire. Advance catheter. Note catheter length at insertion site.		
14. Aspirate and flush the ports with normal saline.	Prevents clotting of line. Helps secure catheter.	
15. Connect to hemodynamic monitoring system (see Procedure 69) or intravenous fluid.	Necessary for pressure monitoring or line patency.	
16. Suture the line in place.	Secures the catheter.	

| Procedure | **for Central Venous Catheter Insertion (Perform)** *Continued* |

Steps	Rationale	Special Considerations

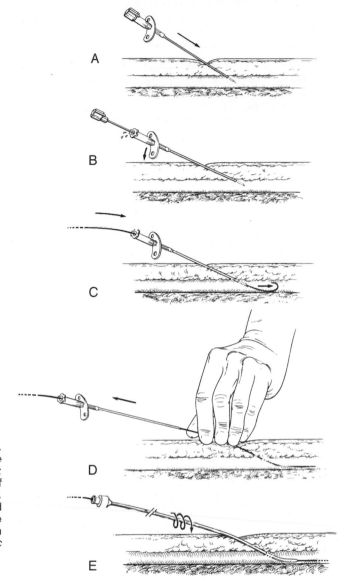

▪ ● **FIGURE 73–2.** Basic procedure for Seldinger technique. *A,* The vessel is punctured with the needle at a 30- to 40-degree angle. *B,* The stylet is removed, and free blood flow is observed; the angle of the needle is then reduced. *C,* The flexible tip of the guidewire is passed through the needle into the vessel. *D,* The needle is removed over the wire while firm pressure is applied at the site. *E,* The tip of the catheter or sheath is passed over the wire and advanced into the vessel with a rotating motion. (From Dailey EK, Schroeder JS. *Techniques in Bedside Hemodynamic Monitoring.* St. Louis, Mo: C.V. Mosby; 1994.)

Steps	Rationale	Special Considerations
17. Apply dry, sterile dressing.	Decreases risk of infection.	
18. Return patient to neutral or head-up position.	Provides comfort.	
19. If monitoring, identify appropriate waveforms (see Procedure 62).	Ensures accurate monitoring of values.[7]	
20. Assess lung sounds and obtain chest x-ray	Confirms placement and assesses for pneumothorax.	The x-ray needs to be read before administration of total parenteral nutrition or chemotherapeutic agents.

Subclavian Vein (Fig. 73–3)

1. Identify the junction of the middle and medial thirds of the clavicle. Needle insertion should be 1 to 2 cm laterally.	Identifies landmarks for catheter placement.	

▪▪ AP   This procedure should be performed only by physicians, advanced practice nurses, and other health care professionals (including critical care nurses) with additional knowledge, skills, and demonstrated competence per professional licensure or institutional standard.

Procedure continued on following page

Procedure	**for Central Venous Catheter Insertion (Perform)** *Continued*	

Steps	**Rationale**	**Special Considerations**
2. Depress the area 1 to 2 cm beneath the junction with the thumb of nondominant hand and the index finger 2 cm above the sternal notch.		To avoid the subclavian artery, select a puncture site away from most lateral course of vein and do not aim too posteriorly.
3. Administer local anesthetic and locate the vein with 21- to 25-G needle directed to index finger at 20- to 30-degree angle. Have the patient turn his or her head to contralateral side.	Provides patient comfort and assists patient cooperation and ease of insertion. Extends vein to ease location.	
4. Use the Seldinger technique for placement of the catheter (see Fig. 73–2).	This technique is the preferred method of cental venous catheter placement. This technique uses a dilator and guidewire.	
5. Insert the needle under the clavicle and "walk down" until it slips below the clavicle into the vein while maintaining negative pressure within the syringe until free flowing blood is returned (Fig. 73–4).	Decreases risk of pneumothorax. Slight negative pressure helps to ensure placement into the vein and decreases the risk of air embolism and pneumothorax.	Insert at 45-degree angle to prevent pneumothorax. If it is difficuilt to depress the needle down, the needle may be bent to form an arc. For the elderly: the subclavian vein may be more inferior.
6. When free flow of blood is returned, turn the bevel to the 3 o'clock position. Once in the vein, remove the syringe and insert the flexible guidewire after asking patient to hum or hold his or her breath.	Free flow of blood indicates a vein is entered. Turning the bevel helps the guidewire advance to the correct position. Holding the breath or humming decreases the risk of air embolus.	Risk of pneumothorax can be reduced by avoiding a too lateral or too deep a needle insertion.

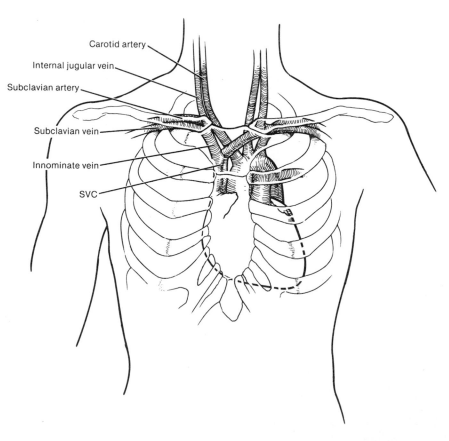

Carotid artery
Internal jugular vein
Subclavian artery
Subclavian vein
Innominate vein
SVC

■ ● **FIGURE 73–3.** Anatomic location of subclavian vein and surrounding structures. The subclavian vein joins the internal jugular vein to become the innominate vein at about the manubrioclavicular junction. The innominate vein becomes the superior vena cava (SVC) at about the level of the midmanubrium. (From Dailey EK, Schroeder JS. *Techniques in Bedside Hemodynamic Monitoring.* St. Louis, Mo: C.V. Mosby; 1994.)

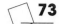

Procedure **for Central Venous Catheter Insertion (Perform)** *Continued*		
Steps	**Rationale**	**Special Considerations**

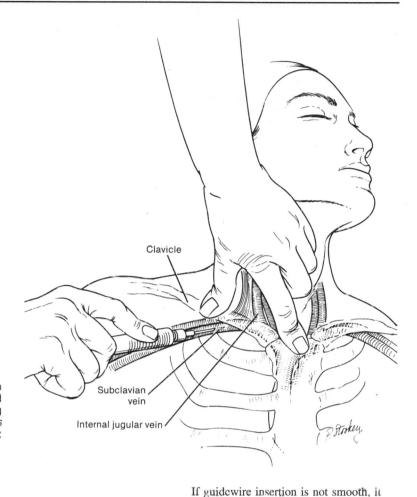

■ ● **FIGURE 73–4.** Puncture of the subclavian vein with the needle inserted beneath the middle third of the clavicle at a 20- to 30-degree angle aiming medially. (From Dailey EK, Schroeder JS. *Techniques In Bedside Hemodynamic Monitoring.* St. Louis, Mo: C.V. Mosby; 1994.)

Steps	Rationale	Special Considerations
7. Insert the guidewire 10 to 15 cm through the needle and remove the needle.		If guidewire insertion is not smooth, it may be in the internal jugular vein.
8. Advance the dilator over the guidewire into the vein, using a light twisting motion.	This aids dilation of subcutaneous tissue to ease insertion and prevents the formation of a false channel.	
9. Remove the dilator from the wire.		
10. Insert the catheter of choice over the guidewire, then remove the guidewire.		Aspirate and flush the ports with normal saline.
11. Suture the line in place.	Secures the catheter.	
12. Connect the catheter to the hemodynamic monitoring system (see Procedure 69) or to intravenous fluid.	Necessary for pressure monitoring or line patency.	
13. Apply an occlusive, sterile dressing to site.	Decreases risk of infection.	
14. If monitoring, identify appropriate waveforms (see Procedure 62).	Ensures accurate monitoring of values.[7]	

AP This procedure should be performed only by physicians, advanced practice nurses, and other health care professionals (including critical care nurses) with additional knowledge, skills, and demonstrated competence per professional licensure or institutional standard.

Procedure continued on following page

Procedure	**for Central Venous Catheter Insertion (Perform)** *Continued*

Steps	Rationale	Special Considerations
15. Assess lung sounds and obtain a chest x-ray.	Confirms placement and assesses for pneumothorax.	X-ray must be read before administration of total parenteral nutrition or chemotherapeutic agents.

Femoral Vein (Fig. 72–2)

Steps	Rationale	Special Considerations
1. Identify anatomy, including femoral artery (remember NAVEL).	NAVEL is an acronym for remembering anatomy (*N*erve, *A*rtery, *V*ein, *E*mpty space, *L*igament; from lateral to medial).	
2. Administer local anesthetic and locate the vein with a 21- to 25-G needle lateral to femoral artery. Aim the needle at a 20- to 30-degree angle.	Anesthetizes the area to provide patient comfort.	
3. Attach a 3- or 5-mL syringe with 2 or 3 mL 1% lidocaine to the 18-G needle.	Anesthetizes the area to provide patient comfort.	
4. Use the Seldinger technique for placement of the catheter (see Fig. 73–2).	This technique is the preferred method of central venous catheter placement. This technique uses a dilator and guidewire.	
5. Puncture the skin and advance the needle while maintaining slight negative pressure until free flow of blood is obtained.	Negative pressure helps to identify free flow of blood and ensure proper placement into the vein.	If free flow of blood is not obtained, remove and redirect the needle 5 to 10 degrees more laterally.
6. After free flow of blood is obtained, detach the syringe and insert a soft-tipped guidewire through the needle 10 to 15 cm. Remove the needle and wipe the guidewire with sterile 4 × 4 gauze.	Free flow of blood indicates that the vessel has been accessed.	
7. With a number 11 blade, make a small (2- to 3-mm) stab wound at insertion site.	Eases insertion of the introducer through the skin.	
8. Insert the dilator over the guidewire until 10 to 15 cm of wire extends beyond the sheath. Advance the dilator through the skin.	Dilator dilates the vessel and skin to assist in the ease of the introducer insertion.	
9. Remove the dilator.		
10. Insert the catheter of choice over the guidewire and into the vein, then remove the guidewire.	Aspirate and flush the ports with normal saline.	
11. Suture the catheter in place.	Secures the catheter.	
12. Connect to hemodynamic monitoring system or to intravenous fluid.	Necessary for pressure montioring or line patency.	
13. Apply an occlusive, sterile dressing.	Decreases risk of infection.	
14. Identify appropriate waveforms (see Procedure 62).	Ensures accurate monitoring of values.[7]	

Arm Vein (Fig. 73–5)

Steps	Rationale	Special Considerations
1. Identify the median basilic vein.	Identifies site for catheter placement.	The basilic vein is deeper and ascends along the unlar surface of the forearm, joined by median cubital vein in front of the elbow.

Procedure	**for Central Venous Catheter Insertion (Perform)** *Continued*

Steps	Rationale	Special Considerations

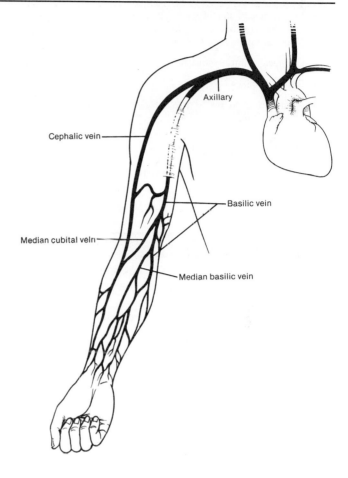

■ ● FIGURE 73–5. Anatomy of arm veins. (From Dailey EK, Schroeder JS. *Techniques in Bedside Hemodynamic Monitoring.* St. Louis, Mo: C.V. Mosby, 1994.)

Steps	Rationale	Special Considerations
2. Further patient preparation includes applying a tourniquet to locate the vein. Abduct the selected arm 30 to 45 degrees and secure it on a flat, padded arm board resting on a flat surface.	Aids preparation.	
3. Use the Seldinger technique for placement of the catheter (see Fig. 73–2).	This technique is the preferred method of central venous catheter placement. This technique uses a dilator and guidewire.	
4. Apply a venous tourniquet to upper arm. Maintain traction on the skin distal to the insertion with one hand; puncture the vein with the needle bevel up at a 15- to 20-degree angle.	Allows for better visualization of veins. Helps with insertion and prevents the needle from penetrating too deeply.	Do not attempt to place a central venous catheter in a vein that cannot be seen or palpated.
5. When blood appears in the needle, insert the guidewire into the vein approximately 2 to 4 cm beyond the tip.		If resistance is met, do not force the catheter to advance. Withdraw the catheter 2 to 3 cm, rotate it, and readvance it.
6. Release tourniquet and advance the guidewire several centimeters. Remove the needle; wipe the guidewire with sterile 4 × 4 gauze.		

Procedure continued on following page

Procedure	**for Central Venous Catheter Insertion (Perform)** *Continued*	
Steps	**Rationale**	**Special Considerations**
7. Insert the catheter of choice over the guidewire. Remove the guidewire. Note centimeter mark at skin.		Aspirate and flush the ports with normal saline.
8. Connect to intravenous fluid.	Maintains line patency.	
9. Suture in place.	Secures the line.	
10. Apply an occlusive, sterile dressing to insertion site.	Reduces the incidence of infection.	
11. Immobilize on arm board.	Ensures that minimal movement of catheter and sheath occurs.	
12. Discard supplies, and wash hands.	Reduces transmission of microorganisms; standard precautions.	

Expected Outcomes

- Placement of central venous catheter is successful.
- If infusing IV solution, the solution infuses without problems.
- The a, c, and v waves are identified on hemodynamic monitoring.
- CVP measurement is determined via hemodynamic monitoring.

Unexpected Outcomes

- Pain or severe discomfort during the insertion procedure
- Pneumothorax, tension pneumothorax, or hemothorax
- Nerve injury
- Sterile thrombophlebitis
- Infection
- Cardiac dysrhythmias
- Misplacement (eg, carotid artery, subclavian artery)
- Hemorrhage
- Hematoma
- Venous air embolism
- Pulmonary embolus
- Cardiac tamponade
- Sepsis
- Heparin-induced thrombocytopenia or thrombosis

Patient Monitoring and Care

Patient Monitoring and Care	Rationale	Reportable Conditions
		These conditions should be reported if they persist despite nursing interventions.
1. Perform cardiovascular, peripheral vascular, and hemodynamic assessments immediately prior to and following the procedure and as the patient's condition necessitates.		
○ Level of consciousness	Assess for signs of adequate perfusion; air embolism may present with restlessness; patient may present with decreased level of consicousness if the catheter is advanced into carotid artery.	• Change in level of consciousness

Patient Monitoring and Care *Continued*

Patient Monitoring and Care	Rationale	Reportable Conditions
○ Vital signs, central venous waveform, central venous pressure	Changes in pressures may indicate change in volume status. Changes in waveforms may indicate change in right ventricular function or catheter migration.	• Changes in vital signs • Abnormal waveforms or pressures
2. Monitor site for hematoma and hemorrhage.	If patient is coagulopathic, a pressure dressing may be required.	• Bleeding that does not stop • Hematoma and expanding hematoma
3. Assess heart and lung sounds.	Abnormal heart or lung sounds may indicate cardiac tamponade, pneumothorax, or hemothorax.	• Diminished or muffled heart sounds • Absent or diminished breath sounds unilaterally
4. Assess results of chest x-ray.	Ensures adequate placement in the right atrium and identification of pneumothorax, if present.	• Abnormal x-ray results
5. Monitor for signs of complications.	May decrease mortality if recognized early.	• Signs and symptoms of complications

Documentation

Documentation should include the following:

- Patient and family education
- Informed consent
- Insertion of central venous catheter
- Insertion site of central venous catheter
- Vein selected and type and size of catheter placed
- Right atrial pressure and CVP waveform
- Central venous pressure values after insertion
- Centimeter mark at skin
- Patient tolerance
- Confirmation of placement (ie, chest x-ray)
- Occurrence of unexpected outcomes
- Additional nursing interventions

References

1. Dailey EK, Schroeder JS. *Techniques in Bedside Hemodynamic Monitoring.* 5th ed. St. Louis, Mo: C.V. Mosby; 1994.
2. Hurford WE, Zapol WM. The right ventricle and critical illness: a review of anatomy, physiology, and clinical evaluation of its function. *Intens Care Med.* 1988;14:448–457.
3. Sibbald WJ, Driedger AA. Right ventricular function in acute disease states: pathophysiologic consideration. *Crit Care Med.* 1983;11(5):339–345.
4. Venus B, Mallory DL. Vascular cannulation. In: *Critical Care.* 2nd ed. Philadelphia, Pa: J.B. Lippincott, 1992.
5. Silver D, Kapsch DN, Tsoi EK. Heparin-induced thrombocytopenia, thrombosis, and hemorrhage. *Ann Surg.* 1983;198:301–306.
6. Ahrens TS, Taylor LK. *Hemodynamic Waveform Analysis.* Philadelphia, Pa: W.B. Saunders; 1992.
7. Ahrens TS. Hemodynamic monitoring. *Crit Care Clin.* 1999;11:19–31.

Additional Readings

AACN. Evaluation of the effects of heparinized and nonheparinized flush solutions on the patency of arterial pressure monitoring lines: The AACN Thunder Project. *Am J Crit Care.* 1993;2:3–15.
Darovic GO. *Hemodynamic Monitoring Invasive and Noninvasive Clinical Application.* Philadelphia, Pa: W.B. Saunders, 1995.
Friesinger GC, Williams SV, the ACP/AHA Task Force on Clinical Privileges in Cardiology. Clinical competence in hemodynamic monitoring. *J Am Coll Cardiol.* 1990;15:1460.
Hilton E. Central catheter infections: single- versus triple-lumen catheters. *Am J Med.* 1988;84:667–672.
Marion PL. *The ICU Book.* Philadelphia, Pa: Lea & Febiger; 1991.

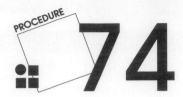

74

Central Venous Catheter Insertion (Assist)

P U R P O S E : Central venous catheters are inserted to measure and obtain right atrial pressure (RAP) and central venous pressure (CVP). Clinically useful information can be obtained about right ventricular function, cardiovascular status, and fluid balance in patients who do not require pulmonary artery pressure monitoring. Central venous catheters also are placed for infusion of vasoactive medications, total parenteral nutrition, and hemodialysis access.[1, 2] In addition, central venous catheters are used to administer medication and intravenous (IV) products to patients with limited peripheral IV access. The critical care nurse's role is to assist the physician or advanced practice nurse in the process of central venous catheter insertion.

Marie Arnone

PREREQUISITE NURSING KNOWLEDGE

- Understanding of the normal anatomy and physiology of the cardiovascular system is needed.
- Knowledge of the anatomy and physiology of the vasculature and adjacent structures of the neck is necessary.
- Basic dysrhythmia interpretation should be understood.
- Advanced cardiac life support knowledge and skills are needed.
- Indications for a central venous catheter include the following:
  ❖ Blood loss
  ❖ Hypotension following major surgery
  ❖ Right ventricular ischemia or infarction
  ❖ Hemodialysis access
  ❖ Total parenteral nutrition
  ❖ Lack of peripheral venous access
  ❖ Assessment of hypovolemia or hypervolemia
- Relative contraindications of CVP line insertion include the following:
  ❖ Fever
  ❖ Coagulopathies
  ❖ Presence of a pacemaker
- Site selection is based on vasculature of the patient. The most common sites include the internal jugular veins, subclavian veins, and the femoral veins.[1, 3, 4]
- Type of catheter inserted and purpose of insertion should be considered. Catheters may be single lumen or multiple lumen. Central venous catheters may be inserted for monitoring, infusion of medications, or parenteral nutrition.
- Principles of aseptic technique should be understood. Prevention of infection is a significant concern for patients with indwelling catheters.
- CVP can be measured using a water manometer system

(see Procedure 62) or via a hemodynamic monitoring system (see Procedures 62 and 69).
- The CVP provides information regarding right heart filling pressures and right ventricular function and volume.
- The normal CVP value is 2 to 6 mm Hg.
- ECG monitoring is essential in determining accurate interpretation of the CVP.
- Understanding of a, c, and v waves: the a wave reflects right atrial contraction; the c wave reflects closure of the tricuspid valve; the v wave reflects right atrial filling during ventricular systole (Fig. 74–1).
- Dysrhythmias may alter CVP or RAP waveforms.
- Complications may occur during or after insertion of a central venous catheter (Table 74–1).

EQUIPMENT

- Basic phlebotomy kit or CVP insertion kit
- Face masks, surgical caps, goggles (shield and mask combination may be used), sterile gloves and sterile gowns
- Moisture-proof underpad
- Antiseptic solution
- Nonsterile gloves
- Sterile towels
- Catheter of choice (single, dual, or triple lumen), usually supplied with insertion needle, syringe, and guidewire
- Number 11 scalpel
- Syringes: one 10- to 12-mL syringe, two 3- to 5-mL syringes, two 22-G, 1 ½-in needles
- Large package of 4×4 gauze sponges
- Three-way stopcock
- Suture kit (hemostat, scissors, needle holder)
- 3-0 or 4-0 nylon suture with curved needle
- Package of alcohol pads or swabsticks
- Package of povidone-iodine pads or swabsticks

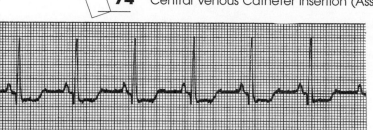

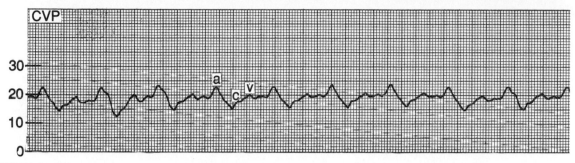

■ ● **FIGURE 74–1.** CVP waveform with *a*, *c*, and *v* waves present. The *a* wave is usually seen just after the P wave of the ECG. The *c* wave appears at the time of the RST junction on the ECG. The *v* wave is seen in the TP interval. CVP, central venous pressure; ECG, electrocardiogram.

- 1% lidocaine vial without epinephrine
- One 25-G ⅝-in needle
- 0.9% sodium chloride, 10 to 30 mL

- Skin protectant pads or swabsticks
- Roll of 2-in tape
- 2 × 2 gauze pad or transparent dressing

Additional equipment as needed includes the following:

- Hemodynamic monitoring system (see Procedure 69)
- IV solution with Luer-Lok administration set for IV infusion

- Luer-Lok extension tubing
- Bedside monitor and oscilloscope

PATIENT AND FAMILY EDUCATION

- Explain the procedure to the patient and family, and reinforce information given. ➤*Rationale:* Prepares the patient and family and reduces anxiety.
- Explain the required positioning for the procedure and the importance of not moving during the insertion. ➤*Rationale:* Encourages cooperation and reduces anxiety.
- Explain the need for sterile technique and that the patient's face may be covered. ➤*Rationale:* Decreases patient anxiety and elicits cooperation.

PATIENT ASSESSMENT AND PREPARATION
Patient Assessment

- Assess vital signs and pulse oximetry. ➤*Rationale:* Provides baseline data.
- Assess cardiac and pulmonary status. ➤*Rationale:* Some patients may not tolerate a supine or Trendelenburg position for extended periods.
- Assess coagulopathic status or recent anticoagulant or thrombolytic therapy. ➤*Rationale:* These patients are more likely to have complications related to bleeding.

Patient Preparation

- Ensure that the patient and family understand preprocedural teaching. Answer questions as they arise and reinforce information as needed. ➤*Rationale:* Evaluates and reinforces understanding of previously taught information.
- Ensure that informed consent was obtained. ➤*Rationale:* Protects the rights of the patient and makes a competent decision possible for the patient; however, under emergency circumstances, time may not allow for this form to be signed.
- If needed, perform endotracheal or tracheostomy suctioning on ventilated patients before the procedure. ➤*Rationale:* Minimizes the risk of contamination of the sterile field and the need to interrupt the procedure for suctioning.

Table 74–1 ●■■ **Complications of Central Venous Catheter Insertion**

Complication	Clinical Manifestation	Treatment	Prevention

Pneumothorax	Sudden respiratory distress
	Chest pain
	Hypoxia/cyanosis
	Decreased breath sounds
	Resonance to percussion
		Confirmation by chest x-ray
		Symptomatic treatment
		Small pneumothorax:
		  Bed rest
		  O_2
		Pneumothorax > 25%:
		  Chest tube
		  Cardiopulmonary support
			Proper patient preparation
			Sedation as necessary
			Proper patient positioning
			Adequate hydration status
			Low acuity of the angle of the needle on venipuncture
			Avoid multiple passes with the needle
			Clinician skilled and experienced in insertion technique
			Use of peripherally inserted central venous catheter

Tension pneumothorax	Most likely to occur in patients on ventilatory support
	Respiratory distress
	Rapid clinical deterioration:
	  Cyanosis
	  Venous distension
	  Hypotension
	  Decreased cardiac output
		Treatment must be rapid and aggressive
		Immediate air respiration followed by chest tube
		Cardiopulmonary support
			Proper patient preparation
			Sedation as necessary
			Proper patient positioning
			Adequate hydration status
			Reduction of PEEP $\leq$ 5 cm H_2O at time of venipuncture
			Low acuity of the angle of the needle on venipuncture
			Avoid multiple passes with the needle
			Clinician skilled and experienced in insertion technique
			Use of peripherally inserted central venous catheter

Delayed pneumothorax	Slow onset of respiratory symptoms Subcutaneous emphysema Persistent pleuritic chest or back pain	Confirmation by chest x-ray Chest tube Cardiopulmonary support	Proper patient preparation Sedation as necessary Proper patient positioning Adequate hydration status Low acuity of the angle of the needle on venipuncture Avoid multiple passes with the needle Clinician skilled and experienced in insertion technique Use of peripherally inserted central venous catheter
Hydrothorax hydromediastinum	Dyspnea Chest pain Muffled breath sounds High glucose level of chest drainage Low-grade fever	Stop infusion Confirmation by chest x-ray; contrast injection may be helpful Cardiopulmonary support	Proper patient preparation Sedation as necessary Proper patient positioning Adequate hydration status Low acuity of the angle of the needle on venipuncture Avoid multiple passes with the needle Clinician skilled and experienced in insertion technique Use of peripherally inserted central venous catheter Placement of catheter tip in lower superior vena cava
Hemothorax	Respiratory distress Hypovolemic shock Hematoma in the neck with jugular insertions	Confirmation by chest x-ray Chest tube Thoracotomy for arterial repair if indicated	Correct coagulopathies before insertion Adequate hydration status Avoid multiple passes with the needle Evaluation by venogram of suspected thrombosis from prior cannulation before insertion

Arterial puncture/laceration	Return of bright red blood in the syringe under high pressure
	Pulsatile blood flow on disconnection of the syringe
	Deterioration of clinical status:
	  Hemorrhagic shock
	  Respiratory distress
	Bleeding from catheter site may or may not be observed
	Deviation of trachea with large hematoma in the neck
	Hemothorax may be detected on chest x-ray
		Application of pressure for 3 to 5 minutes following removal of the needle
		Elevate head of bed
		Chest tube as indicated
		Thoracotomy for arterial repair if indicated
			Correct coagulopathies before insertion
			Adequate hydration status
			Avoid multiple passes with the needle
			Evaluation by venogram of suspected thrombosis from prior cannulation before insertion
			Use of small-gauge needle to first locate the vein

Table 74–1 ●■■ **Complications of Central Venous Catheter Insertion** *Continued*

Complication	Clinical Manifestation	Treatment	Prevention
Bleeding/hematoma, venous or arterial bleeding	Bleeding from insertion site Hematoma formation; not likely to be seen with subclavian approach Bleeding may occur internally without visible evidence Tracheal compression Respiratory distress Carotid compression	Application of pressure to the insertion site Thoracotomy for arterial repair Tracheostomy for tracheal deviation from hematoma	Correct coagulopathies before insertion Adequate hydration status Avoid multiple passes with the needle at venipuncture Use of small-gauge needle to first locate the vein

Cardiac dysrhythmias	Cardiac dysrhythmias:
	   Premature ventricular contractions
	   Supraventricular trachycardia
	   Ventricular trachycardia
	   Premature atrial contractions
	   Refractory atrial flutter
	   Sudden cardiovascular collapse
		Withdraw the guidewire or catheter from the heart
		Pharmacologic treatment of persistent arrhythmias
			Avoid entry into the heart with guidewire to catheter
			Observe cardiac monitor; tall peaked P waves can be identified as the catheter tip enters the right atrium
			Palpation of peripheral pulse (if not on ECG monitor)

Air embolism	Symptoms dependent on amount of air drawn in Sudden cardiovascular collapse Tachypnea, apnea, tachycardia Hypotension, cyanosis, anxiety Diffuse pulmonary wheezes "Mill wheel" churning heart murmur Neurologic deficits, paresis, stroke, coma Cardiac arrest	Stop airflow Position patient on left side with head down (Durant position) Oxygen administration Air aspiration; transthoracic needle or intracardiac catheter Cardiopulmonary support	Adequate hydration status Head-down tilt or Trendelenburg position during catheter insertion Use of small-bore needle for insertion Application of thumb over needle or catheter hub during disconnection; needle or hub should not be exposed longer than 1 second Advancement of catheter during positive-pressure cycle in patients on ventilatory support Avoid nicking of catheter with careful suturing technique Avoid catheter exchange from large-bore catheter (Swan-Ganz) to smaller catheter Use of Luer-Lok connections Minimal risk with peripherally inserted central venous catheter
Catheter malposition	Pain in ear or neck Swishing sound in ear with infusion Sharp anterior chest pain Pain in ipsilateral shoulder blade Cardiac dysrhythmia Observation on chest x-ray Signs or symptoms may be absent No blood return on aspiration	Position the patient in a high Fowler's position to allow gravity to correct jugular tip malposition Repositioning of catheter with guidewire under fluoroscopy or new venipuncture Catheter removal	Proper patient positioning Anthropometric measurement for accurate intravascular catheter length Avoid use of force when advancing the catheter Use of a guidewire or blunt-tipped stylet
Catheter embolism	Cardiac dysrhythmias Chest pain Dyspnea Hypotension Tachycardia May be clinically silent	Location of fragment on x-ray Transvenous retrieval of catheter fragment Thoracotomy	Use of "over a guidewire" (Seldinger) insertion technique Extreme caution with use of through-the-needle catheter designs; *never* withdraw a catheter through the needle Use of guidewire or stylet within a catheter that is inserted through a needle
Pericardial tamponade	Retrosternal or epigastric pain Dyspnea Venous engorgement of face and neck Restlessness, confusion Hypotension, paradoxical pulse Muffled heart sounds Mediastinal widening Pleural effusion Cardiac arrest	Treatment must be rapid and aggressive Discontinuation of infusions Aspiration through the catheter Emergency pericardiocentesis Emergency thoracotomy Slow withdrawal of catheter with contrast injection to detect residual myocardial leak	Catheter tip position: Parallel to the walls of the superior vena cava 1 to 2 cm above the junction of the superior vena cava and right atrium Use of soft, flexible catheters Minimal risk with peripherally inserted central venous catheter
Tracheal injury	Subcutaneous emphysema Pneumomediastinum Air trapping between the chest wall and the pleura Respiratory distress with puncture of endotracheal tube cuff	Emergency reintubation (for punctured endotracheal tube cuff) Aspiration of air in mediastinum	Clinician skilled and experienced in insertion techniques Use of peripherally inserted central venous catheter

Table continued on following page

Table 74–1 ● ■ ■   **Complications of Central Venous Catheter Insertion** *Continued*

Complication	Clinical Manifestation	Treatment	Prevention
Nerve injury	Patient complaints of tingling/ numbness in arm or fingers Shooting pain down the arm Paralysis Diaphragmatic paralysis (phrenic nerve injury)	Remove catheter if suspected brachial plexus injury	Clinician skilled and experienced in insertion technique Minimal risk with peripherally inserted central venous catheter
Sterile thrombophlebitis	Potential complication of the peripherally inserted central venous catheter Redness, tenderness, swelling along the course of the vein Pain in the upper extremity or shoulder	Application of heat for 48 to 72 hours Removal of catheter	Thorough washing of gloves prior to handling Silastic catheters Strict aseptic technique during catheter insertion Adequate skin preparation Atraumatic insertion
Pulmonary embolism	Potential complication of catheter exchange Often clinically silent Chest pain Dyspnea Coughing Tachycardia Anxiety Fever	Chest x-ray Lung perfusion scan Cardiopulmonary support	Avoid catheter exchange in veins with thrombosis

Procedure for Central Venous Catheter Insertion (Assist)

Steps	Rationale	Special Considerations
1. Wash hands, and don gloves.	Reduces the transmission of microorganisms; standard precautions.	
2. Prepare IV solution or flush solution.	Prepares infusion system.	
3. Prime IV tubing or hemodynamic monitoring system (see Procedure 69).	Prepares infusion system or monitoring system.	
4. Don surgical cap, face mask, sterile gown, and sterile gloves.	Reduces transmission of microorganisms; standard precautions.	
5. Place moisture-proof pad under the selected site of insertion.	Avoids soiling of the bed.	
6. Assist, if needed, with cleansing of the intended insertion site with antiseptic solution (Fig. 74–2). A. Subclavian insertion: scrub shoulder to contralateral nipple line and from neck to nipple line. B. Jugular vein insertion: scrub midclavicle to opposite border of the sternum and ear to a few inches above the nipple line.	Mechanical friction physically removes microbes. Antiseptics chemically destroy microbes.	The patient's skin should be physically clean before the application of an antiseptic solution. Organic material may inactivate antiseptic agents. Antiseptic scrub solutions may include povidone-iodine solution, 7.5% chlorhexidine, gluconate 4%, and isopropyl alcohol 70%.
7. Allow area to dry and cover with a sterile towel.	Protects the cleansed area from contamination until the insertion procedure begins.	
8. Ensure that all individuals in the immediate area of the bedside wear a face mask.[4]	Prevents transmission of microorganisms.	
9. Turn or instruct the patient to turn his or her head away from the insertion site.	Prevents transmission of microorganisms.	
10. Remove the sterile towel from the insertion site.	Exposes the area for the sterile preparation.	

Procedure **for Central Venous Catheter Insertion (Assist)** *Continued*		
Steps	**Rationale**	**Special Considerations**
11. While the physician or advance practice nurse completes the skin preparation, ensure patient comfort by explaining what is happening at the time. A. Application of the antiseptic solution will be cold and wet. B. Injection of local anesthetic may burn or sting as the tissue is being infiltrated.	Reduces anxiety and encourages cooperation.	Continue providing support and comfort throughout the procedure.
12. Place the bed in a 15- to 25-degree Trendelenburg position.	Provides venous dilatation and increases central venous pressure to reduce the risk of air embolism.	May be contraindicated in certain patients (eg, those with increased intracranial pressure, elevated venous pressure, respiratory or cardiac compromise).
13. Monitor the heart rate, respiratory rate and rhythm, and any patient response to the procedure.	Assessment may indicate occurrence of complications (see Table 74–1) or inadequate pain control.	
14. During insertion, again ensure that the patient's head is turned away from the side where the guidewire and the catheter are being advanced.	Reduces contamination and may avoid malpositioning of the catheter.	

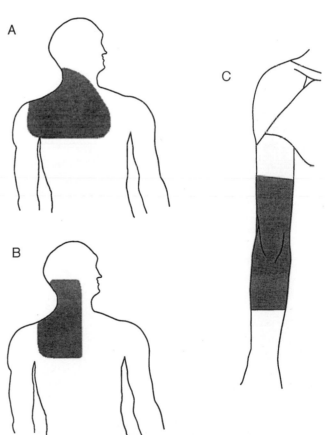

■ ● **FIGURE 74–2.** Area of preoperative skin preparation for central venous catheter insertions. *A, Subclavian insertions:* Scrub from shoulder to contralateral nipple line and neck to nipple line. *B, Jugular insertions:* Scrub midclavicle to opposite border of the sternum and from the ear to a few inches above the nipple line. *C, Peripherally inserted central venous catheters (PICC):* Scrub the entire arm circumference from midforearm to midupper arm. (Courtesy of Suredesign.)

Procedure continued on following page

Procedure for Central Venous Catheter Insertion (Assist) *Continued*

Steps	Rationale	Special Considerations
15. Observe the cardiac monitor while the guidewire and catheter are advanced, and inform the physician or advanced practice nurse immediately if a dysrhythmia occurs.	Advancement of the guidewire or catheter into the heart may induce cardiac dysrhythmias.	Tall, peaked P waves may be identified as the catheter tip enters the right atrium or if the guidewire has been advanced too far into the right atrium. Dysrhythmias may resolve with withdrawal of the guidewire or catheter. If the dysrhythmia continues, antidysrhythmic medications may be required.
16. Assist with connection of IV administration or monitoring tubing to the catheter. If monitoring, observe the waveform.	Maintains aseptic technique. Immediate connection of the IV or monitoring system to the catheter prevents air embolism.	Ensure a tight connection to prevent accidental disconnection. Luer-Lok devices prevent an accidental disconnection.
17. Obtain a chest x-ray.	Ensures that the catheter is properly placed and that there is no pneumothorax present.	Infusions (especially total parenteral nutrition and chemotherapeutic agents) should not be initiated until tip placement is confirmed.
18. Reposition the patient in a supine or low semi-Fowler position.	Head-tilt position is no longer necessary.	Remove the towel roll, if used.
19. Apply sterile, occlusive dressing.	Prevents catheter-related infections.	
20. If a triple-lumen catheter has been inserted, withdraw blood to remove air in the catheter, then irrigate additional lumens of the catheter or initiate infusion therapy as prescribed.	Prevents clotting of lumens.[2]	Common dosage is 2 to 3 mL of heparin, 100 U/mL.
21. Discard used supplies, and wash hands.	Reduces transmission of microorganisms; standard precautions.	

Expected Outcomes	Unexpected Outcomes
• Placement of central venous catheter is successful. • If infusing IV solution, the solution infuses without problems. • The a, c, and v waves are identified if hemodynamic monitoring is used. • CVP measurement is determined if hemodynamic monitoring is used.	• Pain or severe discomfort during the insertion procedure • Pneumothorax, tension pneumothorax, hemothorax • Nerve injury • Sterile thrombophlebitis • Infection • Cardiac dysrhythmias • Misplacement (eg, carotid artery, subclavian artery) • Hemorrhage • Hematoma • Venous air embolism • Pulmonary embolus • Cardiac tamponade • Sepsis • Heparin-induced thrombocytopenia or thrombosis

Patient Monitoring and Care

Patient Monitoring and Care	Rationale	Reportable Conditions
		These conditions should be reported if they persist despite nursing interventions.
1. Monitor the patient's vital signs and assess level of consciousness before the procedure, after the procedure, and as needed during the procedure.	Identifies signs and symptoms of complications and allows for immediate interventions.	• Abnormal vital signs • Changes in level of consciousness
2. If the catheter was placed for obtaining CVP measurement, assess the waveform.	Ensures that catheter is in the proper location for monitoring. Allows assessment of a, c, and v waves and measurement of pressure.	• Abrupt and sustained changes in pressure • Abnormal waveforms
3. Observe the catheter site for bleeding or hematoma every 15 to 30 minutes for the first 2 hours after insertion.	Postinsertion bleeding may occur in a patient with coagulopathies or arterial punctures, multiple attempts at vein access, or with the use of through-the-needle introducer designs for insertion.	• Bleeding or hematoma
4. Assess heart and lung sounds before and after the procedure.	Abnormal heart or lung sounds may indicate cardiac tamponade, pneumothorax, or hemothorax.	• Diminished or muffled heart sounds • Absent or diminished breath sounds unilaterally
5. Monitor for signs and symptoms of complications (see Table 74–1).	May decrease mortality if recognized early.	• Signs and symptoms of complications

Documentation

Documentation should include the following:

- Patient and family education
- Vital signs
- Catheter location
- Medications administered
- Date and time of procedure
- Catheter type
- Lumen size
- Length inserted and length remaining outside the insertion site

- Nursing interventions
- Fluids administered
- Hard copy of the waveform with analysis, if possible
- Patient tolerance of procedure
- Type of dressing applied
- Any unexpected outcomes encountered and the interventions taken

References

1. Andris DA, Krzywda EA. Central venous access: clinical practice issues. *Nurs Clin North Am.* 1997;32(4):719–740.
2. Darovic G. Monitoring central venous pressure. In: *Hemodynamic Monitoring: Invasive and Noninvasive Clinical Applications.* 2nd ed. Philadelphia, Pa: W.B. Saunders; 1995.
3. Krzywda EA. Central venous access—catheters, technology and physiology. *MEDSURG Nurs.* 1998;7(3):132–139.
4. Pearson ML. Special communication guideline for prevention of intravascular device-related infections. Part I: intravascular device-related infections: an overview. *Am J Infect Control.* 1996;24:262–293.

Additional Readings

Larsen L, Thurston NE. Research utilization: development of a central venous catheter procedure. *Appl Nurs Res.* 1997;10(1)44–51.
Levins T. Central intravenous lines: your role. *Nursing96.* 1996;26(4):48–49.

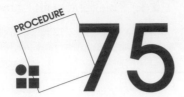

75

Peripheral Intravenous Line Insertion

P U R P O S E: A peripheral intravenous (IV) line is inserted for a variety of purposes: to provide a route for the administration of IV fluids, medications, and blood products; to maintain a patent venous route for use during emergency situations; to obtain venous blood samples for laboratory tests; and to provide nutritional supplements and hydration for patients unable to obtain them by other means.

Linda Bucher

PREREQUISITE NURSING KNOWLEDGE

- Nurses must be adequately prepared to insert a peripheral IV line. This preparation should include specific educational content regarding the indications for and the complications and maintenance of IV therapy. Opportunities to demonstrate clinical competency in the insertion of a peripheral IV line should also be included.
- Principles of aseptic technique should be understood.
- Knowledge of the anatomy and physiology of the vasculature and adjacent structures in the upper extremities is important. The most commonly used veins are located on the forearm; specifically the cephalic, basilic, and median veins in the lower arm, and the metacarpal veins in the dorsum of the hand (see Figs. 77–1 and 77–2).[1–3]
- Superficial veins lie in loose connective tissue under the skin and are best suited for venous cannulation. Peripheral IV therapy can be maintained longer by selecting the most distal site on the extremity; by using the smallest gauge catheter appropriate to vein size and prescribed therapy; by avoiding areas of flexion such as the antecubital fossa and the wrist; by using the nondominant hand, if possible; and by choosing sites that are located above previous insertion sites and sites that are phlebitic, infiltrated, or bruised.[2, 3]
- Indications for the insertion of a peripheral IV line will vary and can include patients experiencing fluid and electrolyte imbalances, malnutrition, shock, trauma, sepsis, surgery, endocrine disorders, cardiovascular disease, and cancer.
- Complications associated with the insertion of a peripheral IV can be local or systemic. Common local complications include phlebitis, thrombophlebitis, infiltration, and catheter occlusion. Systemic complications occur less frequently than local complications and include septicemia, thromboembolism, and embolism (air, catheter). Circulatory overload, speed shock, and allergic/anaphylactic reactions are systemic complications that are related di-

rectly to intravenous therapy. Systemic complications, when they occur, are often life-threatening.[4, 5]
- The most common type of IV catheter used for short-term intravenous therapy (7 days or less) is the over-the-needle, plastic catheter (Fig. 75–1).[6] The winged infusion set, or "butterfly," is recommended for use in patients who require IV therapy for less than 24 hours (Fig. 75–2).[7] Through-the-needle peripheral catheters are usually restricted to long-term intravenous use.
- The length and gauge of catheters used for peripheral IV therapy vary. Over-the-needle plastic catheters range from 5/8 in to 2 in in length and from 27 G to 12 G in size. The most common adult sizes are 22 G, 20 G, and 18 G.[6]
- A variety of safety IV devices are available and should be used to reduce the risk of needlestick injury.

EQUIPMENT

- IV catheter of appropriate type, size, and length
- IV fluid as prescribed with IV administration set and short extension tubing attached and primed (for continuous IV infusion); an intermittent infusion cap/adapter may be attached per institutional policy
- Short extension tubing with an intermittent infusion cap/adapter attached and primed with normal saline (NS) (for intermittent infusion device [IID])
- Single-use tourniquet
- Two to three alcohol prep pads or swabsticks
- Two to three povidone-iodine pads or swabsticks
- 2-in × 2-in sterile gauze pad
- One roll of 1-in, nonallergenic tape
- Transparent semipermeable dressing (small)
- One pair of examination gloves
- Biohazard container

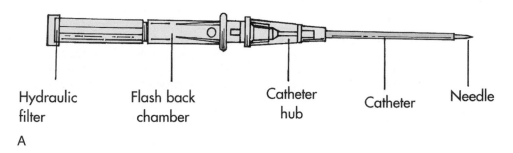

Hydraulic filter   Flash back chamber   Catheter hub   Catheter   Needle

A

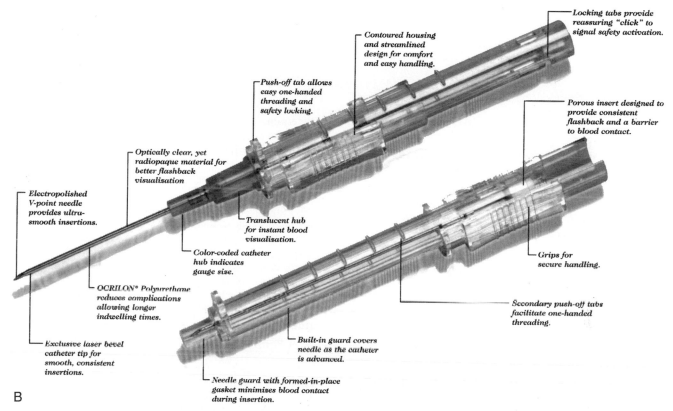

Locking tabs provide reassuring "click" to signal safety activation.

Contoured housing and streamlined design for comfort and easy handling.

Push-off tab allows easy one-handed threading and safety locking.

Porous insert designed to provide consistent flashback and a barrier to blood contact.

Optically clear, yet radiopaque material for better flashback visualisation.

Electropolished V-point needle provides ultra-smooth insertions.

Translucent hub for instant blood visualisation.

Color-coded catheter hub indicates gauge size.

Grips for secure handling.

OCRILON® Polyurethane reduces complications allowing longer indwelling times.

Secondary push-off tabs facilitate one-handed threading.

Built-in guard covers needle as the catheter is advanced.

Exclusive laser bevel catheter tip for smooth, consistent insertions.

Needle guard with formed-in-place gasket minimises blood contact during insertion.

†Membrane used in tests simulated human skin.
**Trademark of Becton Dickinson.
†Source: EPINet data.
*Trademark

B

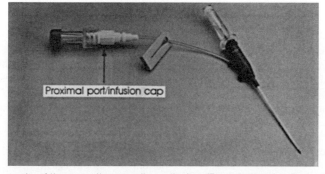

Proximal port/infusion cap

C

■ ● **FIGURE 75–1.** **A,** Components of the over-the-needle catheter. (From Potter PA, Perry AG, eds. *Basic Nursing: A Critical Thinking Approach.* 4th ed. St. Louis, Mo: Mosby; 1999:863.) **B,** PROTECTIV* PLUS IV Catheter Safety System. (Courtesy of Johnson & Johnson.) **C,** Multilumen peripheral (over-the-needle) catheter. (Courtesy of Arrow International, Inc.)

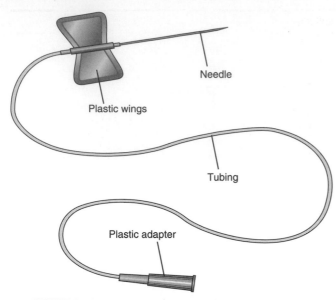

■ ● **FIGURE 75–2.** Components of the winged infusion (butterfly) set.

Additional equipment as needed includes the following:

- 3 to 5 mL of NS (flush for IID)
- IV pole
- VACUTAINER® with Luer-Lok adapter and collecting tubes (if venous sampling is needed); a 10-mL syringe may be used in place of the VACUTAINER® system

- Lidocaine or eutectic mixture of local anesthetics (EMLA) cream (optional)

PATIENT AND FAMILY EDUCATION

- Explain the purpose of the peripheral IV line and include the patient in the selection of the site (if possible). ➡️*Rationale:* Clarification of information is an expressed patient and family need and helps to diminish anxiety, enhance acceptance, and encourage questions. Patients often request that their nondominant hand or arm be used for IV line placement.
- Explain the overall steps of the procedure, including the patient's role during the procedure. ➡️*Rationale:* Decreases patient anxiety, enhances cooperation, and provides an opportunity for the patient to voice concerns; limits risk of accidental movement during the procedure.
- Instruct the patient and family on the signs and symptoms that should be reported to the nurse (eg, discomfort, burning, swelling, wetness). ➡️*Rationale:* Enables the patient and family to recognize possible complications related to the IV line and includes them in the plan of care.

PATIENT ASSESSMENT AND PREPARATION

Patient Assessment

- Assess current anticoagulation therapy, thrombolytic therapy, or known blood dyscrasias. ➡️*Rationale:* Anticoagulation and thrombolytic therapies or blood dyscrasias could increase the risk of hematoma formation or excessive bleeding at the insertion site. Patients who are receiving thrombolytic therapy should have adequate peripheral access established prior to initiation of therapy.
- Assess allergy history (eg, lidocaine, EMLA cream, antiseptic solutions, adhesives). ➡️*Rationale:* Reduces the risk of allergic reactions by avoiding known allergenic products.
- Assess history of mastectomy, fistula, shunt, neurovascular injury, cellulitis, thrombosis. ➡️*Rationale:* These conditions predispose patients to IV-related complications. Insertion of a peripheral IV line should be avoided in extremities affected by these conditions.
- Assess the patient's age, general size, skin condition, and anatomy of venous system. ➡️*Rationale:* Assists in the determination of the most appropriate catheter size and insertion site. Small-gauge catheters (eg, 24 to 22 G) are less traumatizing to veins. If large-gauge catheters are required (eg, 20 to 14 G), the selected vein should be able to accommodate the catheter. Edematous areas or sites of previous hematoma or infection and veins that are very small, sclerosed, scarred, or tortuous should be avoided, because these conditions can inhibit successful insertion of an IV line and can contribute to complications.
- Determine whether or not venous sampling is needed. ➡️*Rationale:* Accurate laboratory samples can be obtained during the process of initiating a peripheral IV line.[6] Concurrent collection of venous blood for laboratory testing during this procedure limits the number of venipunctures required by the patient.

Patient Preparation

- Ensure that the patient and family understand preprocedural teaching. Answer questions as they arise and reinforce information as needed. ➡️*Rationale:* Evaluates and reinforces understanding of previously taught information.
- Position the patient in a supine position with the head slightly elevated and arms at side. ➡️*Rationale:* Proper positioning of the patient enhances accessibility to the venipuncture site and promotes patient comfort.
- Extend the patient's upper extremity to form a straight line from the shoulder to the wrist. A pillow can be placed under the arm for support, if needed. ➡️*Rationale:* Proper positioning of the extremity enhances accessibility to the venipuncture site and reduces the risk of patient movement during the procedure.

Procedure for Peripheral Intravenous Line Insertion

Steps	Rationale	Special Considerations
1. Wash hands.	Reduces transmission of microorganism; standard precautions.	
2. Prepare the IV infusion and prime the tubing or the intermittent infusion cap or adapter, as indicated. If a multiple-lumen peripheral catheter is used, flush the proximal port through the infusion cap with NS.	Allows procedure to be completed expeditiously and reduces risk of occlusion once the IV line is established. Avoids infusion of air into the patient.	Short extension tubing attached to the administration set or intermittent infusion cap/adapter facilitates access to the IV line and limits manipulation at the catheter hub.
3. Wash hands, and don clean gloves.	Reduces transmission of microorganisms; standard precautions.	
4. Apply tourniquet proximal to proposed puncture site. Tie in a manner such that the tourniquet can be released by pulling on one end. If veins are not prominent, instruct patient to open and close hand (make a fist) several times.	Impedes venous return to the heart and produces venous distention. Proper application of the tourniquet allows for the quick, one-handed release of the tourniquet.	Arterial blood flow should not be impeded. Arterial perfusion should be verified by palpating for the radial pulse. For patients with large, prominent veins, a tourniquet is not recommended. Alternative approaches to facilitating venous distention include gentle tapping of the skin over the venipuncture area with the index and second fingers and permitting the arm to hang dependently below the level of the heart. Warm compresses can also be applied to facilitate venous distention.
5. Select appropriate venipuncture site and use the most distal branch of the vein selected.	Multiple factors determine the success of securing and maintaining a patent venous access site.	Vein size, elasticity, and distance below the skin should be considered. Shorter and smaller catheters may be needed in the elderly and very young patients.
6. Release tourniquet	Prolonged vein distension causes undue patient discomfort and impairs circulation to the extremity. In addition, a tourniquet left on for more than 1 to 2 minutes may result in hemoconcentration or variation in blood test values if blood is to be collected during the procedure.	In some cases (eg, tortuous or sclerosed veins), a tourniquet may increase venous pressure such that the vein may rupture when punctured.
7. If lidocaine or EMLA cream is to be used, then apply to site selected for insertion of the IV line. *(Level V: Clinical studies in more than one or two different patient populations and situations to support recommendations)*	Provides relief from pain associated with venipuncture and may reduce or eliminate anxiety associated with procedure.[9–11]	Research on length of time from application of lidocaine or EMLA to procedure has produced inconclusive results.[9–11] If used, the manufacturer's recommendations for application should be followed. The time from application to procedure varies from 5 to 60 minutes.
8. Prepare site beginning with the alcohol pad or swabstick. Starting at the insertion site, cleanse outward, using a circular motion while applying friction. After the area dries, cleanse in a similar fashion using the povidone-iodine pad or swabstick.	Limits the introduction of potentially infectious skin flora into the vessel during the puncture. Combination of cleansing solutions enhances the antimicrobial actions of the agents.	Never remove the povidone-iodine solution with alcohol because alcohol cancels the effect of the povidone-iodine.[1] Application time (a *minimum* of 30 seconds) is the chemical kill.[5] If you must palpate the area once cleansing has been performed, you must use sterile gloves or recleanse the area.

Procedure continued on following page

| Procedure | **for Peripheral Intravenous Line Insertion** *Continued* |

Steps	Rationale	Special Considerations
9. Reapply the tourniquet.	Produces venous distention.	
10. Draw the skin just below the insertion site taut, using the thumb of the nondominant hand.	Immobilizes the vein for insertion of the IV line.	
11. Puncture the skin parallel to the path of the vein with the bevel up and the needle at a 30- to 45-degree angle.	Causes least amount of discomfort.	Before puncturing the patient's skin, inform patient that you are about to insert the device.
12. Advance the needle until resistance is met. Next, reduce the angle of the needle and slowly pierce the vein. Observe for blood in the catheter hub (flashback chamber) or tubing of winged infusion set. Continue to insert the needle approximately ¼ in into the vein.	Limits the risk of puncturing the posterior wall of the vein. Establishes entry into the vein. Ensures full entry of the catheter into the vein, because the catheter is slightly shorter than the stylet (needle).	A "pop" may or may not be felt when the needle enters the vein. Winged infusion sets can be used to collect venous samples for laboratory testing. When this is the case, the tubing of the infusion set is *not* primed and retrograde blood flow will be observed upon entry of the needle into vein.
13. Release the tourniquet.	Reduces the risk of rupturing the vein.	Keep tourniquet in place if blood for laboratory testing is to be collected. If blood flow is found to be sluggish during collection process, the tourniquet should be kept in place until collection of blood is completed and then removed.
14. Advance the device, following the appropriate procedure for the needle type: A. Catheter-over-needle (Figs. 75–3 and 75–4): ○ Holding the device stable, advance the catheter into the vein until hub rests at insertion site.	Stabilization of the device reduces the risk of puncturing the posterior wall of the vein.	Procedures for advancing the catheter will vary according to the device used. It is recommended that safety devices be used to reduce the risk of needlestick injuries.[12–14]
○ Place a 2-in × 2-in gauze pad under the catheter hub and remove the stylet (or needle guard) while holding the hub securely.	Provides absorption of any blood that may escape when stylet is removed. Prevents dislodgment of the catheter.	Never reinsert the needle into the catheter, because the needle could cut the catheter, resulting in catheter embolus. The application of digital pressure to the vein just above the tip of the catheter limits the escape of blood.

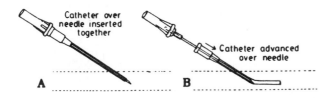

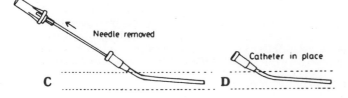

■ ● FIGURE 75–3. Insertion of catheter-over-needle. (Courtesy of Johnson & Johnson.)

| Procedure | **for Peripheral Intravenous Line Insertion** *Continued* |

Steps	Rationale	Special Considerations
○ Properly dispose of sharp.	Limits risk of needlestick injury and exposure to bloodborne pathogens.	If blood for laboratory testing is required, attach the VACUTAINER® and collect appropriate blood samples before connecting IV or IID (Fig. 75–5). A 10-mL syringe can be used in lieu of the VACUTAINER® system.
		Procedure continued on following page

One-Handed Technique

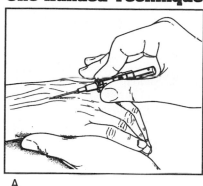

A

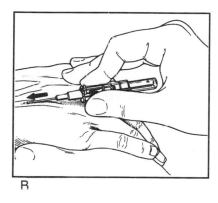

R

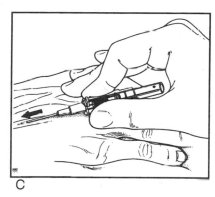

C

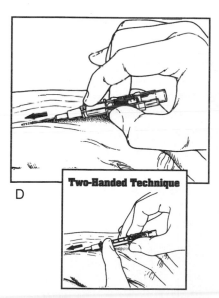

D

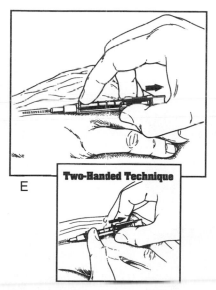

E

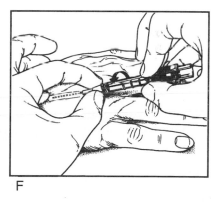

F

■ ● **FIGURE 75–4.** Insertion of PROTECTIV* PLUS IV Catheter Safety System. *A,* One- or two-handed technique: Hold device by the ribbed needle housing with thumb and fingers on opposite sides. *B,* With bevel and push-off tabs in the "up" position, insert the needle through the skin into the vein. Observe for blood in the flashback chamber. *C,* Slightly advance the catheter and needle together to assume full catheter entry into the vein lumen. *D,* One-handed technique: Holding the device stable, place finger on the primary push-off tab and thread the catheter to the desired length. Two-handed technique: Holding the device stable with one hand, place thumb of the other hand behind the primary push-off tab, and thread catheter to the desired length. As you thread the catheter, the needle guard begins to cover the needle. *E,* One-handed technique: Using a finger to stabilize the device at the push-off tab, draw the needle into the needle guard by retracting the ribbed needle housing until it locks securely in place. Two-handed technique: With thumb behind the primary push-off tab to stabilize the device, retract the ribbed needle housing with the other hand until it locks securely in place. Listen for a "click" indicating that the needle is locked. *F,* Secure the hub and remove the needle guard by twisting slightly and pulling it out of the catheter hub.

Procedure **for Peripheral Intravenous Line Insertion** *Continued*

Steps	Rationale	Special Considerations
○ Connect primed IV administration set or IID to catheter hub.	Prompt connection maintains patency of vein and sterility. Provides direct entrance for IV fluids or access for the intermittent administration of IV fluids, medications, and so on.	Use of safety devices reduces needlestick injury.[12]
○ Initiate proper IV flow rate or flush port of IID with 3 mL of NS flush; assess for signs of infiltration. *(Level VI: Clinical studies in a variety of patient populations and situations to support recommendations)*	If sylet has punctured posterior wall of vein, fluid or blood will infuse into surrounding tissue, as evidenced by local edema or hematoma formation.	Use of NS flush is recommended over heparin flush for maintaining the patency of peripheral IV lines in adults.[15, 16]
○ Secure catheter with transparent semipermeable dressing, gauze and tape, or adhesive bandage. If transparent semipermeable dressing is used, do *not* cover the connection between tubing and catheter hub (Fig. 75–6).	Prevents early access of microorganisms to bloodstream and stabilizes catheter, thereby reducing irritation of the intimal lining of the vein by the catheter. Facilitates changing of IV tubing if necessary before catheter change.	Procedures for covering peripheral IV sites will vary. Research is mixed regarding the efficacy of applying antimicrobial ointment at the insertion site. Similarly, research varies regarding the efficacy of transparent semipermeable dressing, gauze and tape, and adhesive bandages as IV site dressings.[16–20]

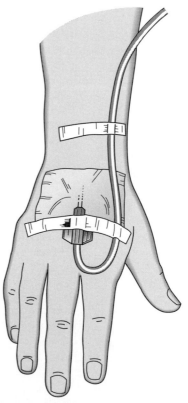

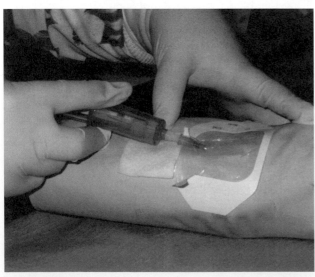

■ ● **FIGURE 75–5.** Collection of blood specimens during the insertion of a peripheral IV using the VACUTAINER® system. (Courtesy of Becton Dickinson.)

■ ● **FIGURE 75–6.** Transparent semipermeable dressing over the catheter insertion site. An additional ½-in tape is placed over the connection between the catheter hub and the tubing. Note intravenous tubing is looped in a "J" loop and secured with additional tape. It is not recommended that tape be placed under the transparent dressing. (From Farley KL. Taping and dressing suggestions and tips for use with non-winged IV catheters. Courtesy of Johnson & Johnson.)

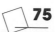

Procedure **for Peripheral Intravenous Line Insertion** *Continued*

Steps	Rationale	Special Considerations
B. Winged infusion set (or "butterfly"): ○ Prime the device with NS if IV line or IID is to be established.	Avoids the entrance of air into the vein.	If blood for laboratory testing is required, the device should *not* be primed.
○ Advance the needle fully, if possible, into the vein.	Increases the stabilization of the device in the vein.	If the device is primed, retrograde blood flow usually will *not* be observed in the tubing.
○ Release the tourniquet and connect the IV tubing or the injection port to the end of the tubing.	Prompt connection maintains patency of vein and sterility. Provides direct entrance for IV fluids or access for the intermittent administration of IV fluids, medications, and so on.	If blood for laboratory testing is required, attach VACUTAINER® (or a 10-mL syringe) and collect appropriate blood samples before connecting IV line or injection port (see Procedure 77).
○ Initiate proper IV flow rate or flush port of IID with 3 mL of NS flush; assess for signs of infiltration. *(Level VI: Clinical studies in a variety of patient populations and situations to support recommendations)*	If needle has punctured posterior wall of vein, fluid or blood will infuse into surrounding tissue, as evidenced by local edema or hematoma formation.	Use of NS flush is recommended over heparin flush for maintaining the patency of peripheral IV lines in adults.[15, 16]
○ Secure catheter with transparent semipermeable dressing, gauze and tape, or adhesive bandage.	Prevents early access of microorganisms to bloodstream and stabilizes catheter, thereby reducing irritation of the intimal lining of the vein by the catheter. Follow institutional policy for dressing and catheter changes.	Procedures for covering peripheral IV sites will vary. Research is mixed regarding the efficacy of applying antimicrobial ointment at the insertion site. Similarly, research varies regarding the efficacy of transparent semipermeable gauze and tape, or adhesive bandages as IV dressings.[16–20]
15. Label dressing with date, time, catheter gauge and length, and initials.	Provides information related to catheter insertion.	
16. Discard supplies in appropriate container, and wash hands.	Reduces tranmission of microorganisms; standard precautions.	Expedite delivery of blood specimens to laboratory, if collected.

Expected Outcomes

- Patent venous access
- Insertion site free of local complications (eg, pain, edema, tenderness, erythema, blanching, catheter occlusion)
- Patient free of systemic complications (eg, fever, chills, malaise, tachycardia, respiratory distress, hemoptysis, hypotension, cyanosis)

Unexpected Outcomes

- Pain/severe discomfort during the procedure
- Local complications during or after the procedure (eg, hematoma, phlebitis, thrombophlebitis, infiltration, catheter occlusion)
- Systemic complications following the procedure (eg, septicemia, thromboembolus, catheter embolus)

Patient Monitoring and Care	Rationale	Reportable Conditions
		These conditions should be reported if they persist despite nursing interventions.
1. Observe peripheral IV site for signs and symptoms of local complications every hour (continuous infusion) or every 4 hours (IID).	Local complications occur more frequently than systemic complications. The catheter (or needle) can become dislodged and can cause infiltration of the infusing substances or blood into the surrounding tissues. Causative factors related to phlebitis can be chemical (related to the infusing solutions), bacterial (related to contamination), or mechanical (related to the catheter).[4] Thrombophlebitis can result from trauma to the vein and venous stasis. Catheter occlusion usually results from inadequate flushing procedures (IID), obstruction to free-flowing infusion (eg, positional catheter, flexion of extremity), dry solution containers, or precipitate from incompatible solutions or medications.	• Edema around the IV site • Pain, tenderness, erythema, blanching • Hardness along path of vein, when palpated • Drainage from insertion site
2. For IID, assess catheter for venous blood return and patency before initiating infusions.	Verifies position of the catheter in the vascular space and patency before initiating infusions.	
3. Assess patient for signs and symptoms of systemic infection.	Insertion of peripheral IV lines causes trauma to the surrounding tissues and the intimal layer of the vessel wall. Proper insertion technique and surveillance will minimize the risk of septicemia. Incidence of infection related to the catheter may result from failure to maintain asepsis during insertion, failure to comply with dressing change protocols, immunosuppression, frequent access to the catheter, and long-term use of a single peripheral IV access site.	• Fever, chills, malaise, headache (early signs of septicemia)[4] • Tachycardia, hypotension, nausea or vomiting, backache (late signs of septicemia)[4]
4. Assess for signs or symptoms of emboli.	Emboli can result from the release of a preexisting thrombus, from a portion of the IV catheter, and from the inadvertent introduction of air into the venous system.	• Pulmonary embolus: sudden onset of dyspnea, apprehension, unexplained hemoptysis, tachycardia, shock, cardiac arrest[4] • Catheter embolus: cyanosis, hypotension, tachycardia, jugular venous distension (JVD), loss of consciousness, shock, cardiac arrest • Air embolus: chest pain, shortness of breath, shoulder or back pain, cyanosis, shock, cardiac arrest.[4] Air embolism is a rare complication of peripheral IV lines. It is more common with centrally placed cathters. If suspected, place patient in the left lateral recumbent position (to trap air in the right heart) and notify physician immediately.[4]

Patient Monitoring and Care *Continued*

Patient Monitoring and Care	Rationale	Reportable Conditions
5. Follow institution standard for frequency and type of dressing change.	Decreases risk of infection at catheter site. The CDC has made no recommendation for the frequency of routine peripheral catheter dressing change, but recommends replacing the dressing when the dressing becomes damp, loosened, or soiled or when inspection of the site is necessary.[16]	
6. Rotate the IV site every 48 to 72 hours.	The CDC recommends rotating the IV site every 48 to 72 hours to minimize the risk of phlebitis.[16] Heparin locks should be replaced at least every 96 hours.[16]	

Documentation

Documentation should include the following:

- Patient and family education
- Known allergies
- Date and time of procedure
- Catheter type, gauge, and length
- Type and amount of local anesthetic (if used)
- Location of peripheral IV insertion site and vein accessed
- Problems encountered during or after procedure and nursing interventions
- Patient tolerance of procedure
- Assessment of insertion site
- Disposition of specimens, if appropriate

References

1. Krozek C, Millam D, Pelikan R. Intravascular therapy. In: *Nursing Procedures.* 2nd ed. Springhouse, Pa: Springhouse Corp; 1996:380–395.
2. Perucca R. Obtaining vascular access. In: Terry J, Baranowski L, Lonsway RA, Hedric C, eds. *Intravenous Therapy: Clinical Principles and Practice.* Philadelphia, Pa: W.B. Saunders; 1995:379–385.
3. Speakman E. Fluid, electrolyte, and acid-base balances. In: Potter PA, Perry AG, eds. *Basic Nursing: A Critical Thinking Approach.* 4th ed. St. Louis, Mo: Mosby; 1999:857–890.
4. Perdue M. Intravenous complications. In: Terry J, Baranowski L, Lonsway RA, Hedric C, eds. *Intravenous Therapy: Clinical Principles and Practice.* Philadelphia, Pa: W.B. Saunders; 1995:419–443.
5. Perucca R. Intravenous monitoring and catheter care. In: Terry J, Baranowski L, Lonsway RA, Hedrick C, eds. *Intravenous Therapy: Clinical Principles and Practice.* Philadelphia, Pa: W.B. Saunders; 1995:392–399.
6. Jensen BL. Intravenous therapy equipment. In: Terry J, Baranowski L, Lonsway RA, Hedrick C, eds. *Intravenous Therapy: Clinical Principles and Practice.* Philadelphia, Pa: W.B. Saunders; 1995:303–319.
7. Olson KL, Gomes V. Intravenous therapy needle choices in ambulatory cancer patients. *Clin Nurs Res.* 1996;5:543–461.
8. Kennedy C, Angermuller S, King R, et al. A comparison of hemolysis rates using intravenous catheters versus venipuncture tubes for obtaining blood samples. *J Emerg Nurs.* 1996;22:566–569.
9. Hussey VM, Poulin MV, Fain JA. Effectiveness of lidocaine hydrochloride on venipuncture sites. *AORN J.* 1997;66:472–475.
10. Lander J, Nazarali S, Hodgins M, et al. Evaluation of a new topical anesthetic agent: a pilot study. *Nurs Res.* 1996;45:50–52.
11. Nott M, Peacock J. Relief of injection pain in adults: EMLA cream for 5 minutes before venepuncture. *Anaesthesia.* 1990;45:772–774.
12. National Committee on Safer Needle Devices. *Using Safer Needle Devices: The Time Is Now.* Washington, DC: Author; 1997.
13. Jagger J. Reducing occupational exposure to bloodborne pathogens: where do we stand a decade later? *Infect Control Hosp Epidemiol.* 1996;17:573–575.
14. Jagger J, Hunt EH, Brand-Elnaggar J, Pearson RD. Rates of needle-stick injury caused by various devices in a university hospital. *N Engl J Med.* 1988;319:284–288.
15. Goode CJ, Titler M, Rakel B, et al. A meta-analysis of effects of heparin flush and saline flush: quality and cost implications. *Nurs Res.* 1991;40:324–330.
16. Pearson ML. Hospital infection control practices advisory committee: guideline for prevention of intravascular device-related infections. *Infect Control Hosp Epidemiol.* 1996; 17:438–473.
17. Zinner SH, Denny-Brown BC, Braun P, et al. Risk of infection with intravenous indwelling catheters: effect of application of antibiotic ointment. *J Infect Dis.* 1969;120:616–619.
18. Craven DE, Lichtenberg DA, Kunches LM, et al. A randomized study comparing a transparent polyurethane dressing to

a gauze dressing for peripheral intravenous catheter sites. *Infect Control*. 1985;6:361–366.

19. Pettit DM, Kraus V. The use of gauze versus transparent dressings for peripheral intravenous catheter sites. *Nurs Clin North Am*. 1995;30:495–506.

20. VandenBosch TM, Cooch J, Treston-Aurand J. Research utilization: adhesive bandage dressing regimen for peripheral venous catheters. *Am J Infect Control*. 1997;25:513–519.

Additional Readings

Potter PA, Perry AG, eds. *Basic Nursing: A Critical Thinking Approach*. 4th ed. St. Louis, Mo: Mosby; 1999.

Schull PD, ed. *Nursing Procedures*. Springhouse, Pa: Springhouse Corp; 1996.

Terry J, Baranowski L, Lonsway RA, Hedrick C, eds. *Intravenous Therapy: Clinical Principles and Practice*. Philadelphia, Pa: W.B. Saunders; 1995.

76

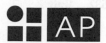

Peripherally Inserted Central Catheter

P U R P O S E : Peripherally inserted central catheters (PICCs) are used to deliver central venous therapy for 5 days to 12 months and to provide venous access for patients who require multiple venipunctures. PICCs are used to administer long-term antibiotic therapy, chemotherapy, total parenteral nutrition, analgesia, intermittent inotropic (eg, dobutamine) therapy, and fluids.[1, 2]

Linda Bucher

PREREQUISITE NURSING KNOWLEDGE

- Successful completion of a certification program designed for instruction in PICC insertion is required. In addition, opportunities to demonstrate clinical competency initially and on a regular basis (eg, yearly) may be required.
- Clinical and technical competence in suturing PICC lines in place.
- Understanding of sterile technique is necessary.
- Knowledge of the anatomy and physiology of the vasculature and adjacent structures in the upper extremity, neck, and chest is important. The patient receiving a PICC needs to have a peripheral vein that can accommodate a 14-G or 16-G introducer needle. The basilic and cephalic antecubital fossa veins are the preferred veins for cannulation with a PICC (Fig. 76–1). The basilic vein is the larger of the two veins and is the vein of choice for insertion of a PICC. Once inserted, the PICC is advanced to the superior vena cava or the subclavian vein.
- Patient indications for the insertion of a PICC vary. A PICC is used increasingly for patients receiving intravenous (IV) therapy in the home setting for chronic heart failure, cancer, chronic pain management, nutritional support, and fluid replacement (eg, hyperemesis gravidarum).
- PICCs may be preferred over percutaneously inserted central venous catheters for patients suffering from trauma (eg, burns) of the chest or from certain pulmonary disorders (eg, chronic obstructive pulmonary disease, cystic fibrosis).[1]
- PICCs are contraindicated in patients with sclerotic veins and in extremities affected by a mastectomy, an arteriovenous graft, or a fistula.
- IV therapy via the PICC poses fewer and less severe complications compared to percutaneously inserted central venous catheters. The most common complications associated with the PICC are phlebitis and catheter occlusion.[1]
- A variety of PICCs are available for use. PICCs are flexible catheters that are made of silicone or polyurethane. Catheter diameters range from 23 G to 16 G, and catheter length ranges from 16 in to 24 in. For adults, 18-G or 20-G catheters that are 24 inches in length are the standard. PICCs are available as single- or double-lumen catheters and can be inserted with or without the use of a guidewire. The nurse needs to be familiar with the design, material, and insertion technique, which are unique to the selected catheter.
- Generally, a PICC can be inserted through a breakaway needle or a cannula. The breakaway needle involves passing the catheter through a needle that can be split and peeled from around the catheter once it is properly placed. Alternately, the cannula design involves introducing an over-the-needle plastic cannula. Once the introducer is inserted, the needle is removed and the catheter is threaded through the cannula.[2]
- When a guidewire is used, venous access needs to be achieved with a needle. Once the needle is inserted, the guidewire is threaded through the needle, the needle is removed, and the catheter is inserted over the guidewire. This approach is referred to as the Seldinger method.[2] Care must be taken with the use of a guidewire. Although catheter advancement is enhanced by the firmness provided by the guidewire, the guidewire can inadvertently traumatize the vessel.[1]
- A variety of safety PICCs are available and should be used to reduce the risk of blood exposure and needlestick injury.

AP This procedure should be performed only by physicians, advanced practice nurses, and other health care professionals (including critical care nurses) with additional knowledge, skills, and demonstrated competence per professional licensure or institutional standard.

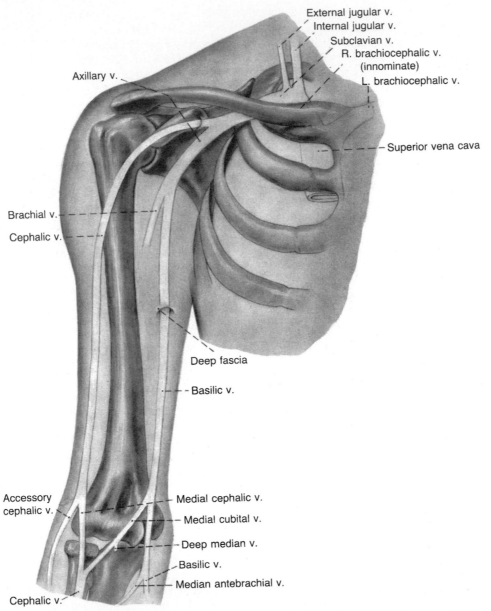

External jugular v.
Internal jugular v.
Subclavian v.
R. brachiocephalic v.
(innominate)
L. brachiocephalic v.

Axillary v.

Superior vena cava

Brachial v.

Cephalic v.

Deep fascia

Basilic v.

Accessory
cephalic v.

Medial cephalic v.

Medial cubital v.

Deep median v.

Basilic v.

Median antebrachial v.

Cephalic v.

■ ● **FIGURE 76–1.** Location of the veins of the right shoulder and upper arm. (From Jacob SW, Francone CA. *Elements of Anatomy and Physiology.* 2nd ed. Philadelphia, Pa: W.B. Saunders, 1989:192.)

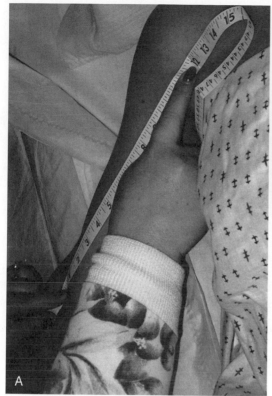

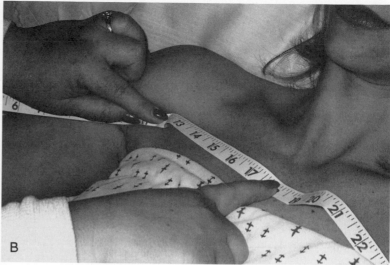

■ ● FIGURE 76–2. Measurement of the catheter length for subclavian vein placement. *A*, First, measure the distance from the selected insertion site to the shoulder. *B*, Continue measuring from the shoulder to the sternal notch.

EQUIPMENT

- Catheter insertion kit
- PICC catheter of choice
- Single-use tourniquet or blood pressure cuff
- Sterile and nonsterile measuring tape
- Waterproof underpad/linen saver
- Sterile gown
- Mask
- Goggles
- Two pairs of nonpowdered, sterile gloves
- Sterile drapes and towels, including one fenestrated drape
- Three alcohol pads or swabsticks
- Three povidone-iodine pads or swabsticks
- 10-mL vial of heparin (concentration per institutional policy)
- 30-mL vial of normal saline (NS)

- Luer-Lok injection port (cap) with short extension tubing
- One 10-mL, 20-G, 1-in needle syringe (blunt needle recommended)
- One 3-mL, 20-G, 1-in needle syringe or one 5-mL, 20-G, 1-in needle syringe if inserting a double-lumen catheter (blunt needle recommended)
- Three to four sterile 4 × 4-in gauze pads or sponges
- 1% lidocaine without epinephrine or 1 to 2 mL of eutectic mixture of local anesthetics (EMLA) cream (optional)
- Two sterile 2 × 2 in gauze pads or sponges
- One skin protectant swabstick
- Sterile, transparent, semipermeable dressing

Additional equipment as needed includes the following:

- One 1-mL, 25-G, 5/8-in needle syringe (if using intradermal lidocaine)
- One 3-0 or 4-0 nylon suture on a small, curved cutting needle (optional)
- One packet of Steri-Strips (if not suturing)

PATIENT AND FAMILY EDUCATION

- Explain the reason for the PICC, as well as the benefits and risks associated with the catheter. ➤*Rationale:* Clarification of information is an expressed patient need and helps to diminish anxiety, enhance acceptance, and encourage questions.
- Describe the major steps of the procedure, including the patient's role in the procedure. ➤*Rationale:* Decreases patient anxiety, enhances cooperation, provides opportunity for patient to voice concerns, and prevents accidental contamination of the sterile field and equipment.
- Instruct patient and family to refuse injections, venipunctures, and blood pressure measurements on the arm with the PICC. ➤*Rationale:* Minimizes the risk of catheter-related complications and catheter damage.
- Provide appropriate patient and family discharge education regarding the care and maintenance of the PICC. ➤*Rationale:* Reduces the risk of catheter-related complications due to lack of knowledge and skills needed to care for the PICC after discharge.

PATIENT ASSESSMENT AND PREPARATION
Patient Assessment

- Assess past medical history for mastectomy, fistula, or shunt. ➤*Rationale:* PICC insertion should be avoided

⬛⬛ AP This procedure should be performed only by physicians, advanced practice nurses, and other health care professionals (including critical care nurses) with additional knowledge, skills, and demonstrated competence per professional licensure or institutional standard.

in extremities affected by these conditions, because the risk of complications is increased.

- Obtain baseline vital signs and cardiac rhythm. ➤*Rationale:* Cardiac dysrhythmias can occur if the catheter is advanced into the heart. Baseline data facilitate the identification of clinical problems and the efficacy of interventions.
- Assess vasculature of the antecubital space of both arms, focusing on the basilic and cephalic veins (see Fig. 76–1). A tourniquet or blood pressure cuff should be applied on the mid-upper arm for vein assessment and then removed. ➤*Rationale:* Proper vein selection increases the success of insertion and decreases the incidence of postinsertion complications.
- Determine allergy history (eg, lidocaine, EMLA cream, antiseptic solutions, tape). ➤*Rationale:* Decreases the risk of allergic reactions by avoiding known, allergenic products.

Patient Preparation

- Ensure that the patient and family understand preprocedural teaching. Answer questions as they arise and reinforce information as needed. ➤*Rationale:* Evaluates and reinforces understanding of previously taught information.
- Ensure that informed consent has been obtained. ➤*Rationale:* Protects the rights of the patient and allows the patient to make a competent decision.
- Place the patient in a semi-Fowler or dorsal recumbent position, depending on the patient's clinical condition and level of comfort. ➤*Rationale:* The upright position allows gravity to assist in directing the catheter downward when advancing the catheter into the innominate vein and superior vena cava. It also may help avoid inadvertent placement of the catheter into the jugular vein.

- Position the selected arm at 45 degrees of extension from the body for anthropometric measurement. For catheter placement in the subclavian vein, use the nonsterile measuring tape to measure the distance from the selected insertion site to the shoulder (Fig. 76–2A) and from the shoulder to the sternal notch (Fig. 76–2B). For catheter placement in the superior vena cava, add 3 inches (7.5 cm) to this number. ➤*Rationale:* Extending the extremity allows for displacement of the catheter with arm movement. Accurate measurement ensures proper tip position within the central vein for the administration of IV solutions and determines the length of the catheter to be inserted.
- Measure the mid-upper arm circumference of the selected extremity. ➤*Rationale:* Provides a baseline for evaluation of suspected thrombosis. Increases greater than 2 cm over baseline are supportive of venous occlusion.
- Stabilize the position of the arm with a towel or pillow. ➤*Rationale:* Increases patient comfort, secures work area, and facilitates access to the selected vein.
- Instruct the patient on proper head positioning. The head is positioned to the contralateral side throughout the procedure, except when advancing the catheter from the axillary vein to the superior vena cava. At this point, the patient is instructed to position his or her head toward the ipsilateral side with the chin dropped to the shoulder. ➤*Rationale:* Limits the risk of inadvertently directing the catheter into the jugular vein.

Procedure for Peripherally Inserted Central Catheter

Steps	Rationale	Special Considerations
1. Wash hands, using antiseptic soap for a minimum of 60 seconds.[2]	Reduces the transmission of microorganisms.	
2. Place waterproof pad under the selected arm.	Avoids soiling bed linens.	
3. Position the tourniquet high on the upper extremity, near the axilla, but do not constrict venous blood flow at this time.	Placement high on the extremity avoids contamination of the sterile field.	A blood pressure cuff may be used in place of a tourniquet.
4. Open PICC insertion tray and drop remaining sterile items onto sterile field.	Maintains aseptic technique; preparation of work area, including procurement of all necessary equipment, avoids interruption of the procedure as well as contamination of the work area.	
5. Don mask, goggles, sterile gown, and clean gloves.	Standard precautions; PICC insertion is a sterile procedure.	Blood splashing may occur with the use of guidewires, stylets, and breakaway or peelaway introducers.
6. Using the sterile measuring tape, cut the catheter to the predetermined length. A. Add 1 in (2.5 cm) to the premeasured length to be left outside the insertion site.	Catheters are provided at various lengths.	

Procedure	**for Peripherally Inserted Central Catheter** *Continued*

Steps	Rationale	Special Considerations

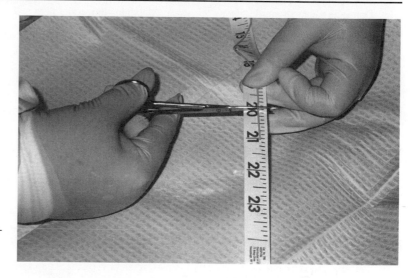

▪ ● **FIGURE 76–3.** Measuring and cutting the catheter tip to premeasured length.

B. Remove the guidewire and cut the tip of the catheter straight across with the sterile scissors (Fig. 76–3).	Prevents the catheter tip from lying flush against the vessel wall, which can increase the incidence of clot formation.	A catheter with a guidewire or stylet is recommended in order to reduce the risk of catheter coiling or knotting in the vein and for the ease in insertion.
7. Reinsert the guidewire so that the tip of the guidewire is covered by approximately 0.5 to 1 cm of the catheter.	Facilitates the removal of the guidewire; provides softness and flexibility at the catheter tip, thus preventing perforation of the vein during insertion.	
8. Fill the 10-mL syringe with NS. Add the injection port (cap) to the short extension tubing and prime with NS. Leave the syringe attached.	Avoids inadvertently introducing air into the system.	If inserting a double-lumen catheter, prime the additional lumen of the catheter with NS.
9. Prepare the venipuncture site, beginning with the alcohol pads or swabsticks. Starting at the insertion site, cleanse outward, using a circular motion, to an area 6 to 8 inches in diameter. Repeat three times. Allow the area to dry and then cleanse in a similar fashion using the three povidone-iodine pads or swabsticks. Allow the area to air dry completely.	Limits the introduction of potentially infectious skin flora into the vessel during the puncture. Combination of cleansing solutions enhances the antimicrobial actions of the agents.	Do not remove the povidone-iodine solution with alcohol, because alcohol cancels the effect of the povidone-iodine.[3] Application time (a *minimum* of 30 seconds) is the chemical kill.[4]
10. Remove gloves and apply the tourniquet (or blood pressure cuff) snugly approximately 6 in (15 cm) above the antecubital fossa.	Provides vasodilatation of the vein for venipuncture.	Constriction should effectively cause venous distention without arterial occlusion. A blood pressure cuff may be used and may be more effective, especially with obese patients. After the cuff is inflated, palpate the radial artery to assess for arterial blood flow. *Procedure continued on following page*

▪▪ AP   This procedure should be performed only by physicians, advanced practice nurses, and other health care professionals (including critical care nurses) with additional knowledge, skills, and demonstrated competence per professional licensure or institutional standard.

Procedure **for Peripherally Inserted Central Catheter** *Continued*

Steps	Rationale	Special Considerations
11. Don a new pair of sterile gloves. Instruct the patient to lift his or her arm, and place a sterile drape underneath and the fenestrated drape over the prepared area, leaving the venipuncture site exposed. Drop a sterile 4-in × 4-in gauze pad over the tourniquet.	Maintains the sterile field and facilitates aseptic technique.	
12. Inject a skin weal of approximately 0.5 mL of 1% lidocaine without epinephrine at or adjacent to the venipuncture site. *(Level V: Clinical studies in more than one or two different patient populations and situations to support recommendations)*	Provides local anesthesia for venipuncture with large-gauge needles and introducers. Research suggests that local anesthesia should be considered when inserting a PICC.	Most patients report less pain when a local anesthetic agent is used before venipuncture.[5] Lidocaine may produce stinging, burning, obliteration of the vein, or venospasm. The use of EMLA, a topical anesthetic cream, before venipuncture has been researched.[6, 7] If used, the manufacturer's recommendations should be followed.
13. Perform the venipuncture according to catheter design and manufacturer's instructions (Fig. 76–4).	Catheters vary according to design and introducing techniques.	
14. Observe for blood return in the flashback chamber and gently advance the introducer sheath until the tip is well within the vein.	Verifies venous access.	If there is no blood return, the procedure should be terminated and an alternate access site should be selected.
15. Withdraw the needle while stabilizing the introducer.	Limits inadvertent trauma to the vein or dislodgment of the introducer.	Use of safety devices minimizes exposure to blood when the introducer needle is removed and protects against needlestick injury (Fig. 76–5).[8]
16. Insert the catheter approximately 6 to 8 in (15 to 20 cm) (Fig. 76–6).	Establishes venous access.	Sterile forceps may be used to insert the catheter into the introducer and advance the catheter into the vein.

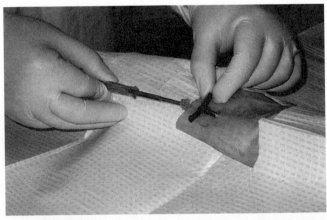

■ ● FIGURE 76–5. Removal of the introducer needle using the PROTECTIV* valved safety introducer system. When the introducer needle is withdrawn, the valve shuts to minimize exposure to blood and the needle tip is covered to help protect against needlestick injuries. (Courtesy of Johnson & Johnson.)

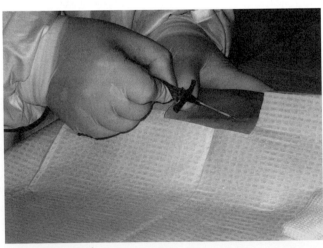

■ ● FIGURE 76–4. Performing the venipuncture.

Procedure **for Peripherally Inserted Central Catheter** *Continued*

Steps	Rationale	Special Considerations

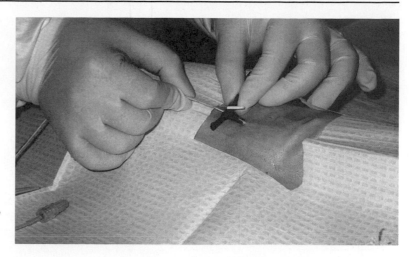

■ ● **FIGURE 76–6.** Catheter is inserted through the introducer. (Courtesy of Johnson & Johnson.)

Steps	Rationale	Special Considerations
17. Release the tourniquet using the sterile 4-in × 4-in gauze pad.	Continued vasodilatation may not be required for catheter advancement.	If a blood pressure cuff is used, it may remain inflated throughout the advancement of the catheter. Leaving the tourniquet in place (or the blood pressure cuff inflated) may facilitate catheter advancement if vascular insufficiency is evident.
18. Instruct the patient to turn his or her head toward the cannulated arm and to drop his or her chin to the chest.	Occludes the jugular vein and avoids malpositioning of the catheter in the jugular vein.	
19. Advance the remainder of the catheter until approximately 4 in (10 cm) remain. Observe (or palpate) the heart rate and rhythm.	Cardiac dysrhythmias may occur if the catheter is advanced into the heart.	Never advance the catheter if resistance is felt. Excessive pushing could lead to perforation of the vein or myocardium.
20. Instruct the patient to return his or her head to the contralateral side.	Prevents contamination of the field by organisms from the patient's respiratory tract.	
21. Pull the introducer sheath out of the vein and away from the insertion site, and remove (Fig. 76–7).	The introducer sheath is not needed once the catheter is in place.	Methods of removing the introducer sheath vary according to the manufacturer.
22. Measure the length of the catheter remaining outside the skin and reposition, if necessary, to the predetermined length. Approximately 1 in (2.5 cm) of the catheter should remain externally.	Ensures proper catheter tip position.	
23. Slowly and gently remove the guidewire.	Prevents recoiling of the catheter.	

Procedure continued on following page

| Procedure | **for Peripherally Inserted Central Catheter** *Continued* |

| **Steps** | **Rationale** | **Special Considerations** |

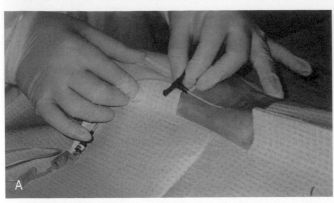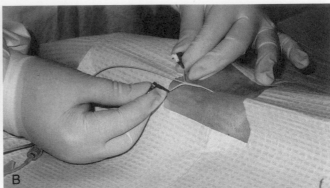

■ ● **FIGURE 76–7.** Removal of the PROTECTIV* valved safety introducer sheath *A*, Introducer sheath is pulled out of the vein. *B*, Valved introducer is split and peeled away from the catheter. (Courtesy of Johnson & Johnson.)

Steps	Rationale	Special Considerations
24. Attach the primed extension tubing (with injection port) to the catheter; aspirate for evidence of blood, and flush with NS.	Affirms patency of the catheter. Use of extension tubing provides easier access to the catheter and reduces local trauma at the insertion site.	
25. Inject recommended amount and concentration of heparin into the catheter, clamp the extension tubing, and remove the syringe. Repeat procedure if using a double-lumen catheter.	Maintains catheter patency and prevents backflow of blood in the catheter.	Recommendations vary regarding the amount and concentration of heparin used to maintain catheter patency.[4, 9] Institutional policies should be followed.
26. Secure the catheter at the insertion site by suturing or by applying Steri-Strips.	Prevents inward or outward migration of the catheter.	Nylon suture is recommended.[9] Procedure should follow institutional guidelines.
27. Cover insertion site with sterile, 2-in × 2-in gauze pad(s). Swab the surrounding skin with the skin protectant swabstick and cover the site with a sterile, transparent, semipermeable dressing.[1]	Decreases catheter-related infections.	Initial dressing should be left in place for 24 hours. After this, assess the insertion site and upper forearm while performing a sterile dressing change. Policies may vary regarding the frequency of dressing changes after the initial dressing change.
28. Discard used supplies and wash hands.	Reduces transmission of microorganisms and body secretions; standard precautions.	
29. Prepare the patient for a chest x-ray.	Confirms placement of the catheter tip and detects any complications.	Some PICCs require contrast media for good visualization. Infusions should not be initiated until catheter tip placement is confirmed.

Expected Outcomes	Unexpected Outcomes
• Catheter tip is positioned in the superior vena cava or subclavian vein. • Catheter remains patent. • Insertion site and upper extremity remain free of phlebitis and thrombophlebitis. • Insertion site, catheter, and systemic circulation remain free of infection.	• Pain or severe discomfort during the procedure • Complications on insertion—cardiac dysrhythmias, pneumothorax, hemothorax, air embolism, catheter embolism, arterial puncture, nerve or tendon damage • Complications following insertion—phlebitis, thrombophlebitis, catheter occlusion, infection (eg, insertion site, catheter, systemic), infiltration

Patient Monitoring and Care

Patient Monitoring and Care	Rationale	Reportable Conditions
		These conditions should be reported if they persist despite nursing interventions.
1. Observe the patient for signs or symptoms of cardiac dysrhythmias during the procedure. If cardiac dysrhythmias occur, pull the catheter back and reassess the patient.	Cardiac dysrhythmias may occur if the catheter is advanced into the heart.	• Cardiac dysrhythmias • Hemodynamic instability (changes in vital signs, level of consciousness, peripheral pulses)
2. Assess the patient and obtain the chest x-ray report confirming proper catheter tip placement before initiating any intravenous solutions.	Ensures accurate catheter tip placement and aids in identifying life-threatening complications.	• Abnormal chest x-ray report • Change in lung sounds • Chest pain • Respiratory distress
3. Observe dressing and insertion site every 30 minutes for the first 4 hours after insertion.	Postinsertion bleeding may occur in patients with coagulopathies, arterial punctures, multiple attempts at venipuncture, or with the through-the-needle introducer designs for insertion.	• Excessive bleeding, hematoma • Changes in vital signs
4. Assess the insertion site and upper extremity every 8 hours for signs and symptoms of thrombophlebitis.	Sterile thrombophlebitis may occur within 0 to 10 days of catheter insertion.	• Pain along vein • Edema at puncture site • Erythema • Ipsilateral swelling of arm, neck, face
5. Assess catheter for venous blood return and patency before initiating infusions. Connect a 5-mL syringe filled with 3 mL of NS to the extension tubing. Release the clamp and aspirate slowly to verify blood return. Flush with 3 mL of NS and then administer the infusion.	Verifies position of the catheter in the vascular space and patency before initiating infusions.	• Venous occlusion (changes in arm circumference greater than 2 cm from baseline) • Catheter occlusion (failure to obtain blood return on aspiration or resistance to irrigation) • Infiltration (infusion continues in spite of restriction to venous blood flow by tourniquet)
6. Assess the catheter for dislodgment or migration by measuring the length of the external catheter.	Catheter may no longer be properly positioned if the length of external catheter is longer or shorter than the length measured at the time of insertion.	• Change in external catheter length • Catheter occlusion • Cardiac dysrhythmias • Pain or burning during infusions • Palpation of catheter in the internal jugular vein • Palpation of coiled catheter • Infiltration

Continued on following page

AP This procedure should be performed only by physicians, advanced practice nurses, and other health care professionals (including critical care nurses) with additional knowledge, skills, and demonstrated competence per professional licensure or institutional standard.

Patient Monitoring and Care *Continued*

Patient Monitoring and Care	Rationale	Reportable Conditions
7. Monitor insertion site and patient for signs and symptoms of local or systemic infection.	Incidence of infection related to the catheter may result from failure to maintain asepsis during insertion, failure to comply with dressing change protocols, immunosuppression, frequent access to the catheter, and long-term use of a single IV access site.	• Redness, warmth, hardness, tenderness or pain, swelling at insertion site • Presence of purulent drainage from insertion site • Local rash or pustules • Fever, chills, elevated white blood cell count • Nausea and vomiting
8. Avoid obtaining blood pressures, performing venipunctures, or administering injections in the extremity with a PICC.	Minimizes the risk of catheter-related complications and catheter damage.	

Documentation

Documentation should include the following:

- Patient and family education
- Signed informed consent
- Known allergies
- Related lab results (white blood cell count, PT, PTT, platelet count)
- Date and time of procedure
- Catheter type, size, and length, including length of catheter remaining outside the insertion site
- Mid-upper arm circumference
- Type and amount of local anesthetic (if used)

- Location of PICC insertion site and vein accessed
- Method of securing catheter (suture, Steri-Strips)
- Confirmation of catheter tip placement
- Problems encountered during or after procedure and nursing interventions
- Patient tolerance of procedure
- Vital signs and cardiac rhythm
- Assessment of insertion site

References

1. Krozek C, Millam D, Pelikan R. Intravascular therapy. In: *Nursing Procedures.* 2nd ed. Springhouse, Pa: Springhouse Corp; 1996:305–311.
2. Perucca R. Obtaining vascular access. In: Terry J, Baranowski L, Lonsway RA, Hedric C, eds. *Intravenous Therapy: Clinical Principles and Practice.* Philadelphia, Pa: W.B. Saunders; 1995:379–391.
3. Krozek C, Millam D, Pelikan R. Intravascular therapy. In: *Nursing Procedures.* 2nd ed. Springhouse, Pa: Springhouse Corp; 1996:380–395.
4. Perucca R. Intravenous monitoring and catheter care. In: Terry J, Baranowski L, Lonsway RA, Hedric C, eds. *Intravenous Therapy: Clinical Principles and Practice.* Philadelphia, Pa: W.B. Saunders; 1995:392–399.
5. Hussey VM, Poulin MV, Fain JA. Effectiveness of lidocaine hydrochloride on venipuncture sites. *AORN J.* 1997;66(3):472–475.
6. Lander J, Nazarali S, Hodgins M, et al. Evaluation of a new topical anesthetic agent: a pilot study. *Nurs Res.* 1996;45(1):50–52.
7. Nott M, Peacock J. Relief of injection pain in adults: EMLA cream for 5 minutes before venepuncture. *Anaesthesia.* 1990;45:772–774.
8. National Committee on Safer Needle Devices. *Using Safer Needle Devices: The Time Is Now.* Washington, DC: Author; 1997.
9. Perdue M. Intravenous complications. In: Terry J, Baranowski L, Lonsway RA, Hedric C, eds. *Intravenous Therapy: Clinical Principles and Practice.* Philadelphia, Pa: W.B. Saunders; 1995:419–443.

Additional Readings

Abi-Nader JA. Peripherally inserted central venous catheters in critical care patients. *Heart Lung.* 1993;22:428–434.

Driscoll M, Buckenmyer C, Spirk M, Molchany C. Inserting and maintaining peripherally inserted central catheters. *MedSurg Nurs.* 1997;6(6):350–355.

Potter PA, Perry AG, eds. *Basic Nursing: A Critical Thinking Approach.* 4th ed. St. Louis, Mo: C.V. Mosby; 1999.

Schull PD, ed. *Nursing Procedures.* 2nd ed. Springhouse, Pa: Springhouse Corp; 1996.

Terry J, Baranowski L, Lonsway RA, Hedrick C, eds. *Intravenous Therapy: Clinical Principles and Practice.* Philadelphia, Pa: W.B. Saunders; 1995.

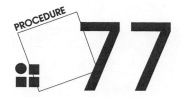

77

Venipuncture

PURPOSE: Venipuncture is performed to obtain a sample of venous blood suitable for a variety of laboratory tests (eg, measurement of serum electrolytes, blood urea nitrogen (BUN), creatinine, prothrombin time (PT), partial thromboplastin time (PTT), cardiac enzymes, complete blood count (CBC), amylase). Proper specimen collection and handling are integral to the accuracy of the results; the likelihood of introducing error is greater in these areas than during the actual laboratory analysis.

Linda Bucher

PREREQUISITE NURSING KNOWLEDGE

- Nurses must be adequately prepared to perform venipuncture. This preparation should include specific educational content regarding venipuncture and opportunities to demonstrate clinical competency.
- Principles of aseptic technqiue should be understood.
- Knowledge of the anatomy and physiology of the vasculature and adjacent structures in the upper extremity is important. The most commonly used veins are located on the forearm (eg, cephalic, basilic, median cubital veins), followed by those on the dorsum of the hand (eg, dorsal venous arch, metacarpal plexus) (Figs. 77–1 and 77–2).[1]
- Superficial veins lie in loose connective tissue under the skin and are best suited for venipuncture.[2] Typically, venipuncture is performed using a vein in the antecubital fossa.[3]
- Patient indications for venipuncture vary and can include patients with suspected electrolyte imbalances, bleeding disorders, infections, and myocardial infarctions (MIs).
- For patients who require frequent venous sampling and who have limited peripheral access, cannulation of a central vein should be considered.
- The most common complication associated with venipuncture is hematoma. Less common complications include excessive pain, excessive bleeding, thrombosis, phlebitis, and cellulitis.[1]
- Modifications to the specimen collection procedure are related to specific laboratory tests. These can include not using a tourniquet and requesting the patient not to clench his or her fist during the venipuncture (eg, lactate levels), placing the specimen on ice immediately after collection (eg, ammonia levels), and avoiding use of alcohol to prep the skin before collection (eg, blood alcohol levels). It is imperative that the nurse performing the venipuncture has a complete knowledge of these modifications.

EQUIPMENT

- One pair of examination gloves
- One 2-in by 2-in gauze pad
- Single-use tourniquet
- VACUTAINER® adapter
- VACUTAINER® needle (20-, 21-, or 22-G) or 23-G butterfly blood collection set
- One alcohol pad or swabstick
- One povidone-iodine pad or swabstick
- One adhesive bandage
- Biohazard box for discarding used needles
- Appropriate color-coded collection tubes (including extras)
- Appropriate specimen labels and laboratory forms

Additional equipment as needed includes the following:

- Plastic bag with ice
- Lidocaine or eutectic mixture of local anesthetics (EMLA) cream (optional)

PATIENT AND FAMILY EDUCATION

- Explain the reason for the venipuncture to the patient and family. ➤*Rationale:* Clarification of information is an

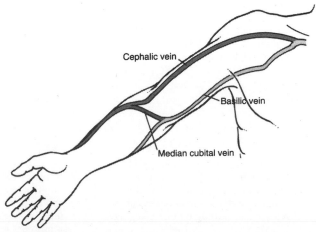

■ ● **FIGURE 77–1.** Superficial veins of the upper extremity. (From Flynn JC. *Procedures in Phlebotomy.* 2nd ed. Philadelphia, Pa: WB Saunders; 1999: 91.)

expressed patient and family need and helps to diminish anxiety, enhance acceptance, and encourage questions.

- Describe the overall steps of the procedure, including the patient's role in the procedure. ⇥*Rationale:* Decreases patient anxiety, enhances cooperation, and provides an opportunity for the patient to voice concerns; prevents accidental movement during the procedure.

PATIENT ASSESSMENT AND PREPARATION

Patient Assessment

- Assess current anticoagulation therapy or blood dyscrasias. ⇥*Rationale:* Anticoagulation therapy or blood dyscrasias could prolong hemostasis at the puncture site and increase the risk of hematoma formation or excessive bleeding.
- Assess allergy history (eg, lidocaine, EMLA cream, antiseptic solutions, adhesives). ⇥*Rationale:* Reduces the risk of allergic reactions.
- Determine history of mastectomy, fistula, shunt, vascular injury. ⇥*Rationale:* Venipuncture should be avoided in extremities affected by these conditions.
- Determine current intravenous (IV) therapy or blood administration. ⇥*Rationale:* Venipuncture should be avoided in extremities with these therapies, because they may alter the accuracy of the test results.[1] If the patient is receiving IV therapy in both arms, venipuncture should be performed below the site of the IV line.
- Determine the best venipuncture site on the patient's arms. ⇥*Rationale:* Lower extremities should be avoided in adults. Hand veins should be avoided, because they lie just beneath the surface of the skin and tend to roll. Avoid edematous areas or sites of previous hematoma, infection, or vascular injury and veins that are very small, sclerosed, scarred, or tortuous, because these conditions inhibit successful venipuncture and can contribute to complications.
- Determine whether IV access (peripheral or central) is to

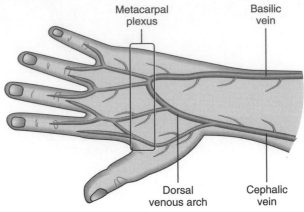

■ ● **FIGURE 77–2.** Superficial veins of the hand.

be initiated in addition to venipuncture. ⇥*Rationale:* Accurate laboratory samples can be collected during the initiation of IV access, thereby limiting the number of venipunctures required.[4]

Patient Preparation

- Ensure that the patient and family understand preprocedural teaching. Answer questions as they arise and reinforce information as needed. ⇥*Rationale:* Evaluates and reinforces understanding of previously taught information.
- Position the patient in a supine position with head slightly elevated and arms at side. ⇥*Rationale:* Proper positioning of patient enhances accessibility to the venipuncture site and promotes patient comfort.
- Extend the patient's upper extremity to form a straight line from the shoulder to the wrist. A pillow can be placed under the arm for support, if needed. ⇥*Rationale:* Proper positioning of the extremity enhances accessibility to the venipuncture site and reduces the risk of patient movement during the procedure.

Procedure for Venipuncture

Steps	Rationale	Special Considerations
1. Gather supplies, including extra tubes, and attach VACUTAINER® needle (20-G, 21-G, or 22-G) to adapter (Fig. 77–3).	Extra tubes avoid interruption of procedure. Proper needle size minimizes trauma to the vein and the risk of hemolysis.[4]	If using a butterfly (23-G), attach a VACUTAINER® adapter to the butterfly blood collection set (Fig. 77–4). A 10-mL syringe with a 20-G or 21-G needle can be used to perform venipuncture if the VACUTAINER® system is not available.
2. Wash hands, and don clean gloves.	Reduces transmission of microorganisms; standard precautions.	
3. Apply tourniquet 2 in above the area chosen for venipuncture. Tie in a manner so that the tourniquet can be released by pulling on one end (Fig. 77–5).	Impedes venous return to the heart and produces venous dilation. Proper application of the tourniquet allows for the quick, one-handed release of the tourniquet when desired.	Arterial blood flow should not be impeded. Arterial perfusion should be verified by palpating for the radial pulse. For patients with large, prominent veins, a tourniquet is not recommended.[1]

Procedure for **Venipuncture** *Continued*

Steps	Rationale	Special Considerations

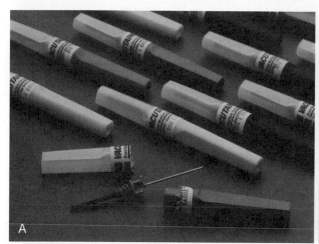 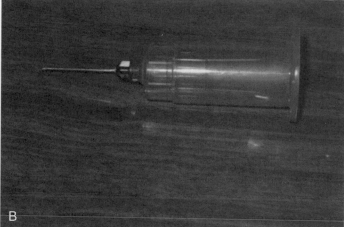

■ ● **FIGURE 77–3.** VACUTAINER® system. *A,* VACUTAINER® needles. *B,* VACUTAINER® needle attached to adapter. (Courtesy of Becton Dickinson.)

4. Use the tip of the index or second finger to palpate the area across the arm at the elbow. If veins are not prominent, instruct patient to open and close hand (make a fist) several times, ending with clenched fist. If a vein still cannot be palpated, remove tourniquet and apply to alternate arm.

Veins should be palpated before venipuncture to improve chance of success. The milking action of opening and closing the hand causes blood to flow into the veins.

Alternative approaches to facilitating venous distention include gentle tapping of the skin over the venipuncture area with the index and second fingers and permitting the arm to hang dependently below the level of the heart. Warm compresses also can be applied to facilitate venous dilation. The tourniquet should not be left on for more than 2 minutes because it may result in hemoconcentration or variation in blood test values.[1,2]

Procedure continued on following page

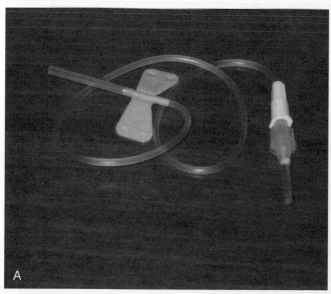 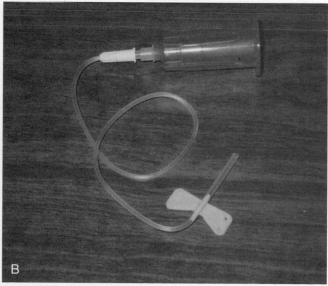

■ ● **FIGURE 77–4.** VACUTAINER® butterfly blood collection system. *A,* VACUTAINER® butterfly blood collection set. *B,* VACUTAINER® blood collection set attached to adapter. (Courtesy of Becton Dickinson.)

Procedure **for Venipuncture** *Continued*

Steps	Rationale	Special Considerations
5. If lidocaine or EMLA cream is to be used, then remove the tourniquet and apply to site selected for venipuncture. *(Level V: Clinical studies in more than one or two different patient populations and situations to support recommendations)*	Provides relief from pain associated with venipuncture and may reduce or eliminate anxiety associated with procedure.[5–7]	Research on length of time from application of lidocaine or EMLA to procedure has produced inconclusive results.[5–7] If used, the manufacturer's recommendations for application should be followed. The time from application to procedure varies from 5 to 60 minutes.
6. Prepare site, beginning with the alcohol pad or swabstick. Starting at the puncture site, cleanse outward, using a circular motion while applying friction. After the alcohol has dried, continue cleansing in a similar fashion using the povidone-iodine pad or swabstick. Allow the prepared area to dry (30 seconds to 2 minutes).[1, 3, 8, 9]	Limits the introduction of potentially infectious skin flora into the vessel during the puncture. Combination of cleansing solutions enhances the antimicrobial actions of the agents.[8, 9]	Never remove the povidone-iodine solution with alcohol, because alcohol cancels the effect of the povidone-iodine.[1] Application time (a *minimum* of 30 seconds) is the chemical kill.[8] If you must palpate the area once cleansing has been performed, you must use sterile gloves or recleanse the area.[3]
7. Draw the skin just below the venipuncture site taut using the thumb of the nondominant hand.	Immobilizes the vein for venipuncture.	
8. Push the stopper of the collecting tube into the needle up to the guideline on the VACUTAINER® adapter.	Prepares the VACUTAINER® system for blood collection and limits the need for manipulation of equipment once the venipuncture is made.	

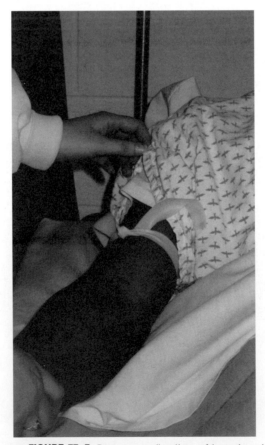

■ ● **FIGURE 77–5.** Proper application of tourniquet.

Procedure **for Venipuncture** *Continued*

Steps	Rationale	Special Considerations

9. Collecting tubes are filled in the following order:
   A. Blood culture tubes
 	
   B. Empty tubes, generally plain, red-top tubes or tubes with gel separators without clot enhancers
 	
   C. Tubes with additives, generally light blue, then heparin, lavender, and gray[3]
	Minimizes the risk of bacterial contamination.[3] Tissue fluids may interfere with coagulation studies.[3]
	
	Additives from the tubes may interfere with the accuracy of the laboratory results if there is any carryover between collection tubes.[3]
		Consult the manufacturer's recommendations and protocols within your institution. If a coagulation tube is the only tube requested, a plain, red-top tube should be collected first and discarded.[3] If a syringe is used, transfer sample to the collecting tubes by detaching the syringe needle, opening the collection tube, and emptying the sample into the tube by allowing it to steadily flow down the sides of the tubes.[1] Blood collected with a syringe should be added to the anticoagulant tubes first, followed by the remaining tubes.[10]

10. Position the needle with the bevel up and the shaft parallel to (along side of) the path of the vein.	Provides least traumatic entry through the skin.	
11. Insert the needle through the skin at a 15- to 30-degree angle and ¼ to ½ in below the intended entry into the vein (Fig. 77–6).	Provides least traumatic entry of needle into vein and limits risk of hematoma.	As the needle pierces the vein, a sensation of resistance may be felt, followed by ease of penetration.
12. Grasp the flange of the needle adapter and push the collecting tube forward until the needle punctures the stopper. Observe for the flow of blood into the collecting tube.	Stabilizes the needle in the vein and activates the vacuum within the collecting tube, thereby facilitating the flow of blood into the tube.	If blood does not flow, move the needle slightly in and out. Change collecting tubes to ascertain whether or not the first tube had vacuum. If blood still does not flow, release the tourniquet, remove the needle, apply pressure with the gauze, and attempt a second venipuncture at a new location and with a new needle.

Procedure continued on following page

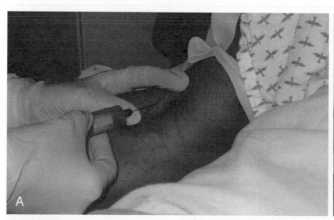
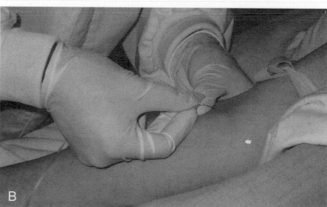

■ ● **FIGURE 77–6.** Venipuncture. *A,* VACUTAINER® system. *B,* VACUTAINER® butterfly blood collection system. (Courtesy of Becton Dickinson.)

| Procedure | **for Venipuncture** *Continued* |

Steps	Rationale	Special Considerations
13. If a butterfly is being used, blood flow will first be observed in the tubing (Fig. 77–7A). Once blood flow is established, grasp the flange of the butterfly needle adapter and push the collecting tube forward until the needle punctures the stopper. Observe for the flow of blood into the collecting tube (Fig. 77–7B).	Activates the vacuum within the collecting tube, thereby facilitating the flow of blood into the tube.	
14. If a syringe is being used, observe for blood in the hub. Withdraw blood slowly by pulling gently on the plunger of the syringe until the required sample is obtained.		
15. Release tourniquet as soon as blood flow is established. Allow blood to fill the collecting tube until the vacuum is exhausted.	Prevents stasis and hemoconcentration, which can impair accuracy of test results.[1]	If blood flow is sluggish, the tourniquet may be kept in place. Once blood flow is established, have patient release clenched fist, if appropriate.
16. While holding adapter steady, remove collecting tube and replace with new tube. Repeat until all required tubes are filled.	Prevents the inadvertent dislodgment of the needle.	For tubes containing an additive (eg, anticoagulant), gently rotate five to ten times by inversion. Do not mix tubes that contain no additive.
17. To remove needle, release tourniquet, if not already done. Place gauze pad over puncture site and gently remove the needle.	Limits the risk of the development of a hematoma.	Last collecting tube must be removed from the adapter to release the vacuum before removing the needle.
18. Place needle and adapter directly into Biohazard container.	Limits risk of accidental puncture by contaminated needle.	Equipment varies and may be designed to provide protection from needlesticks upon removal of needle (Fig. 77–8).
19. Apply continuous pressure to the gauze pad over the puncture site for 2 to 3 minutes.	Prevents extravasation of blood into the surrounding tissues and limits the development of a hematoma.	Continued pressure may be necessary for patients with history of blood dyscrasias or anticoagulation therapy. If bleeding persists, the extremity may be elevated above level of heart while maintaining pressure to the site. Avoid flexing the extremity because this enhances hematoma formation.

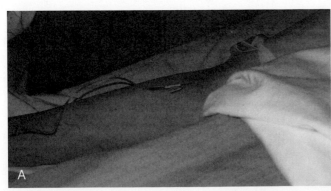
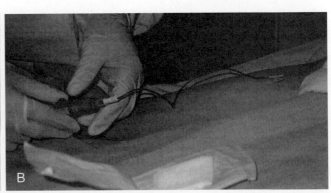

■ ● **FIGURE 77–7.** Venipuncture using the VACUTAINER® butterfly blood collection system. *A,* Flow of blood into tubing of butterfly establishes successful venipuncture. *B,* Flow of blood into collecting tube once vacuum is activated. (Courtesy of Becton Dickinson.)

Procedure for Venipuncture *Continued*

Steps	Rationale	Special Considerations

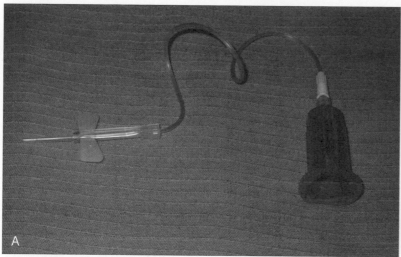
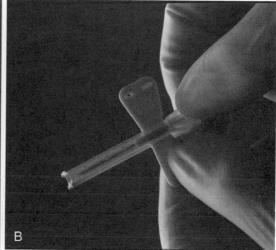

■ ● **FIGURE 77–8.** VACUTAINER® SAFETY-LOK™ Blood Collection Set. *A,* SAFETY-LOK™ blood collection set before use. *B,* SAFETY-LOK™ blood collection set after use and with needle guard activated. (Courtesy of Becton Dickinson.)

20. Once hemostasis has been established, apply an adhesive bandage to venipuncture site.

Limits risk of infection at venipuncture site.

21. Label specimens and verify laboratory requisitions per protocol.

Ensures accuracy of results (eg, right patient, right specimen, right test).

22. Expedite delivery of specimens to laboratory.

Ensures timeliness of laboratory analyses.

23. Dispose of gloves and equipment properly; wash hands.

Reduces the transmission of microorganisms; standard precautions.

Expected Outcomes

- Venous sample is collected such that accuracy of results is maintained.
- Puncture site remains free of complications (eg, hematoma, pain, excessive bleeding, thrombosis, phlebitis, and cellulitis).
- Alterations in laboratory values are identified and treated accordingly.

Unexpected Outcomes

- Excessive pain or severe discomfort during procedure
- Hemolyzed specimens
- Complications following venipuncture: hematoma, excessive bleeding, thrombosis, phlebitis, and cellulitis

Patient Monitoring and Care

Patient Monitoring and Care	Rationale	Reportable Conditions
		These conditions should be reported if they persist despite nursing interventions.
1. Observe venipuncture site for signs of hemostasis after procedure.	Postpuncture hematoma can occur if the needle passes through both walls of the vein, if the needle bevel is not fully seated in the vein, if the extremity is flexed after needle removal, or if insufficient time is spent applying pressure to venipuncture site. Postpuncture bleeding is more likely to occur in patients with coagulopathies or in patients receiving anticoagulation therapy.	• Excessive bleeding, large hematoma • Changes in vital signs
2. Assess venipuncture site and involved extremity for signs of postprocedure complications (eg, thrombosis, phlebitis, cellulitis).	All venipunctures cause trauma to the surrounding tissues and the intimal layer of the vessel wall. This trauma causes cells and platelets to aggregate. The greater the trauma, the greater the risk of complications. Proper technique minimizes these risks.	• Erythema, warmth, hardness, tenderness or pain at venipuncture site or along path of vein • Presence of purulent drainage from puncture site

Documentation

Documentation should include the following:

- Patient and family education
- Date, time, and laboratory tests requested
- Venipuncture site used
- Local anesthetic used (if applicable)
- Patient's tolerance of procedure
- Postvenipuncture site care
- Disposition of specimen(s), results, and analysis
- Unexpected outcomes
- Additional interventions

References

1. Buffington S. Specimen collection and testing. In: *Nursing Procedures.* 2nd ed. Springhouse, Pa: Springhouse Corp; 1996:135–138.
2. Hadaway LC. Anatomy and physiology related to intravenous therapy. In: Terry J, Baranowski L, Lonsway RA, Hedric C, eds. *Intravenous Therapy: Clinical Principles and Practice.* Philadelphia, Pa: W.B. Saunders; 1995:97–100.
3. Flynn JC. Proper procedures for venipuncture. In: Flynn JC, ed. *Procedures in Phlebotomy.* 2nd ed. Philadelphia, Pa: W.B. Saunders; 1999:87–113.
4. Kennedy C, Angermuller S, King R, et al. A comparison of hemolysis rates using intravenous catheters versus venipuncture tubes for obtaining blood samples. *J Emerg Nurs.* 1996;22:566–569.
5. Hussey VM, Poulin MV, Fain JA. Effectiveness of lidocaine hydrochloride on venipuncture sites. *AORN J.* 1997;66:472–475.
6. Lander J, Nazarali S, Hodgins M, et al. Evaluation of a new topical anesthetic agent: a pilot study. *Nurs Res.* 1996;45:50–52.
7. Nott M, Peacock J. Relief of injection pain in adults: EMLA cream for 5 minutes before venipuncture. *Anaesthesia* 1990;45:772–774.
8. Perucca R. Obtaining vascular access. In: Terry J, Baranowski L, Lonsway RA, Hedric C, eds. *Intravenous Therapy: Clinical Principles and Practice.* Philadelphia, Pa: W.B. Saunders; 1995:379–391.
9. Speakman E. Fluid, electrolyte, and acid-base balances. In: Potter PA, Perry AG, eds. *Basic Nursing: A Critical Thinking Approach.* 4th ed. St. Louis, Mo: Mosby; 1999:857–890.
10. Flynn JC. Special collection procedures. In: Flynn JC, ed. *Procedures in Phlebotomy.* 2nd ed. Philadelphia, Pa: W.B. Saunders; 1999:115–134.

Additional Readings

Flynn JC, ed. *Procedures in Phlebotomy.* 2nd ed. Philadelphia, Pa: W.B. Saunders; 1999.

Potter PA, Perry AG, eds. *Basic Nursing: A Critical Thinking Approach.* 4th ed. St. Louis Mo: Mosby; 1999.

Schull PD, ed. *Nursing Procedures.* 2nd ed. Springhouse, Pa: Springhouse Corp; 1996.

Terry J, Baranowski L, Lonsway RA, Hedrick C, eds. *Intravenous Therapy: Clinical Principles and Practice.* Philadelphia, Pa: W.B. Saunders, 1995.

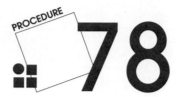

Intracranial Bolt Insertion (Assist), Monitoring, Care, Troubleshooting, and Removal

P U R P O S E: Intracranial bolts are used to measure and continuously monitor intracranial pressure (ICP), calculate cerebral perfusion pressure (CPP), and assess cerebral compliance and autoregulation. Intracranial bolts cannot be used to treat elevated intracranial pressure through cerebrospinal fluid (CSF) removal, because these devices do not provide adequate access for CSF drainage.

Jacqueline Sullivan

PREREQUISITE NURSING KNOWLEDGE

- Knowledge of neuroanatomy and physiology is needed.
- Knowledge of aseptic technique is needed.
- ICP is measured as the pressure of CSF within the intraventricular, subarachnoid, intraparenchymal (brain tissue), epidural, or subdural spaces.
- Cerebral tissue (brain), cerebral blood, and CSF comprise three discrete volumes occupying the closed compartment of the cranium. Increases in any one or a combination of these volumes will result in adjustments in the remaining volumes so that total volume of the intracranium remains constant (Monro-Kellie hypothesis). This description of intracranial compensatory mechanisms is also known as intracranial compliance. Intracranial compliance is defined as an expression of change in ICP resulting from changes in intracranial volumes. Quantitative measurement of ICP and qualitative analysis of ICP waveform morphology reflect this dynamic compliance relationship among the brain, cerebral circulation, and CSF.
- Several concepts related to CSF secretion and pathways may be important to consider when making clinical decisions related to placement and integrity of intracranial bolts. CSF is secreted by the choroid plexus, which

lines the lateral ventricles. There are approximately 90 to 150 mL of CSF circulating within the CSF pathways in the brain and spinal subarachnoid space at any given point in time. There is a total of 20 mL of CSF within the lateral ventricles and the cranial CSF pathways in nonpathologic conditions. The remaining circulating CSF is found within the distensible compartment of subarachnoid space surrounding the spinal cord. CSF is secreted at a rate of 0.35 mL per minute, or approximately 20 mL per hour. In conditions involving cerebral edema, CSF may be shunted from the cranial ventricular compartments to the subarachnoid space surrounding the spinal cord. CSF is reabsorbed by the subarachnoid villi. Although CSF production is relatively unaffected by increased ICP, there is evidence to suggest that rate of CSF reabsorption increases with ICP elevations.
- Cerebral autoregulation is a protective mechanism whereby the cerebral blood flow remains constant despite fluctuations in systemic blood pressure. Cerebral autoregulation is dependent on intact systemic and intracranial pressure regulation, as well as chemical mechanisms. Systemic and intracranial pressure ranges necessary for intact cerebral autoregulation are listed in Table 78–1. Chemical stimuli, including PCO_2, PO_2, and pyruvic acid,

Table 78–1 ●■■	Parameters Required for Cerebral Autoregulation Preservation

Intracranial pressure (ICP) less than or equal to 30 mm Hg
Mean arterial pressure (MAP) within range of 60 to 160 mm Hg
Cerebral perfusion pressure (CPP) within range of 50 to 150 mm Hg

must also be balanced in order to preserve cerebral autoregulation.

- Normal ICP ranges from 0 to 15 mm Hg (or 0 to 20 cm H_2O).
- CPP is a derived mathematical calculation that indirectly reflects the adequacy of cerebral blood flow. CPP is calculated by subtracting ICP from mean systemic arterial blood pressure (CPP = MAP − ICP). Some experts consider CPP to be at least as, if not more, significant than ICP, because this derived calculation reflects both systemic ability to deliver blood to the brain (MAP) and resistance (ICP) that must be overcome in order to perfuse the brain. Normal CPP ranges from 60 to 160 mm Hg. CPP below 50 mm Hg demonstrates inadequate cerebral perfusion. CPP less than 30 mm Hg results in cerebral tissue hypoxia and irreversible neuronal damage. Some experts recommend protecting cerebral perfusion by maintaining CPP within the minimal range of 70 to 90 mm Hg. Loss of cerebral autoregulation may occur when CPP is persistently not within the range of 50 to 150 mm Hg.[1–5]
- Intracranial hypertension may be described as sustained ICP elevations that do not respond to traditional therapeutic methods used for lowering ICP.
- Traditional therapeutic methods used for lowering ICP may include but are not limited to corticosteroid administration, osmotic diuresis, loop diuresis, hyperventilation, sedation, paralysis, normothermia/hypothermia, CSF drainage, and induced therapeutic barbiturate coma. Precise use of these methods varies depending on etiologic origin of elevated ICP and individual patient conditions. Research-based guidelines for management of ICP in traumatic brain injury (TBI) have been widely disseminated and used in recent years.[4, 6]
- Intracranial bolts may be placed in the subdural, subarachnoid, or intraparenchymal (brain tissue) spaces (Fig. 78–1). Because these devices are not located in areas with bountiful access to CSF, they do not possess capabilities for significant CSF removal and cannot be used to treat intracranial hypertension through CSF drainage. Intraventricular catheters, therefore, are the only ICP monitoring devices available with capabilities for both treating and monitoring ICP. However, intracranial bolts have a lower relative risk for infection and hemorrhage because they are less invasive than intraventricular catheters. There are a variety of intracranial bolts currently available for monitoring ICP, including traditional fluid-coupled devices, fiberoptic systems, and microsensors. Fluid-coupled devices require the use of external strain gauge transducers; other systems do not. Accepted placement of external strain gauge transducers for ICP monitoring is at the anatomic reference point for the foramen of Monro (top of the external auditory canal).

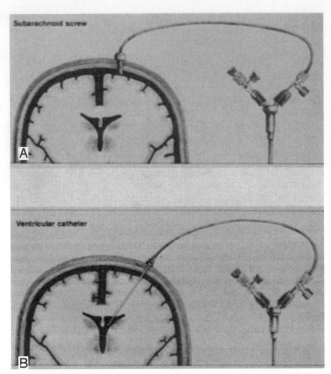

■ ● FIGURE 78–1. Anatomic placement of intracranial monitoring devices. *A,* Subarachnoid bolt. *B,* Intraventricular catheter. (From Cardona VD, Hurn PD, Mason PJ, et al. *Trauma Nursing: From Resuscitation Through Rehabilitation.* Philadelphia: W.B. Saunders; 1988).

- ICP waveform morphology reflects transmission of arterial and venous pressure through CSF and brain parenchyma. A normal ICP waveform has three distinct pressure oscillations or peaks, referred to as P1, P2, and P3. P1, also known as the percussion wave, reflects myocardial systole. P2, also known as the tidal wave, reflects myocardial diastole and ends on the dicrotic notch. P3, the dicrotic wave, is located immediately after the dicrotic notch and slopes into the diastolic baseline position (Fig. 78–2). P3 oscillations are correlated with venous fluctuations. P2 elevations are known to occur with loss of cerebral compliance. P2 pressure oscillation amplitudes approach and surpass P1 pressure oscillations during periods of decompensation and loss of intracerebral compliance (Fig. 78–3). Changes in ICP waveform morphology may also reflect loss of cerebral autoregulation. With loss of cerebral autoregulation, the ICP waveform may assume a mirror-like image of the intra-arterial waveform. These identical ICP and intra-arterial waveforms demonstrate the dependency of cerebral blood flow on systemic arterial blood pressure. As systemic blood

■ ● FIGURE 78–2. Components of the intracranial pressure waveform: P_1, P_2, and P_3.

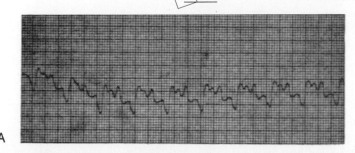

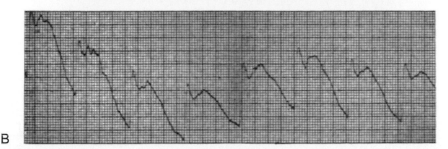

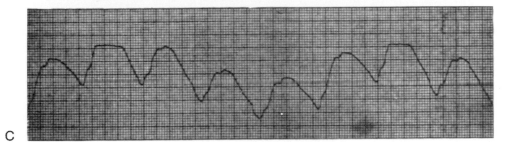

■ ● **FIGURE 78–3.** Example of intracranial pressure waveform with P_2 elevation indicating decreased cerebral compliance.

pressure rises, cerebral blood flow increases and ICP elevates during periods of absent cerebral autoregulation.

- Continuous ICP monitoring data trends may demonstrate three discrete ICP wave trends. These ICP trends are A waves, B waves, and C waves. A waves, also known as plateau waves, occur in severe intracranial hypertension and are characterized by sudden ICP escalations up to 50 to 100 mm Hg, have a duration of 5 to 20 minutes, and frequently are accompanied by neurologic deterioration

or cerebral herniation (Fig. 78–4). B waves are sharp rhythmic oscillations that occur with a frequency of every 30 seconds to 2 minutes; B waves may escalate up to 20 to 50 mm Hg and may precede plateau waves (Fig. 78–5). C waves demonstrate ICP elevations of up to 20 mm Hg and occur with a frequency of every 4 to 8 minutes; they are not thought to be clinically significant (Fig. 78–6).

- Contraindications for intracranial bolt placement may include intracranial infection or coagulopathies.

■ ● **FIGURE 78–4.** A or plateau waves. Open arrows indicate plateau elevations in intracranial pressure. Note that when intracranial pressure falls, it does not return to baseline preceding the first wave *(closed arrow)*. (From Marshall SB, Marshall LF, Vos HR, Chestnut RM. *Neuroscience Critical Care: Pathophysiology and Patient Management.* Philadelphia: W.B. Saunders; 1990.)

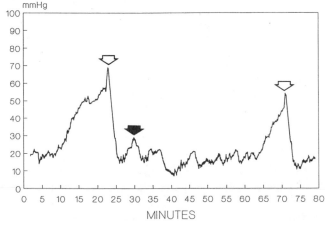

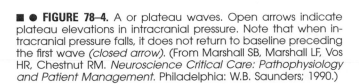

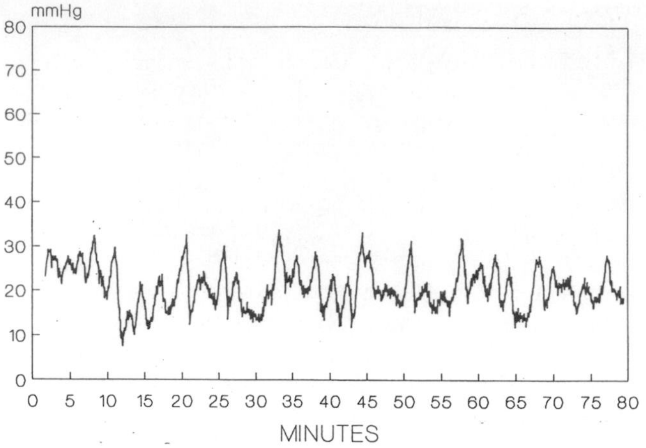

■ ● **FIGURE 78–5.** Elevations in intracranial pressure represent B waves. The intracranial pressure rise is steep and rapid, but to heights less than those observed with A waves and much briefer. (From Marshall SB, Marshall LF, Vos HR, Chestnut RM. *Neuroscience Critical Care: Pathophysiology and Patient Management*. Philadelphia: W.B. Saunders; 1990.)

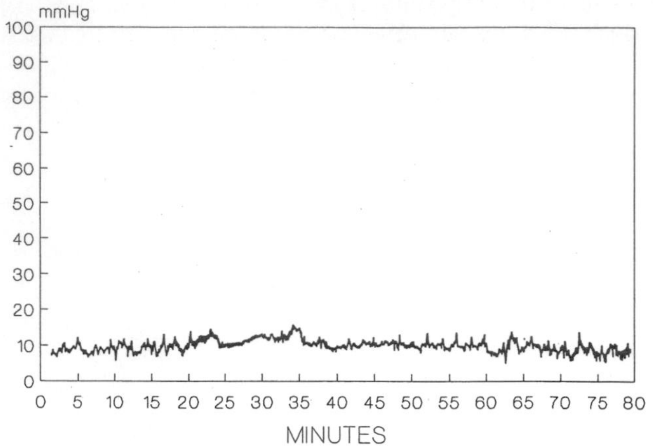

■ ● **FIGURE 78–6.** Lundberg or C waves. The intracranial pressure changes are much less impressive than those in A or B waves and reflect changes in arterial blood pressure. (From Marshall SB, Marshall LF, Vos HR, Chestnut RM. *Neuroscience Critical Care: Pathophysiology and Patient Management*. Philadelphia: W.B. Saunders; 1990.)

EQUIPMENT

- Povidone-iodine scrub solution
- Povidone-iodine pads or swabsticks
- Sterile gloves, surgical caps, masks, goggles, and sterile surgical gowns
- Sterile towels, half-sheets, and drapes
- Local anesthetic (lidocaine 1% or 2% without epinephrine)
- 5- or 10-mL Luer-Lok syringe with 18-G needle (for drawing up lidocaine) and 23-G needle (for administering lidocaine)
- Twist drill and bits (these are provided by a variety of manufacturers in both generic and custom kits, depending on physician preference)
- Sutures (2-0 nylon, 3-0 silk, 4-0 Vicryl)
- Scalpel with No. 11 blade
- Scalp retractor
- Forceps
- Sterile scissors
- Needle holder
- Disposable cautery
- Suction and sterile suction apparatus
- Bone wax or gelfoam
- Light source (headlamp, etc.; optional)
- Intracranial bolt: plastic or metal (for all systems)
- Fiberoptic or microsensor bolt catheter (if using these choices)
- Sterile occlusive dressing (sterile 4×4 gauze pads or bio-occlusive dressing)
- Silk tape (1- and 2-in rolls)

Note: Many of the disposable surgical supplies listed above are available in generic and custom kits supplied by ICP monitoring device manufacturers. Check kit labels for necessary contents.

Additional equipment as neeeded includes the following:

- Two 4-in Kling or Kerlex rolls (optional, needed if performing complete head dressing over insertion site dressing)
- Razor
- Fluid-coupled system: transducer cable, external strain gauge transducer, pressure tubing, three-way stopcock, 0.9% sodium chloride solution without preservative (may use sterile intravenous solution)
- Fiberoptic system: microprocessor (stand-alone monitor), pre-amp connector cable, monitoring cable to "slave"/connect microprocessor (stand-alone monitor) to primary bedside monitoring system, fiberoptic intracranial bolt catheter with calibration screwdriver, sterile CSF drainage system (collection tubing, chamber, and bag)
- Sensor system: microprocessor (stand-alone monitor), microprocessor/sensor cable, monitoring cable to "slave"/connect microprocessor (stand-alone monitor) to primary bedside monitoring system, intracranial bolt sensor catheter with calibration tool, sterile CSF drainage system (collection tubing, chamber, and bag)

Note: A variety of preassembled sterile CSF drainage systems are available in generic and custom kits from ICP monitoring device manufacturers.

PATIENT AND FAMILY EDUCATION

- Assess patient and family understanding of intracranial bolt ICP monitoring and its purpose. ➸***Rationale:*** Clarification and repeat explanation may limit anxiety and stress for the patient and family.
- Explain standard care for insertion, patient monitoring, and care involving intracranial bolt. ➸***Rationale:*** Explanation of expected intervention may allay patient and family anxiety and encourage questions.
- Explain expected outcomes of intracranial bolt use. ➸***Rationale:*** Patient and family may experience less stress if aware of goals, duration, and expectations of intracranial bolt monitoring use.

PATIENT ASSESSMENT AND PREPARATION

Patient Assessment

- Assess baseline neurologic status. ➸***Rationale:*** Knowledge of baseline clinical neurologic status permits recognition of neurologic changes that may occur during or as a result of intracranial bolt placement.

- Observe for early signs of increased intracranial pressure, such as decreased level of consciousness, restlessness, agitation, lethargy, vomiting, motor weakness, or pupillary constriction dysfunction.   ➤*Rationale:* Patients requiring placement of ICP monitoring devices are at risk for or are actually experiencing elevated ICP. Clinical signs of increased ICP should corroborate monitoring data.
- Observe for late signs of increased intracranial pressure, such as loss of consciousness, posturing (decortication, decerebration), sluggish pupillary or absent pupillary light reflex, respiratory pattern changes, Cushing's triad of vital sign changes (bradycardia, increased systolic blood pressure, widening pulse pressure).   ➤*Rationale:* Precise neurologic assessment provides baseline data and establishes clinical correlate for quantitative ICP measurement data.
- Assess current laboratory profile, including CBC, platelet count, prothrombin time (PT), partial thromboplastin time (PTT), bleeding time, and International Normalized Ratio (INR).   ➤*Rationale:* Baseline coagulation studies are necessary to determine degree of risk for bleeding during intracranial bolt insertion.

Patient Preparation

- Ensure that the patient and family understand preprocedural teaching. Answer questions as they arise and reinforce information as needed.   ➤*Rationale:* Evaluates and reinforces understanding of previously taught information.
- Ensure that informed consent has been obtained.   ➤*Rationale:* Protects the rights of the patient and makes a competent decision possible for the patient or family.
- Administer preprocedure analgesia or sedation, as indicated.   ➤*Rationale:* Patients are expected to remain very still during intracranial bolt insertion and may require sedation and analgesia to tolerate the procedure. Alternately, in crisis situations, patients may be unconscious and experiencing cerebral herniation, requiring very little sedation or analgesia for procedural tolerance.
- Assist patient to a supine position with the head of the bed elevated at 30 to 45 degrees with the neck in midline, neutral position.   ➤*Rationale:* This position provides necessary accessibility for intracranial bolt insertion and enhances jugular venous outflow, contributing to possible reduction in intracranial pressure.

Procedure **for Intracranial Bolt Insertion (Assist), Monitoring, Care, Troubleshooting, and Removal**

Steps	Rationale	Special Considerations
1. Wash hands.	Reduces transmission of microorganisms; standard precautions.	
2. Assemble and flush fluid-coupled system with external strain gauge transducer per institutional procedure.	Preparation of external transducer or CSF drainage system promotes efficiency during the insertion procedure and ensures capability of immediate measurement of ICP upon insertion.	A variety of sterile, preassembled external transducer and CSF drainage systems are available in both generic and custom kits from ICP monitoring device manufacturers.
3. Flush system(s), if applicable, with preservative-free 0.9% NaCl solution.	Removes air from the system.	Preserves sterility of systems after preparation, before insertion.
4. Turn on bedside monitor and microprocessor (stand-alone monitor) if using fiberoptic or sensor devices.	Ensures that monitoring equipment is functional and permits immediate recording of ICP on insertion.	
5. Prepare and check suction.	Provides safety during insertion process by confirming suctioning function before procedure.	Suctioning may be needed during ICP bolt placement to control bleeding or remove small fragments of bone or tissue from insertion site.
6. Assist physician in identifying optimal area for placement of device.	Facilitates placement.	Nondominant hemisphere is optimal location for placement of intracranial bolt. However, presence of skull fractures, etiology of intracranial hypertensive process, or nature of cerebral trauma may limit placement options.
7. Wash hands, and don gloves.	Reduces transmission of microorganisms; standard precautions.	
8. Shave and prepare insertion site with povidone-iodine solution.	Reduces microorganisms and minimizes risk of infection.	
9. Drape head and upper thorax with sterile half-sheets and drapes.	Protects insertion site from contamination.	

Procedure continued on following page

Procedure for Intracranial Bolt Insertion (Assist), Monitoring, Care, Troubleshooting, and Removal *Continued*

Steps	Rationale	Special Considerations
10. Open sterile trays and have accessible previously prepared external transducer system.	Facilitates efficiency of insertion and immediate ICP monitoring on insertion.	A variety of preassembled sterile trays containing disposable surgical instruments (as listed on equipment list) are available from ICP monitoring device manufacturers. Check list of sterile tray contents for presence of necessary equipment before opening tray.
11. Zero the monitoring system. Fluid-coupled system: the external transducer system may be zeroed before or immediately after insertion. Anatomic reference point for zeroing and maintaining external transducer is at the level of foramen of Munro (top of external auditory canal). Fiberoptic and sensor systems must be zeroed before insertion using their appropriate microprocessors (stand-alone monitors).	Zero balances to atmospheric pressure and ensures accuracy of monitored data.	Fluid-coupled systems: the external transducer system must be zeroed prior to instituting monitoring and should be rezeroed at periodic intervals. It is also recommended that the monitoring system be rezeroed after any positioning changes occur that alter the location of the transducer from the designated anatomic reference point. Fiberoptic/sensor systems: these systems require the zeroing procedure prior to insertion but do not require periodic zeroing procedures during continued catheter use.
12. Correlation procedure for fiberoptic systems: ensure that slave cable is connecting the microprocessor to the pressure module of the primary bedside monitoring system. Depress "Cal/Step" soft key on fiberoptic microprocessor until number 0 appears on microprocessor monitoring screen. Continue to hold "Cal/Step" soft key in depressed position with one hand while pressing zero option on primary bedside monitoring system. When the number 0 appears on the bedside monitoring screen (it should still be appearing on the microprocessor screen also), release both soft keys on both monitors.	Ensures correlation between fiberoptic microprocessor and primary bedside monitoring system. Integration of ICP data with primary monitoring system data permits use of centralized alarm systems and trending of ICP data with other multisystemic monitored data.	Although this procedure is called "Cal/Step," its purpose is not calibration in the traditional sense. Rather, it is meant to ensure correlation between the fiberoptic microprocessor and the primary bedside monitoring system.
13. Ensure health care providers don surgical caps, masks, goggles, and sterile gloves and gowns.	Provides aseptic environment.	
14. Assist as needed with insertion.	Facilitates insertion process.	
15. Cleanse around the insertion site with a povidone-iodine pad or swabstick. Apply an occlusive dressing. Apply complete head dressing in addition to insertion site dressing if desired.	Protects site from contamination by microorganisms.	
16. Obtain "opening" ICP (initial ICP reading once continuous monitoring is initiated immediately following insertion). Assess ICP waveform morphology (ie, P1, P2, P3). Obtain hard copy recording of ICP waveform and include in medical record/chart.	Provides initial baseline data for quantitative ICP measurement and qualitative assessment of ICP waveform morphology.[7]	Waveform morphology data yield information related to status of cerebral compliance and autoregulation.
17. Calculate and document CPP. $$CPP = MAP - ICP$$	Provides initial, indirect assessment of adequacy of cerebral perfusion through derived mathematical calculation.[1–3, 5, 8]	
18. Discard disposable supplies, and wash hands.	Reduces transmission of microorganisms; standard precautions.	

Procedure **for Intracranial Bolt Insertion (Assist), Monitoring, Care, Troubleshooting, and Removal** *Continued*

Steps	Rationale	Special Considerations
19. Perform a postprocedural clinical neurologic assessment and compare with preprocedure baseline assessment.	Identifies any neurologic changes occurring during procedure and potential need for intervention.	
20. Evaluate integrity of intracranial bolt and functioning of monitoring system.	Ensures accuracy and reliability of monitoring.	

Troubleshooting

1. Assess integrity of intracranial bolt device if dampened ICP waveform appears on monitor display screen. A. Check for air bubbles in fluid-filled pressure tubing and remove if possible. B. Correct ICP monitoring device malfunction according to manufacturers' guidelines and institutional policy. C. Using aseptic technique, change ICP monitoring system setup if indicated by malfunction as per institutional policy.	Fluid-coupled system may develop a leak or air bubbles, requiring changing or flushing of pressure tubing or external strain gauge transducer. Fiberoptic or sensor system may be damaged, requiring replacement of catheter. Brain tissue or blood may occlude any of the various intracranial bolt devices, also resulting in a dampened waveform. Occlusion may require irrigation, manipulation, or replacement.	Responsibility for pressure tubing change and irrigation of intracranial bolt systems may vary according to institutional policy. Intracranial bolt irrigation and manipulation usually is viewed as a physician responsibility in most institutions. Notify physician for intervention as indicated by specific device malfunction and institutional policy.
2. Assess ICP monitors for evidence of mechanical failure or need for zeroing.	Fluid-coupled devices require rezeroing at 2- to 4-hour intervals and with transducer position changes. Fiberoptic devices and sensor devices must be zeroed before insertion and do not subsequently require or permit zeroing attempts. Loose cables and connecting devices may contribute to mechanical failure. Excessively high readings (ie, 888, 999) registered by fiberoptic catheters usually indicate damaged fibers and the need for catheter replacement.	Notify physician If unable to successfully resolve mechanical failure or zeroing issues involving intracranial bolt. Device replacement may be necessary.

Removal of Intracranial Bolt

1. Prepare sterile gloves, suture materials, sterile hemostat, sterile scissors, clamp, or twist drill.	Ensures efficiency of removal procedure.	Sterile, palm-sized twist drill handle may facilitate removal of intracranial bolts. In fiberoptic or microsensor systems, the fiberoptic or microsensor catheter is removed first, followed by the actual intracranial bolt.
2. Wash hands. Don sterile gloves.	Reduces transmission of microorganisms; standard precautions.	
3. Assist the physician with removal of the intracranial bolt as needed.	Facilitates removal process.	
4. Apply povidone-iodine and sterile occlusive or translucent dressing after device is removed.	Prevents contamination by microorganisms.	
5. Dispose of used supplies and wash hands.	Reduces transmission of microorganisms; standard precautions.	

- Accurate and reliable ICP monitoring, CPP calculation, and cerebral compliance and autoregulation assessment
- Maintenance of ICP within range of 0 to 15 mm Hg
- Precise, expeditious management of elevated ICP
- Early detection of elevated ICP trends
- Protection of cerebral perfusion by maintaining CPP within a range of 60 to 160 mm Hg

- CSF infection
- CSF leakage
- Dislodging or occlusion of intracranial bolt
- Pneumoencephalopathy (rare)
- Cerebral hemorrhage (rare)

Patient Monitoring and Care

Patient Monitoring and Care	Rationale	Reportable Conditions
		These conditions should be reported if they persist despite nursing interventions.
1. Monitor patient throughout procedure for neurologic status, vital sign changes, pain, and procedural tolerance.	Assessment of patient for signs of intracranial hypertension, hemodynamic status changes, pain, and procedural tolerance facilitates patient comfort, safety, and success of insertion attempt.	Change in neurologic status, vital signs, or unrelieved discomfort.
2. Assess vital signs, comfort level of patients.	May indicate any unexpected, although rare, multisystem consequences of intracranial bolt insertion.	Changes in vital signs; unrelieved discomfort.
3. Note ICP waveform trends during initial continuous monitoring period.	ICP waveform trends may yield information regarding presence of A, B, or C waveform trends with the associated need for intervention.	Abnormal waveform trends.
4. Set alarm limits slightly above and below the range determined to be acceptable by physician.	Goals for ICP management are individualized for each patient based on etiology, pathophysiology, and management strategies.	
5. Assess ICP and record ICP hourly. ICP should be read on "mean" setting. Perform neurologic assessment at least every hour or more frequently if indicated, including level of consciousness and Glasgow Coma Scale (GCS), pupillary light reflex, motor assessment, and vital signs.	ICP, although continuously monitored, should be assessed and recorded on at least an hourly basis. Neurologic assessment also should be performed and compared with ICP, providing clinical confirmation of and correlation with monitored ICP data.	ICP elevations, deviations, or abnormalities. Sustained ICP elevations of 20 mm Hg or greater require immediate reporting and intervention.
6. Assess for any waveform dampening or abnormalities. Assess morphology of ICP waveform hourly (or more often, if indicated).	Dampening of ICP waveform may indicate air bubbles in fluid-coupled monitoring system. Waveform dampening may reveal inaccurate ICP monitoring data. ICP waveform assessment of P1, P2, and P3 demonstrates status of cerebral compliance and autoregulation.[7]	Dampened ICP waveform may be corrected independently by nursing by removing air bubbles from fluid-filled monitoring system tubing or may require physician intervention, depending on the source of malfunction and institutional policy. ICP waveform changes indicating loss of cerebral compliance or cerebral autoregulation should be reported immediately.
7. Assess ICP waveform trends at least hourly.	Assessment for presence of A, B, or C ICP waveform trends reveals severity of ICP elevation trends and may indicate need for clinical intervention.[2]	A or B waveform trends should be reported to the physician immediately.

Patient Monitoring and Care	Rationale	Reportable Conditions
8. Calculate and record CPP hourly (or more often, if indicated).	CPP calculation provides indirect clinical indication of adequacy of cerebral blood flow.	CPP of less than 60 or 70 mm Hg should be reported to the physician immediately because of the imminent risk of cerebral ischemia or infarction. Each patient may have specific CPP parameters for reporting, depending on cranial etiology, individual clinical condition, and physician preference.
9. Assess integrity, stability, and sterility of intracranial bolt system at least hourly. Fluid-coupled system: external strain gauge transducer should maintain position at the anatomic reference point for foramen of Monro (top of external auditory canal) to ensure system accuracy and reliability.[2, 8, 9] Fluid-coupled system requires re-zeroing of external transducer every 2 to 4 hours and after any repositioning of external transducer.	Hourly system inspection ensures accuracy and safety of monitoring and prevents contamination by microorganisms.	
10. Provide safe environment, preventing unintentional dislodging of ICP monitoring device through repeated explanation, sedation, or analgesia as needed, using mechanical restraints as a last resort.	Patient safety and prevention of unintentional removal of intracranial bolt can be achieved through a variety of measures tailored to meet the individualized patient profile. Unintentional dislodging of the bolt must be avoided, because it can result in pneumoencephalopathy or excessive CSF drainage.	Patient restlessness; device dislodgment.
11. Check integrity of occlusive insertion site dressing and optional full head dressing. Change head dressing and insertion site dressing and assess insertion site as indicated by institutional policy or physician preference.	Permits assessment of device integrity and direct visualization of insertion site. Prevents contamination of insertion site by soiled, wet, or loose dressing. Practices regarding frequency of head dressing change and site care for ICP monitoring devices vary considerably. Responsibility for insertion site dressing change and head dressing change is institutionally specific.	Significant drainage on ICP insertion site dressing or head dressing should be reported to physician, because this may indicate bleeding, infection, or CSF leakage.
12. Change the ICP monitoring system as indicated in institutional policy using aseptic technique. *(Level II: Theory based, no research data to support recommendations; recommendations from expert consensus group may exist)*	Limits risk of infection at insertion site or within CSF pathways. There is considerable variability regarding optimal frequency for ICP monitoring system changes. Some clinicians recommend changing system setup every 24, 48, or even 72 hours. Others prefer not invading or changing system at arbitrary intervals. However, there is little clinical or laboratory research available to guide these decisions.	

Documentation

Documentation should include the following:

- Patient and family education
- Insertion of intracranial bolt, including any difficulties or abnormalities experienced during insertion procedure
- Initial, opening ICP reading
- Initial CPP calculation
- Description of CSF (clarity, color, characteristics, etc) if observed during intracranial bolt insertion
- Patient's tolerance of procedure
- Insertion site assessment

- Recording of ongoing hourly assessment of ICP reading, CPP calculation, ICP waveform morphology (P1, P2, P3, including assessment of cerebral compliance and autoregulation), and ICP waveform trends (including A, B, and C waveform trends)
- Description of expected or unexpected outcomes
- Nursing interventions used to treat ICP or CPP deviations and expected or unexpected outcomes

References

1. Andrews BT. *Neurosurgical Intensive Care.* New York, NY: McGraw-Hill; 1993.
2. Marshall SB, Marshall LF, Vos HR, Chestnut RM. *Neuroscience Critical Care: Pathophysiology and Patient Management.* Philadelphia, Pa: W.B. Saunders; 1990.
3. Ropper AH, ed. *Neurological and Neurosurgical Intensive Care.* 3rd ed. New York, NY: Raven; 1993.
4. Bullock R, Chestnut RM, Clifton G, et al. *Guidelines for Management of Severe Head Injury.* The Brain Trauma Foundation; 1995.
5. Rosner M, Daughton S. Cerebral perfusion pressure management in head injury. *J Trauma.* 1990;30:933–941.
6. Bullock R, Chestnut RM, Clifton G, et al. Guidelines for the management of severe head injury. *J Neurotrauma.* 1996; 13(11):639–734.
7. Germon K. Interpretation of ICP pulse waves to determine intracerebral compliance. *J Neurosci Nurs.* 1988;20:344–349.
8. Germon K. Intracranial pressure monitoring. *Crit Care Nurs Q.* 1994;17:21–32.
9. Hollingsworth-Friedlund P, Vos H, Daily E. Use of fiberoptic pressure transducer for intracranial pressure measurements: a preliminary report. *Heart Lung.* 1988;17:111–120.

Additional Readings

Feldman Z, Kanter MJ, Robertson CS, et al. Effect of head elevation on intracranial pressure, cerebral perfusion pressure, and cerebral blood flow in head injured patients. *J Neurosurg.* 1992;76:201–211.

Hacke W, ed. *NeuroCritical Care.* New York, NY: Springer-Verlag; 1994.

March K, Mitchell P, Grady S, Winn R. Effect of backrest position on intracranial and cerebral perfusion pressure. *J Neurosci Nurs.* 1990;22:375–381.

Schneider GH, Helden AV, Franke R, Lanksch WR, Unterberg A. Influence of body position on jugular venous oxygen saturation, intracranial pressure, and cerebral perfusion pressure. *Acta Neurochir Suppl.* 1993;59:107–112.

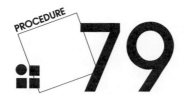

Intraventricular Catheter Insertion (Assist), Monitoring, Care, Troubleshooting, and Removal

PURPOSE: Intraventricular catheters are used to measure and continuously monitor intracranial pressure (ICP), calculate cerebral perfusion pressure (CPP), assess cerebral compliance and autoregulation, and treat elevated intracranial pressure by providing access for cerebrospinal fluid (CSF) drainage.

Jacqueline Sullivan

PREREQUISITE NURSING KNOWLEDGE

- Knowledge of neuroanatomy and physiology is necessary.
- Knowledge of aseptic technique is necessary.
- ICP is measured as the pressure of CSF within the intraventricular, subarachnoid, intraparenchymal (brain tissue), epidural, or subdural spaces.
- Cerebral tissue (brain), cerebral blood, and CSF comprise three discrete volumes occupying the closed compartment of the cranium. Increases in any one or a combination of these volumes will result in adjustments in the remaining volumes so that total volume of the intracranium remains constant (Monro-Kellie hypothesis). This description of intracranial compensatory mechanisms is also known as intracranial compliance. Intracranial compliance is defined as an expression of change in ICP resulting from changes in intracranial volumes. Quantitative measurement of ICP and qualitative analysis of ICP waveform morphology reflect this dynamic compliance relationship among the brain, cerebral circulation, and CSF.
- Several concepts related to CSF secretion and pathways may be important to consider when making clinical decisions related to placement, patency, and integrity of intraventricular catheters. CSF is secreted by the choroid plexus that lines the lateral ventricles. There are approximately 90 to 150 mL of CSF circulating within the CSF pathways in the brain and spinal subarachnoid space at any given point in time. There is a total of 20 mL of CSF within the lateral ventricles and the cranial CSF pathways in nonpathologic conditions. The remaining circulating CSF is found within the distensible compartment of subarachnoid space surrounding the spinal cord.

CSF is secreted at a rate of 0.35 mL per minute, or approximately 20 mL per hour. In conditions involving cerebral edema, CSF may be shunted from the cranial ventricular compartments to the subarachnoid space surrounding the spinal cord. CSF is reabsorbed by the subarachnoid villi. Although CSF production is relatively unaffected by increased ICP, there is evidence to suggest that rate of CSF reabsorption increases with ICP elevations.

- Cerebral autoregulation is a protective mechanism whereby the cerebral blood flow remains constant despite fluctuations in systemic blood pressure. Cerebral autoregulation is dependent on intact systemic and intracranial pressure regulation, as well as chemical mechanisms. Systemic and intracranial pressure ranges necessary for intact cerebral autoregulation are listed in Table 78–1. Chemical stimuli, including P_{CO_2}, P_{O_2}, and pyruvic acid, also must be balanced in order to preserve cerebral autoregulation.
- Normal ICP ranges from 0 to 15 mm Hg (or 0 to 20 cm H_2O).
- CPP is a derived mathematical calculation that indirectly reflects the adequacy of cerebral blood flow. CPP is calculated by subtracting ICP from mean systemic arterial blood pressure (MAP) (CPP = MAP − ICP). Some experts consider CPP to be at least as, if not more, significant than ICP, because this derived calculation reflects both systemic ability to deliver blood to the brain (MAP) and resistance (ICP) that must be overcome in order to perfuse the brain. Normal CPP ranges from 60 to 160 mm Hg. CPP below 50 mm Hg demonstrates inadequate cerebral perfusion. CPP less than 30 mm Hg results in cere-

bral tissue hypoxia and irreversible neuronal damage. Some experts recommend protecting cerebral perfusion by maintaining CPP within the minimal range of 70 to 90 mm Hg. Loss of cerebral autoregulation may occur when CPP is persistently not within the range of 50 to 150 mm Hg.

- Intracranial hypertension may be described as sustained ICP elevations that do not respond to traditional therapeutic methods used for lowering ICP.
- Traditional therapeutic methods used for lowering ICP may include but are not limited to corticosteroid administration, osmotic diuresis, loop diuresis, hyperventilation, sedation, paralysis, normothermia/hypothermia, CSF drainage, and induced therapeutic barbiturate coma. Precise use of these methods varies depending on etiologic origin of elevated ICP and individual patient conditions. Research-based guidelines for management of ICP in traumatic brain injury (TBI) have been widely disseminated and used in recent years.[1, 2]
- Intraventricular catheters, by nature of their placement in the lateral ventricle, provide access for CSF drainage. Intraventricular catheters, therefore, are the only ICP monitoring devices available with capabilities for both treating and monitoring ICP (see Fig. 78–1).
- Intraventricular catheters are the most invasive type of ICP monitoring devices and have the highest relative associated risk for infection and hemorrhage.
- There are a variety of intraventricular catheters currently available for monitoring ICP, including traditional fluid-coupled devices, fiberoptic systems, and microsensors. Fluid-coupled devices require use of external strain gauge transducers; other systems do not. Accepted placement of external strain gauge transducers for ICP monitoring is at the anatomic reference point for the foramen of Monro (top of the external auditory canal). Fiberoptic and sensor ventricular catheter systems are capable of simultaneous ICP monitoring and CSF drainage. Fluid-coupled intraventricular monitoring systems do not provide simultaneous monitoring and drainage capability. Fluid-coupled intraventricular catheters may be used in one of two ways: (1) as continuous ICP monitoring devices with intermittent CSF drainage capabilities, or (2) as continuous CSF drainage devices with intermittent ICP monitoring.
- ICP waveform morphology reflects transmission of arterial and venous pressure through CSF and brain parenchyma. A normal ICP waveform has three distinct pressure oscillations or peaks, referred to as P1, P2, and P3. P1, also known as the percussion wave, reflects myocardial systole. P2, also known as the tidal wave, reflects myocardial diastole and ends on the dicrotic notch. P3, the dicrotic wave, is located immediately after the dicrotic notch and slopes into the diastolic baseline position (see Fig. 78–2). P2 elevations are known to occur with loss of cerebral compliance. P2 pressure oscillation amplitudes approach and surpass P1 pressure oscillations during periods of decompensation and intracerebral compliance loss (see Fig. 78–3). Changes in ICP waveform morphology also may reflect loss of cerebral autoregulation. With loss of cerebral autoregulation, the ICP waveform may assume a mirror-like image of the intra-arterial waveform. These identical ICP and intra-arterial wave-forms demonstrate the dependency of cerebral blood flow on systemic arterial blood pressure. As systemic blood pressure rises, cerebral blood flow increases and ICP elevates during periods of absent cerebral autoregulation.

- Continuous ICP monitoring data trends may demonstrate three discrete ICP wave trends. These ICP trends are A waves, B waves, and C waves. A waves, also known as plateau waves, occur in severe intracranial hypertension and are characterized by sudden ICP escalations up to 50 to 100 mm Hg, have a duration of 5 to 20 minutes, and frequently are accompanied by neurologic deterioration or cerebral herniation (see Fig. 78–4). B waves are sharp rhythmic oscillations that occur with a frequency of every 30 seconds to 2 minutes; B waves may escalate up to 20 to 50 mm Hg and may precede plateau waves (see Fig. 78–5). C waves demonstrate ICP elevations of up to 20 mm Hg and occur with a frequency of every 4 to 8 minutes; they are not thought to be clinically significant (see Fig. 78–6).
- Contraindications for intraventricular catheter placement may include intracranial infection, coagulopathies, and excessive cerebral edema with collapsed ("slit") ventricles.

EQUIPMENT

- Povidone-iodine scrub solution
- Povidone-iodine pads or swabsticks
- Sterile gloves, surgical caps, masks, and sterile surgical gowns
- Sterile towels, half-sheets, and drapes
- Local anesthetic (lidocaine 1% or 2% without epinephrine)
- 5- or 10-mL Luer-Lok syringe with 18-G needle (for drawing up lidocaine) and 23-G needle (for administering lidocaine)
- Twist drill and bits (these are provided by a variety of manufacturers in both generic and custom kits, depending on physician preference)

- Sutures (2-0 nylon, 3-0 silk, 4-0 Vicryl)
- Scalpel with No. 11 blade
- Scalp retractor
- Forceps
- Sterile scissors
- Needle holder
- Disposable cautery
- Suction and sterile suction apparatus
- Bone wax or gelfoam
- Light source (headlamp, etc.; optional)
- Intraventricular catheter (Silastic, fiberoptic, or microsensor)
- Sterile occlusive dressing (sterile 4×4 gauze pads or bio-occlusive dressing)
- Silk tape (1- and 2-in rolls)

Note: Many of the disposable surgical supplies listed above are available in generic and custom kits supplied by ICP monitoring device manufacturers. Check kit labels for necessary contents.

Additional equipment as needed includes the following:

- Razor
- Two 4-inch Kling or Kerlex rolls (optional, needed if performing complete head dressing over insertion site dressing)
- Fluid-coupled system: transducer cable, external strain gauge transducer, pressure tubing, three-way stopcock,

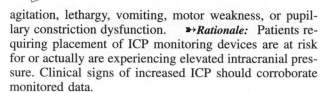

0.9% sodium chloride solution without preservative (may use sterile intravenous solution), sterile CSF drainage system (collection tubing, chamber, and bag)
- Fiberoptic system: microprocessor (stand-alone monitor), pre-amp connector cable, monitoring cable to "slave"/connect microprocessor (stand-alone monitor) to primary bedside monitoring system, fiberoptic intraventricular catheter with calibration screwdriver, sterile CSF drainage system (collection tubing, chamber, and bag)
- Sensor system: microprocessor (stand-alone monitor), microprocessor/sensor cable, monitoring cable to "slave"/connect microprocessor (stand-alone monitor) to primary bedside monitoring system, intraventricular sensor catheter with calibration tool, sterile CSF drainage system (collection tubing, chamber, and bag)

Note: A variety of preassembled sterile CSF drainage systems are now available in generic and custom kits from ICP monitoring device manufacturers.

PATIENT AND FAMILY EDUCATION

- Assess patient and family understanding of intraventricular catheter ICP monitoring and its purpose. **➤Rationale:** Clarification and repeat explanation may limit anxiety and stress for the patient and family.
- Explain standard care for insertion, patient monitoring, and care involving intraventricular catheter. **➤Rationale:** Explanation of expected intervention may allay patient/family anxiety and encourage questions.
- Explain expected outcomes of intraventricular catheter use. **➤Rationale:** Patient and family may experience less stress if aware of goals, duration, and expectations of intraventricular catheter monitoring use.

PATIENT ASSESSMENT AND PREPARATION

Patient Assessment

- Assess baseline neurologic status. **➤Rationale:** Knowledge of baseline neurologic status provides ability to determine occurrence of neurologic changes that may occur during or as a result of intraventricular catheter insertion.
- Observe for early signs of increased intracranial pressure, such as decreased level of consciousness, restlessness,

agitation, lethargy, vomiting, motor weakness, or pupillary constriction dysfunction. **➤Rationale:** Patients requiring placement of ICP monitoring devices are at risk for or actually are experiencing elevated intracranial pressure. Clinical signs of increased ICP should corroborate monitored data.
- Observe for late signs of increased intracranial pressure, such as loss of consciousness, posturing (decortication, decerebration), sluggish pupillary or absent pupillary light reflex, respiratory pattern changes, Cushing's triad of vital sign changes (bradycardia, increased systolic blood pressure, widening pulse pressure). **➤Rationale:** Precise neurologic assessment provides baseline data and establishes clinical correlate for quantitative ICP measurement data.
- Assess current laboratory profile, including CBC, platelet count, prothrombin time (PT), partial thromboplastin time (PTT), bleeding time, and International Normalized Ratio (INR). **➤Rationale:** Baseline coagulation studies are necessary to determine degree of risk for bleeding during intraventricular catheter insertion.

Patient Preparation

- Ensure that the patient and family understand preprocedural teaching. Answer questions as they arise and reinforce information as needed. **➤Rationale:** Evaluates and reinforces understanding of previously taught information.
- Ensure that informed consent has been obtained. **➤Rationale:** Protects the rights of the patient and makes a competent decision possible for the patient or family.
- Administer preprocedure analgesia or sedation, as indicated. **➤Rationale:** Patient is expected to remain very still during intraventricular catheter insertion and may require sedation and analgesia to tolerate the procedure. Alternately, in crisis situations, patients may be unconscious and experiencing cerebral herniation, requiring very little sedation or analgesia for procedural tolerance.
- Assist patient to a supine position with the head of the bed elevated at 30 to 45 degrees with neck in midline, neutral position. **➤Rationale:** This position provides necessary accessibility for intraventricular catheter insertion and enhances jugular venous outflow, contributing to possible reduction in intracranial pressure.

Procedure **for Intraventricular Catheter Insertion (Assist), Monitoring, Care, Troubleshooting, and Removal**

Steps	Rationale	Special Considerations
1. Wash hands.	Reduces transmission of microorganisms; standard precautions.	
2. Assemble and flush fluid-coupled system with external strain gauge transducer as per institutional procedure.	Preparation of external transducer or CSF drainage system promotes efficiency during insertion procedure and ensures capability of immediate CSF drainage, if necessary, in the presence of elevated ICP.	A variety of sterile, preassembled external transducer and CSF drainage systems are available in both generic and custom kits from ICP monitoring device manufacturers.

Procedure continued on following page

| **Procedure** | **for Intraventricular Catheter Insertion (Assist), Monitoring, Care, Troubleshooting, and Removal** *Continued* |

Steps	Rationale	Special Considerations
3. Assemble and flush sterile CSF drainage system that is compatible with specific catheter device as per institutional procedure.		
4. Prepare sterile field, and don sterile gloves.	Prepares for procedure.	
5. Flush system(s) with preservative-free 0.9% NaCL solution. Remove all air bubbles.	Removes air bubbles from the system.	
6. Preserve sterility of systems after preparation, before insertion.		
7. Turn on bedside monitor and microprocessor (stand-alone monitor) if using fiberoptic or sensor devices.	Ensures that monitoring equipment is functional and permits immediate recording of ICP on insertion.	
8. Prepare and check suction.	Provides safety during insertion process by confirming suctioning function prior to procedure.	Suctioning may be needed during intraventricular catheter placement to control bleeding or remove small fragments of bone or tissue from the operative site.
9. Assist physician in identifying optimal area for placement of device.	Facilitates placement.	Nondominant hemisphere is the optimal location for placement of intraventricular catheter. However, presence of skull fractures, etiology of intracranial hypertensive process, or nature of cerebral trauma may limit placement options.
10. Shave and prep insertion site with povidone-iodine solution.	Reduces microorganisms and minimizes risk of infection.	
11. Drape head and upper thorax with sterile half sheets and drapes.	Protects insertion site from contamination.	
12. Open sterile trays and have accessible previously prepared external transducer or CSF drainage system.	Facilitates efficiency of insertion and immediate ICP monitoring on insertion.	A variety of preassembled sterile trays containing disposable surgical instruments (as listed on equipment list) are available from ICP monitoring device manufacturers. Check list of sterile tray contents for presence of necessary equipment before opening tray.

13. Zero transducer. Procedure for fluid-coupled system:
  A. External transducer may be zeroed before or immediately after insertion.
  B. Anatomic reference point for zeroing and maintaining external transducer is at the level of foramen of Monro (top of external auditory canal).
  C. Fiberoptic and sensor systems must be zeroed prior to insertion using their appropriate microprocessors (stand-alone monitors).
	Zero balances to atmospheric pressure and ensures accuracy of monitored data.	Fluid-coupled systems: external transducers must be zeroed before instituting monitoring and should be re-zeroed at periodic intervals. External strain-gauge transducers must also be re-zeroed after any positioning changes occur that alter the location of the transducer from the designated anatomic reference point. Fiberoptic and sensor systems require the zeroing procedure before insertion but do not require periodic zeroing procedures during continued catheter use.

Procedure **for Intraventricular Catheter Insertion (Assist), Monitoring, Care, Troubleshooting, and Removal** *Continued*

Steps	Rationale	Special Considerations
14. Correlation procedure for fiberoptic system: A. Ensure that the slave cable is connecting the microprocessor to the pressure module of the primary bedside monitoring system. B. Depress "Cal/Step" soft key on fiberoptic microprocessor until number 0 appears on microprocessor monitoring screen. C. Continue to hold "Cal/Step" soft key in depressed position with one hand while pressing the zero option on the primary bedside monitoring system. D. When the number 0 appears on the bedside monitoring screen (it should still be appearing on the microprocessor screen also), release both soft keys on both monitors.	Ensures correlation between the fiberoptic microprocessor and the primary bedside monitoring system. Integration of the ICP data with the primary monitoring system data permits use of the centralized alarm systems and trending of ICP data with other multisystemic monitored data.	Although this procedure is called "Cal/Step," its purpose is not calibration in the traditional sense. Rather, it is meant to ensure correlation between the fiberoptic microprocessor and the primary bedside monitoring system.
15. Ensure that health care providers don surgical caps, masks, goggles, and sterile gloves and gowns.	Provides aseptic environment.	
16. Assist as needed with insertion.	Facilitates insertion process.	
17. Attach the sterile CSF drainage system distal to the external transducer in the fluid-coupled system and distal to the insertion end of the catheter in the fiberoptic and the sensor systems.	Intraventricular catheters permit both monitoring and treatment of ICP through capability for CSF drainage.	Fiberoptic and sensor systems provide capability for simultaneous ICP and CSF drainage. These functions must be accomplished in an alternate, not simultaneous, manner when using a fluid-coupled system.
18. Apply povidone-iodine to insertion site and apply an occlusive dressing of choice.	Protects site from contamination by microorganisms.	Apply complete head dressing in addition to insertion site dressing, if desired.
19. Document "opening" ICP (initial ICP reading once continuous monitoring is initiated immediately following insertion). Assess ICP waveform morphology. Obtain hard copy recording of ICP waveform and include in medical record/chart.	Provides initial baseline data for quantitative ICP measurement and qualitative assessment of ICP waveform morphology.	Waveform morphology data yields information related to status of cerebral compliance and autoregulation.
20. Calculate and document CPP: CPP = MAP − ICP	Provides initial, indirect assessment of adequacy of cerebral perfusion through derived mathematical calculation.	
21. Discard disposable supplies, and wash hands.	Reduces spread of microorganisms; standard precautions.	
22. Perform a postprocedural clinical neurologic assessment and compare with preprocedure baseline assessment.	Identifies any neurologic changes occurring during the procedure and the potential need for intervention.	
23. Evaluate patency of CSF drainage system and functioning of monitoring system by checking for adequate CSF drainage in CSF drainage collection system.	Ensures accuracy and reliability of monitoring. Maintains CSF drainage capability if required for treatment of ICP elevation.	

Procedure continued on following page

| Procedure | for Intraventricular Catheter Insertion (Assist), Monitoring, Care, Troubleshooting, and Removal *Continued* |

Steps	Rationale	Special Considerations

Troubleshooting

1. Assess integrity of intraventricular catheter device if dampened ICP waveform appears on monitor display screen.

   A. Check for air bubbles in fluid-filled pressure tubing and remove if possible.

   B. Correct ICP monitoring device malfunction according to manufacturers' guidelines and institutional policy.

   C. Using aseptic technique, change ICP monitoring system setup if indicated by malfunction as per institutional policy.

Fluid-coupled system may develop a leak or air bubbles, requiring changing or flushing of pressure tubing or external strain gauge transducer. Fiberoptic or sensor system may be damaged, requiring replacement of catheter. Brain tissue or blood may occlude any of the various intraventricular catheter devices, also resulting in a dampened waveform. Occlusion may require catheter irrigation, manipulation, or replacement.

Responsibility for pressure tubing change and flushing of intraventricular catheter systems may vary according to institutional policy. Intraventricular catheter irrigation and manipulation is usually viewed as a physician responsibility in most institutions. Notify physician for intervention as indicated by specific catheter malfunction and institutional policy.

2. Assess ICP monitors for evidence of mechanical failure or need for zeroing.

Fluid-coupled devices require re-zeroing at 2- to 4-hour intervals and with transducer position changes. Fiberoptic devices and sensor devices must be zeroed before insertion and do not subsequently require or permit zeroing attempts. Loose cables and connecting devices may contribute to mechanical failure. Excessively high readings (ie, 888, 999) registered by fiberoptic catheters usually indicate damaged fibers and the need for catheter replacement.

Notify physician if unable to successfully resolve mechanical failure or zeroing issues involving intraventricular catheters. Catheter replacement may be necessary.

3. Assess patency of CSF drainage system by ensuring flow of CSF through CSF drainage system. Flush CSF drainage system and change system using aseptic technique, if necessary, as per institutional policy.

CSF drainage system may become occluded by cerebral tissue, blood clots, or sediment as these substances pass through the intraventricular catheter along with CSF.

Notify physician if significant amount of cerebral tissue, blood, or sediment is found in intraventricular catheter or CSF drainage system, indicating possible occurrence of further pathologic conditions.

Removal of Intraventricular Catheter

1. Prepare sterile gloves, suture materials, sterile hemostat, sterile scissors, clamp, or twist drill for assisting with intraventricular catheter removal.

Ensures efficiency of removal procedure.

Sterile, palm-sized twist drill handle may facilitate removal of intraventricular catheters that have been inserted through intracranial bolts.

2. Wash hands, and don sterile gloves and mask with shield or goggles.

Reduces transmission of microorganisms; standard precautions.

3. Assist physician with removal of intraventricular catheter.

Facilitates removal process.

Culture tip of intraventricular catheter as per institutional policy.

4. Apply povidone-iodine and sterile occlusive or translucent dressing after device is removed.

Prevents contamination by microorganisms.

5. Dispose of sterile supplies and device in appropriate container and wash hands.

Reduces transmission of microorganisms; standard precautions.

- Accurate and reliable ICP monitoring, CPP calculation, and cerebral compliance and autoregulation assessment
- Maintenance of ICP within range of 0 to 15 mm Hg
- Precise, expeditious management of elevated ICP
- Early detection of elevated ICP trends
- Protection of cerebral perfusion by maintaining CPP within a range of 60 to 160 mm Hg
- Ability to manage elevated ICP through CSF drainage

- CSF infection
- CSF leakage
- Dislodging or occlusion of the intraventricular catheter
- Pneumoencephalopathy (rare)
- Cerebral hemorrhage (rare)

Patient Monitoring and Care

Patient Monitoring and Care	Rationale	Reportable Conditions
		These changes should be reported if they persist despite nursing interventions.
1. Monitor patient throughout procedure for neurologic status, vital sign changes, pain, and procedural tolerance. Administer sedation and analgesia as indicated.	Assessment of patient for signs of intracranial hypertension, hemodynamic status changes, pain, and procedural tolerance facilitates patient comfort, safety, and success of insertion attempt.	Changes in neurologic status; unrelieved pain
2. Assess ICP and record ICP hourly. ICP should be read on "mean" setting. Adjust pressure scale according to patient's individualized ICP reading to capture ICP waveform and accurate digital reading. Perform neurologic assessment at least every hour or more frequently if indicated, including level of consciousness and Glasgow Coma Scale (GCS), pupillary light reflex, motor assessment, and vital signs.	ICP, although continuously monitored, should be assessed and recorded on at least an hourly basis. Neurological assessment should also be performed and compared with ICP to provide clinical confirmation of and correlation with monitored ICP data.	ICP elevations, deviations, or abnormalities. Sustained ICP elevations of 20 mm Hg or greater require immediate reporting and intervention.
3. Note ICP waveform trends during initial continuous monitoring period.	ICP waveform trends may yield information regarding presence of A, B, or C waveform trends with associated need for intervention.[3-5]	A or B waveform trends
4. Assess ICP waveform trends at least hourly.	Assessment for presence of A, B, or C ICP waveform trends reveals severity of ICP elevation trends and may indicate need for clinical intervention.	A or B waveform trends
5. Calculate and record CPP hourly (or more often if indicated).	CPP calculation provides indirect clinical indication of adequacy of cerebral blood flow.	CPP that is less than 60 or 70 mm Hg due to imminent risk of cerebral ischemia/infarction. Each patient may have specific CPP parameters for reporting depending on cranial etiology, individual clinical condition, and physician preference.
6. Assess integrity, stability, and sterility of intraventricular catheter system at least hourly. ○ Fluid-coupled system: External strain gauge transducer should maintain position at the anatomic reference point for foramen of Monro (top of external auditory canal) to ensure system accuracy and reliability. ○ Fluid-coupled system requires re-zeroing of external transducer every 2 to 4 hours and after any repositioning of the external transducer.	Hourly system inspection ensures accuracy and safety of monitoring and prevents contamination by microorganisms.	

Continued on following page

Patient Monitoring and Care	Rationale	Reportable Conditions
7. Check integrity of occlusive insertion site dressing and optional full head dressing. Change head dressing and insertion site dressing and assess insertion site as indicated by institutional policy or physician preference.	Permits assessment of device integrity and direct visualization of insertion site. Prevents contamination of insertion site by soiled, wet, or loose dressing. Practices regarding frequency of head dressing change and site care for ICP monitoring devices vary considerably. Responsibility for insertion site dressing change and head dressing change is institutionally specific.	Significant drainage on ICP insertion site dressing or head dressing should be reported to physician because this may indicate bleeding, infection, or CSF leakage.
8. Assess vital signs, comfort level of patient.	May indicate any unexpected, although rare, multisystemic consequences of intraventricular catheter insertion. Provides opportunity to evaluate postprocedural/ongoing need for sedation or analgesia.	Changes in vital signs; unrelieved pain
9. Provide safe environment, preventing unintentional dislodging of ICP monitoring device through repeated explanation, sedation, or analgesia as needed, using mechanical restraints only as a last resort.	Patient safety and prevention of unintentional removal of intraventricular catheter can be achieved through a variety of measures tailored to meet the individualized patient needs. Unintentional dislodging of catheter must be avoided because it can result in pneumoencephalopathy or excessive CSF drainage.	Dislodged device
10. Change the ICP monitoring system and CSF drainage system as indicated in institutional policy using aseptic technique.	Limits risk of infection at insertion site and within CSF pathways. There is considerable variability regarding optimal frequency for ICP monitoring system changes. Some recommend changing system setup every 24, 48, or even 72 hours. Others recommend not invading or changing system at arbitrary intervals. Check institutional policy.	
11. With aseptic technique, obtain routine CSF specimen from intraventricular catheter using sampling port on CSF drainage system for access according to manufacturer's recommendations. Send CSF specimen for laboratory analysis, including culture and sensitivity, Gram stain, cell count, glucose, and protein.	Provides early detection and intervention in cases where CSF infection occurs during or as a result of intraventricular catheter monitoring. There are insufficient data to guide/support decisions on necessary frequency of routine CSF sampling from intraventricular catheters. It is therefore recommended to follow institutional policy regarding frequency for routine CSF sampling.	CSF results indicative of intraventricular infection may include elevated white blood cell count, elevated protein, and decreased glucose.

Documentation

Documentation should include the following:

- Insertion of intraventricular catheter, including any difficulties or abnormalities experienced during insertion procedure
- Initial, opening ICP reading
- Initial CPP calculation
- Description of CSF (eg, clarity, color, characteristics) as observed during intraventricular catheter insertion and initial drainage
- Patient's tolerance of procedure
- Insertion site assessment

- Digital and waveform hard copy recording of ongoing hourly assessment of ICP reading, CPP calculation, ICP waveform morphology (including cerebral compliance and autoregulation), and ICP waveform trends (including A, B, and C waveform trends)
- Description of expected or unexpected outcomes
- Nursing interventions used to treat ICP or CPP deviations and expected or unexpected outcomes

References

1. Bullock R, Chestnut RM, Clifton G, et al. *Guidelines for Management of Severe Head Injury.* The Brain Trauma Foundation; 1995.
2. Bullock R, Chestnut RM, Clifton G, et al. Guidelines for the management of severe head injury. *J Neurotrauma.* 1996;13(11):639–734.
3. Germon K. Intracranial pressure monitoring. *Criti Care Nurs Q.* 1994;17:21–32.
4. Hollingsworth-Friedlund P, Vos H, Daily E. Use of fiberoptic pressure transducer for intracranial pressure measurements: a preliminary report. *Heart Lung.* 1988;17:111–120.
5. Marshall SB, Marshall LF, Vos HR, Chestnut RM. *Neuroscience Critical Care: Pathophysiology and Patient Management.* Philadelphia, Pa: W.B. Saunders; 1990.

Additional Readings

Andrews BT. *Neurosurgical Intensive Care.* New York, NY: McGraw Hill; 1993.

Feldman Z, Kanter MJ, Robertson CS, et al. Effect of head elevation on intracranial pressure, cerebral perfusion pressure, and cerebral blood flow in head injured patients. *Neurosurg.* 1992;76:201–211.

Germon K. Interpretation of ICP pulse waves to determine intracerebral compliance. *J Neurosci Nurs.* 1988;20:344–349.

Hacke W, ed. *NeuroCritical Care.* New York, NY: Springer-Verlag; 1994.

March K, Mitchell P, Grady S, Winn R. Effect of backrest position on intracranial and cerebral perfusion pressure. *J Neurosci Nurs.* 1990;22:375–381.

Ropper AH, ed. *Neurological and Neurosurgical Intensive Care.* 3rd ed. New York, NY: Raven; 1993.

Rosner M, Daughton S. Cerebral perfusion pressure management in head injury. *J Trauma.* 1990;30:933–941.

Schneider GH, Helden AV, Franke R, Lanksch WR, Unterberg A. Influence of body position on jugular venous oxygen saturation, intracranial pressure, and cerebral perfusion pressure. *Acta Neurochir Suppl.* 1993;59:107–112.

80

Jugular Venous Oxygen Saturation Monitoring: Insertion (Assist), Care, Troubleshooting, and Removal

P U R P O S E: Jugular venous oxygen saturation ($SjvO_2$) catheters are used to measure and continuously monitor the oxygen saturation of hemoglobin in the internal jugular venous blood supply following emptying of the intracranial venous sinuses. This measurement reflects oxygen saturation of blood volume returned after cerebral perfusion has occurred. $SjvO_2$ data and associated derived mathematical calculations (ie, arteriovenous jugular oxygen content difference ($AVjDO_2$), cerebral extraction of oxygen (CeO_2), global cerebral oxygen extraction ratio (O_2ER)), are used clinically to determine cerebral oxygen use, cerebral metabolic demand, and relative adequacy of cerebral oxygen delivery.

Jacqueline Sullivan

PREREQUISITE NURSING KNOWLEDGE

- Knowledge of neuroanatomy and physiology is necessary.
- Knowledge of aseptic technique is essential.
- $SjvO_2$ monitoring may be used in determining balance or imbalance between cerebral perfusion and cerebral metabolism, including identification of the following cerebral perfusion states: (1) global cerebral luxury perfusion, (2) normal coupling of global cerebral blood flow with global cerebral metabolism, (3) global cerebral hypoperfusion, and (4) global cerebral ischemia.
- Contraindications for placement of $SjvO_2$ catheters include coagulopathies, local infection, cervical spine injury, local neck trauma, and impaired cerebral venous drainage.
- Patients experiencing increased intracranial pressure, potential compromise in cerebral perfusion, and alterations leading to cerebral ischemia are appropriate candidates for $SjvO_2$ catheter monitoring.
- $SjvO_2$ catheters may be used in conjunction with other types of cerebral dynamics monitoring (including but not limited to intracranial pressure monitoring) to provide increased precision in management of increased intracranial pressure and compromised cerebral perfusion (ie, titration of hyperventilation for treatment of intracranial hypertension).

- $SjvO_2$ catheters are available as 4-Fr fiberoptic oximetric catheters from several manufacturers. These fiberoptic catheters are used with optical module cables and stand-alone oximetric monitors (processors) to provide continuous display of $SjvO_2$ values. Pediatric central venous pressure (CVP) catheters may also be used to cannulate the internal jugular vein for $SjvO_2$ monitoring purposes. However, pediatric CVP catheters adapted for this use do not provide continuous oxygen saturation monitoring capabilities. Pediatric CVP catheters require periodic sampling of venous blood supplies to acquire $SjvO_2$ data.
- To provide accurate and reliable data, the $SjvO_2$ catheter tip is positioned at the location of the jugular bulb of the internal jugular vein. The jugular bulb is a dilatation of the rostral internal jugular vein just below the jugular foramen.
- Normally, 80% to 90% of cerebral blood drains from both hemispheres via intracranial sinuses through the sigmoid sinuses and into the right internal jugular vein. For this reason, the right internal jugular vein is the optimal vessel for measuring and monitoring $SjvO_2$. However, simultaneous bilateral jugular bulb saturation measurements have been demonstrated to be equivalent and probably represent drainage from all parts of the brain. In the presence of focal intracranial pathology, patterns of venous drainage may change, resulting in differences in right and left $SjvO_2$ measurements.

Table 80–1 ● ■ ■ **Etiology of SjvO₂ Desaturation**

Anemia
Decreased cardiac output
Systemic hypotension
Arterial oxygen desaturation
Decreased cerebral blood flow
Increased cerebral metabolic demand (increased cerebral
   metabolic rate of oxygen)

- The normal range for SjvO₂ values is between 55% and 70%.
- In the absence of anemia or sudden increases in fraction of inspired oxygen, increases in SjvO₂ values over 75% suggest "luxury perfusion" globally, although areas of regional ischemia or infarction may still be present.
- Reductions in SjvO₂ values below 54% indicate relative cerebral hypoperfusion.
- Reductions in SjvO₂ values below 40% demonstrate global cerebral ischemia and may be associated with increased production of lactic acid.
- SjvO₂ desaturation demonstrates potential systemic or cerebral decompensation and should be dealt with as a clinical emergency (See Table 80–1 for a description of potential causes of SjvO₂ desaturation.)
- Research suggests a significant correlation between repeated SjvO₂ desaturation events and poor outcome in patients with severe traumatic brain injury.[1]
- AVjDO₂ and CeO₂ serve as indirect clinical indicators of cerebral oxygen uptake. AVjDO₂ calculation requires data obtained from both systemic arterial and jugular venous blood gas analysis (ie, PaO₂, PjvO₂). CeO₂ calculation may be derived from continuously monitored data without requiring data from blood gas analysis (ie, continuously monitored SaO₂, SjvO₂). Although AVjDO₂ and CeO₂ measurements are expected to correlate and trend in the same direction, these parameters differ in that AVjDO₂ calculation considers hemoglobin, whereas CeO₂ calculation does not.
- Formulas and normal ranges for SjvO₂ catheter data and calculations (eg, SjvO₂, AVjDO₂, CeO₂) are included in Tables 80–2 and 80–3.
- SjvO₂, AVjDO₂ and CeO₂ data may be used to precisely manage intracranial hypertension and potential cerebral ischemia states by providing capability for titrating clinical interventions according to status of intracranial pressure (ICP) as well as cerebral oxygen uptake and cerebral metabolic demand.
- SjvO₂ values are inversely proportional to CeO₂ and AVjDO₂ values.
- In cases where cerebral blood flow and cerebral oxygen delivery are inadequate to meet cerebral metabolic demand, SjvO₂ decreases while CeO₂ and AVjDO₂ increase.
- In cases where cerebral blood flow and cerebral oxygen delivery are in surplus supply relative to cerebral metabolic demand, SjvO₂ increases while CeO₂ and AVjDO₂ decrease.
- Increases in AVjDO₂ indicate increased oxygen uptake by cerebral cells.
- Decreases in AVjDO₂ indicate decreased oxygen uptake by cerebral cells.
- Increases in CeO₂ indicate increased oxygen uptake by cerebral cells.
- Decreases in CeO₂ indicate decreased oxygen uptake by cerebral cells.
- Given that arterial oxygen saturation, hemoglobin concentration, and position of the oxyhemoglobin dissociation curve remain constant, the ratio of global cerebral blood flow to cerebral metabolism of oxygen (ie, CBF:CMRO₂) is directly proportional to SjvO₂.
- A decision tree for clinical interventions based on SjvO₂, AVjDO₂, and CeO₂ data is included in Table 80–4.

EQUIPMENT

- Povidone-iodine scrub solution
- Povidone-iodine pads or swabsticks
- Surgical caps, masks, goggles, sterile gloves, and gowns
- Sterile towels, half-sheets, and drapes
- Local anesthetic (lidocaine 1% or 2% without epinephrine)
- 5- or 10-mL Luer-Lok syringe with 18-G needle (for drawing up lidocaine) and 23-G needle (for administering lidocaine)
- Central venous catheter insertion tray (various types available from several manufacturers; may be customized per institutional request)
- 5-Fr percutaneous transvenous introducer catheter
- 4-Fr fiberoptic oximetric SjvO₂ catheter (available from several manufacturers)
- Optical module–fiberoptic cable
- Oximetric monitor (processor)
- 500-mL bag of 0.9% sodium chloride intravenous solution (heparinized or nonheparinized, depending on physician preference or institutional standard)
- Bifurcated or dual lumen pressure tubing
- Pressure bag or device
- Sterile occlusive central venous catheter dressing

Table 80–2 ● ■ ■ **Formulas for SjvO₂ Data Calculations**

SjvO₂ Data Calculations	Formula
AVjDO₂ (mL/dL)	CaO₂ (mL/dL) − CjvO₂ (mL/dL)
CaO₂ (mL/dL)	$1.34 \times$ Hgb $\times$ SaO₂ + 0.0031 $\times$ PaO₂
CjvO₂ (mL/dL)	$1.34 \times$ Hgb $\times$ SjvO₂ + 0.0031 $\times$ PjvO₂
CeO₂ (%)	SaO₂ (%) − SjvO₂ (%)
CMRO₂ (mL/100 g/min)	$\dfrac{\text{CBF (mL/100 g/min)} \times \text{AVjDO₂ (mL/dL)}}{100}$
O₂ER (%)	SaO₂ − SjvO₂/SaO₂ or CeO₂/SaO₂
CMRL (mL/100 g/min)	$\dfrac{\text{AVDL (mL/dL)} \times \text{CBF (mL/100 g/min)}}{100}$
AVDL (mL/dL)	Arterial lactate (mL/dL) − jugular Venous lactate (mL/dL)

AVDL, arteriovenous difference of lactate; AVjDO₂, arteriovenous jugular oxygen content difference; CaO₂, arterial oxygen content saturation; CBF, cerebral blood flow; CeO₂, cerebral extraction of oxygen; CjvO₂, jugular venous oxygen content saturation; CMRL, cerebral metabolic rate of lactate; CMRO₂, cerebral metabolic rate of oxygen; Hgb, hemoglobin; O₂ER, global cerebral oxygen extraction ratio; SaO₂, oxygen saturation in arterial blood; SjvO₂, jugular venous oxygen saturation.

Table 80–3 ●■■ **Normal Ranges for SjvO₂ Catheter Data and Calculations**

SjvO₂ Data	Normal Ranges
$SjvO_2$	55%–70%
$AVjDO_2$	3.5–8.1 mL/dL
CeO_2	24%–42%

$AVjDO_2$, arteriovenous jugular oxygen content difference; CeO_2, cerebral extraction of oxygen; $SjvO_2$, jugular venous oxygen saturation.

PATIENT AND FAMILY EDUCATION

- Assess patient and family understanding of $SjvO_2$ catheter monitoring and its purpose. ➤➤*Rationale:* Clarification and repeat explanation may alleviate anxiety and stress for patient and family.
- Explain standard for insertion, patient monitoring, and care involving $SjvO_2$ catheter. ➤➤*Rationale:* Explanation of expected intervention may allay patient and family anxiety and stimulate requests for clarification or additional information.
- Explain expected outcomes of $SjvO_2$ catheter use. ➤➤*Rationale:* Patient and family stress and anxiety may diminish if they are aware of goals, duration, and expectations of $SjvO_2$ catheter use.

PATIENT ASSESSMENT AND PREPARATION

Patient Assessment

- Assess neurologic status. ➤➤*Rationale:* Baseline data provides information necessary to recognize changes occurring during or as a result of catheter insertion.
- Assess patient for evidence of local infection or local neck trauma that may be signs of actual or potential impaired cerebral venous drainage. ➤➤*Rationale:* These conditions are contraindications for $SjvO_2$ catheter placement.
- Obtain current laboratory profile including complete blood count (CBC), platelet count, prothrombin time (PT), partial thromboplastin time (PTT), bleeding time, and International Normalized Ratio (INR). ➤➤*Rationale:* Baseline coagulation studies are necessary to determine degree of risk for excessive bleeding during $SjvO_2$ catheter placement.

Patient Preparation

- Ensure that the patient understands preprocedural teaching. Answer questions as they arise, and reinforce information as needed. ➤➤*Rationale:* Evaluates and reinforces understanding of previously taught information.
- Administer preprocedure analgesia or sedation as indicated. ➤➤*Rationale:* Patients will be expected to remain still during $SjvO_2$ catheter insertion and may require sedation or analgesia to tolerate the procedure. Alternatively, in crisis situations, patients may be unconscious and experiencing severe neurologic depression or instability, requiring little if any sedation or analgesia for procedural tolerance.
- Assist the patient to a supine position with the neck in a neutral position and with the head of the bed elevated at 30 to 45 degrees. Note patient's baseline intracranial pressure (ICP). Turn patient's head laterally, away from selected side for insertion. Again, note patient's ICP. ➤➤*Rationale:* Head elevation provides necessary accessibility for $SjvO_2$ catheter insertion and enhances jugular venous outflow, contributing to possible reduction in ICP. Most patients who are candidates for $SjvO_2$ catheter monitoring are experiencing elevated ICP and require ICP monitoring. Lateral head turning may inhibit jugular venous outflow and cause elevated ICP. Lateral positioning of the patient's head immediately before $SjvO_2$ catheter insertion may demonstrate related effect of insertion procedure on ICP, thereby demonstrating anticipated procedural tolerance. Continuous placement of indwelling $SjvO_2$ catheter may also influence jugular venous outflow and, subsequently, ICP. Baseline, preinsertion ICP data provide necessary information for assessing influence of continuous presence of indwelling $SjvO_2$ catheter on jugular venous outflow and ICP.

Table 80–4 ●■■ **Balancing Cerebral Perfusion and Cerebral Metabolism: Clinical Interventions Based on SjvO₂ Parameters**

SjvO₂	AVjDO₂	CeO₂	O₂ER	CBF Status (relative to CMRO₂)	Clinical Intervention
Decreased	Increased	Increased	Increased	Decreased (cerebral hypoperfusion, ischemia, infarction)	Normalize CO_2 Hypervolemic hemodilution Induced systemic hypertension
Increased	Decreased	Decreased	Decreased	Increased ("luxury perfusion," relative cerebral hyperemia)	Hyperventilation Diuresis

$AVjDO_2$, arteriovenous jugular oxygen content difference; CBF, cerebral blood flow; CeO_2, cerebral extraction of oxygen; $CMRO_2$, cerebral metabolic rate of oxygen; CO_2, carbon dioxide; O_2ER, global cerebral oxygen extraction ratio; $SjvO_2$, jugular venous oxygen saturation.

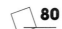

| **Procedure** | **for Assisting with SjvO₂ Catheter Insertion Procedure** |

Steps	Rationale	Special Considerations
1. Wash hands.	Reduces transmission of microorganisms; standard precautions.	
2. Using aseptic technique, assemble and flush bifurcated pressure tubing (see Procedure 69). Remove all air bubbles. Preserve sterility of system after preparation, before insertion.	Prepares monitoring system and eliminates air from system. Bifurcated pressure tubing will provide a joint flush system for both the 5-Fr percutaneous introducer catheter and the 4-Fr fiberoptic SjvO₂ catheter.	Although invasive pressure monitoring is not required for continuous SjvO₂ monitoring, one of the two jugular catheter lumens (preferably the 4-Fr SjvO₂ catheter) may be attached to a continuous invasive monitoring system, providing a continuous recording of jugular venous pressure waves and continuous reading of jugular venous pressures.
3. Turn on oximetric processor (stand-alone monitor). Follow manufacturer instructions regarding performing in vitro calibration before catheter insertion, if required.	Ensures that monitoring equipment is functional and prepares for in vitro calibration procedure if required by particular SjvO₂ catheter and monitor manufacturer.	Unlike SvO₂ catheters, not all SjvO₂ catheters require in vitro calibration before insertion. Check particular manufacturer's instructions regarding in vitro calibration before proceeding with insertion. *All* SjvO₂ catheters *do* require performance of in vivo calibration procedure after insertion.
4. Ensure that the patient is positioned with his or her neck in neutral position and head elevated at 30 to 45 degrees. Note and document patient's baseline ICP in this position.	Head elevation provides necessary accessibility for SjvO₂ catheter insertion and enhances jugular venous outflow, contributing to possible reduction in ICP. Provides baseline preinsertion ICP data necessary for evaluating influence of continuous indwelling SjvO₂ catheter on ICP.	Most patients who are candidates for SjvO₂ catheter monitoring are experiencing elevated ICP and require ICP monitoring.
5. Turn patient's head laterally away from selected side for SjvO₂ catheter insertion. Note and document patient's ICP.	Lateral head position may inhibit jugular venous outflow and cause elevated ICP. Lateral head positioning before insertion procedure demonstrates patient's ability to tolerate the procedure.	Most initial SjvO₂ catheter insertion attempts involve use of right internal jugular vein because 80% to 90% of cerebral venous blood empties into right internal jugular vein.
6. Ensure that health care providers don caps, masks, goggles, sterile gloves, and gowns.	Provides aseptic environment.	
7. Prepare selected insertion site with povidone-iodine scrub solution.	Reduces microorganisms and minimizes risk of infection.	
8. Drape upper thorax and neck with sterile half-sheets and drapes.	Protects insertion site from contamination.	
9. Open sterile CVP insertion tray and set up sterile field using aseptic technique. Add 5-Fr percutaneous introducer catheter and 4-Fr fiberoptic SjvO₂ catheter using aseptic technique. Have bifurcated or dual lumen pressure tubing or flush system available for flushing catheter before insertion.	Facilitates efficiency of insertion and avoids contamination by microorganisms.	CVP insertion trays are available from a variety of manufacturers and may be customized to meet institutional requests. Check contents of tray before opening.
10. Assist the physician as needed with insertion.	Facilitates insertion process.	

Procedure continued on following page

| Procedure | for Assisting with SjvO$_2$ Catheter Insertion Procedure *Continued* |

Steps	Rationale	Special Considerations
11. Monitor patient throughout insertion procedure for neurologic status, vital signs, pain, and increased ICP. Administer analgesia or sedation as indicated.	Assessment of patient for signs of neurologic or hemodynamic compromise and pain facilitates patient comfort, safety, and success of insertion attempt.	Lateral head positioning during SjvO$_2$ catheter insertion may cause elevated ICP.
12. Attach bifurcated or dual lumen pressure tubing flush system to introducer and fiberoptic catheters. Confirm patency of both jugular catheter lumens by aspirating and flushing both lumens.	Promotes catheter patency. Prevents thrombosis or extravasation of catheters.	
13. Apply occlusive dressing to insertion site.	Prevents contamination of insertion site by microorganisms.	
14. Set alarms.	Alarms will signal changes in oxygenation.	
15. Obtain lateral skull or lateral cervical radiographs to confirm SjvO$_2$ catheter placement at the level of the jugular bulb of the internal jugular vein. *(Level VI: Clinical studies in a variety of patient populations and situations to support recommendations)*	Optimum placement of SjvO$_2$ catheter tip is at the level of the jugular bulb of the internal jugular vein. SjvO$_2$ catheter tip position is confirmed radiographically by obtaining lateral skull or lateral cervical films to determine catheter position high in the jugular bulb, preferably above the upper border of the second cervical vertebra.[2-5]	Jugular bulb placement of SjvO$_2$ catheter provides optimal sampling of jugular venous oxygen saturation, reflecting oxygen saturation immediately following cerebral venous outflow and emptying.
16. Obtain jugular venous blood gas sample and perform in vivo calibration procedure, following manufacturer guidelines for particular SjvO$_2$ catheter and monitor.	In vivo calibration ensures reliability between monitored SjvO$_2$ data and SjvO$_2$ data obtained by laboratory analysis.	Although not all varieties of SjvO$_2$ catheters require in vitro calibration, *all* varieties *do* require performance of in vivo calibration immediately following insertion and periodically thereafter.
17. Discard used supplies, and wash hands.	Reduces transmission of microorganisms; standard precautions.	

| Procedure | for Troubleshooting SjvO$_2$ Catheter |

Steps	Rationale	Special Considerations
Problem 1: Poor Light Intensity	Fiberoptic technology permits continuous monitoring of SjvO$_2$ through digital analysis of reflected light signals. Limitations of this technology are demonstrated with poor light intensity signals. Light intensity should be displayed during measurement of SjvO$_2$.	
1. Identify the low light intensity.	Low light intensity may indicate damage to the fiberoptics or catheter occlusion or obstruction.[2, 3]	
2. Check the fiberoptic catheter for occlusion or obstruction.		
3. Aspirate the catheter until blood may be freely sampled and a normal light intensity is displayed.		
4. If unable to aspirate blood or restore normal light intensity, the catheter should be replaced.		

Procedure for Troubleshooting SjvO₂ Catheter *Continued*

Steps	Rationale	Special Considerations
Problem 2: High Light Intensity 1. Identify the high light intensity. 2. Attempt to restore normal light intensity by adjusting or slightly turning the patient's head to restore neutral neck alignment.	High light intensity indicates vessel wall artifact. SjvO₂ readings are characteristically inaccurate and in the range of 85% to 95% in situations of vessel wall artifact, except in cases of brain death. Vessel wall artifact is frequently encountered during repositioning of patient's head or body. This situation is usually corrected by repositioning the patient's head. Occasionally, the catheter itself will need to be repositioned by the physician.[2, 3]	
Problem 3: Sampling and Calibration Errors	In vivo calibration errors may occur if significant changes in saturation are displayed during aspiration of a jugular venous sample or if the sample is contaminated with extracerebral venous blood.	
1. Identify sampling or calibration error. 2. Avoid in vivo calibration errors by *slowly* aspirating (1 mL of blood over 1 minute) the jugular venous sample for in vivo calibration.	Slow aspiration of the jugular venous sample avoids contamination of the sample with extracerebral venous blood.[2, 3] It has also been considered that changes in blood flow characteristics or movement of the catheter tip may occur during aspiration of the jugular venous sample, contributing to in vivo calibration errors. These issues require further investigation.	
Problem 4: Coiling of SjvO₂ Catheter 1. Identify rhythmic fluctuations in SjvO₂ trends. 2. Consider obtaining radiograph to assess if the catheter is coiled in the internal jugular vein. 3. If coiling is confirmed, consider preparing for catheter replacement.	Coiling of the SjvO₂ catheter within the internal jugular vein may cause rhythmic fluctuations in SjvO₂ trends that are unrelated to changes in ICP, cerebral perfusion pressure, and systemic blood pressure. Light intensity may remain within acceptable range even in the presence of coiling of SjvO₂ catheter.	
Problem 5: SjvO₂ Desaturation 1. Identify SjvO₂ desaturations. 2. Confirm the SjvO₂ data by obtaining a jugular venous blood gas sample for laboratory analysis. 3. Perform an in vivo calibration.	SjvO₂ desaturations are emergent events requiring immediate interventions for restoration or enhancement of cerebral blood flow and cerebral oxygen delivery. Monitored desaturations should be confirmed by laboratory analysis to rule out monitor malfunction.[1, 6]	

Procedure for Removal of SjvO₂ Catheter

Steps	Rationale	Special Considerations
1. Prepare sterile gloves, suture removal equipment, sterile hemostat, sterile scissors, etc.	Prepares for procedure.	
2. Wash hands, and don gloves.	Reduces transmission of microorganisms; standard precautions.	

Procedure continued on following page

Procedure for Removal of $SjvO_2$ Catheter *Continued*

Steps	Rationale	Special Considerations
3. Inactivate the alarm system.	Monitoring is no longer needed.	
4. Turn stopcocks on flush system to "off" position and assist with catheter removal.	Facilitates the removal process.	
5. Apply povidone-iodine and sterile occlusive dressing after device is removed.	Prevents contamination by microorganisms.	
6. Dispose of sterile supplies and device in appropriate container, and wash hands.	Reduces transmission of microorganisms; standard precautions.	
7. Observe for signs of excessive bleeding from insertion site (every 15 minutes × 4, every 30 minutes × 2, then 1 hour later).	Identifies complications.	

Expected Outcomes

- Accurate and reliable $SjvO_2$ monitoring and $AVjDO_2$ and CeO_2 calculation
- Preservation and maximization of balance between cerebral perfusion, cerebral oxygenation, and cerebral metabolic demand with stabilization of ICP
- Early detection of compromised cerebral perfusion and impaired cerebral oxygenation
- Precise, expeditious management of impaired cerebral perfusion or compromised cerebral oxygenation

Unexpected Outcomes

- Carotid artery puncture (3% to 4% incidence)
- Excessive bleeding (rare)
- Site of venous infection (line sepsis) (0% to 5% infection rate)
- Impaired cerebral venous drainage or increased ICP
- Internal jugular venous thrombosis (less than 5% incidence)
- Pneumothorax (rare)
- Injury to stellate ganglion, phrenic nerve, or cervical ganglion (rare)

Patient Monitoring and Care

Patient Monitoring and Care	Rationale	Reportable Conditions
		These conditions should be reported if they persist despite nursing interventions.
1. Assess patient's baseline neurologic status, vital signs, and ICP immediately after insertion.	Presence of internal jugular catheter may potentially influence or inhibit jugular venous outflow and subsequently cause increased ICP. Some experts consider a sustained increase in ICP of more than 5 mm Hg over the baseline, preinsertion value as an indication for $SjvO_2$ catheter removal.[2, 3, 5]	- Change in neurologic status, vital signs, and ICP
2. Note and record baseline for continuously monitored $SjvO_2$ value and calculate baseline $AVjDO_2$, CeO_2, and O_2ER.	Baseline $SjvO_2$ monitored and calculated data provide opportunity to track trends in cerebral oxygen extraction and cerebral metabolism within individual patients. Repeated patterns of $SjvO_2$ desaturation have been shown to be predictive of poor outcome in patients with severe head injury.	- Changes in $SjvO_2$ values and $AVjDO_2$, CeO_2, and O_2ER calculations

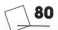

Patient Monitoring and Care *Continued*

Patient Monitoring and Care	Rationale	Reportable Conditions
3. Provide safe environment, preventing unintentional dislodging of SjvO₂ catheter, through repeated explanation and sedation or analgesia as needed, using mechanical restraints only as a last resort.	Patient safety and prevention of unintentional removal of the SjvO₂ catheter may be achieved through a variety of measures tailored to meet individualized patient needs. Unintentional dislodging of SjvO₂ catheter may result in excessive blood loss or jugular venous thrombosis, potentially influencing jugular venous outflow and ICP.	• Catheter dislodgment
4. Continuously monitor SjvO₂.	SjvO₂ trends can reflect patterns in cerebral oxygen extraction and cerebral metabolic demand.	• SjvO₂ values higher than 75% suggest "luxury perfusion" globally, although areas of regional ischemia or infarction may still be present. • Reductions in SjvO₂ values lower than 54% indicate relative cerebral hypoperfusion. • Reductions in SjvO₂ values lower than 40% indicate global cerebral ischemia.
5. Measure ICP hourly and more frequently as indicated.	Assesses trends in ICP monitoring, changes in ICP, and effect of the internal jugular catheter.	• Changes in ICP, sustained increases in ICP of more than 5 mm Hg over baseline preinsertion value • Sustained ICP elevations of over 20 mm Hg indicate potential onset of intracranial hypertension
6. Calculate CeO₂ hourly if indicated. Calculate O₂ER hourly if indicated. Obtain blood gas analysis samples necessary for calculating AVjDO₂ as indicated. Consider calculating cerebral metabolic rate of lactate and cerebral metabolic rate of oxygen, as indicated.	CeO₂, O₂ER, and AVjDO₂ data are used clinically to determine cerebral oxygen use, cerebral metabolic demand, and balance between cerebral perfusion, cerebral oxygen delivery, and cerebral metabolism. These data are used in conjunction with ICP data for precise management of patients who are experiencing intracranial hypertension with potential or actual impaired cerebral perfusion. CeO₂ and O₂ER may be conveniently calculated on an hourly basis because their parameters are derived from continuously monitored data (ie, SaO₂, SjvO₂). AVjDO₂ calculation requires data from both arterial and jugular venous blood gas samples (ie, PaO₂, PjvO₂) and may be calculated on a less frequent basis based on physician preference. Cerebral metabolic rate of lactate is usually calculated during occurrence of SjvO₂ desaturation as confirmatory data. Cerebral metabolic rate of oxygen calculation requires availability of cerebral blood flow measurement.[2, 3, 4, 7–10]	• Increases in CeO₂ (higher than 42%) and increases in AVjDO₂ (higher than 8.1 mL/dL) indicate increased cerebral oxygen uptake and increased cerebral metabolic demand. • Decreases in CeO₂ (below 24%) and decreases in AVjDO₂ (below 3.5 mL/dL) indicate decreased cerebral oxygen uptake and decreased cerebral metabolic demand.

Continued on following page

Patient Monitoring and Care	Rationale	Reportable Conditions
7. Obtain jugular blood gas sample and perform in vivo calibration procedure at regularly scheduled intervals as recommended by manufacturer.	In vivo calibration ensures reliability between monitored $SjvO_2$ data and $SjvO_2$ data obtained from laboratory analysis. Cases of $SjvO_2$ desaturation (as witnessed by continuously monitored data) are usually confirmed by obtaining laboratory analysis of jugular venous blood gas sample and by performing in vivo calibration procedure.[1, 6]	
8. Assess integrity, stability, and sterility of $SjvO_2$ catheter monitoring system at less hourly.	Hourly inspection ensures accuracy and safety of monitoring system and prevents contamination by microorganisms.	
9. Check integrity of occlusive dressing hourly. Using aseptic technique, change dressing if soiled and at minimum frequency indicated for CVP dressing changes as per institutional policy.	Prevents contamination of insertion site by soiled, wet, or loose dressing. Permits assessment of device integrity and direct visualization of insertion site. The Centers for Disease Control and Prevention (CDC) has made no recommendation for the frequency of routine central catheter dressing changes but recommends replacing dressings when the dressing becomes damp, loosened, or soiled or when inspection of the site is necessary.[11]	
10. Change the intravenous flush solution and tubing for $SjvO_2$ catheter per institutional policy.	Prevents contamination of monitoring system by microorganisms. Specific recommendations are not available for $SjvO_2$ monitoring. However, for pulmonary artery catheter monitoring, the CDC states that the hemodynamic flush system can be used safely for 72 hours.[11]	

Documentation

Documentation should include the following:

- Patient and family education
- Insertion of $SjvO_2$ catheter, including any difficulties or abnormalities experienced during insertion, and depth in centimeters of catheter insertion
- Initial $SjvO_2$ recording
- Initial CeO_2 and $AVjDO_2$ calculations
- Patient's tolerance of insertion procedure and ongoing catheter presence
- CVP dressing and insertion site assessment

- Recording of hourly $SjvO_2$, CeO_2, and $AVjDO_2$ (when indicated) data
- Recording of $SjvO_2$, CeO_2, or $AVjDO_2$ deviations and description of interventions used to treat those deviations
- Recording and description of ICP during and after insertion
- Hourly recording of ICP data
- Identification of expected and unexpected outcomes and description of interventions used to treat these outcomes

References

1. Robertson CS. Desaturation episodes after severe head injury: Influence on outcome. *Acta Neurochir.* 1993;59(suppl): 98–101.
2. Cruz J. Jugular-venous oximetry: cerebral oxygenation monitoring and management. *Acta Neurochir.* 1993;59(suppl): 86–90.
3. Dearden NM, Midgley S. Technical considerations in continuous jugular venous oxygen saturation measurement. *Acta Neurochir.* 1993;59(suppl):91–97.
4. Sheinberg M, Kanter MJ, Robertson CS, Contant CF, Narayan RK, Grossman RG. Continuous monitoring of jugular venous oxygen saturation in head-injured patients. *J Neurosurg.* 1992;76:212–217.
5. Sikes PJ, Segal J. Jugular bulb oxygen saturation monitoring for evaluating cerebral ischemia. *Crit Care Nurs Q.* 1994;17(1):9–20.
6. Robertson CS, Narayan RK, Gokaslan ZL, Pahwa R, Grossman RG, Caram P, Allen E. Cerebral arteriovenous oxygen difference as an estimate of cerebral blood flow in comatose patients. *J Neurosurg.* 1989;70:222–230.
7. Cruz J, Gennarelli TA, Alves WM. Continuous monitoring of cerebral oxygenation in acute brain injury: multivariate assessment of severe intracranial "plateau" wave—case report. *J Trauma.* 1992;32:401–403.
8. Douglas Miller J, Piper IR, Jones PA. Integrated multimodality monitoring in the neurosurgical intensive care unit. *Neurosurg Clin N Am.* 1994;5:661–670.
9. Gopinath SP, Robertson CS, Contant CF, Hayes C, Feldman Z, Narayan RK, Grossman RG. Jugular venous desaturation and outcome after head injury. *J Neurol Neurosurg Psychiatry.* 1994;57:717–723.
10. Ritter AM, Robertson CS. Cerebral metabolism. *Neurosurg Clin N Am.* 1994;5:633–645.
11. Pearson ML. Hospital infection control practices advisory committee. Guideline for prevention of intravascular device-related infections. *Infect Control Hosp Epidemiol.* 1996;17: 438–473.

Additional Readings

Cruz J. An additional therapeutic effect of adequate hyperventilation in severe acute brain trauma: normalization of cerebral glucose uptake. *J Neurosurg.* 1995;82:379–385.

Cruz J. Continuous versus global cerebral hemometabolic monitoring: Applications in acute brain trauma. *Acta Neurochir.* 1988;42(suppl):35–39.

Cruz J, Gennarelli TA, Alves WM. Continuous monitoring of cerebral hemodynamic reserve in acute brain injury: relationship to changes in brain swelling. *J Trauma.* 1992;32:629–635.

Cruz J, Hoffstad OJ, Jaggi JL. Cerebral lactate-oxygen index in acute brain injury with acute anemia: assessment of false versus true ischemia. *Crit Care Med.* 1994;22:1465–1470.

Cruz J, Miner ME, Allen SJ, Alves WM, Gennarelli TA. Continuous monitoring of cerebral oxygenation in acute brain injury: injection of mannitol during hyperventilation. *J Neurosurg.* 1990;73:725–730.

Cruz J, Miner ME, Allen SJ, Alves WM, Gennarelli TA. Continuous monitoring of cerebral oxygenation in acute brain injury: Assessment of cerebral hemodynamic reserve. *Neurosurgery.* 1991;29:743–749.

Feldman Z, Kanter MJ, Robertson CS, Contant CF, Hayes C, Sheinberg MA, Villareal CA, Narayan RK, Grossman RG. Effect of head elevation on intracranial pressure, cerebral perfusion pressure, and cerebral blood flow in head-injured patients. *J Neurosurg.* 1992;76:207–211.

Fortune JB, Feustel PJ, Weigle CGM, Popp AJ. Continuous measurement of jugular venous oxygen saturation in response to transient elevations of blood pressure in head-injured patients. *J Neurosurg.* 1994;80:461–468.

Jaggi JL, Cruz J, Gennarelli TA. Estimated cerebral metabolic rate of oxygen in severely brain-injured patients: a valuable tool for clinical monitoring. *Crit Care Med.* 1995;23:66–70.

81

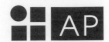

Transcranial Doppler Monitoring

P U R P O S E: Transcranial Doppler (TCD) measures blood flow velocities in the major branches of the circle of Willis through an intact skull. This measurement supports the grading of vasospasm severity, localization of intracranial stenoses or occlusions, monitoring of hemodynamic changes with increasing intracranial pressure, and assessment of the impact of therapeutic interventions on intracranial hemodynamics.[1-8]

Anne W. Wojner
Andrei V. Alexandrov

PREREQUISITE NURSING KNOWLEDGE

- Neuroanatomy and physiology should be understood.
- Clinical and technical competence related to TCD sonography is necessary.
- Noninvasive assessment of the intracranial vasculature is indicated for patients with subarachnoid hemorrhage, ischemic stroke, cerebral circulatory arrest, and other neurovascular disorders.
- Successful ultrasound penetration through the skull is possible through intracranial windows, which either lack bone or consist of thinner bone structure compared with overall cranial bone thickness. Four windows are available for insonation: temporal, orbital, foraminal, and submandibular windows (Fig. 81–1).[1, 2, 6]
- The transtemporal window allows insonation of the middle cerebral artery (MCA), the anterior cerebral artery (ACA), the posterior cerebral artery (PCA), and the anterior and posterior communicating arteries (AComA and PComA).[1, 2, 6]
- The transorbital window allows insonation of the ophthalmic artery (OA) and the internal carotid artery (ICA) siphon.[1, 2, 6]
- The transforaminal window allows insonation of the vertebral arteries (VA) and the basilar artery (BA).[1, 2, 6]
- The submandibular window allows insonation of the ICA as it enters the skull.[1, 2, 6]
- TCD locates both the depth and direction of arterial blood flow relative to transducer position and ultrasonic beam direction. Flow moving toward the transducer is displayed as a waveform with a positive velocity spectrum, whereas flow moving away from the transducer

is displayed as a waveform with a negative velocity spectrum.[1, 2, 6]
- The examination should begin with maximum power and gate settings (ie, power 100%, gate 10 to 15 mm) to expedite identification of the temporal window and various arterial segments and to minimize the time of patient exposure to ultrasound. Transorbital examination should always be performed with minimal power (ie, 10%).[1, 2, 6]
- The highest velocity signals for each arterial segment studied, as well as any abnormal or unusual waveforms, should be measured and stored in the system's computer.[6]
- Criteria for normal insonation depths, flow direction, and mean flow velocities are used to identify arteries appropriately and to diagnose abnormalities[6] (Table 81–1; Fig. 81–2).
- Criteria for determination of a normal examination are listed in Table 81–2.[6]
- Criteria supporting differential diagnosis are listed in Table 81–3.[6]
- *Pulsatility of flow* refers to vessel resistance and is measured by the pulsatility index (PI); normal range for PI is 0.6 to 1.1.[2, 6]
- Hyperventilation increases the PI and decreases mean flow velocity.[6]
- Hypercapnia decreases PI and increases mean flow velocity.[6]
- Anatomic variations in the circle of Willis are common.[2, 6]
- Inability to find an artery by TCD should *not* be interpreted as arterial occlusion in the absence of other abnormal flow findings (ie, secondary signs such as high resistance and flow diversion).[6]
- Clinical conditions and the effects of medications (dehydration or increased blood viscosity, hypertension or hypotension) should correlate with examination findings.[6]
- Although subjective, differentiation of Doppler sounds assists with identification of arterial segments and altered flow patterns.[6]
- Proximal extracranial, focal intracranial, and distal circulatory conditions are determinants of waveform patterns.[6]

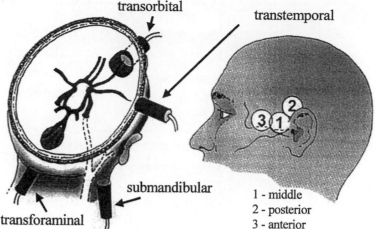

■ ● FIGURE 81–1. Four windows of transcranial Doppler insonation (left image, clockwise): orbital, temporal, submandibular, and foraminal. The temporal window has three aspects (right image): 1, middle; 2, posterior; 3, anterior. (From Alexandrov AV. *Transcranial Doppler Ultrasonography.* Houston, Tx: University of Texas Medical School; 1998.)

transorbital

transtemporal

submandibular

transforaminal

1 - middle
2 - posterior
3 - anterior

EQUIPMENT

- A pulse wave TCD system
- A 2-MHz probe (single or bilateral)
- Acoustic transmission gel

PATIENT AND FAMILY EDUCATION

- Explain the purpose of the diagnostic test and the procedure for testing. ➤*Rationale:* Decreases patient and family anxiety.
- Explain the need for the patient to remain still and quiet during the procedure. ➤*Rationale:* Elicits patient cooperation and facilitates examination.
- Explain that the procedure will not cause any discomfort to the patient. ➤*Rationale:* Decreases patient and family anxiety.

PATIENT ASSESSMENT AND PREPARATION

Patient Assessment

- Note pertinent patient history. ➤*Rationale:* TCD may be used to assist with the diagnosis and management of a number of intracranial arterial conditions, including

⠿ AP This procedure should be performed only by physicians, advanced practice nurses, and other health care professionals (including critical care nurses) with additional knowledge, skills, and demonstrated competence per professional licensure or institutional standard.

vasospasm, hyperemia, stenosis, occlusion, intracranial hypertension, cerebral circulatory arrest, cerebral embolization, and vasomotor or autoregulation testing.
- Obtain arterial blood pressure by arterial line or cuff. ➤*Rationale:* Arterial blood pressure may contribute to flow velocity and waveform pattern.
- Assess preload or hydration state. ➤*Rationale:* Dehydration may alter flow velocity because of an increase in blood viscosity and decreased preload pressures.
- Assess for hyperventilation or hypercapnia ➤*Rationale:* Carbon dioxide level may promote vasoconstriction (hyperventilation) or vasodilation (hypercapnia).
- Measure intracranial pressure (ICP) and determine cerebral perfusion pressure (CPP). ➤*Rationale:* ICP and CPP influence pulsatility of flow and end-diastolic velocities.
- Assess neurologic status. ➤*Rationale:* Provides baseline data.

Patient Preparation

- Ensure that the patient understands preprocedural teaching. Answer questions as they arise and reinforce information as needed. ➤*Rationale:* Evaluates and reinforces understanding of previously taught information.
- Assist the patient with positioning. Supine is the best position for insonation via the transtemporal, transorbital, or submandibular windows. If the patient is alert and hemodynamically and neurologically stable, assist the patient to a sitting position for insonation through the transforaminal window; if the patient is unable to sit for

Table 81–1 ●■■	Depth, Direction, and Mean Flow Velocities for Circle of Willis Arteries		
Artery	Depth (mm)	Flow Direction*	Adults
M1 MCA	45–65	Toward	32–82 cm/s
A1 ACA	62–75	Away	18–82 cm/s
ICA siphon	60–64	Bidirectional	20–77 cm/s
OA	50–62	Toward	Variable
PCA	60–68	Bidirectional	16–58 cm/s
BA	80–100+	Away	12–66 cm/s
VA	45–80	Away	12–66 cm/s

Toward the probe indicates a positive ($+$) waveform; *away* from the probe indicates a negative ($-$) waveform.

Abbreviations: M1 MCA, A1 ACA, first segments of the middle and anterior cerebral arteries; ICA, internal carotid artery; OA, ophthalmic artery; PCA, posterior cerebral artery; BA, basilar artery; VA, vertebral artery.

Adapted with permission from Alexandrov AV. Transcranial Doppler sonography: principles, examination technique and normal values. *Vascular Ultrasound Today.* 1998;10:141–160.

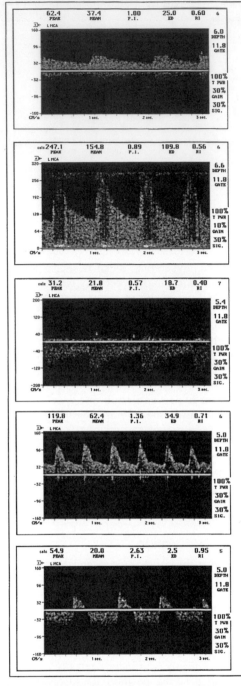

A normal waveform with sharp systolic flow acceleration, stepwise diastolic deceleration, and pulsatility index (PI) range of 0.6 – 1.1.

A focal significant MFV increase, with moderate vasospasm (MCA MFV range 120-200 cm/sec, MCA/ICA MFV ratio 3-6). Severe MCA spasm produces MFV > 200 cm/sec and ratio greater than 6.

A blunted waveform indicates near occlusion with flow diversion to a branching vessel. Differential diagnosis includes the presence of a proximal ICA obstruction.

A high resistance waveform with PI ≥ 1.2 can be found with systemic hypertension, increased cardiac output, distal vasospasm or increased ICP after other reasons are excluded.

A reverberating flow waveform shows diastolic flow reversal due to ICP equal or exceeding CPP. If found in both MCA and BA, this waveform indicates cerebral circulatory arrest.

■ ● **FIGURE 81–2.** Typical middle cerebral artery (MCA) waveforms. Vertical scale is in cm/s; horizontal scale is in seconds. Direction of flow: (+)—toward the probe, (−)—away from the probe. Velocity and pulsatility values (left to right): peak systolic, mean, pulsatility index (PI), end diastolic (ED), resistance index (RI). Depth indicates depth of insonation in cm. Gate is the diameter of sample volume in mm. Power and gain setting are given in percentages.

transforaminal insonation, assist the patient to turn his or her head laterally; if the latter is not feasible, examine the patient supine with a smaller transducer with a removable handle or a monitoring probe.   **➢►Rationale:** The transtemporal, transorbital, and submandibular windows are accessible with the patient in the supine position, whereas the transforaminal window requires a sitting position for proper probe angulation (see Fig. 81–1).

• Ask the patient to close his or her eyes for insonation via the transorbital window.   **➢►Rationale:** The probe is placed lightly, without pressure, on the eyelid and angled slightly medially to detect OA and ICA siphon flow signals.
• If necessary, ask the patient to hold his or her breath during insonation via the submandibular window.   **➢►Rationale:** Breathing may produce audible and visual artifacts, obstructing assessment of the waveform.

Table 81–2 ●■■ **Criteria for Normal TCD Findings**

1. Optimal windows of insonation, permitting identification of all proximal arterial segments
2. Direction of flow and depths consistent with criteria in Table 81–1
3. Difference between flow velocities in homologous arteries is ≤30%
4. Presence of a normal velocity ratio: MCA ≥ ACA ≥ ICA Siphon ≥ PCA ≥ BA ≥ VA
5. Positive end-diastolic flow velocity of 20%–50% of the peak systolic velocity values
6. Low-resistance flow pattern, with PI between 0.6 and 1.1 in all intracranial arteries when $Paco_2$ between 35 and 45 mm Hg
7. High-resistance flow pattern with PI ≥ 1.2 in the OA only
8. High-resistance flow patterns with PI ≥ 1.2 in all arteries during hyperventilation or elevated BP

Reprinted with permission from Alexandrov AV. Transcranial Doppler sonography: principles, examination technique and normal values. *Vascular Ultrasound Today.* 1998;10:141–160.

Table 81–3 ●■■ **Differential Diagnosis**

Problem	Findings	Differential Diagnosis
Arterial stenosis	Focal MFV increase above normal values Turbulence, bruits Flow diversion to adjacent arteries Flow alteration distal to site of stenosis (deceleration, low PIs)	Primary arterial stenosis Compensatory flow increase Adjacent artery occlusion Hyperemia
Arterial near occlusion	Blunted waveform Focal decrease in MFV Slow systolic acceleration Slow flow deceleration Flow diversion to adjacent arteries	Near occlusion at the site of insonation Arterial occlusion proximal to insonation site Incorrect vessel identification
Arterial occlusion	No detectable flow Good unilateral window of insonation High-resistance flow proximal to occlusion Flow diversion to adjacent arteries	Primary arterial occlusion Incorrect vessel identification Mass effect
Arterial vasospasm	Proximal vasospasm: 　Focal or diffuse elevation of MFV without parallel FV increase in feeding extracranial arteries; HI > 3 Distal vasospasm: 　Focal increase in flow pulsatility (PI ≥ 1.2), indicating increased resistance distal to site of insonation 　Increase in MFV in the involved and adjacent arteries may not be present	Vasospasm Hyperemia Vasospasm with hyperemia Altered cerebral autoregulation Increased intracranial pressure
Increased intracranial pressure	Decreased EDV or absent end-diastolic flow Rapid flow deceleration PI ≥ 1.2 Note that these findings may be present in patients with increased cardiac output or elevated blood pressure, as well as in elderly individuals.	The presence of PI ≥ 1.2 and positive end-diastolic flow in all arteries may be caused by the following: Hyperventilation Hypertension Increased ICP Unilateral PI ≥ 1.2 may be caused by the following: 　Compartmental ICP increase 　Stenoses distal to the site of insonation 　PI ≥ 2.0 associated with absent end-diastolic flow is caused by extreme elevations in ICP and possible cerebral circulatory arrest.
Cerebral circulatory arrest	Reversed end-diastolic flow or reverberating flow pattern *or* Minimal systolic flow acceleration with no end-diastolic flow *or* Absent flow signals in all intracranial arterial systems	Possible or probable circulatory arrest; measure both MCA and BA for 30 min, then reassess. (Transient arrest may occur during transient ICP increase or low blood pressure values.)

Abbreviations: BA, basilar artery; EDV, end-diastolic velocity; FV, flow velocity; HI, hemispheric index; ICP, intracranial pressure; MCA, middle cerebral artery; MFV, mean flow velocity; PI, pulsatility index.

●■ AP This procedure should be performed only by physicians, advanced practice nurses, and other health care professionals (including critical care nurses) with additional knowledge, skills, and demonstrated competence per professional licensure or institutional standard.

Procedure for Transcranial Doppler Monitoring

Steps	Rationale	Special Considerations
1. Wash hands, and don gloves.	Reduces transmission of microorganisms and body secretions; standard precautions.	

Transtemporal Insonation

Steps	Rationale	Special Considerations
1. Set the depth at 50 to 56 mm.	Depth of 50 to 56 mm allows insonation of the M1 MCA.	
2. Set the power to maximum or 100%.	Optimizes ability to identify arterial waveforms.	
3. Place the probe above the zygomatic arch and aim slightly upward and anterior to the contralateral ear.	Accesses the transtemporal window (see Fig. 81–1).	No transtemporal window or a suboptimal window can be found in approximately 5% to 15% of the population.
4. Find a flow signal directed toward the probe that meets MCA flow criteria (see Table 81–1).		
5. Follow the signal until it disappears by holding the probe in a constant position and changing the depth setting to a shallow setting of 40 to 45 mm and a deep setting of 65 to 70 mm.	Verifies MCA identification; limits operator error.	
6. Find the ICA bifurcation at 65 mm and obtain both MCA and ACA signals.	ICA bifurcation is visualized at a depth of 65 mm; a bidirectional MCA/ACA waveform is noted.	
7. Follow the ACA signal to a depth of 70 to 75 mm.	ACA insonation begins at a depth of 70 to 75 mm.	The contralateral ACA may be insonated at a depth of more than 75 mm in the case of a unilateral suboptimal transtemporal window.
8. Return to the bifurcation and reset the depth to 62 mm while slowly rotating the probe posteriorly by 10 to 30 degrees to find the PCA.	PCA is commonly detected at depths of 60 to 64 mm.	
9. Find the P1 PCA signal directed toward the probe and the P2 PCA signal directed away from the probe.		
10. Record and print findings, including at least waveforms, mean flow velocities, and PIs for all arteries insonated.		

Transorbital Insonation

Steps	Rationale	Special Considerations
1. Decrease the power to minimum or 10%.	Limits eye exposure to ultrasound.	
2. Set the depth at 52 mm.		
3. Place the transducer gently over the eyelid without applying pressure, and turn the transducer slightly medially.		
4. Determine flow pulsatility and direction in the distal ophthalmic artery.	PI is ≥1.2 because OA is an anastomosis with a high resistance arterial system (extracranial carotid branches).	
5. Confirm findings at a depth of 55 to 60 mm.		
6. Reset the depth to 60 to 64 mm and find the ICA siphon flow signals.	The ICA siphon can have bidirectional low resistance flow signals.	
7. Record and print findings, including peak systolic, end-diastolic, and mean flow velocities, as well as PI for both the ICA and OA.		

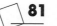

Procedure	for Transcranial Doppler Monitoring *Continued*

Steps	Rationale	Special Considerations
Transforaminal Insonation		
1. Use maximum or 100% power.		
2. Set depth at 75 mm.	The VA/proximal BA junction is insonated at 75 mm.	
3. Place the probe at midline, 1 inch below the edge of the skull; aim toward the bridge of the nose.		
4. Identify flow directed away from the probe.		
5. Increase the depth to 80 mm, then 90 mm, and 100 mm to follow the BA from proximal to distal segments.	The proximal BA is insonated at 80 mm, mid-BA is insonated at 90 mm, and the distal BA is insonated at 95 to 100 mm or more.	
6. Confirm findings while slowly decreasing the depth of insonation.	Tortuous BA may be difficult to insonate; operator errors are common.	
7. Set the depth at 60 mm and reposition the probe laterally, aiming at the eye.		
8. Find the VA flow directed away from the probe and follow it at 40 to 60 mm and 60 to 80 mm; repeat examination on the opposite side.	The intracranial portions of the right and left VA are insonated at depths between 40 and 80 mm.	
9. Record and print findings, including peak systolic, end-diastolic, and mean flow velocities, as well as PI for both the BA and bilateral VA.		
Submandibular Insonation		
1. Set the depth at 50 to 60 mm, place the probe laterally under the jaw, and aim upward and medially.		Calculate the hemispheric index (HI): HI = MFV MCA/MFV ICA. Normal values are <3. HI is used to differentiate between M1-MCA vasospasm after subarachnoid hemorrhage and hyperemia.
2. Find a low-resistance flow directed away from the probe that meets ICA criteria (see Table 81–1).	A high-resistance flow pattern is consistent with the external carotid artery, *not* the ICA.	
3. Repeat the examination on the opposite side.		
4. Record and print findings, including at least waveforms, mean flow velocities, and PIs for both the right and left ICAs.		
5. Clean gel from patient's head.	Promotes comfort.	
6. Discard gloves, and wash hands.	Reduces transmission of microorganisms; standard precautions.	

AP This procedure should be performed only by physicians, advanced practice nurses, and other health care professionals (including critical care nurses) with additional knowledge, skills, and demonstrated competence per professional licensure or institutional standard.

Expected Outcomes	Unexpected Outcomes
• Determination of normal or pathologic flow conditions	• Inability to insonate via temporal window in 2% of patients after subarachnoid hemorrhage, aneurysm, or surgical obliteration and in up to 15% to 20% of other adult patients with intact skulls
• Recommendation, as needed, for definitive angiographic examination and treatment	
• Recognition of technical limitations, including operator skill	• Underestimation of highest detectable velocity because of operator skill

Patient Monitoring and Care

Patient Monitoring and Care	Rationale	Reportable Conditions
		These conditions should be reported if they persist despite nursing interventions.
1. Monitor respiratory and cardiovascular status during procedure; document $PaCO_2$, mean arterial pressure, and cardiac rhythm and the use of vasoactive medications, if any, during procedure.	Velocity is affected by systemic hemodynamics as well as vasomotor response of the resistance vessels in the brain (ie, arterioles). TCD is not associated with the development of changes in respiratory or cardiovascular status; instead, it is influenced by these changes, should they occur.	• Changes that may affect velocity
2. When conducting the examination with a headframe, loosen probe fixation after 1 hour and assess skin.	Tight fixation by headframe may be required to achieve better sound transmission and constant angle of insonation.	• Skin breakdown • Unrelieved discomfort
3. When monitoring for brain embolization, note the timing of events associated with emboli detection (eg, placement or removal of aortic cross clamp during cardiac surgery with cardiopulmonary bypass).	Continuous monitoring with TCD has shown an association between specific operative events during cardiac surgery using cardiopulmonary bypass and the detection of brain emboli on TCD.	• Events that may affect emboli detection

Documentation

Documentation should include the following:

- Patient and family education
- Patient name, age, gender, and medical record number
- Clinical diagnosis (indication for testing)
- Significant, clinically detectable neurologic findings
- Arterial blood pressure, $PaCO_2$, and ICP (when feasible) during examination
- Preload measures as confirmation of hydration status
- Flow velocity spectra (waveforms), MFV, and PI in the arteries insonated
- Hard copies of arterial waveforms
- Presence of suboptimal windows indicated in the report
- Interpretation
- Unexpected outcomes
- Additional interventions

References

1. Aaslid R, Markwalder TM, Nornes H. Noninvasive transcranial Doppler ultrasound recording of flow velocity in basal cerebral arteries. *J Neurosurg.* 1982;57:769–774.

2. Otis SM, Ringelstein EB. The transcranial Doppler examination: principles and applications of transcranial Doppler sonography. In: Tegeler CH, Baikian VL, Gomez CR. *Neurosonology,* St Louis, Mo: C.V. Mosby; 1996:140–155.

3. Lindegaard KF, Nornes H, Bakke SJ, et al. Cerebral vasospasm diagnosis by means of angiography and blood velocity measurements. *Acta Neurochir (Wien).* 1987;100:12–24.

4. Sloan MA. Transcranial Doppler monitoring of vasospasm after subarachnoid hemorrhage. In: Tegeler CH, Baikian VL, Gomez CR, eds. *Neurosonology.* St Louis, Mo: C.V. Mosby; 1996:156–171.

5. Alexandrov AV, Babikian BL, Adams RJ, Tegeler CH, Caplan LR, Spencer MP. The evolving role of transcranial Doppler in stroke prevention and treatment. *J Stroke Cerebrovasc Dis.* 1998;7:101–104.

6. Alexandrov AV. Transcranial Doppler sonography: principles, examination technique and normal values. *Vascular Ultrasound Today.* 1998;10:141–160.

7. Stump DA, Newman SP. Embolus detection during cardiopulmonary bypass. In: Tegeler CH, Baikian VL, Gomez CR. *Neurosonology,* St Louis, Mo: C.V. Mosby; 1996: 252–258.

8. Newell DW. Trauma and brain death. In: Tegeler CH, Baikian VL, Gomez CR. *Neurosonology.* St Louis, Mo: C.V. Mosby; 1996:189–199.

Additional Reading

Wojncr AW. Neurovascular disorders. In: Kinney MR, Dunbar SB, Brooks-Brunn JA, Molter N, Vitello-Cicciu JM, eds. *AACN's Clinical Reference for Critical Care Nursing.* 4th ed. St Louis, Mo: C.V. Mosby; 1998.

PROCEDURE

82

Cerebrospinal Fluid Drainage Assessment

P U R P O S E: This procedure describes the collection and assessment of cerebrospinal drainage. It is important to identify cerebrospinal fluid leaks to decrease the risk of central nervous system (CNS) infection and pneumocephalus.[1-4]

Phyllis Dubendorf

PREREQUISITE KNOWLEDGE

- Neuroanatomy and physiology should be understood.
- Cerebrospinal fluid (CSF) circulates in the subarachnoid space, beneath the dura in the layers of the meninges.
- CSF leaks may occur with any breech of the dura commonly resulting from trauma or surgery. Although rare, CSF leaks can occur spontaneously.

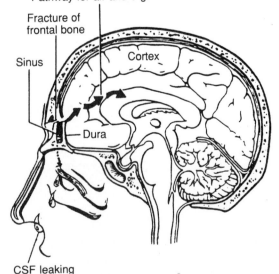

■ ● FIGURE 82–1. Cerebrospinal fluid leak resulting from skull fracture. This diagram depicts a CSF leak from the nose (rhinorrhea), but CSF drainage also may be experienced from the ear (otorrhea), nasopharyngeally (described as postnasal drip), and, rarely, in tears. CSF, cerebrospinal fluid. (From Shyder M, Jackie M. *Neurologic Problems: A Critical Care Nursing Focus.* Englewood, NJ: RJ Brady; 1981.)

- Most CSF leaks spontaneously resolve in 7 to 10 days.
- CSF leaks predispose the individual to CNS infection by allowing the entry of bacteria into the subarachnoid space.
- CSF leaks may predispose the individual to the development of pneumocephalus.
- CSF leaks may manifest as the following (Fig. 82–1):
  - ❖ Rhinorrhea (leakage of fluid from the nose)
  - ❖ Otorrhea (leakage of fluid from the ear)
  - ❖ Postnasal drip
- A CSF leak can sometimes be identified by a characteristic *halo* or *ring sign:* fluid absorbed by linen may create a collection of blood encircled with a larger concentric "halo" of clear fluid. The reliability of the halo sign is controversial.[1, 4]
- CSF can be identified by laboratory assay of quantitative glucose (>30 mg/dL is suggestive of CSF); however, false positives occur frequently. Urine glucose sticks are extremely sensitive to the presence of glucose, and their use also yields a frequent false-positive result.
- CSF can be identified definitively by laboratory assay to detect the presence of beta-2-transferrin, a glycoprotein found in CSF but not in tears, nasal exudates, or serum.[1, 5]

EQUIPMENT

- Nonsterile gloves
- Small sterile container (test tube or specimen cup)
- Gauze
- Tape
- Specimen label
- Laboratory form

PATIENT AND FAMILY EDUCATION

- Explain the procedure and reason for drainage identification. **➡Rationale:** Reinforces need for procedure and allows patient or family to ask questions.

- Review signs and symptoms of meningeal irritation and CNS infection. ➤*Rationale:* Recognition of meningeal signs and symptoms supports diagnosis of CNS infection and facilitates treatment.

PATIENT ASSESSMENT AND PREPARATION

Patient Assessment

- Obtain vital signs. ➤*Rationale:* Vital signs may be used to support the diagnosis of CNS infection.
- Perform a neurologic assessment. ➤*Rationale:* Deterioration of the neurologic assessment may be used to support the diagnosis of CNS infection.
- Assess for the presence of meningeal signs (photophobia, headache, nuchal rigidity). ➤*Rationale:* These signs may be used to support the diagnosis of CNS infection.

Patient Preparation

- Ensure that the patient and family understand preprocedural teaching. Answer questions as they arise and reinforce information as needed. ➤*Rationale:* Evaluates and reinforces understanding of previously taught information.
- Position patient comfortably and in a position that facilitates fluid drainage and collection. ➤*Rationale:* The presence and rate of CSF leakage may depend on the position of the patient's head.

Procedure for Cerebrospinal Fluid Drainage Assessment

Steps	Rationale	Special Considerations
1. Wash hands, and don gloves.	Reduces transmission of microorganisms; standard precautions.	
2. If applicable, remove any sterile dressing the patient has that covers the flow of drainage.	Facilitates the collection of fluid.	
3. Collect fluid at drainage site in small sterile container.	Enables laboratory evaluation.	Obtain at least 1 mL fluid for evaluation. This may be a time-consuming process if the leak is very slow.
4. Apply a new sterile dressing (if applicable).	Absorbs drainage.	
5. Discard gloves and soiled dressings, and wash hands.	Reduces transmission of microorganisms; standard precautions.	
6. Label sample and complete laboratory form for detection of beta-2-transferrin	Identifies patient and test needed.	Beta-2-transferrin is a glycoprotein found in CSF.

Expected Outcomes

- Collection of sample for analysis
- Determination of CSF leak

Unexpected Outcomes

- Inability to obtain sufficient fluid for evaluation
- Laboratory unable to evaluate sample
- Development of CNS infection

Patient Monitoring and Care

Patient Monitoring and Care	Rationale	Reportable Conditions
		These conditions should be reported if they persist despite nursing interventions.
1. Monitor neurologic status (using Glasgow Coma Score) before and after collection and as indicated.	Provides data for ongoing diagnosis and treatment.	• Changes in neurologic status
2. Change sterile dressing every day and as needed.	Provides subjective means of measuring amount of drainage.	• Change in drainage volume or character
3. Monitor for signs and symptoms of meningitis.	Signs and symptoms of meningitis may indicate the need for further testing and evaluation.	• Change in level of consciousness • Temperature greater than 101.5°F • Photophobia • Nuchal rigidity • Seizure • Headache

Continued on following page

Patient Monitoring and Care	Rationale	Reportable Conditions
4. Monitor for signs and symptoms of pneumocephalus.	Signs and symptoms of pneumocephalus may indicate the need for further testing and evaluation.	• Headache • Nuchal rigidity • Photophobia • Change in level of consciousness
5. Patients experiencing rhinorrhea should be encouraged *not* to blow the nose or sneeze.	Blowing the nose or sneezing causes an increase in CSF pressure and can increase drainage.	

Documentation

Documentation should include the following:

- Patient and family education
- Patient's neurologic status
- Area from which drainage is flowing
- Color, amount, and character of drainage
- Date, time, and amount of drainage collected for evaluation
- Unexpected outcomes
- Additional interventions

References

1. Greenberg MS. *Handbook of Neurosurgery.* Lakeland, Fla: Greenberg Graphics; 1997.
2. Barker E. *Neuroscience Nursing.* St Louis, Mo: C.V. Mosby; 1994.
3. Hickey JV. *The Clinical Practice of Neurological and Neuro-surgical Nursing.* 4th ed. Philadelphia, Pa: J.B. Lippincott; 1997.
4. Narayan E, Wilberger J, Povlishock J. *Neurotrauma.* New York, NY: McGraw-Hill; 1996.
5. Knight JA. Advances in the analysis of cerebrospinal fluid. *J Clin Lab Sci.* 1997;27:93–104.

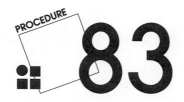

83

External Warming/ Cooling Devices

P U R P O S E: An external warming device is applied to increase an undesirably low body temperature. An external cooling device is applied to reduce an undesirably high body temperature and to decrease cellular metabolism.

Eileen M. Kelly

PREREQUISITE NURSING KNOWLEDGE

- The *hypothalamus* is the primary thermoregulatory center for the body; it maintains normothermia through internal regulation of heat production or heat loss. Superficial or shell-zone temperature information is transmitted by thermal receptors in the skin and subcutaneous tissue to the posterior hypothalamus through the spinal cord. Thermoreceptors in the brain, heart, and other deep organs transmit core-zone temperature. Effective temperature regulation depends on the ability of the posterior hypothalamus to receive and integrate the signals received from the core and shell zones.
- Terms associated with temperature should be known (Table 83–1).
- The hypothalamus regulates temperature in the range of approximately 36.4°C to 37.3°C (97.5°F to 99.4°F). By initiating physiologic responses to changes above or below this range, the hypothalamus coordinates heat loss or gain. Vasoconstriction and vasodilatation control the distribution and flow of blood to the organs, viscera, and skin surface; thus, the amount of heat loss to the environment is influenced by vasomotor activity. In response to heat loss, shivering and vasoconstriction occur, the muscles tense and the extremities are drawn closer to

the body, and the person seeks warmth. In response to heat gain, sweating and vasodilatation occur, muscles relax, and the person seeks coolness.
- Alteration in thermoregulation can result from a primary central nervous system injury or disease (eg, subarachnoid hemorrhage, spinal cord injury, or neoplasm) and metabolic conditions (eg, diabetes mellitus, toxic levels of ethanol alcohol or other drugs, such as barbiturates and phenothiazines).
- *Body temperature* is the measurement of the presence or absence of heat. Body heat is generated, conserved, redistributed, or dissipated during all physiologic processes. Factors such as age, circadian rhythms, and hormones influence body temperature.
- Body temperature may be measured by a variety of thermometers and sites. Electronic or mercury-in-glass thermometers are used to obtain rectal, oral, and axillary temperatures. Thermistors within catheters or probes measure rectal, esophageal, bladder, and pulmonary artery temperatures. Infrared thermometers measure tympanic membrane temperature.
- *Core temperature* represents the temperature of internal sites ranging from the rectum to the tympanic membrane. Variations in temperatures normally occur in the body (Table 83–2).
- Site choice for temperature monitoring is based on the clinical data needed and on the patient's condition, safety, comfort, and environmental factors (eg, room temperature), the indication for catheter or probe (eg, pulmonary artery catheter), and the availability of equipment. A consistent temperature site must be monitored during the application of a warming or cooling device.
- Heat flows from a higher temperature to a lower temperature until the gradient between the two temperatures diminishes. Conduction, convection, radiation, and evaporation transfer heat as follows:
  - ❖ *Conduction* occurs when a warmer object comes in direct contact with one of lower temperature.
  - ❖ *Convection* occurs when air or liquid carries heat away from an object.
  - ❖ *Radiation* occurs when thermal energy passes through air or space.

Table 83–1 ■■■ **Terms Associated with Temperature**

Term	Definition
Euthermia	Range of body temperature associated with health
Hypothermia	Temperature below 36.4°C
Induced hypothermia	Intentional cooling by surface (transfer of heat from the skin to the coolant circulating through the coils of the cooling device) or central means (circulatory heat exchange in a cardiopulmonary bypass machine)
Fever	Response to a pyrogen; the hypothalamus either resets its range higher, maintaining thermoregulation, or there is a change in the sensitivity of hypothalamus neuron activity to warmth and coldness[1]
Hyperthermia	Dysfunction of thermoregulation caused by an injury to the hypothalamus or when a person's heat loss mechanisms are overwhelmed by high environmental heat

Table 83–2 ●■■	**Normal Variations in Body Temperature Based on a Rectal Temperature of 37°C**
Type of Temperature Measurement	Degrees Lower than Rectal Temperature
Oral	0.3–0.5°C
Esophageal	0.2°C
Pulmonary artery	0.2–0.3°C
Tympanic membrane	0.05–0.25°C
Bladder	0.1–0.2°C
Axillary	0.6–0.8°C

❖ *Evaporation* occurs when heat is lost to the surrounding air.

- Refer to Table 83–3 for techniques to increase heat gain.
- *Shivering* is an involuntary shaking of the body. It is caused by contraction or twitching of the muscles, and it is a physiologic method of heat production.
- Shivering increases the metabolic rate, carbon dioxide (CO_2) production, oxygen consumption, and myocardial work. If cardiopulmonary compensation does not occur to meet these demands, anaerobic metabolism occurs, resulting in acidosis.
- Early detection of shivering can be accomplished by palpating mandible vibration as a "humming" vibration and electrocardiogram (ECG) artifact from skeletal muscle.[2, 3] If not detected early, shivering can progress to visible fasciculation of the head or neck, then to visible fasciculation of the pectorals or trunk, and then to generalized shaking of the entire body and teeth chattering.
- At a body temperature below 35°C, the basal metabolic rate can no longer supply sufficient body heat, and an exogenous source of heat is needed.
- *Hypothermia* may be categorized as mild (34°C to 36.5°C), moderate (27.5°C to 33.9°C), deep (17°C to 27.4°C), or profound (less than 16.9°C).
- Hypothermia may be caused by an increase in heat loss, a decrease in heat production, an alteration in thermoregulation, and miscellaneous clinical conditions.
- An increase in heat loss may occur from the following:
  ❖ Environmental exposure
  ❖ Near drowning
  ❖ Induced vasodilatation caused by high levels of ethanol alcohol, barbiturates, and general anesthesia
  ❖ Dermal dysfunction (eg, burns)
  ❖ Iatrogenic conditions (eg, administering cold intravenous fluids, hemodialysis, cardiopulmonary bypass)
- A decrease in heat production is associated with the following:

Table 83–3 ●■■	**Techniques to Increase Heat Gain**
Mechanism of Heat Transfer	Techniques to Increase Heat Gain
Radiation	Warming lights, warm environment, room temperature, blankets
Conduction	Warm blankets, circulating water blanket, continuous arteriovenous rewarming, cardiopulmonary bypass
Convection	Thermal fans, circulating air blanket
Evaporation	Head and body covers; warm, humidified oxygen

❖ Endocrine conditions (eg, hypothyroidism)
❖ Insufficient fuel because of malnutrition
❖ Diabetic ketoacidosis
❖ Neuromuscular insufficiency (eg, that caused by a pharmacologic paralysis from a neuromuscular blocking agent or anesthetic agents)

- Clinical conditions associated with hypothermia are sepsis, hepatic coma, and systemic inflammatory response syndrome.
- The significant physiologic alterations that occur with hypothermia depend on the degree of hypothermia present and the cause of the hypothermia (Table 83–4).
- Severe hypothermia may mimic death; resuscitative efforts should be initiated despite the absence of vital signs.
- Rewarming should not occur faster than 2°C per hour.
- Rapid rewarming can cause a rewarming acidosis, shivering, hypovolemic shock, temperature afterdrop, and temperature overshoot.
- *Afterdrop* is a decrease in core temperature after rewarming is discontinued.

Table 83–4 ●■■	**Physiologic Responses to Hypothermia**

Central Nervous System

Decreased cerebral blood flow
Progressive paralysis of the central nervous system
Reduced cerebral metabolic demand

Cardiovascular System

Decreased heart rate, contractility, and cardiac output
Delayed depolarization in pacemaker tissue
Electrocardiogram characteristics: increased PR, QRS, and QT intervals; J wave (the J wave is a deflection of the QRS-ST junction); ST elevation; and T wave inversion
Decreased transmembrane resting potential resulting in atrial fibrillation or ventricular fibrillation

Pulmonary System

Hypoventilation
Decreased cough reflex
Increased airway secretions
Paralysis of mucociliary mechanism

Gastrointestinal System

Hypomotility
Decreased hepatic metabolism
Decreased insulin release from the pancreas
Stress ulceration

Renal System

Impaired renal tubular transport causing decreased sodium and water reabsorption
Decreased antidiuretic hormone
Fluid shift from vascular compartment to interstitial spaces

Acid-Base Balance

Decreased systemic carbon dioxide production
Early respiratory alkalosis
Eventual metabolic acidosis in severe hypothermia

Hematologic System

Shift of oxyhemoglobin dissociation curve to the left, causing decreased oxygen delivery to tissues
Increased blood viscosity
Coagulopathy caused by inhibition of the enzyme reactions of the coagulation cascade and splenic sequestration of platelets

Immunologic System

Leukocyte sequestration in the spleen
Decreased neutrophil function
Reduced collagen deposition

- *Overshoot* occurs when the thermoregulator mechanisms rebound or overcompensate. Terminating active external rewarming at 36°C to 36.5°C may prevent temperature overshoot.
- *Rewarming acidosis* results from the increase in CO_2 production associated with temperature increase and from the return of accumulated acids in the peripheral circulation to the heart.
- *Rewarming shock* occurs when hypothermic vasoconstriction masks hypovolemia. If the patient's circulating volume is insufficient during rewarming vasodilatation, there is a sudden decrease in blood pressure, systemic vascular resistance (SVR), and preload.
- *Hyperthermia* occurs when the thermoregulator system of the body absorbs or produces more heat than it is able to release.
- *Malignant hyperthermia* is a rare, hereditary condition of the skeletal muscle that occurs on exposure to a triggering agent or agents. The triggering agents most commonly associated with malignant hyperthermia are anesthetic agents, particularly inhalation anesthetics and succinylcholine. Malignant hyperthermia involves instability of the muscle cell membrane that causes a sudden increase in myoplasmic calcium and skeletal muscle contractures.
- The earliest indication of malignant hyperthermia is an increase in end-tidal carbon dioxide ($ETCO_2$) of 5 mm Hg more than the patient's baseline. If the $ETCO_2$ is not being monitored, the earliest sign is tachycardia, occurring within 30 minutes of anesthesia induction. Tachycardia is followed by ventricular ectopy that may progress to ventricular tachycardia and ventricular fibrillation. Muscle rigidity usually begins in the extremities, chest, or jaws.
- A cooling device is used to treat malignant hyperthermia after administration of the triggering agent is stopped, and dantrolene is given. Dantrolene (a muscle relaxant) blocks the release of calcium from the sarcoplasmic reticulum without affecting calcium uptake.[4]
- *Heat stroke* occurs when the outdoor temperature and humidity are excessive, and heat is transferred to the body. The high humidity prevents cooling by evaporation. The rectal temperature is greater than 104°C to 106°C. Other signs are hypotension, tachycardia, tachypnea, mental status changes from confusion to coma, and possibly seizures. The skin is hot and dry, and sweating may occur. Initial interventions include support of airway, breathing, and circulation. Rapid cooling of the patient is the main treatment priority with a goal of reducing the temperature to 101°C to 102°C in 1 hour.
- *Fever* occurs in response to a pyrogen. During fever, the hypothalamus retains its function, and shivering and diaphoresis occur to gain or lose body heat. Fever may be an adaptive response and may be considered beneficial.[1] However, a febrile state increases the heart rate and metabolic rate and may be detrimental to a critically ill patient. The decision to reduce a fever needs to be based on the patient's physical and hemodynamic stability during the fever.
- A cooling or warming device circulates warmed or cooled fluid through coils in a thermal blanket or pad. Warmth or coolness is transferred to the patient by conduction.
- Specific information about controls, alarms, troubleshooting, and safety features is available from each manufacturer and must be understood by the nurse before using the equipment.
- A device used only for warming blows warm air through microperforations on the underside of a blanket that covers the patient. Warm air is directed through the blanket onto the patient's skin. This method of heat transfer is convection.

EQUIPMENT

- Sheet or bath blanket
- Temperature probe, cable, and module (varies with type of site and type of thermometer selected and available) to monitor patient's temperature
- Cardiac monitoring
- Warming and cooling fluid unit (console and hoses) with circulating fluid blanket

Additional equipment to have available as needed includes the following:

- Hemodynamic monitoring
- Warm air unit (console and hose) with circulating air blanket

PATIENT AND FAMILY EDUCATION

- Explain reason for use of a warming or cooling device and standard of care, including monitoring of temperature, expected length of therapy, comfort measures, and parameters for discontinuation of device. ➤*Rationale:* Encourages patient and family to ask questions and verbalize concerns about the procedure.
- Assess patient and family understanding of warming or cooling therapy. ➤*Rationale:* Clarification and reinforcement of information is needed during times of stress and anxiety.
- Encourage patient to notify nurse of any discomfort. ➤*Rationale:* Facilitates early relief and minimizes discomfort.
- If convection warming device will be used, explain rationale for removing patient's sheet or gown or both. Reassure patient and family that privacy will be respected. ➤*Rationale:* Patient and family will know what to expect.

PATIENT ASSESSMENT AND PREPARATION

Patient Assessment

- Assess risk factors, medical history, the cause of the patient's underlying condition, and the type and the length of temperature exposure. ➤*Rationale:* Assists in anticipating, recognizing, and responding to patient's responses and potential side effects to therapy.
- Assess patient medication therapy. ➤*Rationale:* Medications such as vasopressors and vasodilators may affect heat transfer, increase the potential for skin injury, and contribute to an adverse hemodynamic response.
- Obtain a core (pulmonary artery, urinary, or rectal) temperature. ➤*Rationale:* Determines baseline temperature. Determines when a warming or cooling device is needed.
- Obtain vital signs and hemodynamic values (if using

pulmonary artery monitoring). ➟*Rationale:* Determines baseline cardiovascular data. Initially, cold temperatures activate the sympathetic nervous system, resulting in tachycardia, vasoconstriction, and shivering. Rapid rewarming may result in vasodilatation and hypotension. Heart failure may occur with malignant hyperthermia and heat stroke.

- Monitor cardiac rhythm. ➟*Rationale:* Determines baseline cardiac rhythm. Hypothermia has a negative chronotropic effect on pacemaker tissue, which may lead to bradycardia and atrioventricular heart block. Hypothermia may cause repolarization abnormalities, producing ST segment elevation and T wave inversion. A hypothermic heart is susceptible to atrial and ventricular fibrillation. Tachycardia and ventricular dysrhythmias may occur if the patient is hyperthermic.
- Assess electrolytes, glucose, arterial blood gas, and coagulation studies. ➟*Rationale:* Alteration in temperature balance may result in acid-base imbalance, coagulopathy, electrolyte imbalance, and hypoxemia. Hypothermia inhibits insulin release from the pancreas, but glucose levels remain normal in mild hypothermia because shivering increases glucose utilization. Hyperglycemia occurs at temperatures less than 32°C because shivering ceases.
- Assess level of consciousness and neurologic function. ➟*Rationale:* Determines baseline neurologic status. A change in mental status, level of consciousness, and impaired neurologic function may occur because of an undesirable high or low temperature or from the condition causing the alteration in temperature. Fatigue, muscle incoordination, poor judgment, weakness, hallucinations, lethargy, and stupor may occur with hypothermia. Seizures may occur with hyperthermia.

- Assess ventilatory function. ➟*Rationale:* Hypoventilation, suppression of cough, and mucociliary reflexes associated with hypothermia may lead to hypoxemia, atelectasis, and pneumonia. Hypothermia shifts the oxygenation dissociation curve to the left, and less oxygen is released from oxyhemoglobin to the tissues. Because of peripheral vasoconstriction, pulse oximetry is unreliable. Hyperthermia shifts the oxygenation dissociation curve to the right, and oxygen is readily released from oxyhemoglobin.
- Assess bowel sounds, abdomen, and gastrointestinal function. ➟*Rationale:* Determines baseline status. Patients experiencing hypothermia may develop an ileus because of decreased intestinal motility. Vomiting and diarrhea may occur with hyperthermia.
- Assess skin integrity. ➟*Rationale:* Provides baseline data. Externally applied warming or cooling device can cause skin injury or exacerbate skin injury. Preexisting conditions such as diabetes and peripheral vascular disease increase the patient's risk for skin injury.

Patient Preparation

- Ensure that the patient understands preprocedural teaching. Answer questions as they arise, and reinforce information as needed. ➟*Rationale:* Evaluates and reinforces understanding of previously taught information.
- If convection warming device will be used, remove the patient's sheet. ➟*Rationale:* The convection warming device should be in direct contact with the patient for optimal results.
- If the patient is hypothermic, cover the patient's head with a warmed blanket or towel or an aluminum cap. ➟*Rationale:* Minimizes additional heat loss.

Procedure for External Warming/Cooling Devices

Steps	Rationale	Special Considerations
1. Wash hands, and don gloves.	Reduces transmission of microorganisms; standard precautions.	
2. Obtain method for continuously monitoring core temperature.	Continuous core temperature monitoring is necessary when using external warming or cooling devices.	Some warming or cooling devices have an adapter for connecting a rectal temperature probe from the patient directly to the device.
3. Plug the device into a grounded outlet.	Establishes power source.	
To Use Warming or Cooling Device		
1. Apply a dry sheet or bath blanket between the patient and the circulating fluid blanket.	Protects the skin.	Avoid applying additional sheets or blankets because efficient heating or cooling occurs with maximal contact between the thermal pad and skin.
2. Fill the reservoir in the unit with distilled water to the indicated full level.	The reservoir must contain enough water for the machine to function properly.	The manufacturer determines the appropriate fluid level.
3. Attach hoses to the circulating fluid blanket. Check that the clamps are closed before connecting the hoses from the device to the fluid blanket. After connecting the hoses, make sure all connections are tight before unclamping. Check for kinks in the hoses.	Allows the flow of warmed or cooled water to the blanket.	Prevent water spraying.

Procedure	for External Warming/Cooling Devices *Continued*

Steps	Rationale	Special Considerations
4. Press the start switch on.	Activates the device.	
5. Connect the temperature probe to the unit 1 minute before pressing a control mode switch.	Prevents the triggering of the temperature probe alarm.	Most warming or cooling devices sound an alarm if the probe relays a low temperature (30°C), indicative of probe dislodgment.

Manual Control

Steps	Rationale	Special Considerations
1. Press the manual control switch on.		
2. Choose the set point for the temperature of the circulating fluid.	The device maintains the circulating fluid in the blanket at the temperature set point.	The patient's temperature must be continuously monitored by a method other than the cooling or warming device.

Automatic Control

Steps	Rationale	Special Considerations
1. Select automatic mode.	On automatic mode, the unit warms or cools the circulating fluid in the blanket based on the set point (desired temperature) for the patient. A rectal or skin probe connected to the unit monitors the patient's temperature.	On automatic mode, the unit operates only if the patient's temperature probe is connected to the unit. Lights on the display panel indicate whether the unit is heating or cooling at any given time.
2. Obtain patient's temperature from the readout on the display unit.	Indicates patient's temperature.	
3. Take patient's temperature and compare with readout on the display unit.	Ensures the warming or cooling device's temperature probe is functioning and correlating with the patient's temperature obtained by another method.	
4. Warm or cool the blanket before applying to the patient.		
5. Place the circulating fluid blanket over the sheet or bath blanket on the patient. Check that the hoses are free from kinks.	Maintains cooling or warming.	
6. Turn warming or cooling off when desired temperature is reached. Continue to monitor patient's temperature by turning off automatic mode and pressing on monitor only switch.	Detects temperature afterdrop or temperature overshoot.	

To Use Warm Air Device

Steps	Rationale	Special Considerations
1. Connect air blanket to the hose attached to the unit. Turn the unit on and select temperature.	The blanket inflates as the air blows from the hose into it.	
2. Remove patient's gown and blankets or sheet. Apply circulating air blanket.	Device warms the patient by directing warm airstreams onto the patient's skin.	
3. Place a bath blanket or sheet over the circulating air blanket.	Prevents heat loss.	
4. Wash hands.	Reduces transmission of microorganisms; standard precautions.	

- External warming or cooling device applied
- Desirable core body temperature achieved

- Unable to achieve desired core body temperature
- Hemodynamic instability
- Cardiac dysrhythmias
- Acid-base imbalance
- Shivering
- Skin injury

Patient Monitoring and Care

Patient Monitoring and Care	Rationale	Reportable Conditions
		These conditions should be reported if they persist despite nursing interventions.
1. Perform a physical assessment of all systems every 1 to 2 hours.	Alterations in temperature affect every system. The condition causing the change in temperature may worsen or be refractory to treatment.	• Significant changes in assessment
2. Continuously monitor core temperature; set high and low temperature limits as determined by patient's condition. If a rectal probe is contraindicated and a skin probe is applied to the axilla area, take an oral or ear temperature.[5]	Prevents rapid rewarming and cooling. Detects patient's response to intervention. Convective warming devices can increase a patient's temperature 2°C to 3°C per hour. The axilla temperature does not correlate with core temperatures as measured in the pulmonary artery.[5]	• Continued hypothermia or hyperthermia
3. Measure blood pressure every 15 minutes for the first hour and as frequently as indicated by the patient's condition.	Vasodilatation occurs with rewarming and vasoconstriction may occur with cooling.	• Hypotension or hypertension
4. Palpate mandible for "humming" vibration and observe for involuntary skeletal muscle movement that may be first detected as ECG artifact.	Early detection and prompt treatment of shivering.	• Shivering, decreased mixed venous oxygenation saturation, and continued shivering despite prescribed medications
5. Examine skin condition hourly.	Detects skin injury.	• Skin injury such as frostbite or burns
6. Continuous cardiac monitoring.	Detects cardiac dysrhythmias associated with warming or cooling.	• Cardiac dysrhythmias
7. Obtain arterial blood gas as prescribed and as indicated.	Detects hypoxemia and acid-base imbalances.	• Abnormal arterial blood gas results
8. Ensure patient comfort.	Minimizes discomfort.	• Unrelieved discomfort

Documentation

Documentation should include the following:

- Patient and family education
- Patient's temperature and site of temperature assessment
- Vital signs and hemodynamic status
- Physical assessment findings
- Cardiac rhythm
- Type of warming or cooling device used
- Time external warming or cooling initiated and terminated
- Patient's symptoms and degree of comfort
- Unexpected outcomes
- Additional interventions

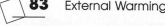

References

1. Henker R, Shaver J. Understanding the febrile state according to an individual adaptation framework. *AACN Clin Iss Crit Care Nurs.* 1994;2:186–193.
2. Holtzclaw B. Monitoring body temperature. *AACN Clin Iss Crit Care Nurs.* 1993;1:44–55.
3. Holtzclaw B. Temperature problems in the postoperative period. *Crit Care Nurs Clin North Am.* 1990;4:589–597.
4. Miranda A, Donovan L, Schuster L, Gerber D. Malignant hyperthermia. *Am J Crit Care.* 1997;5:368–374.
5. Schmitz T, Bair N, Falk M, Levine C. A comparison of five methods of temperature measurement in febrile intensive care patients. *Am J Crit Care.* 1995;4:286–292.

Additional Readings

Cammarano W, Pittet J. Pain management in the intensive care unit. In: *Critical Care Secrets.* 2nd ed. Philadelphia, Pa: Hanley & Belfus; 1998.

Cox A. Ventricular dysrhythmia secondary to select environmental hazards. *AACN Clin Iss Crit Care Nurs.* 1992;1:233–242.

Elixson E. Hypothermia: Cold water drowning. *Crit Care Nurs Clin North Am.* 1991;2:287–292.

Fritsch D. Hypothermia in the trauma patient. *AACN Clin Iss Crit Care Nurs.* 1995;2:196–211.

Ginsberg M, Busto R. Combating hyperthermia in acute stroke: a significant clinical concern. *Stroke.* 1998;2:529–534.

Haskell R, Boruta B, Rotondo M. Hypothermia. *AACN Clin Iss Crit Care Nurs.* 1997;3:368–382.

Janke E, Pilkingtone S, Smith D. Evaluation of two warming systems after cardiopulmonary bypass. *Br J Anaesthesia.* 1996;77:268–270.

Marx J. Hypothermia. In: *Critical Care Secrets.* 2nd ed. Philadelphia, Pa: Hanley & Belfus; 1998.

Osguthorpe S. Hypothermia and rewarming after cardiac surgery. *AACN Clin Iss Crit Care Nurs.* 1993;2:276–292.

Rescorl D. Environmental emergencies. *Crit Care Nurs Clin North Am.* 1995;3:445–456.

Sanford M. Rewarming cardiac surgical patients: warm water vs. warm air. *Am J Crit Care.* 1997;1:39–45.

Schafer Wlody G. Malignant hyperthermia. *Crit Care Nurs Clin North Am.* 1991;1:129–134.

Stevens T. Managing postoperative hypothermia, rewarming, and its complications. *Crit Care Nurs Q.* 1993;1:60–77.

Villamaria F, Baisden C, Hillis A, Rajab H, Rinaldi P. Forced-air warming is no more effective than conventional methods for raising postoperative core temperature after cardiac surgery. *J Cardiothoracic Vasc Anesth.* 1997;6:708–711.

Whitman G. Hypertension and hypothermia in the acute postoperative period. *Crit Care Nurs Clin North Am.* 1991;4:661–673.

84

Iced Caloric Testing for Vestibular Function (Assist)

P U R P O S E: Caloric testing for vestibular function (oculovestibular reflex) is a diagnostic procedure that tests vestibular function in the awake patient and the functional connectivity between the medulla and the midbrain in the comatose patient.[1] Caloric testing can be used as part of brain death evaluation.

Phyllis Dubendorf

PREREQUISITE NURSING KNOWLEDGE

- Neuroanatomy and physiology should be understood.
- The oculovestibular reflex is elicited by introducing iced water or normal saline into the external auditory canal.[2] The vestibular portion of the eighth cranial nerve (acoustic) is stimulated and transmits this impulse via the medial longitudinal fasciculus to two of the cranial nerve nuclei involving extraocular eye movements (cranial

nerves III and VI). Stimulation of this reflex results in deviation of the eyes (Fig. 84–1).
- A *normal response* in the *awake* patient is nystagmus, a slow component toward the irrigated ear, then a faster component *away* from the irrigated ear. If warm water is used for testing, there is a slow component of nystagmus initially *away* from the irrigated side, then a faster component *toward* the irrigated ear, hence the mnemonic COWS—Cold: Opposite; Warm: Same.[1–3]

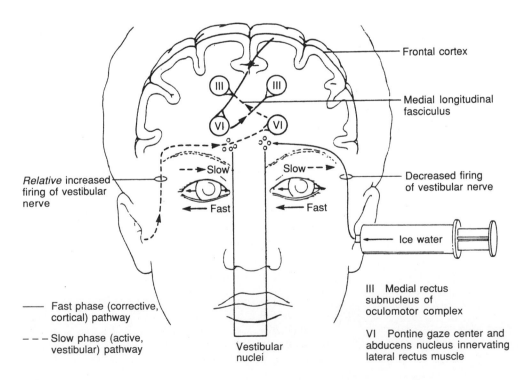

Fast phase (corrective, cortical) pathway

- - - Slow phase (active, vestibular) pathway

Frontal cortex

Medial longitudinal fasciculus

Decreased firing of vestibular nerve

Relative increased firing of vestibular nerve

Slow — Slow

Fast — Fast

Ice water

Vestibular nuclei

III   Medial rectus subnucleus of oculomotor complex

VI   Pontine gaze center and abducens nucleus innervating lateral rectus muscle

■ ● **FIGURE 84–1.** Physiology of the oculovestibular reflex. Cold-water irrigation of a patient will elicit this reflex if both the cerebral hemisphere and the brain stem are intact. The signal passes through the pathways from the medulla to the midbrain, resulting in a slow movement of the eyes toward the irrigated ear. Then, as the impulse travels to the intact ipsilateral hemisphere, a rapid corrective movement of the eyes (nystagmus away from the irrigated ear) can be observed. (From *Patient Care Magazine,* Medical Economics Publishing; 1981:29.)

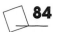

Patient response with intact brainstem

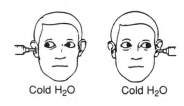

Cold H$_2$O   Cold H$_2$O

Abnormal or absent patient response

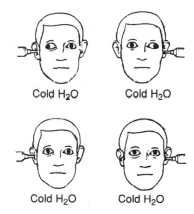

Cold H$_2$O   Cold H$_2$O

Cold H$_2$O   Cold H$_2$O

■ ● **FIGURE 84–2.** Cold-water caloric responses in the comatose patient. If the patient's brain stem is intact, the normal response to cold-water irrigation is slow movement *toward* the irrigated ear. When the brain stem is not intact, an abnormal (dysconjugated) or absent response may be observed. (From Plum F, Posner J. *The Diagnosis of Stupor and Coma.* 3rd ed. Philadelphia: F.A. Davis; 1980.)

- A *normal response* in the *comatose* patient usually results in stimulation of the slow component only and results in reflex conjugate eye movement *toward* the cold-water irrigated ear[3] (Fig. 84–2).
- An abnormal (dysconjugate) or absent response to cold water testing in the unconscious patient *may* indicate brain stem dysfunction and a poor prognosis; however, this test alone is not definitive.
- This test is *contraindicated* in patients with a perforated tympanic membrane.
- Agents or conditions that can potentially interfere with the oculovestibular reflex include the following:
  ❖ Ototoxic medications
  ❖ Neurosuppressant medications, such as barbiturates, phenytoin, sedatives, and tricyclic antidepressants
  ❖ Aminoglycosides
  ❖ Neuromuscular blockade
  ❖ Anticholinergics
  ❖ Preexisting vestibular disease, active labyrinth disease (Meniere's disease)
  ❖ Preexisting cranial nerve disorders involving cranial nerves III and VI (oculomotor and abducens)
  ❖ Facial trauma involving the auditory canal and petrous bone
- This test should be performed bilaterally, if possible, with at least 5 minutes between irrigations.
- This test may produce decorticate or decerebrate postur-

ing in the *unconscious* patient because of the noxious nature of the stimulus. It is extremely uncomfortable and may produce nausea and vomiting in the *awake* patient.
- Additional clinical data, such as lack of spontaneous respirations, doll's eyes (oculocephalic reflex), no response to painful stimulation, nonreactive pupils, absent corneal reflexes, and abnormal diagnostic studies, are required to support the diagnosis of brain death (see Procedure 130).

EQUIPMENT

- 50- to 60-mL irrigating syringe
- Small basin
- Iced water or normal saline
- Towels and protective bedding
- Disposable nonsterile gloves

PATIENT AND FAMILY EDUCATION

- Discuss the purpose of the test with the patient and family. ➥*Rationale:* Prepares the patient and family for what to expect.
- Discuss unpleasant sensations that may be experienced by the awake patient, if applicable. ➥*Rationale:* The awake patient may experience nausea, dizziness, pain, or vomiting.

PATIENT ASSESSMENT AND PREPARATION

Patient Assessment

- Obtain vital signs. ➥*Rationale:* Establishes baseline values for the patient.
- Perform a neurologic assessment including the following: eye opening, verbal, and motor responses, cranial nerve function, and respiratory pattern. ➥*Rationale:* Establishes baseline neurologic function to support the presence or absence of voluntary or reflexive activity.
- Review medications. ➥*Rationale:* Some medications may interfere with the oculovestibular response.
- Assess medical history of cranial nerve dysfunction. ➥*Rationale:* The occurrence of preexisting vestibular disease may produce unreliable results related to oculovestibular testing.
- Assess current medical history. ➥*Rationale:* Identifies medical conditions that may be affecting the patient's responsiveness.
- Ensure that tympanic membranes are intact and that external auditory canals are not blocked with cerumen. ➥*Rationale:* Iced caloric testing is contraindicated in patients with a perforated eardrum. The presence of cerumen may impede or prevent the flow of irrigant to the semicircular apparatus.

Patient Preparation

- Ensure that the patient understands preprocedural teaching. Answer questions as they arise and reinforce information as needed. ➥*Rationale:* Evaluates and reinforces understanding of previously taught information.
- Assist the patient in positioning his or her head in a

neutral position with the head of bed at 30 degrees. ➥*Rationale:* Places the lateral semicircular canals in a vertical position, which allows maximal stimula-

tion and optimizes venous jugular drainage. This position may be deferred if the patient experiences cardiovascular decompensation that demands alternative positioning.

Procedure for Iced Caloric Testing for Vestibular Function (Assist)

Steps	Rationale	Special Considerations
1. Wash hands, and don gloves.	Reduces transmission of microorganisms; standard precautions.	
2. Place protective pad under the patient.	Absorbs iced irrigant.	
3. Verify that the integrity of the tympanic membrane has been assessed.	This test is contraindicated for patients with a perforated tympanic membrane.	
4. Assist with instillation of 50 mL iced water or normal saline into the external auditory canal. The instillation should occur from over 30 seconds to 3 minutes, to allow adequate time for stimulation.	Stimulates oculovestibular reflex.	The physician may elect to use up to 100 mL iced water or normal saline. More than one examiner is needed to simultaneously inject irrigant and ensure that the patient's eyes are open to assess extraocular movements.
5. Observe the patient's eyes for a response for up to 1 minute.	Determines response to instillation.	
6. Assist with irrigation of iced water or normal saline into the opposite external auditory canal.	Both sides must be assessed for responses.	A 5-minute interval between irrigations is recommended.
7. Assess patient's tolerance to procedure.	The noxious stimuli may cause posturing in the comatose patient and dizziness, nausea, pain, and vomiting in the awake patient.	
8. Discard supplies in appropriate receptacles, and wash hands.	Reduces transmission of microorganisms; standard precautions.	

Expected Outcomes
- Successful assessment of brain stem function in the comatose patient
- Successful assessment of vestibular function in the awake patient

Unexpected Outcomes
- Test cannot be completed.
- Ocular movement is dysconjugated.

Patient Monitoring and Care

Patient Monitoring and Care	Rationale	Reportable Conditions
		These conditions should be reported if they persist despite nursing interventions.
1. Monitor vital signs and cardiac rhythm before and after the procedure.	Patients with severe neurologic dysfunction may exhibit changes in cardiovascular and respiratory function because of involvement of brain stem structures.	• Hypotension or hypertension • Bradycardia or tachycardia • Ventricular or atrial dysrhythmias • Changes in breathing patterns
2. Monitor neurologic status before and after the procedure.	Determines neurologic responses.	• Deterioration in neurologic responses

Documentation

Documentation should include the following:

- Patient and family education
- Date and time of testing
- Patient's baseline neurologic status and responses
- Presence of intact tympanic membrane
- Temperature and amount of irrigant
- Time between stimulus and response
- Description of extraocular movement
- Untoward responses
- Neurologic status preprocedure and postprocedure
- Additional interventions

References

1. Barker E. *Neuroscience Nursing.* St Louis, Mo: C.V. Mosby; 1994.
2. Greenberg MS. *Handbook of Neurosurgery.* Lakeland, Fla: Greenberg Graphics; 1997.
3. Samuels M. The evaluation of comatose patients. *Hosp Pract.* 1993;28:165–182.

Additional Readings

Hickey J. *The Clinical Practice of Neurological and Neurosurgical Nursing.* 2nd ed. Philadelphia, Pa: J.B. Lippincott; 1986.
Plum F, Posner J. *The Diagnosis of Stupor and Coma.* 3rd ed. Philadelphia, Pa: F.A. Davis; 1983.

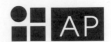

85 Lumbar Puncture (Perform)

PURPOSE: Lumbar puncture (LP) is performed to obtain a cerebrospinal fluid (CSF) sample or to access the subarachnoid space for infusion of medications or contrast agents.[1-5]

Anne W. Wojner
Marc Malkoff

PREREQUISITE NURSING KNOWLEDGE

- Computed tomography (CT) and magnetic resonance imaging supersede the routine use of LP for many diagnoses.[1, 2]
- The anatomy and physiology of the vertebral column, spinal meninges, and CSF circulation, including the location of the lumbar cistern, should be known.
- Technical and clinical competence in performing LPs is necessary.
- Knowledge of sterile technique is essential.
- The presence of meningeal irritation caused by either infectious meningitis or subarachnoid hemorrhage may promote discomfort when the patient is placed in the flexed, lateral decubitus position for LP.
- Indications for LP include the following:[1-4]
  - ❖ Suspected central nervous system infection
  - ❖ Clinical examination suggestive of subarachnoid hemorrhage accompanied by negative CT scan findings
  - ❖ Suspected Guillain-Barré syndrome
  - ❖ Suspected multiple sclerosis
  - ❖ Intrathecal administration of medications
  - ❖ Imaging procedures requiring infusion of contrast agents
  - ❖ Measurement of CSF pressure
  - ❖ CSF drainage
- Contraindications for LP include the following:[1-4]
  - ❖ Increased intracranial pressure with mass effect
  - ❖ Superficial skin infection localized to the site of entry
  - ❖ Bleeding diathesis (relative contraindication)
  - ❖ Platelet count less than 50,000/mm³
- Normal CSF values include the following:[1-4]
  - ❖ Opening pressure 50 to 200 mm H_2O (elevated pressure, >250 mm H_2O)
  - ❖ White blood cells <5/mm³

- ❖ Glucose, 60% to 70% of serum blood glucose
- ❖ Protein, 15 to 45 mg/dL
- ❖ Clear, colorless appearance
- ❖ Negative culture
- Recommended CSF tests include the following:[1, 2]
  - ❖ Tube #1, Biochemistry
    Glucose
    Protein
    Protein electrophoresis (if clinically indicated)
  - ❖ Tube #2, Bacteriology
    Gram stain
    Culture
        Bacterial culture
        Fungal culture (if clinically indicated); requires larger volume
        Tuberculosis culture (if clinically indicated); requires larger volume
  - ❖ Tube #3, Hematology
    Cell count
    Differential
  - ❖ Tube #4, Optional Studies as Indicated
    Venereal Disease Research Laboratory (VDRL) test
    Oligoclonal bands
    Myelin protein
    Cytology

EQUIPMENT

- Sterile gloves, caps, masks with eye shield, and gowns
- Sterile drapes
- Sterile gauze pads
- Povidone-iodine pads or swabsticks
- Alcohol pads or swabsticks
- Fenestrated drape
- Manometer with three-way stopcock
- Lidocaine, 1% to 2% (without epinephrine)
- 3- to 5-mL syringe
- 20-, 22-, and 25-G needles
- 20- or 22-G spinal needles
- Four numbered, capped test tubes

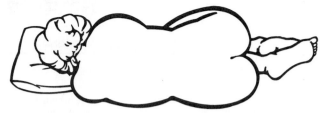

■ ● **FIGURE 85–1.** The lateral decubitus (fetal) position appropriate for lumbar puncture. The patient's knees are drawn up tightly to the chest, and the patient flexes the chin down to the chest. This increases the intraspinous space to facilitate needle insertion.

- Adhesive strip or sterile dressing supplies
- Specimen labels
- Laboratory forms

Additional equipment to have available as needed includes the following:

- Rolled towels or small pillows to support the patient during positioning

PATIENT AND FAMILY EDUCATION

- Explain the purpose of the diagnostic test and the procedure for testing. ➛*Rationale:* Decreases patient and family anxiety.
- Explain the need for the patient to remain still and quiet in a lateral decubitus position with head and neck flexed and knees bent up toward the chest (Fig. 85–1). ➛*Rationale:* Elicits patient cooperation during the examination; the intervertebral space widens in this position, facilitating entry of the spinal needle into the subarachnoid space.[1, 2, 4]
- Explain that the procedure may produce some discomfort and that a local anesthetic agent will be injected to minimize pain. ➛*Rationale:* Prepares the patient and family for what to expect.
- Explain that the patient will need to lie flat for 1 to 4 hours after the LP. ➛*Rationale:* Minimizes postprocedural headache.[1, 2]

PATIENT ASSESSMENT AND PREPARATION

Patient Assessment

- Note pertinent patient history. ➛*Rationale:* LP is performed to assist with the diagnosis and management of a number of neurologic disease processes (see list of indications for LP).
- Obtain a baseline neurologic assessment, including assessment for increased intracranial pressure, before per-

forming LP. ➛*Rationale:* Increased intracranial pressure during LP may place the patient at risk for a downward shift in intracranial contents when the pressure is suddenly released in the lumbar subarachnoid space.[1–5]
- Assess for coagulopathies, local skin infections in close proximity to the site, or pertinent medication or contrast material allergies. ➛*Rationale:* Identifies potential risks for bleeding, infection, and allergic reactions.
- Assess patient's ability to cooperate with procedure. ➛*Rationale:* Sudden, uncontrolled movement may result in needle displacement with associated injury or need for reinsertion.
- Identify through history and clinical examination vertebral column deformities or tissue scarring that may interfere with the ability to successfully carry out the procedure. ➛*Rationale:* Scoliosis, lumbar surgery with fusion, and repeated LP procedures may interfere with successful cannulation of the subarachnoid space.[1]
- Assess for signs and symptoms of meningeal irritation, which include the following:
  ❖ Nuchal rigidity
  ❖ Photophobia
  ❖ Brudzinski or Kernig sign
  ❖ Fever
  ❖ Headache
  ❖ Nausea or vomiting
  ❖ Nystagmus

➛*Rationale:* Establishes a baseline of neurologic function before the introduction of the needle into the subarachnoid space.

Patient Preparation

- Ensure that the patient and family understand preprocedural teaching. Answer questions as they arise and reinforce information as needed. ➛*Rationale:* Evaluates and reinforces understanding of previously taught information.
- Obtain informed consent. ➛*Rationale:* Protects rights of patient and makes competent decision possible for the patient; however, under emergency circumstances, time may not allow form to be signed.
- Position patient in the lateral decubitus position near the side of the bed, with head and neck flexed and knees bent up toward the head. ➛*Rationale:* The intervertebral space widens in this position and facilitates entry of the spinal needle into the subarachnoid space.

■■ AP This procedure should be performed only by physicians, advanced practice nurses, and other health care professionals (including critical care nurses) with additional knowledge, skills, and demonstrated competence per professional licensure or institutional standard.

Procedure	for Lumbar Puncture (Perform)

Steps	Rationale	Special Considerations
1. Wash hands.	Reduces transmission of microorganisms; standard precautions.	
2. With patient in position for examination, identify the intervertebral spaces of L3–L4, L4–L5, and L5–S1; the L3–L4 intervertebral space is level with the iliac crests (Fig. 85–2).	LP is performed below the level of the conus medullaris, which ends at L1–L2. The most common site used for LP is the L4–L5 interspace, but the L3–L4 or the L5–S1 interspace may be used when cannulation of the L4–L5 interspace is not possible.[1, 2]	An imaginary line is drawn by the practitioner between the two iliac crests.
3. Wash hands, and don personal protective equipment.	Reduces transmission of microorganisms; standard precautions.	
4. Set up sterile field on bedside stand. A. Preassemble the manometer, attaching the three-way stopcock; set to the side.	Prepares equipment for use in procedure.	
B. Open test tubes and place in order of use in tray slots.		Have assistant prepare numbered labels for test tubes; ensure that the tubes are labeled in the order in which they are filled to facilitate laboratory differentiation of traumatic tap versus subarachnoid hemorrhage.
C. Draw up approximately 3 mL 1% lidocaine using a 20-G needle. Change to a 25-G needle for superficial injection; change to a 22-G, 1.5-inch needle for deeper injection.[2]		
5. Cleanse the skin over the L4–L5 puncture site, including one intervertebral space above and below the site. Start with alcohol pads or swabsticks; follow with povidone-iodine pads or swabsticks. Use a circular motion, starting from the center and working toward the outside. Allow to air dry; cover with a fenestrated drape.	Prepares site for LP; reduces incidence of infection.	Eliminate povidone-iodine cleansing in cases of reported allergic reaction or sensitivity.

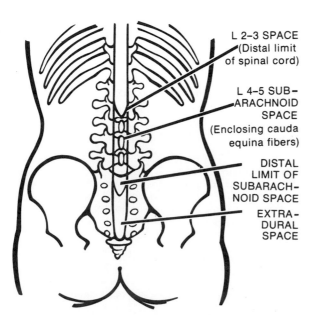

L 2–3 SPACE
(Distal limit of spinal cord)

L 4–5 SUB-ARACHNOID SPACE
(Enclosing cauda equina fibers)

DISTAL LIMIT OF SUBARACH-NOID SPACE

EXTRA-DURAL SPACE

■ ● **FIGURE 85–2.** The body of the spinal cord ends at L2–3. The region below, L4–5, encloses the cauda equina (a bundle of lumbar and sacral nerve roots) within the subarachnoid space. It is this area that is appropriate for lumbar puncture.

Procedure	**for Lumbar Puncture (Perform)** *Continued*

Steps	Rationale	Special Considerations
6. Administer local anesthetic using a 25-G needle, raising a wheal in the skin. Inject a small amount into the posterior spinous region using a 22-G needle.[2]	Reduces discomfort associated with needle insertion.	
7. Insert a 22- or 20-G spinal needle through the skin into the intervertebral space of L4–L5, with the needle at an angle of 15 degrees cephalad, aiming toward the umbilicus and level with the sagittal midplane of the body.	Facilitates passage of the needle between intervertebral spaces toward dura mater.	If bone is encountered on needle insertion, pull back slightly, correct the angle to between 15 and 40 degrees cephalad, and reinsert. Use the interspace above (L3–L4) or below (L5–S1) the original L4–L5 insertion site, should difficulty with advancement of the needle be encountered despite correction of insertion angle.[1,2] Variations in the anatomic configuration of the vertebral column, a history of vertebral column surgery, or repeat LPs may necessitate needle insertion at a different level.
8. Once the needle has been advanced approximately 3 to 4 cm, withdraw the stylus and check the hub for CSF. If CSF is not present, replace the stylus and advance slightly. Once CSF is draining, advance the needle another 1 to 2 mm.	In most adults, a 3- to 4-cm insertion depth is sufficient to enter the subarachnoid space.	A "popping" sensation is often associated with penetration of the dura mater.
9. Attach the stopcock of the manometer to the needle. Have the patient straighten his or her legs and relax his or her position. Measure the opening pressure, and note the color of the fluid in the manometer.	Flexing the legs or straining to maintain position may artificially elevate the CSF pressure.	
10. Consider performing the Queckenstedt test. Ask the critical care nurse to simultaneously compress the jugular veins for 10 seconds; watch for a change in subarachnoid CSF pressure on the manometer.[1,2]	The Queckenstedt test is used to assess for an obstruction of CSF flow in the spinal subarachnoid space; the practitioner must ensure proper placement of the spinal needle for test findings to be accurate. Test findings are often unreliable.[2]	Normal findings reflect a sharp increase in spinal subarachnoid CSF pressure on compression of the jugular veins; on release, pressure returns to precompression levels. A lack of change in CSF pressure indicates an obstruction of CSF flow. The Queckenstedt test is contraindicated in patients with increased intracranial pressure. *Procedure continued on following page*

AP This procedure should be performed only by physicians, advanced practice nurses, and other health care professionals (including critical care nurses) with additional knowledge, skills, and demonstrated competence per professional licensure or institutional standard.

Procedure	**for Lumbar Puncture (Perform)** *Continued*

Steps	Rationale	Special Considerations

11. Obtain laboratory samples:
  A. Position the first test tube over the third stopcock port.
  B. Turn the stopcock, and drain CSF from the manometer into the first test tube.
  C. Return the stopcock to the off position, and discard manometer.
  D. Continue filling test tubes from the hub of the spinal needle; a minimum of 1 to 2 mL CSF should be collected in the first three test tubes. The second and fourth test tubes may require up to 8 mL CSF depending on the tests ordered (eg, fungal or tuberculosis testing).[1, 2]
	By draining CSF from the manometer into the test tubes, the CSF volume withdrawn is minimized.[1] Allows for progressive clearing of CSF blood in the case of a traumatic tap.[1, 4, 5]	In subarachnoid hemorrhage, CSF with the same consistency of blood is drained in all 4 test tubes. In the case of a traumatic tap, progressive clearing of bloody CSF occurs as drainage continues.

12. Cover the opening of the needle with a sterile, gloved finger. Replace the stylus, and withdraw the needle.[1, 2]	Prevents unnecessary CSF loss and facilitates needle withdrawal without traction on the spinal nerve roots. Reduces contamination by microorganisms.	Minimizes postprocedural headache.
13. Cover the puncture site with an adhesive strip or sterile dressing.		
14. Place patient in a supine position immediately after the procedure.[1, 3, 4] Consider using a prone position immediately after the procedure.	Patient's weight acts as site pressure; facilitates dural closure. Some practitioners advocate placing the patient in a prone position for 1 to 4 hours after the LP to facilitate dural closure.[2, 5]	It remains unclear whether prone or supine positioning better expedites closure of the dura mater after the LP.

Expected Outcomes	Unexpected Outcomes
• Determination of characteristics of CSF that support establishment of diagnosis • Recommendation for definitive treatment that promotes restoration of health or optimal functional status • Postprocedure headache may occur in 10% to 25% of patients undergoing LP and is usually self-limiting;[1] the incidence of headache is reduced with the use of smaller-gauge spinal needles and prone positioning for 1 to 4 hours postprocedure.[1, 2] • No change in neurologic status postprocedure	• In cases of supratentorial mass or severely elevated intracranial pressure, a shift in intracranial contents (brain herniation) may be promoted by the sudden decrease in pressure incurred with LP.[1-5] • Injury of the periosteum or spinal ligaments may produce local back pain.[1, 2] • Infectious meningitis may result from improper technique that produces contamination.[1-5] • Traumatic taps may result from inadvertently puncturing the spinal venous plexuses; usually this is a self-limiting process, but it may result in hematoma in patients with bleeding disorders.[1, 2] • Transient lower extremity pain may occur from irritation of a spinal nerve.[1-5] • Persistent CSF leak from the puncture site is associated with nonclosure of the dura. • Inability to obtain CSF specimen because of practitioner skill level, patient intolerance of the procedure, pathologic blockage of CSF flow, or aberrant anatomy.

Patient Monitoring and Care

Patient Monitoring and Care	Rationale	Reportable Conditions
		These conditions should be reported if they persist despite nursing interventions.
1. Monitor the patient's neurologic status, the patient's procedural tolerance, and the development of new onset pain or numbness in the lower extremities throughout the procedure.	Changes in neurologic status may be related to sudden intracranial decompression with brain herniation or local irritation of a spinal nerve by the needle.	• Deterioration in neurologic status related to brain herniation • Transient lower extremity motor or sensory changes associated with spinal nerve irritation
2. Monitor for postprocedural headache, drainage from puncture site, and changes in neurologic status from baseline for 24 hours after completion of LP.	Headache occurs in 10% to 25% of patients after LP. Persistent drainage may indicate an unresolved CSF leak. Lower extremity motor or sensory changes may indicate hematoma at puncture site.	• Intractable postprocedural headache • Dural tear requiring patch or closure • Spinal hematoma requiring emergent surgical evacuation
3. Monitor effectiveness of supine positioning in preventing or treating postprocedural headache. Consider administration of mild analgesic agent and increasing intravenous fluid rate for first 4 hours postprocedure, depending on headache severity, existing preload indices, and ability to tolerate increased intravascular volume.	Additional treatment measures may be necessary to manage postprocedural headache.	• Intractable postprocedural headache • Dural tear requiring patch or closure • Intravascular fluid volume overload associated with increased intravenous volume delivery

Documentation

Documentation should include the following:

- Patient and family education
- Performance of the procedure, significant findings, CSF appearance, and opening pressure
- Patient tolerance of the procedure
- Change in neurologic status associated with the procedure
- CSF specimens obtained
- Unexpected outcomes
- Additional interventions

References

1. O'Brien J. Lumbar puncture. In: Pfenninger JL, Fowler GC. *Procedure for Primary Care Physicians*. St Louis; Mo: C.V. Mosby; 1994:1109–1114.
2. Bleck TP. Clinical use of neurologic diagnostic tests. In: Weiner WJ, Goetz CG, eds. *Neurology for the Non-Neurologist*. 4th ed. Philadelphia, Pa: Williams & Wilkins; 1999: 27–37.
3. Davis AE. Neurological patient assessment. In: Kinney MR, Dunbar SB, Brooks-Brunn JA, Molter N, Vitello-Cicciu JM, eds. *AACN's Clinical Reference for Critical Care Nursing*. 4th ed. St Louis, Mo: C.V. Mosby; 1998:663–683.
4. Hickey JV. *The Clinical Practice of Neurological and Neurosurgical Nursing*. 4th ed. Philadelphia, Pa: J.B. Lippincott; 1997.
5. Barker E. *Neuroscience Nursing*. St Louis, Mo: C.V. Mosby; 1994.

Additional Readings

Abolnik IZ, Perfect JR, Durack DT. Acute bacterial meningitis. In: Wilkins RH, Rengachary SS, eds. *Neurosurgery*. New York, NY: McGraw-Hill; 1996:3299–3306.
Miller DW, Hahn JF. General methods of clinical examination. In: Youmans JR, ed. *Neurological Surgery*. Vol 1. Philadelphia; Pa: W.B. Saunders; 1996:3–43.
Nikas DL. The neurologic system. In: Alspach JAG, ed. *Core Curriculum for Critical Care Nursing*. 5th ed. Philadelphia, Pa: W.B. Saunders; 1998:339–463.
Scheld WM, Whittley RJ, Durach DT. *Infections of the Central Nervous System*. 2nd ed. New York, NY: Raven Press; 1997.

AP This procedure should be performed only by physicians, advanced practice nurses, and other health care professionals (including critical care nurses) with additional knowledge, skills, and demonstrated competence per professional licensure or institutional standard.

Lumbar and Cisternal Punctures (Assist)

PURPOSE: Lumbar and cisternal punctures are procedures that access cerebrospinal fluid to support a diagnosis of subarachnoid hemorrhage or central nervous system (CNS) tumor, infection, or autoimmune disorder. Punctures may also be performed to infuse medications or contrast agents into the subarachnoid space.

Phyllis Dubendorf

PREREQUISITE NURSING KNOWLEDGE

- Neuroanatomy and physiology should be understood.
- Lumbar puncture (L3–L4, L4–L5) is the usual procedure employed to obtain a sample of cerebrospinal fluid.
- Cisternal puncture (C1–C2) is performed if lumbar puncture is not possible or appropriate for the patient because of positioning or anatomic restrictions.
- Indications for lumbar or cisternal puncture are as follows:
  ❖ Cerebrospinal fluid analysis may be indicated in the differential diagnosis of subarachnoid hemorrhage, CNS infection, CNS autoimmune processes, and some CNS tumors.
  ❖ Lumbar punctures may also be used as therapy to treat cerebrospinal fluid fistulas and pseudotumor cerebri or to deliver medications or contrast material into the subarachnoid space.
- Contraindications for lumbar or cisternal puncture are as follows:
  ❖ Lumbar or cisternal punctures are contraindicated if the patient has a known or suspected intracranial mass or elevated intracranial pressure (ICP), has noncommunicating hydrocephalus, has infection in the region that would be used for puncture, or is coagulopathic.[1]
  ❖ Lumbar and cisternal punctures are *cautioned against* in patients suspected of having aneurysmal subarachnoid hemorrhage and in those with complete spinal blocks.
- The preferred positioning for lumbar puncture is side lying with the neck flexed (see Fig. 85–1).
- The preferred positioning for cisternal puncture is side lying with the neck flexed. Proper positioning widens the interspinous process space and facilitates the passage of the needle (Fig. 86–1).

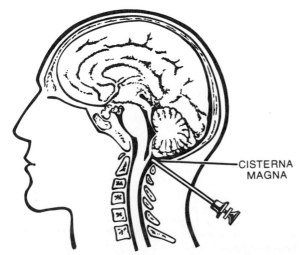

■ ● FIGURE 86–1. The cisterna magna, located at the base of the skull between the second cervical vertebra and under the posterior rim of the foramen magnum.

CISTERNA MAGNA

EQUIPMENT

- Sterile gloves, caps, masks with eye shield, and gowns
- Sterile drapes
- Sterile gauze pads
- Povidone-iodine pads or swabsticks
- Alcohol pads or swabsticks
- Fenestrated drape
- Manometer with three-way stopcock
- Lidocaine, 1% to 2% (without epinephrine)
- 3- to 5-mL syringe
- 20-, 22-, and 25-G needles
- 20- or 22-G spinal needles
- Four numbered, capped test tubes
- Adhesive strip or sterile dressing supplies
- Specimen labels
- Laboratory forms

Additional equipment to have available as needed includes the following:

- Disposable razor (for cisternal puncture)
- Two overbed tables (one for sterile field; one to position patient, if necessary)
- Rolled towels or small pillows to support patient during positioning
- Emergency medications and resuscitative equipment (for cisternal puncture)

PATIENT AND FAMILY EDUCATION

- Assess patient and family understanding of and need for procedure. ➤*Rationale:* Reinforces understanding of procedure and decreases anxiety.
- Explain positioning requirements for lumbar or cisternal puncture. ➤*Rationale:* Compliance with positioning requirements will facilitate procedure.
- Explain that procedure may cause some mild discomfort; the patient will receive local anesthesia and may also receive some mild sedation, if appropriate. ➤*Rationale:* Relieves anxiety about experiencing pain and allows the patient to verbalize concerns.
- Explain positioning requirements for after the procedure. ➤*Rationale:* Compliance with positioning may improve patient comfort.

PATIENT ASSESSMENT AND PREPARATION

Patient Assessment

- Obtain vital signs. ➤*Rationale:* Establishes baseline values for the patient, which are especially important with cisternal puncture.
- Perform a neurologic assessment, including mental status and motor and sensory function. ➤*Rationale:* Establishes baseline neurologic function before the insertion of the needle in proximity to sensitive neurologic tissue.
- Assess current laboratory profile, including complete blood cell count, platelets, prothrombin time, partial thromboplastin time, bleeding time, and international normalized ratio. ➤*Rationale:* To establish baseline values and to identify any coagulopathies that require intervention before puncture.
- Assess for signs and symptoms of meningeal irritation, which include the following:
  - ❖ Nuchal rigidity
  - ❖ Photophobia
  - ❖ Brudzinski or Kernig sign
  - ❖ Fever
  - ❖ Headache
  - ❖ Nausea or vomiting
  - ❖ Nystagmus

➤*Rationale:* To establish a baseline of neurologic function before introduction of the needle into the subarachnoid space.

Patient Preparation

- Ensure that the patient and family understand preprocedural teaching. Answer questions as they arise and reinforce information as needed. ➤*Rationale:* Evaluates and reinforces understanding of previously taught information.
- Ensure that informed consent was obtained. ➤*Rationale:* Protects rights of patient and makes competent decision possible for the patient; however, under emergency circumstances, time may not allow form to be signed.
- Position patient as follows:
  - ❖ For a lumbar puncture, position the patient in a lateral decubitus position with knees tightly drawn to chest and neck flexed, or seat patient on the edge of the bed and support the patient over a bedside table.
  - ❖ For a cisternal puncture, position the patient comfortably in a side-lying position with the head and jaw supported or over a table with the crown of the head and jaw supported.

➤*Rationale:* Facilitates entry of the spinal needle.

Procedure for Lumbar and Cisternal Punctures (Assist)

Steps	Rationale	Special Considerations
1. Wash hands.	Reduces transmission of microorganisms; standard precautions.	
2. Ensure that the patient is in the proper position.	Ensures spinal alignment and allows for access to the area.	The patient should be able to tolerate a side-lying position with his or her head flat. For *lumbar punctures*, to help the patient maintain this position, the nurse should place one arm behind the patient's head and the other arm around the knees. For *cisternal punctures*, to maintain this position, support the crown of the head and the jaw.
3. Wash hands, and don cap, mask, gown, and gloves.	Reduces transmission of microorganisms; standard precautions.	

Procedure continued on following page

Procedure for **Lumbar and Cisternal Punctures (Assist)** *Continued*

Steps	Rationale	Special Considerations
4. Prepare the skin with alcohol, followed by povidone-iodine solution.	Reduces microorganisms and helps prevent infection.	For *cisternal puncture* only, the nape of the neck must be shaved.
5. Assist in draping the area with sterile drapes.	Decreases risk of contamination and provides a sterile field for procedure.	Draping may be deferred during cisternal puncture so as not to obscure anatomic landmarks.
6. Assist in identifying the appropriate anatomic site for puncture.	*Lumbar punctures:* below the level of L3 to prevent damage to the spinal cord. (In the adult, the body of the spinal cord ends at L1–L2.)	An imaginary line is drawn vertically between the iliac crests, and a second line is imagined horizontally across the spinous processes. These lines should intersect the L3–L4 area, and the puncture can be performed here or one level below at L4–L5.
	Cisternal punctures: the skull base is used to select for puncture.	The second cervical vertebra is the *first* palpable spinous process. The needle is inserted slightly above this level.
7. Assist with administration of local anesthesia.	Prevents or decreases pain from needle insertion.	Initially, the skin is injected, then a deeper injection of anesthetic is administered to the interspinous ligament.
8. Once the needle is in place, instruct the patient to relax and breathe normally and to avoid holding his or her breath.	Increased muscle tension or intrathoracic pressure may falsely elevate CSF pressure.	Patients undergoing lumbar puncture may also straighten the legs, because severe leg flexion can increase intrathoracic pressure.
9. Using aseptic technique, assist in attaching the manometer to the spinal needle via a three-way stopcock.	Obtain the CSF pressure measurement while maintaining needle and field sterility.	Readings taken at the cisternal area or with the patient in a sitting position are of little value because of altered pressure mechanics. Normal CSF pressure readings taken at the lumbar area normally range from 50 to 200 mm H_2O.
10. Assist in performing the Queckenstedt test by simultaneously compressing the jugular veins for 10 seconds, while observing for a change in subarachnoid CSF pressure on the manometer.	Used if an obstruction in the spinal subarachnoid space is suspected. A normal response indicates that the pathway between the skull and the lumbar needle is patent. This maneuver is *contraindicated* in patients with known or suspected elevated intracranial pressure; a sudden release of CSF pressure distally can result in herniation.	Normally there is a rapid increase in CSF pressure with resultant decrease when compression is released. If there is a complete or partial spinal block, the level will not rise, or will rise slowly, and will remain elevated when the jugular veins are released. No increase in CSF pressure may be caused by improper needle placement.
11. Assist with the collection of CSF specimens.	The manometer system must be stabilized with one hand, while the other turns the stopcock.	Aseptic technique must be used, and care is taken to avoid rapid loss of CSF.
12. Label each tube with type of specimen, patient name, and order in which the specimen was collected.	Differentiates between subarachnoid hemorrhage and traumatic tap by evaluating each numbered specimen.	Red blood cell (RBC) dissipation through consecutive samples is indicative of traumatic tap; consistent RBC presence is indicative of subarachnoid hemorrhage.
13. Apply a dressing to the puncture site once the needle is removed.	Reduces the incidence of infection.	
14. Discard supplies and wash hands.	Reduces the transmission of microorganisms; standard precautions.	
15. Label and send specimens to laboratory.	Provides specimen for laboratory analysis.	

Expected Outcomes

- Lumbar or cisternal puncture is completed.
- CSF sample is obtained.
- Patient's vital signs and level of consciousness remain stable before, during, and after the procedure.
- The patient does not experience headache, neck stiffness, local pain at puncture site, leg spasms, or elevated temperature related to the procedure.

Unexpected Outcomes

- Significant change in vital signs or level of consciousness
- Inability to void spontaneously (if able to before procedure)
- CSF is not obtained or unable to complete procedure
- Prolonged headache, stiff neck, and photophobia and acute increase in temperature related to procedure
- Excessive drainage at puncture site
- New and persistent complaints of pain, numbness, tingling, weakness, or paralysis in the lower extremities
- Cranial neuropathy
- Spinal or paraspinal abscess
- Implantation of epidermal tumors
- Vasovagal syncope
- Seizure

Patient Monitoring and Care

Patient Monitoring and Care	Rationale	Reportable Conditions
		These changes should be reported if they persist despite nursing interventions.
1. Monitor the patient's neurologic, respiratory, and cardiovascular status during the procedure.	Pain or abnormal sensation radiating down one or both legs may result from spinal nerve irritation, and this may necessitate a change in patient or needle position. Respiratory depression or an altered level of consciousness may result from cisternal needle proximity to the medulla.	• Respiratory depression • Motor or sensory changes • Changes in level of consciousness • Change in vital signs
Assess vital signs and perform systematic neurologic assessments every 15 minutes for the first hour, every 30 minutes twice, then every hour for the next 4 hours, and every 4 hours for the following 24 hours following the procedure (or as prescribed).	A change in vital signs or neurologic assessment could indicate acute hematoma formation, injury to a spinal nerve, infection, or herniation.	
2. Monitor needle puncture site.	Identifies complications at the site.	• Persistent bleeding at the site • Drainage of clear, "serous" fluid
3. Monitor the patient for pain or discomfort.	Identifies traumatic complications of needle placement.	• Severe, persistent back or leg pain not evident before the procedure
4. Instruct the patient to remain flat in bed for 1 to 4 hours or for the length of time prescribed. Patient may turn from side to side.	Postprocedure positioning restrictions remain controversial, but a flat position is helpful in relieving headache associated with CSF withdrawal and leakage at the puncture site.	• Persistent headache

Documentation

Documentation should include the following:

- Patient and family education
- Date and time of procedure
- Status of puncture site
- Amount and character of CSF collected
- Patient's baseline assessment and tolerance of procedure
- Any unexpected outcomes
- Additional interventions

Reference

1. Greenberg MS. *Handbook of Neurosurgery*. Lakeland, Fla: Greenberg Graphics; 1997.

Additional Readings

Barker E. *Neuroscience Nursing*. St Louis, Mo: C.V. Mosby; 1994.

Davis AE. Neurological patient assessment. In: Kinney MR, Dunbar SB, Brooks-Brunn JA, Molter N, Vitello-Cicciu JM, eds. *AACN's Clinical Reference for Critical Care Nursing*. 4th ed. St Louis, Mo: C.V. Mosby; 1998:663–683.

Evans RW. Complications of lumbar puncture. *Neurol Clin.* 1998;16:83–105.

Hickey JV. *The Clinical Practice of Neurological and Neurosurgical Nursing*. 4th ed. Philadelphia, Pa: J.B. Lippincott; 1997.

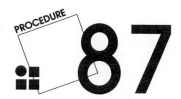

87

Lumbar Subarachnoid Catheter Insertion (Assist) for Cerebral Spinal Fluid Pressure Monitoring and Drainage

---

P U R P O S E: Lumbar subarachnoid catheters may be inserted via a lumbar puncture procedure for use in cerebrospinal fluid (CSF) pressure monitoring and drainage. These catheters may be used for neurologic patients with dural tears, CSF leaks, or pseudotumor cerebri. Lumbar subarachnoid catheters may also be used in the care of intraoperative and postoperative patients having thoracic and thoracoabdominal aortic aneurysm (TAAA) repair.

Jacqueline Sullivan

PREREQUISITE NURSING KNOWLEDGE

- Neuroanatomy and physiology should be understood.
- Knowledge of aseptic technique is essential.
- Normal CSF pressure in the lumbar subarachnoid space ranges from 0 to 15 mm Hg.
- Lumbar subarachnoid catheters (also known as lumbar drains or intrathecal catheters) may be inserted via a lumbar puncture procedure. These catheters may then be used to monitor CSF pressure or drain CSF.
- Intermittent or continuous CSF drainage from the lumbar subarachnoid space may be useful in patients with tears or interruptions in the dura mater who require lower CSF pressure during repair of these dural tears.
- Patients with pseudotumor cerebri ("benign or diffuse intracranial pressure elevations") who require frequent lumbar puncture procedures for CSF removal may benefit from placement of lumbar subarachnoid catheters for CSF pressure monitoring and CSF drainage during acute exacerbation episodes.
- CSF drainage has been reported to protect the spinal cord during surgical procedures requiring thoracic aortic cross clamping.
- Lumbar subarachnoid catheter insertion for CSF pressure monitoring and drainage may reduce the incidence of paraplegia associated with surgical repair of descending TAAA.
- Although still under scrutiny as a relatively new treatment strategy, it has been proposed that monitoring of CSF pressure and drainage of CSF to maintain pressure at 10 to 15 mm Hg or less is associated with reduction of spinal cord deficit in patients having TAAA repair.[1-3]

EQUIPMENT

- Povidone-iodine scrub solution
- Povidone-iodine pads or swabsticks
- Alcohol pads or swabsticks
- Sterile gloves
- Surgical caps and masks
- Sterile surgical gowns
- Sterile towels, half-sheets, and drapes
- Local anesthetic (lidocaine 1% or 2% without epinephrine)
- 5- or 10-mL Luer-Lok syringe for drawing up lidocaine and 23-G needle for administering lidocaine
- Sutures (2-0 nylon, 3-0 silk, 4-0 Vicryl)
- Forceps
- Sterile scissors
- Needle holder
- Lumbar catheter
- Lumbar puncture tray with spinal needle (generic or custom kit available from a variety of manufacturers)
- Sterile occlusive dressing (sterile 4 × 4 gauze pads or bio-occlusive dressing)
- Silk tape (1- and 2-in rolls)
- External transducer with fluid-filled pressure monitoring tubing
- Pressure cable
- External CSF drainage and monitoring system (generic or custom kit available from a variety of manufacturers)

Additional equipment to have available as needed includes the folowing:

• Rolled towels or small pillows to support the patient during positioning

PATIENT AND FAMILY EDUCATION

• Assess patient and family understanding of purpose of lumbar subarachnoid catheter monitoring and drainage system. ➤*Rationale:* Clarification and repeat explanation may limit anxiety and stress for the patient and family.

• Explain standard care for insertion, patient monitoring, and care involving the lumbar subarachnoid catheter. ➤*Rationale:* Explanation of expected intervention may allay patient and family anxiety and encourage questions.

• Explain expected outcomes of lumbar subarachnoid catheter monitoring use. ➤*Rationale:* Patient and family may experience less anxiety if aware of goals, duration, and expectations of lumbar subarachnoid catheter monitoring use.

PATIENT ASSESSMENT AND PREPARATION

Patient Assessment

• Assess baseline neurologic status, including motor function in lower extremities and bowel and bladder function. ➤*Rationale:* Knowledge of baseline neurologic status provides ability to determine the occurrence of neurologic changes that may result from lumbar subarachnoid catheter insertion or neurologic changes that may result from spinal cord damage related to TAAA repair.

• Assess current laboratory profile, including complete blood count (CBC), platelet count, prothrombin time (PT), partial thromboplastin time (PTT), bleeding time, and International Normalized Ratio (INR). ➤*Rationale:* Baseline coagulation studies may be necessary to determine degree of risk for bleeding as a result of lumbar subarachnoid catheter insertion.

Patient Preparation

• Ensure that the patient and family understand preprocedural teaching. Answer questions as they arise and reinforce information as needed. ➤*Rationale:* Evaluates and reinforces understanding of previously taught information.

• Ensure that informed consent has been obtained. ➤*Rationale:* Protects the rights of the patient and makes a competent decision possible for the patient.

• Administer preprocedure analgesia or sedation as prescribed. ➤*Rationale:* Patient will be expected to be very still during lumbar subarachnoid catheter insertion and monitoring and therefore may require sedation or analgesia to tolerate the procedure.

• Position patient in a flat lateral, sidelying position for lumbar subarachnoid catheter insertion (see Fig. 85–1). Patient should remain in a flat supine or flat lateral, sidelying position for the duration of lumbar subarachnoid catheter placement, monitoring, and drainage. ➤*Rationale:* The flat lateral, sidelying position provides necessary anatomic accessibility for subarachnoid catheter insertion. Maintenance of the flat supine or flat lateral, sidelying position protects from excessive loss of CSF during lumbar subarachnoid catheter placement, monitoring, and drainage. For patients post TAAA repair, the drainage system may be turned off to the patient during changes in activity (eg, dangling) as prescribed by the physician.

Procedure **for Lumbar Subarachnoid Catheter Insertion (Assist)**

Steps	Rationale	Special Considerations
1. Wash hands.	Reduces transmission of microorganisms; standard precautions.	
2. Assemble and flush fluid-filled tubing system with external transducer (see Procedure 69).	Preparation of external transducer and CSF drainage system promotes efficiency during catheter insertion procedure and ensures capability of immediate CSF drainage if necessary in the presence of elevated lumbar subarachnoid CSF pressure.	Flush the systems with preservative-free 0.9% NaCl solution. A variety of sterile, preassembled external tranducer and CSF drainage systems are available in both generic and custom kits.
3. Assemble and flush sterile CSF drainage system that is compatible with specific lumbar subarachnoid catheter device as per institutional procedure.		
4. Preserve sterility of systems after preparation, before insertion of catheter.		
5. Turn on bedside monitor.	Ensures that monitoring equipment is functional and readied.	
6. Ensure that the patient is in the flat lateral, sidelying position (see Fig. 85–1).	Lateral sidelying position provides appropriate anatomic access for lumbar subarachnoid catheter insertion.	

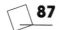

| **Procedure** for Lumbar Subarachnoid Catheter Insertion (Assist) *Continued* |

Steps	Rationale	Special Considerations
7. Prepare insertion site with alcohol followed by povidone-iodine solution. Drape posterior thorax at lumbar area with sterile drapes and half-sheets.	Reduces microorganisms, minimizes risk of infection, and protects insertion site from contamination.	
8. Open sterile trays and have accessible previously prepared external transducer or CSF drainage system.	Facilitates efficiency of insertion and immediate lumbar subarachnoid CSF pressure monitoring upon insertion.	A variety of preassembled sterile trays containing disposable surgical instruments (as listed on equipment list) are available from multiple manufacturers. Check list of sterile tray contents for presence of necessary equipment before opening tray.
9. Zero the system by opening the system to air and zeroing the monitoring system.	Zero balances to atmospheric pressure and ensures accuracy of monitored data.	External transducers for fluid-filled monitoring systems must be zeroed prior to instituting monitoring and should be re-zeroed at periodic intervals. External strain-gauge transducers also must be rezeroed after any positioning changes occur that alter the location of the transducer from the designated anatomic reference point.
10. Perform the zeroing procedure with the air–fluid interface of the monitoring system at the level of the patient's lumbar subarachnoid space (level of lumbar spinal canal).	Anatomic reference point for lumbar subarachnoid CSF pressure monitoring is at the level of the patient's lumbar spinal canal.	
11. Attach the sterile CSF drainage system distal to the external transducer monitoring system.	Dual monitoring and drainage systems provide capability for both monitoring of lumbar subarachnoid CSF pressure and drainage of CSF, if required, for lowering lumbar subarachnoid CSF pressure.	Through stopcock manipulation using dual CSF drainage/monitoring systems, lumbar subarachnoid CSF pressure may be alternately monitored continuously or lowered via intermittent CSF drainage.
12. Assist with the catheter insertion.	Facilitates insertion.	In patients having TAAA repair, the catheter is inserted in the operating room.
13. Measure the initial CSF pressure.	Guides therapy.	
14. Apply occlusive sterile dressing to the catheter insertion site.	Protects site from contamination by microorganisms.	
15. Secure the catheter in place.	Reduces the potential for catheter dislodgment.	
16. Zero the monitoring system.	Ensures accuracy of the system with the established reference point.	
17. Observe the waveform morphology, obtain a strip of the waveform, and measure the CSF pressure.[4, 5]	Provides initial baseline data for quantitative CSF pressure measurement and qualitative assessment of CSF waveform morphology.	Waveform morphology data yield information confirming correct placement of catheter. Lumbar subarachnoid CSF pressure waveform data are similar in morphologic presentation to traditional ICP waveform data generated from intracranial neuroinvasive monitoring devices (ie, ICP monitoring devices such as intracranial bolts or intraventricular catheters).
18. Discard used supplies, and wash hands.	Reduces the transmission of microorganisms; standard precautions.	

Procedure continued on following page

Procedure **for Lumbar Subarachnoid Catheter Insertion (Assist)** *Continued*

Steps	Rationale	Special Considerations
Troubleshooting		
1. If CSF waveform is overdampened: A. Assess the integrity of the lumbar subarachnoid catheter device and correct any problems if possible.	Overdampening of the waveform may indicate catheter occlusion, obstruction, or potential dislodgment of the catheter.	Catheter occlusion may result from precipitate or sediment present in CSF.
B. Check for air bubbles in the fluid-filled pressure tubing and remove air bubbles, if present.	The fluid-coupled system may develop a leak or air bubbles, requiring changing or flushing of the pressure tubing or external strain gauge transducer.	Responsibility for changing the fluid-filled system or flushing the lumbar subarachnoid catheter varies according to institutional standards and policies. Notify the physician for intervention as indicated by specific catheter malfunction and institutional policy.
C. Assess the monitoring system for disconnections or problems and correct the CSF pressure monitoring device malfunctions according to the manufacturer's guidelines and institutional policy.	Ensures functional equipment. Loose cables and connecting devices may contribute to mechanical failure.	
2. Assess lumbar subarachnoid CSF pressure monitor for sudden absence of pressure waveform, significant changes in pressure measurements, or need for re-zeroing. Correct the problem identified.	Ensures accurate measurement of CSF pressure.	Notify the physician if unable to successfully resolve mechanical failure or zeroing issues that involve the lumbar subarachnoid catheter. Catheter replacement may be necessary.
3. Assess patency of CSF drainage/collection system by ensuring flow of CSF through CSF drainage system. Flush CSF drainage system and change system using aseptic technique, if necessary, as per institutional policy.	CSF drainage/collection system may become occluded by precipitate or sediment present in CSF.	Notify the physician if a significant amount of precipitate/sediment is present in CSF, because this is considered abnormal and may indicate the occurrence of infection or another unusual event. Lumbar subarachnoid catheter irrigation and manipulation may be viewed as a physician responsibility. Follow institutional policy.
Removal of Lumbar Subarachnoid Catheter		
1. Prepare sterile gloves, suture materials, sterile hemostat, sterile scissors, and clamp for assisting with lumbar subarachnoid catheter removal.	Ensures efficiency of removal procedure.	
2. Wash hands, and don sterile gloves.	Reduces the transmission of microorganisms; aseptic technique.	
3. Assist the physician or advanced practice nurse with removal of the lumbar subarachnoid catheter. Culture the tip of the lumbar subarachnoid catheter as per institutional policy.	Facilitates catheter removal. Culture of the lumbar subarachnoid catheter may reveal evidence of CSF infection.	
4. Apply sterile occlusive or translucent dressing after the device is removed.	Prevents contamination by microorganisms.	
5. Discard supplies, and wash hands.	Reduces transmission of microorganisms; standard precautions.	

- Accurate and reliable CSF pressure monitoring
- Maintenance of CSF pressure within range of 0 to 15 mm Hg or as indicated by the physician
- Early detection and precise, expeditious management of elevated CSF pressure
- Ability to manage elevated CSF pressure through CSF drainage
- Adequate treatment of dural tears or pseudotumor cerebri through maintenance of lumbar subarachnoid catheter, monitoring of CSF pressure, and drainage of CSF, as indicated
- Prevention of spinal cord damage associated with TAAA repair by maintaining CSF pressure within or below 10 to 15 mm Hg through continuous monitoring and intermittent CSF drainage

- CSF leakage or excessive CSF drainage
- CSF infection
- Dislodgment or occlusion of lumbar subarachnoid catheter
- Change in LOC or development of cranial nerve deficits
- Motor function deficits involving lower extremities or involving myotome distribution of thoracic or lumbar spinal cord
- Tension pneumocranium
- Bladder or bowel dysfunction
- Extreme discomfort or pain involving catheter insertion site or sensory dysfunction involving dermatome distribution of thoracic or lumbar spinal cord

Patient Monitoring and Care

Patient Monitoring and Care	Rationale	Reportable Conditions
		These conditions should be reported if they persist despite nursing interventions.
1. Monitor patient throughout insertion procedure for neurologic status (including level of consciousness, sensation, motor function of lower extremities, bowel and bladder function) and vital sign changes.	Changes in neurologic status may result from irritation of spinal nerves associated with subarachnoid catheter placement or from spinal cord damage related to TAAA repair. Changes in level of consciousness or cranial nerve deficits may be related to subdural hematoma formation, herniation, or tension pneumocranium resulting from overdrainage of CSF.[6][7]	• Changes or abnormal neurologic status, vital signs
2. Administer sedation and analgesia as needed.	Assessment of patient for pain and procedural tolerance facilitates patient comfort, safety, and success of insertion attempt.	• Unrelieved discomfort
3. Assess lumbar subarachnoid CSF pressure and amount of CSF drainage and record hourly. CSF pressure should be measured and monitored on "mean" setting. Adjust the pressure scale on the monitor according to patient's individualized CSF pressure reading to capture the CSF waveform and an accurate digital reading. Assess CSF waveform morphology hourly.[4][5]	Lumbar subarachnoid CSF pressure should be continuously monitored and assessed and recorded on at least an hourly basis. Normal morphology of the CSF pressure waveform confirms accuracy of CSF pressure monitoring.	• Elevations, deviations, or abnormalities in the CSF pressure reading or waveform. Notify physician of need to drain CSF for elevated CSF pressure readings.
4. Assess integrity, stability, and sterility of lumbar subarachnoid catheter system at least hourly.	Hourly system inspection ensures accuracy and safety of monitoring and prevents contamination by microorganisms.	• Lack of integrity in the catheter system
5. Re-zero the fluid-filled pressure monitoring system according to institutional standard or manufacturer recommendation.	Zero balances to atmospheric pressure and ensures accuracy of the monitored data.	

Continued on following page

Patient Monitoring and Care *Continued*

Patient Monitoring and Care	Rationale	Reportable Conditions
6. Check integrity of occlusive insertion site dressing. Change dressing and assess insertion site as indicated by institutional policy or physician preference.	Permits assessment of device integrity and direct visualization of insertion site. Prevents contamination of insertion site by soiled, wet, or loose dressing.	• Responsibility for insertion site dressing change is institutionally specific. Significant drainage on the catheter insertion site should be reported to the physician, because this may indicate bleeding, infection, or CSF leakage.
7. Continue ongoing assessment of neurologic status (including sensation, motor function of lower extremities and bowel and bladder function) and comfort level of the patient.	Changes in neurologic status or comfort level may indicate improper placement/ dislodgment of lumbar subarachnoid catheter, spinal cord damage related to TAAA repair, or underdrainage or overdrainage of CSF.	• Changes in neurologic status (including motor function of lower extremities and bowel and bladder function) or discomfort
8. Maintain patient in flat supine or flat lateral, sidelying position for duration of lumbar subarachnoid catheter placement and monitoring or in position prescribed by the physician.	Maintenance of flat supine or flat lateral, sidelying position protects from inadvertent excessive loss of CSF during lumbar subarachnoid catheter placement, monitoring, and drainage.	• Patients after TAAA may be allowed to dangle at bedside if the system is clamped and off to drainage.
9. Provide safe environment, preventing unintentional dislodgment of the lumbar subarachnoid catheter, through repeated explanation, sedation/analgesia as needed, and the use of mechanical restraints only as a last resort.	Patient safety and prevention of unintentional removal of the lumbar subarachnoid catheter can be achieved through a variety of measures which can be tailored to meet the individualized patient needs. Unintentional dislodgment of the catheter must be avoided, because it may result in inadvertent excessive drainage of CSF or CSF infection.	• Dislodged catheter
10. Change the CSF pressure monitoring and drainage systems, using aseptic technique, as indicated in institutional policy.	Limits risk of infection at insertion site or within CSF pathways. There is considerable variability regarding optimal frequency for changing lumbar subarachnoid catheter monitoring and drainage systems. Some recommend changing system setup every 24, 48, or even 72 hours. Others advise against invading or changing these systems at arbitrary intervals because of the increased associated risk of infection. Check institutional policy.	
11. Using aseptic technique, obtain CSF specimen from the lumbar subarachnoid catheter by accessing sampling port on CSF drainage system according to institutional standard or physician prescription.	Provides early detection and intervention in cases where CSF infection occurs in association with lumbar subarachnoid catheter use. There currently are insufficient data to guide or support decisions on the necessary frequency of routine CSF sampling from lumbar subarachnoid catheters. It is therefore recommended to follow institutional policy regarding frequency of routine CSF sampling.	• Elevated white blood cell (WBC) count, elevated protein, and decreased glucose in CSF fluid

Documentation

Documentation should include the following:

- Patient and family education
- Insertion of lumbar subarachnoid catheter, including any difficulties or abnormalities experienced during insertion procedure
- Initial, opening CSF pressure
- Description of CSF (eg, clarity, color, characteristics) as observed during lumbar subarachnoid catheter insertion, initial drainage, and intermittent drainage as indicated
- Patient's tolerance of procedure

- Insertion site assessment
- Hourly measurement of CSF pressure and amount of CSF drainage
- Hard copy of waveform recording at baseline, every 8 hours, and when significant changes occur
- Description of expected or unexpected outcomes
- Nursing interventions used to treat elevated CSF pressure and expected or unexpected outcomes

References

1. Crawford ES, Svensson LG, Hess KR, et al. A prospective randomized study of cerebrospinal fluid drainage to prevent paraplegia after high-risk surgery on the thoracoabdominal aorta. *J Vasc Surg.* 1991;13:36–45.
2. Murray MJ, Bower TC, Oliver WC, Werner E, Gloviczki P. Effects of cerebrospinal fluid drainage in patients undergoing thoracic and thoracoabdominal aortic surgery. *J Cardiothorac Vasc Anesth.* 1993;7;266–272.
3. Mutch WA. Control of outflow pressure provides spinal cord protection during resection of descending thoracic aortic aneurysms. *J Neurosurg Anesth.* 1995;7:133–138.
4. Marshall SB, Marshall LF, Vos HR, Chestnut RM. *Neuroscience Critical Care: Pathophysiology and Patient Management.* Philadelphia, Pa: W.B. Saunders; 1990.
5. Ropper AH, ed. *Neurological and Neurosurgical Critical Care.* 3rd ed. New York, NY: Raven Press, 1993.
6. Saether OD, Juul R, Aadahl P, Stromholm T, Myhre HO Cerebral haemodynamics during thoracic and thoracoabdominal aortic aneurysm repair. *Eur J Vasc Endovasc Surg.* 1996;12:81–85.
7. Thompson HJ. *American Association of Neuroscience Nurses Clinical Guideline Series: Lumbar Drain Management.* Chicago: American Association of Neuroscience Nurses; 1998.

Additional Readings

Bethel S. Use of lumbar cerebrospinal fluid drainage in thoracoabdominal aortic aneurysm repairs. *J Vasc Nurs.* 1999; XVII(3):53–58.
Nugent M. Pro: cerebrospinal fluid drainage prevents paraplegia. *J Cardiothoracic Vasc Anesth.* 1992;6:366–368.
Safi HJ, Hess KK, Randei M, Hiopoulos DC, Baldwin JC, Mootha RK, Shenaq SS, Sheinbaum R, Green T. Cerebrospinal fluid drainage and distal aortic perfusion: reducing neurologic complications in repair of thoracoabdominal aortic aneurysm types I and II. *J Vasc Surg.* 1996;23:223–229.

PROCEDURE

88

External Fixation Device Insertion (Assist)

PURPOSE: External fixation devices or skeletal cervical traction devices (tongs) are applied to the skull to immobilize and align the cervical spine. Realignment and immobilization provides time for healing of fractures or recovery of supportive structures.

Joanne V. Hickey

PREREQUISITE NURSING KNOWLEDGE

- Neuroanatomy and physiology should be understood.[1]
- Cervical spine immobilization is instituted to stabilize the cervical vertebral column when the cervical vertebral column has become unstable as a result of vertebral fracture, vertebral dislocation, vertebral fracture-dislocation, or injury to the soft tissue ligaments that support the cervical vertebral column.
- Cervical spine immobilization may be required as the definitive treatment or as part of preoperative management. An unstable cervical spinal injury may require long-term cervical traction (approximately 6 to 8 weeks) and immobility to stabilize the spine. Cervical traction may be used preoperatively to reduce a dislocation before going on to surgery. The definitive method used to treat cervical fractures depends on the injury classification, as well as on physician or institutional preference.
- Tongs consist of a stainless steel body with pins attached at each end or a graphite body with titanium pins (used in institutions where magnetic resonance imaging [MRI] is available) (Fig. 88–1).
- Cervical spine traction is provided with the use of tongs that are applied to the outer table of the skull to stabilize the cervical spine when the cervical spine has become unstable as a result of cervical spinal fracture or dislocation, cervical spinal cord injury, degenerative processes of the cervical vertebrae, or spinal surgery (Fig. 88–2).
- Immobilization reduces dislocations and assists in achieving vertebral alignment. It also reduces the risk of further injury to the vertebrae, ligaments, or spinal cord in the case of an unstable vertebral column.
- There are a number of treatment options available to

manage cervical injuries. The specific treatment for a particular patient depends on the type of injury, the level of injury (eg, C2 as compared to C6), and the specific classification of the injury, as well as patient characteristics.
- Cervical tongs are available in a variety of types: Crutchfield, Gardner-Wells, and Vinke tongs and a halo ring. The shape, features, insertion site, and placement vary slightly, but the purpose, principles, and care are the same. Physician preference is an important deciding factor in choosing the specific type of cervical external fixation device to be used.
- The insertion of Crutchfield and Vinke tongs necessitates an incision to expose the skull. Two holes are made in the outer table of the skull with a twist drill, and the pins are inserted and tightened until there is a firm fit. Gardner-Wells tongs are inserted by placing the razor-sharp pin edges to the prepared areas of the scalp and tightening the screws until the spring-loaded mechanism indicates that the correct pressure has been achieved. All types of pins are well seated into the outer table of the skull and angle inward to decrease the possibility of tong displacement.
- Cervical traction also may be applied using a halo ring device. This is a stainless steel or graphite ring that is attached to the skull by four stabilizing pins (two anterior and two posterolateral) (Fig. 88–3). The pins are threaded through holes in the ring, screwed into the outer table of the skull, and locked in place. Direct traction may be applied to the ring device with a rope and pulley or by attaching the ring to a body vest, which allows for mobility of the patient.

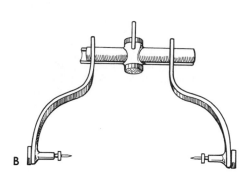

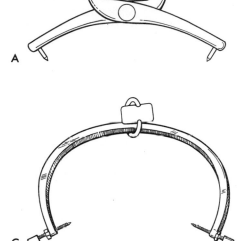

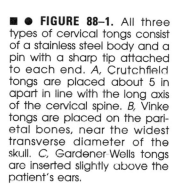

■ ● **FIGURE 88–1.** All three types of cervical tongs consist of a stainless steel body and a pin with a sharp tip attached to each end. *A,* Crutchfield tongs are placed about 5 in apart in line with the long axis of the cervical spine. *B,* Vinke tongs are placed on the parietal bones, near the widest transverse diameter of the skull. *C,* Gardener-Wells tongs are inserted slightly above the patient's ears.

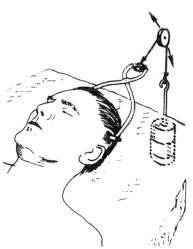

■ ● **FIGURE 88–2.** Continuous traction provided by weight applied to a cervical external fixation device via a rope-and-pulley system. (From McRae R. *Practical Fracture Treatment.* 2nd ed. Edinburgh: Churchill-Livingstone; 1989:184.)

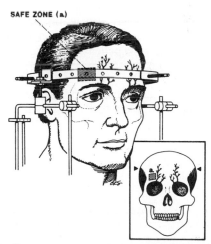

■ ● **FIGURE 88–3.** Placement of halo pins and ring. The anterior pins are placed anterolaterally 1 cm above the orbital ridge. This "safe zone" avoids the temporalis muscle laterally and an orbital nerve plexus and frontal sinus medially. (From Botte M, Garfin S, Byrne T, et al. The halo skeletal fixator: principles of applications and maintenance. *Clin Orthop.* 1989;239:14.)

EQUIPMENT

- Tongs or halo ring
- Insertion tray, including either the specific type of tongs to be used or halo ring with insertion pins
- Local anesthetic: lidocaine 1% to 2% (with or without epinephrine, depending on the physician's preference)
- Sponges (3-mL size)
- Needles (18- and 23-G)
- Sterile gloves, gowns, and protective glasses

- Povidone-iodine scrub or other antimicrobial solution
- Sterile sponges
- Sterile drill and bits
- Traction assembly for bed
- Rope
- S and C hooks (to attach to distal end of rope for weight application)
- Weights to attach to traction
- Torque wrench

Additional equipment as needed includes the following:

- Hair clipper or razor
- Emergency equipment

PATIENT AND FAMILY EDUCATION

- Explain the procedure and reason for cervical traction. Clarify or reinforce information as expressed by the patient or family. Discuss use of any special equipment, such as a special bed, which may be needed.   ➻*Rationale:* Decreases the patient's and family's anxiety.
- Explain the patient's role in assisting with insertion of the tongs.   ➻*Rationale:* Elicits patient cooperation and facilitates insertion.
- Explain that the procedure can be uncomfortable when incisions are made but that an anesthetic will be used. ➻*Rationale:* Prepares the patient for some discomfort and promotes cooperation.

PATIENT ASSESSMENT AND PREPARATION
Patient Assessment

- Conduct a complete neurologic assessment that includes cranial nerves, motor strength of major muscles, sensory (assess light touch and pain, noting highest dermatome level), and deep tendon (biceps, triceps, patella, and Achilles) and superficial reflexes (abdomen, anal wink). ➻*Rationale:* Provides baseline data for comparison of postinsertion assessments to determine neurologic compromise or extension of spinal cord injury.
- Assess vital signs.   ➻*Rationale:* Provides baseline data for comparison of postinsertion assessments.
- Assess respiratory pattern and auscultate lung sounds. Note use of accessory respiratory muscles and any signs or symptoms of dyspnea.   ➻*Rationale:* Establishes baseline data to determine any compromise to respiratory function as a result of the procedure.
- Inspect scalp for abrasions, lacerations, or sites of infection.   ➻*Rationale:* Identifies any potential sites of infection that may contraindicate insertion of cervical fixation device into the infected area.
- Assess level of pain, discomfort, or anxiety.   ➻*Rationale:* Establishes data for decision making regarding the need for analgesia or anxiolytics for comfort and cooperation during the insertion procedure.

Patient Preparation

- Ensure that the patient and family understand preprocedural teaching. Answer questions as they arise and reinforce information as needed.   ➻*Rationale:* Evaluates and reinforces understanding of previously taught information.
- Ensure that the head of the bed is flat and that the patient's head is in a neutral position by whatever approved means (eg, hard collar, manual traction) have been instituted.   ➻*Rationale:* Prevents extension of injury or spinal cord injury.

Procedure **for External Fixation Device Insertion (Assist)**

Steps	Rationale	Special Considerations
1. Order a bed with an orthopedic traction frame that is attached to the bed.	Traction must be ready to reduce the potential for movement of the head and neck.	May require assistance from other departments; therefore, plan ahead to coordinate.
2. Wash hands; don gloves, gowns, and protective glasses.	Reduces transmission of microorganisms; standard precautions.	
3. Cleanse potential pin sites with povidone-iodine solution.	Decreases skin surface bacteria.	

Steps	Rationale	Special Considerations
4. Assist the physician with tong insertion:	Facilitates the procedure.	Because of the high risk for extension of cervical injury, this procedure usually is performed by a neurosurgeon, who can respond rapidly to extension of injury, if it occurs.
A. Assist with local anesthesia administration.	Decreases patient's discomfort during pin insertion.	Cervical stabilization can be maintained with the use of a hard collar, Philadelphia collar, or other
B. Don sterile gloves.	Decreases bacteria in prepared area.	devices that prevent head rotation and neck flexion or extension. A soft
C. Stabilize the patient's head during the procedure.	Maintains alignment of the cervical spine and provides support to the injured areas.	collar is *not* considered a stabilizing device. Utmost care must be taken to prevent head and neck flexion or extension. Be prepared for the possibility of respiratory insufficiency, respiratory arrest, hypotension, or cardiac arrest.
5. Monitor the patient for changes in respiratory function, neurologic deterioration, and pain.	Identifies evidence of untoward effects or complications related to the procedure.	In addition to untoward effects, patient may require additional reassurance, support, sedation, and analgesia.
6. Apply occlusive dressings to pin sites (see Procedure 90).	Maintains asepsis.	
7. Assist with application and connection to traction as needed.	Ensures accurate and safe use of the traction.	
A. Maintain patient's head in neutral position.	Safeguards against extension of injury.	
B. Apply weights as prescribed.	Ensures safe use of equipment and maintains principles of traction.	
C. Ensure that weights are unobstructed.		
8. Discard used supplies, and wash hands.	Reduces transmission of microorganisms; standard precautions.	

Expected Outcomes

- External fixation device is inserted.
- Head and neck are immobilized to allow for alignment, stabilization, and healing of fractures.
- Neurological function (motor and sensory) improves or remains stable.
- Patient discomfort is minimized.

Unexpected Outcomes

- Slippage of tongs, pins, or external fixation device
- Extension or deterioration of neurologic deficits or spinal cord injury
- Respiratory compromise or arrest
- Hypotensive episode
- Pain
- Bleeding at pin site

Patient Monitoring and Care

Patient Monitoring and Care	Rationale	Reportable Conditions
		These conditions should be reported if they persist despite nursing interventions.
1. Neurologic assessment every 5 minutes during the procedure, including level of consciousness, movement or intact function in arms and legs, mastication, and eyelid closure.	Facilitates early recognition of neurologic deterioration. Bitemporal tongs may interfere with these functions.	• Any deterioration or extension of baseline neurologic function (eg, loss of more dermatomal sensation; decrease in motor strength)
2. Assessment of respiratory function (respiratory rate, pulse oximetry, lung sounds) before, during, and after the procedure.	Early identification of hypoxia or respiratory distress from extension of neurologic deterioration. Decrease in peripheral oxygen saturation may be an early indicator of respiratory compromise.	• Changes in respiratory function (eg, decrease in SaO_2, increase or decrease in respiratory rate, abnormal lung sounds)
3. Provide emotional support and reassure patient during procedure.	Decreases anxiety and facilitates patient cooperation.	• Unrelieved anxiety
4. Monitor dressings at pin sites for hemostasis immediately after the procedure, every 15 minutes times four, every 30 minutes times two, then hourly and as indicated.	The scalp is vascular and there may be continued bleeding at pin sites that require assessment and cleansing.	• Evidence of bleeding
5. Check security of traction, bed frame, and bed.	Traction frame is attached to the bed and must be secure. The head of the bed may be placed on shock blocks to provide countertraction.	• Break in the integrity of the traction equipment or bed frame
6. Maintain the patient's head flat on bed and ensure that the bed is flat, although the head of the bed frame may be on shock blocks to provide countertraction.	Head must be flat on the bed to maintain neutral position. Countertraction is often provided to prevent the patient from being pulled toward the top of the bed.	• Neck or head twisted or out of neutral alignment • Evidence of slippage of countertraction
7. Prepare patient for bedside confirmatory x-ray of cervical spine.	X-ray is done to determine or verify alignment of cervical spine.	• Abnormal x-ray results

Documentation

Documentation should include the following:
- Patient and family education
- Type of cervical traction applied
- Date, time, and name of physician applying traction
- Anesthetic used
- Sedation used
- Amount of weight applied to traction
- Ongoing comprehensive assessment data and action taken for abnormal response
- Verification of proper functioning and security of traction equipment
- Occurrence of unexpected outcomes
- Patient response to care
- Additional interventions

Reference

1. Hickey JV. Vertebral and spinal cord injuries. In: Hickey JV, ed. *The Clinical Practice of Neurological and Neurosurgical Nursing.* 4th ed. Philadelphia, Pa: J.B. Lippincott; 1997:420–434.

Additional Readings

Davis A. Sensory and motor disorders. In: Kinney MR, Dunbar SB, Molter N, et al, eds. *AACN Clinical Reference for Critical Care Nursing.* 4th ed. St. Louis, Mo: C.V. Mosby; 1998:711.

Maher AB, Salmond SW, Pellino TA. *Orthopedic Nursing.* 2nd ed. Philadelphia, Pa: W.B. Saunders; 1998:296.

Mollabasby A. Immobilization techniques in cervical spine injury: cervical orthoses, skeletal traction, and halo devices. *Topics Emerg Med.* 1997;12:3.

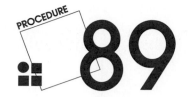

89 Halo Traction Care

P U R P O S E: A halo ring with or without a halo vest is designed to provide immobility to the cervical spine when the cervical spine has become unstable as a result of cervical spinal fracture or dislocation, cervical spinal cord injury, degenerative processes of the cervical vertebrae, or spinal surgery. This procedure focuses on the management of the patient who requires external cervical fixation when a halo vest and struts attached to a halo ring are used.

Joanne V. Hickey

PREREQUISITE NURSING KNOWLEDGE

- Neuroanatomy and physiology should be understood.[1]
- There are a number of treatment options available to manage cervical injuries. The specific treatment for a particular patient depends on the type of injury, the level of injury (eg, C2 as compared to C6), and the specific classification of the injury, as well as patient characteristics.
- Cervical spine immobility and traction are available with the aid of a number of devices. The most common types of cervical devices are Crutchfield, Gardner-Wells, and Vinke tongs and a halo ring with pins. The shape, features, insertion site, and placement vary slightly, but the purpose, principles, and care are the same. Physician preference is an important deciding factor in choosing the specific type of cervical fixation device to be used. The halo approach is very popular because of its versatility.
- A halo ring device is a stainless steel or graphite ring that is attached to the skull by four stabilizing pins (two anterior and two posterolateral) (see Fig. 88–3). The pins are threaded through holes in the ring, screwed into the outer table of the skull, and locked in place. Direct traction may be applied to the ring device with a rope and pulley or by attaching the ring to a body vest with struts, which allows for mobility of the patient.
- After the halo ring and pins are inserted, traction can be applied by the serial addition of weights to a rope-and-pulley device attached to the ring. The physician will use serial x-rays of the cervical spine to assist in determining the optimal amount of traction (measured in pounds) needed to reduce a fracture and provide optimal alignment. Additional weight is added gradually and followed with an x-ray. Excessive traction may cause stretching of and damage to the spinal cord; the addition of traction is managed by the physician.
- With the halo ring and pins in place, traction can be discontinued and a halo vest and struts added for long-term immobilization of the cervical neck (Fig. 89–1). The advantage to this approach is that the patient can ambulate, if he or she is neurologically intact, or his or her head can be elevated and the patient can get up to a chair.
- Patients with a halo ring, pins, and traction applied with weights are cared for similarly to patients in cervical tongs (see Procedure 88).
- The nurse must be familiar with the components of the halo-vest device, including how to access the anterior chest to administer cardiopulmonary resuscitation (CPR)

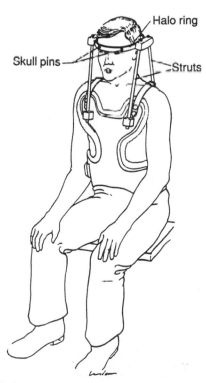

■ ● **FIGURE 89–1.** Halo-vest apparatus. Supportive struts and ring are attached to plastic vest, thereby applying cervical traction while allowing for patient mobility. (From Colbert MF, Kincaide SL. Halo immobilization device. In: Kincaide SL, Lohrman J, eds. *Critical Care Nursing Procedures.* Philadelphia: BC Decker; 1990:286.)

UCSD MEDICAL CENTER

SPINAL CORD INJURY ASSESSMENT

KEY

Sensory:	Motor: (Indicate best response)
S - sharp	0 - none
D - dull	1 - trace
H - hyperesthesia	2 - not greater than gravity
O - absent	3 - greater than gravity
	4 - slight weakness
	5 - normal

Source _____ Date _____

Patient Identification

	TIME		06		07		08		09		10		11		12		13		14		15	
			R	L	R	L	R	L	R	L	R	L	R	L	R	L	R	L	R	L	R	L
MOTOR	Shoulder Abduct	C5																				
	Elbow Flexion	C5-C6																				
	Elbow Extension	C7																				
	Wrist Dorsiflexion	C6-7																				
	Thumb-Index Pinch	C7																				
	Hand Grasp	C8																				
	Hip Flexion	L2-3-4																				
	Knee Flexion	L5-S1																				
	Knee Extension	L2-4																				
	Foot Dorsiflex	L5																				
	Foot Plantarflex	S1																				
SENSORY	Cervical	5																				
		6																				
		7																				
		8																				
	Thoracic	1																				
		2																				
		4																				
		5																				
		12																				
	Lumbar	1																				
		2																				
		3																				
		4																				
		5																				
	Sacral	1																				
		2																				
		3, 4, 5																				
	Position	Big Toe																				
	+ −	Index Finger																				
	Deep Pain Big Toe																					
	Initials of Examiner																					

■ ● **FIGURE 89–2.** Sample of flow sheet documentation form for motor and sensory testing. (From University of California–San Diego Medical Center.)

Table 89–1 ● ■ ■	**Assessment of Muscle Strength**
Motor Score	Indicators
5	Normal muscle strength; can maintain high degree of function against maximal resistance.
4	The muscle can go through its normal range of motion, but it can be overcome by increased resistance.
3	The muscle can go through its normal range of motion against gravity only; it cannot tolerate external resistance.
2	The muscle contracts weakly; it does not have sufficient strength to overcome gravity.
1	Visible or palpable muscle contractions may be seen or felt, but there is no movement in the limb.
0	Complete paralysis; no evidence of motor function.

Adapted from Hickey J. *The Clinical Practice of Neurological and Neurosurgical Nursing.* 4th ed. Philadelphia: JB Lippincott; 1997.

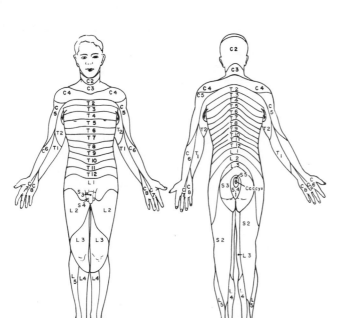

■ ● FIGURE 89–3. Sensory dermatomes; guidelines for sensory testing. (From Barr ML, Kiernan JA. *The Human Nervous System: An Anatomical Viewpoint.* 5th ed. Philadelphia: JB Lippincott; 1988:81.)

in case of cardiac arrest. Refer to information from the manufacturer of the halo vest for specific information on emergency access to the chest.

EQUIPMENT

- Halo device (in place)
- Soap and a basin of warm water
- Wash cloth and towel

PATIENT AND FAMILY EDUCATION

- Explain skin care and turning and positioning procedures and the reason for cervical traction. ➥*Rationale:* Decreases the patient's and family's anxiety.
- If the patient is ambulatory, explain modifications in meeting basic needs such as bathing, toileting, eating, dressing, ambulation precautions, and safety needs. ➥*Rationale:* Develops self-care skills and awareness of special safety precautions.
- For patients who will be discharged home wearing a halo-vest device, begin a comprehensive teaching program with patient and family. ➥*Rationale:* Prepares the patient for self-care in the home environment.

PATIENT ASSESSMENT AND PREPARATION

Patient Assessment

- Perform a complete neurologic assessment (Figs. 89–2 and 89–3 and Table 89–1). ➥*Rationale:* Provides baseline data.
- Obtain vital signs. ➥*Rationale:* Provides baseline data.
- Assess the skin at the edges of the vest and where the vest overlaps for redness or abrasions. ➥*Rationale:* Identifies skin irritation related to the halo-vest device.
- Check fit of vest for tightness or looseness. ➥*Rationale:* Identifies need for change or modification of vest. Patient weight loss may contribute to vest looseness.
- Check vest for loose straps, dirt, odor, or evidence of need to repair vest. ➥*Rationale:* The vest may need to be repaired or the liner changed.

Patient Preparation

- Ensure that the patient and family understand preprocedural teaching. Answer questions as they arise and reinforce information as needed. ➥*Rationale:* Evaluates and reinforces understanding of previously taught information.
- Assist the patient as he or she lies supine in neutral position with proper body alignment. ➥*Rationale:* Keeps the patient safe and accessible for inspection.
- Observe the sides and back of the vest and adjacent skin with the patient standing, if possible. ➥*Rationale:* Provides opportunity to inspect all areas in which the skin and vest come in contact.

Procedure for Halo Traction Care

Steps	Rationale	Special Considerations
1. Wash hands.	Reduces the transmission of microorganisms; standard precautions.	
2. Unbuckle one side of the halo vest while maintaining spinal alignment.	Gains access to underlying skin.	Inadvertent rotation of shoulders or hips may result in torsion of the spinal cord. Follow manufacturer recommendations for unbuckling.
3. Assess skin.	Identifies skin integrity.	Insensate patients may be more vulnerable to skin breakdown. The halo should fit snugly but not cause pain over pressure areas. The fit of the halo is checked daily. The sternum, ribs, scapulae, and clavicle areas are especially at high risk for skin breakdown.
4. Bathe the skin with soap and water.	Cleanses the skin.	Dry skin thoroughly and avoid excessive lotion or powder, because these agents tend to mat the sheepskin liner.
5. Auscultate breath sounds.	Identifies adventitious breath sounds.	Breath sounds may be decreased at the bases in patients with poor diaphragm and intercostal function.
6. Perform anterior and posterior chest physiotherapy, if indicated.	May enhance secretion maintenance and facilitate airway clearance.	There may be a slight decrease in vital capacity related to vest placement.
7. Rebuckle vest.	Maintains cervical traction.	Ensure that the strap is secured for proper fit.
8. Turn the patient to the opposite side, keep the head of the bed flat, and repeat steps 2 through 7.	Facilitates assessment of the opposite side of the patient's body.	
9. Change the anterior sheepskin as needed:	Provides comfort and cleanliness and protects the skin.	Follow the hospital protocol for who changes the liner and the recommended procedure for the change. The anterior portion of the sheepskin liner may require frequent changes because of secretions or drainage from tracheostomy or spills while eating. Note: The halo-vest side panels may be opened simultaneously only when the patient is flat and supine.
A. Place the patient supine with the head of the bed flat.	Provides support and alignment.	
B. Unbuckle both side straps of the vest.	Provides access to sheepskin.	
C. Remove the soiled anterior sheepskin liner.		
D. Match the clean liner to Velcro guides on the anterior vest, and press it into place.	Secures the liner in place.	
E. Buckle both sides of the vest.	Maintains cervical traction.	
10. Change the posterior sheepskin:	Promotes comfort and protects the skin.	Follow the hospital protocol for who changes the liner and the recommended procedure for the change.
A. Position the patient with the head of the bed flat and the patient turned to the sidelying position.	Provides support and protects the skin.	
B. Unbuckle one side of the halo vest.		
C. Roll the soiled liner to the corresponding portion of the posterior vest, and roll the remainder to the center of the vest.	Simplifies the liner change.	
D. Match half the clean liner to the corresponding portion of the posterior vest, and roll the remainder to the center of the vest.	Provides comfort and protects the skin.	
E. Buckle the side strap.	Maintains cervical traction.	

Procedure **for Halo Traction Care** *Continued*		
Steps	**Rationale**	**Special Considerations**
F. Roll the patient to the opposite side.	Accesses the liner.	
G. Unbuckle the side strap, and remove the remainder of the soiled liner.		
H. Unroll the clean liner, and match to the corresponding Velcro strips on the vest.	Secures the liner in place.	
I. Buckle the side strap.	Maintains cervical traction.	
11. Wash hands.	Reduces the transmission of microorganisms; standard precautions.	

Expected Outcomes

- Cervical alignment is maintained.
- Underlying skin remains intact and free of irritation.
- Vest is functional, fits well, and is clean and odorless.
- Mobility is maintained if patient is neurologically intact.
- Patient's safety is maintained.

Unexpected Outcomes

- Slippage of tongs, pins, or external fixation device
- Interruption of continuous traction
- Extension or deterioration of neurological deficits or spinal cord injury
- Infection
- Skin irritation around vest or injury
- Respiratory compromise or arrest
- Injury from fall while ambulating and in halo vest

Patient Monitoring and Care

Patient Monitoring and Care	Rationale	Reportable Conditions
		These conditions should be reported if they persist despite nursing interventions.
1. Monitor motor/sensory function every 2 to 4 hours.	Early recognition of neurologic deterioration.	• Any deterioration or extension of baseline neurologic function (eg, loss of more dermatomal sensation; decrease in motor strength)
2. Monitor for dyspnea, hypoxia, or decreasing tidal volumes (monitor pulse oximetry, and measure tidal volumes).	Early identification of hypoxia or respiratory distress from extension of neurologic deterioration or compromised respiratory function from vest constriction. A decrease in peripheral oxygen saturation or a decrease in tidal volume may be early indicators of respiratory compromise.	• Decreased oxygen saturation • Decreased tidal volumes from baseline • Dyspnea
3. Check fit of vest, especially if the patient has lost or gained significant weight.	Vest may be too big if significant weight loss occurred or too small if improperly fitted originally or with weight gain.	• Vest too loose or too tight
4. Observe skin at edges of vest and where vest overlaps at least each shift. Replace vest liner if it is wet or soiled.	Promotes comfort and skin integrity.	• Skin irritation noted; liner is wet or dirty and needs replacement. Follow the hospital protocol for who changes the liner and the recommended procedure for the change.
5. Wash exposed skin with warm water and soap; rinse well and dry. Be careful not to wet the liner.	Maintains cleanliness of skin and protects the liner.	• Need for liner replacement

Continued on following page

Patient Monitoring and Care	Rationale	Reportable Conditions
6. Provide pin care (see Procedure 90).	Monitors pin sites and prevents infection.	• Evidence of infection
7. Check integrity of halo, pins, struts, and vest.	Provides for safe use of equipment and appropriate therapy.	• Any break in integrity of equipment
8. Move patient and halo vest as a unit to avoid pressure that may dislodge pins. Never use the struts attaching the halo to the vest for moving patients.	Prevents dislodgment of pins and injury.	• Evidence of dislodgment of pins or halo
9. Support patient with pillows when positioning patient in proper body alignment.	Prevents dislodgment of halo-vest device.	• Evidence of dislodgment of pins or halo
10. Discuss change in body image related to the halo-vest device; provide emotional support.	There is a dramatic change in body image with the wearing of the halo-vest device that needs to be acknowledged.	• Maladaption to altered body image
11. Discuss safety in ambulation and fall prevention (eg, scanning with eyes to compensate for inability to move head; walking slower).	Because of the immobilization of the head and neck, the patient is at a high risk for falls.	• Patients that are at high risk for falls

Documentation

Documentation should include the following:

- Patient and family education
- Date, time, and name of physician applying halo vest
- Skin and pin assessment
- Integrity of vest
- Neurologic (motor/sensory assessment) and pulmonary assessment (tidal volume, pulse oximetry)
- Date and time of chest physiotherapy performed
- Occurrence of unexpected outcomes
- Patient response to care
- Additional interventions

Reference

1. Hickey JV. Vertebral and spinal cord injuries. In: Hickey JV, ed. *The Clinical Practice of Neurological and Neurosurgical Nursing*. 4th ed. Philadelphia, Pa: J.B. Lippincott; 1997:420–434.

Additional Readings

Davis A. Sensory and motor disorders. In: Kinney MR, Dunbar SB, Molter N, et al., eds. *AACN Clinical Reference for Critical Care Nursing*. 4th ed. St. Louis, Mo: C.V. Mosby; 1998:711.

Maher AB, Salmond SW, Pellino TA. *Orthopedic Nursing*. 2nd ed. Philadelphia, Pa: W.B. Saunders; 1998:296.

Mollabasby A. Immobilization techniques in cervical spine injury: cervical orthoses, skeletal traction, and halo devices. *Topics Emerg Med*. 1997;12:3.

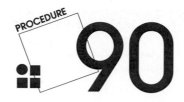

90 Tong and Pin Care

P U R P O S E: Tong and pin care is provided to assess the pin insertion sites for signs and symptoms of infection, loosening, or displacement. In addition, pin care provides for removal of exudate at the pin site and for cleansing of each pin site.

Joanne V. Hickey

PREREQUISITE NURSING KNOWLEDGE

- Neuroanatomy and physiology should be understood.
- The insertion of Crutchfield and Vinke tongs necessitates an incision to expose the skull. Two holes are made in the outer table of the skull with a twist drill, and the pins are inserted and tightened until there is a firm fit. Gardener-Wells tongs are inserted by placing the razor-sharp pin edges on the prepared areas of the scalp and tightening the screws until the spring-loaded mechanism indicates that the correct pressure has been achieved. All types of pins are well seated into the outer table of the skull and angled inward to decrease the possibility of tong displacement.
- Cervical traction also may be applied using a halo ring device, which is a stainless steel or graphite ring that is attached to the skull by four stabilizing pins (two anterior and two posterolateral) (see Fig. 88–3). The pins are threaded through holes in the ring, screwed into the outer table of the skull, and locked in place.
- Once inserted, the cervical fixation devices require special care of the skin at the pin insertion site (called *pin care*) to prevent infection and to monitor for it. Because the pins are inserted through the skin and into the bone, local infections can develop and proliferate and may result in cranial osteomyelitis. Tong and pin care is essentially the same for all devices.
- Definitive guidelines for the specific use of solutions, use or nonuse of a dressing, and frequency of pin care have not been established and depend on institutional guidelines. A solution of hydrogen peroxide (H_2O_2) and normal saline is often used as a cleansing agent. Generally, pin sites do not require a dressing unless there is excessive drainage at the site.

EQUIPMENT

- Approximately eight cotton-tipped applicators
- Nonsterile gloves
- Approximately 60 mL cleansing solution (commonly a solution of half H_2O_2 and half sterile normal saline is used)
- Sterile container for cleansing solution
- Approximately 30 mL normal saline for rinsing pin sites after cleansing (in a sterile container)

Additional equipment to have available as needed includes the following:

- Razor or hair clippers
- Dressings, if included in guidelines

PATIENT AND FAMILY EDUCATION

- Explain the procedure and reason for pin care. **➤➤Rationale:** Decreases patient and family anxiety.
- Explain the patient's role in assisting with the procedure. **➤➤Rationale:** Elicits patient cooperation and facilitates procedure.

PATIENT ASSESSMENT AND PREPARATION
Patient Assessment

- Assess scalp for signs and symptoms of skin irritation; carefully inspect pin sites for signs and symptoms of infection (eg, redness, edema, or drainage). **➤➤Rationale:** Identifies skin breakdown, irritation, or pin-site infection.
- Assess level of pain, discomfort, and anxiety. **➤➤Rationale:** Establishes comfort level and need for intervention to facilitate patient cooperation with pin care.

Patient Preparation

• Ensure that the patient and family understand preprocedural teaching. Answer questions as they arise and reinforce information as needed.   ➤➤**Rationale:** Evaluates and reinforces understanding of previously taught information.

• Assist patient to supine position.   ➤➤**Rationale:** Facilitates access to pins for care.

Procedure **for Tong and Pin Care**

Steps	Rationale	Special Considerations
1. Wash hands, and don gloves.	Reduces the transmission of microorganisms; standard precautions.	
2. Mix 1 oz H_2O_2 with 1 oz normal saline in a sterile container.	Prepares cleansing solution for pin care.	Solutions may be kept in a covered sterile container for 24 hours. Label the date and time the solution was prepared.
3. Place 1 oz normal saline in a second sterile container.	Prepares solution for rinsing off the H_2O_2.	
4. Cleanse the area around each pin and tong with a cotton-tipped swab and half-strength H_2O_2–normal saline solution. Use separate swabs for each site to decrease the chance of cross-contamination.	Removes drainage, prevents excessive exudate, and cleanses area.	Serous drainage may be present the first two to three days after insertion.
5. Rinse site with cotton-tipped swabs and normal saline.	Removes H_2O_2 and any further exudate.	
6. Discard used supplies, and wash hands.	Reduces the transmission of microorganisms; standard precautions.	

Expected Outcomes

• Pin or tong sites will remain intact.
• Pin or tong sites will be free of infection.

Unexpected Outcomes

• Infection at pin or tong site that is local, extends into bone, or becomes systemic
• Skin irritation or injury
• Bleeding at pin site
• Pain at pin site

Patient Monitoring and Care

Patient Monitoring and Care	Rationale	Reportable Conditions
		These conditions should be reported if they persist despite nursing interventions.
1. Administer pin care every 4 to 8 hours and as indicated.	Keeps pin site clean and provides an opportunity for monitoring pin site.	• Evidence of infection
2. Examine each pin site for evidence of bleeding, swelling, drainage, or infection.	Look for evidence of infection or slippage of pins.	• Evidence of bleeding, infection, or drainage; pin dislodgment
3. Obtain a sample of drainage if signs of infection are present.	Identifies presence of infectious organisms for further treatment.	• Positive culture of exudate; signs of infection
4. Monitor for pain or discomfort.	Early evidence of possible infection or slippage of pin.	• Unrelieved pain

Documentation

Documentation should include the following:

- Patient and family education
- Condition of skin of scalp
- Condition of skin at pin or tong sites
- Evidence of redness, drainage, or infection
- Occurrence of unexpected outcomes
- Patient response to care
- Additional interventions

Additional Readings

Davis A: Sensory and motor disorders. In: Kinney MR, Dunbar SB, Molter N, et al., eds. *AACN Clinical Reference for Critical Care Nursing.* 4th ed. St Louis, Mo: C.V. Mosby; 1998:711.

Hickey JV. Vertebral and spinal cord injuries. In: Hickey JV: *The Clinical Practice of Neurological and Neurosurgical Nursing.* 4th ed. Philadelphia, Pa: J.B. Lippincott; 1997:420–434.

Maher AB, Salmond SW, Pellino TA: *Orthopedic Nursing.* 2nd ed. Philadelphia, Pa: W.B. Saunders; 1998:296.

Mollabasby A: Immobilization techniques in cervical spine injury: cervical orthoses, skeletal traction, and Halo devices. *Top Emerg Med.* 1997;12:3.

91

Traction
Maintenance

P U R P O S E: Once the external cervical fixation device (tongs) is applied to the skull, the nurse cares for the patient who is immobilized on complete bedrest. Traction must be maintained on a continuous basis, often for a period of weeks, until realignment or healing is completed.

Joanne V. Hickey

PREREQUISITE NURSING KNOWLEDGE

- Neuroanatomy and physiology should be understood.
- The nurse needs to be knowledgeable about the anatomy and physiology of the spine, spinal cord, and supporting ligaments and especially the special anatomy of the cervical vertebrae, the cervical spinal nerves, and innervated dermatome. In addition, the nurse must understand the pathophysiology of vertebral and spinal cord trauma, especially spinal shock, early ascending edema, and related clinical deterioration of respiratory and vasomotor tone.
- The nurse needs to be knowledgeable about the signs and symptoms of new injury or extension of spinal cord injury and the needed interventions.
- After the cervical tongs are inserted, traction is applied by the serial addition of weights to a rope-and-pulley device attached to the tongs (see Fig. 88–2). The physician will use serial x-rays of the cervical spine to assist in determining the optimal amount of traction (measured in pounds) needed to reduce a fracture and provide optimal alignment. Additional weight may be added gradually, followed with an x-ray. Excessive traction may cause stretching of and damage to the spinal cord; the addition of weight to the traction is managed by the physician.[1]
- Once the cervical tongs are in place, the patient is maintained on strict bedrest. In order to facilitate turning, he or she may be placed on a special bed or turning frame (Fig. 91–1).
- The principles of traction are the foundation of managing any patient in traction. Such key points as never raising the traction weights, never disconnecting the traction, and never allowing the traction weights to rest on the floor or other obstructing objects must be followed.

EQUIPMENT

- Cervical traction system in place
- Pillows
- Positioning devices

PATIENT AND FAMILY EDUCATION

- Explain the procedure and the reason for the traction.
  ➤Rationale: Decreases patient and family anxiety.

- Explain the patient's role in maintaining the traction.
  ➤Rationale: Elicits patient cooperation.
- Explain how the patient's basic needs will be met during the confinement to bed and the maintenance of traction. Explain any special procedures that will be instituted, such as pin care or turning. **➤Rationale:** Reassures the patient and family that the patient will be cared for and his or her needs met.

PATIENT ASSESSMENT AND PREPARATION

Patient Assessment

- Conduct a complete neurologic assessment that includes cranial nerves, motor strength of major muscles, and sensory (assess light touch and pain, noting highest dermatome level), deep tendon (biceps, triceps, patellar, and Achilles), and superficial reflexes. **➤Rationale:** Establishes database to determine any change in neurologic function.
- Assess patient's comfort. **➤Rationale:** Pain in the head, neck, or at the pin sites may suggest malalignment, pin site infection, or slippage of traction.

Patient Preparation

- Ensure that the patient and family understand preprocedural teaching. Answer questions as they arise and reinforce information as needed. **➤Rationale:** Evaluates and reinforces understanding of previously taught information.
- Ensure that body alignment is maintained and that the patient is positioned in the middle of the bed. **➤Rationale:** Facilitates comfort and even distribution of the traction.
- Check the orthopedic traction frame, knots, and pulleys for secure attachment and function. Check the ropes to be sure that they are hanging freely. **➤Rationale:** Maintains function and prevents slippage of orthopedic equipment.

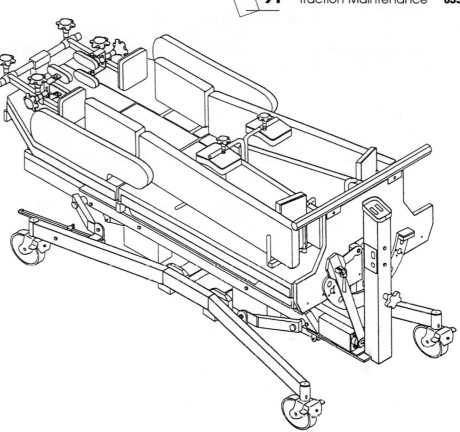

■ ● **FIGURE 91–1.** The Rotating Kinetic Treatment Table®. The patient is positioned and balanced on the table. The motor mechanism allows the patient to be rotated side to side, thereby displacing weight and assisting to relieve pressure areas. Cervical traction may be applied via a tension system at the head of the bed. Kinetic therapy can also facilitate pulmonary care of the patient, allowing easy access to the thoracic area for physiotherapy and coughing. (Courtesy of Kinetic Concepts Incorporated, San Antonio, Texas.)

Procedure	for Traction Maintenance	
Steps	**Rationale**	**Special Considerations**
1. Wash hands.	Reduces the transmission of microorganisms; standard precautions.	
2. Ensure that orthopedic frame and traction equipment are intact.	Promotes patient safety.	
3. Maintain weights so that they hang freely at all times.	Obstruction to free hanging of weights will eliminate traction and could precipitate adverse neurologic responses in the patient.	Inform physician of interruption of traction, because a cervical radiograph may be necessary to assess cervical alignment.
4. Ensure that there are no knots in the rope that could rest on a pulley.	Could interfere with prescriptive adequacy of the weights and traction.	
5. Maintain patient in a straight line (centered on the bed) and in a neutral position and aligned with the pulleys and ropes.	Alignment ensures optimal traction that is balanced (does not pull on one side of the body more than on the other side) and prevents traction slippage and pain.	Reposition as necessary; ensure adequate help to prevent extension of cervical injury.
6. When turning, log roll with three caregivers.	Maintains alignment.	Turning or moving the patient in a neutral position using a triple log-rolling technique requires coordination of turning and preplanning.
7. Use pillows and special positioning devices to maintain the patient in body alignment.	Prevents malalignment and possible extension of cervical injury.	Do not use pillows under the patient's head; maintain patient flat on bed; use pillows to support alignment and neutral position.
8. Wash hands.	Reduces transmission of microorganisms; standard precautions.	

Expected Outcomes	Unexpected Outcomes
• Orthopedic traction frame and all traction equipment are secure and functional. • Proper body alignment of the patient is maintained. • Patient is comfortable and safe.	• Slippage of tongs, pins, or external fixation device • Interruption of continuous traction • Extension or deterioration of neurologic deficits or spinal cord injury • Pain

Patient Monitoring and Care

Patient Monitoring and Care	Rationale	Reportable Conditions
		These conditions should be reported if they persist despite nursing interventions.
1. Frequent neurologic assessment every 2 to 4 hours and as indicated; include cranial nerve assessment, especially mastication and eyelid closure, because bitemporal tongs may interfere with these functions.	Early recognition of neurologic deterioration.	• Any deterioration or extension of baseline neurologic function (eg, loss of more dermatomal sensation; decrease in motor strength)
2. Vital signs every 2 to 4 hours and as indicated.	Determines cardiovascular stability.	• Changes in vital signs
3. Respiratory assessment (lung sounds, use of accessory muscles, etc.) every 2 to 4 hours and as indicated (see Table 91–1).	Early identification of atelectasis, pneumonia, respiratory distress, or extension of neurologic deterioration.	• Decreased lung sounds, increased sputum, yellow-green sputum, elevated temperature, use of accessory muscles
4. Cardiac assessment every 2 to 4 hours (see Table 91–1).	Early identification of cardiac dysrhythmias or decompensation.	• Dysrythmias, abnormal heart sounds, hemodynamic instability
5. Peripheral vascular assessment every 2 to 4 hours; consider deep vein thrombosis (DVT) prophylaxis (anticoagulation, sequential compression boots, etc.).	Early identification of peripheral vascular insufficiency and DVT.	• Peripheral vascular changes and signs of DVT

Continued on following page

Table 91–1 ● ■ ■ **Physiologic Responses to Immobility and Spinal Cord Injury**

Body System	Physiologic Response to Immobility	Physiologic Response to Spinal Cord Injury	Assessment Parameters
Integumentary	Pressure → ischemia → integumentary disruption	Protective motor and sensory functions lost or impaired below the level of the lesion	Inspect bony prominences. Identify preexisting skin disruptions. Assess specific pressure areas related to traction devices and positioning.
Pulmonary	Decreased chest expansion Secretions pool CO_2 retention → respiratory acidosis	Lost or impaired neuromuscular stimulus to diaphragm, internal and external intercostals, abdominal muscles, and accessory muscles	Observe thorax for symmetrical chest expansion. Identify breathing patterns. Auscultate breath sounds. Respiratory parameters (NIF/FVC). Supplemental O_2. ABG/pulse oximetry. Identify associated pulmonary injury.
Cardiovascular	Increased cardiac workload Thrombus formation Orthostasis	Decreased vasomotor tone Loss of sympathetic response Poor venous return Poikilothermia Spinal shock → autonomic dysreflexia	Vital signs and rhythm interpretation. Hemodynamic parameters. Body/skin temperature. Organ perfusion assessment: 　Level of consciousness. 　Urine output.
Musculoskeletal	Muscle atrophy Joint immobility → contractures	Loss/impairment of voluntary motor function Flaccid → spastic paralysis	Identify level of lesion. Serial motor/sensory examinations. Assess joint mobility (flaccidity/spasticity). Identify traction and applied weights.

Patient Monitoring and Care *(Continued)*

Patient Monitoring and Care	Rationale	Reportable Conditions
6. Gastrointestinal assessment every 4 to 8 hours; consider gastric prophylaxis.	Early identification of paralytic ileus and gastric distension; prevention of gastric hemorrhage.	• Abdominal distension, nausea, vomiting, decreased bowel sounds, constipation
7. Genitourinary assessment every 4 to 8 hours.	Early identification of urinary tract infection (UTI), neurogenic bladder.	• Low or high output, distended bladder, signs and symptoms of UTI
8. Skin assessment every 4 hours (Table 91–2).	Early recognition of skin breakdown.	• Evidence of skin breakdown
9. Musculoskeletal assessment every 8 hours (see Table 91–1).	Early recognition of musculoskeletal contractures.	• Increased spasticity or malpositioning of extremity
10. Nutritional assessment every 8 hours.	Early attention to providing a means for nutritional needs, based on condition.	• Decreased intake; poor skin turgor; intolerance of nutrition
11. Assess anxiety level and coping.	Early recognition of anxiety, depression, or agitation.	• Anxiety, depression, agitation, or other untoward responses
12. Pin care every 4 to 8 hours (see Procedure 90).	Monitoring of skin and prevention of infection.	• Evidence of infection
13. Reposition and turn, maintaining neutral body alignment every 2 hours.	Maintains skin integrity. Prevents complications of immobility.	• Impaired skin integrity
14. Respiratory management (deep breathing, suction, incentive spirometer, chest physical therapy, etc.); ventilatory management.	Supports respiratory function and oxygenation of all body organs.	• Decreased or increased respirations • Abnormal lung sounds • Decreased oxygen saturation
15. Consider bladder and bowel programs.	Supports adequate emptying of bladder and pattern of bowel activity.	• Bladder distension, constipation, or decrease in or absence of bowel signs
16. Perform range of motion every 2 to 4 hours and application of splints and other positioners.	Maintains intact motor function.	• Evidence of contractures, deformities, functional loss
17. Offer emotional support.	Supports patient and family through the continuum of care and keeps them actively involved.	• Refer to other team members as needed.

Table 91–2 ■■■ **High-Risk Focus-Area Skin Assessment Guide**

High-Risk Skin Areas

Devices/Positions	Forehead	Occiput	Chin	Ear	Clavicle	Scapula	Shoulder	Upper Arm	Elbow	Forearm	Wrist	Thumb Webbing	Axilla	Sternum	Ribs	Iliac Crest: Anterior	Iliac Crest: Posterior	Sacrum	Groin	Trocanter	Thigh	Knee	Calf	Ankle	Heel	Toe	Pin Sites
Halo-vest device		√			√	√	√						√	√												√	
High-top sneakers																							√	√	√		
Resting arm splints								√	√	√	√																
Resting foot splints																						√	√	√	√		
Rotating kinetic table		√		√	√	√		√					√			√	√	√	√					√	√		
Stryker frame: prone	√		√												√	√				√					√		
Stryker frame: supine		√			√			√									√	√							√		
Tenodesis splints									√	√	√																
Tongs:																											
Gardner-Wells		√																									√
Crutchfield		√																									√
Vinke		√																									√

Documentation

Documentation should include the following:

- Patient and family education
- Ongoing comprehensive assessment data and action taken for abnormal data
- Verification of proper functioning and security of traction equipment

- Occurrence of unexpected outcomes
- Patient response to care
- Additional interventions

Reference

1. Hickey JV. *The Clinical Practice of Neurological and Neurosurgical Nursing.* 4th ed. Philadelphia, Pa: J.B. Lippincott; 1997:419–465.

Additional Readings

Davis A. Sensory and motor disorders. In: Kinney MR, Dunbar SB, Molter N, Vitello-Cicciu JM, eds. *AACN Clinical Reference for Critical Care Nursing.* 4th ed. St. Louis, Mo: C.V. Mosby; 1998:711–732.

Maher AB, Salmond SW, Pellino TA. *Orthopedic Nursing.* 2nd ed. Philadelphia, Pa: W.B. Saunders; 1998:296–350.

Mollabasby A. Immobilization techniques in cervical spine injury: cervical orthoses, skeletal traction, and halo devices. *Topics Emerg Med.* 1997;12:26–33.

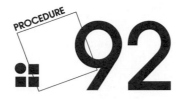

Pain Management Using Epidural Catheters

P U R P O S E: The epidural catheter is used to deliver certain medications or medication combinations directly into the epidural space surrounding the spinal cord, thereby providing site-specific analgesia. Epidural pain management may be employed short term (eg, obstetric (during labor), for postoperative pain management, after trauma), or long term (eg, for chronic pain and advanced cancer pain management).

Robyn Dealtry

PREREQUISITE NURSING KNOWLEDGE

- State boards of nursing may have detailed guidelines involving epidural analgesia. Each institution providing this therapy also has policies and guidelines pertaining to epidural therapy. The nurse should be aware of both of these guidelines and policies.
- The epidural catheter placement and the continuing pain management of the patient should be under the supervision of an anesthesiologist, nurse anesthetist, or the acute pain service.
- The spinal cord and brain are covered by three membranes, called meninges: the outer layer is called the dura mater; the middle layer is the arachnoid, lying just below the dura, and with the dura forms the dural sac; the inner layer, the pia mater, adheres to the surface of the cord and the brain. The epidural space lies between the dura mater and the bone and ligaments of the spinal canal (Fig. 92–1).
- The epidural space (potential space) contains fat, large blood vessels, connective tissue, and nerve roots.
- Analgesia via an epidural catheter may be given by continuous, intermittent, or in a patient-controlled analgesia (PCA) pump system.
- A variety of medication options are available, including local anesthetics, opiates, mixtures of local anesthetics and opiates, and alpha$_2$-adrenergic agonists. All medications should be preservative free for epidural administration.
- The pharmacology of agents given for epidural analgesia, including side effects and duration of action should be understood.

- Knowledge of signs and symptoms of sensory blockade or overmedication is essential. Intravenous (IV) access and immediate availability of opioid antagonist are necessary.
- Assessment of pain, including levels of sensory blockade, should be completed at regular intervals.
- According to the American Pain Society,[1] the most common reason for unrelieved pain in hospitals is the failure of staff to routinely assess pain and pain relief. Many patients silently tolerate unrelieved pain if not specifically asked about it.
- The Agency for Health Care Policy and Research[2] urges health care professionals to accept the patient's self-report as "the single most reliable indicator of the existence and intensity" of pain. Behavioral observations are unreliable indicators of pain levels.
- Pain is an unpleasant sensory and emotional experience that arises from actual or potential tissue damage or is described in terms of such damage.[3, 4] No matter how successful or how deftly conducted, operations produce tissue trauma and release potent mediators of inflammation and pain.[5]
- Pain is just one response to the trauma of surgery. In addition to the major stress of surgical trauma and pain, the substances released from injured tissue evoke "stress hormone" responses in the patient. Such responses promote breakdown of body tissue; increase metabolic rate, blood clotting, and water retention; impair immune function; and trigger a "fight-or-flight" alarm reaction with autonomic features (eg, rapid pulse) and negative emotions.[6–9]

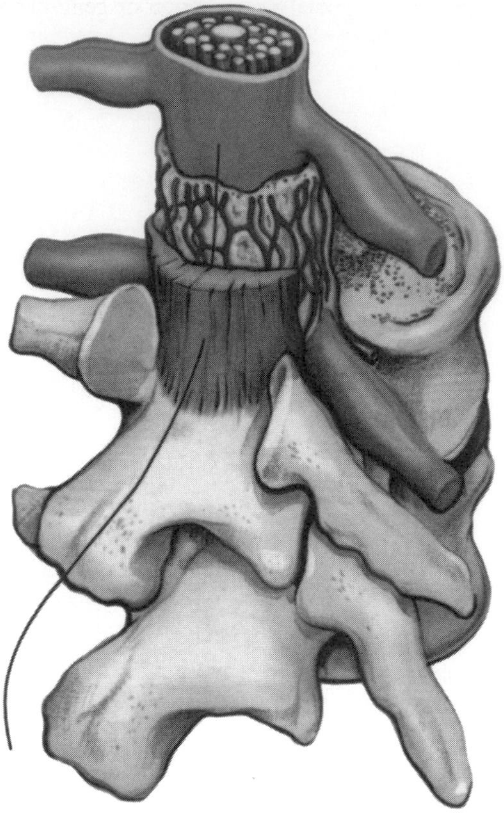

■ ● **FIGURE 92–1.** Epidural catheter positioning. (Courtesy of Astra Pharmaceuticals.)

- Pain itself may lead to shallow breathing and cough suppression in an attempt to "splint" the injured site, followed by retained pulmonary secretions and pneumonia.[10–14] Unrelieved pain also may delay the return of normal gastric and bowel function in the postoperative patient.[15]

EQUIPMENT

- One epidural catheter kit or the following supplies:

  ❖ One 25-G × ⅝-in (0.5 × 16 mm) injection needle
  ❖ One 23-G × 1¼-in (0.6 × 30 mm) injection needle
  ❖ One 18-G × 1½-in (1.2 × 40 mm) injection needle
  ❖ One 5-mL Luer-Lok syringe
  ❖ One 20-mL Luer-Lok syringe
  ❖ One Luer-Lok loss of resistance syringe
  ❖ One 18-G × 3¼-in (1.3 × 80 mm) epidural needle (pink)
  ❖ One 0.45 × 0.85 mm epidural catheter
  ❖ One introducer stabilizing catheter guide
  ❖ One screw-cap Luer-Lok catheter
  ❖ One screw-cap Luer-Lok catheter connector
  ❖ One 0.2 μm epidural flat filter

- Topical skin antiseptic, as prescribed (eg, povidone-iodine, chlorhexodine)
- Sterile towels

- Sterile forceps
- Sterile gauze 4 × 4s
- Sterile gloves, face masks with eye shields, sterile gowns
- 20 mL normal saline
- 5 to 10 mL local anesthetic as prescribed (lidocaine 1%) (local infiltration)
- 5 mL local anesthetic as prescribed (to establish the block)
- Test dose (eg, 3 mL lidocaine 2% with epinephrine 1:200,000)
- Occlusive dressing to cover epidural catheter entry site
- Dressing to secure epidural catheter to the patient's back and over the patient's shoulder
- Labels stating "epidural only"
- Pump for administering analgesia (eg, volumetric pump or patient-controlled analgesia pump)
- Specific observation chart for patient monitoring of epidural infusion
- Prescribed medication analgesics and local anesthetic medications
- Equipment for monitoring BP, heart rate, and SpO₂

  Additional equipment as needed includes the following:

- Ice for demonstrating block, if desired
- Emergency medications
- Respiratory equipment: oxygen mask and tubing, intubation equipment, hand-held resuscitation bag and tubing, and flowmeter

PATIENT AND FAMILY EDUCATION

- Explain the reason and purpose of the epidural catheter. ➤➤*Rationale:* Patient and the family know what to expect; may reduce anxiety.
- Explain to the patient and family that the procedure can be uncomfortable but that local anesthetic will be used to facilitate comfort. ➤➤*Rationale:* Elicits patient's co-operation and comfort and facilitates insertion; decreases anxiety and fear.
- During therapy, instruct the patient to report unwanted side effects or changes in pain management; eg, suboptimal analgesia, numbness of extremities, itching, and nausea and vomiting. ➤➤*Rationale:* Aids patient's comfort level and identifies side effects.

PATIENT ASSESSMENT AND PREPARATION

Patient Assessment

- Observe for local or generalized sepsis. ➤➤*Rationale:* Increases the risk for epidural infection (eg, epidural abscess). Septicemia and bacteremia are contraindications for epidural catheter placement.
- Assess concurrent anticoagulant therapy. ➤➤*Rationale:* Heparin (unfractionated and low-molecular-weight heparin) and heparinoids administered concurrently increase the risk of epidural hematoma and paralysis. Care must be taken with insertion and removal of the epidural catheter when patients are on anticoagulant therapy. Special institutional guidelines must be observed.
- Obtain vital signs. ➤➤*Rationale:* Provides baseline data.

Patient Preparation

- Ensure that the patient and family understand preprocedural teaching. Answer questions as they arise, and reinforce information as needed.   ➛*Rationale:* Evaluates and reinforces understanding of previously taught information.
- Ensure that informed consent has been obtained.   ➛*Rationale:* Protects the rights of the patient and makes a competent decision possible for the patient.
- Wash the patient's back with soap and water and open the gown in the back.   ➛*Rationale:* Cleanses skin and allows easy access to the patient's back.

- Consider NPO, especially if sedation or general anesthesia are to be employed.   ➛*Rationale:* Decreases the risk of vomiting and aspiration.
- Establish IV access or ensure the patency of IV lines.   ➛*Rationale:* The need to treat hypotension or respiratory depression may occur.
- Position the patient on his or her side in the knee-chest position or have the patient sit on the edge of the bed and lean over a bedside table with a pillow for comfort (Fig. 92–2).   ➛*Rationale:* Both positions open up the interspinous spaces, aiding in epidural catheter insertion.
- Reassure the patient.   ➛*Rationale:* May reduce anxiety and fears.

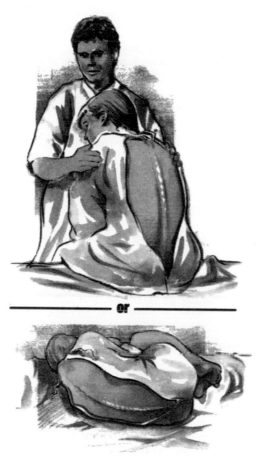

■ ● **FIGURE 92–2.** Epidural patient positioning. (Courtesy of Astra Pharmaceuticals.)

Procedure for Pain Management Using Epidural Catheters

Steps	Rationale	Special Considerations
1. Wash hands, and don gloves, gowns, and masks with eye shields.	Reduces transmission of microorganisms and body secretion; standard precautions.	Check for latex or other allergies.
2. Obtain the prepared epidural fluid with medication from the pharmacy as prescribed.	Medication should be prepared by aseptic technique by the pharmacy under laminar flow or prepared commercially to decrease risk of epidural infection.	All epidural solutions are preservative free to avoid reactions.
3. Connect the epidural tubing to the prepared epidural fluid with medication and prime the tubing.	Removes air from the infusion system.	
4. Ensure that the patient is in position for catheter placement (see Fig. 92–2).	Facilitates ease of insertion of epidural catheter.	
5. Assist as needed with the antiseptic preparation of the intended insertion site.	Reduces the transmission of microorganisms into the epidural space.	
6. Assist with holding the patient in position or consider sedation, if necessary.	Movement of the back may inhibit placement of the catheter.	
7. Assist the physician as needed with epidural catheter placement.	Facilitates catheter insertion.	
8. After the epidural catheter is inserted, assist as needed with application of an occlusive dressing.	Reduces the incidence of infection.	
9. Secure the epidural filter to the patient's shoulder with a gauze padding and an occlusive dressing.	Avoids disconnection between the epidural catheter and filter. Gauze padding prevents discomfort and skin pressure from the filter.	
10. The physician will administer a bolus dose of medication.	Facilitates a therapeutic level of analgesia.	If a local anesthetic is used for the bolus, monitor the blood pressure frequently for 20 minutes, assessing for hypotension. Some analgesics (eg, morphine) may take up to 1 hour to be effective.
11. Connect the prescribed medication infusion system.	Prepares infusion system.	
12. Initiate therapy: A. Place the system in a volumetric pump and set the rate and volume to be infused. B. Attach "epidural only" label to epidural tubing and tape over ports or use a portless system. C. Do not use a burette. D. Lock the key pad on the volumetric pump.	Do not give any other solution or medication (eg, antibiotic or total parenteral nutrition) through the epidural catheter. Inadvertent epidural administration of some medications can precipitate serious adverse reactions, including death.	Responses to epidural analgesia vary individually, and epidural analgesia is tailored according to individual responses.
13. Discard used supplies, and wash hands.	Reduces transmission of microorganisms; standard precautions.	

Expected Outcomes	Unexpected Outcomes
• Epidural catheter is inserted.	• Inability to insert the epidural catheter
• Pain is minimized or relieved.	• Suboptimal pain relief
• The patient experiences little or no sedation.	• Oversedation or drowsiness
• The patient experiences little or no motor loss in limbs.	• Respiratory depression or hypoxia
	• Hypotension
	• Motor blockade of limbs
	• Unilateral block (eg, pain relief on one side of the body only)
	• Patchy block (eg, uneven pain relief at operative site)
	• Urinary retention
	• Epidural hematoma
	• Epidural abscess
	• Pruritus
	• Weakness in upper limbs
	• Tingling around lips
	• Pressure areas (sacrum, heels)
	• High epidural block
	• Occlusion of epidural catheter
	• Epidural catheter tip migration
	• Dysphoria
	• Seizures
	• Accidental epidural catheter dislodgment
	• Leakage from epidural catheter insertion site
	• Cracked epidural filter

Patient Monitoring and Care

Patient Monitoring and Care	Rationale	Reportable Conditions
Observe at a minimum of each hour for the first 6 hours, or as prescribed or as necessary, and thereafter every 2 hours.		*These conditions should be reported if they persist despite nursing interventions.*
1. Sedation score: S = Sleeping, easily aroused; requires no action. 1 = Awake and alert; requires no action. 2 = Occasionally drowsy, easy to arouse; requires no action. 3 = Frequently drowsy, arousable, drifts off to sleep during conversation; decrease the opioid dose. 4 = Somnolent, minimal or no response to stimuli; discontinue opioid and consider use of naloxone (Narcan).	Sedation precedes respiratory depression.	• Increasing sedation and drowsiness or sudden change in sedation score
2. Pain score: Record the patient's subjective level of pain. Numeric pain intensity scale 0 to 10: 0 = No pain. 5 = Moderate pain. 10 = Worst possible pain.	Describes patient response to pain therapy. A low pain score is expected.	• Moderate to severe pain scores

Continued on following page

Patient Monitoring and Care	Rationale	Reportable Conditions
3. Assess respiratory rate.	Provides data for early diagnosis of respiratory depression.	• Increasing respiratory depression or sudden change in respiratory rate combined with increasing somnolence
4. Assess heart rate.	Tachycardia and bradycardia may indicate a condition such as shock or overmedication and sympathetic blockade.	• Change in heart rate
5. Assess blood pressure: If profound hypotension occurs, turn off epidural infusion and call the physician, advanced practice nurse, or the acute pain service. Place the patient in a supine, flat position. Administer IV fluids as prescribed or according to protocol.	Epidural solutions containing local anesthetic may cause peripheral and venous dilation, providing a "sympathectomy." If patient's fluid status is low, hypotension may occur.	• Hypotension
6. Monitor infusion rate hourly. Ensure that the control panel is locked if using the volumetric infusor or ensure that the PCA program is locked in via key or code access.	Ensures that medication is administered safely.	
7. Monitor oxygen saturation continuously.	Assesses oxygenation.	• Oxygen saturation less than 92% or decreasing trend in oxygenation
8. Obtain temperature every 4 hours; assess more frequently if febrile.	Increasing hyperpyrexia could signify epidural space infection.	• Temperature greater than 101°F (38.5°C)
9. Assess epidural catheter site every 4 hours and as needed.	Identifies site complications.	• A change in integrity of epidural insertion site; ie, redness, tenderness or swelling, or presence of exudate on epidural dressing
10. Monitor bladder function.	Provides data regarding urinary retention.	• Urinary incontinence; change in bladder function • Lack of urination for greater than 6 to 8 hours
11. Monitor sensory or motor loss.	Motor or sensory loss may be early warning signs of epidural abscess or hematoma or may indicate excessive dose of local anesthetic.	• Change in sensory or motor function
12. Assess for tingling around lips: check and assess during general conversation with patient during nursing care.	If local anesthetic is used in the epidural solution, tingling around the lips may indicate impending local anesthetic toxicity.	• Tingling around the lips
13. Assess for tinnitus: check and assess during general conversation and during patient care.	If a local anesthetic is used in the epidural solution, ringing in the ears can be a sign of toxicity.	• Decreasing or sudden change in patient's hearing
14. Monitor and check skin integrity of sacrum and heels every 2 hours and as needed. Change patient's position as needed.	If a local anesthetic is used in the epidural solution, check for decubitus ulceration (patient may have sensory loss in lower limbs).	• Increasing redness or blistering of the skin on the sacrum or heels
15. Change the epidural catheter insertion site dressing as prescribed or if soiled.	Provides an opportunity to cleanse the area around the catheter and to assess for signs and symptoms of infection.	• Signs of site infection (eg, swelling, pain, redness or presence of drainage) • Leakage of epidural solution

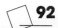

Patient Monitoring and Care *Continued*

Patient Monitoring and Care	Rationale	Reportable Conditions
16. Assess for the presence of nausea or vomiting.	Antiemetics may need to be administered; the medication may need adjustment (eg, opiates may need to be removed).	• Unrelieved nausea and vomiting
17. Assess for presence of pruritus.	Epidural opiates may cause itching. Antihistamines or other medications may be necessary to relieve pruritus.	• Itching, redness, or rashes
18. Label the epidural pump and consider placing the epidural pump on one side of the patient's bed and all other pumps on the other side of the bed.	Aids in minimizing the risk of mistaking the epidural infusion for an IV infusion system.	

Documentation

Documentation should include the following:

- Patient and family education
- Any difficulties in insertion
- Type of dressing used
- Confirmation of epidural catheter placement (eg, decrease in blood pressure, demonstrable block to ice)
- Site assessment
- Pain assessment
- Sedation score assessment
- Vital signs and oxygen saturation
- Epidural analgesic medication and medication concentration being infused
- Bolus dose administration and patient response following bolus dose, including quality of pain relief
- Occurrence of unexpected outcomes
- Nursing interventions taken

References

1. American Pain Society. *Principles of Analgesic Use in the Treatment of Acute and Chronic Cancer Pain: A Concise Guide to Medical Practice.* 2nd ed. Skokie, Il: American Pain Society; 1989.
2. Acute Pain Management Guideline Panel. *Acute Pain Management: Operative or Medical Procedures and Trauma. Clinical Practice Guidelines.* AHCPR Pub. 92-0032. Rockville, Md: Agency for Health Care Policy and Research, Public Health Service, U.S. Department of Health and Human Services, 1992.
3. International Association for the Study of Pain. Pain terms: a list with definitions and notes on usage. *Pain.* 1979;6:249.
4. Merskey H. An investigation of pain in psychological illness. D.M. thesis, Oxford University, 1964.
5. Hargraves KM, Dionne RA. Evaluating endogenous mediators of pain and analgesia in clinical studies. *Advances in Pain Research and Therapy.* 1991;19:579.
6. Dinarello C. Interleukin-1. *Rev Infect Dis.* 1984;6:51–95.
7. Egdahl G. Pituitary-adrenal response following trauma to the isolated leg. *Surgery.* 1959;46:9–21.
8. Kehlet H. The endocrine-metabolic response to postoperative pain. *Acta Anaesth Scand.* 1982;74(suppl):173–175.
9. Kehlet H, Brandt MR, Rem J. Role of neurogenic stimuli in mediating the endocrine-metabolic response to surgery. *J Paren Enterol Nutr.* 1980;4:152–156.
10. Anscombe AR, Buxton RJ. Effect of abdominal operations on total lung capacity and its subdivisions. *Br Med J.* 1958;2:84–87.
11. Hewlett AM, Branthwaite MA. Postoperative pulmonary function. *Br J Anaesth.* 1975;47:102–107.
12. Latimer RG, Dickman M, Day WC, Gunn ML, Schmidt CD. Ventilatory patterns and pulmonary complications after upper abdominal surgery determined by preoperative and postoperative computerized spirometry and blood gas analysis. *Am J Surg.* 1971;122:622–623.
13. Marshall BE, Wyche MQ Jr. Hypoxaemia during and after anesthesia. *Anesthesiology.* 1972;37:178–209.
14. Sydow FW. The influence of anesthesia and postoperative analgesic management on lung function. *Acta Chir Scand.* 1989;550(suppl):159–165.
15. Wattwil M. Postoperative pain relief and gastrointestinal motility. *Acta Chir Scand.* 1989;550(suppl):140–145.

Additional Readings

Ballanytne JC, Carr DB. The comparative effects of postoperative analgesic therapies on pulmonary outcome: cumulative meta-analyses of randomised, controlled trials. *Anesth Analg.* 1998;86:598–612.

Benedetti JC. Intraspinal analgesia: an historical overview. *Acta Anaesth Scand.* 1987;31(suppl 85):17–24.

Cooper DW, Turner G. Patient-controlled extradural analgesia to compare bupivicaine, fentanyl and bupivicaine with fentanyl in the treatment of postoperative pain. *Br J Anaesth.* 1993;70:503–507.

Cousins MJ, Mather LE. Intrathecal and epidural administration of opioids. *Anaesthesiology.* 1984;61:276–310.

Daly S, Ellis RD, et al. Special administration techniques: epidural administration of analgesics. In: Daly S, Ellis R, Falk D, eds. *Nursing Procedures.* Pennsylvania, Pa: Springhouse; 1992:262.

Liu SS, Allen HW, et al. Patient-controlled epidural analgesia with bupivacaine and fentanyl on hospital wards: prospective experience with 1,030 surgical patients. *Anesthesiology.* 1998;3:688–695.

Liu SS, Carpenter RL, et al. Effects of perioperative analgesic technique on rate of recovery after colon surgery. *Anesthesiology.* 1995;83:757–765.

Lubenow TR. Epidural analgesia: considerations and delivery methods. In: Sinatra RS, Hord AH, Ginsberg B, Preble LM, eds. *Acute Pain Mechanisms and Management.* St. Louis, Mo: Mosby Year Book; 1992:233.

Macintyre PE, Ready BL. Epidural and intrathecal analgesia. In: Macintyre PE, Ready BL, eds. *Acute Pain Management: A Practical Guide.* London: W.B. Saunders, 1996:114.

McCaffery M. Practical tips for relieving your patient's pain. *Nursing97.* 1997 April:42–43.

McCaffery M, Ferrell B. Nurses knowledge of pain assessment and management: how much progress have we made? *J Pain Sympt Manage.* 1997;14:175–188.

Sevarino FB, Preble LM. Continuous epidural infusions for postoperative analgesia. In: Sevarino FB, Preble LM, eds. *A Manual for Acute Postoperative Pain Management.* New York, NY: Raven Press; 1992:50.

Stanik-Hutt J. Pain management in the acutely ill. *Clinical practice protocol.* Aliso Viejo, Ca: American Association of Critical-Care Nurses; 1998.

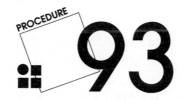

93

Peripheral Nerve Stimulators

P U R P O S E: Peripheral nerve stimulators (PNSs) are used in association with administration of neuromuscular blocking agents (NMBAs) to assess nerve impulse transmission at the neuromuscular junction of skeletal muscle.

Janet G. Whetstone Foster

PREREQUISITE NURSING KNOWLEDGE

- Peripheral nerve stimulators are used to assess neuromuscular transmission (NMT) when NMBAs are given to block skeletal muscle activity.
- Neuromuscular blocking agents are given in the intensive care unit (ICU), along with sedatives and narcotics; most commonly they are administered to facilitate mechanical ventilation and promote ventilator synchrony with newer modes of ventilation in patients with severe lung injury. NMBAs are also used to decrease oxygen consumption and carbon dioxide production during the work of breathing, assist with management of increased intracranial pressure following head injury, and promote healing of surgical wounds that would place the patient at extreme risk if disrupted.[1, 2]
- Neuromuscular blocking agents do not affect sensation or level of consciousness. Because NMBAs lack amnestic, sedative, and analgesic properties, sedatives and analgesics should *always* be given concurrently and should be initiated *before* NMBAs to minimize the patient's awareness of blocked muscle activity. Sedatives and analgesics should also be given prophylactically, because neuromuscular blockade hinders the assessment of pain.[3]
- The muscle twitch response to a small electrical stimulus delivered by the PNS corresponds to the number of nerve receptors blocked by NMBAs and assists the clinician in assessment and titration of medication dosage. The level of blockade is estimated by observing the muscle twitch after stimulating the appropriate nerve with a small electrical current delivered by the PNS.
- The train-of-four (TOF) method of stimulation most commonly is used for ongoing monitoring in the critical care unit. After delivering four successive stimulating currents to a selected peripheral nerve with the PNS, in the absence of significant neuromuscular blockade, four muscle twitches follow. The four twitches signify that 75% or less of receptors are blocked. Three twitches correspond to approximately 80% blockade, and one to two twitches in response to four stimulating currents correlate with approximately 85% to 90% blockade of the neuromuscular junction receptors.[4, 5] This is the recommended level of block, although the appropriate level has not yet been determined through research in the critically ill population.[5] Zero twitches may indicate that 100% of receptors are blocked, which exceeds the desired level of blockade (Table 93–1).

- Titration of the medication according to clinical assessment and muscle twitch response may help provide a sufficient level of blockade without overshooting. Overshooting the level of blockade by using excessive doses of NMBAs is of special concern in the critically ill patient because it may predispose the patient to prolonged paralysis. Prolonged paralysis and severe weakness following termination of NMBAs in critically ill patients has been reported extensively in the literature.[6–8] Monitoring with a PNS during administration of NMBAs results in the use of less medication and hastens the recovery of spontaneous ventilation.[9] Expert opinion holds that exposing nerve receptors to lower medication dosages enables faster recovery of skeletal muscle and helps to prevent persistent paralysis and weakness after termination of the medications.[3]

- The stimulating current is measured in milliamperes (mA). The usual range of mA required to stimulate a peripheral nerve and elicit a muscle twitch is 20 to 50 mA, although it may be necessary to increase the current to 80 mA, the highest setting on the instrument.

- Some stimulators do not indicate the mA. Instead, digital or dialed numbers ranging from 1 to 10 represent the range of mA from 20 to 80 mA. When using these instruments, the usual setting is 2 to 5, although a setting of 10 is sometimes necessary.

Table 93–1 ∎∎∎	Train-of-Four Stimulation as a Correlation of Blocked Nerve Receptors
TOF (Number of Twitches)	% of Receptors Blocked (Approximately)[4, 5]
0/4	100
1/4	90
2/4	85
3/4	80
4/4	75 or less

- The ulnar nerve in the wrist is recommended for testing, although the facial and the posterior tibial nerves may also be used.

EQUIPMENT

- Peripheral nerve stimulator
- Two gelled electrode pads (the same as is used for electrocardiography monitoring)
- Two lead wires packaged with the nerve stimulator

Additional equipment as needed includes the following:

- A ball electrode attachment may be substituted for the electrodes and lead wires

PATIENT AND FAMILY EDUCATION

- Explain the purpose of nerve monitoring; for example, assessing effect and guiding dosage of the medication infusion. ➻*Rationale:* May decrease anxiety.
- Describe the equipment to be used. ➻*Rationale:* May decrease anxiety.
- Describe the experience of the stimuli as a slight prickly sensation. ➻*Rationale:* The use of sensation descriptors is effective in reducing anxiety.
- Explain that the electrodes require periodic changing, which feels like removing a bandage. ➻*Rationale:* May elicit patient and family cooperation.

PATIENT ASSESSMENT AND PREPARATION
Patient Assessment

- Assess the patient for the best location for electrode placement. Consider criteria such as edema, diaphoresis, wounds, dressings, and arterial and venous catheters. ➻*Rationale:* Improves conduction of stimulating current through dermal tissue.
- Assess if burns are present or if topical ointments are being used. ➻*Rationale:* In patients with burns or topical ointments, for whom electrode adherence is difficult, the ball electrodes may be more effective than the electrode pads and lead wires. Poor electrode adherence interferes with conduction of the stimulating current.

Patient Preparation

- Ensure that the patient and family understand preprocedural teaching. Answer questions as they arise and reinforce information as needed. ➻*Rationale:* Evaluates and reinforces understanding of previously taught information.
- If possible, apply the electrodes and test the TOF response to determine adequacy of the location prior to initiating NMBAs. ➻*Rationale:* Improves reliability in interpretation of the TOF response.
- It may be helpful to determine the supramaximal stimulation (SMS) level prior to initiating NMBAs. The SMS is the level at which additional stimulating current elicits no further increase in the intensity of the four twitches. ➻*Rationale:* Helps establish adequate stimulating current; improves reliability.

Procedure for Peripheral Nerve Stimulators

Steps	Rationale	Special Considerations
Testing the Ulnar Nerve		
1. Wash hands.	Reduces transmission of microorganisms; standard precautions.	
2. Extend the arm, palm up, in a relaxed position (Fig. 93–1).	The ulnar nerve is superficial and easy to locate.	
3. Apply two gelled electrodes over the path of the ulnar nerve (see Fig. 93–1). Place the distal electrode on the skin at the flexor crease on the ulnar surface of the wrist. Place the second electrode approximately 1 to 2 cm proximal to the first, parallel to the flexor carpi ulnaris tendon.	Enables stimulation of the ulnar nerve.	
4. Use caution in selecting the site of electrode placement in order to avoid direct stimulation of the muscle rather than the nerve.	Direct muscle stimulation elicits a response similar to the TOF, making it difficult to evaluate blocked nerve impulse transmission.	
5. Plug in the lead wires to the nerve stimulator, matching the black and red leads (negative and positive) to the black and red connection sites.	Necessary for conduction of electrical current.	

Procedure for **Peripheral Nerve Stimulators** *Continued*

Steps	Rationale	Special Considerations

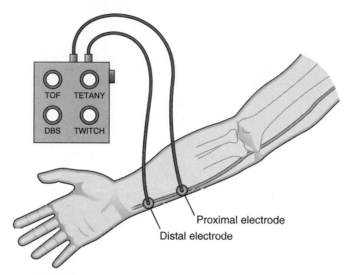

■ ● **FIGURE 93–1.** Placement of electrodes along the ulnar nerve.

Steps	Rationale	Special Considerations
6. Attach the lead wires to the electrodes. The negative and positive leads can be placed on either electrode. *(Level V: Clinical studies in more than one or two different patient populations and situations to support recommendations)*	Polarity usually does not matter when electrodes are placed close together directly over the nerve.[2, 10]	Occasionally twitch height is altered with reversed polarity; place the red lead proximally when a poor twitch response occurs.[10]
7. Turn on the PNS and select a low mA.	Excessive current results in overstimulation and can cause repetitive nerve firing.	
8. Depress the TOF key and observe twitching of the thumb, counting the number of twitches. Do not count finger movements, only the thumb.	Finger movements result from direct muscle stimulation.	Placing the operator's hand over the fingers helps reduce interpretation of artifactual movement.
9. Wash hands.	Reduces transmission of microorganisms; standard precautions.	

Testing the Facial Nerve

Steps	Rationale	Special Considerations
1. Place one electrode on the face at the outer canthus of the eye and the second electrode approximately 2 cm below, parallel with the tragus of the ear (Fig. 93–2).	Stimulates the facial nerve.	When wounds, edema, invasive lines, and other factors interfere with ulnar nerve testing, the facial or posterior tibial nerves may be substituted. The risk of direct muscle stimulation is greater, however, with resulting underestimation of blockade. Also, the alternate nerves correlate less well with the blockade in the diaphragm.[4]
2. Plug the lead wires into the nerve stimulator, matching the black and red leads to the black and red connection sites.	Necessary for conduction of electrical current.	
3. Attach the lead wires to the electrodes.		
4. Turn on the PNS and select a low mA.		

Procedure continued on following page

Procedure **for Peripheral Nerve Stimulators** *Continued*

Steps	Rationale	Special Considerations

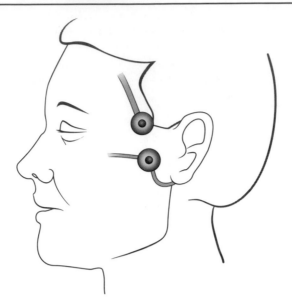

■ ● **FIGURE 93–2.** Placement of electrodes on the face.

5. Depress the TOF key and observe the muscle twitching above the eyebrow, counting the number of twitches.

Determines the neuromuscular blockade at the junction between a branch of the facial nerve and orbicularis muscle.

6. Wash hands.

Reduces transmission of microorganisms; standard precautions.

Testing the Posterior Tibial Nerve

1. Place one electrode approximately 2 cm posterior to the medial malleolus in the foot (Fig. 93–3).

Stimulates the posterior tibial nerve.

2. Place the second electrode approximately 2 cm above the first (see Fig. 93–3).

3. Plug the lead wires into the nerve stimulator, matching the black and red leads to the black and red connection sites.

Necessary for conduction of electrical current.

4. Attach the lead wires to the electrodes.

5. Turn on the PNS and select a low mA.

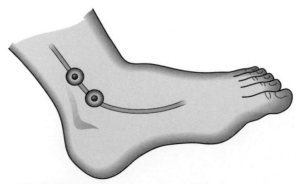

■ ● **FIGURE 93–3.** Placement of electrodes on the foot.

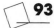

Procedure **for Peripheral Nerve Stimulators** *Continued*

Steps	Rationale	Special Considerations
6. Depress the TOF key and observe the plantar flexion of the great toe, counting the number of twitches.	Determines block at the junction between the posterior tibial nerve and the flexor hallucis brevis muscle.	
7. Wash hands.	Reduces transmission of microorganisms; standard precautions.	

Determine the SMS

1. Increase the mA in increments of 1 until four twitches are observed.		
2. Note the mA that corresponds to four vigorous twitches. Administer one to two more TOFs.	If there is no increase in intensity of the muscle twitch when the mA is increased, the SMS is the level at which four vigorous twitches was observed. For example, if a strong response was observed at 3 mA, raise the current to 4 mA. If there is no increase in intensity of the twitch, the SMS is 3 mA. If there is an increase, raise the mA to 5. If there is an additional increase in twitch intensity, raise it to 6. If the intensity shows no further increase, the SMS is 5 mA.	

Determine the TOF Response During NMBA Infusion

1. Ten to fifteen minutes after a bolus dose and continuous infusion of NMBA is given, retest the TOF.	Evaluates the level of blockade provided.	
2. Retest every 1 to 2 hours until clinically stable and a satisfactory level of blockade is achieved.	Evaluates the level of blockade and avoids under- and overestimation of blockade.	Always assess electrode condition and placement before testing.
3. If more than one or two twitches occurs and neuromuscular blockade is unsatisfactory, increase the infusion rate as prescribed or according to hospital protocol.	Signifies that less than 85% to 90% of receptors are blocked.	

Troubleshooting when There Are Zero Twitches

1. Retest another nerve (the other ulnar nerve or facial or posterior tibial nerves).	Avoids overestimating the level of blockade.	
2. Change electrodes.	Drying of the gel or poor contact compromises conduction.	
3. Check lead connections and PNS for mechanical failure (ie, the battery may need changing).	The most common cause of PNS malfunction is low battery voltage.[10]	
4. Increase the stimulating current.	After troubleshooting leads and PNS, current may be inadequate to stimulate the nerve.	
5. If there are no other explanations for a zero response, check the NMBA infusion for rate, dose, and concentration. Reduce the infusion rate of the NMBA as prescribed or according to hospital protocol.	Excessive neuromuscular blockade produces absence of twitch response.	

- Slight discomfort is experienced during the TOF test.
- The muscles of the thumb twitch, rather than the fingers, when the ulnar nerve is stimulated.
- The twitch response approximates the number of blocked peripheral nerve receptors; for example, four twitches before initiating the NMBA infusion and one to two twitches when a desired level of blockade is achieved.
- The NMBA dosage is titrated according to the TOF test and clinical goals.
- Resumption of four twitches occurs within 2 hours when the NMBA is discontinued.

- Moderate to severe discomfort from the TOF test
- Impaired skin integrity when the electrodes are removed
- The fingers twitch when the ulnar nerve is stimulated
- Resumption of four twitches does not occur within 2 hours of discontinuation of NMBA

Patient Monitoring and Care

Patient Monitoring and Care	Rationale	Reportable Conditions
		These conditions should be reported if they persist despite nursing interventions.
1. Cleanse and thoroughly dry the skin before applying electrodes.	Improves electrode adherence.	
2. Change the electrodes whenever they are loose or when gel becomes dry.	Optimizes conduction of stimulating current.	
3. Select the most accessible site with the smallest degree of edema, with no wounds, catheters, or dressings that impede accurate electrode placement over the selected nerve.	Facilitates ease in testing, electrode adherence, and conduction of current.	
4. Never use the "Single Twitch," "Tetany," or "Double Burst" settings if available on the PNS.	These methods are less accurate and may cause extreme discomfort.[11]	
5. The patient may demonstrate subtle movement of the extremities with an acceptable TOF response.	Clinical decisions should never be made solely on the TOF test results. Assessment of oxygenation and ventilation, neurologic function, tissue perfusion, and other clinical goals should be evaluated when deciding to increase the rate of NMBA infusion.	• Patient movement despite acceptable TOF
6. Microshock hazard may be a risk to patients with external pacing catheters. Extreme caution must be exercised to prevent the PNS lead wires from contacting the pacing catheter or pacing lead wires.	Direct electrical current can be conducted from the PNS through the pacing wires to the heart.	• Cardiac dysrhythmias or change in patient condition
7. Perform TOF testing every 4 to 8 hours during NMBA infusion.	Aids in dosing NMBA.	• Abnormal TOF results

Documentation

Documentation should include the following:

- Patient and family education
- The time, TOF twitch response, the mA, and the nerve site tested
- The TOF response as 0/4, 1/4, 2/4, 3/4, or 4/4

- Unexpected outcomes
- Troubleshooting attempts
- Additional interventions

References

1. Boysen PG. *The Role of Neuromuscular Blockers in Critical Care.* New York, NY: Wellcome Burroughs; 1992.
2. Ford EV. Monitoring neuromuscular blockade in the adult ICU. *Am J Crit Care.* 1995;4:122–132.
3. Shapiro BA, Warren J, Egol AB, et al. Practice parameters for sustained neuromuscular blockade in the adult critically ill patient: an executive summary. *Crit Care Med.* 1995;23:1601–1605.
4. Ali HH, Savarese JJ, Crowley MP. Monitoring the neuromuscular junction. In: Blitt CD, ed. *Monitoring in Anesthesia and Critical Care Medicine.* New York, NY: Churchill Livingstone; 1990:635–650.
5. Sgalio T. Monitoring the administration of neuromuscular blockade in critical care. *Crit Care Nurs Q.* 1995;18:41–59.
6. Leatherman JW, Fluegel WC, David WS, Davies SF, Iber C. Muscle weakness in mechanically ventilated patients with severe asthma. *Am J Respir Care Med.* 1996;153:1686–1690.
7. Segredo V, Caldwell JE, Matthay MA, Sharma ML, Gruenke LD, Miller RD. Persistent paralysis in critically ill patients after long-term administration of vecuronium. *N Engl J Med.* 1992;327:524–528.
8. Watling SM, Dasta JF. Prolonged paralysis in intensive care unit patients after the use of neuromuscular blocking agents: a review of the literature. *Crit Care Med.* 1994;22:884–893.
9. Rudis MI, Sikora CA, Angus E, et al. A prospective, randomized, controlled evaluation of peripheral nerve stimulation versus standard clinical dosing of neuromuscular blocking agents in critically ill patients. *Crit Care Med.* 1997;25:575–583.
10. Neurotechnology, Inc. *Instruction Manual for MicrostimPlus P/N 7100.* Kerrville, Tx: Neurotechnology, Inc.; 1991.
11. Connelly NR, Silverman DG, O'Connor TZ, Brull SJ. Subjective responses to train-of-four and double burst stimulation in awake patients. *Anesth Analg.* 1990;70:650–653.

Additional Readings

Caffrey RR, Warren ML, Becker K. Neuromuscular blockade monitoring comparing orbicularis oculi and adductor pollicis muscles. *Anesthesiology.* 1986;65:95–97.

Davidson JE. Neuromuscular blockade: indications, peripheral nerve stimulation, and other concurrent interventions. *New Horizons.* 1994;2:75–84.

Johnson KL, Cheung RB, Johnson SB, et al. Therapeutic paralysis of critically ill trauma patients: perceptions of patients and their family members. *Am J Crit Care.* 1999;8:490–498.

Saitoh Y, Nakazawa K, Toyooka H, Amaha K. Optimal stimulating current for train-of-four stimulation in conscious subjects. *Can J Anaesth.* 1995;42:992–995.

Tschida S, Hoey J, Lori L, Vance-Bryan K. Inconsistency with train-of-four monitoring in a critically ill paralyzed patient. *Pharmacotherapy.* 1995;15:540–545.

PROCEDURE

94

Esophagogastric Tamponade Tube

PURPOSE: Esophagogastric tamponade therapy is used to provide temporary control of bleeding from gastric or esophageal varices.

Michael W. Day

PREREQUISITE NURSING KNOWLEDGE

- Tamponade therapy exerts direct pressure against the varices with the use of a gastric or esophageal balloon and may be used as the primary treatment or for cases unresponsive to medical therapy. Tamponade therapy also is used to control bleeding pending sclerotherapy.[1]
- Esophagogastric tamponade tubes are used to control bleeding from either gastric or esophageal varices. The suction lumens allow the evacuation of accumulated blood from the stomach or esophagus. The suction lumens also allow for the intermittent instillation of saline to assist in the evacuation of blood or clots.
- There are three types of tubes available for esophagogastric tamponade therapy. The two most common are the Sengstaken-Blakemore and the Minnesota tubes. The three-lumen Sengstaken-Blakemore tube (Fig. 94–1) has a gastric and esophageal balloon and a gastric suction lumen. The four-lumen Minnesota tube (Fig. 94–2) has a gastric and esophageal balloon and separate gastric and esophageal suction lumens. The third, the Linton or Linton-Nachlas tube, has a gastric balloon and separate gastric and esophageal suction lumens and is used only for treatment of bleeding gastric varices. The Sengstaken-Blakemore and Minnesota tubes are considered the standard for esophagogastric tamponade therapy.
- Esophagogastric tamponade tubes may be introduced by either the nasogastric or orogastric routes. The tubes are then advanced through the oropharynx and esophagus and into the stomach.
- Relative contraindications include esophageal strictures or recent esophageal surgery.[2]

EQUIPMENT

- Tamponade tube (Sengstaken-Blakemore, Minnesota, or Linton-Nachlas)
- Irrigation kit (or catheter-tipped, 60-mL syringe and basin)
- Sphygmomanometer or pressure gauge
- Four rubber-shod clamps
- Adhesive tape
- Two suction setups and tubing
- Nasogastric (NG) tube(s)— one for Minnesota or Linton-Nachlas tube; two for Sengstaken-Blakemore tube
- Normal saline (NS)
- Water-soluble lubricant
- Topical anesthetic agent
- Bite block or oral airway
- Stethoscope
- Emergency intubation equipment
- Endotracheal suction equipment
- Cardiac monitor
- Atropine or transcutaneous pacemaker
- Scissors to be kept at bedside

Additional equipment (to have available based on patient need) includes the following:

- Rubber cube sponge (used for nasal intubation)
- Balanced suspension traction apparatus with 1 to 3 pounds of weights, or football helmet with face mask or guard (used for oral intubation)
- Suture material to secure NG tube to the Sengstaken-Blakemore tube

PATIENT AND FAMILY EDUCATION

- Explain the reason and procedure for the tube insertion.[1, 6] **➤Rationale:** Decreases patient anxiety.
- Explain the patient's role in assisting with the passage of the tube and maintenance of tamponade traction.[1] **➤Rationale:** Elicits patient cooperation during the insertion and tamponade therapy.
- Explain that the procedure can be uncomfortable, because the gag reflex may be stimulated, causing the patient to be nauseated or vomit.[1] **➤Rationale:** Elicits patient cooperation during the insertion.

PATIENT ASSESSMENT AND PREPARATION
Patient Assessment

- Signs and symptoms of major blood loss
  - ❖ Tachycardia

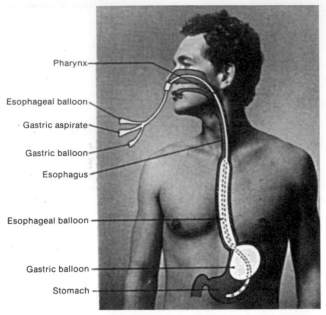

■ ● FIGURE 94–1. Sengstaken-Blakemore tube. (From Swearingen PL. *Photo Atlas of Nursing Procedures.* Reading, Ma: Addison-Wesley; 1991: 228.)

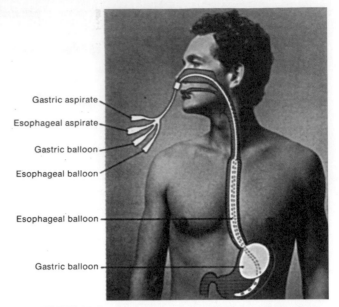

■ ● FIGURE 94–2. Minnesota four-lumen tube. (From Swearingen PL. *Photo Atlas of Nursing Procedures.* Reading, Ma: Addison-Wesley; 1991: 229.)

❖ Hypotension
❖ Decreased urine output
❖ Decreased filling pressures (PAP, PCWP, CVP)
❖ Decreased platelets
❖ Hematocrit and hemoglobin

➻**Rationale:** Esophageal or gastric varices can cause significant blood loss.

• Baseline cardiac rhythm.   ➻**Rationale:** Passage of a large-bore tube down the esophagus may cause vagal stimulation and bradycardia.

• Baseline respiratory status (ie, rate, depth, pattern, and characteristics of secretions).   ➻**Rationale:** Use of topical anesthetic agents in the nares or oropharynx may alter the gag or cough reflex, increasing the risk of aspiration. Passage of a large-bore tube may impair the airway. Large amounts of blood in the stomach predispose a patient to vomiting and potential aspiration.[2]

• If anticipating nasal intubation:
  ❖ Past medical history of nasal deformity, surgery, trauma, or epistaxis.   ➻**Rationale:** Increases the risk of complications with nasal insertion.
  ❖ Evaluate patency of nares. Occlude one naris at a time and ask the patient to breathe through the nose. Select the naris with the best air flow.   ➻**Rationale:** Choosing the most patent naris will ease insertion and may improve patient tolerance of the tube.

• Nausea or vomiting.   ➻**Rationale:** Nausea or vomiting increases the risk of aspiration during insertion of the tube.

• Mental status.   ➻**Rationale:** Patients with altered mental status should be intubated prophylactically to prevent airway complications.[2, 6]

Patient Preparation

• Ensure that patient understands preprocedural teaching. Answer questions as they arise and reinforce information as needed.   ➻**Rationale:** Evaluates and reinforces understanding of previously taught information.

• Measure the tube from the bridge of the nose to the earlobe to the tip of the xyphoid process (see Fig. 97–3). Mark the length of tube to be inserted.   ➻**Rationale:** Estimating the length of tube to be inserted will help place the distal tip in the stomach.

• If alert, place the patient in high-Fowler or semi-Fowler position. If the patient is unconscious or obtunded, place patient head down in the left lateral position.[2] Cover the patient's chest with a towel.   ➻**Rationale:** Facilitates the passage of the tube into the stomach and reduces the risk of aspiration.

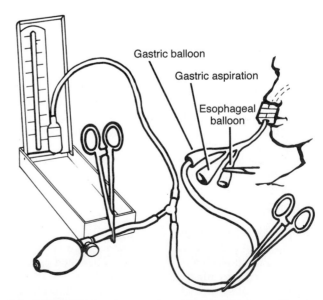

■ ● FIGURE 94–3. Inflation of esophageal balloon. (Courtesy of Davol, Inc.)

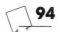

Procedure for Inserting Esophagogastric Tamponade Tube

Steps	Rationale	Special Considerations
1. Wash hands, and don personal protective equipment.	Reduces risk of transmission of microorganisms and body secretions; standard precautions.	
2. Attach the gastric balloon port to the sphygmomanometer or pressure gauge (Fig. 94–3).	Measuring the pressure of the gastric balloon as it is inflated immediately upon insertion may prevent its inflation in the esophagus, causing esophageal rupture.	
3. Test the tamponade tube balloon integrity: A. If applicable, inflate the esophageal balloon with the volume indicated in the package insert. *(Level I: Manufacturer's recommendation only)*	Ensures integrity of esophageal balloon.[3–5]	
B. Inflate the gastric balloon with 100, 200, 300, 400, and 500 mL of air, noting the pressure reading at each stage of inflation. *(Level I: Manufacturer's recommendation only)*	Knowing the pressure required at each stage of inflation may prevent inadvertent perforation of the esophagus after insertion.[3–5]	
C. Hold the air-filled balloon(s) under water to test for air leaks. *(Level I: Manufacturer's recommendation only)*	Ensures integrity of balloon(s).[3–5]	
D. Actively deflate the balloon(s) and clamp. *(Level I: Manufacturer's recommendation only)*	Deflated balloon will ease insertion.[6]	
4. Insert a nasogastric tube (see Procedure 97), lavage the stomach, and remove tube.	Emptying the stomach of blood will decrease the risk of aspiration[6] and blocking the tube with blood clots.	
5. Lubricate balloons and distal 15 cm of tube with water-soluble lubricant. *(Level IV: Limited clinical studies to support recommendations)*	Minimizes mucosal injury and irritation during insertion; facilitates insertion.	Use only water-soluble lubricant. Oil-based lubricants, such as petroleum jelly, may cause respiratory complications if inadvertently aspirated.
6. Apply the topical anesthetic agent to the posterior oropharynx (and nostril if nasally inserted). *(Level IV: Limited clinical studies to support recommendations)*	Decreases discomfort caused by insertion.[3–5]	Caution: gag and cough reflexes may be compromised by topical anesthetic, increasing the risk of aspiration. Keep emergency intubation equipment easily available.
7. Insert oral airway (see Procedure 7) or bite block if patient is to be orally intubated. *(Level II: Theory based, no research data to support recommendations; recommendations from expert consensus group may exist)*	Prevents patient from biting on tube or inserter's fingers.	Remove dentures, if present.
8. Ensure that balloons are completely deflated. *(Level II: Theory based, no research data to support recommendations; recommendations from expert consensus group may exist)*	Eases passage of tube.	

Procedure continued on following page

Procedure **for Inserting Esophagogastric Tamponade Tube** *Continued*

Steps	Rationale	Special Considerations
9. Insert tube into mouth or selected nostril and advance into stomach to at least the 50 cm mark on the tube or 10 cm beyond the estimated length needed to reach the stomach. *(Level I: Manufacturer's recommendation only)*	Ensures placement of entire gastric balloon in stomach.[3–5]	Heart rate may decrease as a result of vagal stimulation. Administer atropine or initiate transcutaneous pacing for symptomatic bradycardia.
10. Lavage stomach via gastric suction port with normal saline until clear of large blood clots. *(Level I: Manufacturer's recommendation only)*	Ensures patency and prevents clots from blocking the tube.[3–5]	
11. Connect gastric suction port to intermittent suction at 60 to 129 mm Hg. *(Level II: Theory based, no research data to support recommendations; recommendations from expert consensus may exist)*	Provides for evacuation of gastric contents and for assessment of continued bleeding.[2, 4]	
12. Connect esophageal suction port to intermittent suction at 120 to 200 mm Hg. *(Level II: Theory based, no research data to support recommendations; recommendations from expert consensus may exist)*	Provides for evacuation of secretions and for assessment of continued bleeding.[2, 4]	
13. Confirm tube placement: A. Aspirate drainage from gastric suction port. *(Level I: Manufacturer's recommendation only)*	Prevents gastric balloon from being inflated in the esophagus, causing rupture.[2] With pH testing, gastric placement will show a pH <5.5. Intestinal placement with show a pH >6.0. Pulmonary secretions have an alkaline pH.[1, 2]	The ability to simply aspirate fluid from the tube is often interpreted as confirmation of gastric intubation. Several reports[3, 4] have shown that fluid can also be aspirated after endotracheal intubation. Common practice for many years has been to evaluate tube placement by placing a stethoscope over the stomach and instilling 20 to 50 mL of air via syringe. There are numerous reports in the literature of false-positive results using this method. *(Level V: Clinical studies in more than one patient population and situation)*
B. *Slowly* inflate the gastric balloon with increments of 100 mL of air, up to a total 500 mL, observing the pressure on the sphygmomanometer or pressure gauge at each increment. (If the pressure exceeds preinflation pressure for a particular volume by more than 15 mm Hg, withdraw all of the air and advance tube an additional 10 cm.) *(Level I: Manufacturer's recommendation only)*	A pressure difference of more than 15 mm Hg indicates that the gastric balloon is in the esophagus.[3–5]	
C. Upon full inflation of the gastric balloon, clamp the gastric balloon lumen with a rubber-shod clamp. Obtain abdominal x-ray. *(Level I: Manufacturer's recommendation only)*	Outline of gastric balloon can be visualized on x-ray. Ensure placement of entire gastric balloon with the stomach.[2, 4, 5]	

Steps	**Rationale**	**Special Considerations**
14. Upon x-ray confirmation of placement, withdraw the tube until slight resistance is met and double clamp with rubber-shod clamp. *(Level I: Manufacturer's recommendation only)*	Inflated balloon fills stomach and creates tamponade effect. Positions gastric balloon at gastroesophageal junction. Clamps prevent air leak from gastric balloon.[3–5]	
15. Place tape marker around tube as it exits the mouth or nose. *(Level III: Laboratory data, no clinical data to support recommendations)*	Reference point to assess movement of tube.	
16. Inflate esophageal balloon if bleeding is not controlled by gastric tamponade. A. Clamp the tube and disconnect the sphygmomanometer or pressure gauge from the gastric balloon port and attach it to the esophageal balloon port. *(Level I: Manufacturer's recommendation only)*	Produces direct pressure on esophageal vessels.	Maintain esophageal balloon pressures as prescribed.
B. Gradually inflate the esophageal balloon to 25 to 45 mm Hg. *(Level I: Manufacturer's recommendation only)*	Higher pressures may cause esophageal necrosis.[3, 4, 7, 8]	Patient may experience chest pain with inflation.
C. Double clamp esophageal balloon port with rubber-shod clamps. *(Level I: Manufacturer's recommendation only)*	Prevents air leaks from esophageal balloon.	
17. If bleeding has not stopped, apply gentle traction on the tube. *(Level II: Theory based, no research data to support recommendations; recommendations from consensus group may exist)* A. Apply gentle traction with 1 to 3 pounds of weight attached to tube using balance suspension traction. (Fig. 94–4) OR B. Tape tube to sponge cube at naris, if tube is passed nasally. C. Apply football helmet to patient and tape tube to chin or faceguard (Fig. 94–5).	Fixes position of gastric balloon and exerts pressure on varices.[1–6]	Pad inside of helmet to prevent pressure ulcer formation on back of head.
18. Place the head of the bed at 30 to 45 degrees. *(Level IV: Limited clinical data support recommendations)*	Promotes comfort and prevents aspiration.[1, 4, 5, 7]	
19. Insert an NG tube (see Procedure 97) to just above esophageal balloon. *(Level II: Theory based, no research data to support recommendations; recommendations from expert consensus group may exist)* A. Secure the NG tube to the tamponade tube with a suture where it exits the mouth. B. Connect to intermittent suction 120 to 200 mm Hg (Sengstaken-Blakemore only).	Removes secretions and accumulated blood.[1, 3]	

Procedure continued on page 661

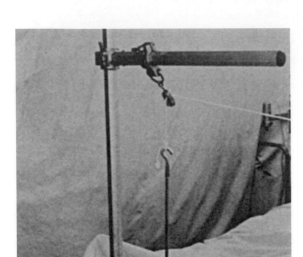

■ ● **FIGURE 94–4.** Balanced suspension traction securing tamponade tube and placement. (From DeGroot KD, Damato M. *Critical Care Skills.* Norwalk, Ct: Appleton & Lange; 1987: 257.)

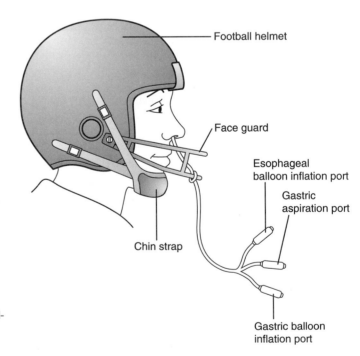

■ ● **FIGURE 94–5.** Tamponade tube secured in position with helmet.

Procedure	**for Inserting Esophagogastric Tamponade Tube** *Continued*	

Steps	Rationale	Special Considerations
Discontinuing Tamponade Therapy		
20. Discontinue tamponade therapy in stages. *(Level I: Manufacturer's recommendation only)*	Provides for gradual reduction in tamponade in order to assess cessation of bleeding.	Never deflate gastric balloon while esophageal balloon remains inflated.[7] A deflated gastric balloon may allow an inflated esophageal balloon to migrate in the airway. *If the airway becomes obstructed, cut both balloon ports to deflate the balloons and remove the tube immediately.*
A. Deflate esophageal balloon by unclamping the esophageal balloon port and aspirating with an irrigation syringe to actively deflate the balloon.		
B. Observe for the recurrence of bleeding over 4 hours. If bleeding recurs, reinflate the esophageal balloon.	Bleeding may recur with the release of pressure on the esophageal varices.[4]	
C. Deflate the gastric balloon by unclamping the gastric balloon port and aspirating with an irrigation syringe to actively deflate the balloon.		
D. Observe for the recurrence of bleeding over 4 hours. If bleeding recurs, reinflate the gastric balloon.	Bleeding may recur with the release of pressure on the gastric varices.[4]	Recurrence of bleeding.
21. Cut the balloon lumens with scissors and remove tube slowly. *(Level I: Manufacturer's recommendation only)*	Ensures complete balloon deflation before removal.[4]	Recurrence of bleeding.

Expected Outcomes	Unexpected Outcomes
• Cessation of variceal bleeding • Gastric decompression and evacuation	• Inappropriate placement of tamponade tube • Gastric or esophageal necrosis • Esophageal rupture • Airway obstruction • Cardiac dysrhythmias (during insertion or removal) • Aspiration of gastric or oropharyngeal contents • Erosion of mucosa around nares

Patient Monitoring and Care

Patient Monitoring and Care	Rationale	Reportable Conditions
		These conditions should be reported if they persist despite nursing interventions.
1. Maintain tamponade therapy as needed; maximum of 24 to 36 hours for esophageal balloon, 48 to 72 hours for gastric balloon. *(Level II: Theory based, no research data to support recommendations; recommendations from expert consensus group may exist)*	Longer inflation time may cause necrosis or ulceration.[1, 3, 4, 6]	• Continued bleeding

Continued on following page

Patient Monitoring and Care	Rationale	Reportable Conditions
2. Provide nares care every 2 hours when tube is inserted nasally. *(Level IV: Limited clinical studies to support recommendations)* A. Remove dried blood or secretions from nasal orifice and proximal narves. B. Apply lubricating ointment or gel to keep mucosa moist.	Prevents drying and ulcerations of mucosa.	• Breakdown of tissue around nares
3. Provide oral care every 2 hours. Swab mouth with cleansing agents and mechanical débriders. *(Level IV: Limited clinical studies to support recommendations)*	Prevents drying and ulcerations of mucosa.	• Mouth, tongue, or lip ulcerations
4. Provide frequent oral suctioning. *(Level II: Theory based, no research data to support recommendations; recommendations from expert consensus group may exist)*	Esophageal balloon prevents swallowing of secretions and saliva.[3]	• Bloody oral secretions
5. Monitor esophageal balloon pressure hourly. Maintain esophageal balloon pressures at 25 to 45 mm Hg (pressures will vary with respirations and may intermittently reach 70 mm Hg). *(Level II: Theory based, no research data to support recommendations; recommendations from expert consensus group may exist)*	Prevents excessive pressure on esophageal tissues.[1, 3, 6] Sudden loss of pressure may indicate rupture of balloon or esophagus.	• Continued esophageal bleeding • Sudden loss of balloon pressure
6. Decrease esophageal balloon pressure by 5 mm Hg every 3 hours until pressure is 25 mm Hg, without evidence of bleeding. *(Level II: Theory based, no research data to support recommendations; recommendations from expert consensus group may exist)*	Using the lowest possible pressure to create tamponade effect will decrease the possibility of necrosis.[4]	• Continued esophageal bleeding
7. Completely deflate the esophageal balloon for 5 minutes every 6 hours. *(Level II: Theory based, no research data to support recommendations; recommendations from expert consensus group may exist)*	Intermittent relief of the pressure may prevent necrosis of esophageal tissue.[6, 7]	• Continued esophageal bleeding
8. Evaluate for recurrence of variceal bleeding. *(Level II: Theory based, no research data to support recommendations; recommendations from expert consensus group may exist)*	Bleeding may occur despite tamponade therapy.	• Continued bleeding
9. Monitor for airway patency and respiratory status. *(Level II: Theory based, no research data to support recommendations; recommendations from expert consensus group may exist)*	Presence or movement of a large-bore tube may impair the upper airway.	• Tachypnea • Stridor • Cough

Patient Monitoring and Care *Continued*

Patient Monitoring and Care	Rationale	Reportable Conditions
10. Maintain scissors at the bedside to immediately deflate the balloons. *(Level II: Theory based, no research data to support recommendations; recommendations from expert consensus group may exist)*	Inadvertent deflation of the gastric balloon may allow blockage of the airway by the esophageal balloon.[1,2,7]	
11. Monitor gastric output. Irrigate gastric suction port with 50 mL of normal saline every 30 minutes, or as needed, to keep lumen patent. *(Level I: Manufacturer's recommendation only)*	Blood clots may occlude the gastric lumen.[3]	• Continued gastric bleeding • Change in characteristics of output (color, quantity)
12. Monitor esophageal output. Irrigate esophageal suction port (or NG with Sengstaken-Blakemore) with 5 to 10 mL of normal saline every 2 to 4 hours, or as needed, to keep patent. *(Level I: Manufacturer's recommendation only)*	Blood clots may occlude the esophageal suction lumen (or NG tube).[3]	• Continued esophageal bleeding • Change in characteristics of drainage (color, quantity)

Documentation

Documentation should include the following:

- Patient and family education
- Date and time of insertion
- Name of tube inserter, if other than nurse documenting
- Tube type
- Any difficulties with insertion
- Patient tolerance of insertion
- Confirmation of placement
- Type and maintenance of traction device
- Amount and type of suction applied to various lumens
- Esophageal or gastric balloon pressures
- Periodic deflation of esophageal balloon
- Appearance and volume of gastric and esophageal drainage, if present
- Nasal or oral care
- Maintenance of traction
- Tube site assessments (nasal or oral)
- Unexpected outcomes
- Nursing interventions
- Deflation sequence of tubes

References

1. Smith SL. Gastrointestinal system. In: Clochesy JM, Breu C, Cardin S, et al. *Critical Care Nursing.* 2nd ed. Philadelphia, Pa: W.B. Saunders; 1996:1048–1090.
2. Pasquale MD, Cerra FB. Sengstaken-Blakemore tube placement. *Crit Care Clin North Am.* 1992;8:743–753.
3. Davol, Inc. *Blakemore Esophageal-Nasogastric Tube: Instructions for Passing the Esophageal Balloon for the Control of Bleeding for Esophageal Varices.* Cranston, Ri: Davol, Inc.; 1985.
4. Davol, Inc. *Minnesota Four Lumen Esophagogastric Tamponade Tube for Control of Bleeding from Esophageal Varices.* Cranston, Ri: Davol, Inc.; 1985.
5. Barefield LB, personal communication, October 7, 1998.
6. Kerber K. The adult with bleeding esophageal varices. *Crit Care Clin North Am.* 1993;5:153–162.
7. Coy DL, Blei AT. Portal hypertension. In: Haubrich WS, Schaffner F, eds. *Bockus Gastroenterology.* 5th ed. Philadelphia, Pa: W.B. Saunders; 1995:1955–1987.
8. Gastrointestinal disorders and therapeutic management. In: Thelan LA, et al. *Critical Care Nursing: Diagnosis and Management.* 3rd ed. St. Louis, Mo: Mosby; 1998;945–972.

Additional Readings

Matloff DS. Treatment of acute variceal bleeding. *Gastroenterol Clin North Am.* 1992;21:103–118.
Navarro VJ, Garcia-Tsao G. Variceal hemorrhage. *Crit Care Clin North Am.* 1995;11:391–414.

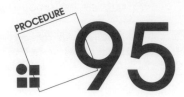

95

Gastric Lavage in Hemorrhage and in Overdose

P U R P O S E: In hemorrhage, gastric lavage is used to localize the site and severity of upper gastrointestinal (GI) bleeding, monitor for continued bleeding, cleanse the stomach of blood and clots in preparation for endoscopy or endoscopic treatments (such as scleral therapy), decrease or prevent absorption of a high nitrogen load, and prevent aspiration of blood. In overdose, gastric lavage is used to evacuate drugs or toxins and therefore prevent or minimize both the serious consequences of systemic absorption of drugs or toxins and damage to the GI tissue.

Robin H. Thomas

PREREQUISITE NURSING KNOWLEDGE

- Major upper GI hemorrhage leads to severe volume loss and significant decrease in oxygen-carrying capacity of the blood, putting the patient at risk for life-threatening complications.
- Signs and symptoms of major blood loss include tachycardia, hypotension, decreased hemodynamic filling pressures, pallor, cold and clammy skin, and decreased urine output.
- Gastric lavage should be carefully considered in patients with esophageal varices or a history of recent gastric surgery because of the risk of GI hemorrhage or perforation.
- Ingestion of large amounts of drugs or toxins into the GI tract can put the patient at risk for potentially lethal consequences, such as cardiac dysrhythmias and respiratory depression.
- Several methods may be used to remove drugs or toxins from the GI tract. These include induced vomiting, gastric lavage, administration of activated charcoal, and whole bowel irrigation.
- Indications for gastric lavage in drug or toxin ingestion include symptomatic patients who
  - ❖ present within one hour of ingestion,
  - ❖ have ingested a life-threatening amount of drug or toxin so that a sufficient dose of activated charcoal cannot be given to absorb the drug, or
  - ❖ are hemodynamically unstable and present with an unknown substance and time of ingestion.[1, 2]
- Gastric lavage following toxin ingestion is contraindicated in patients who have ingested strong corrosives, sharp objects, or hydrocarbons.

- Gastric lavage following overdose or toxin ingestion has variable efficacy. The amount of toxin or drug recovered depends on variables such as time from ingestion, whether liquid or pills were ingested, specific agent ingested, and size of lavage tube used. Even if lavage is performed close to the time of ingestion, not all the ingested toxin will be recovered.
- Lavaging or cleansing of the stomach is accomplished by instilling large amounts of neutral fluid (normal saline [NS] or tap water) into the stomach and then draining the gastric contents and lavage fluid out of the stomach.
- Patients with altered mental status can safely have gastric lavage performed. All patients receiving gastric lavage should be positioned in the left lateral or semi-Fowler position to prevent aspiration. If the gag reflex is not intact, the patient should be endotracheally intubated before gastric lavage.
- Passage of the lavage tube may cause vagal stimulation and precipitate bradydysrhythmias.

EQUIPMENT

- Lavage tube
  - ❖ Number 32- to 40-Fr gastric tube (Ewald or Lavaculator) *or*
  - ❖ Number 16- to 18-Fr Levine tube or Salem sump
- Irrigating kit with 50- to 60-mL irrigating syringe
- Water-soluble lubricant
- Lavage fluid (NS or tap water)
- Disposable basin for aspirate
- Suction source and connecting tubing
- Rigid pharyngeal suction-tip (Yankauer) catheter
- Topical anesthetic agent

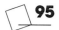

- Bite block or oral airway
- Continuous lavage kit (if available) or the following:
  - ❖ Y connector
  - ❖ Infusion tubing
  - ❖ Tapered connector
  - ❖ Soft latex connecting tubing
  - ❖ Drainage container
  - ❖ Two rubber-shod clamps
  - ❖ Two 1-in pieces of soft latex tubing (if needed)
- Stethoscope
- Emergency intubation equipment
- Endotracheal suction equipment
- Cardiac monitor
- Pulse oximeter
- Automatic blood pressure cuff
- Nonsterile gloves
- Eye and face protection
- Barrier gowns

Additional equipment (to have available based on patient need) includes the following:

- Specimen container for aspirate (for overdose)
- Absorptive agent for instillation (for overdose, if prescribed)
- Atropine, 1 mg (if needed)

PATIENT AND FAMILY EDUCATION

- Explain the indications and procedure for gastric lavage. ➻**Rationale:** Decreases patient and family anxiety.
- Explain the patient's role in assisting with passage of the tube and lavage of the stomach. ➻**Rationale:** Elicits patient's cooperation during the procedure.
- Explain the purpose of the cardiac monitor, automatic blood pressure cuff, and pulse oximeter. ➻**Rationale:** Decreases patient and family anxiety.
- Evaluate patient and family need for information on prevention of accidental ingestion of drugs or toxic agents. ➻**Rationale:** Patient and family may be unaware or uninformed that the agent or drug is (potentially) toxic.
- Evaluate patient and family need for information on emergency treatment for accidental ingestion of drug or toxic agents. ➻**Rationale:** Emergency first aid measures may be helpful with some ingestions to decrease potential toxicity or systemic absorption.

PATIENT ASSESSMENT AND PREPARATION
Patient Assessment

- Baseline respiratory, cardiovascular, and neurologic assessments; hemodynamic status; cardiac rhythm; and vital signs. ➻**Rationale:** Passage of the lavage tube may cause vagal stimulation and precipitate bradydysrhythmias. In the overdose patient, toxic levels of certain classes of drugs (eg, tricyclic antidepressants) can cause electrocardiogram (ECG) changes. Gastric lavage has been shown to cause ECG changes, especially in older smokers.[3]
- Baseline pulse oximetry. ➻**Rationale:** Gastric lavage has been shown to cause changes in oxygen saturation, especially in older smokers.[3]
- Signs and symptoms of major blood loss, as follows:
  - ❖ Tachycardia
  - ❖ Hypotension
  - ❖ Decreased hemodynamic filling pressures
  - ❖ Pallor, cold and clammy skin
  - ❖ Decreased urine output. ➻**Rationale:** Esophageal or gastric varices can cause significant blood loss.
- History of esophageal varices, recent esophageal or gastric surgery. ➻**Rationale:** Varices or recent surgery may predispose the patient to complications during tube insertion.
- Baseline coagulation studies, hematocrit and hemoglobin, and liver function tests (GI hemorrhage patient and overdose cases where toxin ingested is liver toxic). ➻**Rationale:** Provides for baseline information so that patient progress can be more accurately monitored.
- Adequacy of gag reflex. ➻**Rationale:** For the overdose patient, induced vomiting may be the treatment of choice if the patient is alert and awake with an adequate gag reflex, making lavage unnecessary.
- Drugs or toxic substances ingested as well as quantity ingested (for the overdose patient). ➻**Rationale:** Certain substances may require neutralization before attempting tube evacuation. A poison control center should be contacted if the practitioner is unsure that lavage is indicated. Side effects can be anticipated if the drugs or toxins that were swallowed as well as the quantity are known.
- Careful skin assessment (overdose patient). ➻**Rationale:** May give evidence regarding route (needle tracks) and name of drug or toxin ingested. Various drugs can cause cutaneous changes. Changes to look for include diaphoresis, bullae, acneiform rash, flushed appearance, and cyanosis.
- Odors present (overdose patient). ➻**Rationale:** Some toxins have a distinctive odor, aiding in identification of substance ingested.
- 12-lead ECG. ➻**Rationale:** For the overdose victim, the drug or toxin ingested may be cardiotoxic. For the patient with a GI hemorrhage, comorbid disease states may increase risk of tissue hypoxia and ischemia.
- Serum toxicology screen, urinalysis and urine toxicology screen, and anion gap (overdose victim). ➻**Rationale:** Provides baseline information for diagnosis so that intervention can be made appropriately and patient progress can be more accurately monitored.
- Arterial blood gas (ABG). ➻**Rationale:** Overdose victims with hypoventilation and GI hemorrhage patients with significant blood loss or comorbid disease are at risk for hypoxia.

Patient Preparation

- Ensure that patient understands preprocedural teaching. Answer questions as they arise, and reinforce information as needed. ➻**Rationale:** Evaluates and reinforces understanding of previously taught information.
- Place the patient on a cardiac monitor, automatic blood pressure cuff, and pulse oximeter. Set up oropharyngeal suction. ➻**Rationale:** Allows for close cardiovascular

and respiratory monitoring during the procedure and makes suction available for procedure.

- Establish and maintain intravenous (IV) access. For the GI hemorrhage patient, two large-bore (18-G or larger) IVs are essential. →*Rationale:* IV access is necessary for emergency IV medication administration and volume resuscitation in the case of GI hemorrhage.
- Position patient in left lateral or semi-Fowler

position. →*Rationale:* Facilitates passage of the tube into the stomach. The left lateral position is the position of choice if the patient should vomit, to prevent aspiration.

- Apply oxygen by nasal prongs or mask (GI hemorrhage patient or overdose patient as indicated). →*Rationale:* Supplemental oxygen will optimize the patient's oxygen saturation.

Procedure **for Gastric Lavage in Hemorrhage and in Overdose**

Steps	Rationale	Special Considerations
1. Wash hands, and don nonsterile gloves, eye and face protection, and a barrier gown.	Reduces transmission of microorganisms; standard precautions.	
2. Coat 6 to 10 cm of the distal end of the lavage tube with water-soluble lubricant.	Minimizes mucosal injury and irritation during insertion of the tube.	
3. Place the bed in a 15-degree Trendelenburg position.	In cases of toxic ingestion, the slight Trendelenburg position will decrease movement of stomach contents into the duodenum. This position also aids in siphoning contents out of the stomach.	Patients may not be able to tolerate a head-down position because of underlying medical conditions and decreased oxygen-carrying capacity. A semi-Fowler position should be used in these cases.
4. Insert Ewald or Lavaculator tube.	A large-bore tube (number 32 to 40 Fr) is preferred for the evacuation of blood, clots, undigested pills or pill fragments. A smaller-bore tube may become occluded with solid material. The Ewald tube is softer but has only one distal opening. The Lavaculator tube has additional holes along the side of the tube.[4]	Do not pass nasally because severe nasal trauma will occur. If the patient does not have an intact gag reflex, endotracheal intubation should be done first. The patient may require physical restraint to allow passage of the lavage tube.
A. Measure distance from patient's ear to bridge of nose and then from nose to tip of xiphoid process (see Fig. 97–3). Mark this distance on the tube.		
B. Anesthetize posterior oropharynx with topical anesthetic agent, as ordered.	Decreases discomfort caused by passing tube.	The gag reflex may be compromised by topical anesthesia, increasing the risk of aspiration. Have emergency intubation equipment available.
C. Insert oral airway (see Procedure 7) or bite block.	Prevents patients from biting on tube or inserter's fingers.	Remove patient dentures.
D. Position tube toward posterior pharynx over tongue.		Heart rate may decrease as a result of vagal stimulation, especially if the patient has ingested toxic amounts of digoxin. Have atropine (or transcutaneous pacer) ready, and use as necessary.
E. Pass tube slowly into stomach (approximately 20 in). Encourage patient to attempt to swallow while passing tube.	Rapid passage of tube may stimulate vomiting and increase risk of aspiration. The swallowing maneuver causes the epiglottis to close the trachea and directs the tube into the esophagus.	Have oropharyngeal suction available.
5. *Or* insert (number 16 to 18 Fr) Levin tube or Salem sump (see Procedure 97).	The larger lumen helps prevent the drainage ports from becoming occluded with clots or pill fragments. In overdose, a smaller lumen may be used with ingestion of liquid agents or liquefied tablets or capsules.	

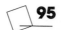

Procedure **for Gastric Lavage in Hemorrhage and in Overdose** *Continued*

Steps	Rationale	Special Considerations
6. Aspirate with syringe for return of stomach contents. The aspirate can be tested with pH paper to confirm gastric placement (acid pH).[5] *(Level V: Clinical studies in more than one patient population and situation)*	The position of the lavage tube must be confirmed to be in the stomach because of the risk of endotracheal placement of the lavage tube and subsequent pulmonary complications. X-ray confirmation of lavage tube placement has been suggested in the literature.[6] With pH testing, gastric placement will show a pH <5.5. Intestinal placement will show a pH >6.0. Pulmonary secretions have an alkaline pH.[5]	
7. After placement is confirmed, aspirate gastric contents through lavage tube using irrigating syringe. In GI hemorrhage, instead of aspirating, stomach contents can be allowed to drain by gravity into a large collection container.	Hand aspiration will withdraw gastric contents and toxic agents or blood and clots out of the stomach.	In cases of overdose, put specimen in specimen container and send to laboratory for analysis.
8. Perform intermittent lavage (using either room-temperature saline or tap water). *(Level III: Laboratory data, no clinical data to support recommendations)*	In overdose, lavage aids in diluting toxic agents and removing them from the stomach before absorption. In GI hemorrhage, lavage aids in breaking up clots and rinsing the stomach of blood. In GI hemorrhage, iced solutions may predispose the patient to hypothermia and will prolong bleeding time.[8, 9] Room-temperature solutions have been shown to be effective in clearing the stomach of clots and promoting hemostasis. No benefit has been shown in using saline over tap water for lavage with GI bleeding.[10]	The use of NS may lead to hypernatremia in patients with renal failure.[7]
A. Instill lavage fluid into lavage tube using irrigating syringe. (For adults, use 100 to 150 mL of fluid.[11])		For the elderly patient, the lavage fluid should be slightly warmed to prevent hypothermia. (Bottles of NS may be submerged in warm water before use as an irrigant.)
B. Aspirate gastric contents through lavage tube using irrigating syringe.	Evacuates stomach contents and clots or ingested toxic agents.	With hemorrhage, lavage fluid may be drained immediately or retained in the stomach for up to 30 minutes to facilitate dissolving of clots. The amount returned should equal the amount instilled.
C. *Or* allow gastric contents to drain by gravity into a large collection container.		
D. *Or* connect lavage tube to <80 mm Hg suction (GI hemorrhage patient).	Low levels of suction should be used to prevent suction-induced mucosal damage.	
E. For GI hemorrhage patients, continue intermittent lavage until returns are clear and free of clots. For overdose patients, lavage should continue once returns are clear for an additional 1 to 2 L of fluid. *(Level IV: Limited clinical studies to support recommendations)*	In overdose patients, lavaging with an additional 1 to 2 L after the aspirate is clear has been shown to allow recovery of more of the ingested materials as compared with lavaging only until the aspirate is clear.[12]	

Procedure continued on following page

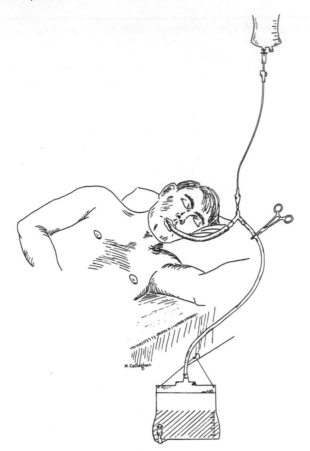

■ ● **FIGURE 95–1.** Continuous lavage system.

Procedure	**for Gastric Lavage in Hemorrhage and in Overdose** *Continued*

Steps	Rationale	Special Considerations
9. *Or* perform continuous lavage (Fig. 95–1).	In overdose, lavage aids in diluting toxic agents and removing them from the stomach before absorption. In GI hemorrhage lavage, it aids in breaking up clots and rinsing the stomach of blood.	
A. Assemble all equipment.		
○ Connect infusion tubing to lavage fluid container.		
○ Connect distal end of infusion tubing to stem of Y connector.		If not using a preassembled lavage kit, a 1-in piece of soft latex tubing may be required to connect the infusion tubing to the stem of the Y connector.
○ Connect one limb of Y connector to lavage tube.		A tapered connector may be needed to fit the tube and the limb of the Y connector. A 1-in piece of soft latex tubing may be required to connect the tapered connector to the Y connector.
○ Attach connecting tubing to other limb of Y connector.		
○ Attach distal end of connecting tubing to drainage container.		

Procedure	**for Gastric Lavage in Hemorrhage and in Overdose** *Continued*

Steps	Rationale	Special Considerations
B. Instill lavage fluid (room-temperature NS or tap water). *(Level III: Laboratory data, no clinical data to support recommendations)*	In GI hemorrhage, research has shown that iced solutions may predispose the patient to hypothermia and will prolong bleeding time.[8, 9] Room-temperature solutions have been shown to be effective in clearing the stomach of clots and promoting hemostasis. No benefit has been shown in using NS over tap water for lavage with GI bleeding.[10]	The lavage fluid should be slightly warmed in the elderly patient to prevent hypothermia. (A fluid or blood warmer may be used to warm the irrigant as it infuses.) The use of NS may lead to hypernatremia in patients with renal failure.[7]
○ Clamp connecting tubing just distal to the Y connector (outflow side of system) with a rubber-shod clamp.		
○ Open clamp on infusion tubing and instill room-temperature NS or tap water in desired amount into stomach (usually 100- to 150-mL increments in adults[11]).		
○ Close clamp on infusion tubing.		Lavage fluid may be retained in stomach for 30 minutes before draining to facilitate dissolving clots.
C. Remove clamp on connecting tubing (outflow side).	Allow fluid to siphon from stomach into drainage container.	Speed and amount siphoned depend on height of siphon column. To increase speed of and amount siphoned, raise height of patient in reference to drainage container.
D. Allow gastric contents to drain by gravity into drainage container.		
E. For the GI hemorrhage patient, repeat Step 9, B through D, until returns are clear. For the patient with an overdose, repeat Step 9, B through D, until returns are free of particulate matter, and then lavage with an additional 1 to 2 L of fluid. *(Level IV: Limited clinical studies to support recommendations)*	In overdose patients, lavaging with an additional 1 to 2 L after the aspirate is clear has been shown to allow recovery of more of the ingested materials as compared with lavaging only until the aspirate is clear.[12]	
10. Remove Ewald or Lavaculator tube, if used. If the lavage tube is not able to be removed easily, the patient may be experiencing esophageal spasm and the tube may be impacted. Glucagon can be administered via the subcutaneous or intramuscular route. *(Level IV: Limited clinical studies to support recommendations)*	Glucagon can decrease esophageal spasm and allow removal of impacted lavage tubes. Contraindications to the use of glucagon include a history of pheochromocytoma, insulinoma, or Zollinger-Ellison syndrome.[13]	
A. Clamp lavage tube with rubber-shod clamp.	Prevents leakage of contents remaining within lumen and possible aspiration of contents during removal.	
B. Pull tube out slowly and steadily.	Minimizes risk of vomiting.	

Procedure continued on following page

| Procedure | **for Gastric Lavage in Hemorrhage and in Overdose** *Continued* |

Steps	Rationale	Special Considerations
11. Insert nasogastric (NG) (see Procedure 97) tube, if needed. Instill medications as ordered. The NG tube should be clamped after medication instillation.	For the overdose victim, an NG tube provides access to the stomach for administration of activated charcoal. Activated charcoal is used for absorption of the residual substance ingested (unable to be removed by lavage). If the patient is alert and has an intact gag reflex, activated charcoal can be swallowed. For the GI hemorrhage patient, the NG tube may also allow for close assessment of further bleeding. However, the presence of an NG tube can cause further mucosal damage during insertion or if connected to suction.	Before administration of activated charcoal, the bottle must be mixed well.
12. Dispose of equipment in appropriate receptacle.	Standard precautions.	
13. Remove barrier gown, face and eye protection, and gloves. Wash hands.	Reduces transmission of microorganisms.	

Expected Outcomes	Unexpected Outcomes

Expected Outcomes

- Evacuation of blood and clots from the stomach
- Prevention of blood aspiration
- Prevention of absorption of high nitrogen load
- Prevention or minimization of systemic complications secondary to the absorption of drugs or toxic agents
- Minimization of mucosal damage by toxic agents

Unexpected Outcomes

- Endotracheal intubation rather than gastric intubation with lavage tube
- Esophageal perforation
- Trauma to the nose, throat, or esophagus
- Epistaxis if NG route is used for lavage
- Hypothermia in the elderly patient
- Bradydysrhythmias
- Pulmonary aspiration of gastric contents
- Movement of gastric contents into the small bowel, potentially increasing the amount of toxin absorbed
- Fluid and electrolyte imbalance

| Patient Monitoring and Care |

Patient Monitoring and Care	Rationale	Reportable Conditions
		These conditions should be reported if they persist despite nursing interventions.
1. Monitor vital signs every 15 minutes throughout the procedure and every hour following lavage for at least 4 hours, longer dependent on patient condition.	Continued blood loss or side effects of drugs or toxins ingested may cause changes in vital signs. Cold lavage fluid may cause hypothermia in the elderly patient.	• Increase in heart rate 10 to 20 beats above baseline • Decrease in blood pressure 20 to 30 mm Hg below baseline • Respiratory rate <8 or >24 breaths per minute • Temperature <97.5°F (36.5°C) or >101°F (38°C)
2. Monitor neurologic status continuously throughout procedure and after lavage.	Side effects from toxic agents ingested or significant blood loss may lead to decrease in level of consciousness.	• Decreasing level of consciousness • Loss of gag reflex

Patient Monitoring and Care *Continued*

Patient Monitoring and Care	Rationale	Reportable Conditions

3. Monitor respiratory status continuously throughout procedure and after lavage.
  ○ Pulse oximetry
  ○ Respiratory rate
  ○ Ease of breathing
	Aspiration is a potential complication because of change in level of consciousness, loss of gag reflex, or vomiting. Pulse oximetry values have been shown to decrease during gastric lavage, especially in older smokers.[3]	• Decrease in oximetry below baseline or 92%
		• Increase in respiratory rate above baseline
		• Complaints of shortness of breath

4. Monitor cardiac status continuously throughout procedure and after lavage.
  ○ Heart rate
  ○ Heart rhythm
  ○ ECG intervals
  ○ Signs and symptoms of decreased cardiac output
	Bradydysrhythmias may be caused by passage of the lavage tube. Toxic effect of drugs ingested may also cause ECG changes, including prolongation of the PR, QRS, and QT intervals. ECG changes have been shown during gastric lavage, especially in older smokers.[3]	• Heart rate less than 60 beats per minute with or without a decrease in blood pressure below baseline or the presence of other symptoms including chest pain, diaphoresis, change in level of consciousness, and shortness of breath
		• Change in ECG rhythm or length of PR, QRS, and QT intervals from baseline

5. Assess for normal pharyngeal function. After lavage, keep patient in left lateral position with slight head elevation until normal gag reflex returns.	Topical anesthesia will decrease the gag reflex and increase the risk of aspiration. The left lateral position is the position of choice to prevent aspiration should the patient not be able to control secretions or vomit.	• Prolonged absence of gag reflex

6. For the GI hemorrhage patient
  ○ Measure blood volume loss.
 	
  ○ Monitor for recurrence of bleeding, color, and consistency of gastric drainage, serial hemoglobin and hematocrit, postural vital signs, urine output, and change in level of consciousness.
	Aids in assessment of fluid balance and fluid resuscitation requirements.
	
	Cessation of bleeding with lavage may be temporary.
		• Bright red emesis or bleeding from the lavage tube or NG tube inserted after lavage
		• Decrease in hemoglobin or hematocrit below baseline
		• Decrease in blood pressure 20 to 30 mm Hg below baseline
		• Increase in pulse 10 to 20 beats per minute above baseline
		• Urine output <30 mL/hr
		• Increasing confusion or decreasing level of consciousness

○ Administer NS or lactated Ringer's injection at 150 to 200 mL/hr. Switch to administration of packed cells or whole blood when available for volume replacement.	Volume replacement and prevention of hemorrhagic shock.	
○ Administer antacids, histamine$_2$ (H$_2$) blockers, sucralfate, or omeprazole as ordered by physician.	Antacids neutralize gastric acid. H$_2$ blockers decrease gastric acid secretion. Sucralfate reacts with gastric acid, forming a paste, which adheres to ulcer sites. Omeprazole inhibits the proton pump in the parietal cells of the stomach, suppressing gastric acid secretion.	
○ In the hours and days following lavage, evaluate blood ammonia levels in patients with liver failure.	The ammonia level provides an estimate of the nitrogen load that has been absorbed and helps determine the need for agents (Lactulose) to prevent the absorption of ammonia from the bowel.	• Rising serum ammonia level • Increasing confusion or decreasing level of consciousness
7. For the overdose victim ○ Evaluate the patient's need for follow-up psychiatric support for suicide ideation.	The drug or toxin ingestion may be a result of suicidal ideations.	• Patient reports intent to harm self • Patient reports that ingestion was a suicide attempt

Continued on following page

Patient Monitoring and Care *Continued*

Patient Monitoring and Care	Rationale	Reportable Conditions
○ Institute suicide precautions until patient has been cleared by psychiatric services. This includes removal of objects from patient's room that could be used by patient to harm self.		
○ In the hours and days following ingestion, repeat laboratory tests, including electrolytes, glucose, blood urea nitrogen and creatinine, liver function, and drug or toxin levels.	Laboratory tests ordered will depend on the drug or toxins ingested. Lavage may cause electrolyte abnormalities. Liver function tests may be necessary if the drug is toxic to the liver. Drug or toxin level tests will validate the clearance of the drug or toxin from the patient's system.	• Variation of various tests outside normal limits

Documentation

Documentation should include the following:

- Patient and family education
- History of ingestion of drug or toxin *or* upper GI bleeding
- Date, time, and reason for lavage
- Type and size of lavage tube inserted
- Patient tolerance of tube placement and lavage procedure
- Verification of lavage tube placement (method used)
- Type and amount of lavage fluid used
- Unexpected outcomes

- Nursing interventions
- Amount and characteristics of aspirate
- Assessment of gastric drainage after lavage
- Name and dose of medications given after the lavage
- Aspirated specimen sent to laboratory for analysis
- Size of NG tube inserted after lavage
- Patient tolerance of NG tube insertion

References

1. Vale JA. Position statement: gastric lavage. American academy of clinical toxicology; European association of poison centres and clinical toxicologists. *J Toxicol Clin Toxicol.* 1997;35:711–719.
2. Hoffman R. The inquiring toxicologist; old myths and new realities. *Emerg Med.* 1997;29:64–78.
3. Thompson AM, Robins JB, Prescott LF. Changes in cardiorespiratory function during gastric lavage for drug overdose. *Hum Toxicol.* 1987;6:215–218.
4. Lanphear WF. Gastric lavage. *J Emerg Med.* 1986;4:43–47.
5. Metheny N, Williams P, Wiersema L, Wehrle MA, Eisenberg P, McSweeney M. Effectiveness of pH measurements in predicting feeding tube placement. *Nurs Res.* 1989;38:280–285.
6. Sabga E, Dick A, Letzman M, Tenenbein M. Direct administration of charcoal into the lung and pleural cavity. *Ann Emerg Med.* 1997;30:695–697.
7. Weinman SA. Emergency management of drug overdose. *Crit Care Nurse.* 1993;13:45–51.
8. Ponsky JL, Hoffman M, Swayngim DS. Saline irrigation in gastric hemorrhage: the effect of temperature. *J Surg Res.* 1980;28:204–205.
9. Waterman NG, Walker JL. The effect of gastric cooling on hemostasis. *Surg Gynecol Obstet.* 1973;137:80–82.
10. Bryant LR, Mobin-Uddin K, Dillon ML, Griffen WO Jr. Comparison of ice water with iced saline solution for gastric lavage in gastroduodenal hemorrhage. *Am J Surg.* 1972;124:570–572.
11. Shannon MW, Haddad LM. The emergency management of poisoning. In: Haddad LM, Shannon MW, Winchester JF, eds. *Clinical Management of Poisoning and Drug Overdose.* 3rd ed. Philadelphia, Pa: WB Saunders; 1998:2–31.
12. Young WF, Bivins HG. Evaluation of gastric emptying using radionuclides: gastric lavage versus ipecac induced emesis. *Ann Emerg Med.* 1993;22:70–74.
13. Thoma MA, Glauser JM. Use of glucagon for removal of an orogastric lavage tube. *Am J Emerg Med.* 1995;13:219–222.

Additional Readings

Bitterman RA. Upper gastrointestinal hemorrhage. *Emerg Med.* 1989;21:77–78, 83–84, 86.
Civetta JM, Taylor RW, Kirby RR. *Critical Care.* 2nd ed. Philadelphia, Pa: JB Lippincott; 1992.
Clochesy JM, Breu C, Cardin S, Whittaker AA, Rudy EB. *Critical Care Nursing.* 2nd ed. Philadelphia, Pa: WB Saunders; 1996.
Deglin JH, Vallerand AH. *Davis's Drug Guide for Nurses.* 5th ed. Philadelphia, Pa: FA Davis; 1997.

Erickson TB. Dealing with the unknown overdose. *Emerg Med.* 1996;28:74, 79–83, 84, 86–88.

Harris CR, Kingston R. Gastrointestinal decontamination: which method is best? *Postgrad Med.* 1992;92:116, 118–122, 125, 128.

Hoffman R. Choices in gastric decontamination. *Emerg Med.* 1992;24:212, 214, 217, 221–224.

Kastrup EK, ed. *Drug Facts and Comparisons.* St. Louis, Mo: Wolters Kluwer Co.; 1998.

Intra-abdominal Pressure Monitoring

PURPOSE: Intra-abdominal pressure (IAP) measurement is indicated in patients who are at risk for the development of intra-abdominal hypertension (IAH) or abdominal compartment syndrome (ACS). IAH and ACS result when the abdominal contents expand in excess of the capacity of the abdominal cavity.[1-5]

John J. Gallagher

PREREQUISITE NURSING KNOWLEDGE

- Gastrointestinal anatomy and physiology should be understood.
- Knowledge of aseptic technique is essential.
- Possible causes of IAH and ACS include the following:
  - ❖ Intraperitoneal blood
  - ❖ Third space resuscitation fluid
  - ❖ Peritonitis
  - ❖ Ascites
  - ❖ Gaseous bowel distention
- Additionally, the presence of intra-abdominal packing, use of pneumatic antishock garments, insufflation of the peritoneum during laparoscopic procedures, and full closure of the abdominal wall in the presence of visceral edema have also been implicated in the development of IAH and ACS[1, 2, 4] (Table 96–1).
- Elevated intra-abdominal compartment pressures may result in decreased blood flow to organs in the abdominal cavity and can adversely affect the functioning of multiple organ systems[1-9] (Table 96–2).

Table 96–1 ● ▊▊	**Patients at Risk for Development of Intra-abdominal Hypertension and Abdominal Compartment Syndrome[1-6]**

1. Trauma/Abdominal Surgery
   Blunt or penetrating abdominal trauma/intraperitoneal hematoma
   Pelvic fractures/retroperitoneal hematoma
   Damage control abdominal surgery/abdominal packing/primary closure
   Visceral tissue edema secondary to ischemia and fluid resuscitation
   Pneumoperitoneum during laparoscopic procedures
   Liver transplant
2. Pneumatic antishock garments
3. Ruptured abdominal aortic aneurysm
4. Cirrhosis/ascites
5. Small bowel obstruction
6. Hemorrhagic pancreatitis
7. Neoplasm
8. Obstetrical
   Preeclampsia
   Pregnancy related disseminated intravascular coagulation/hemorrhage

- IAP measurements should be correlated with associated organ system pathophysiology to determine the presence of IAH/ACS and the need for surgical intervention.
- Several methods are described in the literature to measure IAP.[1, 2, 4, 5, 9, 10] These include direct intraperitoneal measurement using a peritoneal dialysis catheter, the intragastric method via a nasogastric (NG) tube, the rectal route, and through a urinary catheter in the bladder. Measurement of bladder pressures via an indwelling urinary catheter is the most widely accepted method for clinical use and may be performed with equipment readily available in the critical care environment.
- Compartment syndrome can result in any confined anatomical space where there is an increase in pressure.
- The elevation of pressure within the compartment can cause compression or occlusion of arterial blood flow, resulting in ischemia, tissue necrosis, and irreversible organ failure if blood flow is not restored.
- The bladder acts as a passive reservoir and will accurately reflect intra-abdominal pressure (IAP) when the intravesicular volume is 100 mL or less.[11]
- Bladder pressures may be measured using a standard pressure transducer monitoring set connected to the patient's urinary drainage system (see Procedure 69).
- Bladder pressures reflective of the IAP are measured in millimeters of mercury (mm Hg) and may be classified as normal (0 mm Hg to subatmospheric), mildly elevated (10 to 20 mm Hg), moderately elevated (>20 to 40 mm Hg) and severely elevated (>40 mm Hg).[6, 9]
- Pressures between 0 and 15 mm Hg normally are seen after abdominal surgery; however, measurements in the upper portion of this range also may indicate early IAH. Bladder pressures of greater than 15 mm Hg indicate onset of IAH and generally are associated with early organ system pathophysiology.[1, 2] Pressures in the moderate to severe range are associated with marked alterations in cardiovascular function, anuria or oliguria, and impaired respiratory function[1, 3, 7] (see Table 96–2). It is accepted surgical practice to perform surgical decompression of the abdomen in patients who achieve IAPs of 20 to 25 mm Hg, which are associated with clinical assessment findings that indicate IAH/ACS.[1, 11]

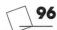

Table 96–2 ● ■ ■ **Physiologic Changes Associated with Intra-abdominal Hypertension and Abdominal Compartment Syndrome**[1–9, 11]

Organ System (IAP range of initial organ system impact)	Rationale
Cardiovascular (IAPs low to moderate range) ⇑ CVP, PAP, PCWP, SVR ⇓ CO (more pronounced with hypovolemia) ⇓ Venous return from lower extremities (risk of DVT)	Increased abdominal pressure prevents venous return (preload reduction) and impedes arterial outflow (increase in afterload). Transmitted backpressure from the abdominal cavity falsely elevates CVP, PAP, PCWP, PVR, and SVR.
Renal (IAPs low to moderate) ⇓ Renal blood flow → ⇓ GFR → ⇓ urine output	Increased intra-abdominal pressure compresses the renal parenchyma, reducing blood flow and urine output.
Pulmonary (IAPs moderate to severe range) ⇑ Intrathoracic pressures ⇑ Peak inspiratory pressures ⇓ Tidal volume → hypercarbia + ⇓ PaO_2 ⇓ Compliance	Increased intra-abdominal pressure causes an increase in intrathoracic pressure and limits diaphragm excursion, resulting in hypoventilation and hypoxia.
Neurological (IAPs low to moderate range) ⇑ ICP ⇓ CPP	Increased intra-abdominal pressure impedes venous outflow from the brain, increasing cerebral venous congestion.
Gastrointestinal/Hepatic Effect (IAPs low to moderate range) ⇓ Celiac and portal blood flow ⇓ Lactate clearance ⇓ Mucosal blood flow → ⇓ intramucosal pH (pHi)	Increased intra-abdominal pressure reduces perfusion to the abdominal organs.

CPP, cerebral perfusion pressure; CVP, central venous pressure; DVT, deep vein thrombosis; GFR, glomerular filtration rate; IAP, intra-abdominal pressure; ICP, intracranial pressure; PAP, pulmonary artery pressure; PCWP, pulmonary capillary wedge pressure; PVR, pulmonary vascular resistance; SVR, systemic vascular resistance.

EQUIPMENT

- Nonsterile gloves
- Cardiac monitor and pressure cable for interface with the monitor
- 500- or 1000-mL IV bag of normal saline solution with appropriate-size pressure bag
- Pressure transducer system including pressure tubing with flush device, transducer, and two stopcocks
- 60-mL Luer-Lok syringe
- Clamp
- Povidone iodine pads or swab-sticks
- 18-G needle or angiocatheter

PATIENT AND FAMILY EDUCATION

- Explain the procedure of bladder pressure measurement and its purpose to the patient and family. **➤Rationale:** Decreases patient and family anxiety. Understanding of how the procedure is done will assist in the patient's ability to cooperate.
- Inform the patient that he or she will feel a "fullness" in the bladder when saline is injected into the bladder during the procedure. **➤Rationale:** Decreases patient anxiety. Prepares patient for what to expect.

PATIENT ASSESSMENT AND PREPARATION

Patient Assessment

- Obtain a patient health history to uncover risk factors predisposing the patient to IAH or ACS. These conditions are outlined in Table 96–1. **➤Rationale:** Patients with these conditions may experience an increase in abdominal cavity fluid collection or tissue edema, placing them at risk for IAH and ACS.
- Assess the patient for signs of IAH or ACS, including decreased cardiac output and blood pressure, oliguria and anuria, increased peak inspiratory pressures (PIPs), hypercarbia and hypoxia, increased intracranial pressure (ICP), increase in abdominal girth, and abdominal wall rigidity (see Table 96–2). **➤Rationale:** These physical findings indicate pathophysiologic organ system changes associated with the onset and presence of IAH and ACS.

Patient Preparation

- Ensure that the patient and family understand preprocedural teaching. Answer questions as they arise and reinforce information as needed. **➤Rationale:** Evaluates and reinforces understanding of previously taught information.
- Ensure the presence of a conventional (single-lumen) urinary catheter connected to a closed drainage system. **➤Rationale:** A urinary catheter with a closed drainage system is required to obtain bladder pressure measurements. Multi-lumen irrigation urinary catheters also may be used, but are not required.
- Place the patient in the supine, flat position (if this can be tolerated) in preparation for bladder pressure measurement. **➤Rationale:** The supine, flat position reduces the effect of downward pressure from the abdominal organs on the bladder, reducing the chance that IAP will be falsely elevated. Patients who cannot tolerate the supine position (head injury, respiratory compromise) may have measurements taken with the head of the bed elevated; however, the same position should be used for all subsequent measurements to obtain comparable readings.

Procedure	for Intra-abdominal Pressure Monitoring

Steps	Rationale	Special Considerations
1. Wash hands, and don gloves.	Reduces the transmission of microorganisms; standard precautions.	
2. Assemble the entire pressure transducer system as shown (Fig. 96–1), flush the system with normal saline, and pressurize the system to 300 mm Hg using the pressure bag.	Ensure all air is out of the system. Pressurizing the system will allow for easier filling of the syringe.	Do not pressurize the system before flushing the tubing with fluid to minimize air bubbles in the system.
3. Attach the 60-mL syringe to the distal stopcock and attach the needle to the end of the tubing (see Fig. 96–1).	The syringe is used to fill the bladder with saline from the IV bag.	If an angiocatheter is used, do not attach it to the end of the tubing until after step 7, when it has been threaded into the urinary drainage system sampling port.
4. Connect the pressurized system to the pressure module of the monitoring system with the transducer cable. Select a 30- or 60-mm Hg scale.	Connects the system for monitoring. The 30- or 60-mm Hg scale will be sufficient to measure the majority of IAP ranges.	
5. Level the fluid interface (zeroing stopcock) to the symphysis pubis.	The symphysis pubis approximates the level of the bladder and should be used as the reference point.	Marking the position ensures consistent use of the same reference point. The transducer may be secured to an IV pole beside the patient and leveled in the standard fashion or it may be placed on the patient at the level of the symphysis pubis.

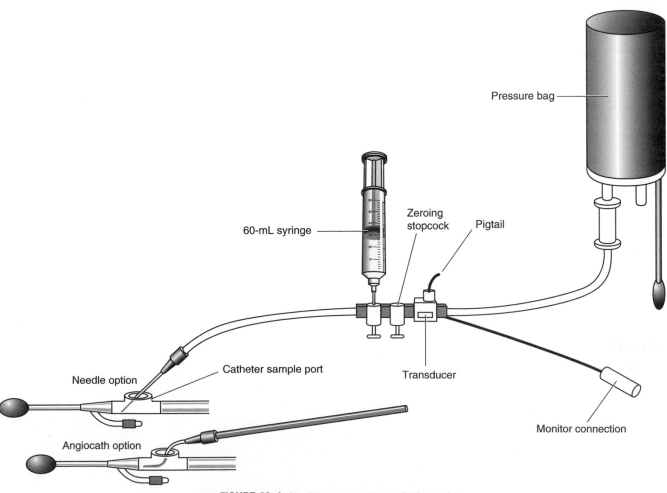

Pressure bag

60-mL syringe

Zeroing stopcock

Pigtail

Needle option

Catheter sample port

Transducer

Angiocath option

Monitor connection

■ ● **FIGURE 96–1.** Bladder pressure monitoring setup.

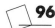

Procedure **for Intra-abdominal Pressure Monitoring** *Continued*

Steps	Rationale	Special Considerations
6. Zero the intra-abdominal pressure monitoring system (see Procedure 69).	Negates the effect of atmospheric pressure. Ensures accuracy of the system with the established reference point.	
7. Clamp the bladder drainage system just distal to the catheter and drainage bag connection on the drainage bag tubing.	Prevents drainage of saline out of the bladder during bladder filling.	
8. Cleanse the sampling port on the urinary drainage system with povidone and aseptically insert the needle or angiocatheter into the sampling port. *If using the angiocatheter, insert the angiocatheter and thread the catheter into the port; remove the needle and connect the catheter to the pressure tubing.*	Cleansing the sampling port reduces the incidence of nosocomial urinary tract infection (UTI) from system contamination.	Either a needle for intermittent connection of the pressure transducer to the catheter system or an angiocatheter threaded through the sampling port that remains in place continuously can be used. The angiocatheter method prevents the need for repeated punctures of the sampling port and may reduce the chance of needle stick injury.[1] It has also been hypothesized that this technique may reduce the incidence of UTI.
9. Turn the stopcock attached to the syringe off to the patient and open to the pressure bag and syringe. Activate the fast-flush mechanism (pigtail) while pulling back on the syringe plunger to fill the syringe to 50 mL.		
10. Turn the stopcock off to the pressure bag and open to the syringe and patient. Inject the 50 mL of saline into the bladder.	The fluid-filled bladder will accurately reflect IAP. Using a volume of 50 mL will prevent overdistention of the bladder and false elevation of the bladder pressure.	
11. Expel any air seen between the clamp and the urinary catheter by opening the clamp and allowing the saline to flow back past the clamp; then reclamp.	Air in the system may dampen the pressure reading.	
12. Run a strip of the waveform.	Intra-abdominal pressure should be determined from the graphic strip, because the effect of ventilation can be identified.	Use of the numeric IAP pressure displayed on the monitor should not be used. This numeric reading is a "mean" pressure value reflecting the average of both inspiratory and expiratory IAP, rather than just the expiratory IAP.
13. Measure the intra-abdominal pressure at end expiration (Fig. 96–2).	Measurement is most accurate as the effects of pulmonary pressures are minimized.	

Procedure continued on following page

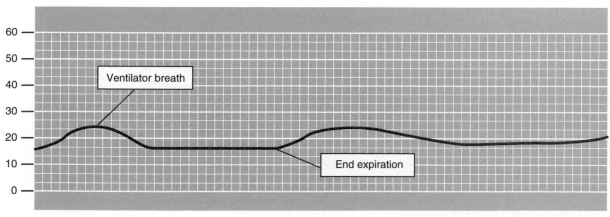

■ ● **FIGURE 96–2.** IAP waveform. The IAP read at end-expiration is 16 mm Hg in this mechanically ventilated patient.

Steps	Rationale	Special Considerations
14. Once a reading has been obtained, remove the needle from the sampling port and unclamp the drainage system. If an angiocatheter has been used, it should be left in the sampling port with the entire transducer system left connected. *The urinary drainage system should be left unclamped between readings.*	Removing the needle and unclamping the drainage system will discontinue pressure measurement and resume the normal urinary drainage function of the catheter system.	Although the angiocatheter/transducer system remains attached, bladder pressures cannot be continuously measured. Monitoring requires clamping the drainage system and filling the bladder to obtain a reading. Continuous connection of the system simply prevents repeated punctures of the sampling port.
15. Record the bladder pressure on the patient flow sheet and remember to subtract the 50 mL of instilled saline from the hourly urine output.	The volume of instilled normal saline will falsely elevate hourly urine output if it is not subtracted.	
16. Report IAP readings as per patient care prescriptions, if they are trending upward or if they are associated with other assessment findings indicating the development of IAH and ACS.	Early detection and surgical intervention to relieve high IAPs is essential to reduce the morbidity and mortality associated with IAH and ACS.	
17. Discard used supplies, and wash hands.	Reduces transmission of microorganisms; standard precautions.	

Expected Outcomes

- Intra-abdominal pressure monitoring is achieved.
- Compartment pressure is within normal limits.
- Elevated compartment pressure is detected.

Unexpected Outcomes

- Inability to monitor intra-abdominal pressure
- Inaccurate pressure readings obtained
- Development of a nosocomial UTI secondary to urinary drainage system manipulation
- Patient discomfort

Patient Monitoring and Care

Patient Monitoring and Care	Rationale	Reportable Conditions
		These conditions should be reported if they persist despite nursing interventions.
1. Assess the patient for signs of increasing intra-abdominal pressure, including ○ Decrease in blood pressure and cardiac output ○ Oliguria or anuria ○ Increase in peak inspiratory pressures ○ Hypoxia and hypercarbia ○ Elevated intracranial pressure (ICP) ○ Increase in abdominal girth ○ Increase in the tenseness of the abdomen wall	Patients may develop symptoms slowly over time. The symptoms may mimic other clinical conditions such as acute respiratory distress syndrome (ARDS), acute renal failure, congestive heart failure, and intracranial hypertension.	• Decrease in blood pressure and cardiac output • Oliguria or anuria • Increase in peak inspiratory pressures • Hypoxia and hypercarbia • Elevated intracranial pressure • Increase in abdominal girth • Increase in the tenseness of the abdomen wall
2. Monitor intra-abdominal pressures every 2 to 4 hours or more frequently, depending on clinical need.	Serial measurements will detect a trended increase in IAPs, reflecting development of ACS.	• IAPs >15 mm Hg • IAPs <15 mm Hg if associated with other clinical findings suggestive of IAH/ACS
3. Monitor for signs and symptoms of UTI.	Frequent breaks in the integrity of the urinary drainage system may contribute to the development of UTI.	• Temperature elevation • Elevated white blood cell count • Increased sediment or cloudiness of urine

Documentation

> Documentation should include the following:
>
> - Patient and family education
> - Assessment findings before obtaining intra-abdominal pressures
> - Intra-abdominal pressure value
> - Postprocedure assessment
> - Changes in the patient's assessment indicating onset of IAH/ACS
> - The amount of fluid instilled into the bladder to be subtracted from the hourly urine output
> - Unexpected outcomes
> - Additional interventions

References

1. Cheatham ML. Intraabdominal hypertension. *New Horiz.* 1999;7:96–115.
2. Lozen Y. Intraabdominal hypertension and abdominal compartment syndrome in trauma: pathophysiology and interventions. *AACN Clin Iss.* 1999;10:104–112.
3. Losanoff JE. Abdominal compartment syndrome: prompt recognition and treatment. *Am Surg.* 1999;65:93–94.
4. Cheatham ML, Safcak K. Intraabdominal pressure: a revised method for measurement. *J Am Coll Surg.* 1998;186:594–595.
5. Nayduch DA, Sullivan K, Reed RL II. Abdominal compartment syndrome. *J Trauma Nurs.* 1996;4:5–11.
6. MacDonnell SP. Comments on the abdominal compartment syndrome: the physiological and clinical consequences of elevated intraabdominal pressure. *J Am Coll Surg.* 1996;183:419–420.
7. Stein M, et al. The abdominal compartment syndrome: the physiological and clinical consequences of elevated intraabdominal pressure. *J Am Coll Surg.* 1995;180:745–753.
8. Ridings P, et al. Cardiopulmonary effects of raised intraabdominal pressure before and after intravascular volume. *J Trauma.* 1995;39:1071–1075.
9. Cullen D, et al. Cardiovascular, pulmonary, and renal effects of massively increased intraabdominal pressure in critically ill patients. *Crit Care Med.* 1989;17:118–122.
10. Lameier D, DeCamp D. Measuring intraabdominal pressure. *Crit Care Nurs.* 1995;10:54–66.
11. Kron I, Harman K, Nolan SP. The measurement of intraabdominal pressure as a criterion for abdominal re-exploration. *Ann Surg.* 1984;199:28–30.

Additional Reading

Gallagher JJ. Ask the expert: describe the procedure for monitoring intra-abdominal pressure via an indwelling urinary catheter. *Crit Care Nurs.* 2000;20:87–91.

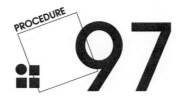

97

Orogastric and Nasogastric Tube Insertion, Care, and Removal

P U R P O S E: Orogastric or nasogastric (NG) tube insertion is performed to decompress the stomach; to remove blood, secretions, ingested drugs or toxins; or to instill medications, feedings, lavage fluids, or warmed lavage fluids to correct hypothermia.

Karen K. Carlson

PREREQUISITE NURSING KNOWLEDGE

- Knowledge of anatomy of the upper gastrointestinal tract is needed.
- Orogastric or NG tubes are used for both diagnostic and therapeutic purposes. They are frequently indicated for stomach decompression and gastric contents evacuation when a patient has overdosed or hemorrhaged or has an ileus. Gastric content samples may be obtained for laboratory analysis, and medications, fluids, or feedings can be instilled.
- Orogastric or NG intubation is performed by passing a tube through either a nostril (NG) or the oral cavity (orogastric), advancing it through the oropharynx and esophagus and into the stomach.
- Orogastric intubation is specifically recommended for patients with anterior fossa skull fracture or maxillofacial injury. These patients have increased potential for inadvertent tube placement into the brain via the cribriform plate or ethmoid bone, if the tube is inserted nasally. Additionally, patients needing extra-large caliber tubes (30 to 36 Fr) for gastric emptying in drug overdoses should be orally intubated.
- A variety of tubes are available for gastric intubation. Tubes have single or double lumens, are weighted or nonweighted, and are vented or nonvented. The Levine tube is a nonvented, single-lumen tube (Fig. 97–1). This tube, used primarily for decompression, lavage, or feeding, should not be connected to suction because it may cause the tube to adhere to the mucosal surface, causing irritation. The Salem sump (Fig. 97–2), a vented, nonweighted double-lumen tube, is more commonly used when suction is desired. The second lumen of the sump tube is the air vent, allowing air to continually irrigate the distal tip of the tube. This continual air irrigation decreases the likelihood of tube adherence to the gastric mucosa and resultant irritation.

- Small-bore, weighted, single-lumen tubes are preferred for enteral feedings (see Procedure 128).

EQUIPMENT

- Orogastric or NG tube (size range is 12 to 18 Fr for adults)
- Water-soluble lubricant
- Nonsterile gloves
- 20 to 50 mL syringe with catheter tip or adapter
- Normal saline (NS) for irrigation
- Two emesis basins
- Ice
- Ice chips or cup of tap water with straw
- Suction source with connecting tubing
- Rubber band
- Safety pin
- Pink tape or tube attachment device
- pH test paper
- Tongue blade

Additional equipment (to have available depending on patient need) includes the following:

- Tincture of benzoin
- Guaiac test materials

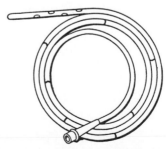

■ ● FIGURE 97–1. Nonvented single-lumen (Levin) tube. (From Norton BA, Miller AM. *Skills for Professional Nursing Practice.* Norwalk, Ct: Appleton-Century-Crofts; 1986.)

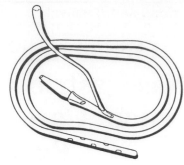

■ ● FIGURE 97–2. Vented double-lumen (Salem sump) tube. (From Norton BA, Miller AM. *Skills for Professional Nursing Practice.* Norwalk, Ct: Appleton-Century-Crofts; 1986.)

PATIENT AND FAMILY EDUCATION

- Explain the procedure and the reason for tube insertion. ➥*Rationale:* Decreases patient anxiety.
- Explain the patient's role in assisting with passage of the tube. ➥*Rationale:* Elicits patient cooperation and facilitates insertion.
- Explain that the procedure can be uncomfortable because the gag reflex may be stimulated, causing the patient to feel nauseated or to vomit. ➥*Rationale:* Elicits patient cooperation and facilitates insertion.

PATIENT ASSESSMENT AND PREPARATION

Patient Assessment

- Obtain past medical history of nasal deformity, epistaxis, surgery, trauma, varices, or recent esophageal or gastric surgery. ➥*Rationale:* Increases the risk of complications from tube placement.
- Ensure patency of nares, if NG intubation is planned. This can be done by occluding one nostril at a time, asking the patient to breathe, and selecting the nostril with the best airflow. ➥*Rationale:* Choosing the most patent nostril will ease insertion and may improve patient tolerance of tube.
- Obtain immediate history of ingestion of drugs or toxins. ➥*Rationale:* Allows preparation for immediate evacuation or neutralization of gastric contents to prevent absorption and tissue damage.
- Obtain immediate history of facial or head injury. ➥*Rationale:* To decrease risk of inadvertent tube placement into the brain, orogastric tube placement should be used.
- Signs of gastric distention include the following:
  ❖ Nausea
  ❖ Vomiting
  ❖ Absence of or hypoactive bowel tones

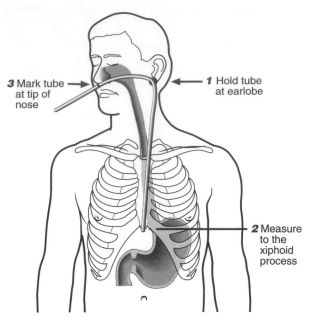

3 Mark tube at tip of nose

1 Hold tube at earlobe

2 Measure to the xiphoid process

■ ● FIGURE 97–3. (From Luckmann J. *Saunders Manual of Nursing Care.* Philadelphia: WB Saunders; 1997: 1262.)

➥*Rationale:* Accumulation of secretions or air in the stomach increases the risk of vomiting and aspiration and provides baseline for later comparison.
- Determine need for analysis of gastric contents (eg, pH, guaiac, drug screen). ➥*Rationale:* Knowing before the procedure is initiated if samples are needed will allow the practitioner to have necessary supplies available and to obtain samples in a timely manner.

Patient Preparation

- Ensure that patient understands preprocedural teaching. Answer questions as they arise, and reinforce information as needed. ➥*Rationale:* Evaluates and reinforces understanding of previously taught information.
- If patient is alert, place patient in high Fowler or semi-Fowler position. If patient is obtunded or unconscious, place patient head down in the left lateral position. Cover the chest with a towel. ➥*Rationale:* Facilitates passage of tube into the stomach and minimizes risk of aspiration. Inserting an NG tube into an obtunded patient may require the assistance of an additional person.
- Measure the tube from the bridge of the nose to the earlobe to the tip of the xiphoid process (Fig. 97–3). Mark the length of tube to be passed (a small piece of tape works well and can be easily removed). ➥*Rationale:* Estimates the length of the tube to be passed to ensure placement into the stomach.

Procedure	**for Orogastric and Nasogastric Tube Insertion, Care, and Removal**

Steps	Rationale	Special Considerations
1. Wash hands. If tape will be used to secure the tube, prepare the tape by tearing a piece 1.5 to 2 in long. Split the last 1 in of the tape. Set aside.	Once the tube is in place, it will be easier to secure immediately if the tape is ready to apply.	
2. Wash hands, and don personal protective equipment.	Reduces transmission of microorganisms and body secretions; standard precautions.	Immersing a rubber tube in iced water for several minutes before insertion has been recommended as a means to stiffen the tube, facilitating placement, but it may make placement more uncomfortable for the patient. Immersing a plastic tube in warm water will make the tube more flexible, facilitating placement.
3. Lubricate 6 to 10 cm of distal end of tube, using water-soluble lubricant.	Minimizes mucosal injury and irritation during insertion; facilitates insertion.	It is important that only water-soluble lubricants be used in tube placement. Oil-soluble lubricants, such as petroleum jelly, cannot be absorbed by the pulmonary mucosa should the tube be inadvertently placed in the lungs. The lubricant could then cause respiratory complications.
For Orogastric Intubation		
4. Position curved edge of the tube downward, inserting the tube into the oral cavity over the tongue. Aim the tube back and down toward the pharynx. When the tube hits the pharynx, have the patient flex the head forward. If appropriate, ask the patient to take sips of water through a straw while tube is being advanced. Proceed to step 6.	Flexing the head of an unconscious patient will also facilitate tube placement. Having the patent take sips of water or mimic a swallowing motion causes the epiglottis to close the trachea and directs the tube toward the esophagus.	If patient is uncooperative, place an oral airway (see Procedure 7) or bite block in the mouth before attempting to place the tube to prevent the patient from biting on the tube. Having the patient flex his or her head may be especially helpful in intubated patients.
For NG Intubation		
5. Using the more patent nare, insert the tube through the nose, aiming down and back. When the tube hits the pharynx, if patient is able, have him or her flex the head forward and swallow. Advance tube as patient swallows.	If the patient gags, coughs, or begins choking, withdraw slightly and stop insertion, allowing the patient to rest.	If resistance is met, do not force insertion because this could damage the nasal turbinates and mucosa and cause bleeding. Having the patient flex her or his head may be especially helpful in intubated patients.
6. If resistance is met, rotating the tube may facilitate placement.	If unable to advance tube after several attempts, notify physician or nurse practitioner.	
7. Continue to advance the tube until the marked position on the tube is reached.	Advances tube into stomach.	

Procedure continued on following page

Procedure	for Orogastric and Nasogastric Tube Insertion, Care, and Removal *Continued*

Steps	Rationale	Special Considerations
8. Confirm tube placement in stomach. A. Aspirate fluid and evaluate the pH. *(Level V: Clinical studies in more than one patient population and situation)* B. Attach a pressure gauge (negative inspiratory force spring gauge manometer) to distal tip of tube. *(Level IV: Limited clinical studies to support recommendations)*	With pH testing, gastric placement will show a pH <5.5. Intestinal placement will show a pH >6.0. Pulmonary secretions have an alkaline pH.[1–3] Tubes placed in the gastrointestinal tract will yield positive pressures (0 or greater), whereas tubes placed in the pulmonary tract will yield negative pressures (less than 0).[4]	Common practice for many years has been to evaluate tube placement by placing a stethoscope over the stomach and instilling 20 to 50 mL of air via syringe. There are numerous reports in the literature of false-positive results using this method, including reports of serious pulmonary complications because of tracheal tube placement.[3, 5–8] The ability to simply aspirate fluid from the tube is often interpreted as confirmation of gastic intubation. Several reports[8, 9] *(Level V: Clinical studies in more than one patient population and situation)* have shown that fluid can also be aspirated after endotracheal intubation. As well, some authors have suggested that placement can be confirmed by placing the tip of the NG tube under water and observing for bubbles. Bubbles would indicate endotracheal intubation. Although logical, this method is also unreliable.[3, 10] If a tube were lodged in the mucosal wall of either the esophagus or the lung, no bubbles would result, yet placement would be incorrect.
9. Secure tube in position, using pink tape (Fig. 97–4), clear or adhesive tape, or a commercially available tube holder. *(Level IV: Limited clinical studies to support recommendations)*	Maintains tube in correct position and prevents inadvertent dislodgment. Use of pink tape (Plastic Adhesive Tape; Hy-tape Surgical Products Corporation, Yonkers, NY) was found to be superior to two other methods.[11]	A variety of methods are used to secure the tube in place, including use of different types of tape, clear adhesive dressings, and commercially available tube holders. Whatever means employed should be used to avoid exerting pressure against the rim of the nare because ulceration may occur.
10. Attach primary lumen to suction or gravity drainage, as ordered.	Initiates therapy.	
11. Secure tube to patient's gown 10 to 12 in from nose. Loop rubber band around tube, and pin rubber band to gown.	Prevents tube from pulling and putting pressure against the rim of the nose; provides additional protection against tube dislodgment.	
12. Reassess position of tube per institutional standards and patient condition and before instillation of any medication, irrigant, or feeding.	Incorrect position of tube increases risk of aspiration.	
13. Irrigate tube per institutional standards and patient condition and as needed with 20 to 30 mL NS or air.	Ensure tube patency.	

Procedure	**for Orogastric and Nasogastric Tube Insertion, Care, and Removal** *Continued*

Steps	Rationale	Special Considerations

Tube Removal

14. Wash hands, and don personal protective equipment.

Reduces transmission of microorganisms and body secretions; standard precautions.

15. Cover patient's chest with a towel.

Drainage from the tube may be present on the tube as it is removed. Covering the chest with a towel prevents soiling of patient gown and covers.

16. Remove tape or tube holder. If tube is pinned to gown, remove pin.

Allows for easy removal of tube.

17. Using smooth, constant motion, withdraw tube completely out of patient.

18. Wrap tube in towel and discard tube and suction canister according to institutional standard.

Provides a means for collecting any drainage on tube and moving it to a correct disposal receptacle.

19. Provide oral or nasal care as needed.

Cleanse area where tube was in place; increases patient comfort.

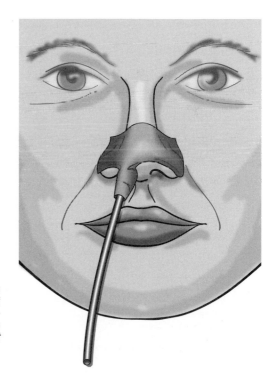

■ ● **FIGURE 97–4.** Pink tape method. One half of a 1.5-in strip was applied to the nose, and the lower portion was split up to the tip of the nose. Each half of the tape was then wrapped around the tube and the strip of white waterproof tape. (Adapted from Burns SM, et al. Comparison of nasogastric tube securing methods and tube types in medical intensive care patients. *Am J Crit Care.* 1995;4(3):201.)

Expected Outcomes	Unexpected Outcomes
• Decompression of stomach • Evacuation of stomach and proximal small intestine contents • Instillation of fluid, medications, or feedings	• Tube placement into trachea, bronchus, or esophagus • Bleeding from nose, mouth, esophagus, or stomach • Vagal response during insertion or from gag reflex stimulation • Skin ulceration, sinusitis, esophageal-tracheal fistula, gastric ulceration, or oral infections • Vomiting or aspiration

Patient Monitoring and Care

Patient Monitoring and Care	Rationale	Reportable Conditions
		These conditions should be reported if they persist despite nursing interventions.
1. Maintain and check tube patency every 2 hours and as needed.	Prevents gastric distention and associated patient discomfort.	• Inability to establish patency.
2. Monitor output (color, amount, type, pH, guaiac) every 2 hours and as needed.	Provides data for diagnosis and fluid balance.	• Increasing output or sudden change in output (increase or decrease) • Frank blood or "coffee-ground," black, or brown returns • Positive guaiac • Abnormal pH
3. Calculate output into patient's overall intake and output record.	Volume loss from gastric secretions can cause patients to become hypovolemic; large volumes may need to be replaced with appropriate intravenous fluids.	• Increasing output or sudden change in output (increase or decrease)
4. Assess oral cavity and perform oral care every 2 hours and as needed.	Patients with orogastric or NG tubes in place tend to mouth breathe, drying their mouths and increasing the risk of mucosal breakdown and ulceration. Tube presence may also predispose a patient to sinusitis or oral infections.	• Ulceration, drainage, foul odor
5. Monitor insertion site of tube for redness, swelling, drainage, bleeding, or skin breakdown. Use only water-soluble lubricants at site.	Many critically ill patients have fragile skin and have associated conditions that predispose them to skin breakdown. Frequent monitoring and subsequent repositioning of the tube can prevent serious damage.	• Redness • Swelling • Drainage • Bleeding • Skin breakdown at insertion site
6. Irrigate the tube, using air or NS, per institutional standards and as needed.	Assists in maintaining patency of tube and facilitates drainage.	• Inability to irrigate tube
7. If using a sump tube, position pigtail above the level of the patient's stomach. Irrigate with 5 to 10 mL of air per institutional standards.	Prevents backflow of gastric secretions; antireflux valves are available.[12]	• Backflow of gastric contents
8. Maintain tube to suction as ordered.	Low (20 to 80 mm Hg), intermittent suction is recommended to minimize gastric mucosal irritation yet provide for adequate drainage.	
9. Monitor vital signs per unit standards. Perfom respiratory and gastrointestinal assessment every 2 hours.	Change in vital signs or respiratory or gastrointestinal assessments may be early warning signs of the development of complications.	• Sudden change in vital signs • Unexplained respiratory distress • Increased abdominal distention, change in bowel tones
10. Reposition and retape tube every 24 hours or when tape is soiled.	Decreases risk of tissue damage to mouth or nares.	

Documentation

Documentation should include the following:

- Patient and family education
- Insertion of orogastric or NG tube
- Tube type and size
- Any difficulties in insertion
- Patient toleration
- How placement was confirmed
- Appearance and volume of gastric secretions, if present
- Amount and type of irrigation fluid (if appropriate)
- Oral care
- Tube site assessments
- Unexpected outcomes
- Nursing interventions

References

1. Metheny N, Williams P, Wiersema L, Wehrle MA, Eisenberg P, McSweeney M. Effectivenss of pH measurements in predicting feeding tube placement. *Nurs Res.* 1989;38:280–285.
2. Metheny N, Reed L, Wiersema L, McSweeney M, Wehrle MA, Clark J. Effectiveness of pH measurements in predicting feeding tube placement: an update. *Nurs Res.* 1993;43:324–331.
3. Metheny N, McSweeney M, Wehrle MA, Wiersema, L. Effectiveness of the auscultatory method in predicting feeding tube location. *Nurs Res.* 1990;5:262–267.
4. Swiech K, Lancaster DR, Sheehan R. Use of a pressure gauge to differentiate gastric from pulmonary placement of nasoenteral feeding tubes. *Appl Nurs Res.* 1994;4:183–189.
5. Metheny N. Measures to test placement of nasogastric and nasoenteric feeding tubes: a review. *Nurs Res.* 1988;37:324–329.
6. Hand RW, Kempster M, Levy J, Rogal PR, Spirn P. Inadvertent transbronchial insertion of narrow bore feeding tubes into the pleural space. *JAMA.* 1984;251:2396–2397.
7. Lipman TO, Kessler T, Arabian A. Nasopulmonary intubation with feeding tubes: case reports and review of the literature. *J Parenter Enteral Nutr.* 1985;5:618–620.
8. Theodore AC, Frank JA, Ende J, Snider G, Beer D. Errant placement of nasoenteric tubes: a hazard in obtunded patients. *Chest.* 1984;86:931–933.
9. Nakao MA, Killam D, Wilson R. Pneumothorax secondary to inadvertent nasotracheal placement of a nasoenteric tube past a cuffed endotracheal tube. *Crit Care Med.* 1983;11:210–211.
10. Chang J, Melnick B, Bedger R, Bleyaert A. Inadvertent endobronchial intubation with nasogastric tube. *Arch Otolaryngol.* 108:528–529.
11. Burns SM, Martin M, Robbins V, Friday T, Coffindaffer M, Burns SC, Burns JE. Comparison of nasogastric tube securing methods and tube types in medical intensive care patients. *AJCC.* 1995;4:198–203.
12. Tucker K, Kaiser S, Ahrens T. Clinical effectiveness of a GI antireflux valve. *Heart Lung.* 1991;20:304.

Additional Reading

Boyes R, Kruse JA. Nasogastric and nasoenteric intubation. *Crit Care Clin.* 1992;10:865–878.

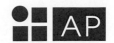

Performing Abdominal Paracentesis

P U R P O S E: Abdominal paracentesis is performed to remove fluid from the peritoneal cavity for diagnostic or therapeutic purposes.

Peggy Kirkwood

PREREQUISITE NURSING KNOWLEDGE

- Peritoneal fluid is normally straw-colored, serous fluid secreted by the cells of the peritoneum. Grossly bloody fluid in the abdomen is abnormal.
- The peritoneal fluid collected is used to evaluate and diagnose the cause of ascites, acute abdominal conditions such as peritonitis or pancreatitis, and blunt or penetrating trauma to the abdomen.
- Therapeutic paracentesis is used to reduce intra-abdominal and diaphragmatic pressures in order to relieve dyspnea and respiratory compromise and prevent peritoneal rupture.
- Ascitic fluid is produced as a result of a variety of conditions. These may include interference in venous return because of heart failure, constrictive pericarditis, or tricuspid valve insufficiency; obstruction of flow in the vena cava or portal vein; disturbance in electrolyte balance such as sodium retention; depletion of plasma proteins, because of nephrotic syndrome or starvation; lymphoma, leukemia, or neoplasms involving the liver or mediastinum; chronic pancreatitis; or cirrhosis of the liver.
- Knowledge of anatomy and physiology of the abdomen is important in order to avoid unexpected outcomes.
  - ❖ Intestines and bladder lie immediately beneath the abdominal surface.
  - ❖ Large volumes of ascitic fluid will tend to float the air-filled bowel toward the midline, where it may be easily perforated during the procedure.
  - ❖ The cecum is relatively fixed and is much less mobile than the sigmoid colon. Therefore, bowel perforations are more frequent in the right lower quadrant than in the left.
- Paracentesis is contraindicated in patients with an acute abdomen, who require immediate surgery. Both coagulopathies and thrombocytopenia are considered relative contraindications.

- Caution should be used when paracentesis is performed in patients with severe bowel distention, previous abdominal surgery (especially pelvic surgery), pregnancy (use open technique after first trimester), distended bladder that cannot be emptied with a Foley catheter, or obvious infection at intended site of insertion (cellulitis or abscess).
- Insertion site should be midline one third the distance from the umbilicus to the symphysis (2 to 3 cm below the umbilicus; Fig. 98–1). Alternate position is a point one third the distance from the umbilicus to the anterior iliac crest (left side preferred).[1]
- Ultrasound can be used prior to paracentesis to locate fluid and during the procedure to guide insertion of catheter[2, 3] (Level V: clinical studies in more than one patient population and situation).

EQUIPMENT

- Commercially prepared kit or the following:
  - ❖ Sterile gloves and mask
  - ❖ Skin-cleansing solution (povidone-iodine)
  - ❖ Sterile marking pen
  - ❖ Sterile towels or sterile drape
  - ❖ Local anesthetic for injection: 1% or 2% lidocaine with epinephrine
  - ❖ 5- or 10-mL syringe with 21- or 25-G needle for anesthetic
  - ❖ Trocar with stylet, needle (16-, 18-, or 20-G), or angiocatheter, depending on abdominal wall thickness
  - ❖ 25- or 27-G 1½-in needle
  - ❖ 20- or 22-G spinal needles
  - ❖ 20-mL syringe for diagnostic tap
  - ❖ 50-mL syringe if using stopcock technique
  - ❖ Four sterile tubes for specimens
  - ❖ Scalpel and no. 11 knife blade
  - ❖ Three-way stopcock
  - ❖ Sterile 1-L collection bottles with connecting tubing
  - ❖ Nylon skin suture material on cutting needle (4-0 or 5-0) and needle holder
  - ❖ Mayo scissors and straight scissors

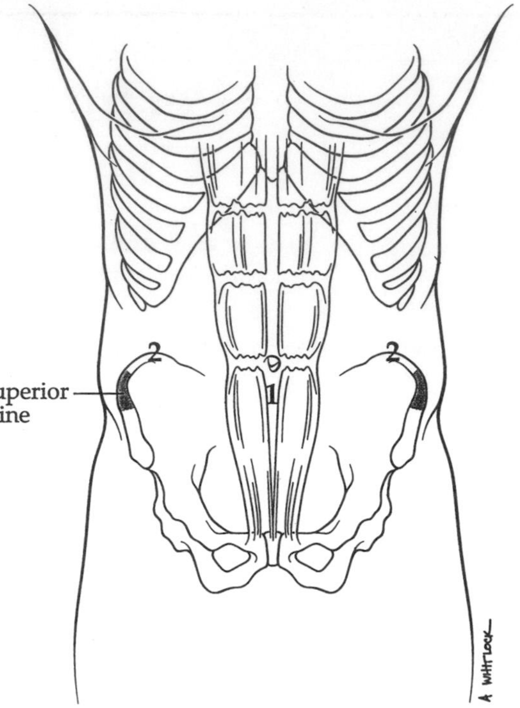

■ ● **FIGURE 98–1.** Preferred sites for paracentesis: *1,* Primary site is infraumbilical in midline through linea alba. *2,* Preferred alternate (lateral rectus) site is in either lower quadrant, approximately 4 to 5 cm cephalad and medial to the anterior superior iliac spine. (From Roberts JR, Hedges JR. *Clinical Procedures in Emergency Medicine.* Philadelphia, WB Saunders; 1998: 744.)

- ❖ Hemostat
- ❖ Four to six sterile 4 × 4 gauze pads
- ❖ Sterile gauze dressing with tape or adhesive strip

PATIENT AND FAMILY EDUCATION

- Explain the indications, procedure, and risks to the patient and family. ➻*Rationale:* Decreases patient anxiety and encourages patient and family cooperation and understanding of the procedure.
- Explain the patient's role in assisting with the procedure and postprocedure care. ➻*Rationale:* Elicits patient cooperation during and after the procedure.
- Explain the signs and symptoms to report, such as fever, abdominal pain, decreased urine output, bleeding, and leakage of fluid from surgical wound site. ➻*Rationale:* Unexpected outcomes may not manifest themselves for a period of time following the procedure.

PATIENT ASSESSMENT AND PREPARATION

Patient Assessment

- Past medical history and review of systems for abdominal injury, major gastrointestinal pathology, liver disease, and portal hypertension. ➻*Rationale:* Certain conditions of the gastrointestinal tract may be diagnosed and treated with paracentesis. Contraindications to paracentesis may be identified.
- Respiratory status (ie, rate, depth, excursion, gas exchange, and use of accessory muscles). ➻*Rationale:* Paracentesis may be indicated to decrease work of breathing.
- Baseline fluid and electrolyte status. ➻*Rationale:* Removal of peritoneal fluid may cause compartment shifting of intravascular volume, electrolytes, and proteins, leading to a decreased circulating volume.
- Bowel or bladder distention. ➻*Rationale:* Distension increases the risk of bowel or bladder perforation during the procedure.
- Abdominal girth. ➻*Rationale:* Provides information on changes in fluid accumulation within the peritoneal cavity.
- Coagulation studies (ie, prothrombin time [PT], partial thromboplastin time [PTT], and platelets). ➻*Rationale:* Abnormal clotting studies may increase the risk of bleeding during and after the procedure. Therapy may be necessary to correct clotting abnormalities before the procedure.

Patient Preparation

- Ensure that patient understands preprocedural teaching. Answer questions as they arise and reinforce information as needed. ➻*Rationale:* Evaluates and reinforces understanding of previously taught information.
- Obtain a written informed consent form. ➻*Rationale:* Paracentesis is an invasive procedure, requiring a signed informed consent form.
- Decompress the bladder either by having the patient void or by inserting a Foley catheter. ➻*Rationale:* A distended bladder increases the risk of bladder perforation during the procedure.
- Obtain plain and upright x-rays of the abdomen before performing the procedure. ➻*Rationale:* Air is introduced during the procedure and may confuse the diagnosis later.
- Place the patient in the supine position (may tilt to side of collection slightly for improved fluid positioning). ➻*Rationale:* Fluid accumulates in the dependent areas.
- Examine abdomen for areas of shifting dullness. Find landmarks and mark appropriately. ➻*Rationale:* Shifting dullness indicates fluid.
- If the patient has altered mental status, soft wrist restraints may be needed. ➻*Rationale:* It is imperative that the patient not move his or her hands into the sterile field once it has been established.

Procedure for Performing Abdominal Paracentesis

Steps	Rationale	Special Considerations
1. Wash hands, and don personal protective equipment.	Reduces transmission of microorganisms and body secretions; standard precautions.	
2. Prepare equipment and sterile field.	Facilitates easy access to needed equipment.	Maintain aseptic technique.
3. Cleanse insertion site with povidone-iodine solution.	Reduces risk of infection.	Use sterile technique.
4. Determine the site for trochar insertion.	Site should be midline one third the distance from the umbilicus to the symphysis (2 to 3 cm below the umbilicus; see Figure 98–1). Alternate position is a point one third the distance from the umbilicus to the anterior iliac crest (left side preferred).[1]	
5. Apply sterile drapes to outline the area to be tapped.	Provide sterile field to decrease risk of infection.	Avoid the rectus muscle because of increased risk of hemorrhage from epigastric vessels; surgical scars because of increased risk of perforation caused by adhesion of bowel to the wall of the peritoneum; and upper quadrants because of the possibility of undetected hepatomegaly.[4]
6. Inject area with local anesthetic (lidocaine with epinephrine preferred). Initially infiltrate skin and subcutaneous tissues, then direct needle perpendicular to the skin and infiltrate the peritoneum.	Local anesthesia minimizes pain and discomfort. Epinephrine helps eliminate unwanted abdominal wall bleeding and false-positive results.	Maximum dose of lidocaine is 30 mL of 1% or 15 mL of 2%. Assess for anesthesia of area. Resistance will be felt as the needle perforates the peritoneum.
7. Using the no. 11 blade and scalpel holder, create a skin incision large enough to allow threading a 3- to 5-mm catheter.	Allows ease of entry for the catheter.	If necessary to lavage, the opening will be large enough to thread the lavage catheter.
8. Insert an 18-gauge needle attached to a 20-mL or 50-mL syringe through the anesthetized tract into the peritoneum. Apply slight suction to the syringe as it is advanced. Grasp the needle close to the skin as it is advanced.	Provides access to peritoneal fluid for evacuation. Slight suction is applied to indicate when the peritoneum is entered and if a blood vessel is entered. Grasping the needle as it is advanced prevents accidental thrusting into the abdomen and possible viscous perforation.	Inserted through small stab wound at midline below umbilicus. A small pop is felt as needle advances through anterior and posterior muscle fascia and enters peritoneum.
9. Once in the cavity, direct the needle at a 60-degree angle toward the center of the pelvic hollow. When fluid returns, fill the syringe (Fig. 98–2).	Collection of fluid for laboratory studies to provide information about the patient's status.	Usual diagnostic tests ordered include tube 1: lactate dehydrogenase (LDH), glucose, albumin; tube 2: protein, specific gravity; tube 3: cell count and differential; tube 4: save until further notice. If indicated, Gram stain, acid-fast bacillus (AFB) stain, bacterial and fungal cultures, amylase and triglycerides.[4]
10. Attach syringes or stopcock and tubing and gently aspirate or siphon fluid by gravity or vacuum into collection device.	Initiates therapy.	Monitor amount of fluid removed. Removal of large amount of fluid (>1 L) may cause hypotension. If large amounts are removed or hypotension seen, consider IV albumin to maintain intravascular volume.[5, 6] *(Level V: Clinical studies in more than one patient population and situation)*

Procedure continued on following page

 This procedure should be performed only by physicians, advanced practice nurses, and other health care professionals (including critical care nurses) with additional knowledge, skills, and demonstrated competence per professional licensure or institutional standard.

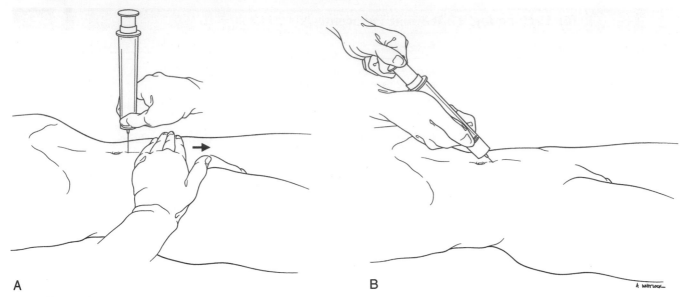

A   **B**

■ ● **FIGURE 98–2.** *A,* Z-tract method of paracentesis. The skin is pulled approximately 2 cm caudad in relation to the deep abdominal wall by the non–needle-bearing hand while the paracentesis needle is slowly being inserted directly perpendicular to the skin. *B,* After penetrating the peritoneum and obtaining fluid return, the skin is released. Note that the needle is angulated caudally. (From Roberts JR, Hedges JR. *Clinical Procedures in Emergency Medicine.* Philadelphia: WB Saunders; 1998:745.)

Procedure | **for Performing Abdominal Paracentesis** *Continued*

Steps	Rationale	Special Considerations
11. After the fluid is removed, gently remove the catheter and apply pressure to the wound. If the wound is still leaking fluid after 5 minutes of direct pressure, suture the puncture site using a mattress suture (see Procedure 120) and apply a pressure dressing.	Keeps insertion site clean. Reduces risk of infection.	Inspect catheter to ensure it is intact.
12. Apply sterile dressing to wound site.	Provides a barrier to infection and collects fluid that may leak from wound site.	
13. Dispose of equipment and soiled material in appropriate receptacle.	Standard precautions.	
14. Wash hands.	Reduces transmission of microorganisms.	

Expected Outcomes | **Unexpected Outcomes**

- Evacuation of peritoneal fluid for laboratory analysis
- Decompression of peritoneal cavity
- Relief of respiratory compromise
- Relief of abdominal discomfort

- Perforation of bowel, bladder, or stomach
- Lacerations of major vessels (mesenteric, iliac, aorta)
- Abdominal wall hematomas
- Laceration of catheter and loss in peritoneal cavity
- Incisional hernias
- Local or systemic infection
- Hypovolemia, hypotension, shock
- Bleeding from insertion site
- Ascitic fluid leak from insertion site
- Peritonitis

Patient Monitoring and Care

Patient Monitoring and Care	Rationale	Reportable Conditions
		These conditions should be reported if they persist despite nursing interventions.
1. Evaluate changes in abdominal girth.	Provides evidence of fluid reaccumulation.	• Increasing abdominal girth
2. Monitor for changes in respiratory status.	Removal of ascitic fluid should relieve pressure on the diaphragm and the resulting respiratory distress.	• Respiratory rate >24 breaths per minute or significant increase from baseline • Increased depth of breathing • Irregular breathing pattern • Pulse oximetry <92%, or significant decrease from baseline
3. Monitor for potential complications, including bowel or bladder perforation, bleeding, and intravascular volume loss.	Paracentesis interrupts the integrity of the skin and underlying peritoneum.	• Hematuria • Hypotension • Tachycardia
4. Monitor vital signs, temperature, insertion site for drainage or evidence of infection.	Infection is a complication of paracentesis.	• Increased temperature • Purulent drainage from insertion site • Redness, swelling at insertion site • Abnormal laboratory results (increased white blood cells [WBCs])
5. Monitor intake and output.	Provides data for evaluation of fluid balance status.	• Inappropriate fluid balance or changes from baseline fluid status
6. Evaluate laboratory data when returned.	Provides for evaluation of condition and aids in diagnosis.	• Red blood cells (RBCs) >100,000/mm³ • Amylase >2.5 times normal • Alkaline phosphatase >5.5 mg/dL • WBCs >100/mm³ • Positive culture results

Documentation

Documentation should include the following:

- Patient and family education
- Date and time of procedure
- Patient tolerance of procedure
- Assessment of insertion site after procedure
- Amount and characteristics of fluid removed
- Specimens sent for laboratory analysis
- Postprocedure vital signs, respiratory status, and abdominal girth
- Unexpected outcomes
- Nursing interventions

References

1. Brown ML. Abdominal paracentesis and peritoneal lavage. In: Pfenninger JL, Fowler GC, eds. *Procedures for Primary Care Physicians.* St. Louis, Mo: Mosby–Year Book; 1994:892–897.
2. Bode PJ, van Vugt AB. Ultrasound in the diagnosis of injury. *Injury.* 1996;27:379–383.
3. Goletti O, Ghiselli G, Lippolis PV, et al. The role of ultrasonography in blunt abdominal trauma: results in 250 consecutive cases. *J Trauma.* 1994;36:178–181.
4. Ferri FF. Paracentesis. In: Ferri F, ed. *The Care of the Medical Patient.* 4th ed. St. Louis, Mo: Mosby; 1998:810–812.
5. Panos MZ, Moore K, Vlavianos P, et al. Single, total paracentesis for tense ascites: sequential hemodynamic changes and right atrial size. *Hepatology.* 1990;11:662–667.
6. Tito L, Gines P, Arroyo V, et al. Total paracentesis associated with intravenous albumin management of patients with cirrhosis and ascites. *Gastroenterology.* 1990;98:146–151.

Additional Readings

Marx JA. Peritoneal procedures. In: Roberts JR, Hedges JR, eds. *Clinical Procedures in Emergency Medicine.* Philadelphia, Pa: W.B. Saunders; 1998:733–749.

Vila MC, Dola R, Molina L, et al. Hemodynamic changes in patients developing effective hypovolemia after total paracentesis. *J Hepatology.* 1998;28:639–645.

⠿ AP This procedure should be performed only by physicians, advanced practice nurses, and other health care professionals (including critical care nurses) with additional knowledge, skills, and demonstrated competence per professional licensure or institutional standard.

Assisting with Abdominal Paracentesis

P U R P O S E: Abdominal paracentesis is performed to remove fluid from the peritoneal cavity for diagnostic or therapeutic purposes.

Peggy Kirkwood
Karen K. Carlson

PREREQUISITE NURSING KNOWLEDGE

- Peritoneal fluid is normally straw-colored, serous fluid secreted by the cells of the peritoneum. Grossly bloody fluid in the abdomen is abnormal.
- The peritoneal fluid collected is used to evaluate and diagnose the cause of ascites, acute abdominal conditions such as peritonitis or pancreatitis, and blunt or penetrating trauma to the abdomen.
- Therapeutic paracentesis is used to reduce intra-abdominal and diaphragmatic pressures in order to relieve dyspnea and respiratory compromise and prevent peritoneal rupture.
- Ascitic fluid is produced as a result of a variety of conditions. These may include interference in venous return because of heart failure, constrictive pericarditis, or tricuspid valve insufficiency; obstruction of flow in the vena cava or portal vein; disturbance in electrolyte balance such as sodium retention; depletion of plasma proteins because of nephrotic syndrome or starvation; lymphoma, leukemia, or neoplasms involving the liver or mediastinum; chronic pancreatitis; or cirrhosis of the liver.
- Knowledge of anatomy and physiology of the abdomen is important in order to avoid unexpected outcomes.
  - ❖ Intestines and bladder lie immediately beneath the abdominal surface.
  - ❖ Large volumes of ascitic fluid will tend to float the air-filled bowel toward the midline, where it may be easily perforated during the procedure.
  - ❖ The cecum is relatively fixed and is much less mobile than the sigmoid colon. Therefore, bowel perforations are more frequent in the right lower quadrant than in the left.
- Paracentesis is contraindicated in patients with an acute abdomen, who require immediate surgery. Both coagulopathies and thrombocytopenia are considered relative contraindications.
- Caution should be used when paracentesis is performed in patients with severe bowel distention, previous abdominal surgery (especially pelvic surgery), pregnancy (use open technique after first trimester), distended bladder that cannot be emptied with a Foley catheter, or obvious infection at intended site of insertion (cellulitis or abscess).
- Insertion site should be midline one third the distance from the umbilicus to the symphysis (2 to 3 cm below the umbilicus; see Figure 98–1). Alternate position is a point one third the distance from the umbilicus to the anterior iliac crest (left side preferred).[1]
- Ultrasound can be used before paracentesis to locate fluid and during the procedure to guide insertion of catheter[2, 3] (Level V: clinical studies in more than one patient population and situation).

EQUIPMENT

- Commercially prepared kit or the following:
  - ❖ Sterile gloves and mask
  - ❖ Skin-cleansing solution (povidone-iodine)
  - ❖ Sterile marking pen
  - ❖ Sterile towels or sterile drape
  - ❖ Local anesthetic for injection: 1% or 2% lidocaine with epinephrine
  - ❖ 5- or 10-mL syringe with 21- or 25-G needle for anesthetic
  - ❖ Trocar with stylet, needle (16-, 18-, or 20-G), or angiocatheter, depending on abdominal wall thickness
  - ❖ 25- or 27-G 1½-in needle
  - ❖ 20- or 22-G spinal needles
  - ❖ 20-mL syringe for diagnostic tap
  - ❖ 50-mL syringe if using stopcock technique
  - ❖ Four sterile tubes for specimens
  - ❖ Scalpel and no. 11 knife blade
  - ❖ Three-way stopcock
  - ❖ Sterile 1-L collection bottles with connecting tubing
  - ❖ Nylon skin suture material on cutting needle (4-0 or 5-0) and needle holder
  - ❖ Mayo scissors and straight scissors
  - ❖ Hemostat

* ❖ Four to six sterile 4 × 4 gauze pads
* ❖ Sterile gauze dressing with tape or adhesive strip.

PATENT AND FAMILY EDUCATION

* Explain the indications, procedure, and risks to the patient and family. ➺*Rationale:* Decreases patient anxiety and encourages patient and family cooperation and understanding of the procedure.
* Explain the patient's role in assisting with the procedure and postprocedure care. ➺*Rationale:* Elicits patient cooperation during and after the procedure.
* Explain the signs and symptoms to report, such as fever, abdominal pain, decreased urine output, bleeding, and leakage of fluid from surgical wound site. ➺*Rationale:* Unexpected outcomes may not manifest themselves for a period of time following the procedure.

PATIENT ASSESSMENT AND PREPARATION

Patient Assessment

* Past medical history and review of systems for abdominal injury, major gastrointestinal pathology, liver disease, and portal hypertension. ➺*Rationale:* Certain conditions of the gastrointestinal tract may be diagnosed and treated with paracentesis. Contraindications to paracentesis may be identified.
* Respiratory status (ie, rate, depth, excursion, gas exchange, and use of accessory muscles). ➺*Rationale:* Paracentesis may be indicated to decrease work of breathing.
* Baseline fluid and electrolyte status. ➺*Rationale:* Removal of peritoneal fluid may cause compartment shifting of intravascular volume, electrolytes, and proteins, leading to a decreased circulating volume.
* Bowel or bladder distention. ➺*Rationale:* Distention increases the risk of bowel or bladder perforation during the procedure.

* Abdominal girth. ➺*Rationale:* Provides information on changes in fluid accumulation within the peritoneal cavity.
* Coagulation studies (ie, prothrombin time [PT], partial thromboplastin time, [PTT] and platelets). ➺*Rationale:* Abnormal clotting studies may increase the risk of bleeding during and after the procedure. Therapy may be necessary to correct clotting abnormalities before the procedure.

Patient Preparation

* Ensure that patient understands preprocedural teaching. Answer questions as they arise and reinforce information as needed. ➺*Rationale:* Evaluates and reinforces understanding of previously taught information.
* Ensure written informed consent has been obtained. ➺*Rationale:* Paracentesis is an invasive procedure, requiring a signed informed consent form.
* Decompress the bladder either by having the patient void or by inserting a Foley catheter. ➺*Rationale:* A distended bladder increases the risk of bladder perforation during the procedure.
* Obtain plain and upright x-rays of the abdomen before the procedure is performed. ➺*Rationale:* Air is introduced during the procedure and may confuse the diagnosis later.
* Place the patient in the supine position (may tilt to side of collection slightly for improved fluid positioning). ➺*Rationale:* Fluid accumulates in the dependent areas.
* Examine abdomen for areas of shifting dullness. Find landmarks and mark appropriately. ➺*Rationale:* Shifting dullness indicates fluid.
* If the patient has altered mental status, soft wrist restraints may be needed. ➺*Rationale:* It is imperative that the patient not move his or her hands into the sterile field once it has been established

---

Procedure for Assisting with Abdominal Paracentesis

Steps	Rationale	Special Considerations
1. Wash hands, and don personal protective equipment.	Reduces transmission of microorganisms and body secretions; standard precautions.	
2. Assist to prepare equipment and sterile field.	Facilitates easy access to needed equipment.	Maintain aseptic technique.
3. Assist physician or nurse practitioner to cleanse insertion site with povidone-iodine solution.	Reduces risk of infection.	Use sterile technique.
4. Apply sterile drapes to outline the area for trochar insertion.	Provides sterile field to decrease risk of infection.	Avoid the rectus muscle due to increased risk of hemorrhage from epigastric vessels; surgical scars due to increased risk of perforation caused by adhesion of bowel to the wall of the peritoneum; and upper quadrants due to the possibility of undetected hepatomegaly.[4]
5. Assist physician or nurse practitioner to draw up local anesthetic (lidocaine with epinephrine preferred).	Local anesthesia minimizes pain and discomfort. Epinephrine helps eliminate unwanted abdominal wall bleeding.	Maximum dose of lidocaine is 30 mL of 1% or 15 mL of 2%.

Procedure continued on following page

Procedure	**for Assisting with Abdominal Paracentesis** *Continued*

Steps	Rationale	Special Considerations
6. Assist in collection of peritoneal fluid for laboratory analysis.	Collection of fluid for laboratory studies to provide information about the patient's status.	Usually diagnostic tests ordered include tube 1: lactate dehydrogenase (LDH) glucose, albumin; tube 2: protein, specific gravity; tube 3: cell count and differential; tube 4: save until further notice. If indicated, Gram stain, acid-fast bacillus (AFB) stain, bacterial and fungal cultures, amylase, and triglycerides.[4]
7. Assist to attach syringes or stopcock and tubing and gently aspirate or siphon fluid by gravity or vacuum into collection device.	Initiates therapy.	Monitor amount of fluid removed. Removal of large amount of fluid (>1 L) may cause hypotension. If large amounts are removed or hypotension seen, consider IV albumin to maintain intravascular volume.[5, 6] *(Level V: Clinical studies in more than one patient population and situation)*
8. After the fluid and catheter are removed, apply pressure to the wound.	Keeps insertion site clean. Reduces risk of infection. If the wound is still leaking fluid after 5 minutes of direct pressure, the site may need to be sutured.	Inspect catheter to ensure it is intact.
9. Assist with suturing (see Procedure 120) as needed and apply a pressure dressing.		
10. Apply sterile dressing to wound site.	Provides a barrier to infection and collects fluid that may leak from wound site.	
11. Dispose of equipment and soiled material in appropriate receptacle.	Standard precautions.	
12. Wash hands.	Reduces transmission of microorganisms.	

Expected Outcomes	Unexpected Outcomes
• Evacuation of peritoneal fluid for laboratory analysis • Decompression of peritoneal cavity • Relief of respiratory compromise • Relief of abdominal discomfort	• Perforation of bowel, bladder, or stomach • Lacerations of major vessels (mesenteric, iliac, aorta) • Abdominal wall hematomas • Laceration of catheter and loss in peritoneal cavity • Incisional hernias • Local or systemic infection • Hypovolemia, hypotension, shock • Bleeding from insertion site • Ascitic fluid leak from insertion site • Peritonitis

Patient Monitoring and Care

Patient Monitoring and Care	Rationale	Reportable Conditions
		These conditions should be reported if they persist despite nursing interventions.
1. Evaluate changes in abdominal girth.	Provides evidence of fluid reaccumulation.	• Increasing abdominal girth

Patient Monitoring and Care *Continued*

Patient Monitoring and Care	Rationale	Reportable Conditions
2. Monitor for changes in respiratory status.	Removal of ascitic fluid should relieve pressure on the diaphragm and the resulting respiratory distress.	• Respiratory rate >24 breaths per minute or significant increase from baseline • Increased depth of breathing • Irregular breathing pattern • Pulse oximetry <92%, or significant decrease from baseline
3. Monitor for potential complications, including bowel or bladder perforation, bleeding, and intravascular volume loss.	Paracentesis interrupts the integrity of the skin and underlying peritoneum.	• Hematuria • Hypotension • Tachycardia
4. Monitor vital signs, temperature, insertion site for drainage or evidence of infection.	Infection is a complication of paracentesis.	• Increased temperature • Purulent drainage from insertion site • Redness, swelling at insertion site • Abnormal laboratory results (increased white blood cells [WBCs])
5. Monitor intake and output.	Provides data for evaluation of fluid balance status.	• Inappropriate fluid balance or changes from baseline fluid status
6. Evaluate laboratory data when returned.	Provides for evaluation of condition and aids in diagnosis.	• Red blood cells (RBCs) >100,000/mm³ • Amylase >2.5 times normal • Alkaline phosphatase >5.5 mg/dL • WBCs >100/mm³ • Positive culture results

Documentation

Documentation should include the following:

- Patient and family education
- Date and time of procedure
- Patient tolerance of procedure
- Assessment of insertion site after procedure
- Amount and characteristics of fluid removed

- Specimens sent for laboratory analysis
- Postprocedure vital signs, respiratory status, and abdominal girth
- Unexpected outcomes
- Nursing interventions

References

1. Brown ML. Abdominal paracentesis and peritoneal lavage. In: Pfenninger JL, Fowler GC, eds. *Procedures for Primary Care Physicians.* St. Louis, Mo: Mosby–Year Book; 1994:892–897.
2. Bode PJ, van Vugt AB. Ultrasound in the diagnosis of injury. *Injury.* 1996;27:379–383.
3. Goletti O, Ghiselli G, Lippolis PV, et al. The role of ultrasonography in blunt abdominal trauma: results in 250 consecutive cases. *J Trauma.* 1994;36:178–181.
4. Ferri FF. Paracentesis. In: Ferri F, ed. *The Care of the Medical Patient.* 4th ed. St. Louis, Mo: Mosby; 1998:810–812.
5. Panos MZ, Moore K, Vlavianos P, et al. Single, total paracentesis for tense ascites: sequential hemodynamic changes and right atrial size. *Hepatology.* 1990;11:662–667.
6. Tito L, Gines P, Arroyo V, et al. Total paracentesis associated with intravenous albumin management of patients with cirrhosis and ascites. *Gastroenterology.* 1990;98:146–151.

Additional Readings

Marx JA. Peritoneal procedures. In: Roberts JR, Hedges JR, eds. *Clinical Procedures in Emergency Medicine.* Philadelphia, Pa: W.B. Saunders; 1998:733–749.
Vila MC, Dola R, Molina L, et al. Hemodynamic changes in patients developing effective hypovolemia after total paracentesis. *J Hepatology.* 1998;28:639–645.

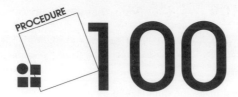
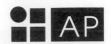

100

Performing Percutaneous Peritoneal Lavage

P U R P O S E: Percutaneous peritoneal lavage is performed for both therapeutic and diagnostic purposes.

Peggy Kirkwood

PREREQUISITE NURSING KNOWLEDGE

- Diagnostic lavage is used after blunt abdominal trauma, or in trauma patients with head injuries, those who are unconscious, or those with preexisting paraplegia to determine the presence of the following:
  - ❖ Hemoperitoneum (blood in lavage returns)
  - ❖ Organ injury (intestinal enzymes or microorganisms in lavage returns).
- Therapeutic lavage is used to
  - ❖ Irrigate and cleanse purulent exudate in patients with peritonitis or intra-abdominal abscess
  - ❖ Warm the abdominal cavity in hypothermic patients
  - ❖ Remove unwanted or toxic chemicals through peritoneal dialysis.
- Computed tomography (CT) frequently is used in hemodynamically stable trauma patients as the diagnostic procedure of choice; however, in hemodynamically unstable patients, diagnostic peritoneal lavage (DPL) is preferred.[1, 2] DPL is quick, inexpensive, safe, and highly sensitive to the presence of blood in the peritoneal cavity.
- Knowledge of anatomy and physiology of the abdomen is important in order to avoid unexpected outcomes.
  - ❖ Intestines and bladder lie immediately beneath the abdominal surface. In children, the bladder is an abdominal organ. In adults, a full bladder is raised out of the pelvis.
  - ❖ The cecum is relatively fixed and is much less mobile than the sigmoid colon. Therefore, bowel perforations are more frequent in the right lower quadrant than in the left.
  - ❖ A distended stomach can extend to the anterior abdominal wall.

- Peritoneal fluid is normally straw-colored, serous fluid secreted by the cells of the peritoneum. Grossly bloody fluid, a red blood cell (RBC) count of greater than $100,000/mm^3$, or the presence of bacteria or bile in the return fluid in the abdomen is abnormal.
- Peritoneal lavage is absolutely contraindicated in an acute abdomen that requires immediate surgery as indicated by free air on x-ray or penetrating abdominal trauma.
- Relative contraindications for DPL include the following[3, 4]:
  - ❖ Thrombocytopenia
  - ❖ Coagulopathy
  - ❖ Severe bowel distension
  - ❖ Previous abdominal surgery, especially pelvic surgery
  - ❖ Distended bladder that cannot be emptied with a Foley catheter
  - ❖ Obvious infection at intended site of insertion (cellulitis or abscess).
- Use caution when performing DPL in patients with suspected pelvic fractures (may use a supra-umbilical site), or pregnancy (use open technique with supra-umbilical approach after first trimester).
- Insertion site should be midline one third the distance from the umbilicus to the symphysis, 2 to 3 cm below the umbilicus (see Fig. 98–1). Alternate position is a point one third the distance from the umbilicus to the anterior iliac crest (left side preferred).[5]
- Ultrasound can be used prior to peritoneal lavage to locate fluid and during the procedure to guide insertion of catheter.[6, 7]

EQUIPMENT

- Commercially prepared kit or
- Sterile gloves and mask or face shield
- Skin cleansing solution (povidone-iodine)
- Sterile marking pen
- Sterile towels or sterile drape
- Razor to shave area, if necessary

AP This procedure should be performed only by physicians, advanced practice nurses, and other health care professionals (including critical care nurses) with additional knowledge, skills, and demonstrated competence per professional licensure or institutional standard.

- Local anesthetic for injection: 1% or 2% lidocaine with epinephrine
- 5- or 10-mL syringe with 25- or 27-G needle for anesthetic
- Scalpel and no. 11 knife blade
- Mayo scissors and straight scissors
- Trocar with stylet, or needle (16-, 18-, or 20-G), or angiocatheter, depending on abdominal wall thickness, guidewire with floppy tip, and 9- to 18-Fr peritoneal lavage catheter
- Hemostat
- 20-mL syringe for diagnostic tap
- Sterile intravenous (IV) tubing (without valves) with appropriate sterile connectors for lavage catheter and IV bags
- Sterile tubes for specimens
- Warmed Ringer's lactate (RL), normal saline (NS), or antibiotic solution for infusion into abdomen
- Three-way stopcock for therapeutic lavage
- Nylon skin suture material on cutting needle (4-0 or 5-0) and needle holder
- Four to six sterile 4 × 4 gauze pads
- Sterile gauze dressing with tape or adhesive strip.

PATIENT AND FAMILY EDUCATION

- Explain the indications, the procedure, and the risks to the patient and family. ⟶*Rationale:* Decreases patient anxiety and encourages patient and family cooperation and understanding of procedure.
- Explain the patient's role in assisting with the procedure and postprocedure care. ⟶*Rationale:* Elicits patient cooperation during and after the procedure.
- Explain the signs and symptoms to report, such as fever, abdominal pain, decreased urine output, bleeding, and leakage of fluid from wound site. ⟶*Rationale:* Unexpected outcomes may not manifest themselves for a period of time following the procedure.

PATIENT ASSESSMENT AND PREPARATION

Patient Assessment

- Past medical history and review of systems for abdominal injury, peritonitis, intra-abdominal abscess, or pregnancy. ⟶*Rationale:* Certain conditions of the gastrointestinal tract may be diagnosed and treated with peritoneal lavage. Contraindications to peritoneal lavage may be identified.

- Bowel or bladder distension. ⟶*Rationale:* Distension increases the risk of bowel or bladder perforation during the procedure.
- Coagulation studies (ie, prothrombin time [PT], partial thromboplastin time [PTT], and platelets). ⟶*Rationale:* Abnormal clotting studies may increase the risk of bleeding during and after the procedure. Therapy may be necessary to correct clotting abnormalities before performing the procedure.
- Plain and upright x-rays of the abdomen (before the procedure). ⟶*Rationale:* Air is introduced during the procedure and may confound the diagnosis later.

Patient Preparation

- Ensure that patient understands preprocedural teaching. Answer questions as they arise and reinforce information as needed. ⟶*Rationale:* Evaluates and reinforces understanding of previously taught information.
- Obtain a written informed consent form, if possible. In a trauma situation or unresponsive patient, this may be implied consent. ⟶*Rationale:* Peritoneal lavage is an invasive procedure, requiring a signed consent form.
- Have patient void or insert a Foley catheter. ⟶*Rationale:* A distended bladder increases the risk of bladder perforation during the procedure.
- Insert a nasogastric tube (see Procedure 97) and attach to low intermittent suction. ⟶*Rationale:* A distended stomach increases the risk of perforation during the procedure.
- Place the patient in the supine position (may tilt to side of collection slightly for improved fluid positioning). ⟶*Rationale:* Fluid accumulates in the dependent areas.
- Examine abdomen for landmarks and mark appropriately. Shave area, if necessary. ⟶*Rationale:* Correct placement of catheter for peritoneal lavage will minimize complications.
- If the patient has altered mental status, soft wrist restraints may be needed. ⟶*Rationale:* It is imperative that the patient not move his or her hands into the sterile field once it has been established.

⊞ AP This procedure should be performed only by physicians, advanced practice nurses, and other health care professionals (including critical care nurses) with additional knowledge, skills, and demonstrated competence per professional licensure or institutional standard.

| Procedure | for Performing Percutaneous Peritoneal Lavage |

Steps	Rationale	Special Considerations
1. Wash hands, and don personal protective equipment.	Reduces transmission of microorganisms and body secretions; standard precautions.	
2. Prepare equipment and sterile field.	Facilitates easy access to needed equipment.	Maintain aseptic technique.

Procedure continued on following page

Procedure **for Performing Percutaneous Peritoneal Lavage** *Continued*

Steps	Rationale	Special Considerations

3. Set up lavage equipment.
  A. Attach IV tubing to lavage fluid and clear tubing of air.
  B. Attach IV tubing to one port of three-way stopcock and attach drainage collector to second port of three-way stopcock.
  OR
  C. Use IV tubing with a roller clamp and use the lavage fluid bag as the drainage bag.
	Provides closed system for instillation and drainage of lavage fluid.	

4. Prepare insertion site with povidone-iodine solution.	Reduces risk of infection.	Use sterile technique.
5. Apply sterile drapes to outline the insertion site. Site should be in the midline about one third the distance from the umbilicus to the symphysis (usually 2 to 3 cm below the umbilicus; see Figure 98–1). Alternate position is a point about one third the distance from the umbilicus to the anterior iliac crest (with the left side preferred).		Avoid rectus muscle because of increased risk of hemorrhage from epigastric vessels; surgical scars because of increased risk of perforation caused by adhesion of bowel to the wall of the peritoneum; and upper quadrants because of possibility of undetected hepatomegaly.[8]
6. Inject area with local anesthetic (lidocaine with epinephrine preferred). Initially direct needle perpendicular to the skin and infiltrate the peritoneum with anesthetic.	Local anesthesia minimizes pain and discomfort. Epinephrine helps eliminate unwanted abdominal wall bleeding and false-positive results.	Maximum dose of lidocaine is 30 mL of 1% or 15 mL of 2%. Assess for anesthesia of area. Resistance will be felt as the needle perforates the peritoneum.
7. Using the no. 11 blade scalpel, create a vertical skin incision large enough to allow threading a 3- to 5-mm lavage catheter. Spread the subcutaneous tissue and incise the fascia to expose the peritoneum. Nick the peritoneal membrane to pass the catheter.	To create an opening large enough to thread the lavage catheter.	When the subcutaneous tissue is nicked with the scalpel, a tough, gritty sensation will be felt.
8. Insert an 18-G needle attached to a 20-mL or 50 mL syringe perpendicular through the anesthetized tract into the peritoneum. Apply slight suction to the syringe as it is advanced. Grasp the needle close to the skin as it is advanced (see Fig. 98–2).	Provides access to peritoneal space. Slight suction is applied to indicate when the peritoneum is entered and if a blood vessel is entered. Grasping the needle as it is advanced prevents accidental thrusting into the abdomen and possible viscous perforation.	Inserted through small incision at midline below umbilicus. A small pop is felt as needle advances through anterior and posterior muscle fascia and enters peritoneum.
9. Once in the cavity, direct the needle at a 60-degree angle toward the center of the pelvic hollow. If fluid returns, fill the syringe.	Collection of fluid for laboratory studies.	A free return of 10 mL of blood is a strong positive finding for a hemoperitoneum. If blood is returned, remove the needle and prepare for immediate surgical intervention.
10. If the tap is dry, perform the lavage technique.	Accurately assesses for hemoperitoneum.	

Procedure **for Performing Percutaneous Peritoneal Lavage** *Continued*

Steps	Rationale	Special Considerations
11. Introduce guidewire through the 18-G needle.	Provides access for insertion of the peritoneal lavage catheter.	The wire should insert easily. If there is any resistance, advance or redirect the needle until the wire feeds easily. Difficulty in advancing the catheter may indicate the stylet is not in the peritoneal cavity or there may be adhesions.
12. Insert about half of the wire into the pelvis and remove the needle. Hold onto the guidewire continuously.	Letting go of the guidewire could allow the wire to inadvertently migrate into peritoneum.	
13. Slide the peritoneal lavage catheter over the wire, using gently twisting motions (Fig. 100–1).	Twisting motion minimizes visceral perforation and displaces abdominal contents.	Always keep a firm hold on the wire to prevent it from slipping into the peritoneal cavity.
14. Remove the wire after the catheter is in the peritoneal cavity.		Aspiration may be attempted. If it is dry, proceed to lavage.
15. Attach lavage catheter to remaining port of stopcock and tubing to withdraw peritoneal fluid.	Fluid may be gently aspirated, siphoned by gravity, or collected into a vacuum device.	Retain first 100 mL of fluid for laboratory analysis.

16. Instill lavage fluid:
  A. If drainage collector is used, turn stopcock off to drainage collector.
  B. Open clamp on IV tubing.
  C. Instill 700 to 1000 mL of warmed RL, NS, or antibacterial fluid.
	Directs lavage fluid into peritoneal space.	Infuse over 10 to 15 minutes. This may be done with a pressure bag to decrease time.

┇┇ AP This procedure should be performed only by physicians, advanced practice nurses, and other health care professionals (including critical care nurses) with additional knowledge, skills, and demonstrated competence per professional licensure or institutional standard.

Procedure continued on following page

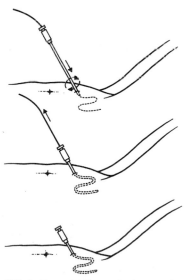

■ ● **FIGURE 100–1.** The plastic catheter is placed over the guidewire and inserted into the peritoneal cavity by means of a twisting motion at the skin level. After the catheter has been advanced, the guidewire is removed. (From Pfenninger JL, Fowler GC, eds. *Procedures for Primary Care Physicians.* St. Louis: Mosby–Year Book; 1994:896.)

Steps	Rationale	Special Considerations
17. Rotate patient side to side (if not contraindicated).	Facilitates sampling of fluid that may accumulate in pockets on either side. Mixes solution with any free material in abdominal cavity.	
18. Drain lavage fluid: A. If drainage collector is used, turn stopcock off to IV tubing. B. If drainage collector is not used, lower IV bag to a level below the patient. C. Allow fluid to drain into drainage collector or lowered IV bag.	Directs lavage fluid from peritoneal space to drainage collector.	In therapeutic lavage, consider dwell time of fluid prior to drainage (usually 5 to 10 minutes). When draining fluid, be careful that there is not tension on the tubing.
19. Rotate patient side to side (if not contraindicated).	Facilitates drainage of fluid that may accumulate in pockets on either side.	Lavage fluid may be absorbed into intravascular space, creating a potential fluid volume excess. Twisting catheter may free the catheter from adhering to peritoneum and facilitate drainage of fluid.
20. Repeat steps 16 to 19 as needed.	Continued lavage may be needed to cleanse peritoneal space.	
21. If lavage is positive, prepare patient for immediate surgery. Leave incision open and cover with sterile, NS-soaked dressing.	Immediate repair of bleeding site is needed.	
22. After the fluid is removed, gently remove the catheter and apply pressure to the wound. Suture the puncture site using a mattress suture with 4-0 nylon (see Procedure 120), and apply a dressing.	Keeps insertion site clean. Reduces risk of infection. Provides a barrier to infection and collects fluid that may leak from wound site.	Inspect catheter to ensure it is intact.
23. Prepare and send fluid specimens for laboratory analysis.	Provides information about patient status.	Have the first 100 mL of fluid analyzed for RBCs, white blood cells (WBCs), amylase, lipase, alkaline phosphate, and culture and sensitivity.
24. Dispose of equipment and soiled material in appropriate receptacle.	Standard precautions.	
25. Wash hands.	Reduces transmission of microorganisms.	

Expected Outcomes

- Lavage fluid returns are obtained for diagnostic evaluation.
- Peritoneum is cleansed of purulent exudate and microorganisms.

Unexpected Outcomes

- Perforation of bowel, bladder, or stomach
- Lacerations of major vessels (mesenteric, iliac, aorta)
- Laceration of catheter or guidewire with loss in peritoneal cavity
- Local or systemic infection
- Hypovolemia, hypotension
- Bleeding from insertion site
- Inadequate drainage of lavage fluid
- Respiratory compromise

Patient Monitoring and Care

Patient Monitoring and Care	Rationale	Reportable Conditions
		These conditions should be reported if they persist despite nursing interventions.
1. Monitor for changes in respiratory status (ie, rate, depth, and pattern).	Retained lavage fluid puts pressure on diaphragm and intra-abdominal organs, causing difficulty breathing.	• Respiratory rate >24 breaths per minute • Increased depth of breathing • Irregular breathing pattern • Pulse oximetry <92%, or significant decrease from baseline
2. Monitor for potential complications, including bowel or bladder perforation, bleeding, and intravascular volume loss.	Peritoneal lavage interrupts the integrity of the skin and underlying peritoneum.	• Acute abdominal pain, distention, rigidity, and guarding • Decreased bowel sounds • Fever, chills • Blood in urine • Hypotension • Tachycardia
3. Monitor vital signs and insertion site for drainage or evidence of infection.	Infection is a complication of peritoneal lavage.	• Increased temperature • Purulent drainage from insertion site • Redness, swelling at insertion site • Labile blood pressure
4. Monitor intake and output.	Provides data for evaluation of fluid balance status.	• Inappropriate fluid balance
5. Evaluate laboratory data when returned.	Provides for evaluation of condition and aids in diagnosis.	• RBCs >100,000/mm³ • Amylase >2.5 times normal • Alkaline phosphate >5.5 mg/dL • WBCs >100/mm³ • Positive culture results

Documentation

Documentation should include the following:

- Patient and family education
- Date and time of procedure
- Patient tolerance of procedure
- Assessment of insertion site after procedure
- Type and amount of fluid instilled and dwell time
- True drainage (total drainage minus lavage fluid input)
- Amount and characteristics of fluid removed
- Specimens sent for laboratory analysis
- Postprocedure vital signs, respiratory status
- Unexpected outcomes
- Nursing interventions

References

1. Coleridge ST. Peritoneal lavage. In: Howell JM, ed. *Emergency Medicine.* Philadelphia, Pa: W.B. Saunders; 1998:73–78.
2. Colucciello SA, Marx JS. Blunt abdominal trauma. In: Harwood-Nuss AL, ed. *The Clinical Practice of Emergency Medicine.* 2nd ed. Philadelphia, Pa: Lippincott-Raven; 1996:460–464.
3. Marx JA. Peritoneal procedures. In: Roberts JR, Hedges JR, eds. *Clinical Procedures in Emergency Medicine.* Philadelphia, Pa: W.B. Saunders; 1998:733–749.
4. Lindsay MC. Abdominal trauma. In: Aghababian RV, ed. *Emergency Medicine: The Core Curriculum.* Philadelphia, Pa: Lippincott-Raven; 1998:1239–1245.
5. Brown ML. Abdominal paracentesis and peritoneal lavage.

This procedure should be performed only by physicians, advanced practice nurses, and other health care professionals (including critical care nurses) with additional knowledge, skills, and demonstrated competence per professional licensure or institutional standard.

In: Pfenninger JL, Fowler GC, eds. *Procedures for Primary Care Physicians.* St. Louis, Mo: Mosby Year Book; 1994:892–897.

6. Bode PJ, van Vugt AB. Ultrasound in the diagnosis of injury. *Injury.* 1996;27:379–383.

7. Goletti O, Ghiselli G, Lippolis PV, et al. The role of ultrasonography in blunt abdominal trauma: results in 250 consecutive cases. *J Trauma.* 1994;36:178–181.

8. Ferri FF. Paracentesis. In: Ferri E, ed. *The Care of the Medical Patient.* 4th ed. St. Louis, Mo: Mosby; 1998:810–812.

Additional Readings

Kemmeter PR, Senagor AJ, Smith D, Oostendorp L. Dilemmas in the diagnosis of blunt enteric trauma. *Am Surg.* 1997;64:750–754.

Simon RR, Brenner BE. Peritoneal lavage. In: *Emergency Procedures and Techniques.* Baltimore, Md; Williams & Wilkins; 1994:557–568.

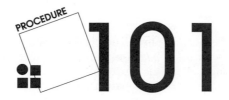

101

Assisting with Percutaneous Peritoneal Lavage

P U R P O S E : Percutaneous peritoneal lavage is performed for both therapeutic and diagnostic purposes.

Peggy Kirkwood
Karen K. Carlson

PREREQUISITE NURSING KNOWLEDGE

- Diagnostic lavage is used after blunt abdominal trauma, or in trauma patients with head injuries, those who are unconscious, or those with preexisting paraplegia to determine the presence of the following:
  - ❖ Hemoperitoneum (blood in lavage returns)
  - ❖ Organ injury (intestinal enzymes or microorganisms in lavage returns).
- Therapeutic lavage is used to
  - ❖ Irrigate and cleanse purulent exudate in patients with peritonitis or intra-abdominal abscess
  - ❖ Warm the abdominal cavity in hypothermic patients
  - ❖ Remove unwanted or toxic chemicals through peritoneal dialysis.
- Computed tomography (CT) is frequently used in hemodynamically stable trauma patients as the diagnostic procedure of choice; however, in hemodynamically unstable patients, diagnostic peritoneal lavage (DPL) is preferred.[1, 2] DPL is quick, inexpensive, safe, and highly sensitive to the presence of blood in the peritoneal cavity.
- Knowledge of anatomy and physiology of the abdomen is important in order to avoid unexpected outcomes.
  - ❖ Intestines and bladder lie immediately beneath the abdominal surface. In children, the bladder is an abdominal organ. In adults, a full bladder is raised out of the pelvis.
  - ❖ The cecum is relatively fixed and is much less mobile than the sigmoid colon. Therefore, bowel perforations are more frequent in the right lower quadrant than in the left.
  - ❖ A distended stomach can extend to the anterior abdominal wall.
- Peritoneal fluid is normally straw-colored, serous fluid secreted by the cells of the peritoneum. Grossly bloody fluid, a red blood cell (RBC) count of greater than 100,000/mm³, or the presence of bacteria or bile in the return fluid in the abdomen is abnormal.

- Peritoneal lavage is absolutely contraindicated in an acute abdomen that requires immediate surgery as indicated by free air on x-ray or penetrating abdominal trauma.
- Relative contraindications for DPL include the following[3, 4]:
  - ❖ Thrombocytopenia
  - ❖ Coagulopathy
  - ❖ Severe bowel distension
  - ❖ Previous abdominal surgery, especially pelvic surgery
  - ❖ Distended bladder that cannot be emptied with a Foley catheter
  - ❖ Obvious infection at intended site of insertion (cellulitis or abscess).
- Use caution when performing DPL in patients with suspected pelvic fractures (may use a supra-umbilical site), or pregnancy (use open technique with supra-umbilical approach after first trimester).
- Insertion site should be midline one third the distance from the umbilicus to the symphysis, 2 to 3 cm below the umbilicus (see Fig. 98–1). Alternate position is a point one third the distance from the umbilicus to the anterior iliac crest (left side preferred).[5]
- Ultrasound can be used prior to peritoneal lavage to locate fluid and during the procedure to guide insertion of catheter.[6, 7]

EQUIPMENT

- Commercially prepared kit or
- Sterile gloves and mask or face shield
- Skin cleansing solution (povidone-iodine)
- Sterile marking pen
- Sterile towels or sterile drape
- Razor to shave area, if necessary
- Local anesthetic for injection—1% or 2% lidocaine with epinephrine
- 5- or 10-mL syringe with 25- or 27-G needle for anesthetic

- Scalpel and no. 11 knife blade
- Mayo scissors and straight scissors
- Trocar with stylet, or needle (16-, 18-, or 20-G), or angiocatheter, depending on abdominal wall thickness, guidewire with floppy tip, and 9 to 18 Fr peritoneal lavage catheter
- Hemostat
- 20-mL syringe for diagnostic tap
- Sterile intravenous (IV) tubing (without valves) with appropriate sterile connectors for lavage catheter and IV bags
- Sterile tubes for specimens
- Warmed Ringer's lactate (RL), normal saline (NS), or antibiotic solution for infusion into abdomen
- Three-way stopcock for therapeutic lavage
- Nylon skin suture material on cutting needle (4-0 or 5-0) and needle holder
- Four to six sterile 4 × 4 gauze pads
- Sterile gauze dressing with tape or adhesive strip.

PATIENT AND FAMILY EDUCATION

- Explain the indications, the procedure, and the risks to the patient and family.   ➺*Rationale:* Decreases patient anxiety and encourages patient and family cooperation and understanding of procedure.
- Explain the patient's role in assisting with the procedure and postprocedure care.   ➺*Rationale:* Elicits patient cooperation during and after the procedure.
- Explain the signs and symptoms to report, such as fever, abdominal pain, decreased urine output, bleeding, and leakage of fluid from wound site.   ➺*Rationale:* Unexpected outcomes may not manifest themselves for a period of time following the procedure.

PATIENT ASSESSMENT AND PREPARATION

Patient Assessment

- Past medical history and review of systems for abdominal injury, peritonitis, intra-abdominal abscess, or pregnancy.   ➺*Rationale:* Certain conditions of the gastrointestinal tract may be diagnosed and treated with peritoneal lavage. Contraindications to peritoneal lavage may be identified.

- Bowel or bladder distension.   ➺*Rationale:* Distension increases the risk of bowel or bladder perforation during the procedure.
- Coagulation studies (ie, prothrombin time [PT], partial thromboplastin time [PTT], and platelets).   ➺*Rationale:* Abnormal clotting studies may increase the risk of bleeding during and after the procedure. Therapy may be necessary to correct clotting abnormalities before performing the procedure.
- Plain and upright x-rays of the abdomen (before the procedure).   ➺*Rationale:* Air is introduced during the procedure and may confound the diagnosis later.

Patient Preparation

- Ensure that patient understands preprocedural teaching. Answer questions as they arise and reinforce information as needed.   ➺*Rationale:* Evaluates and reinforces understanding of previously taught information.
- Ensure that a written informed consent form has been obtained, if possible. In a trauma situation or unresponsive patient, this may be implied consent.   ➺*Rationale:* Peritoneal lavage is an invasive procedure, requiring a signed consent form.
- Have patient void or insert a Foley catheter.   ➺*Rationale:* A distended bladder increases the risk of bladder perforation during the procedure.
- Insert a nasogastric tube (see Procedure 97) and attach to low intermittent suction.   ➺*Rationale:* A distended stomach increases the risk of perforation during the procedure.
- Place the patient in the supine position (may tilt to side of collection slightly for improved fluid positioning).   ➺*Rationale:* Fluid accumulates in the dependent areas.
- Examine abdomen for landmarks and mark appropriately. Shave area, if necessary.   ➺*Rationale:* Correct placement of catheter for peritoneal lavage will minimize complications.
- If the patient has altered mental status, soft wrist restraints may be needed.   ➺*Rationale:* It is imperative that the patient not move his or her hands into the sterile field once it has been established.

| **Procedure** | **for Assisting with Percutaneous Peritoneal Lavage** |

Steps	Rationale	Special Considerations
1. Wash hands, and don personal protective equipment.	Reduces the transmission of microorganisms and body secretions; standard precautions.	
2. Prepare equipment and sterile field.	Facilitates easy access to needed equipment.	Maintain aseptic technique.

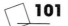

| Procedure | **for Assisting with Percutaneous Peritoneal Lavage** *Continued* |

Steps	Rationale	Special Considerations

3. Set up lavage equipment.
  A. Attach IV tubing to lavage fluid and clear tubing of air.
  B. Attach IV tubing to one port of three-way stopcock and attach drainage collector to second port of three-way stopcock.
  OR
  C. Use IV tubing with a roller clamp and use the lavage fluid bag as the drainage bag.
	Provides closed system for instillation and drainage of lavage fluid.	

4. Assist to prepare insertion site with povidone-iodine solution.	Reduces risk of infection.	Use sterile technique.
5. Apply sterile drapes to outline the insertion site. Site should be in the midline about one third the distance from the umbilicus to the symphysis (usually 2 to 3 cm below the umbilicus; see Fig. 98–1). Alternate position is a point about one third the distance from the iliac crest (with the left side preferred).		Avoid rectus muscle because of increased risk of hemorrhage from epigastric vessels; surgical scars because of increased risk of perforation caused by adhesion of bowel to the wall of the peritoneum; and upper quadrants because of the possibility of undetected hepatomegaly.[8]
6. Assist to draw up local anesthetic (lidocaine with epinephrine preferred).	Local anesthesia minimizes pain and discomfort. Epinephrine helps eliminate unwanted abdominal wall bleeding and false-positive results.	Maximum dose of lidocaine is 30 mL of 1% or 15 mL of 2%. Assess for anesthesia of area. Resistance will be felt as the needle perforates the peritoneum.
7. If fluid returns, fill the syringe and send specimens to laboratory as ordered.	Collection of fluid for laboratory studies.	A free return of 10 mL of blood is a strong positive finding for a hemoperitoneum. If blood is returned, needle should be removed and the patient prepared for immediate surgical intervention.
8. If the tap is dry, assist with insertion of lavage catheter.	Accurately assesses for hemoperitoneum.	
9. Attach lavage catheter to remaining port of stopcock and tubing to withdraw peritoneal fluid.	Fluid may be gently aspirated, siphoned by gravity, or collected into a vacuum device.	Retain first 100 mL of fluid for laboratory analysis.

10. Instill lavage fluid.
  A. If drainage collector used, turn stopcock off to drainage collector.
  B. Open clamp on IV tubing.
  C. Instill 700 to 1000 mL of warmed RL, NS, or antibacterial fluid.
	Directs lavage fluid into peritoneal space.	Infuse over 10 to 15 minutes. This may be done with a pressure bag to decrease time.

11. Rotate patient side to side (if not contraindicated).	Facilitates sampling of fluid that may accumulate in pockets on either side. Mixes solution with any free material in abdominal cavity.	

Procedure continued on following page

Procedure for Assisting with Percutaneous Peritoneal Lavage *Continued*

Steps	Rationale	Special Considerations
12. Drain lavage fluid. A. If drainage collector is used, turn stopcock off to IV tubing. B. If drainage collector is not used, lower IV bag to a level below the patient. C. Allow fluid to drain into drainage collector or lowered IV bag.	Directs lavage fluid from peritoneal space to drainage collector.	In therapeutic lavage, consider dwell time of fluid before drainage (usually 5 to 10 minutes). When draining fluid, be careful that there is no tension on the tubing.
13. Rotate patient side to side (if not contraindicated).	Facilitates drainage of fluid that may accumulate in pockets on either side.	Lavage fluid may be absorbed into intravascular space, creating a potential fluid volume excess. Twisting catheter may free the catheter from adhering to peritoneum and facilitate drainage of fluid.
14. Repeat steps 11 to 13 as needed.	Continued lavage may be needed to cleanse peritoneal space.	
15. If lavage is positive, prepare patient for immediate surgery. Leave incision open and cover with sterile, NS-soaked dressing.	Immediate repair of bleeding site is needed.	
16. After the fluid and catheter are removed, apply pressure to the wound. Assist with suturing (see Procedure 120) as needed and apply a dressing.	Keep insertion site clean. Reduces risk of infection. Provides a barrier to infection and collects fluid that may leak from wound site.	Inspect catheter to ensure it is intact.
17. Prepare and send fluid specimens for laboratory analysis.	Provides information about patient status.	Have the first 100 mL of fluid analyzed for RBCs, white blood cells (WBCs), amylase, lipase, alkaline phosphate, and culture and sensitivity.
18. Dispose of equipment and solid material in appropriate receptacle.	Standard precautions.	
19. Wash hands.	Reduces transmission of microorganisms.	

Expected Outcomes

- Lavage fluid returns are obtained for diagnostic evaluation.
- Peritoneum is cleansed of purulent exudate and microorganisms.

Unexpected Outcomes

- Perforation of bowel, bladder, or stomach
- Lacerations of major vessels (mesenteric, iliac, aorta)
- Laceration of catheter or guidewide with loss in peritoneal cavity
- Local or systemic infection
- Hypovolemia, hypotension
- Bleeding from insertion site
- Inadequate drainage of lavage fluid
- Respiratory compromise

Patient Monitoring and Care

Patient Monitoring and Care	Rationale	Reportable Conditions
		These conditions should be reported if they persist despite nursing interventions.
1. Monitor for changes in respiratory status (ie, rate, depth, and pattern).	Retained lavage fluid puts pressure on diaphragm and intra-abdominal organs, causing difficulty breathing	• Respiratory rate >24 breaths per minute • Increased depth of breathing • Irregular breathing pattern • Pulse oximetry <92% or significant decrease from baseline
2. Monitor for potential complications, including bowel or bladder perforation, bleeding, and intravascular volume loss.	Peritoneal lavage interrupts the skin and underlying peritoneum.	• Acute abdominal pain, distension, rigidity, and guarding • Decreased bowel sound • Fever, chills • Blood in urine • Hypotension • Tachycardia
3. Monitor vital signs and insertion site for drainage or evidence of infection.	Infection is a complication of peritoneal lavage.	• Increased temperature • Purulent drainage from insertion site • Redness, swelling at insertion site • Labile blood pressure
4. Monitor intake and output.	Provides data for evaluation of fluid balance status.	• Inappropriate fluid balance
5. Evaluate laboratory data when returned.	Provides for evaluation of condition and aids in diagnosis.	• RBCs >100,000/mm³ • Amylase >2.5 times normal • Alkaline phosphate <5.5 mg/dL • WBCs >100/mm³ • Positive culture results

Documentation

Documentation should include the following:

- Patient and family education
- Date and time of procedure
- Patient tolerance of procedure
- Assessment of insertion site after procedure
- Type and amount of fluid instilled and dwell time
- True drainage (total drainage minus lavage fluid input)
- Amount and characteristics of fluid removed
- Specimens sent for laboratory analysis
- Postprocedure vital signs, respiratory status
- Unexpected outcomes
- Nursing interventions

References

1. Coleridge ST. Peritoneal lavage. In: Howell JM. *Emergency Medicine.* Philadelphia, Pa: W.B. Saunders; 1998:73–78.
2. Colucciello SA, Marx JS. Blunt abdominal trauma. In: Harwood-Nuss AL, ed. *The Clinical Practice of Emergency Medicine.* 2nd ed. Philadelphia, Pa: Lippincott-Raven; 1996;460–464.
3. Marx JA. Peritoneal procedures. In: Roberts JR, Hedges JR, eds. *Clinical Procedures in Emergency Medicine.* Philadelphia, Pa.: W.B. Saunders, 1998:733–749.
4. Lindsay MC. Abdominal trauma. In: Aghababian RN, ed. *Emergency Medicine: The Core Curriculum.* Philadelphia, Pa: Lippincott-Raven, 1998:1239–1245.
5. Brown ML. Abdominal paracentesis and peritoneal lavage. In: Pfenninger JL, Fowler GC, eds. *Procedures for Primary Care Physicians.* St. Louis, Mo: Mosby Year Book; 1994;892–897.
6. Bode PJ, van Vugt AB. Ultrasound in the diagnosis of injury. *Injury.* 1996;27:379–383.
7. Goletti O, Ghiselli G, Lippolis PV, et al. The role of ultrasonography in blunt abdominal trauma: results in 250 consecutive cases. *J Trauma* 1994;36:178–181.
8. Ferri FF. Paracentesis. In: Ferri F, ed. *The Care of the Medical Patient.* 4th ed. St. Louis, Mo: Mosby; 1998;810–812.

Additional Readings

Kemmeter PR, Senagor AJ, Smih D, Oostendorp L. Dilemmas in the diagnosis of blunt enteric trauma. *Am Surg.* 1997;64:750–754.

Simon RR, Brenner BE. Peritoneal lavage. In: *Emergency Procedures and Techniques.* Baltimore, Md: Williams & Wilkins; 1994;557–568.

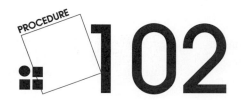

102

Scleral Endoscopic Therapy

P U R P O S E: Scleral endoscopic therapy is performed to control or prevent bleeding from esophageal varices, gastric or duodenal ulcer sites, or other selected causes of upper gastrointestinal (GI) bleeding.

Robin H. Thomas

PREREQUISITE NURSING KNOWLEDGE

- A fiberoptic endoscope is passed through the esophagus and into the stomach and duodenum. Once the site of bleeding is found, a sclerosing agent can be injected through an injector needle, inserted through a port in the endoscope. The sclerosing agent is injected into the bleeding vessel, esophageal varix, or the tissue surrounding the vessel or varix. There are several proposed mechanisms of action of the various sclerosing agents, including esophageal or vascular smooth muscle spasm, compression of the bleeding vessel by submucosal edema or by the volume of sclerosing agent used, arterial constriction, and actual coagulation of the vessel.[1, 2] Ultimately, vessel thrombosis occurs.
- Scleral therapy can be combined with a number of other endoscopic therapies to promote hemostasis, including esophageal band ligation, laser therapy, and thermal coagulation.
- A variety of sclerosing agents are available (Table 102–1). The physician performing the endoscopy will order the agents used.
- Passage of the large-bore therapeutic endoscope may stimulate the vagal response in the patient and precipitate bradydysrhythmias.
- Due to the sedation and topical anesthetic that is used, the patient's gag reflex may be diminished or absent, putting the patient at risk for aspiration.

- Sedation that is used can put the patient at risk for respiratory depression. It is recommended that a conscious sedation protocol be used to monitor the patient.

EQUIPMENT

- Endoscope (rigid or flexible; however, the flexible scope is the usual type used for upper endoscopy)
- Endoscopic injector needle (23- to 26-G, 2- to 5-mm needle)[1, 2] (as ordered by physician)
- Three 10-mL syringes filled with sclerosing agent, as ordered by physician
- Suction setup with connecting tubing
- Rigid pharyngeal suction-tip (Yankauer) catheter
- Safety goggles for each assistant and the patient
- Nonsterile gloves

- Barrier gowns
- Nonsterile 4-in × 4-in gauze or washcloth
- Water-soluble lubricant
- Topical anesthesia
- Premedications (as ordered by physician)
- Two 30- to 60-mL syringes
- Normal saline (NS) or tap water for irrigation
- Oral airway or bite block
- Cardiac monitor
- Pulse oximeter
- Automatic blood pressure cuff
- Emergency intubation equipment

Table 102–1 ● ■ ■ **Sclerosing Agents**

Sclerosants Used for Bleeding Varices[1, 3]	Sclerosants Used for Other Causes of Upper Gastrointestinal Bleeding[2, 3]
Sodium morrhuate (5%)	Epinephrine (1:10,000–1:20,000)
Sodium tetradecyl sulfate (1.5%, 2%, or 3% solutions); can cause higher rates of esophageal ulcerations, dysphagia, and stricture formation than other agents	Ethyl alcohol; volumes greater than 1–2 mL can lead to tissue damage
	Thrombin
	Hypertonic saline
Ethanolamine oleate	Polidocanol
Polidocanol	Other variceal sclerosants can be used
Ethanol; can cause ulceration	
Histoacryl	

Additional equipment (to have available based on patient need) includes the following:

- Nasogastric (NG) tube, Minnesota tube, or Sengstaken-Blakemore tube for esophagogastric tamponade

PATIENT AND FAMILY EDUCATION

- Explain the procedure and indication for scleral therapy, as well as the patient's role in the procedure. ➤*Rationale:* Assists in decreasing patient and family anxiety.
- Explain that the patient will be sedated for comfort and for ease in passing the endoscope. ➤*Rationale:* Assists in decreasing patient and family anxiety.
- Explain that the patient will be monitored closely during and after the procedure. ➤*Rationale:* Assists in decreasing patient and family anxiety.

PATIENT ASSESSMENT AND PREPARATION

Patient Assessment

- Past history of upper GI bleeding and source of bleeding, baseline hematocrit, and hemoglobin. ➤*Rationale:* Used as a basis for assessing bleeding or continued bleeding following scleral therapy.
- Baseline cardiac rhythm. ➤*Rationale:* Passage of a large-bore tube may cause vagal stimulation and bradydysrhythmias.
- Baseline coagulation studies (ie, prothrombin time [PT], partial thromboplastin time [PTT], platelet count). ➤*Rationale:* Abnormal coagulation values increase the potential for bleeding after scleral therapy.
- Respiratory, hemodynamic, and neurologic assessment before the administration of any sedative agent(s). ➤*Rationale:* Baseline assessment data provide information to use as a comparison for further assessment once medications have been administered.
- Baseline vital signs and pulse oximeter reading. ➤*Rationale:* Close monitoring of vital signs and pulse oximetry during the procedure and comparison to baseline are essential to assess patient's tolerance of the procedure.
- Sedation score (Aldrete score, Ramsay scale, or the Conscious Sedation Scale are commonly used) based on blood pressure, pulse, oxygen saturation, level of consciousness, and respiratory status. ➤*Rationale:* Using a scoring system standardizes assessment of the patient's tolerance of conscious sedation.

Patient Preparation

- Ensure that patient understands preprocedural teaching. Answer questions as they arise and reinforce information as needed. ➤*Rationale:* Evaluates and reinforces understanding of previously taught information.
- Ensure that informed consent has been obtained. ➤*Rationale:* Informed consent is necessary prior to invasive procedures and before the administration of conscious sedation.
- Place the patient on a cardiac monitor and apply a pulse oximeter and automatic blood pressure cuff. ➤*Rationale:* Allows for close cardiovascular and respiratory monitoring during the procedure.
- Ensure venous access is in place. ➤*Rationale:* Venous access is needed for premedications and emergency medications.
- Ensure that the patient has been NPO for at least 4 hours before procedure. ➤*Rationale:* Undigested material in the stomach increases the risk of aspiration and decreases visualization of the GI tract.
- Have sedatives (common sedatives used include midazolam, diazepam, meperidine, and fentanyl) available (as ordered) and administer when requested. Naloxone and Romazicon should be available for narcotic or sedative reversal. ➤*Rationale:* Sedation decreases patient anxiety and allows cooperation during the procedure.
- Set up suction with connecting tubing and rigid pharyngeal suction tip attached and a catheter ready. ➤*Rationale:* Necessary for suctioning the patient's oral secretions during the procedure.
- Have atropine available at the bedside. ➤*Rationale:* Necessary if a vagal reaction occurs with the insertion and passage of the endoscope.
- Remove patient dentures. ➤*Rationale:* Dentures interfere with safe passage of the endoscope.
- Protect patient's eyes with goggles or a waterproof covering. ➤*Rationale:* Provides protection against accidental exposure to blood or the sclerosing agents. Sclerosing agents are eye irritants.

Procedure	**for Assisting with Scleral Endoscopic Therapy**	
Steps	**Rationale**	**Special Considerations**
1. Wash hands, and don barrier gown and nonsterile gloves.	Reduces transmission of microorganisms; standard precautions.	
2. Don protective goggles.	Provides protection against accidental spraying with blood or sclerosing agent.	
3. Position patient in the left lateral position. *(Level II: Theory based, on research data to support recommendations: recommendations from expert consensus group may exist)*	The left lateral position allows predictable views of the stomach as the scope is advanced.[3] This position allows secretions to collect in the dependent areas of the mouth for ease of suctioning[3] and is the position of choice to prevent aspiration should the patient vomit.	
4. Perform or assist the physician with gastric lavage (see Procedure 95).	Large amounts of blood or clots in the stomach or esophagus can impair visualization of varices and increase the risk of aspiration during the procedure.	

Procedure	for Assisting with Scleral Endoscopic Therapy *Continued*	

Steps	Rationale	Special Considerations
5. Administer premedications as ordered.	Allows patient cooperation during the endoscopy and facilitates passage of the endoscope.	
6. Assist physician or nurse practitioner with insertion of the endoscope.		
A. Anesthetize the posterior pharynx with topical agent as requested.	Decreases discomfort caused by passage of endoscope.	
B. Insert oral airway (see Procedure 7) or bite block.	Prevents patient from biting the endoscope or inserter's fingers.	
C. Lubricate 20 to 30 cm of distal end of endoscope with water-soluble lubricant. (Many physicians or nurse practitioners prefer to lubricate the scope themselves.)	Minimizes mucosal injury and irritation and facilitates ease of passage of the endoscope.	
D. Encourage patient to simulate swallowing while tube is being passed.	Swallowing maneuver causes epiglottis to close trachea and directs endoscope into esophagus.	
E. Suction oral pharynx as needed.	Due to diminished gag reflex and the presence of the endoscope in the patient's pharynx, oral secretions may not be able to be swallowed. Blood from the GI tract may be vomited and could be aspirated due to the diminished gag reflex.	Gag and cough reflexes may be compromised by topical anesthetics and the patient may vomit as the endoscope is passed, increasing the risk of aspiration. Have emergency intubation equipment available. Monitor heart rate, rhythm, and respiratory status during endoscopy.
7. Inject irrigant via endoscope as requested.	Cleanses area to increase visualization of the tissue.	
8. Manipulate sclerosing needle as requested (Fig. 102–1).	Ensures that the sclerosing needle is in proper position for injection and does not injure tissue during movement of endoscope.	Needle must be retracted prior to manipulation of endoscope.

Procedure continued on following page

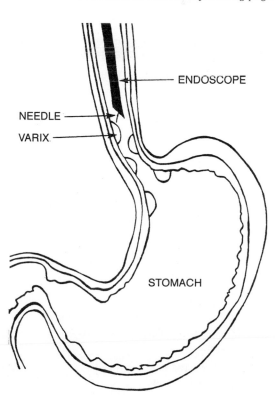

■ ● **FIGURE 102–1.** Injection of sclerosing agent into the engorged varix. (From Pierce JD, Wilkerson E, Griffiths SA. Acute esophageal bleeding and endoscopic injection therapy. *Crit Care Nurse.* 1990;10:67–72.)

Procedure for Assisting with Scleral Endoscopic Therapy *Continued*

Steps	Rationale	Special Considerations
9. Inject sclerosing agent as requested.		The volume of sclerosant used varies depending on the agent used and condition being treated.
10. Insert NG (see Procedure 97) or esophagogastric tamponade tube (see Procedure 94) after removal of endoscope, as requested.	NG tube provides assessment of continued or recurrent bleeding. Esophagogastric tamponade tube may be used to apply pressure to oozing varices.	Suction applied to a NG tube can cause muscosal damage and or disrupt fragile varices and initiate bleeding. A chest x-ray may be performed to rule out aspiration or esophageal perforation.
11. Dispose of equipment in appropriate receptacles. The endoscope should be returned to the GI laboratory for proper disinfection.	Standard precautions.	
12. Wash hands.	Reduces transmission of microorganisms.	

Expected Outcomes

- Hemostasis at site of GI bleeding without recurrent bleeding or prevention of bleeding from esophageal varices
- Stabilization of hematocrit and hemoglobin

Unexpected Outcomes

- Continued or recurrent bleeding from injected varices or ulcer site
- Esophageal sloughing or ulceration
- Esophageal perforation
- Substernal chest pain
- Fever
- Temporary dysphagia
- Allergic response to sclerosing agent
- Aspiration pneumonia
- Pleural effusion
- Atelectasis
- Bacteremia/sepsis

Patient Monitoring and Care

Patient Monitoring and Care	Rationale	Reportable Conditions
		These conditions should be reported if they persist despite nursing interventions.
1. Monitor cardiovascular, respiratory, and neurologic status every 15 min during and after endoscopy until patient returns to preprocedure status then every 30 min to 1 hour for 2 to 4 hours. ○ Level of consciousness ○ Vital signs ○ Oximetry ○ Electrocardiogram	Changes in vital signs, heart rhythm, and oximetry may indicate complications related to the procedure.	- Altered level of consciousness from baseline - Oximetry reading below baseline - Pulse above or below baseline - Fever greater than 101°F - Decrease in blood pressure 20 to 30 mm Hg below baseline
2. Assess pain status.	May indicate continued bleeding or reaction to sclerosant.	- Same pain as experienced before procedure - New onset of chest pain
3. Monitor output from NG tube or any vomitus.	Signs of continued or recurrent bleeding.	- Bright red vomitus or NG drainage
4. Monitor serial hematocrit and hemoglobin results.	Continued fall in the hematocrit and hemoglobin indicates continued or recurrent bleeding.	- Decreasing hematocrit and hemoglobin below baseline

Patient Monitoring and Care *Continued*

Patient Monitoring and Care	Rationale	Reportable Conditions
5. Monitor postural vital signs once the patient is able to be out of bed.	Postural changes indicate volume loss.	• Decrease in blood pressure 20 to 30 mm Hg below baseline • Increase in pulse 10 to 20 beats per minute above baseline
6. Assess for return of normal pharyngeal function. Keep patient on left side with slight head elevation until gag, swallow, and cough reflexes are intact.	Scleral therapy can cause transient dysphagia. Topical anesthesia decreases the gag reflex and increases the risk of aspiration. The left lateral position is the position of choice to prevent aspiration should the patient not be able to control secretions or vomit.	• Prolonged absence of gag, swallow, or cough reflex
7. Provide clear liquids when ordered after return of pharyngeal function. Diet should be progressed slowly to solid food.	Food may act as an irritant to sclerosed ulcer or variceal sites.	• Nausea • Vomiting of bright red blood
8. Administer antacids, histamine$_2$ (H$_2$) blockers, sulcralfate, omeprazole, somatostatin, or octreotide as ordered.	Antacids neutralize gastric acid. Histamine blockers decrease gastric acid secretion. Sulcralfate reacts with gastric acid, forming a paste that adheres to ulcer sites. Omeprazole inhibits the proton pump in the parietal cells of the stomach, suppressing gastric acid secretion. Somatostatin and octreotide (synthetic somatostatin) lower portal pressure by splanchnic vasoconstriction.[4, 5]	
9. Continue patient and family education. ○ Explain signs and symptoms to report (fever, chest pain, difficulty swallowing, vomiting bright red blood, difficulty breathing). ○ Explain diet progression. ○ Explain medication therapy.	Unexpected outcomes can occur within hours or may be delayed days or weeks after scleral therapy. Improves patient compliance and decreases risk of aspiration of liquid or food before patient is ready for swallowing. Improves patient compliance.	

Documentation

Documentation should include the following:

- Patient and family education
- Date and time of procedure
- Initial patient assessment
- Pre- and postprocedure patient and family education
- Baseline vital signs
- Baseline pulse oximetry
- Premedications administered
- Gastric lavage (if performed) and patient's tolerance
- Vital signs and pulse oximetry during scleral therapy
- Sclerosing agents administered and amount

- Time of insertion of NG or tamponade tube (if inserted) and patient's tolerance, characteristics of any drainage from NG tube, x-ray documentation of placement of tamponade tube, and initial pressure applied
- Postscleral therapy vital signs and pulse oximetry
- Position of patient after procedure
- Assessment of gag, swallow, and cough reflexes
- Postprocedure medications administered
- Unexpected outcomes
- Nursing interventions

References

1. Young HS, Matsui SM, Gregory PB. Endoscopic control of variceal upper gastrointestinal hemorrhage. In: Yamada T, ed. *Textbook of Gastroenterology.* Vol. 2, 2nd ed. Philadelphia, Pa: J.B. Lippincott; 1995:2969–2991.

2. Jenson DM. Endoscopic control of upper gastrointestinal nonvariceal bleeding. In: Yamada T, ed. *Textbook of Gastroenterology.* Vol. 2, 2nd ed. Philadelphia, J.B. Lippincott; 1995: 2991–3011.

3. Cotton PB, Williams CB. *Practical Gastrointestinal Endoscopy.* 3rd ed. Oxford: Blackwell Scientific; 1990:23–55.

4. Jenkins SA, Kingsnorth AN, Ellenbogen S, Copeland G, Davis N, Sutton R, Shields R. Octreotide in the control of postsclerotherapy bleeding from oesophageal varices, ulcers and oesophagitis. *HPB Surgery.* 1996;10:1–6.

5. Sieber CC, Mosca PG, Groszmann RJ. Effect of somatostatin on mesenteric vascular resistance in normal and portal hypertensive rats. *Am J Physiol.* 1992;262:G274–277.

Additional Readings

Bryon RJ. Administering conscious sedation. *Crit Care Nurs Clin North Am.* 1997;9:289–299.

Deglin JH, Vallerand AH. *Davis's Drug Guide for Nurses.* 5th ed. Philadelphia, Pa: F.A. Davis; 1997.

Heaton ND. Complications and limitations of injection sclerotherapy in portal hypertension. *Gut.* 1993;34:7–10.

Jenkins SA, Baxter JN, Critchley M, Kingsnorth AN, Makin CA, Ellenbogen S, Grime JS, Love JG, Sutton R. Randomised trial of octreotide for long term management of cirrhosis after variceal haemorrhage. *BMJ.* 1997;315:1338–1341.

Kastrup EK, ed. *Drug Facts and Comparisons.* St. Louis, Mo: Wolters Kluwer Co.; 1998.

McGuirk TD, Coyle WJ. Upper gastrointestinal bleeding. *Emerg Med Clin North Am.* 1996;14:523–545.

Pierce JD, Wilkerson E, Griffiths SA. Acute esophageal bleeding and endoscopic injection therapy. *Crit Care Nurse.* 1990;10: 67–72.

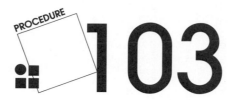

103

Continuous Renal Replacement Therapies

P U R P O S E: Continuous renal replacement therapies (CRRT) are used in the inpatient setting for volume regulation, acid-base control, electrolyte regulation, management of azotemia and, in some cases, immune modulation. These methods are most often used in critically ill patients whose hemodynamic status will not tolerate the rapid fluid and electrolyte shifts associated with hemodialysis.

Karen K. Giuliano

PREREQUISITE NURSING KNOWLEDGE

- CRRT can be accomplished through a variety of methods, as listed. The specifics of the different therapies are outlined in Table 103–1.
  - ❖ Slow continuous ultrafiltration (SCUF)
  - ❖ Continuous arteriovenous hemofiltration (CAVH)
  - ❖ Continuous arteriovenous hemodialysis (CAVHD)
  - ❖ Continuous arteriovenous hemodiafiltration (CAVHDF)
  - ❖ Continuous venovenous hemofiltration (CVVH)
  - ❖ Continuous venovenous hemodialysis (CVVHD)
  - ❖ Continuous venovenous hemodiafiltration (CVVHDF)
- Basic knowledge of the principles of diffusion, ultrafiltration (UF), osmosis, oncotic pressure, and hydrostatic pressure as they pertain to fluid and solute management during dialysis.
  - ❖ Diffusion: The passive movement of solutes through a semipermeable membrane from an area of higher to lower concentration.
  - ❖ Convective transport: When water moves across a membrane along a pressure gradient, some solutes are carried along with the water and do not require a solute concentration gradient (also called solute drag). Convective transport occurs as a result of the friction forces between the solute and water. Convective transport is most effective for the removal of large–molecular-weight solutes.

- ❖ Ultrafiltration. The bulk movement of solute and solvent through a semipermeable membrane using a pressure movement. The size of the solute molecules as compared to the size of molecules that can move through the semipermeable membrane determines the degree of UF.
- ❖ Osmosis: The passive movement of solvent through a semipermeable membrane from an area of higher to lower concentration
- ❖ Oncotic pressure: The pressure exerted by plasma proteins favoring intravascular fluid retention, as well as movement of fluid from the extravascular to the intravascular space.
- ❖ Hydrostatic pressure: The force exerted by arterial blood pressure that favors the movement of fluid from the intravascular to the extravascular space.
- ❖ Absorption: The process by which drug molecules pass through membranes and fluid barriers and into body fluids.
- CRRT uses an artificial kidney (hemofilter, dialyzer) with a semipermeable membrane to create two separate compartments: the blood compartment and the dialysis solution compartment. The semipermeable membrane allows the movement of small molecules (eg, electrolytes) from the patient's blood into the dialysis solution but is impermeable to larger molecules (red blood cells [RBCs], plasma proteins).

Table 103–1 Continuous Renal Replacement Therapies

Mode	Principles Involved	Access	Pump Assisted	Indications	Advantages	Complications/Disadvantages*
Ultrafiltration Therapies						
SCUF (Slow, continuous ultrafiltration)	Ultrafiltration Convection	Arteriovenous	No	Diuretic resistant, volume overloaded, hemodynamically unstable patient who cannot tolerate rapid fluid shifts	Continuous, gradual treatment (fewer high and low extremes)	**Anticoagulation, bleeding** **Hypotension** **Hypothermia** **Access complications (bleeding, clotting, infection)** **Requires strict monitoring of fluid and electrolyte replacement to avoid deficits or overload** **Air embolism** **ICU setting only** **Requires 1:1 nurse/patient ratio** Prolonged, large-bore arterial cannulation required Ideally need MAP of 60 mm Hg to drive extracorporeal circuit Poor control of azotemia, may need dialysis Minimal solute clearance Poor emergent treatment of hyperkalemia/acidosis Loss of limb (distal arterial ischemia)
CAVH (Continuous arteriovenous hemofiltration)	Ultrafiltration Convection	Arteriovenous	No	Diuretic resistant, volume overloaded, hemodynamically unstable patient who cannot tolerate rapid fluid shifts Parenteral or enteral alimentation in volume overloaded patient	Continuous, gradual treatment (fewer high and low extremes) High rate of fluid removal/replacement allows flexibility in fluid balance	**Anticoagulation, bleeding** **Hypotension** **Hypothermia** **Access complications (bleeding, clotting, infection)** **Requires strict monitoring of fluid and electrolyte replacement to avoid deficits or overload** **Air embolism** **ICU setting only** **Requires 1:1 nurse/patient ratio** Prolonged, large-bore arterial cannulation required Ideally need MAP of 60 mm Hg to drive extracorporeal circuit Poor control of azotemia, may need dialysis Poor emergent treatment of hyperkalemia/acidosis Loss of limb (distal arterial ischemia)

Therapy	Functions	Access		Indications	Advantages	Complications/Disadvantages
CVVH (Continuous venovenous hemofiltration)	Ultrafiltration Diffusion Solute removal	Venovenous	Yes	Diuretic resistant, hemodynamically unstable, volume overloaded patient who cannot tolerate rapid fluid shifts Parenteral or enteral alimentation in volume overloaded patient	Precise fluid control Can be done in patient with low MAP Ease of initiation Large volume of parenteral nutrition may be administered No arterial cannulation Better solute clearance than CAVH	**Anticoagulation, bleeding** **Hypotension** **Hypothermia** **Access complications (bleeding, clotting, infection)** **Requires strict monitoring of fluid and electrolyte replacement to avoid deficits or overload** **Air embolism** **ICU setting only** **Requires 1:1 nurse/patient ratio** Waste product removal not as efficient as CVVHDF Requires special pump to augment blood flow through extracorporeal circuit Requires training of ICU nurses in use of pump
Dialysis Therapies						
CAVHD (Continuous arteriovenous hemodialysis) CAVHDF (Continuous arteriovenous hemodiafiltration)	Ultrafiltration Diffusion Solute removal Convection	Arteriovenous	No	Volume overloaded hemodynamically unstable patient with azotemia or uremia Catabolic acute renal failure Electrolyte imbalances and acidosis Parenteral and enteral alimentation in volume overloaded, catabolic patient	Precise fluid control Ease of initiation Large volume of parenteral nutrition may be administered	Same as CAVH Hyperglycemia
CVVHD (Continuous venovenous hemodialysis) CVVHDF (Continuous venovenous hemodiafiltration)	Ultrafiltration Diffusion Solute removal	Venovenous	Yes	Volume overloaded hemodynamically unstable patient with azotemia or uremia Catabolic acute renal failure Electrolyte imbalances and metabolic acidosis Parenteral and enteral alimentation in volume overloaded, catabolic patient	No arterial cannulation Precise fluid control Ease of initiation Large volume of parenteral nutrition may be administered Better solute clearance than CAVHDF Can be done in patient with low MAP	**Same as CVVH** **Hyperglycemia**

*Complications appearing in boldface are common to CAVH/CAVHD/CVVH/CVVHD.

Abbreviations: ICU, intensive care unit; MAP, mean arterial pressure.

From Giuliano K, Pysznik E. Renal replacement therapy in critical care: implementation of a unit-based CVVH program. Crit Care Nurse. 1998;18:40-51.

- Each dialyzer has four ports: two end ports for blood (in one end and out the other) and two side ports for dialysis solution (also in one end and out the other). In most cases, the blood and dialysate are run through the dialyzer in opposite or countercurrent directions.
- With hollow-fiber dialyzers, the blood flows through the center of hollow fibers and the dialysis solution (dialysate) flows around the outside of the hollow fibers. The advantages of hollow-fiber filters include a low priming volume, low resistance to flow, and high amount of surface area. The major disadvantage is the potential for clotting secondary to the small fiber size.
- Parallel-plate dialyzers are designed as sheets of membrane over supporting structures. Blood and dialysis solutions pass through alternate spaces of the dialyzer.
- All dialyzers have UF coefficients; thus, the dialyzer selected will vary in different clinical situations. The higher the UF coefficient, the more rapid the fluid removal. UF coefficients are determined by in vivo measurements done by each dialyzer manufacturer.
- Clearance refers to the ability of the dialyzer to remove metabolic waste products from the patient's blood. The blood flow rate, the dialysate flow rate, and the solute concentration affect clearance. Clearance occurs by the processes of diffusion, convection, and UF.
- The dialysate (when used during CRRT) is composed of water, a buffer (eg, acetate or bicarbonate), and various electrolytes. Most solutions also contain glucose. The buffer helps neutralize acids that are generated as a result of normal cellular metabolism and that usually are excreted by the kidney. The concentration of electrolytes is usually the normal plasma concentration, helping to create a concentration gradient for removal of excess electrolytes. The glucose promotes the removal of plasma water and is available in various concentrations.
- Heparin or citrate is often used during CRRT to prevent clotting of the circuit during treatment.
- Continuous renal replacement therapy can be done by either a pumped or nonpumped system. In a nonpumped system, the patient's arterial pressure provides the gradient that propels the blood through the circuit. In pumped systems, a mechanical roller pump propels the blood

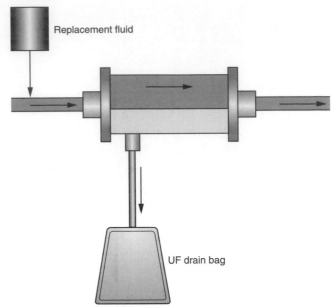

■ ● FIGURE 103–2. Continuous arteriovenous hemofiltration (CAVH). Fluid removal and fluid replacement (© Rhonda K. Martin. All rights reserved. Used with permission.)

through the circuit. The patient's volume status and serum electrolytes are changed gradually so that patients experience fewer problems than they do with hemodialysis. Specifics of all of these therapies are outlined in Table 103–1.

- SCUF (Fig. 103–1), CAVH (Fig. 103–2), CAVHD (Fig. 103–3), and CAVHDF (Fig. 103–4) are all performed using unpumped systems. For all of these therapies, the force generated by arterial pressure drives the system; a mean arterial pressure (MAP) of 60 mm Hg is generally required for adequate UF. Both arterial and venous access are required.

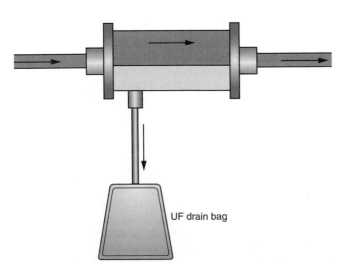

■ ● FIGURE 103–1. Slow continuous ultrafiltration (SCUF). Fluid removal, no fluid replacement. (© Rhonda K. Martin. All rights reserved. Used with permission.)

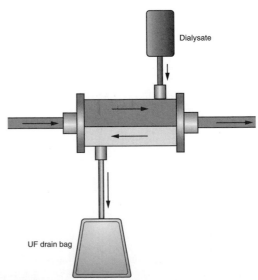

■ ● FIGURE 103–3. Continuous arteriovenous hemodialysis (CAVHD). Fluid and solute removal with dialysate. (© Rhonda K. Martin. All rights reserved. Used with permission.)

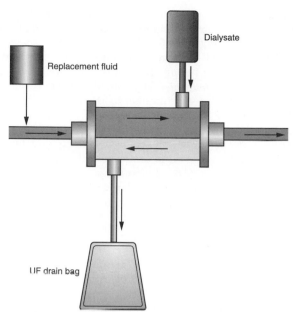

- SCUF and CAVH are used primarily to remove plasma water in small amounts (150 to 300 mL/hr). A hemofilter with a large surface area, high sieving coefficient, and low resistance is used to facilitate slow, continuous fluid removal. Replacement fluid is generally not used.
- CAVHD and CAVHDF are used to remove both plasma water and solutes. Dialysate solution is part of the setup; flow of the dialysate is countercurrent to the blood flow. Intravenous (IV) replacement fluid is used continuously based on the amount of UF removed each hour and net fluid removal goals for each patient.

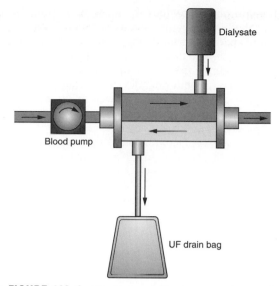

- CAVVH (Fig. 103–5), CVVHD (Fig. 103–6), and CVVHDF (Fig. 103–7) use pumped systems. These therapies are used to remove both plasma water and solutes and are generally more effective than SCUF or CAVH. These therapies require venous access, most commonly provided by a double-lumen catheter (although an external arteriovenous [AV] hemodialysis shunt or a surgically created AV hemodialysis anastomosis may be used). Common sites for the double-lumen catheter include the internal jugular vein, the subclavian vein, or the femoral vein. Common sites for the external shunt include the forearm (radial artery to cephalic vein) or the leg (posterior tibial artery to long saphenous vein).

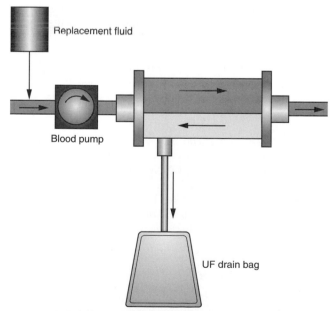

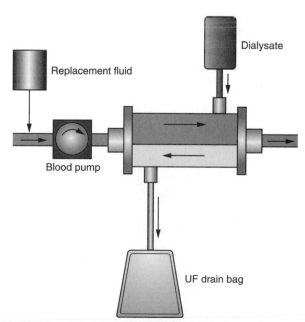

❖ A blood pump provides the pressure driving the system; the blood circuit consists of blood lines, a blood pump, and various monitoring devices. The blood lines carry the blood to and from the patient. The blood pump controls the speed of the blood through the circuit. The monitoring devices include arterial and venous pressure monitors, as well as an air detection monitor to prevent air that may have entered the circuit from being returned to the patient.

❖ Intravenous replacement fluid is used continuously based on the amount of UF removed each hour and net fluid removal goals for each patient.

❖ Dialysate solution can be used as part of the setup, and when it is used with replacement fluid, is referred to as CVVHDF. It is set to flow in a countercurrent direction to the blood flow.

EQUIPMENT

- Masks, goggles, and head coverings
- Sharps container
- 10-mL syringes and 20-mL syringe
- Sterile normal saline (NS), 3 L
- Dressing supplies (sterile barrier, gauze pads, transparent dressing, tape)
- Povidone-iodine solution/swabs
- Heparin (1000 U/mL) (both for priming and infusion, as ordered)
- Sterile bowl
- Two 19-G needles
- Two fistula needles (usually 14 to 16 G)
- 1% lidocaine and two tuberculin syringes

- Antiseptic soap
- Hemostats
- Hemofilter system/setup
- Infusion pumps and blood pump (not needed for SCUF)
- 4 × 4 gauze/tape/sterile barrier
- Replacement fluid, as ordered
- Fluid warmer
- Dialysate fluid, as ordered
- Sterile gloves, clean gloves, masks, goggles
- Alcohol wipes
- Sterile towels
- Drainage bag

Equipment for termination includes the following:

- Hemostats
- Gauze pads, tape, povidone-iodine, sterile barrier, sterile gloves
- NS, 1000 mL

- Clean gloves, goggles, mask
- Heparin, heparin lock caps, syringes (if using vascular catheters), labels

Additional equipment (to have available depending on patient need) includes the following:

- One tourniquet (AV fistula only)

PATIENT AND FAMILY EDUCATION

- Explain the purpose of CRRT. ➤*Rationale:* The patient and family should understand that CRRT is necessary to perform the physiologic functions of the kidneys when fluid overload or renal failure is present.
- Explain the procedure and review any questions the patient may have. ➤*Rationale:* Provides information and decreases patient anxiety.
- Explain the need for careful sterile technique for the

duration of treatment. ➤*Rationale:* It is important for the family to know the importance of sterile technique to decrease the likelihood of systemic infection.

- Explain the need for careful monitoring of the patient during the treatment for fluid and electrolyte imbalance. ➤*Rationale:* The patient and family should understand that careful monitoring is a routine part of CRRT.
- Explain the signs and symptoms of possible complications during CRRT. ➤*Rationale:* Patients and family should be fully prepared in case one of the complications occurs (eg, hypotension, hemorrhage, manifestations of fluid/electrolyte/acid-base imbalance).
- Explain the CRRT circuit setup to the patient and family. ➤*Rationale:* It is important for the patient and family to know that blood will be removed from his or her body and will be visible during the CRRT treatment.

PATIENT ASSESSMENT AND PREPARATION

Patient Assessment

- Baseline vital signs/weight, laboratory values (blood urea nitrogen [BUN]/creatinine/electrolytes/hemoglobin/hematocrit), neurologic status. ➤*Rationale:* Patients in renal failure often have altered baseline assessments, both in physical assessment and in the laboratory values. Having this information before treatments are started is helpful so that interventions, including the dialysate fluid, can be individualized. Alterations during treatment are common due to the rapid removal of fluid and solutes.
- Patency and the ability to easily aspirate blood from both ports. ➤*Rationale:* Adequate blood flow is necessary during a treatment in order to facilitate optimal fluid and solute removal. Patent catheter lumens are necessary for adequate blood flow.
- Catheter insertion site/vascular access site for signs and symptoms of infection. ➤*Rationale:* Catheter insertion sites provide a portal of entry for infection, which may result in septicemia if unrecognized or untreated. If the catheter insertion site appears to be infected, further interventions (eg, site change, culture, antibiotic treatment) may be necessary.
- Check site for presence of bruit and quality of blood flow (if using an AV fistula). ➤*Rationale:* Physical assessment of the fistula can indicate patency of the graft, as well as the possible presence of infection.
- Adequate circulation to the distal parts of the access limb. ➤*Rationale:* The placement of a vascular access may compromise circulation.
- Maintenance of the CRRT circuit (arterial and venous pressures, clotting, blood leaks, or breaks in the closed system). ➤*Rationale:* CRRT treatments pose a risk to the patient if the circuit is not carefully monitored for technical problems in the system and untoward patient responses.

Patient Preparation

- Ensure that patient understands preprocedural teaching. Answer questions as they arise and reinforce information as needed. ➤*Rationale:* Evaluates and reinforces understanding of previously taught information.

- Position the patient in a comfortable position (that will also facilitate optimal blood flow through the vascular access). ➤**Rationale:** It is important for the patient and family to understand that movement during the procedure may effect the blood flow through the system, so getting into a comfortable position before the initiation of therapy is important. They should also understand that different catheter sites may require different patient positions to facilitate optimal blood flow. Chose a position that will allow for setup of the sterile field. It is important for the nurse who is setting up the sterile field and initiating therapy can easily reach all the necessary supplies.

| Procedure | for Initiating and Terminating Continuous Renal Replacement Therapy |

Steps	Rationale	Special Considerations
Nonpumped Systems (SCUF, CAVH, CAVHD, CAVHDF)		
1. Wash hands.	Reduces transmission of microorganisms; standard precautions.	
2. Remove hemofilter and lines from package, and check that protective caps are properly placed at the end of the arterial and venous blood lines.	Maintains a closed system for sterility.	Review the hemofilter and observe the minimal distance between the priming solution and the hemofilter and the collection/measuring device. By raising the priming solution higher than the rest of the system, the amount of time required to prime the system is decreased.
3. Check that blood line connections to hemofilter are secure.	Avoids accidental leaks or disconnections.	
4. Place the hemofilter with arterial end down (blood inlet) in the holder, and lock the holder.	Positions hemofilter for priming procedure.	
5. Connect 1000 mL of heparinized NS to the end of the venous line (blood outlet) and position bag at the level of the hemofilter.	Used as a flushing solution to flush sterilant from filter.	
6. Attach on end of the UF line to the uncapped port on the hemofilter (across from arterial inlet port).	Provides a closed system for collection of ultrafiltrate.	Maintains aseptic technique.
7. Connect the other end of the UF line to the closed collection/measuring device.	Completes assembly of system and facilitates measurement of the priming solution.	
8. Hang the collection system approximately 20 inches (no less than 16 inches) below the level of the hemofilter.	Priming position enhances movement of the priming solution across the membrane of the hemofilter.	
9. Check that all lines are securely connected.	Prevents leaks or disconnections.	Check that the cap on the dialysate inlet port (across from the venous line) is secure.
10. Close clamp on arterial blood line, and keep venous line, UF line, and rinsing bag clamps open.	Primes the system.	Bulldog clamps—nonserrated cannulated clamps that prevent cutting of tubing—can be used if roller clamps are lost.
11. Prepare 2 L of heparinized NS: instill 5000 U heparin per 1000 mL of 0.9% NS.	Primes the system.	Heparin may vary. Check the institutional protocol or order.
12. Hang the heparinized NS at least 48 inches above the level of the hemofilter.	Facilitates priming of the hemofilter by gravity.	
13. Connect infusion pump to arterial line.	Prevents clotting of hemofilter.	

Procedure continued on following page

Procedure **for Initiating and Terminating Continuous Renal Replacement Therapy** *Continued*

Steps	Rationale	Special Considerations
14. Wash hands.	Reduces transmission of microorganisms; standard precautions.	
15. Unclamp the arterial line, and flush all connecting lines with heparinized NS.	Initiates priming of the system.	Ensure that whenever there is fluid, either priming solution or blood, moving through the blood compartment of the hemofilter, the UF line remains unclamped. If the UF line is clamped during the priming procedure, there may be inadequate removal of air or collapse of some or all the layers of the hemofilter, rendering it nonfunctional.
16. Intermittently clamp and unclamp the venous line for 3 to 5 seconds.	Enhances removal of air from the blood compartment.	Some NS may appear in the UF line; this is normal.
17. When 1000 mL of priming solution has flowed into system, clamp the venous line, and rotate the hemofilter so that the arterial line is up.	Initiates thorough priming of the ultrafiltrate compartment.	Hemofilter must be rinsed to remove glycerin coating, ethylene oxide (from sterilization), and all air bubbles.
18. Hang another 1000 mL of heparinized NS.	For priming ultrafiltrate compartment.	
19. Continue priming with heparinized NS until 400 mL has collected in the UF collection/measuring device.	Ensures that ultrafiltrate compartment is thoroughly primed.	
20. Rotate the hemofilter so that the arterial line end is down.	Completes priming of the hemofilter.	
21. Unclamp the venous line.	Allows drainage of fluid from the hemofilter.	
22. Infuse 500 mL through the venous blood site, and intermittently clamp and unclamp the venous line.	Promotes purging of air bubbles from the hemofilter.	
23. When 100 mL of the heparinized NS remains in the IV bag, clamp the arterial line.	Prevents introduction of air into the system.	If air bubbles persist, continue flushing the system with heparinized NS.
24. Clamp the venous and UF lines.	Prevents loss of priming solution from system and potential for air accumulation.	
25. Drain and discard the NS in UF collection device. The system is now ready for patient use.	Excludes NS priming solution from ultrafiltrate volume.	Label hemofilter/tubing with time and date.
26. Wash hands.	Reduces transmission of microorganisms.	
27. Establish vascular access.	Provides route for hemofiltration.	Subclavian and venipuncture access may be initiated, depending on established protocols. Ensure that patient has both an arterial access and a venous access, if needed.
28. Position hemofilter parallel to the patient's access and secure.		
29. Don goggles and gloves.	Standard precautions.	
30. Administer initial heparin dose, if ordered, per institutional standard.	Provides anticoagulation to prevent clotting of hemofilter.	

Procedure **for Initiating and Terminating Continuous Renal Replacement Therapy** *Continued*

Steps	Rationale	Special Considerations
31. Connect setup lines to access.	Establishes closed system for hemofiltration.	Secure access sites and filter for safety.
32. Position the UF collection/measuring device below the level of the patient.	Encourages flow of ultrafiltrate by gravity.	Level of collection device helps determine rate of UF. Raising the level decreases the negative pressure and rate of UF; lowering the collection devices increases the negative pressure and rate of UF.
33. Securely tape all connections.	Prevents leaks or disconnections.	
34. Ensure that system is working.	Validates effectiveness of hemofiltration.	
35. Dispose of soiled material in appropriate receptacle.	Standard precautions.	
36. Wash hands.	Prevents transmission of microorganisms.	

Termination

Steps	Rationale	Special Considerations
1. Wash hands.	Reduces transmission of microorganisms.	
2. Don gloves, mask, and goggles.	Standard precautions.	
3. Clamp the arterial lines.	Stops the patient's blood from entering the system.	
4. Flush the patient's blood back using the replacement fluid.	Returns the blood that is in the circuit to the patient.	
5. Clamp the venous line.		
6. Clamp fluid replacement line.	Prevents further administration of fluid.	
7. Clamp the arterial access line and remove tape.	Prevents further flow of blood.	
8. Clean connection site with 1-minute povidone-iodine scrub.	Reduces transmission of microorganisms.	
9. Disconnect arterial access line from arterial system line.	Breaks system to terminate from the arterial side.	
10. Repeat steps 6 and 7 for venous system line.	Breaks system to terminate from the venous side.	
11. Instill heparin into both the arterial and venous access ports according to institutional protocol.	Maintains patency of vascular access.	
12. Dispose of soiled material in the biohazardous waste receptacle.	Standard precautions.	
13. Wash hands.	Reduces transmission of microorganisms.	

Pumped Systems (CVVH, CVVHD, CVVHDF)

Steps	Rationale	Special Considerations
1. Wash hands.	Reduces transmission of microorganisms; standard precautions.	
2. Verify orders, which should include type of dialyzer, orders for heparin or citrate anticoagulant, replacement fluid, hourly net fluid removal goal, dialysate solution and rate (if used), pump speed, and laboratory testing.	Familiarizes nurse with the individualized patient treatment and reduces the possibility of error.	Ensure patient weight and laboratory values are recorded before initiation of therapy.

Procedure continued on following page

Procedure for Initiating and Terminating Continuous Renal Replacement Therapy *Continued*

Steps	Rationale	Special Considerations
3. Set up system according to manufacturer's instructions, attach any prescribed solutions, and prepare heparin/citrate infusion (if ordered). *(Level V: Clinical studies in more than one patient population and situation)*	Correct system setup is imperative for safety and optimal functioning. Use of anticoagulants prolongs the function of the hemofilter.[1, 2]	Pump must be plugged into a generator outlet because some pumps do not have battery power. Heparin, if ordered, is usually administered via the postpump infusion port; citrate is administered at the arterial port of the vascular access catheter (VAC). Replacement solutions are administered through the arterial or venous infusion port as ordered (usually arterial) using blood tubing. Connect 1 liter NS to arterial infusion port (for flushing system). Dialysate solution (if using CVVHDDF) is connected to the outlet port of the hemofilter near the venous end using blood tubing.
4. Turn on pump and ensure air detector is activated.	Prevents an air embolus.	
5. Place the hemofilter in a vertical position, with the venous side up. Place the UF drain bag below the level of the patient's heart.	Lowering the UF bag promotes drainage.	
6. Place the priming drainage bag (with venous tubing still connected to it), along with empty priming solution bag, at the arterial end on the patient's bed. Clamp the arterial tubing near the priming solution bag.	Promotes priming of the system.	
7. Drape access with a sterile drape and open two 10-mL syringes onto the sterile field. Place povidone-iodine–soaked gauze on connection tubing and on arterial and venous access ports of VAC. *(Level V: Clinical studies in more than one patient population and situation)*	Maintains sterile technique.[3, 4]	
8. Put on a mask and sterile gloves and scrub connections for 1 minute. *(Level V: Clinical studies in more than one patient population and situation)*	Maintains sterile technique.[3, 4]	
9. With both the arterial and venous access ports clamped, remove their caps, and withdraw 5 mL from each port of the access catheter.	Removes the heparin from the ports so that it will not be infused into the patient.	
10. Disconnect the arterial tubing from the priming solution bag, connect it to the arterial access, and make sure all connections are secure.	Loose connections anywhere will introduce air into the circuit.	The venous side is not hooked up yet, so the priming solution can be discarded instead of given to the patient.
11. Open arterial and venous circuit line clamps and then open the arterial vascular access clamp.	Opens the system in preparation of extracorporeal circulation.	

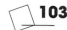

Procedure **for Initiating and Terminating Continuous Renal Replacement Therapy** *Continued*

Steps	Rationale	Special Considerations
12. Turn the pump on and administer the heparin bolus prefilter as the blood is starting to pass by. Begin heparin/citrate infusions.	Anticoagulates the hemofilter.	It is important to begin anticoagulants as soon as the blood enters the hemofilter in order to prolong optimal function of the hemofilter.
13. Turn the pump off as the blood approaches the priming drainage bag. Clamp venous line near drainage bag.	Prevents the patient's blood from entering the priming bag and being discarded.	
14. Don a new pair of sterile gloves.	Maintains sterile technique.	
15. Disconnect the venous tubing from the priming solution drainage bag, connecting it to the venous access.		
16. Open the venous access clamp and the venous line clamp.		
17. Turn the blood pump on and turn the blood pump flow rate up slowly to the ordered rate.	If the rate is turned up too quickly, hypotension may occur.	
18. Start the ordered infusions.		Fluids should be warmed to prevent hypothermia. Ambient room temperature may also need to be increased.
19. Start dialysate for CVVHDF, if ordered.	This begins the process of hemodialysis/diafiltration.	
20. Document pump flow rate, arterial and venous monitor pressures, color of UF, and vital signs at a frequency according to institutional standards.		Watch venous pressure. It will rise slowly over time, which is one of the indications of system clotting.

Flushing

1. Connect NS to arterial infusion port, and shut off replacement solution, heparin/citrate drip, and any other fluid running.		
2. Open the NS flush while the pump continues to run.	Flushing allows the nurse to assess the patency of the system.	Flushing contributes to the patient's IV intake; the volume of fluid should be documented. When the circuit is flushed of blood, clots may be observed. Flushing will not dissolve existing clots.
3. Clamp the arterial side of the circuit (proximal to the arterial infusion port) and the UF tubing.		Prevents any more blood from entering the circuit via the arterial port during flushing. However, make sure that NS flush is running freely in order to prevent rupture or backfiltration. Hemostasis and clot formation in the arterial limb of the tubing is also a possibility if the flushing procedure is prolonged.
4. If no clots are observed, turn the saline off and unclamp the arterial circuit to allow hemofiltration to continue.		If numerous clots are observed, the hemofilter may need to be replaced.

Procedure continued on following page

Procedure	for Initiating and Terminating Continuous Renal Replacement Therapy *Continued*

Steps	Rationale	Special Considerations
Termination		
1. Turn off all infusions into the circuit.		
2. Open NS flush solution attached to arterial infusion port. Clamp the UF line.		
3. With pump still running, open the flush solution (clamp off the arterial line near the patient, place hemofilter with arterial end up) and return the patient's blood.	The blood should be flushed through the circuit to prevent unnecessary blood loss.	If clots are identified beyond the venous bubble trap, *stop* the pump; do *not* return blood to patient. Blood from the arterial limb of the catheter is not returned to the patient because of the possibility of clot formation, because the machine will not detect clots in that location.
4. Once hemofilter is flushed, stop the pump.		
5. When the entire circuit is clear of blood, turn off the pump and clamp off both the arterial and venous access ports and the patient's arterial line.		
6. If the line is to be discontinued, remove it now.		If the line is not being discontinued, flush both ports with heparin.
7. Instill heparin into both the arterial and venous access ports according to institutional standard.	Maintains catheter patency.	
8. Clamp the access line clamps and place sterile caps on the arterial and venous access ports. Secure the catheter and label the dressing with heparin medication label.		
9. Change dressing over catheter site according to institutional standard.		
10. Remove and discard the tubing and filter in an appropriate biohazardous waste container.	Standard precautions.	
11. Wash hands.	Reduces transmission of microorganisms; standard precautions.	
Emergency Termination		
1. Clamp arterial and venous lines.		Emergency termination is used for serious complications, including blood leak, hemofilter rupture, clotting, circuit disconnection, dialyzer reaction.
2. Disconnect from the patient.		
3. Instill heparin into both the arterial and venous access ports according to institutional protocol.	Maintains patency of vascular access.	
4. Dispose of soiled material in the biohazardous waste receptacle.	Standard precautions.	
5. Wash hands.	Reduces transmission of microorganisms.	

Expected Outcomes	Unexpected Outcomes
• Catheter/AV fistula is accessed without any complications.	• Clotting/decreased patency of the AV fistula or the catheter lumens
• Blood is easily aspirated from the access site.	• Crack in the catheter or endcaps
• Accumulated fluid and waste products are removed.	• Bleeding from insertion site or access site
• Acid-base balance is restored.	• Signs and symptoms of infection at the insertion or access site
• BUN and creatinine are restored to baseline levels.	• Dislodgment of the catheter
• Electrolytes are within baseline values.	• Decreased circulation in the vascular access limb
• Hemodynamic stability and maintenance of optimal intravascular volume exist.	• Hematoma formation at the access site
	• Physiologic complications (dysrhythmias, chest pain, fluid or electrolyte imbalance, complications related to anticoagulation, air embolism, hypotension, seizures, nausea and vomiting, headaches, muscle cramping, dyspnea)
	• Introduction of pathogens into the circuit
	• Technical problems with the blood pump during (blood leak, air leak, clotting, disconnection of circuit, hemolysis, hemofilter rupture)
	• Hypothermia

Patient Monitoring and Care

Patient Monitoring and Care	Rationale	Reportable Conditions
		These conditions should be reported if they persist despite nursing interventions.
1. Perform and record a predialysis and daily weights. *(Level V: Clinical studies in more than one patient population and situation)*	Predialysis weight is an important factor in deciding how much UF is needed during treatment. It also helps to guide ongoing treatment.[5, 6]	• Abnormal increase or decrease in weight
2. Perform a baseline and ongoing assessments, including the following: ○ Vital signs ○ Jugular vein distention ○ Presence of edema ○ Intake and output ○ Neurologic assessment *(Level V: Clinical studies in more than one patient population and situation)*	Important to establish a baseline before initiation of treatment.[5, 6] Monitors for complications.	• Hypotension • Hypertension • Tachycardia/bradycardia • Tachypnea/bradypnea • Fever • Hypothermia • Jugular vein distension • Crackles • Edema • Change in level of consciousness, dizziness • Change in cardiac rhythm
3. Monitor the circulation to the extremity where the graft is located. *(Level V: Clinical studies in more than one patient population and situation)*	To assess for any decrease in perfusion distal to the graft site.[5, 6]	• Diminished capillary refill • Diminished or absent peripheral pulses • Pale, mottled, or cyanotic • Cool to touch • Diminished or absent movement • Pain

Continued on following page

Patient Monitoring and Care	Rationale	Reportable Conditions
4. Monitor electrolytes and glucose during treatment as per institutional standard.	Must be monitored because of continued fluid and electrolyte shifts during treatment.	• Hyper/hypokalemia • Hyper/hyponatremia • Hyper/hypocalcemia • Hyper/hypoglycemia
5. Administer medications to correct electrolyte abnormalities as ordered during treatment. *(Level V: Clinical studies in more than one patient population and situation)*	Patients with renal failure are predisposed to many electrolyte abnormalities. During CRRT, several medications/electrolyte replacements may be given as ordered for individual patients.[5, 6]	
6. Monitor the CRRT circuit (eg, occlusions; kinks in UF, blood, or vascular access lines; position of hemofilter). *(Level V: Clinical studies in more than one patient population and situation)*	Disconnections or introduction of air into the circuit are always possible during treatment. Bleeding or exsanguination also can occur.[5, 6] Level of collection device should be approximately 16 to 20 inches below the level of the filter to allow for best gravity drainage. Clotting of the circuit is a potential complication. If hemofilter becomes excessively clotted, the extracorporeal blood volume should be returned to the patient quickly. Blood leaks from the dialyzer into the dialysate may occur and necessitate termination of treatment. Venous or arterial pressures that are out of range may indicate dialyzer or access malfunction.	• Disconnections, cracks, or leaks • Excessive clotting • Blood leaks/hemofilter rupture • Malfunction of dialyzer or access
7. Monitor UF for rate, clarity, and air bubbles. *(Level V: Clinical studies in more than one patient population and situation)*	A decrease in UF production can occur due to clotting of the dialyzer.[1, 5, 6] Pink or blood-tinged UF is indicative of filter leak or rupture.	• Decrease in UF production • Change in color or characteristics of UF • Air in UF
8. Administer heparin or citrate as ordered. *(Level V: Clinical studies in more than one patient population and situation)*	Heparin or citrate often is used to prevent clotting of the circuit.[1, 2] Heparin/citrate dose varies according to patient condition and laboratory values.	• Suspicion of clotting in the circuit
9. Monitor anticoagulation as per institutional standard.	Because heparin or citrate commonly are used to prevent system clotting, coagulation studies should be routinely monitored.	• Abnormal coagulation studies
10. Monitor the vascular access. *(Level V: Clinical studies in more than one patient population and situation)*	Bleeding can occur from either the venous or arterial catheter or AVF. Clotting of the access can occur.[5, 6]	• Decrease in access function or patency
11. Monitor condition of access site. *(Level V: Clinical studies in more than one patient population and situation)*	Bleeding or infection can be access site complications.[5, 6]	• Bleeding • Site redness/edema • Warmth • Bleeding • Purulent drainage • Pain or tenderness • Fever

Patient Monitoring and Care	Rationale	Reportable Conditions
12. Initiate and monitor rate of replacement fluids.	Prevents hypotensive episodes. Replacement fluids are dependent on patient's baseline assessment. Ringer's lactate commonly is used and infused as follows: Amount of previous hour's UF plus previous hour's total output (TO) minus previous hour's IV fluids (IV) plus desired net hourly fluid loss (FL) equals amount of replacement fluid (RF) (UF + TO) − (IV + FL) = RF.	
13. Monitor the patient for complications associated with CRRT treatment. *(Level V: Clinical studies in more than one patient population and situation)*	Several complications are possible with CRRT.[5, 6]	• Muscle cramps • Dialysis disequilibrium (headache, nausea and vomiting, hypertension, decreased sensorium, convulsions, coma) • Air embolism • Dialyzer reaction (hypotension, pruritis, back pain, angioedema, anaphylaxis) • Hypoxemia
14. Monitor the blood pump for proper functioning.	Any type of equipment is subject to malfunctioning. It is important for the nurse operating the blood pump to be competent with its operation, troubleshooting methods, and know when to take the pump out of service to be checked by the biomedical department.	• Problems with the blood pump

---

Documentation

Documentation should include the following:

- Patient and family education
- Date and time of treatment initiation
- Condition of catheter/AV fistula regarding patency, quality of blood flow, ease of access procedure
- Date and time of dressing
- Condition of insertion site and any signs or symptoms of infection
- Presence of bruit if using an AV fistula
- Needle gauge size used for cannulation if using AV fistula
- Vital signs
- Hourly fluid balance calculation
- Patient's response to CRRT and daily progress toward treatment goals
- Unexpected outcomes
- Nursing interventions
- Daily weight
- Laboratory assessment data

References

1. Mehta RL. Anticoagulation strategies for continuous renal replacement therapies: what works? *Am J Kid Dis.* 1996;30:S8–S14.
2. Davenport A. The coagulation system in the critically ill patient with acute renal failure and the effect of an extracorporeal circuit. *Am J Kid Dis.* 1997;30:S20–S27.
3. Goldstein MB. Prevention of sepsis from central venous dialysis catheters. *Semin Dialysis.* 1992;5:106–107.
4. Centers for Disease Control, Hospital Infection Control Advisory Council. Guideline for the prevention of intravascular device-related infections. Part 1: Intravascular device-related infections: an overview. *Am J Infect Control.* 1996;24:262–276.
5. American Nephrology Nurses Association. *Core Curriculum for Nephrology Nursing.* Pitman, NJ: ANNA; 1999:323–345.
6. American Nephrology Nurses Association. *ANNA Standards of Clinical Practice for Nephrology Nurses.* 3rd ed. Pitman, NJ: ANNA; 1999:61–70.
7. Giuliano K, Pysznik E. Renal replacement therapy in critical care: implementation of a unit-based CVVH program. *Crit Care Nurse.* 1998;18:40–51.

Additional Reading

Parker J. *Contemporary Nephrology Nursing.* Pitman, NJ: American Nephrology Nurses Association; 1998:577–588.

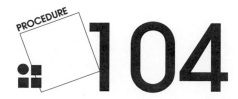

104

Hemodialysis

> **PURPOSE:** Hemodialysis is performed for volume regulation, acid-base control, electrolyte regulation, and management of azotemia.

Karen K. Giuliano

PREREQUISITE NURSING KNOWLEDGE

- Hemodialysis (Fig. 104–1) may be needed for the onset of acute renal failure, as well as for maintenance therapy for patients with chronic renal failure.
- Basic knowledge is necessary of the principles of diffusion, ultrafiltration (UF), osmosis, oncotic pressure, and hydrostatic pressure as they pertain to fluid and solute management during dialysis:
  - ❖ Diffusion is the passive movement of solutes through a semipermeable membrane from an area of higher to lower concentration.
  - ❖ Ultrafiltration is the bulk movement of solute and solvent through a semipermeable membrane using a pressure movement. The size of the solute molecules as compared to the size of molecules that can move through the semipermeable membrane determines the degree of UF.
  - ❖ Osmosis is the passive movement of solvent through a semipermeable membrane from an area of higher to lower concentration.
  - ❖ Oncotic pressure is the pressure exerted by plasma proteins, which favors intravascular fluid retention and movement of fluid from the extravascular to the intravascular space.
  - ❖ Hydrostatic pressure is the force exerted by arterial blood pressure, which favors the movement of fluid from the intravascular to the extravascular space.
- Venous access is needed to perform hemodialysis and can be provided by a double-lumen catheter, an external arteriovenous (AV) shunt, or a surgically created AV anastomosis (eg, fistula or graft). Common sites for the double-lumen catheter include the internal jugular, the subclavian, or the femoral vein. Common sites for the external shunt include the forearm (radial artery to cephalic vein) or the leg (posterial tibial artery to long saphenous vein). The AV fistula or graft is used for long-term dialysis management.
- Hemodialysis uses an artificial kidney (hemofilter, dialyzer) with a semipermeable membrane to create two separate compartments: the blood compartment and the dialysis solution (dialysate) compartment. The semipermeable membrane allows the movement of small molecules (eg, electrolytes) from the patient's blood into the dialysate but is impermeable to larger molecules (red blood cells, plasma proteins).

- Each dialyzer has four ports: two end ports for blood (in one end and out the other) and two side ports for dialysis solution (also in one end and out the other). In most cases, the blood and dialysate are run through the dialyzer in opposite or countercurrent directions.
- The hollow-fiber dialyzer is the most commonly used dialyzer. Using this dialyzer, the blood flows through the center of hollow fibers and the dialysate flows around the outside of the hollow fibers. The advantages of hollow-fiber filters include a low priming volume, low resistance to flow, and high amount of surface area. The major disadvantage is the potential for clotting secondary to the small fiber size.
- Parallel-plate dialyzers are designed as sheets of membrane over supporting structures. Blood and dialysate pass through alternate spaces of the dialyzer. This type of dialyzer is used less frequently because of the higher tendency for allergic dialyzer reactions.
- All dialyzers have UF coefficients; thus, the dialyzer selected will vary in different clinical situations. The higher the UF coefficient, the more rapid the fluid removal. UF coefficients are determined by in vivo measurements done by each dialyzer manufacturer.
- Clearance refers to the ability of the dialyzer to remove metabolic waste products from the patient's blood. The blood flow rate, the dialysate flow rate, and the solute concentration affect clearance. Clearance occurs by the processes of diffusion, convection, and UF.
- The blood circuit consists of blood lines, a blood pump, and various monitoring devices. The blood lines carry the blood to and from the patient. The blood pump controls the speed of the blood through the circuit. The monitoring devices include arterial and venous pressure monitors, as well as an air detection monitor, to prevent air entering the circuit from being returned to the patient.
- The dialysate is composed of water, a buffer (eg, acetate or bicarbonate), and various electrolytes. Most solutions also contain glucose. The buffer helps neutralize acids that are generated as a result of normal cellular metabolism and usually are excreted by the kidney. The concentration of electrolytes is usual normal plasma concentrations, helping to create a concentration gradient for removal of excess electrolytes. The glucose, available in

733

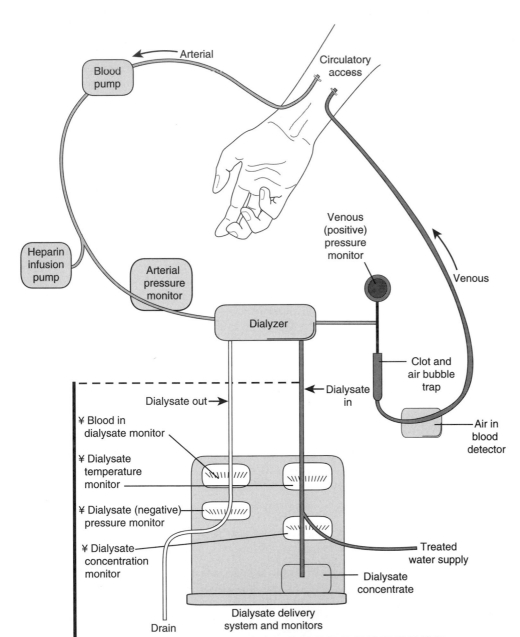

Arterial

Blood pump

Circulatory access

Heparin infusion pump

Arterial pressure monitor

Dialyzer

Venous (positive) pressure monitor

Venous

Clot and air bubble trap

Dialysate in

Dialysate out

Air in blood detector

¥ Blood in dialysate monitor

¥ Dialysate temperature monitor

¥ Dialysate (negative) pressure monitor

¥ Dialysate concentration monitor

Treated water supply

Dialysate concentrate

Drain

Dialysate delivery system and monitors

■ ● FIGURE 104–1. Components of a typical hemodialysis system. (From Thompson JM, McFarland GK, Hirsch JE, Tucker SM, Bowers AC, eds. *Mosby's Manual of Clinical Nursing.* St. Louis, MO: CV Mosby; 1989.)

various concentrations, promotes the removal of plasma water.

- Heparin is usually used during dialysis to prevent clotting of the circuit.
- Because large volumes of water are used during treatments, the water must be purified prior to patient use, preventing patient exposure to potentially harmful substances present in the water supply (eg, calcium carbonate, sodium chloride, and iron).

EQUIPMENT

- Masks
- Sharps container
- Goggles
- Sterile gloves
- Four 10-mL syringes and one 20-mL syringe
- Sterile normal saline (NS)

- Dressing supplies (sterile barrier, gauze pads, transparent dressing, tape)
- Antiseptic soap
- Povidone-iodine solution
- Heparin in 1000-U/mL concentration
- Sterile bowl
- Nonsterile gloves

Additional equipment for graft cannulation includes the following:

- Two 10-mL syringes
- Two 19-G needles
- NS for injection
- Two fistula needles

- Povidone-iodine swabs
- 1% lidocaine and two tuberculin syringes
- Two hemostats

Additional equipment for initiation of hemodialysis includes the following:

- Dialysis machine, tubing, dialyzer and dialysate solution

- Two hemostats
- One 30-mL syringe
- One 18-G needle

Additional equipment (to have available depending on patient need) includes the following:

- One tourniquet (AV fistula only)
- Loading dose of heparin (if ordered)

Equipment for termination of hemodialysis includes the following:

- Four hemostats
- 2 × 2 gauze pads
- NS, 1000 mL
- Nonsterile gloves

- Goggles
- Four bandages
- Sharps container

PATIENT AND FAMILY EDUCATION

- Explain the procedure and review any questions the patient may have. ➤➤*Rationale:* Provides information and decreases patient anxiety.
- Explain the need for careful sterile technique for the duration of treatment. ➤➤*Rationale:* Decreases the chance of systemic infection, because pathogens can be transported throughout the entire body via the circulation.
- Explain the purpose of hemodialysis. ➤➤*Rationale:* Hemodialysis is necessary to perform the physiologic functions of the kidneys when renal failure is present.
- Explain the need for careful monitoring of the patient during the treatment for fluid and electrolyte imbalance. ➤➤*Rationale:* Dialysis treatment puts the patient at risk of imbalance because of the rapid movement of fluid and electrolytes from the patient during treatment.
- Explain the importance of input from the patient on how he or she is feeling during the treatment. ➤➤*Rationale:* Hypotension is a common occurrence during treatment; the patient may experience lightheadedness or dizziness if hypotension is present. Letting the patient know to expect this as a possibility should help decrease patient anxiety.
- Explain the hemodialysis circuit setup to the patient. ➤➤*Rationale:* It is important for the patient and family to know that blood will be removed from his or her body and will be visible during the hemodialysis treatment.

PATIENT ASSESSMENT AND PREPARATION

Patient Assessment

- Baseline vital signs, weight, neurologic status, physical assessment of all body systems, fluid and electrolyte status. ➤➤*Rationale:* Patients in renal failure often have altered baseline assessments, both in physical assessment and in the laboratory values. Having this information before treatments are started is helpful so that interventions, including the dialysate, can be individualized. Alterations during treatment are common due to the rapid removal of fluid and solutes.
- Graft, fistula, or catheter insertion site for signs or symptoms of infection. ➤➤*Rationale:* Because dialysis access sites are used frequently, infection is always a potential risk. Dialysis access sites should only be used for dialysis, and not for other intravenous access needs, except in an emergency situation. Catheter insertion sites provide a portal of entry for infection, which may result in septicemia if unrecognized or untreated. If the catheter insertion site appears to be infected, further interventions (eg, site change, culture, and antibiotic treatment) may be necessary.
- Catheter patency and the ability to easily aspirate blood from both ports. ➤➤*Rationale:* Adequate blood flow is necessary during a treatment in order to facilitate optimal fluid and solute removal. Patent catheter lumens are necessary for adequate blood flow.
- If using an AV fistula, assess the site for presence of bruit, erythema, swelling, and quality of blood flow. ➤➤*Rationale:* Physical assessment of the fistula can indicate patency of the graft, as well as the possible presence of infection.
- Adequate circulation to the distal parts of the access limb. ➤➤*Rationale:* The placement of a vascular access may compromise circulation.

Patient Preparation

- Ensure that patient understands preprocedural teaching. Answer questions as they arise and reinforce information as needed. ➤➤*Rationale:* Evaluates and reinforces understanding of previously taught information.

• Position the patient in a comfortable position (that will also facilitate optimal blood flow through the catheter and allow for the setup of a sterile field). ➤**Rationale:** Facilitating patient comfort will help to minimize the amount of patient movement during treatment, which can change the amount of blood flow through the catheter.

Different catheter sites may require different patient positions to facilitate optimal blood flow.

• If using an AV fistula, ask the patient if he or she wants lidocaine used on the access site prior to accessing the fistula. ➤**Rationale:** Promotes patient comfort and reduces anxiety.

Procedure **for Hemodialysis**

Steps	Rationale	Special Considerations
Cannulation of AV Fistula or Graft		
1. Wash hands.	Reduces transmission of microorganisms; standard precautions.	
2. Wash access arm for 1 full minute with antiseptic soap using a 4 × 4 gauze pad; rinse off with water.	Reduces the transmission of microorganisms.	
3. Place arm on sterile barrier.	Maintains aseptic technique.	
4. Starting at the site for insertion, moving out in concentric circles for 2 to 3 inches, wash access area with povidone-iodine swabs or soaked 2 × 2 gauze pad for 1 full minute. (*Level V: Clinical studies in more than one patient population and situation*)	Povidone-iodine solution serves as a bactericidal agent.[1-3]	Skin asepsis is crucial; however, the most effective method for skin cleansing has not yet been established.
5. Repeat step 4 with second, new swab or 2 × 2 gauze pad.		
6. Using two 10-mL syringes and two 19-G needles, draw up prescribed flush solution in each syringe.	Prepares syringes for flushing fistula/graft.	Use an amount of heparinized saline that is consistent with institutional policy. In some cases, only saline will be used. Activated clotting times (ACTs) will provide information regarding the patient's anticoagulation status.
7. Attach flush to fistula needle tubing, and prime fistula needles.	Prevents clotting of blood in fistula needles.	
8. Clamp catheter/tubing.	Prevents loss of heparinized solution and backflow of blood.	
9. Apply tourniquet to upper portion of access limb (AV fistula cannulation).	Facilitates site determination for cannulation.	
10. Don nonsterile gloves and goggles.	Standard precautions.	
11. Select site to be used.	Decreases recirculation of dialyzed blood.	Arterial site should be at least 3 in from arterial anastomosis. Venous needle must be in the direction of venous flow and, if possible, 3 in or more from the arterial needle.
12. Grasp butterfly wings or hub of fistula needle between thumb and index finger of dominant hand with needle tip bevel up.	Provides secure grasp of needle upon cannulation.	Optional: Before insertion of fistula needle, lidocaine may be injected intradermally to make a small wheal, per patient preference.
13. Remove needle guard.	Exposes fistula needle.	
14. Hold skin taut with nondominant hand.	Prevents rolling of vessel.	Prevents contamination of area to be punctured.

Procedure **for Hemodialysis** *Continued*

Steps	Rationale	Special Considerations
15. With dominant hand, insert needle at a 45-degree angle to the skin (if lidocaine was used, use same puncture site for needle).		
A. *AV fistula:* Advance bevel up to hub of the needle.	Accesses arterial vascular system.	Prevents shearing of graft material.
B. *AV graft:* As soon as tip is through the graft, rotate needle 180 degrees, and advance needle to hub, bevel down.	Accesses arterial vascular system. Bevel-down position prevents shearing of graft.	
16. Remove tourniquet before infusing NS or heparin (AV fistula).	Prevents clotting.	
17. Unclamp needle/tubing clamp and aspirate blood.	Verifies correct placement and patency of access.	
18. Infuse flush solution; reclamp catheter.	Prevents clotting and backflow of blood.	
19. Secure needle with adhesive tape over insertion site.	Maintains angle of needle so that it floats freely in the vessel/graft.	
20. Repeat steps 12 through 18 for insertion of second needle.	Cannulation of venous site.	Hemodialysis can now be initiated.
21. Discard soiled material in appropriate receptacle.	Standard precautions.	
22. Wash hands.	Reduces transmission of microorganisms.	
Accessing a Catheter		
1. Wash hands, and don mask and cap.	Reduces transmission of microorganisms; standard precautions.	
2. Prepare sterile field with sterile barriers, 2 × 2 pads, 4 × 4 pads and transparent dressing.	Prepares material and maintains aseptic technique.	
3. Open sterile needles and syringes. Place on sterile field.	Readies equipment and maintains aseptic technique to prevent transmission of microorganisms.	
4. Attach 19-G needles to 10-mL syringes; prepare flush solution according to institutional standard.	Prepares syringe for catheter flushing.	Quinton catheters recommend 20 to 30 mL per lumen flushes for hemocaths and permacaths.[4] *(Level I: Manufacturer's recommendations only)*
5. Add povidone-iodine solution to sterile basin.	Prepares solution used to cleanse catheter.	
6. Remove dressing from exit site, taking care not to contaminate or dislodge cannula.	Allows access to exit site.	Inspect for signs and symptoms of exit-site infection: drainage, crusting, swelling, redness, exudate, or complaints of pain at the site.
7. Discard soiled dressing in appropriate container.	Standard precautions.	
8. Wash hands.	Reduces transmission of microorganisms.	
9. Don sterile gloves.	Maintains aseptic technique.	

Procedure continued on following page

Procedure	**for Hemodialysis** *Continued*

Steps	Rationale	Special Considerations
10. Place sterile barrier beneath catheter.	Sets up sterile field.	Do not touch catheter with gloves. Should gloves accidentally touch the catheter, a glove change is necessary to maintain aseptic technique.
11. Saturate four of the 4 × 4 pads in povidone-iodine solution and perform a 1-minute scrub of the arterial limb of the catheter.	Povidone-iodine serves as a bactericidal agent.	Make sure to remove any crust or drainage.
12. Wrap second povidone-iodine–soaked 4 × 4 pad around arterial limb and leave in place for approximately 3 to 5 minutes.	Reduces transmission of microorganisms.	
13. After 3 to 5 minutes, remove povidone-iodine–soaked 4 × 4 pad and discard in appropriate receptacle.	Standard precautions.	
14. Remove cap from arterial limb of catheter and discard appropriately.	Provides access to arterial side of catheter. Standard precautions.	Be sure slide clamp is closed before removing arterial limb catheter cap.
15. Attach an empty 3-mL syringe to the arterial limb, open the slide clamp, and gently aspirate 3-mL of blood. Close the slide clamp, remove syringe, and discard in appropriate receptacle.		If you have difficulty aspirating blood, notify physician or nurse practitioner. If serum laboratory work is required, attach another empty syringe to the arterial limb and aspirate required amount of blood.
16. Repeat steps 11 through 15 on the venous limb.	Verifies patency of venous limb; decreases transmission of microorganisms.	Observe for clots.
17. Attach flush syringe to arterial limb, open slide clamp, and gently aspirate 2 to 3 mL of blood; slowly flush catheter, then close slide clamp.	Positive pressure prevents backup of blood into the catheter after flushing.	Syringe should be left attached to catheter limb until replaced with dialyzer tubing connector.
18. Repeat step 17 on venous limb.	Prevents clotting of blood until dialysis is initiated.	Syringe should be left attached to catheter limb until replaced with dialyzer tubing connector.
19. Soak two 2 × 2 pads in povidone-iodine solution and cleanse connection site.	Cleanses connection site.	
20. Remove flush syringe from arterial limb. Attach arterial line from dialysis machine securely to the arterial limb.	Connects to dialysis machine.	
21. Tape connections securely.	Prevents accidental separation of lines.	
22. Open slide clamp on the arterial limb and turn on blood pump.	Primes the blood lines with blood.	
23. When the venous drip chamber located on the hemodialysis machine is pink, turn off the blood pump; clamp the venous line. Remove flush syringe from the venous limb; securely attach to the venous tubing.	Indicates blood has circulated through dialyzer to the venous line.	The venous limb should be left in clamped position.
24. Secure connections.	Prevents accidental separation of lines.	

Procedure **for Hemodialysis** *Continued*

Steps	Rationale	Special Considerations
25. Remove gloves, and discard soiled material in appropriate receptacle.	Standard precautions.	
26. Wash hands. Proceed to initiation of hemodialysis.	Reduces transmission of microorganisms.	

Disconnecting from Catheter

Steps	Rationale	Special Considerations
1. Wash hands, and don mask and cap.	Reduces transmission of microorganisms; standard precautions.	
2. Open syringes, caps, needles, and 2 × 2 gauze pads, and place on sterile field.	Maintains aseptic technique.	
3. Fill two syringes with desired amount of heparin, depending on type of catheter used. Fill 10-mL syringe with NS. *(Level I: Manufacturer's recommendations only)*	Heparin is used to maintain patency of access.[4]	
4. Wrap both catheter limbs with povidone-iodine soaked 2 × 2 pads and scrub for 1 minute.	Povidone-iodine acts as a bactericidal agent.	Be sure to remove any crust or drainage.
5. Place sterile barrier under catheter limbs.	Sets up a sterile field.	
6. Don sterile gloves.	Maintains aseptic technique.	
7. Clamp arterial and venous limbs.	Prevents blood loss from catheters.	
8. Using the same povidone-iodine–soaked 2 × 2 pad to handle the dialysis tubing, disconnect arterial line from the limb and attach the NS-filled syringe.	Prevents blood from entering the tip of the catheter.	
9. Attach a 3- or 5-mL syringe with heparin, unclamp slide clamp; inject prescribed amount of heparin.	Maintains catheter patency by preventing clotting of blood.	Heparin dosage will vary depending on type of catheter used and unit policy. In some cases, catheter may be flushed with NS only.
10. Clamp, disconnect syringe, and cap the arterial limb.	Prevents loss of blood.	
11. Repeat steps 8 through 10 on venous limb.	Maintains patency by preventing clotting of blood.	
12. Apply dressing to catheter site at each hemodialysis treatment or when the dressing become damp, loosened, or soiled. *(Level IV: Limited clinical studies to support recommendations)*	Prevents contamination of catheter exit site.[1, 2]	Dressing should be maintained and changed at least weekly.
13. Apply povidone-iodine ointment to the catheter insertion site at each dressing change. *(Level IV: Limited clinical studies to support recommendations)*	Lowers incidence of catheter-related infections.[1]	
14. Discard soiled material in appropriate receptacle.	Standard precautions.	
15. Wash hands.	Reduces transmission of microorganisms.	

Procedure continued on following page

Procedure	for Hemodialysis *Continued*

Steps	Rationale	Special Considerations
Initiation and Termination of Hemodialysis[5, 6] *(Level IV: Limited clinical studies to support recommendations)*		
1. Verify dialysis orders.	Familiarizes nurse with the individualized patient treatment and reduces the possibility of error.	Orders should include type of dialyzer, number of hours for dialysis treatment, orders for heparin, ultrafiltration, laboratory testing and dialysate solution, and appropriate consents.
2. Set up dialysis machine according to manufacturer's instructions.	Ensures safe and proper assembly and allows for testing of all patient alarms and the proper functioning of the machine prior to accessing the catheter/fistula.	
3. Wash hands, and don examination gloves and goggles.	Reduces transmission of microorganisms; standard precautions.	
4. Access catheter, graft, or fistula.		
5. Wash access arm for 1 full minute with antiseptic soap and a sterile 4 × 4 gauze pad, and place arm on sterile barrier.	Reduces transmission of microorganisms and establishes a sterile field.	
6. Connect arterial access to arterial blood line.	Provides a circuit between the patient and the dialyzer.	
7. Place the venous dialyzer tubing line into the retaining clamps of the fluid catch-all of the side of the dialysis machine.	Prevents contamination of venous tubing.	Be careful not to immerse the end of the venous line below the fluid level.
8. Tape arterial cannula connections securely.	Prevents accidental disconnection.	
9. Remove clamp from arterial line.	Permits flow of blood.	
10. Adjust blood pump to 100 mL/min until blood reaches the venous drip chamber.	Slow rate prevents symptoms of rapid blood loss and allows for assessment of blood flow from the arterial limb.	Heparin loading dose, if ordered, may be given via bolus in arterial line.
11. Turn off blood pump.	Prevents blood loss from dialyzer and cannula.	
12. Clamp the end of the venous tubing below the drip chamber with a bulldog clamp.	Prevents introduction of air.	
13. Remove venous line tubing from fluid catch-all and connect to the venous patient cannula.	Completes pathway circuit for return of blood from the dialyzer to the patient.	
14. Tape venous connections securely.	Prevents accidental separation.	
15. Remove clamp from venous tubing.	Permits flow of blood.	
16. Turn on blood pump and adjust blood flow rate.	Initiates flow of blood from patient to the dialyzer.	
17. Immediately turn on foam detector switch from bypass to alarm position.	Sets the foam detector alarm monitor to on.	The air/foam monitor detects minute air leaks.
18. Adjust the blood level in the arterial and venous drip chambers to three-quarters full.	Prevents accumulation of air in tubing and dialyzer.	
19. Turn dialyzer over so that arterial (red) port is at the top.	Establishes countercurrent flow.	

Procedure **for Hemodialysis** *Continued*

Steps	Rationale	Special Considerations
20. If patient is receiving systemic heparinization, set parameters on heparin infusion pump as prescribed.	Provides anticoagulation.	
21. Secure cannula connections and blood.	Additional precaution against accidental disconnection.	
22. Slowly increase blood pump speed to prescribed rate while continuing to assess patient (level of consciousness, complaints of chest pain, dysrhythmias, and changes in hemodynamic variables).	Prevents complications of rapid removal of blood.	If there is any question as to how well the patient will tolerate hemodialysis, the pump speed should be started at 100 mL/min and gradually increased to goal.
23. Set arterial and venous alarm parameters.	Sets the safety alarm system.	
24. Observe the patient's transmembrane pressure (TMP) display.	Removes desired UF.	To calculate TMP, the following formula may be used: Formula: Weight to be removed × 500 mL − KUF = TMP. (KUF is the coefficient of ultrafiltration of the dialyzer. Each type/size of dialyzer has a different KUF, which can be obtained from the package insert.)
25. Set TMP or negative pressure.	Allows for UF.	Most machines will automatically adjust based on treatment time and volume removal goal.
26. Wash hands.	Reduces transmission of microorganisms.	
27. Continuously monitor patient status and machine function throughout treatment.	Prevents complications and minimizes effects of fluid and electrolyte shifts.	Patient assessment should include vital signs and symptoms related to fluid and electrolyte shifts (eg, cramping, hypotension, nausea, vomiting). Monitor the machine for blood flow rate, arterial and venous pressure readings, dialysate pressure, and blood circuit for clotting or air.

Termination

Steps	Rationale	Special Considerations
1. Wash hands, and don nonsterile gloves and goggles.	Reduces transmission of microorganisms; standard precautions.	
2. Move the arterial, venous, and dialysate pressure alarms to the maximum low/high limits.	Prevents machine from alarming when terminating dialysis as pressures drop.	
3. Turn TMP or negative pressure off.	Removes negative pressure, thereby stopping UF.	
4. Turn off the heparin infusion pump.	Discontinues heparinization prior to the end of dialysis, thus allowing clotting times to return to normal shortly after treatment.	May be done 30 minutes to 1 hour prior to termination of treatment, depending on institutional standard.
5. Decrease the blood pump flow rate.	Reduces blood flow.	
6. Check amount of NS; hang a new bag if necessary.	Minimizes the danger of air embolism on return of blood to patient.	NS (100 mL) or air rinse is used to return blood to patient.
7. Maintain the blood level in the arterial and venous drip chambers at three-quarters full.	Prevents air in tubing and dialyzer.	

Procedure continued on following page

Procedure for Hemodialysis *Continued*

Steps	Rationale	Special Considerations
8. Turn off the blood pump.	Stops blood flow.	
9. Clamp the arterial tubing between patient and blood pump.	Prevents loss of blood if the tubing becomes separated.	
10. Disconnect tubing from vascular access device.	Terminates dialysis.	
11. Turn on blood pump; simultaneously unclamp the patient end connector of the arterial tubing.	Promotes slow return of blood in tubing back to patient.	
12. When blood level is just above the arterial chamber, clamp the tubing above the arterial chamber.	Minimizes the danger of air embolism on return of blood to the patient.	
13. Unclamp the NS IV line.	Flushes the tubing.	
14. Clear the blood tubing and dialyzer with saline until rinse-back is achieved.	Promotes rinse-back of blood to patient.	Satisfactory rinse-back is achieved when venous chamber has pink-tinged NS return.
15. Turn off blood pump.	Terminates flow of blood.	
16. Clamp venous access.	Prevents backflow of blood.	
17. If using a central venous catheter, flush the catheter with heparin or NS (see Procedure 61).	Discontinues vascular access.	
18. AV fistula/AV graft: when fistula needles are used, remove both cannulas from patient's access site, one at a time. Using a sterile 2 × 2 gauze pad, apply moderate pressure to access site until bleeding has stopped.	Discontinues vascular access.	
19. Dress access site(s) with remaining sterile 2 × 2 gauze pad and bandages.	Provides protective barrier.	
20. Dispose of soiled material and equipment in appropriate disposal receptacle.	Standard precautions.	
21. Sanitize single-patient machine according to established procedure. *(Level I: Manufacturer's recommendation only)*	Reduces transmission of microorganisms and readies it for future use.	
22. Wash hands.	Reduces transmission of microorganisms.	

Expected Outcomes	Unexpected Outcomes
• Catheter is accessed without any complications.	• Clotting or decreased patency of the AV fistula or the catheter lumens
• Blood is easily aspirated from the access site.	• Poor blood flow
• Pulsating blood flow exists in the dialysis tubing set.	• Bleeding from the insertion site or access site
• Accumulated waste products are removed.	• Signs or symptoms of infection at the insertion or access site
• Restoration of acid-base balance occurs.	• Dislodgment of the catheter
• Blood urea nitrogen (BUN) and creatinine are restored to baseline levels.	• Decreased circulation in the vascular access limb
• Electrolytes are restored to baseline levels.	• Hematoma formation at the access site
• Accumulated fluid is removed, and dry weight is restored.	• Physiologic complications (dysrhythmias, chest pain, fluid-electrolyte imbalance, hypotension, seizures, nausea and vomiting, headaches, muscle cramping, dyspnea)
	• Technical problems with the dialysis machine

Patient Monitoring and Care

Patient Monitoring and Care	Rationale	Reportable Conditions
		These conditions should be reported if they persist despite nursing interventions.
1. Perform and record a predialysis and daily weights. *(Level V: Clinical studies in more than one patient population and situation)*	Predialysis weight is an important factor in deciding how much UF is needed during treatment. It also helps to guide ongoing treatment.[5, 6]	• Abnormal increase or decrease in weight
2. Perform a baseline and ongoing assessments, including the following: ○ Vital signs ○ Jugular vein distension ○ Presence of edema ○ Intake and output ○ Neurologic assessment *(Level V: Clinical studies in more than one patient population and situation)*	It is important to establish a baseline before initiation of treatment.[5, 6] Monitors for complications.	• Hypotension • Hypertension • Tachycardia/bradycardia • Tachypnea/bradypnea • Fever • Hypothermia • Jugular vein distension • Crackles • Edema • Change in level of consciousness, dizziness • Change in cardiac rhythm
3. Monitor the circulation to the extremity where the graft/fistula is located. ○ Capillary refill ○ Pulses distal to access ○ Color/temperature of extremity ○ Sensation *(Level V: Clinical studies in more than one patient population and situation)*	To assess for any decrease in perfusion distal to the graft site.[5, 6]	• Diminished capillary refill • Diminished or absent peripheral pulses • Pale, mottled, or cyanotic • Cool to touch • Diminished or absent movement • Pain
4. Monitor electrolytes and glucose during treatment as per institutional standard.	Must be monitored because of continued fluid and electrolyte shifts during treatment.	• Hyper/hypokalemia • Hyper/hyponatremia • Hyper/hypocalcemia • Hyper/hypoglycemia

Continued on following page

Patient Monitoring and Care	Rationale	Reportable Conditions
5. Administer medications to correct electrolyte abnormalities as ordered during treatment. *(Level V: Clinical studies in more than one patient population and situation)*	Patients with renal failure are predisposed to many electrolyte abnormalities. During dialysis, several medications/electrolyte replacements may be given, as ordered for individual patients.[5, 6]	
6. Monitor the dialysis circuit (eg, occlusions, kinks, or leaks; blood or clots in vascular access lines). *(Level V: Clinical studies in more than one patient population and situation)*	Disconnections or introduction of air into the circuit are always possible during treatment. Bleeding or exsanguination also can occur.[5, 6] Clotting of the circuit is a potential complication. If hemofilter becomes excessively clotted, the extracorporeal blood volume should be returned to the patient quickly. Blood leaks from dialyzer into the dialysate may occur and would necessitate termination of treatment. Venous or arterial pressures, which are out of range, may indicate dialyzer or access malfunction.	• Disconnections, cracks, or leaks • Bleeding • Excessive clotting • Blood leaks/hemofilter rupture • Malfunction of dialyzer or access
7. Monitor UF for rate, clarity, and air bubbles. *(Level V: Clinical studies in more than one patient population and situation)*	A decrease in UF production can occur due to clotting of the dialyzer.[3, 5, 6] Pink or blood-tinged UF is indicative of filter leak or rupture.	• Decrease in UF production • Change in color or characteristic of UF • Air in UF
8. Administer heparin as ordered. *(Level V: Clinical studies in more than one patient population and situation)*	Heparin is often used to prevent clotting of the circuit.[2, 3] Heparin dose varies according to patient condition and laboratory values.	• Suspicion of clotting in the circuit
9. Monitor anticoagulation as per institutional standard.	Because heparin is commonly used to prevent system clotting, coagulation studies should be routinely monitored.	• Abnormal coagulation studies
10. Monitor the patency of vascular access. ○ Gently palpate along entire length of graft or over access for a thrill (feeling of vibration or purring under fingers). ○ Auscultate for the presence of bruit (sounds like rushing water). *(Level V: Clinical studies in more than one patient population and situation)*	Bleeding can occur from either the venous or arterial catheter or AV fistula. Clotting of the access can occur.[5, 6] Absence of a bruit does not confirm occlusion. Use Doppler if unable to hear a bruit with a stethoscope.	• Decrease in access function or patency • Absence of bruit or thrill
11. Monitor the patient for complications associated with dialysis treatment. *(Level V: Clinical studies in more than one patient population and situation)*	Several complications are possible with dialysis.[5, 6]	• Muscle cramps • Dialysis disequilibrium (headache, nausea/vomiting, hypertension, decreased sensorium, convulsions, coma) • Air embolism • Dialyzer reaction (hypotension, pruritis, back pain, angioedema, anaphylaxis) • Hypoxemia
12. Place a sign above patient's bed indicating which limb has the vascular access (AV graft or fistula).	Blood pressures and blood draws should not be done on the access arm.	

Documentation

Documentation should include the following:

- Patient and family education
- Date and time of treatment initiation
- Condition of catheter or AV fistula regarding patency, quality of blood flow, ease of access procedure
- Condition of insertion site and any signs or symptoms of infection
- Presence of bruit if using an AV fistula
- Needle gauge size used for cannulation
- Type of machine used for dialysis

- Arterial and venous pressures during treatment
- Pump speed
- Length of dialysis treatment
- Vital signs throughout the treatments
- Unexpected outcomes
- Any medications/IV fluids given during treatment
- Nursing interventions
- Pre- and postdialysis weight
- Laboratory assessment data

References

1. Centers for Disease Control, Hospital Infection Control Advisory Council. Guideline for the prevention of intravascular device-related infections. Part 1: intravascular device-related infections: an overview. *Am J Infec Control.* 1996;24:262–276.
2. Centers for Disease Control, Hospital Infection Control Advisory Council. Guideline for the prevention of intravascular device related infections. Part 2: recommendations for the prevention of nosocomial intravascular device-related infections. *Am J Infec Control.* 1996;24:277–293.
3. Thomas-Hawkins C. Nursing interventions related to vascular access infections (review). *Adv Renal Replace Ther.* 1996;3:218–221.
4. Manufacturer's recommendations. Bothell, Wa: Quinton Instrument Co.:1999.
5. American Nephrology Nurses Association. *Core Curriculum for Nephrology Nursing.* Pitman, NJ: ANNA; 1993:207–258.
6. Parker J. *Contemporary Nephrology Nursing.* Pitman, NJ: American Nephrology Nurses Association; 1998:525–576.

Additional Readings

Brunier G. Care of the hemodialysis patient with a new permanent vascular access: review of assessment and teaching. *ANNA J.* 1996;23:547–558.

Carbone V. Heparin and dialyzer membranes during hemodialysis: a literature review. *ANNA J.* 1995;22:452–455.

Dinwiddle LC, Frquman AC, Jaques PF, Mauro MA, Hogan SL, Falk RJ. Comparison of measure for prospective identification of venous stenosis. *ANNA J.* 1996;23:593–600.

Dubose TD, Warnock DG, Mehta RL, et al. Acute renal failure in the 21st century: recommendations for management and outcomes assessment. *Am J Kid Dis* 1997;29:793–799.

Handley J. Rebound hypertension during hemodialysis. *ANNA J.* 1994;21:279.

Hartigan MF. Vascular access and nephrology nursing practice: existing views and rationale for change. *Adv Renal Replace Ther.* 1994;1:155–162.

Himmelfarb J, Hakim RM: The use of biocompatible dialysis membranes in acute renal failure. *Adv Renal Replace Ther.* 1997;4(2 suppl 1):72–80.

Kirby S, Davenport A. Haemofiltration/dialysis treatment in patients with acute renal failure. *Care Critically Ill.* 1996;12:54–58.

Sherman RA, Matera JJ, Novik L, Cody RP. Recirculation assessed: the impact of blood flow rate and low-flow method reevaluated. *Am J Kid Dis.* 1994; 23:846–848.

Wiseman KC. Clinical consult: appropriate nursing care for hemodialysis patients with uncomplicated hypotensive events. *ANNA J.* 1996;23:404–405.

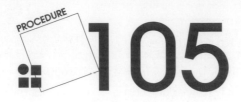
105

Peritoneal Dialysis

P U R P O S E: Peritoneal dialysis (PD) is used for the removal of fluid and toxins, the regulation of electrolytes, and the management of azotemia.

Karen K. Giuliano

PREREQUISITE NURSING KNOWLEDGE

- Basic knowledge of the principles of diffusion and osmosis is necessary.
  - ❖ *Diffusion* is the passive movement of solutes through a semipermeable membrane from an area of higher concentration to one of lower concentration.
  - ❖ *Osmosis* is the passive movement of solvent through a semipermeable membrane from an area of higher concentration to one of lower concentration.
- PD uses the peritoneal membrane as the semipermeable membrane for both fluid solutes.
- Dialysate fluid (dialysate) is infused into the peritoneal cavity through a flexible abdominal catheter (Fig. 105–1).
- A small-framed adult can usually tolerate 2 L to 2.5 L dialysate, whereas a large-framed adult may be able to tolerate up to 3 L in the abdominal cavity. The larger the volume of dialysate, the more effective the removal of blood urea nitrogen (BUN) and creatinine. The most limiting factor is compromise of respiratory excursion by direct pressure on the diaphragm.
- PD involves repeated fluid exchanges or cycles; each cycle has three phases: instillation, dwell, and drain.
  - ❖ During the *instillation phase,* the dialysate is infused by gravity into the patient's abdominal cavity through an abdominal catheter.

- ❖ During the *dwell phase,* the dialysate remains in the patient's abdominal cavity allowing osmosis and diffusion to occur. Dwell time varies based on the patient's clinical need. Using dialysate with a high concentration of glucose enhances fluid removal.
- ❖ During the *drain phase,* the dialysate and excess extracellular fluid, wastes, and electrolytes are drained by gravity from the abdominal cavity via the abdominal catheter.
- PD can be performed either manually by using a single tubing and bag setup or by using a cycler machine (Fig. 105–2). When using a cycler machine, multiple exhanges are programmed into the machine and run automatically. Cycler machines are frequently found in the hospital setting and are often used by outpatients for their evening and night exchanges.

EQUIPMENT

- Masks
- Goggles
- Sterile gloves
- Sterile gauze
- Sterile container
- Hydrogen peroxide
- Povidone-iodine solution
- Tape
- Sterile barriers
- Hemostats

Additional equipment (to have available depending on patient need) includes the following:

- Equipment for culture (if ordered)

Additional equipment for initiation of PD includes the following:

- PD tubing with drainage bag
- Warmed dialysate solution
- Cycler with tubing (if being used)

Additional equipment for termination of PD includes the following:

- Catheter caps
- Labels for catheter

PATIENT AND FAMILY EDUCATION

- Explain the purpose of PD.   ➻*Rationale:* PD is necessary to perform the physiologic functions of the kidneys when renal failure is present.

![Diagram of Tenckhoff catheter placement showing Dacron cuffs, Tenckhoff catheter, Skin, Subcutaneous layer, Peritoneal membrane (Parietal layer), Muscle, Stomach, and Large bowel]

■ ● FIGURE 105–1. Tenckhoff catheter used in peritoneal dialysis. (From Lewis SM, Collier IC. *Medical-Surgical Nursing Assessment and Management of Clinical Problems.* 2nd ed. New York: McGraw-Hill; 1987.)

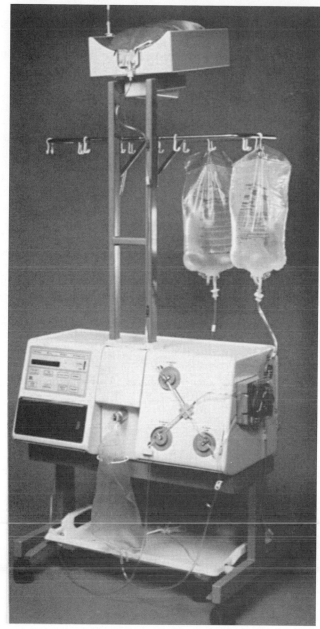

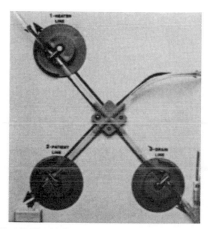

■ ● **FIGURE 105–2.** Automated cycling machine. Peritoneal automated cycler with X-connector set. (Courtesy of Travenol Laboratories.)

- Explain the procedure and review any questions. ➤*Rationale:* Provides information and decreases patient anxiety.
- Explain the need for careful sterile technique when accessing the abdominal catheter. ➤*Rationale:* Sterile technique is used to decrease the chance of peritoneal infection because pathogens can be introduced into the abdominal cavity via the catheter.
- Explain the three phases of PD. ➤*Rationale:* Because each phase is different, it is important for the patient to be informed of all three phases as well as possible interventions associated with each phase.
- Explain the potential for feelings of fullness and possibly shortness of breath during the dwell phase. ➤*Rationale:* The pressure of the dialysate fluid on the diaphragm may cause the patient to have these feelings, which are normal for the dwell phase.

PATIENT ASSESSMENT AND PREPARATION
Patient Assessment

- Baseline vital signs, respiratory status, abdominal assessment, blood glucose level, pertinent laboratory results (potassium, sodium, calcium, phosphorus, magnesium, renal function tests). ➤*Rationale:* Patients in renal failure often have altered baseline assessments, according to both physical assessment and laboratory values. Having this information before treatments are started is helpful so that interventions, including the type and amount of dialysate fluid, can be individualized.

- Volume status, as indicated by the following:
  - ❖ Skin turgor
  - ❖ Edema
  - ❖ Breath sounds
  - ❖ Weight
  - ❖ Intake and output
- ➤*Rationale:* PD is often initiated for the control of hypervolemia. Knowing a patient's pretreatment volume status is essential to allow for the individualization of treatment goals and interventions.
- PD catheter and abdominal exit site for signs and symptoms of infection, leakage or drainage, or signs and symptoms of peritonitis:
  - ❖ Cloudy dialysate solution
  - ❖ Abdominal pain
  - ❖ Fever
  - ❖ Chills
  - ❖ Rebound tenderness
- ➤*Rationale:* Catheter insertion site provides a portal of entry for infection resulting in septicemia or peritonitis.

If the insertion site or effluent appears to be infected, further interventions (eg, site change, culture, antibiotics) may be necessary.
- Peritoneal catheter and tubing for kinking, puncture sites, and loose connections. ➤*Rationale:* Adequate flow is essential for optimal treatment success. A dysfunctional catheter can alter outcomes.

Patient Preparation

- Ensure that patient understands preprocedural teaching. Answer questions as they arise and reinforce information as needed. ➤*Rationale:* Evaluates and reinforces understanding of previously taught information.
- Assist the patient in applying the mask. ➤*Rationale:* Decreases the risk of airborne pathogens.
- Reposition patient to a comfortable position. ➤*Rationale:* Proper positioning is important to ensure patient comfort, optimize respiratory status, and facilitate optimal flow through the abdominal catheter.

Procedure	for Peritoneal Dialysis

Steps	Rationale	Special Considerations
PD Initiation and Discontinuation		
1. Verify PD orders.		Familiarizes nurse with the individualized patient treatment and reduces the possibility of error.
2. Wash hands, and don mask.	Reduces transmission of microorganisms; reduces contamination from airborne pathogens; standard precautions.	
3. Remove dialysate bag from protective pouch; check for expiration date, clarity, and leaks.	Assesses for contamination of dialysate.	
4. Connect and prime tubing with dialysate; clamp tubing.	Fills tubing with dialysate; decreases chance of introducing air into the abdominal cavity.	
5. Wash hands, and don personal protective equipment.	Reduces transmission of organisms; standard precautions.	
6. Prepare sterile field.		
7. Pour povidone-iodine into a sterile container or onto sterile 4 × 4 gauze pads.	Maintains aseptic technique.	
8. Remove old dressing and discard.		Note odor or drainage on the old dressing.
9. Don sterile gloves.	Maintains aseptic technique.	
10. Saturate four of the 4 × 4 gauze pads in povidone-iodine solution and perform a 1-minute scrub catheter-cap connection.	Povidone-iodine serves as a bactericidal agent.	Make sure to remove any crust or drainage.
11. Wrap second povidone-iodine–soaked 4 × 4 gauze pad around catheter-cap connection; leave in place for approximately 3 to 5 minutes.	Reduces transmission of microorganisms.	

Procedure for Peritoneal Dialysis *Continued*

Steps	Rationale	Special Considerations
12. After 3 to 5 minutes, remove povidone-iodine soaked 4 × 4 gauze pad and discard in appropriate receptacle.	Standard precautions.	
13. Using the nondominant hand, pick up the PD catheter with a sterile 4 × 4 gauze pad; remove cap.		
14. Connect catheter to dialysate tubing.	Ensures a tight connection.	
Instillation Cycle		
15. Unclamp and remove any clamps present on the catheter or tubing.	Provides open access between catheter and PD tubing. Allows inflow of dialysate.	
16. Set flow rate as prescribed.		Time for inflow depends on the height of the dialysate bag, position of patient, and the patency of the catheter.
17. When inflow is complete, clamp the dialysate tubing.	Helps prevent backflow.	
Dwell Cycle		
18. Begin dwell cycle.		Dwell time is determined by the number of cycles needed in a 24-hour period. If using a cycler, the cycles will be preprogrammed. Drainage is often routed directly into a toilet or appropriate container.
19. Discard dialysate bag.	Standard precautions.	
Outflow Cycle		
20. Wash hands.	Standard precautions.	
21. Place drainage bag below midabdominal area.	Enhances gravity outflow.	If using a cycler, follow manufacturer's instructions for system setup.
22. Unclamp to permit drainage from peritoneal cavity.		Allow 15 to 20 minutes for outflow; record amount of outflow.
23. Clamp when effluent is completely drained.	Decreases leakage and contamination.	
24. Repeat steps 14 to 23 as ordered.		
Discontinuation of PD		
25. Wash hands.	Reduces the transmission of microorganisms; standard precautions.	
26. Observe outflow of last PD cycle.	Turning the patient from side to side ensures that patient's abdomen is empty of dialysate.	
27. Don clean gloves.		
28. Clamp both the catheter and the PD tubing.	Prevents leakage and contamination.	
29. Prepare sterile field.		

Procedure continued on following page

Procedure **for Peritoneal Dialysis** *Continued*

Steps	Rationale	Special Considerations
30. Pour povidine-iodine into a sterile container with sterile catheter cap.	Acts as a bactericidal agent for cap; some institutions do not use a povidone soak for new caps but instead just attach a new sterile cap.	
31. Don sterile gloves.	Standard precautions.	
32. Remove catheter cap and place on sterile field.		
33. Using sterile 4 × 4 gauze pads, disconnect the catheter from the PD tubing.		
34. Carefully connect catheter cap to catheter.	Maintains aseptic technique.	
35. Securely tape catheter to abdomen.	Prevents accidental dislodgment.	
36. Apply dressing.		Dressing should be changed on a routine basis.
37. Discard soiled materials in an appropriate receptacle.	Standard precautions.	
38. Wash hands.	Reduces transmission of microorganisms.	

Exit Site Care

Steps	Rationale	Special Considerations
1. Wash hands, and don personal protective equipment.	Reduces transmission of microorganisms; standard precautions.	
2. Prepare sterile field.	Prevents contamination of sterile supplies.	
3. Open 4 × 4 gauze pads onto sterile field.	Maintains aseptic technique.	
4. Pour hydrogen peroxide and povidone-iodine into sterile containers.	Reduces transmission of microorganisms.	
5. Remove and discard old dressing into appropriate receptacle.		Be careful not to tug or dislodge the catheter. Note any odor or drainage on old dressing.
6. Inspect catheter exit site and surrounding area for leakage, infection, or trauma.	Provides assessment for complications.	Note any pain, warmth, crusting, bleeding, tenderness, redness, or swelling that may indicate infection.
7. Gently palpate subcutaneous catheter segments and cuff.	Check for pain or accumulated drainage.	Obtain culture if drainage is present.
8. Don sterile gloves.		
9. Use a sterile 4 × 4 gauze pad to hold the catheter off the skin.	Helps prevent contamination of catheter by skin flora.	
10. Use a hydrogen peroxide–soaked 4 × 4 gauze pad to cleanse the catheter and surrounding skin.	Hydrogen peroxide is helpful in removing old secretions.	When cleansing skin, begin at exit site and move outward in concentric circles.
11. Use povidone-iodine–soaked 4 × 4 gauze pads to cleanse both catheter and exit site, and allow them to air dry.	Acts as a bactericidal agent.	
12. Proceed with initiation of PD, or apply a new dressing.		
13. Discard soiled supplies in an appropriate receptacle.	Standard precautions.	
14. Wash hands.	Reduces transmission of organisms.	

Expected Outcomes	Unexpected Outcomes
• Catheter and exit site will be maintained without any complications.	• Drainage from the exit site
• Instillation and drainage of dialysate will occur without problems.	• Poor dialysate flow during instillation or drainage
• Respiratory status will not be compromised during treatment.	• Signs and symptoms of peritonitis
• BUN and creatinine will be restored to baseline levels.	• Inability to drain the total amount of instilled dialysate
• Electrolytes and glucose will be restored to baseline levels.	• Signs or symptoms of infection at the insertion or access site
• Accumulated fluid will be removed.	• Dislodgment of the abdominal catheter
	• Tubing disconnection
	• Physiologic complications during treatment
	• Introduction of pathogens into the abdominal catheter

Patient Monitoring and Care

Patient Monitoring and Care	Rationale	Reportable Conditions
		These conditions should be reported if they persist despite nursing interventions.
1. Perform and record a predialysis and daily weight. *(Level V: Clinical studies in more than one patient population and situation)*	Predialysis weight is an important factor in deciding how much PD is needed during treatment. It also helps to guide ongoing treatment.[1-4]	• Abnormal increase or decrease in weight
2. Perform baseline and ongoing assessments, including the following: ○ Vital signs ○ Jugular vein distention ○ Presence of edema ○ Intake and output ○ Abdominal assessment *(Level V: Clinical studies in more than one patient population and situation)*	Important to establish a baseline before initiation of treatment.[1-4] Monitors for complications.	• Hypotension • Hypertension • Fever • Hypothermia • Jugular vein distention • Crackles • Edema • Abdominal distention or tenderness
3. Monitor electrolytes during treatment at a frequency determined by your institutional standard. *(Level V: Clinical studies in more than one patient population and situation)*	Fluids and electrolytes shift during treatment.[1-4]	• Hyperglycemia • BUN or creatinine levels abnormal for patient • Hyperkalemia or hypokalemia • Hypernatremia or hyponatremia • Hypercalcemia or hypoacalcemia
4. Administer medications to correct metabolic abnormalities as ordered. *(Level V: Clinical studies in more than one patient population and situation)*	Patients with renal failure are predisposed to many metabolic abnormalities. Common medications administered to patients with renal failure include the following[1-4]: ○ Vitamin D and calcium carbonate to increase the serum calcium level and prevent or treat bone disease ○ Erythropoietin and iron to treat anemia ○ Deferoxamine mesylate to remove excessive iron ○ Stool softeners, because constipation can impair drainage of PD fluid ○ Phosphate binders to treat hyperphosphatemia	• Hypercalcemia or hypocalcemia • Abnormal hemoglobin or hematocrit • Hyperphosphatemia or hypophosphatemia

Continued on following page

Patient Monitoring and Care *Continued*

Patient Monitoring and Care	Rationale	Reportable Conditions
5. Monitor serum glucose at the beginning of the treatment and at frequencies throughout the treatment according to institutional standard. *(Level V: Clinical studies in more than one patient population and situation)*	The glucose in the dialysate solution predisposes patients to hyperglycemia, especially diabetic patients.[1-4]	• Hyperglycemia or hypoglycemia
6. Monitor the integrity of the PD setup. *(Level V: Clinical studies in more than one patient population and situation)*	Disconnections in the setup provide a portal of entry for pathogen that can lead to peritonitis.[1-4]	• Fever • Tachycardia • Cloudy dialysate
7. Monitor for signs and symptoms of infection at catheter exit site.		• Site redness or edema • Warmth • Bleeding • Purulent drainage • Pain or tenderness • Fever
8. Monitor the ease with which the dialysate is both instilled and drained through the abdominal catheter.	Patients may need repositioning to facilitate flow through the abdominal catheter. Catheters may also become kinked or occluded. Fibrin clots can obstruct outflow; heparin may be added to the dialysate solution. If clotting is suspected, urokinase may also be used to clear the catheter.	• Inability to instill or drain fluid through the abdominal catheter
9. Ensure proper functioning of cycler (if used).	A cycler can be programmed to perform multiple PD cycles.	• Any problems with cycler function.

Documentation

Documentation should include the following:

- Patient and family education
- Date and time of treatment initiation
- Condition of abdominal catheter and exit site at time of treatment
- Date and time of dressing application
- Patient weight before and after treatment
- Intake and output
- Length and parameters of treatment
- Vital signs throughout the treatment
- Unexpected outcomes
- Nursing interventions
- Laboratory assessment data

References

1. American Nephrology Nurses Association. *Core Curriculum for Nephrology Nursing.* Pitman, NJ: American Nephrology Nurses Association; 1999:281–322.
2. American Nephrology Nurses Association. Peritoneal dialysis. In: *ANNA Standards of Clinical Practice for Nephrology Nurses.* 3rd ed. Pitman, NJ: American Nephrology Nurses Association; 1999:71–84.
3. Bernardini J. Nursing application: established protocols of patient care based on published research. *Perit Dial Int.* 1998;18(1):11–33.
4. Parker J. *Contemporary Nephrology Nursing.* Pitman, NJ: American Nephrology Nurses Association; 1998:603–660.

Additional Readings

Albee B. CAPD catheter exit site healing and clean dressing techniques. *ANNA J.* 1995;22:482–483.
Gokal R, Alexander S, Ash S, et al. Peritoneal catheters and exit-site practices toward optimum peritoneal access: 1998 update. *Perit Dial Int.* 1998;18(1):11–13.
Martis L, Chen C, Moberly JB. Peritoneal dialysis solutions for the 21st century. *Artif Organs.* 1998;22(1):13–16.
Pastan S, Bailey J. Dialysis Therapy. *N Engl J Med.* 1998;338 (20):1428–1437.

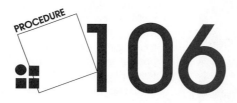

PROCEDURE

106

Assisting with Plasmapheresis

PURPOSE: Plasmapheresis is used to remove plasma from the blood. It is an adjunctive treatment in many diseases, especially in antibody-mediated conditions that produce autoantibodies.

Karen K. Giuliano

PREREQUISITE NURSING KNOWLEDGE

- Apheresis is a technique for separating blood into its various components. There are different apheresis techniques; their names vary according to the component of the blood removed.
  - ❖ Plasmapheresis is the process of removing plasma and proteins from the blood.
  - ❖ Plasma exchange is the process of replacing the plasma removed with an equal amount of either plasma or another fluid.
  - ❖ Leukapheresis is the removal of white blood cells from the blood. It has been used experimentally in the treatment of autoimmune disorders (eg, rheumatoid arthritis and systemic lupus erythematosus). It is also used to remove excess proteins from the blood.
  - ❖ Therapeutic red cell exchange is the process of removing red blood cells (RBCs) from the circulation.
- The plasma removed must be replaced; the most common replacement fluids are plasma, albumin, and normal saline. Because clotting factors are transiently reduced by plasmapheresis, fresh-frozen plasma (FFP) can also be used as a fluid replacement in patients when bleeding is a problem.
- Treatment usually involves plasma exchanges two or three times weekly for up to 6 weeks. The total amount of plasma to be exchanged is used as a guide for treatment. A single treatment, referred to as a plasma exchange, usually takes 2 to 3 hours.
- Plasmapheresis, although commonly performed in critical care units, is most often performed by health care professionals with special knowledge and skills in the plasmapheresis process, such as local blood bank personnel.
- The most commonly used plasmapheresis system (Fig. 106–1) uses either two peripheral venous catheters or a double-lumen central venous catheter to access the vascu-

lar system. A hollow-fiber cell separator, permeable to plasma proteins, is used to remove the patient's plasma via a sophisticated apheresis machine.

- The system should be primed with an anticoagulant (eg, heparin or citrate) to prevent clotting. If citrate is used, the patient must be monitored closely for hypocalcemia. Citrate works as an anticoagulant by binding calcium (Ca^{++}), therefore decreasing the amount of Ca^{++} available for normal clotting.
- Plasmapheresis is used to treat antibody-mediated disorders, because the pathogenic antibodies are contained in the plasma. Removal of these antibodies through plasmapheresis reduces the number of circulating antibodies, temporarily decreasing the patient's symptoms.
- Conditions treated by plasmapheresis may include the following:
  - ❖ Myasthenia gravis
  - ❖ Guillain-Barré syndrome
  - ❖ Various hematologic disorders
  - ❖ Nephrologic disorders
  - ❖ Rhematologic disorders
  - ❖ Poisoning
  - ❖ Drug overdose
- Potential complications of plasmapheresis include the following:
  - ❖ Thrombocytopenia
  - ❖ RBC lysis
  - ❖ Air embolism
  - ❖ Blood leak
  - ❖ Hypotension
  - ❖ Hypothermia

EQUIPMENT

- Blood cell separator machine
- Blood cell separator tubing set

753

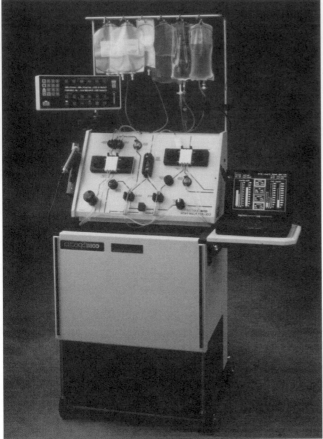

■ ● FIGURE 106–1. COBE® Spectra Apheresis System. (© COBE Laboratories Inc. Photo courtesy of COBE® BCT™ Inc.)

- Replacement fluids
- Hemostats
- Appropriate laboratory specimen tubes

PATIENT AND FAMILY EDUCATION

- Explain the procedure and review any questions the patient may have. ➤➤*Rationale:* Provides information and decreases patient anxiety.
- Explain the purpose of plasmapheresis and specifically why this treatment is being performed. ➤➤*Rationale:* Plasmapheresis is used to treat antibody-mediated disorders.
- Explain the need for careful sterile technique for the duration of treatment. ➤➤*Rationale:* Sterile technique is important in order to decrease the chance of systemic infection, because pathogens can be transported throughout the entire body via the circulation.

- Explain the need for careful monitoring of the patient during the treatment for complications. ➤➤*Rationale:* Hypocalcemia, hypotension, bleeding, and hypothermia are all potential complications of plasmapheresis.
- Explain the importance of the patient letting the nurse know how he or she is feeling during the treatment. ➤➤*Rationale:* Patient symptoms can be important signs of complications related to the procedure. Examples include lightheadedness as a sign of hypotension and numbness and tingling as a sign of hypocalcemia.
- Explain the plasmapheresis circuit setup to the patient and family. ➤➤*Rationale:* Blood will be removed from his or her body and will be visible during the plasmapheresis treatment.

PATIENT ASSESSMENT AND PREPARATION

Patient Assessment

- Baseline vital signs, body system assessment, hemodynamic parameters (if appropriate), and pretreatment fluid balance. ➤➤*Rationale:* Total body assessment should be based specifically on the patient's diagnosis and reason for treatment. Pretreatment assessment provides a baseline for comparison once the treatment is started, allowing for appropriate modification of intervention as needed. Changes in weight during and after treatment are an indicator of fluid balance.
- Pretreatment laboratory values. ➤➤*Rationale:* Coagulation parameters are particularly important; activated clotting time (ACT) and partial thromboplastin time (PTT), if using heparin; ACT and ionized Ca^{++}, if using citrate. Serum sodium and serum bicarbonate levels/pH also should be evaluated in patients when citrate will be used as the anticoagulant.
- Vascular access. ➤➤*Rationale:* A properly functioning vascular access is necessary in order to perform plasmapheresis.

Patient Preparation

- Ensure that patient understands preprocedural teaching. Answer questions as they arise and reinforce information as needed. ➤➤*Rationale:* Evaluates and reinforces understanding of previously taught information.
- Assist the patient to a position of comfort that also facilitates optimal blood flow through the vascular access. ➤➤*Rationale:* Facilitating patient comfort helps to minimize the amount of patient movement during treatment. Movement can change the blood flow through the catheter. Different catheter sites may require different patient positions to facilitate optimal blood flow.

Procedure for Assisting with Plasmapheresis

Steps	Rationale	Special Considerations
1. Verify plasmapheresis orders/consent.	Familiarizes nurse with the individualized patient treatment and reduces the possibility of error.	
2. Gather supplies for vascular access.		The process of vascular access depends on whether the site is central or peripheral.
3. Assist in gathering the supplies for plasmapheresis.		Obtaining and sending laboratory specimens may be part of the plasmapheresis setup as the vascular bed is accessed.
4. Ensure that appropriate replacement fluid is available. Warm replacement fluids. *(Level V: Clinical studies in more than one patient population and situation)*	Avoids chilling patient.[1–5]	Replacement fluids should be slightly warmed before infusion. Never use a microwave to warm fluids. Some patients also may require an increase in the ambient room temperature to avoid hypothermia.
5. Assist with set up and priming of the plasmapheresis circuit as needed.	Ensures safe and proper assembly and complete removal of air from the circuit.	
6. Tape and secure all connections.	Important to prevent inadvertent disconnection of the system.	

Expected Outcomes

- Therapeutic goals are achieved.
- The access site functions properly.

Unexpected Outcomes

- Complications related to the treatment (eg, hypotension, hypocalcemia, hypothermia, hypokalemia, hypernatremia, metabolic alkalosis, air embolism, blood leak, bleeding)
- Poor blood flow through the vascular access
- Bleeding from the access site
- Dislodgment of the catheter
- Hematoma formation at the access site
- Technical problems with plasmapheresis circuit
- Hemolysis

Patient Monitoring and Care

Patient Monitoring and Care	Rationale	Reportable Conditions
		These conditions should be reported if they persist despite nursing interventions.
1. Monitor the patient throughout and after the course of the plasmapheresis treatment. ○ Vital signs ○ Plasmapheresis circuit ○ Laboratory values as ordered *(Level V: Clinical studies in more than one patient population and situation)*	Patients can experience complications such as hypotension, hypothermia, blood leak, air embolism, hypocalcemia, RBC hemolysis, thrombocytopenia, and bleeding that may require intervention.[1–5]	• Hypocalcemia • Hypotension • Hypothermia • Blood leak • Hemolysis • Thrombocytopenia
2. Monitor serum ionized Ca^{++}, serum sodium, and serum bicarbonate levels/pH (if citrate is used as an anticoagulant).	Citrate binds with Ca^{++} and can cause hypocalcemia. It also metabolizes to sodium and bicarbonate, which may cause hypernatremia and metabolic alkalosis.	• Hypocalcemia • Hypernatremia • Metabolic alkalosis

Continued on following page

Patient Monitoring and Care *Continued*

Patient Monitoring and Care	Rationale	Reportable Conditions
3. Monitor ACT/PTT (if heparin is used as an anticoagulant).	These values primarily reflect the activity of the intrinsic clotting pathway.	• Prolonged ACT/PTT
4. Administer replacement fluid as needed.	Replacement fluids are important during the treatment to maintain adequate intravascular volume.	• Hypotension • Tachycardia • Decreased pulmonary artery pressures • Decreased urine output
5. Hold medication administration. *(Level V: Clinical studies in more than one patient population and situation)*	Many medications are removed during treatment, especially those that are protein bound.[1-5] Some medications, such as antihypertensive agents, anticholinergic agents, Ca^{++} supplements, analgesics, and antipyretics, may be indicated during a treatment.	
6. Monitor the access and dressing sites after the termination of plasmapheresis.	Bleeding or signs or symptoms of infection can be complications of the vascular access.	• Bleeding • Redness, tenderness, pain, or warmth at the catheter insertion site • Generalized bleeding or fever

Documentation

Documentation should include the following:

- Patient and family education
- Date and time of treatment initiation
- Condition of vascular access
- Date and time of application
- Vital signs throughout the plasmapheresis treatment
- Daily weight
- Patient's response to plasmapheresis and daily progress toward treatment goals
- Unexpected outcomes
- Nursing interventions
- Laboratory assessment data

References

1. American Nephrology Nurses Association. *Core Curriculum for Nephrology Nursing.* Pitman, NJ: ANNA; 1999:347–365.
2. American Nephrology Nurses Association. Therapeutic plasma exchange. In: *ANNA Standards of Clinical Practice for Nephrology Nurses.* 3rd ed. Pitman, NJ: ANNA; 1999:97–107.
3. Mokrzycki M, Kaplan A. Therapeutic plasma exchange: complications and management. *Am J Kid Dis.* 1994;23:817–827.
4. Price C, McCarley P. Technical considerations of therapeutic plasma exchange as a nephrology nursing procedure. *ANNA J.* 1993;20:41–46.
5. Price C, McCarley P. Physical assessment for patients receiving therapeutic plasma exchange. *ANNA J.* 1994;21:149–154, 201.

Additional Readings

Parker J. *Contemporary Nephrology Nursing.* Pitman, NJ: American Nephrology Nurses Association; 1998:589–602.

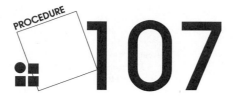

PROCEDURE

107

Blood and Blood Component Administration

PURPOSE: The standard practice in transfusion therapy is to prescribe specific blood components based on the respective appropriate criteria, the patient's clinical picture, and underlying pathophysiology. Although institutions establish criteria for blood component administration, Table 107–1 presents criteria in which a transfusion would be considered reasonable although not mandatory. While not addressed here, additional criteria specific for neonatal and pediatric patients generally are developed by the institution. This procedure will address administration of blood products.

Maribeth Wooldridge-King

PREREQUISITE NURSING KNOWLEDGE

- The Joint Commission on Accreditation of Healthcare Organizations (JCAHO) requires all hospitals to have policies and procedures that address the prescription of appropriate blood and blood components; the distribution, handling, and dispensing of blood and blood components; the administration of blood and blood components; and the monitoring of the effects of blood and blood components on patients.
- Important information about blood and blood components includes the following:
  - ❖ Whole blood rarely is transfused, except in the case of life-threatening hemorrhage.
  - ❖ Red blood cells are transfused to improve oxygen-carrying capacity.
  - ❖ Platelet transfusions are administered to prevent or control the bleeding associated with thrombocytopenia or platelet function defects.
  - ❖ Fresh-frozen plasma (FFP) is administered to treat bleeding or prepare patients for surgery in the presence of single or multiple coagulation factor abnormalities when specific factor concentrates are not available.
  - ❖ Granulocytes are given in rare situations to treat bacterial infections unresponsive to antibiotic therapy in a patient with severe neutropenia or neutrophil dysfunction.

- ❖ Cryoprecipitate is administered for the prevention or treatment of dysfibrinogenemia and hypofibrinogenemia, von Willebrand disease, and in certain situations, factor VII deficiency.
- For each transfusion episode, the medical record should reflect a prescription for the transfusion, documentation of the indication for the transfusion or expected outcome, appropriate laboratory studies pre- and posttransfusion, and the appropriateness of the transfusion with respect to the institution's guidelines for that component.
- White cell-reduced components, cytomegalovirus (CMV)-negative products, irradiated blood components, washed red cells and platelets, frozen-thawed-deglycerolized red cells, and human leukocyte antigen (HLA)-matched platelets are specially processed components that are expensive and time-consuming to prepare, although certain situations exist in which these products are indicated. See Table 107–2 for guidelines for specially processed components.
- Donor blood for allogeneic use is required to undergo testing with U.S. Food and Drug Administration (FDA)–licensed tests for antibodies to the human immunodeficiency virus (anti-HIV), hepatitis C virus (anti-HCV), human T-cell lymphotropic virus (anti-HTLV-I/II), hepatitis B core antigen (anti-HBc), human immunodeficiency virus antigen (HIV-1A), and hepatitis B surface antigen

Table 107–1 ●■■ **Guidelines for Blood and Blood Component Administration**

Whole blood	**Fresh frozen plasma**
Symptomatic anemia with large volume deficit	Management of bleeding in preoperative patients that requires replacement of plasma coagulation factors when specific corrective factors are not available
	Abnormal coagulation assays associated with massive transfusion
	Immediate reversal of warfarin effect
	Thrombotic thrombocytopenic purpura
Red blood cells	**Cryoprecipitate**
Treatment of symptomatic deficit in oxygen-carrying capacity	Control of bleeding associated with fibrinogen deficiency
	Factor VIII deficiency
	Treatment of von Willebrand's disease ONLY if viral-inactivated factor VIII concentrates are not available
Platelets	**Granulocytes**
Thrombocytopenic bleeding due to decreased circulating platelets or functionally abnormal platelets	Neutropenic patients with documented infections (especially gram-negative bacteria and fungi) who have not responded to antibiotics
Patients with platelet counts of <10,000 µL secondary to cancer or chemotherapy	
Management of postoperative bleeding when the platelet count is <50,000/µL	

(HbsAg) and must be found to be negative. A serologic test for syphilis also is performed and must be found to be negative. Units intended for autologous use that test positive for one of the above antibodies/antigens are acceptable to transfuse but are labeled with a biohazard label that indicates the specific reactivity.

- The label on the blood/blood product contains the following information: product name; method by which the product was prepared; temperature range for storage; preservatives and anticoagulant used in the preparation; a standard volume is assumed unless otherwise indicated on the label; number of units in a pooled component; the name, address, and registration number of the collection and processing center; expiration date (and time if applicable—if the time is not indicated, the product expires at midnight); the unit identification number; the donor category; ABO group and Rh type; special handling information, if indicated; and statements regarding recipient identification, infectious disease risk, prescrip-

tion requirement, and mention of the "Circular of Information for the Use of Human Blood and Blood Components."[1]

- No blood container may be vented.
- All blood components must be administered through a filter; a standard filter (170 to 260 microns) is generally used. A leukocyte reduction filter is recommended for all hematology/oncology patients.
- No medications or intravenous (IV) solutions may be added to or infused through the tubing with blood or blood components, with the exception of 0.9% sodium chloride injection (USP). Dextrose-containing solutions should never be used, because glucose induces red cell aggregation. Other IV solutions may be used in the administration set or added to the blood or blood components under the following conditions: (1) the solution(s) have been approved for use by the FDA, and (2) documentation exists that demonstrates that the addition to the component is safe and efficacious.

Table 107–2 ●■■ **Guidelines for Specially Prepared Blood and Blood Components**

Leukocyte-reduced components	**CMV-negative blood**
Prevention of recurrent nonhemolytic febrile transfusion reactions to red cells	CMV-seronegative pregnant women and their fetuses
Beneficial in preventing HLA alloimmunization and platelet refractoriness in selected patients who require long-term transfusion therapy	Low-birthweight infants born to seronegative mothers
	CMV-seronegative bone marrow transplant recipients
Frozen-thawed-deglycerolized red cells	CMV-seronegative solid organ transplant recipients
Frozen red blood cells can be stored for 10 years or longer; appropriate red blood cells to be stored in this manner include the following:	Severely immunocompromised CMV-seronegative recipients
	CMV-seronegative asplenic patients
Autologous red blood cells units collected 42 days before infusion	CMV-seronegative, HIV-infected patients
Units for transfusion to alloimmunized patients when suitable antigen-negative units are not available	**Irradiated blood components**
	Prevents the proliferation of T lymphocytes that cause graft-versus-host disease:
Washed red blood cells and platelets	Bone marrow transplant or peripheral blood progenitor cell transplant recipients
History of anaphylactic reaction to blood component	Patients with immune deficiency syndromes
IgA deficiency with documented IgA antibodies	Neonatal infants who received an intrauterine transfusion or an exchange transfusion following intrauterine transfusion
Recurrent severe urticarial reactions not prevented by pretransfusion administration of antihistamines	Patients with Hodgkin's disease
Febrile reactions associated with red blood cell administration not prevented by white blood cell reduction	Recipients of donor units known to be from a blood relative

Abbreviations: CMV, cytomegalovirus; HIV, human immunodeficiency virus; HLA, human leukocyte antigen; IgA, immunoglobulin A.

- All blood and blood components should be inspected for the presence of excessive hemolysis, a color change in the blood bag when compared to the tubing segments, floccular material, cloudy appearance, or other problems; if any of these situations exist, the unit must be returned to the blood bank for further evaluation.

- Once the integrity of the unit is violated, the component expires 4 hours after entry if the unit is maintained at room temperature (20 to 24°C), or 24 hours after entry if the unit is refrigerated (1 to 6°C).

- In situations that require exchange or massive transfusion, or in patients with cold-reactive antibodies, blood components may be warmed to no more than 42°C during the transfusion (see Procedure 110).

EQUIPMENT

- Blood or component as prescribed
- Appropriate administration set for the blood or component to be transfused
- 0.9% sodium chloride solution for IV administration

- One alcohol pad
- One 19-G needle or needleless connecting device
- Nonsterile gloves
- Thermometer

Additional equipment as needed includes the following:

- Blood pump
- Blood warmer

PATIENT AND FAMILY EDUCATION

- Explain the procedure and reason for administration of the blood or component. ➥*Rationale:* Decreases anxiety and provides an opportunity to ask questions and seek clarification.

- Explain the signs and symptoms of a transfusion reaction and the need to notify the nurse if detected. ➥*Rationale:* The patient may be the first to sense the signs and symptoms of a transfusion reaction. Prompt notification of the nurse facilitates immediate intervention, decreasing the likelihood of serious sequelae.

- Evaluate the patient's need for long-term blood or blood component therapy. ➥*Rationale:* The patient may need to carry a record of transfusion, history/severity of transfusion reactions, and the requirement for premedication(s) or irradiated blood or blood components to reduce the risk of a transfusion reaction.

PATIENT ASSESSMENT AND PREPARATION

Patient Assessment

- Assess for evidence of massive hemorrhage with respect to recent surgery or trauma. ➥*Rationale:* Signs and symptoms of hypovolemic shock with significant blood loss (hemoglobin <8 g/dL) requires replacement with whole blood or packed red blood cells.

- Assess for evidence of deficit in oxygen-carrying capacity: hemoglobin <8 g/dL in the presence of a compromised respiratory status and arterial blood gases. ➥*Rationale:* Significant improvement may be seen in the respiratory status, arterial blood gases, and performance of activities of daily living (ADLs) when the hemoglobin is increased to 10 g/dL or greater. The hematocrit is a less sensitive indicator of oxygen-carrying capacity, because it fluctuates with fluid status.

- Assess for evidence of coagulopathies. ➥*Rationale:* The indications for the transfusion of FFP are limited. FFP should not be administered when a coagulopathy can be corrected more effectively with specific therapy; ie, vitamin K (for patient on warfarin), cryoprecipitate AHF, or factor VIII:C concentrates.

- Assess for evidence of bleeding due to decreased circulating platelets or functionally abnormal platelets (platelet count <20,000/μL) or low platelet counts of <10,000/μL in patients with cancer or undergoing chemotherapy. ➥*Rationale:* Platelets are necessary for normal hemostasis.

- Note transfusion history for presence and severity of transfusion reactions or the necessity of premedications. ➥*Rationale:* A direct relationship exists between the number of transfusions a patient has had and the number of circulating antibodies and thus the likelihood of a transfusion reaction.

- Assess pretransfusion vital signs, including temperature, blood pressure, heart rate, respiratory rate, breath sounds and, if applicable, filling pressures (ie, central venous pressure [CVP], pulmonary artery pressure [PAP], pulmonary capillary wedge pressure [PCWP]). ➥*Rationale:* Establishes baseline values when monitoring for transfusion reaction or fluid overload.

Patient Preparation

- Ensure that the patient and family understand preprocedural teaching. Answer questions as they arise and reinforce information as needed. ➥*Rationale:* Evaluates and reinforces understanding of previously taught information.

- Ensure that informed consent has been obtained. ➥*Rationale:* Protects the rights of the patient and makes a competent decision possible for the patient.

- Establish or ensure the patency of a peripheral intravenous line (bore size minimum is 20 G; an 18-G catheter is preferred) or central venous access device. Blood or blood components are never administered through a pulmonary artery catheter. ➥*Rationale:* Flow of blood at high pressures through a smaller-gauge catheter/needle may damage red blood cells.

- Assess the vascular access line for the possibility of incompatible IV fluids. If necessary, flush the line with normal saline before and after the transfusion. ➥*Rationale:* Only a 0.9% normal saline solution may be infused through the same tubing used with blood or blood components.

Procedure for Blood and Blood Component Administration

Steps	Rationale	Special Considerations
1. Verify the written prescription for transfusion.	Required before initiation of the transfusion.	The prescription should include the name of the blood component, the amount to be transfused, duration of the infusion, and pretransfusion medications, if appropriate.
2. Validate that a current type (ABO and Rh) and screen (all other antibodies) is available in the blood bank.	Type and screen specimens usually are valid for 24 to 72 hours. Check your institution's policy for the number of days the type and screen is valid.	The specimen is typed for ABO and Rh antibodies and screened for all other antibodies. Crossmatching of the donor and recipient blood is done when the blood is ordered. Determine if the patient, family, or friends have donated blood for transfusion. If so, alert the blood bank that a "directed unit" should be available.
3. If a type and screen is not available or outdated, obtain a blood specimen for type and screen and send to blood bank.	The blood bank must have a current specimen for testing the patient and donor blood for reactions.	
4. If indicated, administer pretransfusion medications.	Patients who have a history of a transfusion reaction may require premedication.	Premedications are prescribed by the physician or advanced practice nurse. Patients with a history of a febrile reaction may have their symptoms reduced by premedicating with antipyretics; mild allergic reactions are premedicated with antihistamines; severe allergic reactions are premedicated with antipyretics, antihistamines, and hydrocortisone.
5. Obtain blood or blood component from the blood bank.	Blood or blood components must be initiated within 20 minutes of arrival on the unit.	Blood components may be stored in a special refrigerator where the temperature is maintained between 1 and 6°C. Platelets, cryoprecipitate, and granulocytes *must* be stored at room temperature.
6. With another registered nurse, check the blood or blood component record against the patient's identification band, verifying the following information: A. Exact spelling of the patient's first and last name and medical record number B. Type of blood component C. Compatibility of patient's blood group and Rh type with the donor's blood group and Rh type (Table 107–3, "ABO Blood System with ABO and Rh Compatibility") D. Whether the unit has undergone any special processing E. Unit number F. Expiration date G. Any abnormal color or appearance of the blood or blood component	Verifying this information reduces the risk of an identification error that results in the administration of an incompatible blood/blood component.	If any errors or inconsistencies are noted, *do not puncture the unit or administer the blood or blood component. Notify the blood bank immediately.* Review your institution's policies and procedures for checking blood or blood components. Some patients may require special processing of blood or blood components to reduce the risk of transfusion reaction. See Table 107–2, "Guidelines for Specially Prepared Blood and Blood Components."
7. Ensure that both registered nurses sign the transfusion record.	Validates that proper validation/identification procedures were completed.	
8. Discard supplies, wash hands, and don nonsterile gloves.	Reduces transmission of microorganisms; standard precautions.	

Procedure for Blood and Blood Component Administration *Continued*

Steps	Rationale	Special Considerations
9. Prepare the administration set: A. For Y-type administration set: ○ Close both roller clamps. ○ Spike a 250-mL bag of 0.9% normal saline and prime tubing. Close roller clamp. ○ Attach a 19-G needle or needleless connector to the distal end of the tubing. ○ Spike the unit of blood or blood components.	Y-tubing is used for transfusing whole blood or red blood cells. Prevents spillage. Reduces risk of air emboli. For insertion/connection to primary administration set. Accesses unit for administration.	A Y-type administration set can be used to administer a maximum of two units of whole blood or packed RBC. Make certain the drip chamber is filled so that the filter is saturated with IV solution to prevent hemolysis as blood drips from the bag.

Table 107–3 ●■■ ABO Blood System with ABO and Rh Compatibility

Blood Type	Antigens on Red Cell	Antibodies in Serum
A	A	Anti-B
B	B	Anti-A
AB	A, B	Neither Anti-A nor Anti-B
O	Neither A nor B	Anti-A and Anti-B

Whole Blood

Recipient	A	B	O	AB	Rh Positive	Rh Negative
A	X					
B		X				
O			X			
AB				X		
Rh Positive					X	X
Rh Negative						X

Red Blood Cells

Recipient	A	B	O	AB	Rh Positive	Rh Negative
A	X		X			
B		X	X			
O			X			
AB	X	X	X	X		
Rh Positive					X	X
Rh Negative						X

Plasma

Recipient	A	B	O	AB	Rh Positive	Rh Negative
A	X			X		
B		X		X		
O	X	X	X	X		
AB				X		
Rh Positive					X	X
Rh Negative					X	X

From *Transfusion Therapy Guidelines for Nurses.* Washington, DC: NIH Publication; 1990.

Procedure continued on following page

Procedure for Blood and Blood Component Administration *Continued*

Steps	Rationale	Special Considerations
B. For single-tubing administration set: ○ Close roller clamp. ○ Spike the unit of blood or blood components. ○ Open the roller clamp between the unit and drip chamber; prime the drip chamber, making sure the filter is covered. ○ Prime the remaining length of the tubing. ○ Close the roller clamp. ○ Attach a 19-G needle or needleless connector to the distal end of the tubing.	Prevents spillage. Accesses the unit. Primes drip chamber to prevent damage to constituents in the blood or blood components. Reduces the risk of air emboli. Prevents spillage. For insertion into primary administration set.	Commonly used for the administration of FFP. Platelets, cryoprecipitate, albumin, and granulocytes have product-specific administration sets that are supplied by either the blood bank or pharmacy.
10. Cleanse Y-port injection site proximal to the insertion site with an alcohol wipe.	Reduces transmission of microorganisms.	The IV piggyback port most proximal to the IV insertion site reduces the risk for precipitation or hemolysis in the primary tubing. FFP and platelets should be administered directly into the IV catheter; *do not piggyback.*
11. Insert the needle into the proximal port or attach the blood tubing to the needleless connector of the primary tubing. Clamp off the primary infusion.	Decreases potential for hemolysis or precipitation in primary administration.	Primary infusion set may need to be flushed with normal saline before initiating the transfusion to prevent hemolysis or precipitation in the primary administration set.
12. Release the roller clamp between the unit and the filter.	Allows the transfusion to proceed.	
13. Adjust the rate to infuse 10 to 15 drops per minute for the first 15 minutes.	Ensures patient receives only a small amount of blood or blood components, should a transfusion reaction occur.	
14. Adjust the rate to infuse as prescribed. Transfusion should be completed within maximum of 4 hours of initiating the infusion.	Likelihood of bacterial contamination markedly increases after 4 hours of hang time.	
15. At the completion of whole blood or packed RBC transfusions, flush the administration set with 0.9% normal saline.	Allows for the infusion of the blood in the tubing.	
16. Clamp off the blood administration set and adjust the flow of the primary infusion to the prescribed rate.	Continues primary infusion.	
17. Discard supplies, and wash hands.	Reduces transmission of microorganisms; standard precautions.	
18. Calculate the amount of normal saline, blood or blood components infused and document on the intake and output record. Complete the transfusion record.	Maintains accuracy of intake for evaluation of fluid balance.	

Expected Outcomes

- Complete infusion of blood or blood components
- Restoration of normovolemic status
- Improved oxygen-carrying capacity
- Correction of coagulopathies
- Restoration of hemostasis

Unexpected Outcomes

- Immediate immunologic complications, including hemolytic transfusion reaction, immune-mediated platelet destruction, febrile nonhemolytic reaction, allergic or anaphylactoid reactions, and transfusion-related acute lung injury (see Procedure 111)
- Delayed immunologic complications, including delayed hemolytic reaction, graft-versus-host disease, alloimmunization
- Nonimmunologic complications, including transmission of infectious disease or CMV, bacterial contamination, circulatory overload, hypothermia, and electrolyte disturbances

Patient Monitoring and Care

Patient Monitoring and Care	Rationale	Reportable Conditions
		These conditions should be reported if they persist despite nursing interventions.
1. Monitor the patient continuously for the first 15 minutes of the transfusion.	Acute transfusion reactions usually occur within the first 15 minutes of the infusion.	• If signs and symptoms of a transfusion reaction occur, *stop the transfusion.* See Procedure 111.
2. Monitor the vital signs every 15 minutes for the first hour, then every 30 minutes until the unit is infused.	Detects changes that suggest a transfusion reaction.	• Mild transfusion reaction: temperature rise <1°C above baseline, minimal itching or localized urticaria, chills
		• Moderate transfusion reaction: temperature rise >1 to 2.5°C above baseline, itching unresolved with antihistamines, urticaria unresolved with antihistamines, chills with fever unresolved with antipyretics
		• Severe transfusion reaction: temperature rise >2.5°C above baseline; progressive, confluent, or extensive urticaria; shock, hypotension; cyanosis; hemoglobinuria; dyspnea; back (flank) pain
3. At the completion of the transfusion, calculate the amount of normal saline, blood or blood components infused and document on the intake and output record. Complete the transfusion record.	Maintains accuracy of intake for evaluation of fluid balance.	
4. Obtain posttransfusion laboratory values.	Determines efficacy of transfusion. One unit of PRBC should raise the nonbleeding adult's hemoglobin by 1 g/dL and the hematocrit by 3%. For FFP: monitor the prothrombin time (PT), partial thromboplastin time (PTT) or specific factor assays as prescribed. For platelets: Evaluate platelet count at 1 hour and 24 hours after transfusion to assess patient's response.	• Laboratory results

▌ D o c u m e n t a t i o n

Documentation should include the following:

- Patient and family education
- Pretransfusion assessment
- Informed consent (if required by institution)
- Date and time transfusion was initiated and terminated
- Baseline and serial vital sign measurements

- Transfusion record validated by two registered nurses
- Type and amount of blood or component administered
- Appropriate laboratory values pre- and posttransfusion
- Patient's tolerance of transfusion
- Occurrence of unexpected outcomes and interventions taken

Reference

1. American Association of Blood Banks, America's Blood Centers and the American Red Cross. *Circular of Information for the Use of Human Blood and Blood Components.* ARC; July 1998:3.

Additional Readings

Contreas M, Ala FA, Greaves M, British Committee for Standards in Hematology, Working Party of the Blood Transfusion Task Force, et al. Guidelines for the use of fresh frozen plasma. *Transfus Med.* 1992;2:57–63.

Murphy MF, Brozovic W, Murphy W, Ouwehand W, Waters AH, British Committee for Standards in Hematology, Working Party of the Blood Transfusion Task Force. Guidelines for platelet transfusions. *Transfus Med.* 1992;2:311–318.

National Institutes of Health. *National Blood Resource Education Program's Transfusion Therapy Guidelines for Nurses* (NIH Publication No. 90-2668). Washington, DC: U.S. Government Printing Office; 1990.

Prezepiorka D, LeParc GF, Stovall MA, Werch J, Lichtiger B. Use of irradiated blood components. *Am J Clin Pathol.* 1996;106:6–11.

Przepiorka D, LeParc GF, Werch J, Lichtiger B. Prevention of transfusion-associated cytomegalovirus infection. *Am J Clin Pathol.* 1996;106:163–169.

Stehling L, Luban NLC, Anderson KC, et al. Guidelines for blood utilization review. *Transfusion.* 1994;34:438–448.

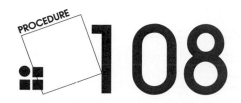

108

Blood Pump Use

PURPOSE: An external pressure infusion cuff or blood pump is used to administer a large amount of blood or plasma to a patient with massive, life-threatening hemorrhage or to infuse viscous whole blood or packed red blood cells within a prescribed period of time.

Maribeth Wooldridge-King

PREREQUISITE NURSING KNOWLEDGE

- External pressure cuffs should only be used with central line catheters or large-bore (18 gauge or larger) peripheral intravenous (IV) catheters. Caution must be exercised when applying a pressurized cuff to a peripheral IV catheter in order to avoid damaging the vein.
- The applied pressure should not exceed 300 torr when pressure-transfusing components that contain red blood cells.[1] Only external pressure cuffs specifically designed for blood or blood component infusions should be used. A standard sphygmomanometer cuff should never be used to administer large-volume transfusions or infusions.
- A rapid infusion (1 unit every 5 minutes) of cold blood (1 to 6°C) may lower the temperature of the sinoatrial node to less than 30°C, at which point ventricular fibrillation can occur.[2]

EQUIPMENT

- Blood administration set
- External pressure infusion cuff or blood pump
- Blood or blood components for transfusion
- 0.9% normal saline for infusion (for whole blood or packed red blood cell transfusions)
- Blood pressure cuff/sphygmomanometer
- Stethoscope
- Thermometer
- Cardiac monitor
- Nonsterile gloves

PATIENT AND FAMILY EDUCATION

- Explain the rationale for using an external pressure infusion cuff. ➤*Rationale:* Informs patient and family regarding the purpose of the device.

- Explain that the patient may feel discomfort in his or her extremity or IV insertion site if the external pressure infusion cuff is used with a peripheral IV catheter. ➤*Rationale:* Pressure applied to a peripheral vein may be uncomfortable to the patient.
- Instruct patient to report any signs or symptoms of a transfusion reaction to the nurse. ➤*Rationale:* Facilitates prompt and immediate intervention by the nurse.

PATIENT ASSESSMENT AND PREPARATION

Patient Assessment

- If using a peripheral IV catheter, assess the IV site for redness, swelling, or pain. ➤*Rationale:* Signs and symptoms of an infiltration that necessitate the insertion of a new peripheral intravenous catheter.
- For peripheral administration, ascertain that the venous catheter is 18 gauge or larger. ➤*Rationale:* External pressure cuffs cannot be used on peripheral venous catheters smaller than 18 G.

Patient Preparation

- Ensure that the patient and family understand preprocedural teaching. Answer questions as they arise and reinforce information as needed. ➤*Rationale:* Evaluates and reinforces understanding of previously taught information.
- Take pretransfusion vital signs, including temperature, pulse, respiration, and blood pressure. Note filling pressures, (central venous pressure [CVP], pulmonary artery pressure [PAP], and pulmonary capillary wedge pressure [PCWP]) if available. ➤*Rationale:* Establishes baseline data.

Procedure for Blood Pump Use

Steps	Rationale	Special Considerations
1. Wash hands, and don nonsterile gloves.	Reduces transmission of microorganisms; standard precautions.	
2. Obtain and set up blood or blood components for administration (see Procedure 107).	Blood or blood components should be assembled before inserting the unit into the pump.	
3. Prime the tubing and piggyback into the primary IV line.	Allows transfusion to proceed.	
4. Open the roller clamp on the administration set.	Rate of infusion is dependent on the amount of pressure applied to the unit, not the position of the roller clamp.	
5. Deflate the external pressure infusion cuff.	Allows for easy placement of unit of blood or blood components into the cuff.	
6. Guide the unit of blood or blood components through the mesh or plastic covering of the cuff so that the entire unit remains within the mesh or plastic panel.	Allows pressure to be evenly applied to blood or blood components bag.	Do not allow the top of the unit to appear above the mesh or plastic covering, because this will interfere with flow.
7. Secure the unit of blood or blood components in place with fabric strap or Velcro closure and hang the cuff from the IV pole.	Prevents unit from slipping out of the cuff when hung from the IV pole.	
8. Inflate the external pressure infusion cuff to achieve the desired rate of flow.	Pressure of blood pump is used to adjust flow, not the position of the roller clamp.	The pressure should not exceed 300 mm Hg to avoid damaging the red blood cells, rupturing the blood bag, dislodging the IV catheter or injuring the vein. The patient may complain of discomfort in his or her extremity if a peripheral catheter is used; if appropriate, decrease the pressure to maintain patient comfort.
9. When the transfusion is complete, deflate the external pressure cuff, close the roller clamp to the blood bag, and open the roller clamp to the 0.9% normal saline solution.	Pressure is usually not needed to infuse the normal saline.	
10. Flush the primary infusion tubing with normal saline.	Allows the patient to receive blood sequestered in the tubing.	
11. Transfuse additional units of blood, if prescribed.	Multiple transfusions may be necessary for life-threatening hemorrhage.	
12. When all of the transfusions are completed, don nonsterile gloves, deflate the cuff, and remove the unit of blood or blood components. Discard the administration setup into the appropriate receptacle or as per institutional policy.	Standard precautions.	
13. Regulate the primary IV infusion at the prescribed rate.	Continues fluid resuscitation.	Administration of crystalloid and colloids can be used in conjunction with blood replacement therapy to provide cardiovascular support.
14. Discard used supplies, and wash hands.	Reduces the transmission of microorganisms; standard precautions.	

Expected Outcomes	Unexpected Outcomes
• Improved or rapid flow of blood or blood components • Infusion completed within prescribed time limit	• Dislodgment of IV catheter • Rupture of blood or blood components bag • Discomfort

Patient Monitoring and Care

Patient Monitoring and Care	Rationale	Reportable Conditions
		These conditions should be reported if they persist despite nursing interventions.
1. Assess the peripheral IV site for redness, swelling, and pain at least every 15 min during the transfusion. If signs and symptoms of infiltration occur, stop the transfusion immediately, remove the catheter, and initiate another IV catheter infusion site.	Pressurized infusion can cause catheter dislodgment.	
2. Monitor the patient's blood pressure, filling pressures (CVP, PAP, and PCWP), heart/rhythm, urine output, and respiratory rate every 15 min for the first hour, then every 30 min until the transfusion is completed.	Monitors patient response to rapid blood administration.	• Changes in vital signs, cardiac rhythm, filling pressures, and fluid status
3. Monitor the patient for signs and symptoms of a transfusion reaction. If a transfusion reaction is suspected, stop the administration of blood.	Blood or blood components replacement therapy constitutes the infusion of a foreign substance into the recipient.	• Signs and symptoms of a transfusion reaction (see Procedure 111)

Documentation

Documentation should include the following:

- Patient and family education
- Pretransfusion assessment
- Date and time infusion is initiated and completed
- Transfusion record validated by two RNs
- Baseline and serial vital sign measurements
- Use of an external pressure cuff or blood pump
- The type and amount of the blood or blood components infused under pressure
- Appropriate laboratory value(s) pre- and posttransfusion
- Patient's tolerance of the transfusion
- Unexpected outcomes and interventions taken

References

1. National Institutes of Health. *National Blood Resource Education Program's Transfusion Therapy Guidelines for Nurses* (NIH Public No. 90-2688). Washington DC: U.S. Government Printing Office, 1990.

2. Snyder EL. Transfusion reactions. In: Hoffman R, Benz EJ Jr, Shattil SJ, Furie B, Cohen HJ, Silberstein LE, eds. *Hematology: Basic Principles and Practice.* 2nd ed. New York, NY: Churchill Livingstone; 1995:2050.

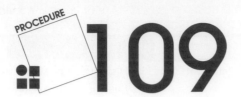

Continuous Arteriovenous Rewarming

PURPOSE: Continuous arteriovenous rewarming (CAVR) is used to rapidly rewarm severely hypothermic patients, reverse hypothermia-induced coagulopathy, prevent or treat adverse physiologic effects of severe hypothermia, and assist with massive fluid resuscitation in hypovolemic patients who are hypothermic.[1] The patient populations CAVR is most frequently used for include critically injured trauma patients, near-drowning patients, patients with massive gastrointestinal (GI) hemorrhage, patients with abdominal aortic aneurysm, and environmental exposure patients.

Christine S. Schulman

PREREQUISITE NURSING KNOWLEDGE

- Knowledge of aseptic technique is essential.
- Severe hypothermia poses a number of adverse physiologic consequences in critically ill or injured patients. Cardiovascular, neurologic, GI, metabolic, and pulmonary disturbances that occur as a result of hypothermia predispose patients to numerous complications and may interfere with the patient's ability to respond to illness or trauma.
- Hypothermia-induced coagulopathies are especially life threatening to patients with ongoing hemorrhage and are an all too-frequent complication of aggressive fluid resuscitation with inadequately warmed fluids and blood products. Hypothermia-induced coagulopathies begin to appear when the patient's body temperature falls below 34.5°C and worsen any preexisting hemorrhage the patient may have.
- Progressive hypothermia causes a left shift of the oxygen-hemoglobin dissociation curve as the patient cools. In the presence of hypothermia, hemoglobin increases its affinity for oxygen and will not release oxygen to the tissues. The resulting cellular hypoxia places additional demands on cells that are already under great physiologic stress from critical illness or injury.[2, 3]
- CAVR is an arteriovenous circuit in which blood is diverted from the patient's femoral artery into special heparin-coated tubing through a rewarming chamber and filter, and then it is returned to the patient via either the subclavian, femoral, or internal jugular vein (Fig. 109–1). The system is driven by the patient's blood pressure. Patients can be rewarmed from 32°C to 36°C in as little as 45 minutes. By being rapidly rewarmed, coagulopathies are reversed, the use of blood products and IV fluids is decreased, and patient mortality is improved.[4]

- The physician or advanced practice nurse inserts the arterial and venous catheters, but it is the nurse's responsibility to maintain patency of the circuit and troubleshoot the system. Nine-French catheters included in the CAVR vascular access kit are the only catheters used; pulmonary artery (PA) catheters and angiography introducers are not large enough for the system to function properly. No stopcocks, reflux valves, or additional connection tubing can be used, because they will slow bloodflow and potentiate clotting of the system. Hemodynamic and laboratory monitoring, fluid and blood product resuscitation, and all other aspects of patient care can occur concurrent to CAVR.[1]
- Contraindications to CAVR include patients with a systolic blood pressure of less than 80 mm Hg, patients weighing less than 90 pounds, and patients with known vascular occlusive disease or compartment syndrome of the lower extremities. Systolic blood pressure usually can be supported to stay above 80 mm Hg by infusion of additional IV fluids, blood products, and vasopressors.[1]
- As patients warm, vasodilation occurs and additional IV fluids often are necessary to reverse hypovolemia. Cold, hyperkalemic, and acidotic blood returns from the previously hypoperfused lower extremities to the core circulation and can cause "reperfusion injury." This is manifested by cardiac dysrhythmias, hypotension, and acidosis and can result in adult respiratory distress syndrome, acute tubular necrosis, and multisystem organ failure.[2] This is more common with peripheral warming, such as warmed cotton blankets and warm air blankets, rather than with central warming, such as warmed peritoneal lavage, CAVR, and cardiac bypass.

EQUIPMENT

- Pulmonary artery catheter, tympanic thermometer, or bladder temperature probe to effectively monitor the patient's core temperature
- Level 1 fluid warmer (Model H-500 or H-250) or Level 1 fluid management system H-1025 (Sims Level 1 Technologies, Rockland, MA)
- Vascular access insertion tray for CAVR via Gentilello technique (Sims Level 1 Technologies, Rockland, MA)
- Nonsterile gloves
- Disposable tubing for CAVR
- Replacement filter with gas vent
- Replacement IV infusion set
- Two central line dressing kits
- Sterile or distilled water for water chamber
- Normal saline or lactated Ringer's IV solution

Additional equipment as needed includes the following:

- Doppler
- Additional massive fluid infusers as indicated by the patient's volume depletion

PATIENT AND FAMILY EDUCATION

- Explain the reason for CAVR. ➡️*Rationale:* Helps the patient and family understand the consequences of hypothermia as well as the plan of care.
- Explain the procedure and explain the equipment. ➡️*Rationale:* Decreases patient and family anxiety about the procedure and unfamiliar equipment at the bedside.

PATIENT ASSESSMENT AND PREPARATION

Patient Assessment

- Obtain the patient's medical history, including the length of exposure to cold, surgical procedure, or types of injuries. ➡️*Rationale:* Assists in anticipating severity of hypothermia, coagulopathy, and potential multisystem complications.
- Assess core temperature using either a tympanic thermometer, bladder probe, or pulmonary artery catheter. ➡️*Rationale:* Assesses severity of hypothermia and efficacy of therapy.
- Obtain vital signs. ➡️*Rationale:* Provides baseline data.
- Obtain hemodynamic parameters to include cardiac output (CO) and index (CI), central venous pressure (CVP), pulmonary artery pressure (PAP), pulmonary capillary wedge pressure (PCWP), and systemic vascular resistance (SVR). If monitoring system is available, measurement of the right ventricular ejection fraction, oxygen delivery, and oxygen consumption also should occur. ➡️*Rationale:* Identifies baseline oxygen transport and tissue perfusion.
- Assess arterial blood gas, hemoglobin, hematocrit, and coagulation studies. ➡️*Rationale:* Measures oxygenation, presence of metabolic acidosis, severity of hemorrhage, and severity of coagulopathy so that effectiveness of interventions can be assessed and additional interventions initiated.

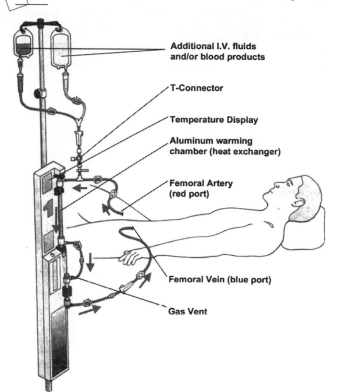

■ ● **FIGURE 109–1.** Continuous arteriovenous rewarming. (Courtesy of SIMS Level 1, Inc., Rockland, Ma.)

Labels: Additional I.V. fluids and/or blood products; T-Connector; Temperature Display; Aluminum warming chamber (heat exchanger); Femoral Artery (red port); Femoral Vein (blue port); Gas Vent

- Assess patency of current IV large-bore sites. ➡️*Rationale:* Infusion of IV fluids in addition to those infused through the CAVR circuit most likely will be necessary. Multiple IV sites will be needed for infusion for supplementary blood products and resuscitation fluids.
- Assess distal pulses, color, and temperature of extremities. ➡️*Rationale:* Provides baseline data.

Patient Preparation

- Ensure that the patient and family understand preprocedural teaching. Answer questions as they arise and reinforce information as needed. ➡️*Rationale:* Evaluates and reinforces understanding of previously taught information.
- Place additional IV sites. ➡️*Rationale:* Aggressive fluid resuscitation will require more access than what is provided by the CAVR circuit. Hypothermia-induced coagulopathy increases the patient's tendency to bleed, necessitating replacement of fluids and blood components.
- If not already in place, assist the physician or advanced practice nurse with placement of central venous access or a pulmonary artery catheter. ➡️*Rationale:* Allows for assessment of volume status in response to fluids, assessment of core temperature with PA catheter, and provides central venous access in the event vasoactive medications are needed.
- Remove any fluids from the patient's skin and change linens frequently to keep dry linens next to the patient. Cover the patient with warm blankets or a warm air blanket; cover the patient's head with an aluminum cap. ➡️*Rationale:* Minimizes additional heat loss via radiation and convection.

Procedure	for Continuous Arteriovenous Rewarming

Steps	Rationale	Special Considerations
1. Wash hands, and don gloves.	Reduces transmission of microorganisms; standard precautions.	
2. Verify the physician's prescription for CAVR and infusion of additional IV fluids or blood products.	Prevents unnecessary blood product or IV fluid administration.	Physician's prescription should include additional IV fluids and blood products, laboratory studies, and temperature at which therapy should be discontinued.
3. Assist the physician or advanced practice nurse with placing arterial and venous access sites.	Establishes arterial and venous access.	Access sites must be large to accommodate the 9-Fr catheters in the CAVR vascular access kit. Angiography and PA catheter introducers are too small for adequate blood flow through the circuit and should not be used. No stopcocks or extension tubing should be added to the system, because they also restrict flow.[1]
4. Push the bottom end of the heat exchanger rod *firmly* into the bottom socket and snap the heat exchanger into the guide (Fig. 109–2).	The bottom of the heat exchanger must be firmly placed, otherwise it will not fit into the top socket.	Being too gentle will result in improper placement of the tubing and the warmer will not run.

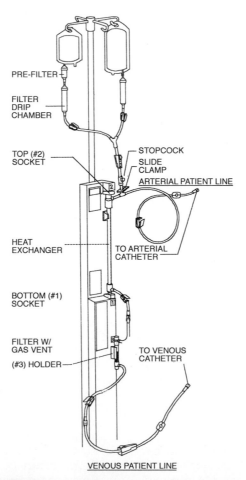

■ ● **FIGURE 109–2.** Insertion of CAVR tubing into Level 1 Rapid Infuser. (Courtesy of SIMS Level 1, Inc., Rockland, Ma.)

Procedure **for Continuous Arteriovenous Rewarming** *Continued*

Steps	Rationale	Special Considerations
5. Slide the top socket up and place the top end of the exchanger into the placement tract.	Prepares the system.	
6. Slide the top heat exchanger socket down over the heat exchanger tube until the pole latch clicks into place.	Locks the warming chamber into place at both the top and bottom sockets.	
7. Snap the air eliminator filter into the holder on the lower portion of the pole assembly with the orange end up.	Filters air and blood clots from the tubing.	It will only fit one way, because the tubing is not long enough if placed incorrectly.
8. Plug the device into the outlet and turn it on.	Activates warmer.	Disposable tubing must be in place in order for the machine to turn on without alarming. If the "Check Disposable" alarm sounds despite tubing being in place, make sure that all pieces fit firmly into their holders.
9. Perform all function and alarm checks as per manufacturer's instructions.	Safety precaution. Validates proper equipment function.	
10. Wait for temperature readout to reach operating temperature of 41°C.	Prevents cooling of the patient's blood by directing it through the warming chamber before it reaches operational temperature.	
11. Close all tubing clamps.	Prevents flow through the circuit before everything is warmed and ready.	
12. Spike one of the sides of the Y-connector with normal saline.	Prepares the tubing system.	This can be done while the infuser is warming to 41°C.
13. Open the main tubing clamp at distal end of tubing to prime with IV fluid.	Prevents air embolus and facilitates blood flow through the system when the CAVR circuit is first opened.	Priming the tubing is optional; the tubing can also be primed with the patient's blood when the arterial catheter clamp is opened.
14. Flush to the end of the line.	Removes air from the tubing.	
15. Close all clamps.		
16. Connect the arterial patient line to the arterial catheter and open the arterial catheter clamp.	Blood will fill the tubing, driven by the patient's blood pressure.	CAVR should be withheld in patients with a systolic blood pressure (SBP) <80 mm Hg. However, additional IV fluids, blood products, and vasopressors usually can maintain the BP above 80 mm Hg.[1]
17. Completely open the distal roller clamp.		
18. Flush the tubing with the patient's blood to the end of the line.	Allows blood to move through the system.	All clamps must be wide open for CAVR to function properly. Priming the system outside of the patient allows for assessment of equipment function and arterial flow before the system is connected to the patient.
19. Close the distal roller clamp.		
20. Attach the venous patient line into the venous catheter and open the roller clamp.	At this point, patient rewarming is occurring.	

Procedure continued on following page

Procedure	for Continuous Arteriovenous Rewarming *Continued*

Steps	Rationale	Special Considerations
21. Infuse additional fluids and blood products into the T-connector.	Supports patient's BP and hematocrit. Helps keep system patent by ensuring good flow of fluid.	Additional IV fluids and blood products may be necessary to speed up blood flow through the circuit to keep it open, as well as to support the patient's blood pressure. May need to use pressure chambers to facilitate forward flow of the piggybacked fluids and prevents back flow into the arterial catheter.
22. Tape the disposble tubing to the patient's leg.	Prevents the catheters from kinking and from being pulled out.	
23. Apply dry, occlusive dressings to the sites.	Prevents infection.	
24. Discard used supplies, and wash hands.	Reduces tranmission of microorganisms; standard precautions.	

Patient Transportation

1. Turn the rewarmer/rapid infuser machine off.	The machine will not operate when the clamps are closed.	Fluid from the water chamber will spill out of the chamber and the aluminum heat exchanger if the machine is on when the tubing is removed from the holders.
2. Clamp the CAVR circuit at the arterial side and backflush into the patient with normal saline until clear. Clamp the arterial catheter.	The Level 1 infuser does not have a battery and rewarming cannot continue when the machine is not plugged in.	It is essential that the unwarmed CAVR fluid does not cool the patient again, so CAVR must be briefly interrupted during actual transport and resumed when the patient arrives at his or her destination.
3. Flush the remainder of the tubing clear of the patient's blood through the venous side with a warmed crystalloid solution. Clamp the venous side of the tubing and the venous catheter.	Returns blood back to the patient. Clears blood from the circuit so that it does not clot while the system is off.	
4. Remove the heat exchanger from the warming device and lay it in the bed alongside the patient.	Keeps the tubing set close to the patient and prevents it from being pulled out.	The Level 1 infuser can now be transported separately from the patient, simplifying transport.
5. Replace the heat exchanger into the infuser on reaching destination.	Readies the circuit for resumption of blood flow.	
6. Plug in the machine and let it warm to 41°C.	Lets the machine reach appropriate temperature before circuit is re-opened.	
7. Open arerial, venous, and distal clamps.	Opens the circuit to blood flow, allowing rewarming to resume.	
8. Assess blood flow through the circuit.	Ensures that catheters or tubing did not clot off during transport.	Patency of the circuit is dependent on brisk blood flow and effective flushing of catheters when not in use.
9. Discard supplies, and wash hands.	Reduces transmission of microorganisms; standard precautions.	

Procedure	**for Continuous Arteriovenous Rewarming** *Continued*

Steps	Rationale	Special Considerations
Troubleshooting CAVR		
1. Check arterial and venous catheter insertion sites for kinking.	Kinking will obstruct flow.	May need to support catheters with folded gauze dressings to keep them straight.
2. Check the filter for clotting.	Continuous flow of patient blood or banked blood can put the system at risk for clotting.	Change whenever flow becomes sluggish and clots are noted in the filter.
A. Change the filter by briefly clamping both arterial and venous clamps on either side of the filter and removing the filter from its holder.	Clamps tubing so that blood will not spill when the tubing is taken apart.	CAVR blood flow will be interrupted.
B. Attach the arterial end of the new filter to the tubing, invert the filter, and slowly release the arterial clamp to prime the filter with the patient's blood. Return the filter to the upright position (orange end up) and place in the holder.	Less air will be trapped in the filter if it is filled in the inverted position.	
C. Unclamp the venous clamp, allow flow through to the end of the filter. Connect the venous end of the filter to the venous tubing. Release the clamp, allowing blood to flow into the patient. Make sure all clamps are open and that the circuit is flowing briskly.	Allows circuit to be reestablished.	Keep additional CAVR filters close at hand if the patient is being massively transfused. CAVR filters are *not* compatible with regular Level 1 infusion tubing.
3. If alarm sounds and "Check Disposable" light is illuminated, check to make sure the disposable tubing is properly placed in all of the holders.	The system will not run if the disposable tubing is not completely set into the machine.	Set can become easily dislodged.
4. If the alarm sounds and "Water Level" light is illuminated, check water level in chamber and replace as needed with sterile or distilled water.	System will not operate if water level is too low.	
5. If the alarm sounds and the "Overtemp" light is illuminated, then turn the machine off and use a different rapid infuser.		
6. Maintain the patient's systolic BP above 80 mm Hg with warmed crystalloids, blood products, and vasopressors as prescribed.	Systolic blood flow drives the CAVR circuit; hypotension causes the circuit to clot.	If the patient is persistently hypotensive despite fluids, blood, and vasopressors, the CAVR circuit may need to be backflushed and discontinued. Fluids can be directly infused into the T-connector through the warmer and into the patient. A second fluid warmer to deliver fluids via another access site often is used in addition to CAVR for patients requiring massive fluid resuscitation.

Procedure continued on following page

Procedure **for Continuous Arteriovenous Rewarming** *Continued*

Steps	Rationale	Special Considerations
Discontinuing CAVR		
	CAVR is discontinued when the patient's temperature reaches 36.5°C and stabilizes there for at least 2 hours.	Once the patient's temperature has reached 36.5°C, his or her temperature is considered back to normal and hypothermia-induced coagulopathies have resolved. Patients can cool down again, however, after CAVR is stopped when cool blood from the distal circulation beds returns to the core circulation. It is important to not discontinue the catheters until the core temperature has been stable for at least 2 hours.[1]
1. Wash hands, and don gloves.	Reduces transmission of microorganisms, standard precautions.	
2. Clamp the arterial end of the circuit.	Turns off the circuit flow.	
3. Backflush the arterial catheter into the patient with normal saline until clear. Clamp the arterial catheter to the patient.	Prevents clotting of the arterial catheter in case it needs to be used again before it is discontinued.	
4. Flush the remaining patient blood through the system into the patient using crystalloids from the T-connector until the tubing is clear.	Returns blood in the tubing back into the patient.	
5. Clamp the venous catheter clamp.	Closes off the CAVR circuit to the patient.	
6. Assist as needed with application of direct pressure to the catheter sites for 15 min after the catheters have been removed by the physician.	Minimizes hematoma development.	Pressure may need to be held longer if the patient has coagulation abnormalities.
7. Apply occlusive dressings to sites.	Reduces incidence of infection.	
8. Discard supplies, and wash hands.	Reduces transmission of microorganisms; standard precautions.	

Expected Outcomes

- Return of patient's core temperature to 36.5°C within 3 hours[4]
- Systolic BP remaining above 80 mm Hg
- Restoration of intravascular volume as patient rewarms and coagulopathy reverses[4]
- Vital signs remaining stable throughout CAVR

Unexpected Outcomes

- Patient does not rewarm to 36.5°C within 3 hours.
- Coagulopathies remain unchanged despite rewarming.
- Inability exists to restore intravascular volume despite return to normothermia.
- Systolic blood pressure remains below 80 mm Hg, so that the CAVR system does not run and clots off.
- Kinking occurs of arterial or venous catheters, occluding blood flow and predisposing the tubing to developing clots.
- Clotting of the filter occurs because of administration of additional blood products, leading to no flow through the CAVR circuit.
- Hematoma development occurs at the catheter insertion sites.
- There is loss of pulses in distal extremities in which the CAVR catheters have been placed.

Patient Monitoring and Care

Patient Monitoring and Care	Rationale	Reportable Conditions
		These conditions should be reported if they persist despite nursing interventions.
1. Assess the patient's core temperature using a consistent route every 15 to 30 min.	Use of a consistent route is essential in correctly trending temperature changes, monitoring efficacy of therapy, and helping to determine when to stop CAVR.	• Unchanging temperature
2. Monitor vital signs, cardiac rhythm, and hemodynamic parameters a minimum of every 15 min.	Cardiac dysrhythmias ranging from bradycardia to premature ventricular contractions (PVCs) and ventricular fibrillation may occur with rapid rewarming. Hypotension also can occur as warming vessels dilate in the face of inadequate intravascular volume. Helps to guide additional infusions of fluids, blood products, and vasopressors to support systolic BP above 80 mm Hg.	• Changes in vital signs, cardiac rhythm, and hemodynamic parameters
3. Assess blood flow through the CAVR circuit every 15 min. Briefly slow the infusion of crystalloid infusing into the T-connector by barely closing the roller clamp. This allows the patient's blood to flow by the T-connector and show a pulsatile backflash of blood backward into the crystalloid line. Open the clamp back up to infuse crystalloids as needed to support the patient's BP and maintain a brisk flow through the circuit. If no flash is seen, the blood flow coming from the patient is sluggish or stopped.	Ensures that system has not clotted off. Immediate troubleshooting for the cause of sluggish or stopped flow is critical to prevent clotting of the circuit.	• Unsuccessful troubleshooting attempts
4. Monitor hemoglobin, hematocrit, PT, PTT, and International Normalized Ratio (INR) at least every hour.	Guides resuscitation of blood and clotting factors to reverse hypothermia induced coagulopathy. Helps determine presence of continued coagulopathy. Helps assess if coagulopathy is improving as the patient's temperature rises.	• Abnormal hemoglobin, hematocrit, or coagulation values
5. Monitor urine output hourly.	Establishes perfusion status of major viscera that may be diminished during hypothermia and shock. As the patient warms and intravascular volume is restored, urine output should increase.	• Urine output less than 0.5 mL/kg/h
6. Assess catheter insertion sites a minimum of every 30 min.	Evaluates for presence of catheter kinking or hematoma development that can compromise flow through the circuit to the extremities.	• Bleeding or hematoma development
7. Assess distal pulses at least every 15 min.	Ensures that distal circulation to and from the extremities is patent around the catheters. All patients will have a femoral artery catheter. Venous sites can be jugular, subclavian, or femoral.	• Distal pulses that cannot be palpated or obtained with a Doppler, or pallor in the distal extremity; pain in the extremity, decreased ability to sense or move the extremity

Documentation

Documentation should include the following:

- Patient and family education
- Time CAVR started and ended
- Temperature throughout duration of CAVR and every hour for at least 4 hours after CAVR has been stopped
- Vital signs, hemodynamic parameters, laboratory values, and urine output throughout CAVR
- Any difficulties with insertion of catheters
- Any difficulties in keeping adequate blood flow through the CAVR circuit that are not resolved with troubleshooting
- Presence of distal pulses in extremities
- Appearance of arterial and venous catheter insertion sites throughout CAVR and on removal of catheters
- Amount of IV fluids and blood products infused during CAVR
- Patient's hemodynamic and temperature response after CAVR is discontinued
- Unexpected outcomes
- Additional interventions

References

1. Gentilello LM: Practical approaches to hypothermia. *Adv Trauma Crit Care.* 1994;9:39.
2. Fritsch DE: Hypothermia in the trauma patient. *AACN Clin Issues Adv Pract Acute Crit Care.* 1995;6:196.
3. Gubler KD, Gentilello LM, Hassantash SA, et al. The effect of hypothermia on dilutional coagulopathy. *J Trauma.* 1994;36:847.
4. Gentilello LM, Jurkovich GJ, Stark MS, et al. Is hypothermia in the victim of major trauma protective or harmful? *Ann Surg.* 1997;226:439.

Additional Readings

Guyton AC, Hall JE. *Textbook of Medical Physiology.* 9th ed. Philadelphia, Pa: W.B. Saunders; 1996:911.
Rohrer MJ, Natale AM. Effect of hypothermia on the coagulation cascade. *Crit Care Med.* 1992;20:1402.
Stevens T. Managing post-op hypothermia, rewarming, and its complications. *Crit Care Nurs Q.* 1993;16:60.

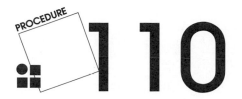

110 Rapid Infuser for Massive Fluid Resuscitation

P U R P O S E: Rapid infusers are used to warm and quickly infuse multiple units of blood and large amounts of intravenous (IV) fluids into patients who are hemodynamically unstable. Patients with trauma, severe gastrointestinal hemorrhage, postoperative hemorrhage, and severe intravascular losses, such as occurring from septic shock and burns, may require rapid administration of IV fluids to maintain homeostasis.

Christine S. Schulman

PREREQUISITE NURSING KNOWLEDGE

- Knowedge of asceptic technique is essential.
- Use of a rapid infusion device, such as the one described in this procedure (see Fig. 110–1), can warm and infuse fluids at rates from 75 to 30,000 mL/h (Sims Level 1, Inc., Rockland, Ma). The tubing is made of soft plastic that expands to allow rapid infusion of fluids under pressure. Some rapid infusers include automated pressure chambers to compress IV bags. They allow for fast and easy bag changes and can accommodate both 1-L IV bags and 500-mL blood product bags. Pressure is maintained at a constant 300 mmHg and is turned on and off via a simple toggle switch at the top of each pressure chamber. Older infusers simply have an IV pole from which to hang fluids, and separate inflatable pressure bags must be used.
- IV catheters for aggressive fluid resuscitation should have a large bore and short diameter to facilitate the rapid infusion of large volumes of IV fluids and blood products. Usually multiple IVs are used, including both peripheral and central sites. Venous access may also be obtained surgically via a venous cutdown of the basilic or saphenous veins when peripheral access cannot be obtained.[1]
- Both crystalloid and colloid solutions are the IV solutions used for resuscitating hypovolemic, hemodynamically unstable patients. Whereas crystalloids directly increase the intravascular volume, colloids will expand plasma volume by pulling interstitial fluid back into the vascular space via osmosis. Numerous crystalloid and colloid preparations are available in isotonic, hypotonic, and hypertonic preparations.
- Crystalloids and colloids must be replaced along with blood and blood products in the patient with ongoing hemorrhage. Preference for using either crystalloids or colloids varies among physicians and geographic regions around the United States.[1]
- Crystalloids most commonly used in aggressive fluid

resuscitation for trauma and other severe hemorrhage are 0.9% normal saline and Ringer's lactated solution. Although both of these solutions are isotonic and suitable for restoring intravascular volume, the latter contains multiple electrolytes, similar in concentration to that of plasma, so that the patient's electrolytes remain more within normal limits.
- The use of colloids such as albumin, dextran, and hetastarch will allow the effective restoration of intravascular volume with smaller amounts of fluid; however, these colloids coat red blood cells and platelets, which may result in type and crossmatch difficulties as well as clotting problems. Even slight overresuscitation with colloids risks fluid overload and pulmonary edema.[1, 2]
- Blood and blood products are naturally occurring colloids that are used to replace lost blood and restore coagulation factors. In the patient with significant ongoing hemorrhage, infusing blood and clotting factors is critical to restoring intravascular volume. Type O negative blood is the universal donor for all patients and can be given in extreme emergencies before the completion of typing and crossmatching. Packed red cells and whole blood are used to replace oxygen-carrying components; fresh frozen plasma, platelets, and cryoprecipitate are used to replace essential clotting factors (see Procedure 107).[1]
- When large volumes of IV fluids are being infused into patients, the fluids must be warmed to prevent hypothermia. (Although institutions vary in what constitutes large volumes, a good rule of thumb to consider is to institute fluid rewarming measures when more than 2 L of fluid are required in less than 1 hour.)
- Hypothermia is a common consequence of aggressive fluid resuscitation and has serious physiologic consequences. Infusion of cold fluids can rapidly cool the patient's body temperature to the point at which cardiovascular, neurologic, gastrointestinal, metabolic, and pulmonary disturbances result. Hypothermia-induced coagu-

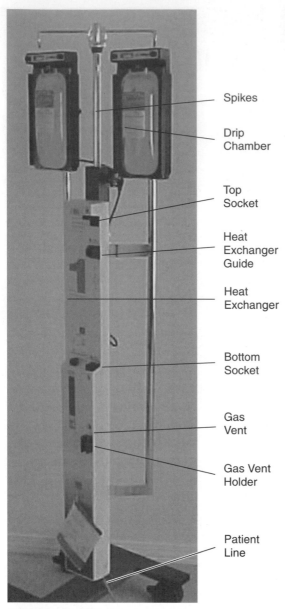

Spikes

Drip Chamber

Top Socket

Heat Exchanger Guide

Heat Exchanger

Bottom Socket

Gas Vent

Gas Vent Holder

Patient Line

■ ● **FIGURE 110–1.** Level 1 Rapid Infuser. (Courtesy of SIMS Level 1, Inc., Rockland, Ma.)

lopathies will exacerbate any ongoing hemorrhage and contribute to intravascular volume loss. Also, a left shift of the oxygen–hemoglobin dissociation curve occurs in hypothermic patients and in patients who receive large amounts of banked blood; thus, hemoglobin increases its affinity for oxygen and will not release it to the tissues, potentially resulting in cellular hypoxia. Continuous arteriovenous rewarming (CAVR) and other interventions to minimize or reverse heat loss may be necessary if the patient's core temperature drops below 34.5°C[2, 3] (see Procedures 83 and 109).

- Patients who have received multiple transfusions and aggressive fluid resuscitation are at risk for multiple complications as a result of being in shock as well as from the fluids and blood products themselves. These sequelae may include fluid overload, adult respiratory distress syndrome, acute tubular necrosis, hypothermia,

hypokalemia, hypocalcemia, hemolytic and allergic reactions, and air embolism.[4]

EQUIPMENT

- Rapid infuser (Fig. 110–1)
- Disposable fluid administration sets (Fig. 110–2)
- Replaceable filter with gas vent (Fig. 110–3)
- IV fluids or blood products as prescribed
- Sterile or distilled water for warmer
- Nonsterile gloves

PATIENT AND FAMILY EDUCATION

- Explain the purpose of warming the fluids and how the equipment operates. ➤➤*Rationale:* Decreases patient and family anxiety about unfamiliar equipment at the bedside.
- Explain that preventing hypothermia is among the top priorities in the resuscitation of the patient. ➤➤*Rationale:* Helps the patient and family understand the plan of care.

PATIENT ASSESSMENT AND PREPARATION

Patient Assessment

- Assess blood pressure, heart rate, respiratory rate, peripheral pulses, and level of consciousness. ➤➤*Rationale:* Necessary to determine the severity of the patient's volume depletion and shock.
- Assess core temperature using either a tympanic thermometer, bladder probe, or pulmonary artery catheter. ➤➤*Rationale:* Necessary to assess for the development of

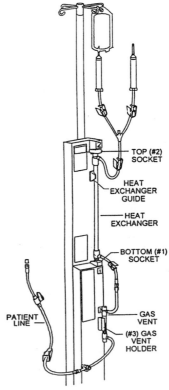

TOP (#2) SOCKET

HEAT EXCHANGER GUIDE

HEAT EXCHANGER

BOTTOM (#1) SOCKET

PATIENT LINE

GAS VENT

(#3) GAS VENT HOLDER

■ ● **FIGURE 110–2.** Placement of tubing in Level 1 Rapid Infuser. (Courtesy of SIMS Level 1, Inc., Rockland, Ma.)

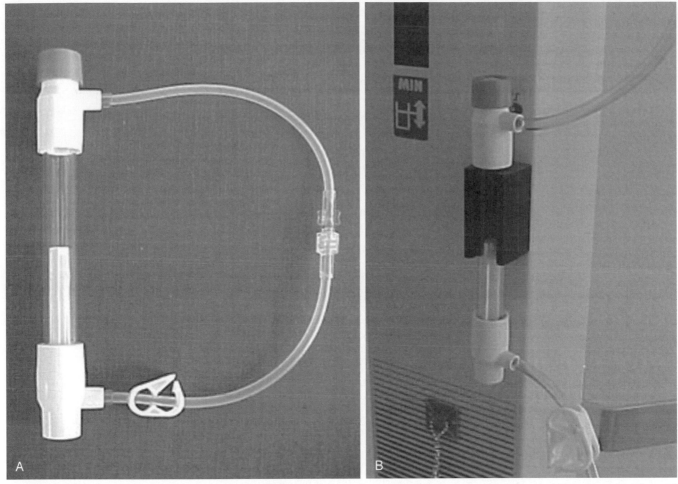

■ ● **FIGURE 110–3.** *A,* Rapid infuser filter showing male/female connecting ends on the right. *B,* Insertion of the filter in the Level 1 Rapid Infuser with the clamp open. (Courtesy of SIMS Level 1, Inc., Rockland, Ma.)

hypothermia while large volumes of fluids are infused. Core temperatures most accurately reflect true body temperature.

- Assess patient history including precipitating events, surgical and medical interventions thus far, and history of cardiac problems. ➤*Rationale:* Identifies potential or actual need for massive fluid resuscitation and risk of fluid overload.

- Assess hemodynamic parameters including baseline central venous pressure (CVP), pulmonary artery pressure (PAP), pulmonary capillary wedge pressure (PCWP), cardiac output (CO) and cardiac index (CI), systemic vascular resistance (SVR), and mixed venous oxygen saturation (Svo_2). Assessment of right ventricular ejection fraction, oxygen delivery and consumption, and oxygen extraction ratio should also be included if the technology is available. ➤*Rationale:* Provides baseline information about patient's preload, afterload, and cardiac contractility.

- Assess laboratory values to include arterial blood gases, serum electrolytes, hemoglobin, hematocrit, and coagulation studies. ➤*Rationale:* Measures baseline oxygenation, presence of metabolic acidosis, severity of ongoing hemorrhage, and severity of coagulopathy so that the

need for intervention and the effectiveness of interventions can be determined.

- Assess patency of multiple large-bore IV sites. ➤*Rationale:* Multiple sites are often necessary to infuse enough fluids and blood products to support the patient's vital signs. Extra sites in addition to those used for rapid infusion should be kept patent in the event one of the other sites becomes nonfunctional or is accidentally pulled out.

Patient Preparation

- Ensure that the patient and family understand preprocedure teaching. Answer questions as they arise, and reinforce information as needed. ➤*Rationale:* Evaluates and reinforces understanding of previously taught information.

- Place additional peripheral IV sites. ➤*Rationale:* Aggressive fluid resuscitation will require additional IV access besides the one site being used with the rapid infuser. Back-up IV sites can be used if other sites infiltrate or become pulled out; extra sites may also be used to infuse medications, such as vasopressors, that should be kept separate from rapid infusion lines. Ideal sites for large

IV catheter access are the antecubital fossae, saphenous veins, and the veins of the forearm and upper arm.
- Assist the physician or advanced practice nurse with placement of central venous access or pulmonary artery catheter or both. ➡**Rationale:** Allows for the assessment of volume status before and after infusing fluids and blood products. Allows for assessment of core temperature with pulmonary artery catheter thermistor. Provides central venous access in the event vasoactive medications are needed.
- Place an automatic blood pressure monitor on the patient's arm that is not being infused with the rapid infusion device. Set it to check blood pressure every 5 minutes. ➡**Rationale:** Provides assessment of patient's hemodynamics and response to fluid replacement. This is used temporarily until an arterial line can be placed by the physician or advanced practice nurse.

- Assist the physician or advanced practice nurse with placement of an arterial line. ➡**Rationale:** Allows for continuous assessment of the blood pressure during resuscitation and provides convenient access for blood sampling.
- Cover the patient with warm cotton blankets or a warm-air blanket. Cover the patient's head with a warmed blanket, a towel, or an aluminum cap. ➡**Rationale:** Minimizes additional heat loss.
- Place a Foley catheter. ➡**Rationale:** Patients who require aggressive fluid resuscitation should have a Foley catheter placed to determine volume status and end-organ perfusion.
- Obtain a blood sample for type and crossmatch. Two tubes should be sent if a large volume of blood is expected to be transfused. ➡**Rationale:** Prepares blood for transfusion.

Procedure for Rapid Infuser for Massive Fluid Resuscitation

Steps	Rationale	Special Considerations
1. Wash hands, and don gloves.	Reduces transmission of microorganisms; standard precautions.	
2. Verify prescription for infusion of IV fluids and blood products and use of a fluid warmer.	Prevents unnecessary blood product or IV fluid administration.	The physician's or advanced practice nurse's prescription should include volume and type of additional IV fluids and blood products, laboratory work, and rationale for using a fluid warmer or rapid infuser.
3. Open Y-set fluid administration package provided by the manufacturer and close all clamps.	Prevents accidental spillage of blood or fluid. Prevents flow of fluid through circuit before machine is warmed.	
4. Spike fluid or blood with both sides of the Y-set.	Allows for smooth transition from an empty bag to the next bag.	
5. Hang fluid bags on small hooks inside the rapid infuser pressure chambers, leaving the chamber doors open (see Fig. 110–1). Or place fluid bags in separate pressure bags.	It is easier to clear the tubing of air if the tubing is primed while the bags are still unpressurized.	Autotransfusion bags will not fit into the pressure chambers.
6. Push the bottom end of the heat exchanger rod *firmly* into the bottom socket, and snap the heat exchanger into the guide (see Fig. 110–2).	The bottom of the heat exchanger must be firmly placed or it will not fit into the top socket.	Being too gentle will result in improper placement of the tubing and the warmer will not run.
7. Slide the top socket up, and place the top end of the exchanger into the placement tract.	Locks the warming chamber into place at both the top and bottom sockets.	
8. Slide the top heat exchanger socket down over the heat exchanger tube until the pole latch clicks into place.		
9. Snap the air eliminator filter into the holder on the lower portion of the pole assembly with the orange end up (see Fig. 110–3).	Filters air and blood clots from tubing.	Will only fit into the machine one way because the tubing is not long enough to be placed incorrectly.
10. Squeeze drip chambers so that they are half full.	Minimizes entrapment of bubbles in the tubing. Allows visualization of the drip chamber so that drip rate can be assessed.	

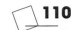

Procedure **for Rapid Infuser for Massive Fluid Resuscitation** *Continued*

Steps	Rationale	Special Considerations
11. Open the clamp on one side of the Y-set.	Make sure that only one side of the Y tubing is open during priming; otherwise, fluid will be pumped from one bag to the other and not through the tubing.	
12. Remove the male luer cap at the end of the IV tubing, and open the clamps.	Will not prime unless the end cap has been removed.	
13. Remove the filter from its holder and invert it. Prime the tubing, then close the roller clamp. Turn the filter back over, and replace it in its holder.	Prevents entrapment of large amounts of air.	
14. Tap the filter or air eliminator against the cabinet several times. Monitor fluid line for bubbles during use.	Releases any residual trapped air.	Never administer fluids if there are air bubbles between the filter chamber and the patient connection. Run IV fluid into the trash container to rid tubing of any residual air. When no more bubbles are observed leaving the heat exchanger, all the air has been vented from the filter or air eliminator.
15. Open the roller clamp partially, and slowly infuse fluid.	Infusing slowly will allow for assessment of any air bubbles. The air filter will eliminate bubbles in the tubing.	If unable to clear line of air and there is more than ¼ in of air at the top of the filter, replace the filter.
16. Replace male luer cap at the end of the tubing, and close the clamps.		
17. Close the pressure chamber doors and latch.	Positions fluid bags for pressurization when the machines are turned on and the pressure switch is activated.	Be certain that the latch is secure before the chamber is pressurized.
18. Plug the device into the outlet and turn it on. Ensure that the green system operational light on the display panel is illuminated.		
19. Perform all function and alarm checks as per manufacturer's instructions.	Validates proper equipment function.	
20. Wait for the temperature readout to reach the operating temperature of 41°C.	Prevents hypothermia by making sure the chamber is warm before fluids are run through it and into the patient.	
21. Flip the toggle switch at the top of the pressure chamber to ON/+ or inflate the separate pressure bags.	Pressurizes the chambers.	The pressure automatically inflates to 300 mm Hg. Fluids will infuse via gravity flow without being pressurized; however, high flow rates cannot be achieved unless the pressure bags are inflated.
22. Connect the distal end of the tubing to the patient IV.	Prepares for infusion.	
23. Open the roller clamp to infuse the fluid.	Fluids or blood products will now infuse under pressure.	It is best to infuse one side at a time, especially when blood products are infusing, to prevent mixing of fluids and blood products. The pressure system is designed to leave a small volume remaining to prevent air emboli.
24. Set the rate by gradually opening the clamp.	Fluids given via rapid infusers are administered as boluses over short periods; roller clamps are usually left wide open until the bolus is complete.	If a slower bolus is desired, adjust the roller clamp to decrease the flow of fluid.

Procedure continued on following page

Procedure	for Rapid Infuser for Massive Fluid Resuscitation *Continued*

Steps	Rationale	Special Considerations
Changing the Bags		
1. Close the top clamp on the side of the Y-connector with the empty fluid bag.		
2. Open the clamp on the side of the Y-connector with the full fluid bag, and infuse the fluid.	Keeping one side of the Y-connector spiked with fluid ready to infuse is helpful when patients are severely unstable and need immediate boluses of fluid.	
3. Turn the ON/+ switch below the pressure chamber to the OFF position and remove the empty bag.	Releases pressure from the pressure chamber.	
4. Replace the empty fluid bag with a full one.	It is important to have the next bag of IV fluid ready to infuse to avoid delays in infusion in the event the patient's blood pressure precipitously falls.	
5. Close the pressure chamber door and latch, and flip the control switch below the pressure chamber to ON/+.	Repressurizes chamber.	
Replacing the Filter or Air Eliminator		
1. Close the clamps on the disposable fluid administration set just proximal to the filter and between the filter and the patient connection.	The filter should be replaced after 3 hours of use, after 4 units of blood, or if fluid rate slows secondary to clotting.	
2. Remove the old filter or air eliminator from the holder and place the new filter or air eliminator in the holder.	Keep the old filter or air eliminator connected to the disposable fluid administration set until ready to change to new one to minimize potential for contaminating exposed tubing ends.	
3. Disconnect the old filter or air eliminator at the upper luer lock and connect the tubing to the new filter.		
4. Disconnect the patient line luer lock from the old filter or air eliminator and connect to the new one.		
5. Open the clamp just proximal to the filter or air eliminator to restart fluid. Invert the filter until completely filled with fluid, then turn back to proper position and replace in holder. Open the clamp between the filter and the patient connection.	Infusion of fluid will resume.	
6. Remove the filter or air eliminator from the holder and tap until all bubbles are eliminated and reinsert. Check patient line for bubbles before opening the roller clamp.	Facilitates removal of bubbles.	If air bubbles are present, disconnect the tubing from the patient and infuse into the trash container until the line is clear of air. Reconnect to the patient and resume the infusion.

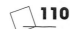

Procedure	for Rapid Infuser for Massive Fluid Resuscitation *Continued*

Steps	Rationale	Special Considerations
Troubleshooting Alarms		
1. If the alarm sounds and the disposable light is illuminated, check to make sure the disposable tubing set is properly placed in the machine.	The system will not run if the disposable tubing is not completely set into the machine.	The tubing set can become inadvertently dislodged.
2. If the alarm sounds and the water level light is illuminated, check the water level in the chamber and replace as needed with sterile or distilled water.	The system will not run if the water level is too low.	
3. If the system alarms "overtemp," turn the machine off and use a different rapid infuser.	Fluids inadequately warmed will cause hypothermia. Fluids overly warmed will cause hemolysis of red blood cells.	Notify biomedical engineering of the problem.
Transporting a Patient with a Rapid Infuser		
1. Turn the rapid infuser off.	If the infuser is still on when the administration set is removed from its holder, water will spurt out of the warming chamber and aluminum tube.	
2. Remove the disposable administration set from its holder on the infuser and place it in the bed alongside the patient or hang it on the transport IV pole.	The rapid infusers described here do not operate on a battery. Fluids will infuse via gravity or separate pressure bags can be used.	Fluids will run briskly via gravity drainage. If pressure is still necessary to infuse fluids, separate pressure bags will need to be used as long as the machine is not plugged in. Interventions to minimize heat loss must be in place while the infuser is not plugged in: aluminum head covering, warmed cotton blankets, and warm-air blankets will help prevent heat loss. Removing the administration set from the machine and transporting the patient separately from the infuser is less awkward and will minimize the risk of pulling out the IV lines during transport.
3. Plug the infuser into an electric outlet on reaching the intended destination.	Establishes power source.	
4. Return administration set into the infuser. Turn the machine on. Return fluid bags to pressure chambers.	The infuser is now ready to repressurize the chambers and warm the fluid. Any bubbles will be eliminated by the filter.	If bubbles are not removed and more than ¼ in of air is at the top of the filter, then the filter must be replaced.

Expected Outcomes	Unexpected Outcomes
• Patient's blood pressure is maintained above 90 mm Hg.	• Blood pressure remains below 90 mm Hg despite multiple liters of fluid and blood products.
• Patient's core temperature remains above 36.0°C.	• Core temperature falls below 36.0°C so that more aggressive rewarming interventions become necessary.
• Urine output is 0.5 to 1 mL/kg/h.	• Hypothermia-induced coagulopathy develops as temperature falls below 34.5°C.
• CVP, PAP, PCWP, CO, CI, and SVR reflect return of normovolemia and hemodynamic stability.	• Inability to restore normal intravascular status occurs as seen by CVP <6, PCWP <6, CO <4 L/m, CI <2 L/m/m², or SVR >1500 dynes/s.
• IV sites remain patent and infuse fluids easily.	• Anuria or oliguria with urinary output <0.5 mL/kg/h occurs.
	• Infiltration of IV sites occurs.
	• Clotting of filter occurs.

Patient Monitoring and Care	Rationale	Reportable Conditions
		These conditions should be reported if they persist despite nursing interventions.
1. Monitor the patient's vital signs every 5 to 15 minutes as indicated. As the patient becomes more stable, assessment of vital signs may be done less frequently, that is, every 15 to 30 minutes until the blood pressure remains stable for more than 2 hours.	Determines severity of shock, responsiveness to fluids and blood products, and the need for additional fluids.	• Systolic blood pressure below 90 mm Hg despite fluid administration • Abnormal vital signs
2. Assess the patient's core temperature every 15 to 30 minutes.	Patients who are in severe shock have impaired thermogenesis. This, in combination wth the infusion of inadequately warmed fluids, will lead to hypothermia. Hypothermia-induced coagulopathies begin at a core temperature of 34.5°C and will exacerbate any hemorrhage already occurring. Also, severe physiologic complications from hypothermia, such as cardiovascular instability, electrolyte changes, urine concentration problems, and shifts in the oxygen-hemoglobin dissociation curve, will affect the patient's ability to respond to physiologic stress. Prevention of hypothermia is a critical goal for patients undergoing massive fluid resuscitation.[2, 5]	• Worsening hypothermia or unrelieved hypothermia
3. Assess the integrity of IV sites every 15 minutes.	IV sites under pressure are at higher risk for infiltration. Also, lines can be inadvertently pulled out during x-ray filming, turning, and other aspects of patient care during a massive resuscitation. It is recommended that multiple IV sites be available at all times in the event an IV infiltrates or is pulled out.	
4. Assess hemodynamic parameters every 15 to 30 minutes.	Determines intravascular volume status and responsiveness to interventions. New research suggests that patients may still be inadequately resuscitated even though vital signs, urine output, and hemodynamic parameters have returned to normal. Recent studies suggest that a complete clinical picture that includes laboratory tests in conjuction with vital signs, urine output, and hemodynamic parameters is the best way to determine if a patient has been adequately resuscitated.[6]	• Abnormal trends in hemodynamic monitoring
5. Assess urine output every 30 to 60 minutes.	Urine output is an assessment of end-organ perfusion. If there is little or no urine being produced, it is assumed that the kidneys are not being perfused, and therefore, other major viscera are also probably not being adequately perfused. Trauma to the urinary tract may interfere with accurate assessment of urine output because clots may block urine drainage and laceration to ureters may result in extravasation of urine into the peritoneum.	• Urine output less than 0.5 mL/kg/h

Patient Monitoring and Care *Continued*

Patient Monitoring and Care	Rationale	Reportable Conditions
6. Draw hemoglobin, hematocrit, and coagulation studies as prescribed by the physician or advanced practice nurse. These are usually measured every 30 to 60 minutes or after transfusion of blood and blood components.	Determines presence of ongoing blood loss and coagulopathy.[2–5]	• Abnormal hemoglobin, hematocrit, and coagulation results
7. Draw arterial blood gases and lactic acid as prescribed and indicated.	Determines persistence of metabolic acidosis and identifies need for additional interventions to improve perfusion to major organs.[6]	• Abnormal laboratory results
8. Draw elecltrolytes as prescribed and indicated.	Patients undergoing large-volume resuscitation are at risk for hypokalemia, hypomagnesemia, hypocalcemia, and hypophosphatemia.[2]	• Abnormal laboratory results

Documentation

Documentation should include the following:

- Patient and family education
- Rationale for using the rapid infuser
- Blood pressure, heart rate, respiratory rate, lung sounds, and peripheral pulses throughout the resuscitation
- The patient's core temperature while the rapid infusers are used
- Hemodynamic parameters to include CVP, PAP, PCWP, CO, CI, and SVR

- Urine output, estimated blood loss, other measured output
- Laboratory results to include arterial blood gases, hematocrit, hemoglobin, electrolytes, and lactic acid
- Appearance of IV sites
- IV insertions
- Total IV fluids and blood products in intake and output record
- Unexpected outcomes
- Additional interventions

References

1. Koran Z, Newberry L: Vascular access and fluid replacement. In: Newberry L, ed. *Sheehy's Emergency Nursing.* 4th ed. St. Louis, Mo: C.V. Mosby; 1998:147.
2. McQuillan KA: Initial management of traumatic shock. In: Cardona VD, Hurn PD, Mason PB, Scanlon AM, Veise-Berry SW: *Trauma Nursing: From Resuscitation Through Rehabilitation.* 2nd ed. Philadelphia, Pa: W.B. Saunders; 1994:151.
3. Fritsch DE: Hypothermia in the truama patient. *AACN Clin Issues Adv Pract Acute Crit Care.* 1995;6:196.
4. Gentilello LM: Practical approaches to hypothermia. *Adv Trauma Crit Care.* 1994;9:39.
5. Gubler KD, Gentilello LM, Hassantash SA, et al: The effect of hypothcrmia on dilutional coagulopathy. *J Trauma.* 1994;36:847.
6. Porter JM, Ivatury RR. In search of the optimal end points of resuscitation in trauma patients: A review. *J Trauma.* 1998;44:908.

Additional Readings

Guyton AC, Hall JE: *Textbook of Medical Physiology.* 9th ed. Philadelphia, Pa: W.B. Saunders; 1996:911.
Stevens T. Managing post-op hypothermia, rewarming, and its complications. *Crit Care Nurs Q.* 1993;16:60.

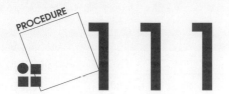

111

Transfusion Reaction Management

P U R P O S E: Prompt recognition and treatment of a transfusion reaction may minimize the development of life-threatening sequelae. Although blood transfusions have become safer than in the past, considerable risk still exists. Twenty percent of all transfusions result in an adverse reaction.[1]

Maribeth Wooldridge-King

PREREQUISITE NURSING KNOWLEDGE

- A *transfusion reaction* may be defined as "any untoward reaction that occurs as a consequence of infusion of blood or one of its components."[2] Transfusion reactions are classified as acute or delayed. *Acute transfusion reactions* occur during the transfusion or within several hours after the transfusion has been completed.

- Increased antibody levels in the recipient increase the likelihood of developing a transfusion reaction on exposure to donor antigens. Factors that increase circulating antibody levels include a history of multiple transfusions and multiparity. With each transfusion, a recipient is exposed to additional donor antigens to which the recipient produces antibodies, thus increasing the circulating antibody levels.

- In multiparity, if an Rh negative mother carries an Rh positive fetus, the mother produces antibodies and continues to do so for any subsequent pregnancy with an Rh positive fetus, again increasing her antibody load.

- Three mechanisms are generally responsible for the majority of transfusion reactions:
  - ❖ An immune response in which the recipient produces antibodies to antigens on the surface of the donor's leukocytes
  - ❖ A bacterial contamination of the component (most common with platelet concentrates as they are stored at room temperature to retain function) secondary to inadequate cleansing of the donor's venipuncture site, contamination during processing, or storage or incubation of an undetected organism[3]
  - ❖ The release of cytokines (tumor necrosis factor and interleukin-6) from leukocytes during the storage of platelets

- Acute transfusion reactions include acute hemolytic reactions, febrile nonhemolytic reactions, an allergic or urticarial reaction, an anaphylactic reaction, transfusion-related acute lung injury and bacterial contamination. See Table 111–1 for a summary of acute transfusion reactions.

- Other potentially adverse effects of a transfusion include hypervolemia, hypothermia, electrolyte imbalances, and transmission of transfusion-related diseases.

- Hypervolemia is associated with a rapid infusion of blood or blood components. The acute expansion of the intravascular volume may exceed the ability of the cardiovascular system to compensate. Signs and symptoms include the onset of a sudden, severe headache; dyspnea; tachycardia; tachypnea; crackles; and increased filling pressures (central venous pressures [CVP], pulmonary artery pressure [PAP], and pulmonary capillary wedge pressure [PCWP]). If the symptoms occur, the patients should be given diuretics to decrease intravascular volume; in some cases, the transfusion may need to be stopped. For patients at risk or with a history of fluid overload, have the blood bank divide the unit into smaller aliquots; the entire unit of blood then can be administered over a longer period.

- Hypothermia can occur with the rapid infusion of refrigerated (1°C to 6°C) blood. Ventricular fibrillation may occur if the temperature of the sinoatrial node is lowered to <30°C.[4] Blood should be warmed only via an electronic blood warmer, in which the temperature is continuously monitored and maintained at 38°C. Hot tap water and microwaves should never be used to warm blood.

- Decreased ionized calcium levels may occur with the infusion of large amounts of citrate-containing blood products. Citrate is a component of the preservative used in blood storage that chelates calcium and interferes with the coagulation cascade. This complication is usually mild and self-limiting; however, if prolonged Q-T intervals or signs of tetany are observed, calcium levels can be monitored and calcium replacement can be administered if indicated. Calcium should never be added to the unit of blood. Patients with severe liver disease or those with inadequate hepatic blood flow receiving rapid, large-volume transfusions are at risk for citrate toxicity.

Table 111-1 ● ▮▮ Summary of Acute Transfusion Reactions

Transfusion Reaction	Frequency of Reaction	Potential Causes	Symptoms	Prevention	Treatment
Febrile nonhemolytic transfusion reaction	1:5 platelets 1:10 RBCs	Recipient antibodies to donor leukocytes Bacterial contamination Inflammatory cytokine release	Increase in temperature 1°C (1.8°F) or greater within 2 h after transfusion	Premedicate with antipyretics	Antipyretics Antihistamines
Bacterial contamination	1:350 platelets 1:2,500,000 RBCs	Contamination of the blood product during procurement, storage, preparation, or administration of product	Chills Fever Chills Sepsis	Use aseptic technique when collecting the blood product Properly store product Change blood tubing or filter every 4 h Ensure transfusion takes no longer than 4 h	Antibiotics Antipyretics
Transfusion-related acute lung injury	1:10,000 RBCs also with cryoprecipitate	Activation of complement and histamine release, resulting in increased pulmonary capillary permeability	Respiratory distress, which may be accompanied by: • Fever • Chills • Cyanosis • Hypotension	No known prevention exists; antihistamines and steroids may be helpful	Standard treatment of acute respiratory distress syndrome: • Antipyretics • Antihistamines • Oxygen • Fluid resuscitation • Mechanical ventilation • Vasopressors
Acute hemolytic reaction	1:25,000 RBCs	Administration of incompatible blood Preexisting antibodies against transfused RBCs, resulting in massive hemolysis Improper administration (ie, with dextrose solution)	Fever Chills Nausea Dyspnea Low back pain Hemoglobinuria Pain at infusion site Tachycardia Hypotension Cardiovascular collapse Renal failure Disseminated intravascular coagulopathy	Strictly adhere to institutional policy regarding collection of patient samples and administration of blood products Initiate transfusion of blood product slowly for the first 15 min Administer only with normal saline	Antipyretics Antihistamines Steroids Fluid resuscitation If progression to shock: • Oxygen • Epinephrine • Diuretics • Vasopressors
Urticarial reaction	1:1000 blood products	Recipient responds to donor proteins	Flushing Hives Itching	Transfuse plasma-free blood products Premedicate with antipyretics or antihistamines or both	Antipyretics Antihistamines
Anaphylaxis	1:1,150,000 blood products	Severe immune response to a foreign substance	Generalized flushing Dyspnea Stridor Chest pain Hypotension Nausea Abdominal cramps Loss of consciousness	Transfuse plasma-free blood products	Epinephrine Code management

Abbreviation: RBC, red blood cell
Adapted from Labovich TM. Transfusion therapy: nursing implications. *Clin J Oncol Nurs.* 1997;3:63–64.

EQUIPMENT

- Intravenous solution (0.9% normal saline)
- Intravenous administration set (macrodrip tubing)
- Stethoscope
- Blood pressure cuff or arterial line
- Electrocardiogram (ECG) monitor
- Pulse oximeter
- Urine specimen container
- Vacutainer holder and needle
- Blood specimen tubes
- Thermometer
- Nonsterile gloves
- Specimen labels
- Laboratory forms

Additional equipment to have available if needed includes the following:

- Flowmeter for oxygen
- Nasal cannula or Venturi mask
- Emergency drug box
- Emergency cart

PATIENT AND FAMILY EDUCATION

- Explain that the patient may be experiencing a transfusion reaction. ➛***Rationale:*** Promotes patient and family understanding of transfusion reaction.
- Once the patient is stabilized, instruct the patient and family to include the occurrence of a transfusion reaction on the patient's medical history. ➛***Rationale:*** Alerts health care providers to potential need for premedication, the need for specially prepared component therapy, or the increased risk of transfusion reactions with future transfusions.
- Evaluate the patient's need for long-term blood or blood component administration. ➛***Rationale:*** Patient may need to carry a record of transfusions, history of severity of transfusion reactions, and requirement for specially processed blood or blood components or premedications to prevent or minimize a transfusion reaction.

PATIENT ASSESSMENT AND PREPARATION

Patient Assessment

- Note the severity of previous transfusion reactions and the treatment to which patient responded. ➛***Rationale:*** Allows the nurse to anticipate what treatment modalities may be required to interrupt this reaction.
- Assess for signs and symptoms of a transfusion reaction (see Table 111–1). ➛***Rationale:*** Severity of a transfusion reaction depends partly on the amount of blood transfused.
- Assess oxygenation (Sao_2) via pulse oximeter or arterial blood gas (ABG). ➛***Rationale:*** Catecholamine release as a response to the antigen-antibody reaction produces vasoconstriction in the lungs; the resulting ventilation-perfusion abnormality may require oxygen administration or intubation with mechanical ventilation.
- Assess vital signs, including temperature, blood pressure, heart rate, respiratory rate, breath sounds, and if applicable, filling pressures (ie, CVP, PAP, PCWP). ➛***Rationale:*** Transfusion reactions will cause deviations from baseline (pretransfusion) vital signs (see Table 111–1).

Patient Preparation

- Ensure that the patient and family understand preprocedural teaching. Answer questions as they arise and reinforce information as needed. ➛***Rationale:*** Evaluates and reinforces understanding of previously taught information.
- Ensure or reestablish patency of the peripheral intravenous line or central venous access device. ➛***Rationale:*** Allows for infusion of crystalloid solution to support the patient's cardiovascular system and increases renal blood flow to prevent the development of acute tubular necrosis.

Procedure for Transfusion Reaction Management

Steps	Rationale	Special Considerations
1. Stop the transfusion.	Prevents additional blood or blood components from being infused.	Severity of the reaction is due in part to the amount of blood infused.
2. Wash hands, and don nonsterile gloves.	Reduces transmission of microorganisms; standard precautions.	
3. Disconnect the blood administration set from the primary intravenous line and cap with a sterile cap.	The remaining contents of the unit of blood are sent back to the blood bank with the administration set attached.	Institution policies and procedures regarding the disposition of the remaining unit contents may vary. Check with your blood bank.
4. Replace primary intravenous tubing with a new macrodrip intravenous administration set.	Prevents the patient from receiving additional blood or blood component that may still be in the primary tubing.	Macrodrip tubing is used for rapid volume replacement if needed.
5. Infuse crystalloid intravenous solution, usually 0.9% normal saline, to maintain a urine output of 100 mL/h for 24 hours or as prescribed.	Supports blood pressure, heart rate, and renal blood flow.	In acute hemolytic reactions, the patient is at risk for developing acute tubular necrosis.

Procedure for Transfusion Reaction Management *Continued*

Steps	Rationale	Special Considerations
6. Obtain a urine specimen.	Determines presence of red blood cells or free hemoglobin.	A urine specimen is usually sent to blood bank with the suspect unit of blood or blood components. Indicate "Possible Transfusion Reaction" on the laboratory form.
7. Obtain two blood specimens (one red top tube and one purple top tube) from a site other than the transfusion site.	The first sample (red top) is crossmatched with the pretransfusion sample to determine if the correct blood was administered. The second sample (purple top) is examined for hemolysis.	Usually, blood specimens are sent to the blood bank with the suspect unit of blood or blood component. Indicate "Possible Transfusion Reaction" on the laboratory form.
8. Recheck blood or blood component label, transfusion slip, and patient's identification band to detect possible error.	The majority of acute hemolytic reactions are caused by the administration of incompatible blood caused by the incorrect identification of the recipient or the patient sample.	
9. Complete the specific forms for a transfusion reaction.	Documents possibility of a transfusion reaction and the actions taken.	Most institutions have specific forms that are completed when a transfusion reaction is suspected.
10. Return the blood or the blood component to blood bank.	Allows the blood bank to confirm the presence or absence of a transfusion reaction.	Patients receiving multiple transfusions over time (eg, patients with cancer or AIDS) may demonstrate signs and symptoms of a transfusion reaction; however, laboratory analysis may not verify that a reaction has occurred. You may be instructed to rehang the unit of blood or the blood component and monitor the patient closely.
11. Discard used supplies, and wash hands.	Reduces transmission of microorganisms; standard precautions.	

Expected Outcomes

- Vital signs remain stable and within patient's baseline values.
- Laboratory values remain within normal limits.
- Renal function remains normal.

Unexpected Outcomes

- Impaired renal function
- Hemodynamic instability
- Abnormal laboratory values
- Cardiopulmonary arrest

Patient Monitoring and Care

Patient Monitoring and Care	Rationale	Reportable Conditions
		These conditions should be reported if they persist despite nursing interventions.
1. Monitor the patient's vital signs and oxygenation every 5 to 15 minutes until stable.	Detects further compromise in cardiovascular status.	• Vital sign and SaO$_2$ abnormalities
2. Monitor urinary output every hour.	Diminished renal blood flow or renal vasoconstriction may result in acute tubular necrosis.	• Decreasing urine output, increasing blood urea nitrogen (BUN) and creatinine
3. Monitor international normalized ratio (INR), prothrombin time (PT), partial thromboplastin time (PTT), and fibrinogen levels.	Extensive destruction of red blood cells may result in disseminated intravascular coagulopathy (DIC).	• Abnormal PT, PTT, INR, or fibrinogen levels

Continued on following page

Patient Monitoring and Care	Rationale	Reportable Conditions
4. Monitor levels of lactate dehydrogenase (LDH).	LDH levels may rise markedly with lysis of red blood cells.	• Elevated lactate levels
5. Should the patient develop signs or symptoms of shock or cardiovascular collapse, perform the following: ○ Insert another large-bore intravenous catheter.	Maintains blood pressure and renal blood flow. Supports cardiovascular and renal systems.	• Signs and symptoms of shock and cardiovascular collapse
○ Prepare and administer emergency medications as prescribed.		
○ If bacterial contamination is suspected, obtain a blood specimen for culture and sensitivity testing. Administer broad-spectrum antibiotics intravenously as prescribed.	An infusion of a contaminated unit of blood or blood components will result in immediate signs and symptoms of cardiovascular collapse.	
○ Administer oxygen therapy as prescribed. Initiate advanced cardiac life support (ACLS) protocol in the event of respiratory or cardiac arrest.	Corrects hypoxemia. Life-preserving intervention.	

Documentation

Documentation should include the following:

- Patient and family education
- Date and exact time signs and symptoms of a transfusion reaction were observed
- Date and time infusion was discontinued
- Assessment findings

- Name of the physician or advanced practice nurse notified
- Unexpected outcomes
- Interventions taken
- Patient's response to the interventions

References

1. Welborn JL, Hersch J. Blood transfusion reactions: which are life-threatening and which are not? *Postgrad Med.* 1991;90:125.
2. Snyder EL. Transfusion reactions. In: Hoffman R, Benz EJ Jr, Shattil SJ, Furie B, Cohen HJ, eds. *Hematology: Basic Principles and Practice.* New York, NY: Churchill Livingstone; 1995:2045.
3. Anderson KC, Lew MA, Gorgone BC, et al. Transfusion-related sepsis after prolonged platelet storage. *Am J Med.* 1986;81:405.
4. Boyan CP, Howland WS. Blood temperature: a critical factor in massive transfusion. *Anesthesiology.* 1961;22:559.

Additional Readings

Coffland FI, Shelton DM. Blood component replacement therapy. *Crit Care Clin North Am.* 1993;5:543–556.
Gloe D. Common reactions to transfusions. *Heart Lung.* 1991;20:506–514.
Labovich TM. Transfusion therapy: nursing implications. *Clin J Oncol.* July 1997;61–72.
National Institutes of Health. National Blood Resource Education Program's Transfusion Therapy Guidelines for Nurses (NIH Publication No. 90-2668). Washington, DC: U.S. Government Printing Office; 1990.
Popovsky MA, Chaplin HC, Moore SB. Transfusion-related acute lung injury: a neglected, serious complication of chemotherapy. *Transfusion.* 1992;32:589–592.

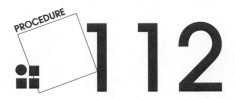

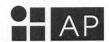

Bone Marrow Biopsy and Aspiration (Perform)

P U R P O S E: Bone marrow biopsy and aspiration are used to diagnose various hematopoietic diseases, to check for residual disease after therapy, to identify metastatic disease to the bone marrow, to ascertain disease status before continued therapy, and to perform chromosome analysis.

Dolores Grosso

PREREQUISITE NURSING KNOWLEDGE

- Anatomy of the bilateral posterior iliac crests and of the sternum should be understood.
- Knowledge of sterile technique is essential.
- Clinical and technical competence in performing a bone marrow biopsy is necessary.
- Bone marrow biopsy and aspiration are diagnostic tests that are used to ascertain various genetic and malignant entities.
- Bone marrow aspirate is used to morphologically identify normal and abnormal hematopoietic elements. The aspirate is also used to identify malignant clones by flow cytometry and is used to identify chromosomal abnormalities that occur in hematologic malignancies. In addition, bone marrow aspirate can be used to perform chimerism studies in patients after allogenic transplant.
- The bone marrow biopsy is used for morphologic analysis of hematopoietic cells and for assessing the architecture of the bone marrow that may be abnormal in certain disease states.
- Indications for bone marrow aspiration and biopsy include the following:

❖ Diagnosing a hematologic abnormality
❖ Monitoring a hematologic disease state after therapy
❖ Ruling out bone marrow metastasis before stem cell collection and for staging in various malignant states
❖ In all patients after bone marrow transplant, assessing the status of engraftment
❖ In patients after allogeneic transplant, assessing for chimerism and immune reconstitution
❖ Harvesting stem cells for donation

- Contraindications to bone marrow biopsy and aspirate include *severe* bleeding dyscrasias.

EQUIPMENT

- Bone marrow biopsy and aspiration kit that includes the following:
  ❖ Sterile drape
  ❖ Betadine swabsticks
  ❖ Biopsy container
  ❖ Laboratory slides with an area to write on each slide
  ❖ Sterile gauze
  ❖ Sterile adhesive strip
  ❖ Lidocaine needles of appropriate lengths to anesthetize both skin and periosteum
  ❖ Scalpel
- Mask with face shield, cap, sterile gown, and sterile gloves
- 1-mL vial EDTA calcium (edetate calcium disodium) to help prevent specimen clotting

- 1-mL vial 1000 U/mL heparin
- One vial 1% lidocaine
- 10-mL sterile water
- Three or four 3-mL syringes
- Three or four 18-G needles
- Two or three sodium heparin blood tubes (green tops)
- 1 EDTA blood tube (purple top)
- Normal saline solution

Additional equipment to have available as needed includes the following:

- One 22-G 3½-in sternal needle may be needed for deep lidocaine placement
- One Jamshidi biopsy needle
- One sternal aspiration needle
- One spinal needle

PATIENT AND FAMILY EDUCATION

- Assess patient and family understanding of the bone marrow biopsy and aspiration procedure and the reason for it. ➤*Rationale:* Clarification of the procedure and reinforcement of information are expressed patient and family needs in times of stress and anxiety.
- Explain the actual procedure to the patient and family. ➤*Rationale:* Prepares the patient and family for what to expect and may decrease anxiety.
- Encourage the patient to remain still during the procedure, and assure the patient that more lidocaine or other pain or anxiety medications will be given as necessary. ➤*Rationale:* Patient movement may cause inappropriate placement or movement of the marrow needles, resulting in tissue trauma or pain.
- Encourage the patient to verbalize any pain experienced during the procedure. ➤*Rationale:* Additional lidocaine or pain medication can be administered.
- Inform the patient and family that the results will be shared with them as soon as they are available. ➤*Rationale:* The patient and family are usually anxious about the results.
- Inform the patient that he or she needs to lie still for 10 to 15 minutes after the procedure (or longer if the patient is severely thrombocytopenic) to prevent bleeding. Ask the patient to report a wet or warm feeling around the site. ➤*Rationale:* Promotes early detection of bleeding.

PATIENT ASSESSMENT AND PREPARATION

Patient Assessment

- Assess coagulation studies and platelet count. ➤*Rationale:* Obtains baseline coagulation results. Provides data regarding the patient's ability to form a clot after the procedure.
- Assess the need for antianxiety or pain medication. ➤*Rationale:* If the patient is very anxious before the procedure, or has experienced severe pain with previous bone marrow procedures, small doses of analgesia or sedation will promote patient comfort.
- Assess vital signs and oxygenation status. ➤*Rationale:* Provides baseline data. Ensures that the blood pressure and oxygenation status can be maintained if the patient is placed on his or her side or prone.
- Assess the ability of the patient to lie on his or her stomach or side, with the head of the bed at no greater than a 25-degree elevation. ➤*Rationale:* Access to, and control of, the posterior iliac crest is best obtained with the patient lying flat, or with the head of the bed only slightly raised, in a side-lying or prone position.
- Assess for recent bone marrow aspiration and biopsy sites. ➤*Rationale:* It may be painful for the patient if an additional biopsy is performed at a site that has not yet healed from a previous procedure.
- Assess the posterior iliac crest by palpation. Choose an area that is firm and not near the edge of the bone. If using the sternum (aspirate only), palpate the sternum, and use the area slightly above the manubrium. Avoid the xiphoid area. ➤*Rationale:* Identifies area for bone marrow biopsy and aspiration. During a sternal aspiration, the xiphoid is avoided as pressure on this part of the sternum may cause it to break and be pushed into the chest cavity.

Patient Preparation

- Ensure that the patient and family understand preprocedural teaching. Answer questions as they arise and reinforce information as needed. ➤*Rationale:* Evaluates and reinforces understanding of previously taught information.
- Obtain informed consent. ➤*Rationale:* Protects rights of patient and makes a competent decision possible for the patient; however, under emergency circumstances, time may not allow form to be signed.
- Prescribe analgesia or sedation if needed. ➤*Rationale:* Patient may need analgesia or sedation to ensure adequate cooperation and minimize discomfort during the procedure.
- Assist the patient to a side-lying or prone position depending on the patient's comfort and the practitioner's style. ➤*Rationale:* Ensures good visualization and control of the posterior iliac crest.

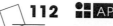

Procedure for Bone Marrow Biopsy and Aspiration (Perform)

Steps	Rationale	Special Considerations
1. Wash hands.	Reduces transmission of microorganisms; standard precautions.	
2. Open the bone marrow biopsy and aspiration kit in a manner that preserves sterility.	Maintains sterility of the procedure.	
3. Open the sterile needles, syringes, and marrow needles and place them on the kit.	Prepares sterile supplies.	
4. Open the vials of lidocaine, heparin, and EDTA, and set them aside.	Readies solutions before donning sterile gloves.	
5. Don mask, cap, sterile gown, and sterile gloves.	Maintains sterility; minimizes risk of infection.	
6. Use an antiseptic solution to prepare and cleanse the intended site.	Minimizes the transmission of microorganisms.	
7. Numb the skin using the sterile lidocaine in the kit.	Numbing the skin and the periosteum is very important for patient comfort.	If additional lidocaine is needed, ask the critical care nurse to assist by inverting the extra vial.
8. After numbing the skin, use a longer needle to feel for and numb the periosteum. The lidocaine needle can help map the geography of the bone.	If the periosteum is not numb, the patient will experience extreme discomfort. Also, it is often difficult to assess the area of the posterior iliac crest in an obese patient. Use of the spinal needle will help the practitioner "tap out" a firm site.	If the lidocaine needles in the kit do not reach the bone, use the spinal needle to reach the bone. The spinal needle can also be used to assess the geography of the posterior iliac crest
9. With the help of the critical care nurse: A. Withdraw 0.5 mL EDTA into a 5- to 10-mL syringe. B. Divide 1.0-mL heparin into two 5- to 10-mL syringes.	EDTA aspirate is used to make the slides and to place in the purple-top tubes for clot sections or polymerase chain reaction (PCR) studies. Heparinized aspirate is used for flow cytometry, chromosome analysis, and chimerism studies.	
10. Place a sterile gauze pad on the drape, and make a small incision in the skin.	Allows smooth entry of the marrow needles into the skin.	
11. Perform aspiration: A. Place the aspiration marrow needle into the incision and push in until the bone is reached.	Aspirate can be obtained without deep penetration.	In some disease states, aspirate cannot be obtained because the marrow is too densely packed with cells or too fibrotic.
B. With a twisting motion, allow the needle to enter the bone just until purchase is achieved. C. Remove the center piece of the needle, so that only the hollow tube is in the bone. D. Screw the EDTA syringe into the aspiration needle and pull back on the syringe. E. If aspirate is not obtained, put the center piece back in and reposition the needle. F. When aspirate is obtained, use a sterile slide from the kit and place a few drops of aspirate on it.		If the patient is obese, it may be necessary to use the longer Jamshidi needle to obtain the aspirate. A connector in the Jamshidi package allows aspirate to be obtained. The connection is not as tight and it may be difficult to obtain aspirate in this manner.
G. Look for spicules on the slide.	Spicules are tiny, white particles that contain the hematopoietic elements.	

Procedure continued on following page

Procedure	for Bone Marrow Biopsy and Aspiration (Perform) *Continued*

Steps	Rationale	Special Considerations
12. Pull 2 to 3 mL of bone marrow aspirate into the syringe containing the EDTA. Take off the EDTA syringe, and screw on the heparin-filled syringe. Pull 3 to 5 mL of aspirate into each heparinized syringe. With each pull, rotate the needle slightly.	Twisting the needle with each aspirate helps obtain aspirate from different angles, thereby getting a less dilute specimen. If more aspirate is needed, the aspirate needle should be removed and placed in a different section of the bone, using the same incision site and moving the skin over.	
13. Pull the aspiration needle out of the site and apply pressure with the sterile gauze.	Minimizes bleeding.	
14. With the help of the critical care nurse, process the aspirate obtained in the EDTA and heparin syringes immediately. A. The aspirate in the EDTA syringe should be used to make the slides. Place a very thin layer of aspirate on each slide, ensuring that spicules are on each slide. B. The remaining aspirate in the EDTA syringe should be placed in a purple-top tube for clot analysis or PCR studies. C. The aspirate in the heparinized syringes should be placed into green-top heparin sodium tubes.	Aspirate in the syringes can clot if it is not placed on the slides and in the appropriate tubes soon after it is obtained. If there are no spicules on the slides, there will be no hematopoietic elements for morphologic analysis.	
15. Insert the Jamshidi needle into the incision and push gently into the tissue until the needle hits the bone.	More lidocaine may be applied to the bone before Jamshidi insertion. The lidocaine needle may be used to "tap out" a firm part of the crest that is not too close to the edge of the bone.	The needle should be placed on a part of the crest that is not too close to the edge so that the needle does not slide off the bone and cause pain or bleeding.
16. Twist the needle just until it catches in the bone.		
17. Pull out the inner rod of the Jamshidi needle, and continue to gently screw it into the bone by using a twisting motion. The inner rod may be placed back into the Jamshidi needle to gauge how far into the bone the needle is.		
18. When the inner rod protrudes about 0.5 to 0.75 cm out of the Jamshidi needle, it can be removed.		
19. Before removal, the Jamshidi needle should be turned by 360 degrees a few times. Place the thumb over the top of the Jamshidi needle and gently pull the needle out.	Giving the Jamshidi needle a few 360-degree turns, and creating a vacuum by placing a finger over the top of the needle during removal, increases the likelihood that a piece of bone core will come out within the needle.	
20. Use the obturator provided with the Jamshidi needle to push the bone core into the specimen container. The core is removed from the Jamshidi needle by pushing the obturator into the bottom of the Jamshidi needle so that the core falls out at the handle end of the needle. If the core was not obtained, repeat the above steps, on a slightly different part of the bone.	Removing the core sample this way prevents damage to the bone by not forcing it through the narrower, "drill" end of the needle. To repeat core sampling, a new incision is not necessary. After the Jamshidi needle is reinserted, it can be used to push the skin over to find a suitable section of bone.	

Procedure for Bone Marrow Biopsy and Aspiration (Perform)

Steps	Rationale	Special Considerations
21. The core sample is placed in a container with normal saline-soaked sterile gauze.	Normal saline helps keep the bone from drying out and sticking to the gauze or container.	
22. Hold pressure over the site with a sterile gauze for at least 5 minutes.	Bleeding may occur under the skin and may not be visible around the puncture site. Because many patients who need a bone marrow procedure are thrombocytopenic, it is important to ensure that all bleeding has stopped after the procedure.	
23. Place a dressing over the site.	Prevents infection.	
24. Discard supplies, and wash hands.	Reduces transmission of microorganisms; standard precautions.	

Expected Outcomes

- Adequate bone marrow aspirate and core biopsy specimens are obtained.
- The aspirate contains spicules (unless the patient is aplastic) and is not clotted.
- Minimal bleeding and discomfort occur.
- The patient may feel a dull ache for a few days after the procedure.

Unexpected Outcomes

- At times it is difficult to obtain a bone marrow aspirate. Difficulty can occur if a patient is aplastic or if the marrow space is packed by disease. In these cases, the practitioner should try to obtain a good core biopsy specimen for pathology analysis. A touch preparation can be made from the biopsy by pressing the biopsy between two slides. This can sometimes help the pathologist obtain information if aspirate smears cannot be obtained.
- Some sections of bone are extremely hard, making placement of the Jamshidi needle difficult. If hard bone is encountered, another section of bone should be used. If a section of bone is extremely soft, it is often difficult to obtain an adequate biopsy, and again, another section of bone should be chosen.
- If the patient experiences excessive pain or feels a pain radiating down the leg, it is recommended that the needle be placed in another section of bone and that additional lidocaine be applied to the outer surface of the bone.

Patient Monitoring and Care

Patient Monitoring and Care	Rationale	Reportable Conditions
		These conditions should be reported if they persist despite nursing interventions.
1. Prescribe analgesia or sedatives as needed before and during the procedure.	Promotes patient comfort.	• Unrelieved discomfort
2. Assess vital signs, oxygenation, and electrocardiogram (ECG) rhythm during the procedure.	Monitors patient response to positioning and the procedure.	• Changes in vital signs, decreases in SaO_2, or changes in cardiac rhythm
3. Assess the site after the procedure.	Monitors for signs and symptoms of complications.	• Bleeding, hematoma, and infection

 This procedure should be performed only by physicians, advanced practice nurses, and other health care professionals (including critical care nurses) with additional knowledge, skills, and demonstrated competence per professional licensure or institutional standard.

Documentation

Documentation should include the following:

- Patient and family education
- Informed consent
- The date and time of the procedure
- The indication for the procedure
- The preparation for the procedure

- Any complications that may have occurred
- Any medications used
- Specimens obtained
- Additional interventions

Additional Readings

Bartl R, Frisch B, Wilmanns W. Bone and marrow findings in multiple myeloma and related disorders. In: Wiernick P, Canellos G, Dutcher J, Kyle R, eds. *Neoplastic Diseases of the Blood.* 3rd ed. New York, NY: Churchill Livingstone; 1996.

Demko SG. Transplantation procedures. In: Burt KR, Keeg HJ, Lothian SC, Santos GW, eds. *On Call in Bone Marrow Transplantation.* Austin, Tx: R.G. Landes; 1996.

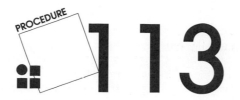

113

Bone Marrow Biopsy and Aspiration (Assist)

PURPOSE: Bone marrow biopsy and aspiration are used to diagnose various hematopoietic diseases, to check for residual disease after therapy, to identify metastatic disease to the bone marrow, to ascertain disease status prior to continued therapy, and to perform chromosome analysis.

Dolores Grosso

PREREQUISITE NURSING KNOWLEDGE

- Knowledge of sterile technique is essential.
- Bone marrow biopsy and aspiration are diagnostic tests that are used to ascertain various genetic and malignant entities.
- Bone marrow aspirate is used to morphologically identify normal and abnormal hematopoietic elements. The aspirate is also used to identify malignant clones by flow cytometry and is used to identify chromosomal abnormalities that occur in hematologic malignancies. In addition, bone marrow aspirate can be used to perform chimerism studies in patients after allogenic transplant.
- The bone marrow biopsy is used for morphologic analysis of hematopoietic cells and for assessing the architecture of the bone marrow that may be abnormal in certain disease states.
- Indications for bone marrow aspiration and biopsy include the following:
  - ❖ Diagnosing a hematologic abnormality
  - ❖ Monitoring a hematologic disease state after therapy
  - ❖ Ruling out of bone marrow metastasis before stem cell collection and for staging in various malignant states
  - ❖ Assessing the status of engraftment in all patients after bone marrow transplant
  - ❖ Assessing for chimerism and immune reconstitution in patients after allogeneic transplant
  - ❖ Harvesting stem cells for donation
- Contraindications to bone marrow biopsy and aspiration include *severe* bleeding dyscrasias.

EQUIPMENT

- Bone marrow biopsy and aspiration kit that includes the following:
  - ❖ Sterile drape
  - ❖ Betadine swabsticks
  - ❖ Biopsy container
  - ❖ Laboratory slides with an area to write on each slide
  - ❖ Sterile gauze
  - ❖ Sterile adhesive strip
  - ❖ Lidocaine needles of appropriate lengths to anesthetize both skin and periosteum
  - ❖ Scalpel
- Mask with face shield, cap, sterile gown, and sterile gloves
- 1-mL vial EDTA calcium (edetate calcium disodium) to help prevent specimen clotting
- 1-mL vial 1000 U/mL heparin
- One vial 1% lidocaine
- 10 mL sterile water
- Three or four 3-mL syringes
- Three or four 18-G needles
- Two or three heparin sodium blood tubes (green tops)
- 1 EDTA blood tube (purple top)
- Normal saline solution
- Specimen labels and laboratory forms

Additional equipment to have available as needed includes the following:

- One 22-G 3½-in sternal needle may be needed for deep lidocaine placement
- One Jamshidi biopsy needle
- One sternal aspiration needle
- One spinal needle

PATIENT AND FAMILY EDUCATION

- Assess patient and family understanding of the bone marrow biopsy and aspiration procedure and the reason for it. ➤**Rationale:** Clarification of the procedure and reinforcement of information is an expressed patient and family need in times of stress and anxiety.

- Explain the actual procedure to the patient and family. ➤*Rationale:* Prepares the patient and family for what to expect and may decrease anxiety.
- Encourage the patient to remain still during the procedure, and assure the patient that more lidocaine or other pain or anxiety medications will be given as necessary. ➤*Rationale:* Patient movement may cause inappropriate placement or movement of the marrow needles, resulting in tissue trauma or pain.
- Encourage the patient to verbalize any pain experienced during the procedure. ➤*Rationale:* Additional lidocaine or pain medication can be administered.
- Inform the patient that he or she needs to lie still for 10 to 15 minutes after the procedure (or longer if the patient is severely thrombocytopenic) to prevent bleeding. Ask the patient to report a wet or warm feeling around the site ➤*Rationale:* Promotes early detection of bleeding.

PATIENT ASSESSMENT AND PREPARATION

Patient Assessment

- Assess coagulation studies and platelet count. ➤*Rationale:* Obtains baseline coagulation results. Provides data regarding the patient's ability to form a clot after the procedure.
- Assess the need for antianxiety or pain medication. ➤*Rationale:* If the patient is very anxious before the procedure, or has experienced severe pain with previous bone marrow procedures, small doses of analgesia or sedation will promote patient comfort.

- Assess vital signs and oxygenation status. ➤*Rationale:* Provides baseline data. Ensures that the blood pressure and oxygenation status can be maintained if the patient is placed on his or her side or prone.
- Assess the ability of the patient to lie on his or her stomach or side with the head of the bed at no greater than a 25-degree elevation. ➤*Rationale:* Access to, and control of, the posterior iliac crest is best obtained with the patient lying flat, or with the head of the bed only slightly raised, in a side-lying or prone position.

Patient Preparation

- Ensure that the patient and family understand preprocedural teaching. Answer questions as they arise and reinforce information as needed. ➤*Rationale:* Evaluates and reinforces understanding of previously taught information.
- Ensure that informed consent was obtained. ➤*Rationale:* Protects rights of the patient and makes a competent decision possible for the patient; however, under emergency circumstances, time may not allow form to be signed.
- Administer prescribed analgesia or sedation if needed. ➤*Rationale:* Patient may need analgesia or sedation to ensure adequate cooperation and minimize discomfort during the procedure.
- Assist the patient to a side-lying or prone position depending on the patient's comfort and the practitioner's style. ➤*Rationale:* Ensures good visualization and control of the posterior iliac crest.

Procedure	for Bone Marrow Biopsy and Aspiration (Assist)

Steps	Rationale	Special Considerations
1. Wash hands.	Reduces transmission of microorganisms; standard precautions.	
2. Ensure that the patient is positioned appropriately.	Prepares patient for the procedure.	
3. Assist the physician or advanced practice nurse with obtaining necessary supplies.	Prepares supplies.	
4. Don mask, cap, sterile gown, and sterile gloves.	Maintains sterility; minimizes risk of infection.	
5. Assist the physician or advanced practice nurse with skin preparation.	Reduces the transmission of microorganisms.	
6. Assist the physician or advanced practice nurse with the administration of local anesthesia as needed.	Numbing the skin and the periosteum is very important for patient comfort.	
7. Assist the physician or advanced practice nurse with syringe preparation: A. Withdraw 0.5 mL EDTA into a 5- to 10-mL syringe. B. Divide 1.0 mL heparin into two 5- to 10-mL syringes.	EDTA aspirate is used to make the slides and to place in the purple-top tubes for clot sections or polymerase chain reaction (PCR) studies. Heparinized aspirate is used for flow cytometry, chromosome analysis, and chimerism studies.	

Steps	Rationale	Special Considerations
8. Assist with processing the aspirate obtained in the EDTA and heparin syringes immediately.	Aspirate in the syringes can clot if it is not placed on the slides and in the appropriate tubes soon after it is obtained.	
A. The aspirate in the EDTA syringe should be used to make the slides. Place a very thin layer of aspirate on each slide, ensuring that spicules are on each slide.	If there are no spicules on the slides, there will be no hematopoietic elements for morphologic analysis.	
B. The remaining aspirate in the EDTA syringe should be placed in a purple-top tube for clot analysis or PCR studies.		
C. The aspirate in the heparinized syringes should be placed into green-top heparin sodium tubes.		
9. Assist as needed with placement of the core sample in a container with normal saline–soaked sterile gauze.	Normal saline helps keep the bone from drying out and sticking to the gauze or container.	
10. Assist with placing a dressing over the site as needed.	Prevents infection.	
11. Label and send samples for laboratory analysis.	Ensures accuracy of results and ensures timeliness of laboratory analyses.	
12. Discard supplies, and wash hands.	Reduces transmission of microorganisms; standard precautions.	

Expected Outcomes

- Adequate bone marrow aspirate and core biopsy specimens are obtained.
- The aspirate contains spicules (unless the patient is aplastic) and is not clotted.
- Minimal bleeding and discomfort occur.
- The patient may feel a dull ache for a few days after the procedure.

Unexpected Outcomes

- Inability to obtain specimens
- Unrelieved pain

Patient Monitoring and Care

Patient Monitoring and Care	Rationale	Reportable Conditions
		These conditions should be reported if they persist despite nursing interventions.
1. Administer analgesia or sedatives as needed before and during the procedure.	Promotes patient comfort.	• Unrelieved discomfort
2. Monitor vital signs, oxygenation, and electrocardiogram (ECG) rhythm during the procedure.	Determines the patient response to positioning and the procedure.	• Changes in vital signs; decreased SaO_2; cardiac dysrhythmias
3. Assess the site after the procedure.	Monitors for signs and symptoms of complications.	• Presence of bleeding, hematoma, infection

Documentation

Documentation should include the following:

- Patient and family education
- Informed consent
- The date and time of the procedure
- The indication for the procedure
- The preparation for the procedure

- Any complications that may have occurred
- Any medications used
- Specimens obtained
- Additional interventions

Additional Readings

Bartl R, Frisch B, Wilmanns W. Bone and marrow findings in multiple myeloma and related disorders. In: Wiernick P, Canellos G, Dutcher J, Kyle R, eds. *Neoplastic Diseases of the Blood.* 3rd ed. New York, NY: Churchill Livingstone; 1996.

Demko SG. Transplantation procedures. In: Burt KR, Keeg HJ, Lothian SC, Santos GW, eds. *On Call in Bone Marrow Transplantation.* Austin, Tx: R.G. Landes; 1996.

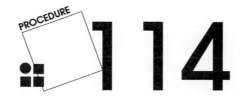

114

Determination of Microhematocrit via Centrifuge

P U R P O S E: Determining the microhematocrit via centrifuge is a point-of-care test commonly performed within the critical care unit. A capillary tube of blood is used to obtain the hematocrit value. Turnaround time, from drawing the blood to obtaining the results, is minimal because the procedure is completed within 5 minutes.

Maribeth Wooldridge-King

PREREQUISITE NURSING KNOWLEDGE

- The hematocrit measures the percent of the total volume of red blood cells within a given blood sample. It is the ratio of the volume of red blood cells to that of whole blood expressed as a percentage.
- A microhematocrit is determined by centrifuging an anticoagulated specimen of blood under standardized conditions.
- A patient's hematocrit is useful in evaluating fluid status, in evaluating volume status after fluid resuscitation, and in classifying various types of anemia. The hematocrit provides a relative indication of the degree of anemia or hemorrhage; the hemoglobin level is more accurate for measuring the red blood cell count.

EQUIPMENT

- Two heparinized capillary tubes (75 × 1.55 mm internal diameter)
- Standardized high-speed centrifuge
- Sealing clay
- Hematocrit linear scale for direct reading (Fig. 114–1)
- Nonsterile gloves

Additional equipment to have available as needed includes the following:

- One 3-mL syringe and one 5-mL syringe and 21-G needle (for sample from arterial line)
- Lancet device (for fingerstick)
- Tourniquet (for venipuncture if necessary)

PATIENT AND FAMILY EDUCATION

- Explain why the microhematocrit is being performed. **➤Rationale:** Promotes patient and family understanding of the treatment plan and encourages the patient and family to ask questions.
- Explain how the procedure is done and discomfort the patient may experience. **➤Rationale:** Elicits patient cooperation, although anxiety may be heightened by knowledge that the patient may need a fingerstick or venipuncture if an arterial line sample is not available.

PATIENT ASSESSMENT AND PREPARATION
Patient Assessment

- Assess for signs and symptoms of fluid volume deficit, including dry mucous membranes, decreased skin turgor, lethargy, hyperventilation, decreased pulmonary artery pressures, increased urine specific gravity, and hypotension. **➤Rationale:** The hematocrit is increased with dehydration.
- Assess for signs and symptoms of fluid volume excess, including edema, dyspnea, crackles, jugular vein distention, hypertension, decreased urine specific gravity, and elevated pulmonary artery pressures. **➤Rationale:** The hematocrit is below normal in the presence of fluid volume excess.
- Note past medical history of massive hemolysis (eg, major burns). **➤Rationale:** Massive red blood cell hemolysis increases the hematocrit.
- Assess for signs and symptoms of anemia or a decreased circulating volume caused by hemorrhage or "third-spacing" of fluid from the intravascular compartment to the

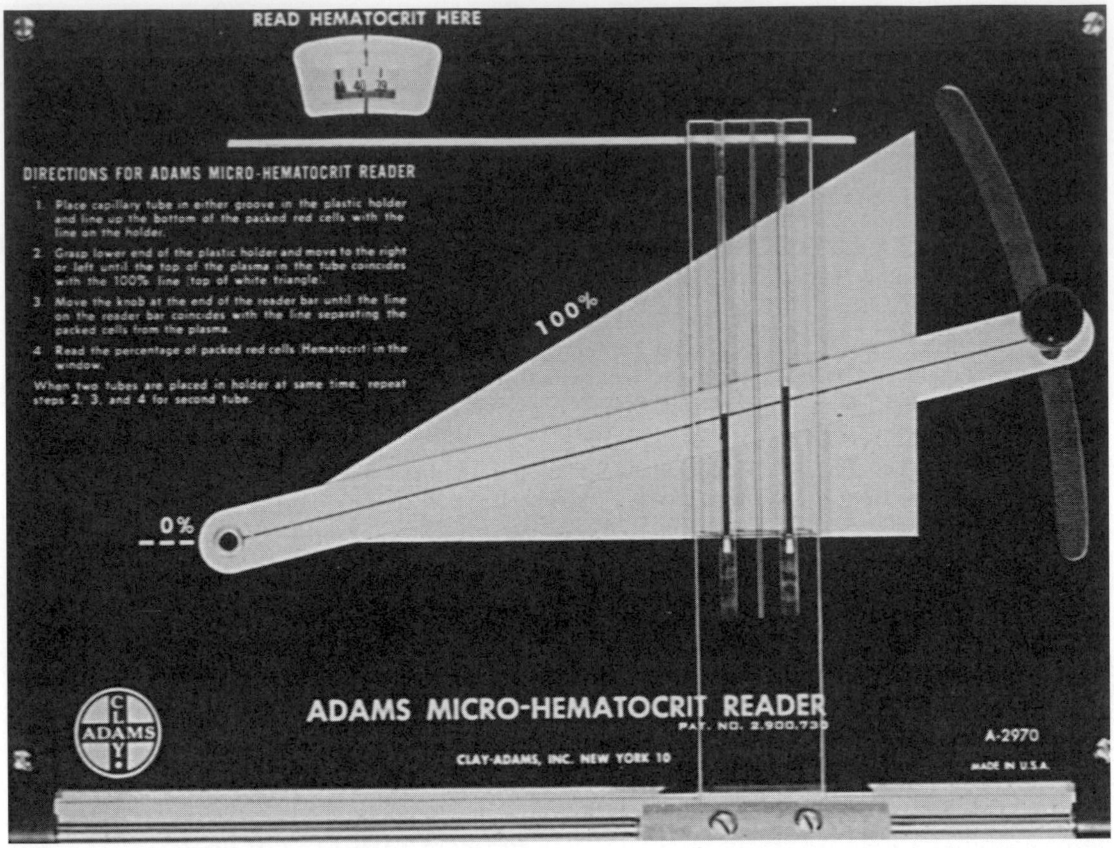

■ ● **FIGURE 114–1.** Adams Micro-Hematocrit Reader. (From Simmons A. *Hematology: A Combined Theoretical and Technical Approach.* Philadelphia, Pa: WB Saunders; 1989:205.)

extravascular compartment. These symptoms include restlessness, dizziness, syncope, severe headaches, disorientation, pallor, diaphoresis, rapid thready pulse, hypotension, and rapid, deep respirations progressing to shallow respirations. ➻***Rationale:*** The hematocrit provides a relative indication of the degree of anemia or decreased circulating volume.

- Assess for evidence of increased intravascular volume caused by congestive heart failure, an overinfusion of intravenous fluids, or the return of "third-spaced" fluids to the intravascular compartment. ➻***Rationale:*** These clinical states commonly have a dilutional effect on the hematocrit and are considered when evaluating the patient's fluid and electrolyte status or effects of transfusion therapy.

Patient Preparation

- Ensure that the patient and family understand preprocedural teaching. Answer questions as they arise and reinforce information as needed. ➻***Rationale:*** Evaluates and reinforces understanding of previously taught information.
- If performing a fingerstick, either wash the patient's hands or have the patient wash his or her hands with soap and water. ➻***Rationale:*** Reduces risk of infection. Warm water dilates peripheral vessels and facilitates the process of obtaining a specimen.
- Assist the patient to hold his or her arm in a dependent position for at least 30 seconds. ➻***Rationale:*** Encourages increased blood flow into fingertips.

Procedure for Determination of Microhematocrit via Centrifuge

Steps	Rationale	Special Considerations
1. Wash hands, and don gloves.	Reduces transmission of microorganisms; standard precautions.	
2. Obtain blood sample. If patient does not have an arterial line, perform venipuncture (see Procedure 77) or fingerstick.	Provides blood for analysis.	The pink lancet (1.4 mm) is used for all pediatric patients and most adult patients. The blue lancet (1.9 mm) is used for adults with thick or callused skin or when an inadequate amount of blood is obtained using the pink lancet.

Procedure	for Determination of Microhematocrit via Centrifuge *Continued*

Steps	Rationale	Special Considerations
3. Keeping the index finger of your dominant hand over one end of the capillary tube, place the other end to the hub of the syringe or the puncture site of the fingerstick to fill with blood. Remove your index finger and reposition it, and continue to repeat until the capillary tube is filled to within 5 to 10 mm of the end of the tube.	Placing your finger over the small diameter of the capillary tube creates a pressure gradient, which causes the tube to fill.	
4. Fill the second capillary tube in the same fashion.	Two tubes are necessary to balance within the centrifuge.	
5. Place one end of each capillary tube into the special sealing clay.	Capillary tubes must be sealed before they are centrifuged.	Make sure the sealing clay forms a straight edge across the interior of the tube.
6. Place one capillary tube on the centrifuge head with the sealed end directed outward; place the second tube directly opposite the first tube.	Avoids spillage of blood and balances the tubes within the machine.	
7. Place the cover on the centrifuge, set the automatic timer to 5 minutes at 10,000 to 15,000 × gravity, then turn the machine on.	Separates red blood cells from plasma so that the hematocrit can be determined.	
8. When the machine stops, remove the capillary tubes from the centrifuge and obtain the graphic reader (see Fig. 114–1).	The graphic reader is used to read hematocrit.	
9. Place a capillary tube in the holder on the graphic reader.	Correct placement of the tube is necessary to obtain an accurate reading.	
10. Align the bottom of the red blood cells with the line on the holder (Figs. 114–1 and 114–2).	The tube is now adjusted for the amount of blood in this specific tube.	
11. Take the plastic capillary tube holder and move it until the top of the plasma (not the red blood cells) coincides with the 100% line that is at the top of the white triangle (see Figs. 114–1 and 114–2).	Prepares tube so hematocrit can be read.	

Procedure continued on following page

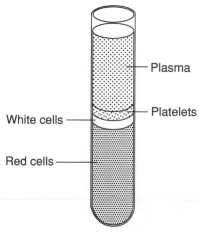

■ ● **FIGURE 114–2.** Cell layers in centrifuged whole blood.

Procedure	**for Determination of Microhematocrit via Centrifuge** *Continued*

Steps	Rationale	Special Considerations
12. Turn the knob to the right of the reader, and move it until the line coincides with the line where the plasma and red blood cells separate (see Figs. 114–1 and 114–2).	Identifies the microhematocrit.	
13. Read the microhematocrit in the window.	This is the microhematocrit measurement that is to be documented.	
14. Validate the microhematocrit obtained with the second capillary tube.	Duplicate results should agree to within ±1%.	
15. Remove and discard gloves, and wash hands.	Reduces transmission of microorganisms; standard precautions.	

Expected Outcomes	Unexpected Outcomes
• Accurate identification of hematocrit	• Inability to identify hematocrit level
	• Continued bleeding from fingerstick site

Patient Monitoring and Care

Patient Monitoring and Care	Rationale	Reportable Conditions
		These conditions should be reported if they persist despite nursing interventions.
1. Monitor the microhematocrit as prescribed and as needed.	Provides data for future interventions.	• Abnormal hematocrit
2. Assess hematocrit levels in relation to blood loss.	Contributes to decision making with regard to blood or blood component transfusion requirements.	• Signs and symptoms correlating with hematocrit level
3. If a fingerstick was performed, examine the puncture site to determine if the bleeding has stopped. If the site continues to bleed, apply continuous pressure and elevate the extremity until bleeding has stopped.	Establishes that hemostasis has occurred.	• Unresolved bleeding

Documentation

Documentation should include the following:

- Patient and family education
- Date and time the procedure was performed
- Microhematocrit obtained by centrifuge
- Pertinent assessment findings that correlate with microhematocrit
- Unexpected outcomes
- Interventions taken based on the assessed findings and patient's response

Additional Readings

Dirk JL. Diagnostic blood analysis using point of care technology. *AACN Clin Iss.* 1996;7:249–259.

Lamb LS, Parrish RS, Goran SF, Bill MH. Current nursing practice of point of care laboratory diagnostic testing in critical care units. *Am J Crit Care.* 1995;4:429–434.

Simmons A. *Hematology: A Combined Theoretical and Technical Approach.* Philadelphia, Pa: W.B. Saunders; 1989.

Across the United States, there is diversity among burn units about policy, practice, and procedure in the care of the thermally injured population. This in no way intimates that the diversity in practice corresponds with diversity in quality. The burn community, consisting of 135 burn units, regularly benchmarks among themselves, both formally and informally. This is done to compare outcomes and update practice to ensure that our patients receive the quality of care they deserve. As is true with any specialty, the effects of research and the trial of new techniques and products will always be part of the search for best practice. Therefore, what is included in this manual is the result of the efforts of this author to describe care of the thermally injured patient, but this does not preclude the fact that practice in individual burn units may vary. If your institution does not have a formal burn unit, Table 116–2 outlines the criteria for appropriate transfer to a burn center.

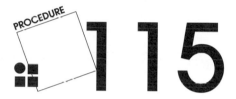

PROCEDURE

115

Care of Donor Sites

P U R P O S E: Care of the donor site is performed to promote wound healing and maintenance of function. Pain control is a priority during donor site care.[1,2]

Eileen E. Pysznik

PREREQUISITE NURSING KNOWLEDGE

- The donor site is a new, superficial partial-thickness wound created surgically for the purpose of providing skin graft coverage for deeper areas of burn (deep partial-thickness or full-thickness burns).[3]
- Donor sites normally heal in 7 to 14 days without infection (Fig. 115–1).[3-4]
- Donor sites may be reharvested for new skin grafts in 7 to 14 days. Each time the same donor site is reharvested, it will take longer to heal and the graft will decrease in quality.[4]
- Donor sites have a high risk of bleeding in the first 24 hours after surgery (Fig. 115–2). A compression dressing is sometimes used for the first 12 to 24 hours to ensure stasis.
- Donor sites are covered in the operating room with both inner and outer dressings. The inner dressing either creates a moist environment (eg, in the case of hydrogel dressing, calcium alginate, hydrocolloid dressing, or thin-film dressing) or requires a dry environment for the

dressing to adhere properly, reducing the chance for infection (eg, in the case of Biobrane, Xeroform gauze, scarlet red, fine-mesh gauze, or biologic dressing). Biologic dressings include homografts or allografts (human skin from donors) and heterografts or xenografts (nonhuman skin, which is usually from pigs).[4] Topical antimicrobials are usually reserved for donor sites that become infected.
- The moist-environment inner dressings are wrapped with a bulky outer dressing for the first 24 hours; some continue to be wrapped for 5 to 10 days.
- The dry-environment inner dressing is usually covered with gauze roll (the outer dressing) for the first 12 to 24 hours until the dressing is adherent; then the outer dressing is removed, and the inner dressing is left to dry. It is vital that the inner dressing remains dry to reduce the chance of infection. Methods used to attain this goal include leaving the dressing uncovered to encourage drying, using a single-layer outer dressing to allow moisture from the inner dressing to evaporate, keeping the patient positioned so that the donor area is exposed to the air at

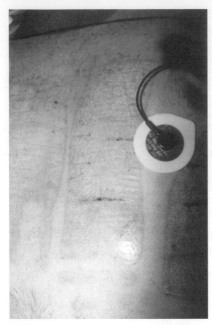

■ ● **FIGURE 115–1.** Donor sites in various stages of healing.

all times, keeping linens and clothing off the donor site until it is dry (inspect the site frequently to be sure it stays dry), possibly using a low-wattage heat lamp or hair dryer on a cool setting, or considering the use of high air–flow cushions if patient positioning requires the patient to lie on the donor site. The wound edges of the dressing will heal first.[5] With a dry dressing, the edges are trimmed back as they separate from the healing skin at the wound edges.

- The inner dressing is left intact until the wound heals, unless it becomes displaced or the wound becomes infected.[6] If the dressing is displaced, it should be replaced. If the wound becomes infected, the dressing must be removed, and dressings are resumed with an antimicrobial cream, solution, or ointment. Wound care now needs to be provided on the same schedule as care to the other burn wounds.
- Most burn centers use clean technique for dressing removal and donor-site cleansing, using sterile technique only for sterile dressing application.[7]
- The wound must be vigilantly assessed for infection because the donor site dressing is not antimicrobial[8];

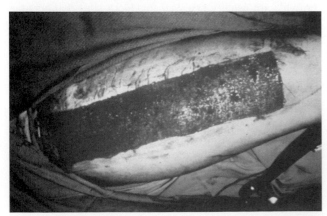

■ ● **FIGURE 115–2.** Fresh donor site.

however, some of the newer dressings have slow-release silver that may provide sufficient protection for a donor site. An infection could lead to prolonged healing or the conversion of the wound to a deeper wound.

- Healing donor sites are painful because they have exposed nerve endings and tightened skin. Epithelialization of the donor site occurs secondary to the deep epithelial cells remaining in this partial-thickness wound. After healing, the donor site should be able to sweat and regrow hair.
- An individualized plan for pain control should be in place for both background pain (ie, pain that is continuously present) and procedural pain (ie, increased intermittent pain related to procedures and routine care). Unrelieved pain can lead to stress-related immunosuppression, an increased potential for infection, delayed wound healing, and depression.[1, 2] Subcutaneous and intramuscular injections should be avoided because absorption will be poor and unreliable because of edema.[9] Intravenous administration of medication is preferred in critically ill patients, and oral medication is preferred in noncritical patients who have functioning gastrointestinal systems. As the wound heals, the patient will experience more discomfort from being itchy and less from pain. A water-based lotion will prevent drying and reduce urticaria.
- The burn patient is hypermetabolic until burn wounds are closed and healing is complete.[4, 10] This is important to note because the patient's baseline body temperature will be higher than normal by 1°F to 2°F[3, 11] (observe for temperature spikes rather than an absolute number), and the patient will be catabolic (resting energy expenditure can increase by as much as 100%),[4] requiring an increased caloric and protein intake for wound healing. It is important to keep the patient warm during wound care because a large amount of heat is lost from the wound, further increasing the metabolic rate.[3, 10]
- The donor site should not be exposed to the sun for a year after the burn. Skin discoloration can be present for up to a year.

EQUIPMENT

- Personal protective equipment
- Examination gloves
- Sterile gloves
- Scissors and forceps (clean and sterile)
- Warm tap water
- Basin
- Clean washcloths
- Replacement dressing (whatever is already being used on the donor site)
- Gauze rolls
- Towels or waterproof pads

Additional equipment (to have available depending on patient need) includes the following:

- Mild liquid soap
- Extra supplies and equipment as needed for burn wound care (see Procedure 116)

PATIENT AND FAMILY EDUCATION

- Teach the patient and family about donor site care. ➤*Rationale:* Diminishes fear of the unknown; increases knowledge about care.
- Teach the patient and family that donor sites generally

heal in 7 to 14 days with minimal scarring (unless the patient has a tendency toward hypertrophic scarring) and tell them why donor sites hurt so much and that the pain will soon be replaced with urticaria. ➤*Rationale:* Decreases anxiety about pain and appearance.

- Discuss the importance of continuing mobility and proper positioning despite the new wound created by the donor site. Self-care and range-of-motion exercises should be encouraged during the healing phase. ➤*Rationale:* Prevents contractures associated with healing skin and loss of function.[5-6]
- Assess the family's ability to provide care at home. ➤*Rationale:* Continued care of the wound will be required after discharge.
- As appropriate, provide detailed wound care instructions in writing, and review them with the patient and family. Demonstrate exactly what to do, and have the patient and family perform the demonstration a week before the planned discharge. Continue to involve the patient and family in the wound care for the remainder of the admission and encourage them to ask questions. Provide positive feedback. Arrange for home care or clinic visits to follow up on dressings and wound care. ➤*Rationale:* Validates the patient's and family's understanding and ability to perform wound care and allows time for them to develop a level of comfort. Provides the opportunity to reinforce important points.
- Teach the patient and family about pain and pruritus medications, as needed, and provide the name of a water-based lotion to apply to healed areas. ➤*Rationale:* Supports comfort at home.
- Teach the patient and family about signs and symptoms of infection and the importance of reporting any of these in a timely manner. ➤*Rationale:* Patient and family will recognize problems early so that appropriate measures can be instituted by the health care professional.
- Stress the importance of wearing pressure garments and splints. ➤*Rationale:* Reduces scar formation and contractures.[3, 8, 10]
- Inform the patient and family that the donor site should not be exposed to the sun for a year after the burn and that discoloration can be present for up to a year. ➤*Rationale:* Prepares the patient and family for changes that will be present after hospital discharge.
- Provide the patient and family with follow-up appointments and a contact to call if there is a problem. ➤*Rationale:* Provides necessary information for further care and follow-up.

PATIENT ASSESSMENT AND PREPARATION
Patient Assessment

- Vital signs, including temperature; then continue to monitor vital signs throughout donor site care. ➤*Rationale:*

Baseline vital signs will allow for comparison during and following the procedure to evaluate patient tolerance of pain and the need for pain medication.
- Evaluate for signs of healing, as follows:
  ❖ Decreased pain
  ❖ Dressing separating at wound edges with reepithelialization beneath it
  ❖ Decreased edema
- Compare level of healing to expected level of healing for number of days since skin harvested. ➤*Rationale:* Healing should occur within 7 to 14 days unless there are complications.
- Evaluate for signs and symptoms of infection, as follows:
  ❖ Foul odor
  ❖ Purulent drainage
  ❖ Increased pain
  ❖ Increasing edema
  ❖ Cellulitis
  ❖ Fever
  ❖ Development of eschar
- ➤*Rationale:* Healing should occur within 7 to 14 days unless there are complications.
- Evaluate the adequacy of the pain control regime by asking the patient to rate the pain on a scale of 0 to 10, both before donor site care (background pain) and during wound care.[1, 2, 9] ➤*Rationale:* An individualized plan for pain control should be in place for background and procedural pain. In addition to the traditional use of pain and anxiety medications, alternative therapies should be included (eg, relaxation techniques, massage therapy, music therapy). The patient's medication requirements should decrease as the donor site heals.
- Evaluate the patient's level of function in the area involving the donor site. ➤*Rationale:* Burns contract during the healing phase[5] and immobility causes loss of function. The patient should be encouraged to continue normal movement and range-of-motion exercises.

Patient Preparation

- Ensure that patient understands preprocedural teaching. Answer questions as they arise and reinforce information as needed. ➤*Rationale:* Evaluates and reinforces understanding of previously taught information.
- Premedicate the patient for pain and anxiety, as needed. Wait until medication has had time to work.[1, 2] ➤*Rationale:* Allows time for medication to take effect and promotes optimal comfort for the patient. Reduces pain and anxiety. Encourages patient trust and compliance with procedure.[9]

Procedure for Care of Donor Sites

Steps	Rationale	Special Considerations
1. Prepare all necessary equipment and supplies.	Preparation facilitates efficient wound care and prevents needless delays.	
2. Wash hands, and don cap, mask, gown, and examination gloves for each health care provider involved in the procedure.	Reduces transmission of microorganisms to the patient; standard precautions.	
3. Remove gauze roll and any padding covering inner dressing (if there is a supportive dressing in place); place a towel or waterproof pad under involved area.	Inner dressing is left in place until the wound heals unless there is a problem with infection.	Gauze roll or outer supportive dressing is usually removed after 24 hours when dry inner dressing is adherent, but gauze roll or outer supportive dressing may be used for 5 to 10 days with moist inner dressing.
4. Assess the donor site for progression of healing and complications; assess whether the inner dressing needs to be changed. Proceed to step 8 if inner donor dressing needs to be changed.	Validates the healing process and identifies complications.	If inner dressing was stapled in place by surgeon, staples will need to be removed as wound heals and dressing is trimmed back.
5. Remove and discard gloves, and don a pair of clean gloves.	Handling the burn dressing contaminates examination gloves, and clean gloves are needed for wound care.	
6. Gently wash exudate from wound edges with warm tap water and pat dry.	Clears exudate that can harbor microorganisms from area of donor site.[5]	
7. With dry inner dressing, use scissors to trim loose edges of donor site dressing. If inner dressing does not need to be changed, proceed to step 14 to complete donor site care.	Because dry inner dressing is not covered, loose edges of dressing can snag and displace inner dressing.	Assess need for outer dressing and apply as needed.

Inner Dressing Change

8. Remove inner dressing and discard it.		If dressing is adherent, soak with warm tap water to loosen.
9. Remove and discard gloves and don a pair of clean gloves.	Handling the burn dressing contaminates examination gloves, and clean gloves are needed for wound care.	
10. Gently wash wound with mild soap solution (if ordered), rinse with warm tap water, and pat dry.	Cleanses donor site.	Cleanse beyond donor site to reduce microbial count on surrounding tissue. Patients may do better if allowed to cleanse their own wounds.
11. Assess the donor site for progression of healing and complications; outline any inflammation with a marking pen.	Validates the healing process and identifies complications.	Notify health care providers from other disciplines who need to observe the wound ahead of time so that they can be present while the wound is uncovered.
12. Remove and discard gloves. Don a pair of sterile gloves.	Gloves are contaminated from contact with donor site. Sterile gloves are used for the sterile dressing.	
13. Cut dressing to the size of donor site with sterile scissors, apply, and secure in place.	Ensures correct fit and adherence.	
14. Remove and discard gloves. Wash hands.	Reduces transmission of microorganisms.	
15. Continue with other burn wound care as needed.	Donor sites are newer wounds and they are created in a sterile environment; therefore, they are likely to be cleaner than other wounds.	Cover donor sites with towel or waterproof pad to protect them from contamination during burn wound care, as needed.

Expected Outcomes	**Unexpected Outcomes**

Expected Outcomes

- Donor site heals in 7 to 14 days without complications.
- Patient maintains a self-identified, acceptable level of pain relief.
- Patient maintains comfort from measures taken for anxiety and itching.
- Patient and family verbalize knowledge of patient condition and plan of care.
- An optimal level of function is maintained or attained.
- Patient and family response and interactions demonstrate adaptation to injury.
- Patient and family collaborate in management of care.
- At the time of discharge, patient and family verbalize and demonstrate an understanding of posthospital care.

Unexpected Outcomes

- Bleeding
- Infection
- Conversion of donor site to deep partial-thickness or full-thickness wound

Patient Monitoring and Care

Patient Monitoring and Care	Rationale	Reportable Conditions
		These conditions should be reported if they persist despite nursing interventions.
1. Evaluate and treat the patient for pain.[1, 2] Ask the patient to rate his or her pain on a scale of 0 to 10; check the orders for pain and sedation for donor site care; check to see what the patient's medication requirements were with previous donor site care and have that amount of medication available in the room before starting the care; assess the need for more medication throughout the donor site care. Incorporate alternative pain relief techniques (eg, relaxation techniques, massage therapy, music, visual imaging).	The burn patient will have baseline pain that requires pain medication; the pain from the donor site will be minimized by use of an intact dressing that does not require dressing changes and protects the nerve endings from contact with the air; the patient will have increased pain medication requirements if the dressing needs to be changed; attention to the patient's pain will foster the patient's trust in health care personnel to control pain and will promote cooperation with future donor site care.	• Increased heart rate • Increased or decreased blood pressure • Increased respiratory rate • Verbalization of pain • Nonverbal indications of pain (eg, restlessness, grimacing, teeth clenching) • Unable to cooperate with donor site care
2. Obtain baseline vital signs before procedure, monitor them throughout procedure, and check them for 30 minutes after procedure is complete.	Changes in vital signs can be a sign that the patient is experiencing pain or anxiety. Decreasing blood pressure, heart rate, and respiratory rate can be complications of pain medication (especially after dressing change is complete and stimulation has stopped).	• Increased or decreased heart rate • Increased or decreased blood pressure • Increased or decreased respiratory rate • High peak pressures on ventilator
3. Assess the donor site for appearance (eg, dressing wet or dry, dressing adherent, presence of drainage or bleeding, redness at edges) and progression toward healing (eg, reepithelialization at wound edges).	Observe for usual progression of wound healing versus complications of infection, progression of donor site to deeper wound, and bleeding.	• Foul odor • Purulent or increased amounts of drainage • Cellulitis or edema • Healing tissue developing eschar • Discoloration of wound • Bleeding
4. Encourage exercise and activities of daily living; place patient in position of optimal function, using splints to maintain position as needed.[8] Use pain medication as needed to facilitate mobility.[1, 2]	Donor site wounds contract during the healing phase if not correctly splinted and exercised.[5] Pain inhibits patients from moving.	• Loss of function

Continued on following page

Patient Monitoring and Care *Continued*

Patient Monitoring and Care	Rationale	Reportable Conditions
5. Monitor patient's toleration of tube feedings or patient's ingestion of a high-calorie and high-protein diet with supplements[8]; encourage nutritious diet and discourage empty calories.	Good nutrition is necessary for wound healing; burn patients are hypermetabolic.	• Poor wound healing

Documentation

Documentation should include the following:

- Patient and family education
- Date and time of donor site care
- Appearance (eg, dressing wet or dry, dressing adherent, presence of drainage or bleeding, redness at edges)
- Progression toward healing (eg, reepithelialization at wound edges)
- Assessment of pain before, during, and after procedure
- Medications given for pain and sedation
- Other comfort measures used
- Patient's tolerance of the procedure
- Unexpected outcomes
- Nursing interventions

References

1. Ashburn MA. Burn pain: the management of procedure-related pain. *J Burn Care Rehabil.* 1995;16:365–371.
2. Ulmer JF. Burn pain management: a guideline-based approach. *J Burn Care Rehabil.* 1998;19:151–159.
3. Jordan BS, Harrington DT. Management of the burn wound. *Nurs Clin North Am.* 1997;32:251–273.
4. Greenfield E. Integumentary disorders. In: Kinney MR, Dunbar SB, Brooks-Brunn J, Molter N, Vitello-Cicciu JM, eds. *AACN's Clinical Reference for Critical Care Nursing.* 4th ed. St. Louis, Mo: C.V. Mosby; 1998:1065–1087.
5. Ward RS, Saffle JR. Topical agents in burn and wound care. *Phys Ther.* 1995;75:526–538.
6. Monafo WW. Initial management of burns. *N Engl J Med.* 1997;335:1581–1586.
7. Herndon DN, ed. *Total Burn Care.* London: W.B. Saunders Ltd; 1996:548.
8. Rose JK, Barrow RE, Desai MH, Herndon DN. Advances in burn care. *Adv Surg.* 1996;30:71–95.
9. Gordon M, Goodwin CW. Burn management. Initial assessment, management, and stabilization. *Nurs Clin North Am.* 1997;32:237–249.
10. Cortiella J, Marvin JA. Management of the pediatric burn patient. *Nurs Clin North Am.* 1997;32:311–329.
11. Nguyen TT, Gilpin DA, Meyer NA, Herndon DN. Current treatment of severely burned patients. *Ann Surg.* 1996;223:14–25.

Additional Readings

Bettinger D, Gore D, Humphries Y: Evaluation of calcium alginate for skin graft donor sites. *J Burn Care Rehabil.* 1995;16:59–61.

Cadier MA, Clarke JA. Dermasorb versus Jelonet in patients with burns: skin graft donor sites. *J Burn Care Rehabil.* 1996;17:246–251.

Griswold JA, Tepica T, Rossi L, et al. A comparison of Xeroform and Skin Temp dressings in the healing of skin graft donor sites. *J Burn Care Rehabil.* 1995;16:136–140.

Young T, Fowler A. Nursing management of skin grafts and donor sites. *Br J Nurs.* 1998;7:326, 328, 330.

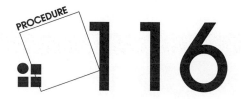

116

Care of Burn Wounds

P U R P O S E: Burn wound care is performed to promote healing, maintain function, and prevent infection and burn wound sepsis. A major focus must be on pain control.[1, 2]

Eileen E. Pysznik

PREREQUISITE NURSING KNOWLEDGE

- Burn injuries disrupt the normal functions of the skin, which include fighting infection, maintaining fluid and electrolyte balance, controlling temperature and pain, and maintaining structural integrity.
- The skin is composed of two layers, the epidermis and the dermis, and is supported by a subcutaneous layer that is rich in blood vessels (Fig. 116–1).
  - ❖ The outermost layer, the epidermis, contains melanocytes (protection from the sun) and Langerhans cells (protection against foreign organisms). The epidermis is capable of rapid regeneration.
  - ❖ The dermis contains collagen and elastin (structure), hair follicles, blood vessels, nerve endings, sebaceous and sweat glands, and fibroblasts (necessary for healing). An epidermal layer lines hair follicles and other structures that extend to the surface; these epidermal elements provide the ability for the skin to regenerate

(the more epidermal elements, the faster the wound heals).

- The depth of the burn is classified as superficial, partial thickness, or full thickness (Table 116–1).
  - ❖ A superficial (first-degree) burn involves only the epidermis and is not included when estimating the size of the burn[3] because it does not activate a systemic inflammatory reaction. The protective barrier of the skin remains intact.
  - ❖ Partial-thickness (second-degree) burns (Fig. 116–2) can be superficial (loss of the epidermis and part of the dermis) or deep (destruction of most of the dermis). Superficial partial-thickness burns have many epidermal elements remaining that allow the wound to heal in 7 to 14 days. Deep partial-thickness burns take longer to heal, have more scarring, and have a higher risk of complications. Therefore, these wounds are frequently treated with skin grafts because healing would otherwise take more than 2 weeks.[4, 5]

Table 116–1 ■■■ **Depth Characteristics of Burn Wounds**

Type	Physical Characteristics	Healing
Superficial burn (first degree): destruction of epidermis	Red, sunburnlike, no blisters, relatively mild pain (compared with partial-thickness burn), uncomfortable to touch	Rapid regeneration, heals within 3 to 7 days, no scarring, no loss of function
Superficial partial-thickness burn (superficial second degree): destruction of epidermis and upper dermis	Pink or red, blisters, wet, exquisitely painful, capillary refill intact	Heals in 7 to 14 days, hypertrophic scars are rare, may be some mild scarring, discoloration for up to 1 year, return to full function
Deep partial-thickness burn (deep second degree): destruction of epidermis through to lower dermis	Red or mottled pink to white, moist (dryer than superficial partial-thickness burn), painful but less sensitive to pinprick, slow or absent capillary refill, may have thin white eschar, blisters drier if present, hair follicles and sweat glands intact	Slow regeneration from epidermal elements that line hair follicles and sweat glands (21 to 60 days in absence of grafting), possible conversion to full-thickness injury, hypertrophic scars and contracture formation common with primary healing, frequently treated with split-thickness skin grafts to reduce healing time and complications, fewer functional limitations with early excision and grafting
Full-thickness burn (third degree): destruction of epidermis and all of dermis	Dry; black, charred, white, tan, or brown; leathery, firm eschar; thrombosed vessels; does not blanch to pressure; insensitive to light touch or pinprick	Incapable of self-regeneration, preferred treatment is early excision and grafting with autograft, functional limitations more frequent

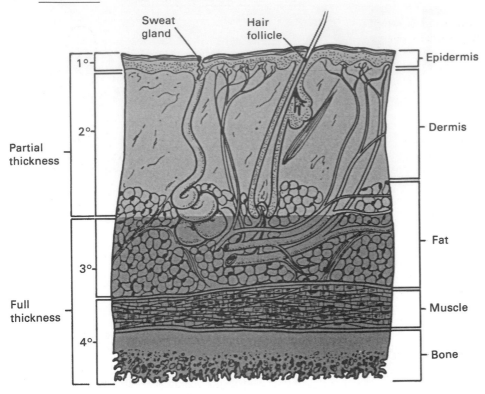

Sweat gland

Hair follicle

1°

2°

3°

4°

Partial thickness

Full thickness

Epidermis

Dermis

Fat

Muscle

Bone

■ ● **FIGURE 116–1.** Cross-section of skin with areas affected by partial- and full-thickness burns. (From Lewis SM, Cox IC. *Medical-Surgical Nursing: Assessment and Management of Clinical Problems.* 2nd ed. New York: McGraw-Hill; 1987:408. Copyright CV Mosby, St. Louis.)

❖ A full-thickness (third-degree) burn involves complete destruction of the dermis (Fig. 116–3). Because the skin is unable to regenerate, the only way to permanently close the wound is with an autograft.

• The depth of the burn wound is directly related to the temperature intensity and the duration of contact with the burning agent. The burning agent can be thermal, chemical, or electrical. Additionally, an inhalation injury should always be suspected if the patient was in an enclosed space with a fire (as many as a third of patients with major burns have an associated inhalation injury).[6]

• Care of the burn wound and associated healing is determined by the extent and depth of the injury and the overall condition of the patient.

• Criteria that indicate that the burn patient should be transferred to a specialized burn care facility are outlined in Table 116–2. These criteria include patients who are likely to have an increased chance of morbidity and mortality.[7]

• The rule of nines is a method used to rapidly assess the size or extent of the burn by dividing the body into various anatomic regions, each of which represents 9% of the total body surface area (TBSA). However, the Lund-Browder chart method[5] should be used once the

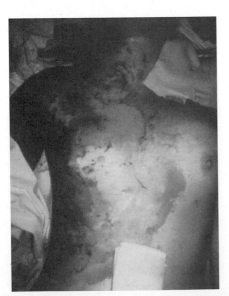

■ ● **FIGURE 116–2.** A fresh burn that is partial thickness toward the patient's left side and progresses to full thickness on the patient's right side.

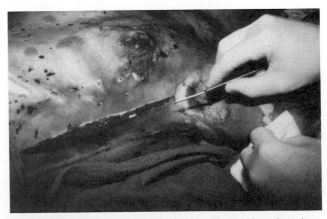

■ ● **FIGURE 116–3.** Full-thickness burn with chest escharotomy to improve chest expansion.

patient is stabilized to determine a more accurate estimation of size (Fig. 116–4).[3] This method allows for changes in body proportion associated with aging. Neither of these methods work for scattered burn areas; however, the extent of the burn can be estimated by using the entire palmar surface of the patient's hand to represent approximately 1% of the patient's TBSA.[8, 9]

- The three zones of cellular destruction are coagulation (cellular death), stasis (vascular impairment, potentially reversible tissue injury), and hyperemia (increased blood flow and inflammatory response, analogous to a first-degree burn, heals rapidly).[3, 4] Decreased circulation in the burn wound can cause areas of stasis to progress to necrosis (eg, deep partial-thickness burn converts to full-thickness wound). This progressive destruction can be minimized with adequate oxygenation and fluid resuscitation, decreasing pressure on the injured tissue, not applying ice, and decreasing edema by elevating the burned area.[10]

- The inflammatory response causes a massive fluid shift to the interstitial space during the first 24 to 48 hours,[4] with mobilization of fluid starting after 72 hours. Large amounts of evaporative water, along with plasma proteins, are lost through the burn wound until the wound is closed.[3, 11]

- Eschar is a thick layer of dead tissue that covers full-thickness burns. Eschar separation is a natural process that happens over 3 to 5 weeks.[11] With early excision and grafting, this is no longer seen unless bacterial proliferation accelerates the process.

- Patients with circumferential full-thickness burns are at high risk for circulatory complications. Eschar acts as a tourniquet while edema forms in the subeschar tissue.[3] Classic signs are pain, paresis, puffiness, pallor, and pulselessness. The most reliable indicator of severe circulatory compromise is a decrease in the Doppler ultrasound signal of the palmar arch vessel in the upper extremities and the posterior tibial artery pulse in the lower extremities.[3, 4] The treatment is escharotomy (Fig. 116–5).[10] This is performed at the bedside without anesthesia because the incision is through eschar only; sedation and a small amount of pain medication are given.[3] A common complication is bleeding, so electrocautery may be used. Compartment syndrome should be suspected if the muscle compartment is rigid or if there are

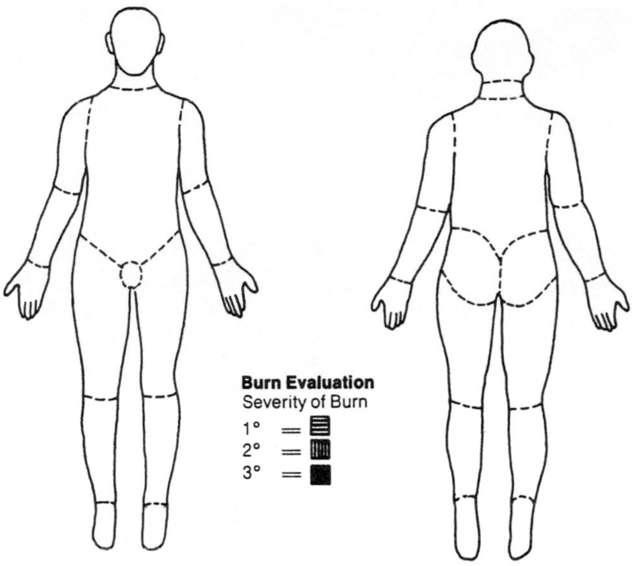

Burn Evaluation
Severity of Burn

1° =
2° =
3° =

AREA	0–1	1–4	5–9	10–15	ADULT	% 2°	% 3°	% TOTAL
Head	19	17	13	10	7			
Neck	2	2	2	2	2			
Ant. Trunk	13	17	13	13	13			
Post. Trunk	13	13	13	13	13			
R. Buttock	2 1/2	2 1/2	2 1/2	2 1/2	2 1/2			
L. Buttock	2 1/2	2 1/2	2 1/2	2 1/2	2 1/2			
Genitalia	1	1	1	1	1			
R.U. Arm	4	4	4	4	4			
L. U. Arm	4	4	4	4	4			
R.L. Arm	3	3	3	3	3			
L.L. Arm	3	3	3	3	3			
R. Hand	2 1/2	2 1/2	2 1/2	2 1/2	2 1/2			
L. Hand	2 1/2	2 1/2	2 1/2	2 1/2	2 1/2			
R. Thigh	5 1/2	6 1/2	8 1/2	8 1/2	9 1/2			
L. Thigh	5 1/2	6 1/2	8 1/2	8 1/2	9 1/2			
R. Leg	5	5	5 1/2	6	7			
L. Leg	5	5	5 1/2	6	7			
R. Foot	3 1/2	3 1/2	3 1/2	3 1/2	3 1/2			
L. Foot	3 1/2	3 1/2	3 1/2	3 1/2	3 1/2			
					Total			

■ ● **FIGURE 116–4.** The Lund and Browder chart is used to assess and graphically document size and depth of the burn wound.

Table 116–2 ● ■ ■ **Criteria for Patient Transfer to a Specialized Burn Care Facility**

Inhalation injury
Burns >20% of the total body surface area (TBSA)
Full-thickness burns >5% TBSA
Burns >10% TBSA in children younger than 10 years and adults older than 50 years
Burns of the face, hands, or genitalia
Chemical burns
Electrical burns

Data from Kinney MR, Dunbar SB, Brooks-Brunn J, Molter N, Vitello-Cicciu JM, eds. *AACN's Clinical Reference for Critical Care Nursing.* 4th ed. St. Louis, Mo: Mosby; 1998. Gordon M, Goodwin CW. Burn management. Initial assessment, management, and stabilization. *Nurs Clin N Am.* 1997;32:237–249.

signs of nerve compression, especially with an electrical injury. The treatment is a fasciotomy.[4]

- Small, intact blisters are sometimes left at the discretion of the burn team; if they are larger than 1 in or broken, they should be débrided to decrease the risk of infection (Fig. 116–6).[3]

- Survival rates for burn patients are markedly improved with early excision and grafting.[4–6, 12] However, the most important indicators of mortality continue to be patient age and the extent of the burn, with the presence of inhalation injury and comorbidity being crucial factors.[6, 9, 13] Even though the burn wound has the most obvious

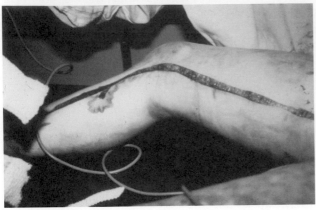

■ ● **FIGURE 116–5.** Escharotomy of the leg to improve circulation.

potential for infection, the lower respiratory tract is the most common site of infection and carries the highest incidence of sepsis and death.[6]

- Topical antimicrobial agents limit bacterial proliferation and fungal colonization in burn wounds.[3, 12] The three most commonly used agents are mafenide acetate (Sulfamylon), silver sulfadiazine (Silvadene), or 0.5% silver nitrate solution (Table 116–3). Nystatin is sometimes added to mafenide acetate to reduce the incidence of candidal growth.

- Attention to specialty areas includes the following: Hair on and around the burn wound, except the eyebrows, should be shaved for infection control purposes;[3, 4] ears are prone to infection and so require careful attention to prevent pressure that will inhibit perfusion. Sulfamylon cream is used because it penetrates eschar well;[3, 4] a burn of the eyelid or other eye involvement requires an ophthalmology consult and the application of artificial tears or ointment to keep the corneas moist.

- The two methods of wound care are the open method and the closed method.

  ❖ Open method—antimicrobial without dressing. Advantages include continuous wound observation and no bulky dressings to inhibit movement of joints.

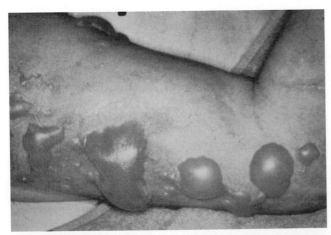

■ ● **FIGURE 116–6.** Blisters of a partial-thickness burn wound on the arm.

Disadvantages include the need to reapply antimicrobial frequently to keep wound covered, that the sight may be more upsetting for the patient and the family, that more caution is needed not to contaminate the uncovered wound, and that the exposure of the wound to air is more painful. This is not a good option for a patient who can get out of bed.

  ❖ Closed method—antimicrobial with dressing. Advantages include the reduction of evaporative water loss, reduction of heat loss, and reduction of pain secondary to nerve endings being exposed to air. Disadvantages include a longer time for wound care, a warm moist environment for bacterial growth, and a decrease in the patient's mobility. This method is necessary if wet dressings are being used.[4]

- Most burn centers use clean technique for dressing removal and wound cleansing, using sterile technique for sterile dressing application only.[14]

- An autograft (skin graft taken from the same person) is the only treatment that can heal a full-thickness burn wound. Deep partial-thickness burn wounds may be surgically converted to full-thickness wounds and covered with an autograft to reduce healing time and thus the risk of complications.[5]

- Artificial skin and other options for wound coverage are currently under study. Growth hormones show promise in reducing wound healing time.[3, 5, 11]

- Granulation tissue refers to a pink, healthy wound bed. This tissue is ready to accept an autograft. If there is a need to wait for grafting, a biologic dressing may be used to protect the wound and promote further vascularization. Biologic dressings include homografts or allografts (human skin from donors) and heterografts or xenografts (nonhuman skin, usually from pigs).[4]

- The burn patient is hypermetabolic until burn wounds are closed and healing is complete.[4, 15] This is important to note because the patient's baseline body temperature will be higher than normal by 1°F to 2°F[3, 11] (observe for temperature spikes rather than an absolute number). The patient will also be catabolic (resting energy expenditure can increase by as much as 100%),[4] requiring an increased caloric and protein intake for wound healing. It is important to keep the patient warm during wound care because a large amount of heat is lost from the wound and this, plus shivering, will further increase the metabolic rate.[3, 15]

- An individualized plan for pain control should be in place for both background pain (pain that is continuously present) and procedural pain (increased intermittent pain related to procedures and routine care). Unrelieved pain can lead to stress-related immunosuppression, an increased potential for infection, delayed wound healing, and depression.[1, 2] Subcutaneous and intramuscular injections should be avoided because absorption will be poor and unreliable as a result of edema.[7] Intravenous administration of medication is preferred in critically ill patients; oral medication is preferred in noncritical patients with a functioning gastrointestinal system. As the wound heals, the patient will experience more discomfort from itchiness and less discomfort from pain. A water-based lotion will prevent drying and reduce urticaria.

Table 116–3 ●■■ **Topical Antimicrobial Agents**

Agent	Activity	Advantages	Disadvantages
Mafenide acetate (Sulfamylon)	Broad spectrum against gram-positive and gram-negative organisms	Highly soluble and penetrates eschar well (agent of choice for ears); persistent activity against *Pseudomonas*	Painful for 20 to 30 min after application; may cause metabolic acidosis (through carbonic anhydrase inhibition) and hyperventilation; systemic absorption; infrequent hypersensitivity; may see yeast overgrowth; do not use with sulfa allergy
Silver nitrate 0.5%	Effective against a wide spectrum of pathogens including fungal infections	Painless application; evaporative heat loss is decreased by use of dressings; no resistant organism reported	Poor eschar penetration. Stains unburned tissue and any object with which it comes in contact brown-black. May be associated with alkalosis, water loading, and loss of electrolytes through wound (eg, hyponatremia). Dressings need to be resoaked about every 2 hr
Silver sulfadiazine (Silvadene)	Good activity for both gram-positive and gram-negative organisms and fungus	Painless application; convenient for outpatient use	Transient leukopenia; only partial eschar penetration; infrequent hypersensitivity; may macerate surrounding tissues; contraindicated for pregnant women, nursing mothers, and infants younger than 2 mo

- Burn wounds contract during the healing phase.[16] Continuing mobility and proper positioning are vital to prevent contractures and loss of function. Self-care and range-of-motion exercises should be encouraged. Once the wounds heal, pressure garments need to be worn at all times, except during bathing, to reduce scar formation.[11, 12]

- The burn wound should not be exposed to the sun for a year. Some scarring will be present; skin discoloration will slowly improve over the first year.

- Emergency treatment of thermal burns includes removal of the burning agent, removal of any clothes near the burn, and covering of the burned area with a clean dry sheet. Towels with cool water can be applied for 5 to 10 minutes; longer application can lead to hypothermia and further damage by causing vasoconstriction.

- Chemical burns can be caused by contact with acids or bases, or fumes can cause an inhalation injury. The type of agent and duration of contact determine depth of burn. Immediate treatment is removing the chemical agent from contact with the skin (removing contaminated clothes), brushing off any dry chemical, and rinsing with copious amounts of water for at least 30 minutes or until the pain has stopped.[10] No attempt should be made to neutralize the agent because this creates a chemical reaction that releases heat, further damaging the skin. Certain chemicals present the additional complication that they can be absorbed into the central circulation, causing further damage.[4] The local poison control center should be contacted to see if further treatment is indicated.

- The entry site of an electrical burn is usually small (Fig. 116–7), whereas the tremendous force at the exit site creates a larger wound. In between, electricity causes destruction while traveling through the body via nerves and blood vessels. Although electrical injuries are much less common than thermal injuries, electrical injuries are much more complex and are associated with higher morbidity and mortality.[4] Because most destruction is internal, it is more difficult to judge the extent of damage and fluid resuscitation. The patient needs to be monitored for 24 hours for cardiac dysrhythmias.[4] Myoglobin, from the breakdown of damaged muscle, can clog nephrons and lead to renal failure. Myoglobinuria is characterized by port wine–colored urine. The urine output should be kept greater than 100 mL per hour until the urine is negative for myoglobin to help flush the myoglobin through the kidneys.[4]

EQUIPMENT

- Personal protective equipment
- Examination gloves
- Sterile gloves
- Warm tap water
- Mild liquid soap, as ordered
- Normal saline (NS)
- Basins
- Washcloths
- Waterproof pads or towels
- Scissors and forceps (clean and sterile)
- Topical agents, as ordered
- Tongue depressors
- Sterile dressings as needed (eg, fine mesh gauze, Exu-dry)
- Gauze rolls
- Linen
- Pillows or elastic net sling
- Pain and sedation medication (as prescribed)

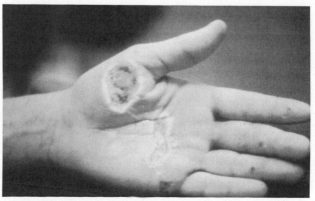

■ ● **FIGURE 116–7.** Entry site of an electrical burn.

Additional equipment (to have available depending on patient need) includes the following:

- Tracheostomy ties or other method to hold endotracheal tube or tracheostomy tube in place
- Cotton-tipped swabs to clean crevices of ears

PATIENT AND FAMILY EDUCATION

- Explain the procedure for wound care to patient and family. ➨*Rationale:* Diminishes fear of the unknown; patient is knowledgeable about care.
- Teach patient and family about pain control; assess the patient's personal acceptable level of pain. ➨*Rationale:* Decreases concerns about pain, facilitates individualized pain relief plan, and fosters cooperation with care.
- Inform patient and family that superficial partial-thickness burns generally heal in 7 to 14 days with minimal scarring[3] but that the burn wound should not be exposed to the sun for a year after the burn. Also, discoloration may be present for up to a year after the burn. ➨*Rationale:* Reduces anxiety about appearance.
- Discuss the importance of mobility and proper positioning (ie, splinting) on function. Self-care (activities of daily living) and range-of-motion exercises should be encouraged during the healing phase. ➨*Rationale:* Prevents contractures associated with healing skin, improper positioning, and immobility.[12, 16]
- Assess the family's ability to provide care at home. ➨*Rationale:* Continued care of the wound will be required after discharge.
- Provide detailed wound care instructions in writing, and review them with patient and family. Demonstrate exactly what to do, and have patient and family return the demonstration a week before the planned discharge. Continue to involve patient and family in wound care for the remainder of the admission and encourage them to ask questions. Provide positive feedback. Arrange for home care or clinic visits to follow up on wound care. ➨*Rationale:* Validates patient and family understanding and ability to perform wound care and allows time for them to develop a level of comfort. Provides the opportunity to reinforce important points.
- Teach patient and family about pain and pruritus medications as needed. Provide the name of a water-based lotion to apply to healed areas. ➨*Rationale:* Supports comfort at home.
- Teach patient and family about signs and symptoms of infection and the importance of reporting these in a timely manner. ➨*Rationale:* Patient and family will recognize problems early so that appropriate measures can be instituted by the health care professional.
- Stress the importance of wearing pressure garments and splints. ➨*Rationale:* Reduces scar formation.[3, 11, 12]
- Inform patient and family that nightmares, alterations in body image, and psychologic disturbances are experienced by many burned patients. Provide resources, including someone to follow up with, if desired. ➨*Rationale:* Increases awareness of these problems and reassures patient and family that what patient is experiencing is not abnormal.

- Provide patient and family with follow-up appointments and someone to call if there is a problem. ➨*Rationale:* Provides necessary information for further care and follow-up.

PATIENT ASSESSMENT AND PREPARATION

Patient Assessment

- Assess vital signs, including temperature. ➨*Rationale:* Baseline vital signs will allow for comparison during and following the procedure to evaluate patient tolerance and need for pain medication.
- Evaluate for signs of healing.
  - ❖ Decreased pain
  - ❖ Dressing separating at wound edges with reepithelialization beneath
  - ❖ Decreased edema
- Compare level of healing with expected level of healing for number of days post burn. ➨*Rationale:* Healing should occur within a predictable time frame determined by the depth of burns unless there are complications.
- Evaluate for signs and symptoms of infection.
  - ❖ Foul odor
  - ❖ Purulent drainage
  - ❖ Increased pain
  - ❖ Increasing edema
  - ❖ Cellulitis
  - ❖ Fever
  - ❖ Development of eschar or early eschar separation
  - ❖ Increase in burn size or depth
  - ❖ Blurring of wound edges

  ➨*Rationale:* Healing should occur within a predicted time frame depending on depth of burns unless there are complications.

- Monitor for distal circulation (pulses, pain, color, sensation, movement, and capillary refill) to areas with circumferential burns and increased edema. ➨*Rationale:* Edema and circumferential burns impede distal circulation and cause worsening tissue perfusion and cell death.
- Determine acceptable level of pain for the patient through discussion with the patient. Then, evaluate the adequacy of the pain control regimen by asking the patient to rate the pain on a scale of 0 to 10, both before wound care (background) and during the dressing change.[1, 2, 7] ➨*Rationale:* An individualized plan for pain control should be in place for background and procedural pain. In addition to the traditional use of pain and anxiety medications, alternative therapies should be included (eg, relaxation techniques, massage therapy, music therapy). The patient's needs will change based on changes in the wound (eg, healing, debridement, conversion to deeper wound).
- Evaluate patient's general level of function, particularly in burned areas. ➨*Rationale:* An individualized plan for range-of-motion exercises, positioning, and splinting should be made to optimize the patient's level of function. Burns contract during the healing phase, and immobility enhances loss of function.[12, 16]

Patient Preparation

- Ensure that patient understands preprocedural teaching. Answer questions as they arise, and reinforce information as needed.   ➥*Rationale:* Evaluates and reinforces understanding of previously taught information.
- Notify other appropriate health care professionals who need to assess the burn wound (eg, physician) or perform a task (eg, quantitative wound biopsies, range-of-motion exercises by physical therapist) of time of dressing change.

➥*Rationale:* Organization of care allows important assessment and intervention to take place without causing extra pain and stress to the patient.
- After checking what was previously needed for patient comfort during the dressing change, premedicate the patient with pain medication and any sedation that is ordered an appropriate amount of time before starting wound care.   ➥*Rationale:* Allows time for medication to take effect and promotes optimal comfort for the patient.[1, 2]

| Procedure | for Care of Burn Wounds |

Steps	Rationale	Special Considerations
1. Prepare all necessary equipment and supplies.	Preparation facilitates efficient wound care and prevents needless delays.	
2. Wash hands, and don cap, mask, goggles, gown, and examination gloves for each health care person involved in the procedure.	Reduces transmission of microorganisms to the patient; standard precautions.	
3. Remove old dressings, and discard them in barrier waste. Place towel or pad under exposed extremity.	Old dressings can contain large amounts of body secretions and blood. A field under the extremity will allow the patient a place to rest the extremity during care.	Remove dressings only from areas that can be redressed within 20 to 30 minutes at one time. Finish wound care to these areas before moving to new areas (decreases heat loss and pain related to nerve endings being exposed to air).
4. Remove and discard gloves, and don a pair of clean gloves.	Used gloves are contaminated by handling of the burn dressing. Clean gloves are needed for wound care.	
5. Wash wound with mild soap solution (if ordered), rinse with warm tap water, and pat dry.	Cleanses wound of debris by mechanical débridement and reduces microorganisms.[16]	Cleanse beyond wound to reduce microbial count on surrounding tissue. Patients may do better if allowed to cleanse their own wounds.
6. Use scissors and forceps to remove loose necrotic tissue and to remove any tissue over broken blisters.	Bacteria proliferate in necrotic tissue.[16]	Typically, physicians perform this function in hospitals that do not specialize in burn wound care.
7. Assess the burn wound for color, size, odor, depth, drainage, bleeding, edema, cellulitis, epithelial budding, eschar separation, sensation, movement, peripheral pulses, and any signs of pressure areas from splints. For wet dressings, proceed to step 10.	Validates the healing process and identifies complications.	Other disciplines that need to observe the wound should be notified ahead of time so that they can be present while the wound is uncovered.
8. Remove and discard gloves. Apply sterile gloves.	Gloves are contaminated from burn wound care. Sterile gloves should be used for application of the sterile dressing.	
9. Use sterile tongue depressor to remove required amount of topical agent from container. Place on sterile surface before applying ⅛-in layer directly to burn wound and covering with burn dressing, or apply ⅛-in layer on burn dressing and cover wound. Proceed to step 13 to continue wound care.	Using sterile tongue depressor and removing only what is needed from container prevent contamination of topical agent.	If the area to be covered has folds and crevices, or if the wound consists of scattered areas, topical agents should be placed directly on the wound, rather than on the burn dressing (ensures good coverage without applying unnecessary amounts of an absorbable topical agent to uninjured areas).

Procedure continued on following page

Procedure for Care of Burn Wounds *Continued*

Steps	Rationale	Special Considerations
10. Pour prescribed solution into sterile bowl, and drop in sterile gauze pads.		Wet dressings must be moistened every 4 hours. Wet-to-dry dressings over eschar are removed dry every 8 to 12 hours. If dressing is adherent to epithelial buds or granulation tissue, wet the dressing with sterile NS to loosen.
11. Remove and discard gloves. Apply sterile gloves.	Gloves are contaminated from burn wound care. Sterile gloves should be used for application of the sterile dressing.	
12. Squeeze excess solution from gauze, and place dressing on wound.		
13. Loosely wrap extremities with gauze rolls.	Holds dressings in place.	Wrap extremities from distal to proximal. Check pulses and capillary refill after wrapping to ensure circulation is not compromised.
14. Assess need for more pain medication before continuing. *(Level II: Theory based, no research data to support recommendations; recommendations from expert consensus group may exist)*	Patients have a right to good pain control. The success or failure of pain control for the current dressing change will affect the way the patient responds to future dressing changes.[1, 2, 10]	
15. Repeat steps starting at step 3 until all burn wounds have been cared for.	Isolating areas for dressing changes prevents unnecessary temperature loss, pain from increased nerve ending exposure to air movement, and cross-contamination of wounds.	The size of the team doing the dressing and the amount of débridement time required will determine how much of the wound should reasonably be exposed at any given time.
16. Apply splints as needed and elevate burned extremities with pillows or elastic net sling or both; elevate head of bed. *(Level II: Theory based, no research data to support recommendations; recommendations from expert consensus group may exist)*	Maintains position of function, prevents contractures, and reduces edema and pain.[3, 10]	Do not "gatch" knees if popliteal space is burned. Do not put pillow under head if neck or ears are burned. Do not inhibit movement with splints if patient is awake and able to use involved extremity.
17. Remove and discard gloves. Wash hands.	Reduces transmission of microorganisms.	

Expected Outcomes

- Wounds heals without infectious complications.
- Patient maintains a self-identified acceptable level of pain relief.
- Patient attains comfort from measures taken for anxiety and itching.
- Patient and family verbalize knowledge of patient condition and plan of care.
- An optimal level of function is maintained or attained.
- Patient and family response and interactions demonstrate adaptation to injury.
- Patient and family collaborate in management of care.
- At the time of discharge, patient and family verbalize and demonstrate an understanding of posthospital care.

Unexpected Outcomes

- Wound converts to deeper injury.
- Wound sepsis occurs.
- Wound heals with unnecessary loss of function.

Patient Monitoring and Care

Patient Monitoring and Care	Rationale	Reportable Conditions
		These conditions should be reported if they persist despite nursing interventions.
1. Evaluate and treat the patient for pain. Ask the patient to rate on a scale of 0 to 10 what his or her pain is, check the orders for pain and sedation for dressing changes, check to see what the patient's medication requirements were with previous dressing changes and have that amount of medication available in the room before starting the dressing, assess the need for more medication throughout the dressing change. Incorporate alternative pain relief techniques (eg, relaxation techniques, massage therapy, music, visual imaging).	The burn patient will have baseline pain requiring pain medication and increased pain medication requirements and possibly sedation requirements for the pain involved in dressing changes.[1, 2] Attention to the patient's pain will foster the patient's trust in health care personnel to control pain and will promote cooperation with future burn wound care.	• Increased heart rate • Increased or decreased blood pressure • Increased respiratory rate • Verbalization of pain • Nonverbal indications of pain (restlessness, grimacing, teeth clenching) • Inability to cooperate with dressing change
2. Obtain baseline vital signs before procedure, monitor throughout procedure, and check for 30 minutes after procedure is complete.	Changes in vital signs can be an indication that the patient is experiencing pain or anxiety. Decreasing blood pressure, heart rate, and respiratory rate can be complications of pain medication (especially after dressing change is complete and stimulation has stopped).	• Increased or decreased heart rate • Increased or decreased blood pressure • Increased or decreased respiratory rate • High peak pressures on ventilator
3. Check patient's temperature before dressing change. Make sure patient environment is warm, keep portions of patient's body covered where not doing dressing change, and check temperature at end of dressing change.	Heat is lost through burn wounds.	• Hypothermia
4. Monitor peripheral pulses and circulation in the burned extremity during the dressing change, within 1 hour after applying dressing, and every 2 hours thereafter. Keep extremities elevated, and assess for increased edema.[10]	Circumferential burns can decrease or prevent blood flow to involved extremity; the dressing can be too tight, especially if edema increases.	• Increased peripheral edema • Decreased or absent pulses • Pain or numbness in extremity • Prolonged or absent capillary refill in extremity • Conversion to deeper burn wound
5. Assess the burn wound for color, size, odor, depth, drainage, bleeding, pain, early eschar separation, healing, and cellulitis in the surrounding tissue.	Observe for usual progression of wound healing versus complications of infection, progression of burn to deeper wound, and bleeding.	• Foul odor • Purulent or increased amounts of drainage • Patient spiking temperatures • Cellulitis • Healthy granulation tissue developing eschar • Increasing necrosis • Blurring of burn wound edges • Discoloration of wound • Early eschar separation • Bleeding

Continued on following page

Patient Monitoring and Care	Rationale	Reportable Conditions
6. Encourage exercise and activities of daily living; perform range-of-motion exercises during dressing changes; place patient in position of optimal function, using splints as needed to maintain. Use pain medication as needed to facilitate mobility.	Burns contract during the healing phase if not correctly splinted and exercised;[16] loss of function is a complication of immobility.[12] Pain inhibits patients from moving.[1,2]	• Contractures • Loss of function
7. Monitor patient's toleration of tube feedings or patient's ingestion of a high-calorie and high-protein diet with supplements; encourage nutritious diet and discourage empty calories.	Nutrition is necessary for wound healing; burn patients are hypermetabolic.[12]	• Refusal to eat or inability to ingest adequate amount of nutrition • Poor wound healing

Documentation

Documentation should include the following:

- Patient and family education
- Date and time of wound care
- Graph areas of burn, other wounds, and pressure ulcers
- Appearance of the wound (color, size, odor, depth, drainage, bleeding)
- Assessment of wound areas for level of pain (appropriate for depth and level of healing)
- Progression toward healing (eg, presence of epithelial budding)
- Evidence of cellulitis around the wound (red, warm, tender)
- Assessment of peripheral pulses; color, movement, sensation, and capillary refill distal to a circumferential wound or an extremity wrapped in dressings
- Assessment of pain before, during, and after procedure
- Medications given for pain and sedation
- Other comfort measures used
- Dressings and topical agents applied
- Patient's tolerance of the procedure
- Unexpected outcomes
- Nursing interventions

References

1. Ashburn MA. Burn pain: the management of procedure-related pain. *J Burn Care Rehabil.* 1995;16:365–371.
2. Ulmer JF. Burn pain management: a guideline-based approach. *J Burn Care Rehabil.* 1998;19:151–159.
3. Jordan BS, Harrington DT. Management of the burn wound. *Nurs Clin N Am.* 1997;32:251–273.
4. Greenfield E. Integumentary disorders. In: Kinney MR, Dunbar SB, Brooks-Brunn J, Molter N, Vitello-Cicciu JM, eds. *AACN's Clinical Reference for Critical Care Nursing.* 4th ed. St. Louis, Mo: Mosby; 1998:1065–1087.
5. Monafo WW. Initial management of burns. *N Engl J Med.* 1997; 335:1581–1586.
6. Mann R, Heimbach D. Prognosis and treatment of burns. *West J Med.* 1996;165:215–220.
7. Hooyman TG. Estimates of the probability of death from burn injuries. *N Engl J Med.* 1998; 338:1849–1850.
8. Nagel TR, Schunk JE. Using the hand to estimate the surface area of a burn in children. *Pediatr Emerg Care.* 1997;13:254–255.
9. Perry RJ, Moore CA, Morgan BD, Plummer DL. Determining the approximate area of a burn: an inconsistency investigated and re-evaluated. *BMJ.* 1996;313:690.
10. Gordon M, Goodwin CW. Burn management. Initial assessment, management, and stabilization. *Nurs Clin N Am.* 1997;32:237–249.
11. Nguyen TT, Gilpin DA, Meyer NA, Herndon DN. Current treatment of severely burned patients. *Ann Surg.* 1996;223:14–25.
12. Rose JK, Barrow RE, Desai MH, Herndon DN. Advances in burn care. *Adv Surg.* 1996;30:71–95.
13. Covington DS, Wainwright DJ, Parks DH. Prognostic indicators in the elderly patient with burns. *J Burn Care Rehabil.* 1996;17:222–230.
14. Herndon DN, ed. *Total Burn Care.* London: WB Saunders Company Ltd; 1996:548.
15. Cortiella J, Marvin JA. Management of the pediatric burn patient. *Nurs Clin N Am.* 1997;32:311–329.
16. Ward RS, Saffle JR. Topical agents in burn and wound care. *Phys Ther.* 1995;75:526–538.

Additional Readings

Carleton SC. Cardiac problems associated with burns. *Cardiol Clin.* 1995;13:257–262.

Herndon DN. Perspectives in the use of allograft. *J Burn Care Rehabil.* 1997;18:S6.

Kealey GP. Opioids and analgesia. *J Burn Care Rehabil.* 1995;16:363–364.

Kealey GP. Pharmacologic management of background pain in burn victims. *J Burn Care Rehabil.* 1995;16:358–362.

Monafo WW. Physiology of pain. *J Burn Care Rehabil.* 1995;16:345–347.

Sheridan RL, Petras L, Lydon M, Salvo PM. Once-daily wound cleansing and dressing change: efficacy and cost. *J Burn Care Rehabil.* 1997;18:139–140.

Ward CG. Burns. *J Am Coll Surg.* 1998;186:123–126.

Yeong EK, Mann R, Goldberg M, Engrav L, Heimbach D. Improved accuracy of burn wound assessment using laser Doppler. *J Trauma.* 1996;40:956–961.

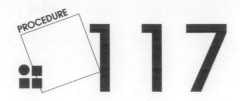
117

Care of Skin Grafts

PURPOSE: Skin-graft care is performed to promote graft take and function and to prevent infection.

Eileen E. Pysznik

PREREQUISITE NURSING KNOWLEDGE

- An autograft is a skin graft taken from the burn patient. It is the surgical removal of the epidermis and superficial dermis, creating a new, superficial, partial-thickness wound called a donor site.[1] The graft, a split-thickness skin graft (STSG), is applied over a clean, excised wound.
- An autograft is the only treatment that can heal a large, full-thickness burn wound. Autografts are frequently used over deep partial-thickness burn wounds after surgically converting the wound to full thickness to reduce healing time and thus the risk of complications.[1]
- It is common to mesh the STSG (Fig. 117–1) so that it can be stretched to cover approximately 1.5 to 3 times more surface area than the original donor site. The goals following a meshed graft placement are to protect the wound bed from infection and drying and to ensure that there is no movement of the graft while it is becoming vascularized. Either a barrier dressing (eg, Biobrane, allograft) protects the wound with or without a bulky dressing added, or a minimal stick-layer dressing (eg, Xeroform) is used with a bulky dressing acting as the barrier to infection and drying. The spaces created by meshing, the interstices, fill in with epithelial cells from the graft. Because of cosmetic and functional concerns related to

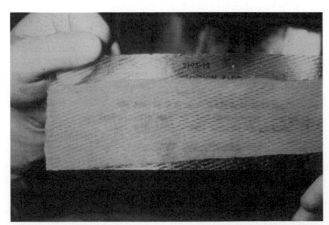

■ ● FIGURE 117–1. Meshed split-thickness skin graft.

appearance and increased shrinkage, meshed grafts are not used on the face and are avoided over joints.
- If the STSG is not meshed, it is called a sheet graft. A sheet graft covers the same amount of surface area as the donor site and is used for cosmetic or functional reasons. Pockets of serous fluid or blood tend to accumulate under these grafts (the interstices of meshed grafts allow the fluid to escape), separating the graft from the wound bed that is vital for blood supply. It is imperative to evacuate this fluid. If the sheet graft has been in place for less than 48 hours and the fluid is near the edge of sheet graft, the fluid can be rolled to the edge and out. However, doing this with a graft beginning to vascularize can disrupt the attachment. Therefore, practice should be to make a small nick in the sheet graft over the area of fluid accumulation and gently express the fluid through the hole.[2] In either case, the fluid should be gently wiped away with gauze dampened with sterile normal saline (NS) or sterile water.
- Cultured epidermal autografts are commercially available and are an option when the patient does not have enough unburned tissue for donor sites to cover the burn in a reasonable period of time.[1] Cultured epidermal autografts are grown from a sample of the patient's own epidermal cells in a laboratory. However, the cost is prohibitive, and successful take of the graft is much more likely if the burn team has experience with this treatment.[1, 3]
- Artificial skin and other options for wound coverage are currently under study.[4, 5]
- In the operating room, all nonviable tissue is surgically excised to create a wound bed able to support a skin graft (Fig. 117–2). Therefore, the grafted area should be observed for bleeding for the first 24 hours.
- The graft is usually stapled or sutured in place or secured with Steri-Strips, covered with a nonadherent dressing, and padded with a bulky dressing to prevent displacement of the graft.
- The first dressing change is usually done after 3 to 5 days. Most burn centers use clean technique for dressing removal and donor-site cleansing and use sterile technique for dressing application only.[6]
- Leg grafts must be supported with Ace wraps or other compressive dressings for the first 3 to 5 days after

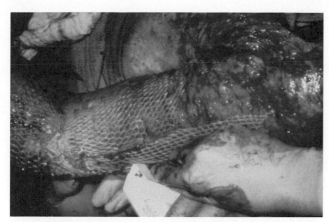

■ ● FIGURE 117–2. Meshed split-thickness skin graft covering the arm, with the remainder of the wound bed ready to be grafted.

surgery to prevent capillary engorgement and hematoma formation beneath the graft.

- Initial healing of the grafted area should occur in 7 to 10 days, with vascularization occurring in the first 4 to 5 days. The graft area is immobilized for 4 to 5 days to prevent dislocation and shearing.
- Signs of graft take include vascularization of the graft, reepithelialization of the interstices, decreased pain, and adherence of the graft. Signs of complications include graft necrosis, graft loss, cellulitis, purulent drainage, and fever.
- Skin grafts contract during the healing phase.[7] Continuing mobility and proper positioning are vital to prevent contractures and loss of function. Self-care and range-of-motion exercises should be encouraged as soon as the graft is adherent. Once the wounds heal, pressure garments need to be worn at all times, except during bathing, to reduce scar formation.[3, 5]
- An individualized plan for pain control should be in place for both background pain (pain that is continuously present) and procedural pain (increased intermittent pain related to procedures and routine care). Unrelieved pain can lead to stress-related immunosuppression, increased potential for infection, delayed wound healing, and depression.[8, 9] Subcutaneous and intramuscular injections should be avoided when edema is present because absorption will be poor and unreliable.[10] Intravenous administration of medication is preferred in critically ill patients; oral medication is preferred in noncritical patients with a functioning gastrointestinal system. As the wound heals, the patient will experience more discomfort from itchiness and less discomfort from pain. A water-based lotion will prevent drying and reduce urticaria.
- The burn patient is hypermetabolic until burn wounds are closed and healing is complete.[1, 11] This is important to note because the patient's baseline body temperature will be higher than normal by 1°F to 2°F[2, 5] (observe for temperature spikes rather than an absolute number), and the patient will be catabolic (resting energy expenditure can increase by as much as 100%),[1] requiring an increased caloric and protein intake for wound healing. It is important to keep the patient warm during wound care

because a large amount of heat is lost from the wound, further increasing the metabolic rate.[2, 11]

- The skin graft should not be exposed to the sun for a year. Some scarring will be present, and skin discoloration will slowly improve over the first year.

EQUIPMENT

- Personal protective equipment
- Examination gloves
- Sterile gloves
- Scissors and forceps
- Warm tap water (sometimes sterile water or sterile NS are used for first dressing change)
- Basin
- Clean washcloths
- Staple remover
- Nonadherent gauze (eg, Adaptic, Xeroform)
- Bulky or thin dressings, as needed
- Pain and sedation medication (as prescribed)

Additional equipment (to have available depending on patient need) includes the following:

- Splints secured with gauze roll or Velcro
- Towels or waterproof pads

PATIENT AND FAMILY EDUCATION

- Explain the procedure for skin graft care to patient and family. ➶*Rationale:* Diminishes fear of the unknown; ensures that patient and family are knowledgeable about graft care.
- Inform patient and family that the grafted area needs to be immobilized for 5 to 7 days to foster graft take and reduce the risk of shearing. ➶*Rationale:* Increases patient's and family's assistance in maintaining immobilization.
- Inform patient and family that the skin graft should not be exposed to the sun for a year after the burn; there will be some scarring and discoloration that will improve over the first year. ➶*Rationale:* Prepares patient and family for changes that will be present after hospital discharge and addresses anxieties about body image.
- Discuss the importance of proper positioning. Explain the need for continuing mobility through self-care and range-of-motion exercises as soon as the graft is adherent and throughout the healing phase. ➶*Rationale:* Prevents contractures and loss of function associated with healing skin grafts.[3, 7]
- Assess family's ability to provide care at home. ➶*Rationale:* Continued care of the wound will be required after discharge.
- As appropriate, provide detailed wound care instructions in writing and review with patient and family. Demonstrate exactly what to do and have patient and family return the demonstration before the planned discharge. Continue to involve patient and family in the wound care for the remainder of the admission, and encourage them to ask questions. Provide positive feedback. Arrange for home care or clinic visits to follow up on dressings and wound care. ➶*Rationale:* Validates patient's and family's understanding and ability to perform wound care and allows time for them to develop a level of comfort. Provides the opportunity to reinforce important points.
- Teach patient and family about pain and pruritus medica-

tions as needed, and provide the name of a water-based lotion to apply to healed areas. ➤**Rationale:** Supports comfort at home.
- Teach patient and family about signs and symptoms of infection and the importance of reporting in a timely manner. ➤**Rationale:** Patient and family will recognize problems early so that appropriate measures can be instituted by the health care team.
- Stress the importance of wearing pressure garments and splints. ➤**Rationale:** Reduces scar formation and contractures.[2, 3, 5]
- Provide patient and family with follow-up appointments and the name of someone to call if there is a problem. ➤**Rationale:** Provides necessary information for further care and follow-up.

PATIENT ASSESSMENT AND PREPARATION

Patient Assessment

- Assess vital signs, including temperature. ➤**Rationale:** Baseline vital signs will allow for comparison during and following the procedure to evaluate patient tolerance and need for pain medication.
- Evaluate graft take.
  - ❖ Vascularization of the graft
  - ❖ Reepithelialization of the interstices
  - ❖ Decreased pain
  - ❖ Adherence of the graft
- Monitor for signs of complications.
  - ❖ Graft necrosis
  - ❖ Graft loss
  - ❖ Cellulitis
  - ❖ Purulent drainage
  - ❖ Fever
- Compare level of healing to expected level of healing for number of days after skin graft. ➤**Rationale:** Initial healing of grafted area should occur in 7 to 10 days.

- Determine adequacy of the pain control regimen by asking the patient to rate the pain on a scale of 0 to 10, both before wound care (background) and during the dressing change.[8-10] ➤**Rationale:** An individualized plan for pain control should be in place for background and procedural pain. In addition to the traditional use of pain and anxiety medications, alternative therapies should be included (eg, relaxation techniques, massage therapy, music therapy). The patient's medication requirements should decrease as the grafted area heals.
- Assess patient's level of function in the grafted area. ➤**Rationale:** Skin grafts contract during the healing phase, and immobility enhances loss of function. The patient should be encouraged to continue normal movement and range-of-motion exercises after graft take has been established.[3]

Patient Preparation

- Ensure that patient understands preprocedural teaching. Answer questions as they arise, and reinforce information as needed. ➤**Rationale:** Evaluates and reinforces understanding of previously taught information.
- Notify other appropriate health care professionals who need to assess the burn wound (eg, physician) or perform a task (eg, range-of-motion exercises by physical therapist) of the time of dressing change. ➤**Rationale:** Organization of care allows important assessment and intervention to take place without causing extra pain and stress to the patient.
- After checking what was previously needed for patient comfort during the dressing change, premedicate the patient with pain medication and any sedation that is ordered an appropriate amount of time before starting wound care.[8, 9] ➤**Rationale:** Allows time for medication to take effect and promotes optimal comfort for the patient. Reduces pain and anxiety. Encourages patient trust and compliance with procedure.[10]

Procedure **for Care of Skin Grafts**

Steps	Rationale	Special Considerations
1. Prepare all necessary equipment and supplies.	Preparation facilitates efficient wound care and prevents needless delays.	
2. Wash hands, and don cap, mask, gown, and examination gloves for each health care person involved in the procedure.	Reduces transmission of microorganisms to the patient; standard precautions.	
3. Remove bulky, outer dressings and discard. Place sterile towel or pad under exposed extremity.	Old dressings can contain large amounts of body secretions and blood. Sterile towel allows a place for patient to rest extremity during care.	Initial dressing is commonly left in place for 3 to 5 days, or bulky, outer dressings are changed while leaving nonadherent gauze in place (check orders).
4. Remove and discard gloves, and don a pair of clean gloves.	Examination gloves are contaminated by handling the burn dressing, and clean gloves are needed for wound care.	
5. Gently lift nonadherent gauze from grafted site, anchoring graft in place as needed. Note: surgeon may staple on dressing that is to remain in place until skin graft heals (eg, Biobrane).	Grafts are not firmly attached to the wound bed and can be pulled loose for up to 5 days after grafting.	Warm tap water may be used to loosen dressings stuck to graft area.

Steps	Rationale	Special Considerations
6. Gently rinse graft site and surrounding tissue with warm tap water and gauze or wash cloths.	Cleanses wound of exudate and reduces microorganisms.[7]	Special care is necessary not to displace skin graft.
7. Use scissors and forceps to remove loose necrotic tissue.[2] If it is a sheet graft, check for and remove any pockets of fluid under the graft.	Clears debris that can harbor microorganisms.[7] Pockets of fluid will separate the graft from the wound bed that is vital for blood supply, causing the graft not to take in that area.	Remove pockets of fluid. If the sheet graft has been in place for less than 48 hours and the fluid is near the edge of sheet graft, roll the fluid to the edge and out; otherwise, make a small nick in the sheet graft over the area of fluid accumulation and gently express the fluid through the hole.[2] Gently remove exudate with gauze dampened with sterile NS or sterile water.
8. Remove staples that are no longer needed to hold graft or dressing in place.	Prevents embedding of staples, local irritation, and infection.[2]	Staples can gradually be removed starting 4 to 5 days after grafting.
9. Assess graft for progression of healing and for complications.	Validates the healing process and identifies complications.	Notify other disciplines that need to observe the wound ahead of time so that they can be present while the wound is uncovered.
10. Apply nonadherent dressing (if interstices are open), cover with bulky dressings, and secure; or apply moisturizer to healed adherent graft areas where interstices are closed and cover with thin dressings to promote mobility.	Protects graft while healing.	A water-based lotion is used to prevent drying and reduce itching when interstices are closed.
11. Apply splints and elevate hands with pillows or elastic net sling; elevate head of bed.	Maintains position of function,[10] prevents contractures, and reduces edema[2] and pain.	If possible, prevent patient from lying on grafted areas. After the intitial period of immobilization, splints are used only when the patient is unable to participate in range-of-motion exercises or self-care.
12. Remove and discard gloves. Wash hands.	Reduces transmission of microorganisms.	

- Graft take of >90% is attained.
- Patient maintains a self-identified acceptable level of pain relief.
- Patient attains comfort from measures taken for anxiety and itching.
- Patient and family verbalize knowledge of patient condition and plan of care.
- An optimal level of function is maintained or attained.
- Patient and family response and interactions demonstrate adaptation to injury.
- Patient and family collaborate in management of care.
- At the time of discharge, patient and family verbalize and demonstrate an understanding of posthospital care.

- Bleeding
- Infection
- Graft loss

Patient Monitoring and Care

Patient Monitoring and Care	Rationale	Reportable Conditions
		These conditions should be reported if they persist despite nursing interventions.
1. Evaluate and treat the patient for pain. Ask the patient to rate on a scale of 0 to 10 what her or his pain is; check the orders for pain and sedation for dressing changes; check to see what the patient's medication requirements were with previous dressing changes and have that amount of medication available in the room before starting the dressing; assess the need for more medication throughout the dressing change. Incorporate alternative pain relief techniques (eg, relaxation techniques, massage therapy, music therapy, visual imaging). *(Level II: Theory based, on research data to support recommendations; recomendations from expert consensus group may exist)*	The patient with new skin grafts will have some baseline pain that requires pain medication and increased pain medication requirements and possibly sedation requirements for the procedural pain involved in graft care.[8, 9] Attention to the patient's pain fosters the patient's trust in health care personnel to control pain and promotes cooperation with future graft care.	• Increased heart rate • Increased or decreased blood pressure • Increased respiratory rate • Verbalization of pain • Nonverbal indications of pain (restlessness, grimacing, teeth clenching) • Inability to cooperate with dressing change
2. Obtain baseline vital signs before graft care, monitor throughout procedure, and check for 30 minutes after procedure is complete.	Changes in vital signs can be an indication that the patient is experiencing pain or anxiety. Decreasing blood pressure, heart rate, and respiratory rate can be complications of pain medication (especially after dressing change is complete and stimulation has stopped).	• Increased or decreased heart rate • Increased or decreased blood pressure • Increased or decreased respiratory rate • High peak pressures on ventilator
3. Assess graft site for appearance (eg, color, drainage, bleeding, graft necrosis, graft loss, cellulitis) and progression toward healing (eg, vascularization of the graft, reepithelialization of the interstices, decreased pain, adherence of the graft).	Observe for usual progression of wound healing verus complications.	• Foul odor • Purulent or increased amounts of drainage • Cellulitis • Hematoma or fluid collection under sheet grafts • Graft necrosis • Sloughing • Bleeding
4. Place patient in position of optimal function during initial period of immobilization of newly grafted areas, using splints to maintain. After the first 5 days, encourage exercise, activities of daily living, and range-of-motion exercises during dressing changes. Use pain medication as needed to facilitate mobility.	Grafted skin contracts during the healing phase if not correctly splinted and exercised;[3, 7] loss of function is a complication of immobility. Pain inhibits patients from moving.[8, 9]	• Contractures • Loss of function
5. Monitor patient's tolerance of tube feedings or patient's ingestion of a high-calorie and high-protein diet with supplements; encourage nutritious diet and discourage empty calories.	Nutrition is necessary for wound healing;[3] burn patients are hypermetabolic.	• Poor wound healing • Graft loss

Documentation

> Documentation should include the following:
>
> - Patient and family education
> - Date and time of graft care
> - Appearance (eg, color, drainage, bleeding, graft necrosis, sloughing, cellulitis)
> - Progression toward healing (eg, adherence and vascularization of the graft, reepithelialization of the interstices, decreased pain)
>
> - Dressings and topicals applied
> - Assessment of pain before, during, and after procedure
> - Medications given for pain and sedation
> - Other comfort measures used
> - Patient's tolerance of the procedure
> - Unexpected outcomes
> - Nursing interventions

References

1. Greenfield E. Integumentary disorders. In: Kinney MR, Dunbar SB, Brooks-Brunn J, Molter N, Vitello-Cicciu JM, eds. *AACN's Clinical Reference for Critical Care Nursing.* 4th ed. St. Louis, Mo: Mosby; 1998:1065–1087.
2. Jordan BS, Harrington DT. Management of the burn wound. *Nurs Clin North Am.* 1997;32:251–273.
3. Rose JK, Barrow RE, Desai MH, Herndon DN. Advances in burn care. *Adv Surg.* 1996;30:71–95.
4. Mann R, Heimbach D. Prognosis and treatment of burns. *West J Med.* 1996;165:215–220.
5. Nguyen TT, Gilpin DA, Meyer NA, Herndon DN. Current treatment of severely burned patients. *Ann Surg* 1996;223:14–25.
6. Herndon DN, ed. *Total Burn Care.* London: WB Saunders Company Ltd; 1996:548.
7. Ward RS, Saffle JR. Topical agents in burn and wound care. *Phys Ther.* 1995;75:526–538.
8. Ashburn MA. Burn pain: the management of procedure-related pain. *J Burn Care Rehabil.* 1995;16:365–371.
9. Ulmer JF. Burn pain management: a guideline-based approach. *J Burn Care Rehabil.* 1998;19:151–159.
10. Gordon M, Goodwin CW. Burn management. Initial assessment, management, and stabilization. *Nurs Clin North Am.* 1997;32:237–249.
11. Cortiella J, Marvin JA. Management of the pediatric burn patient. *Nurs Clin North Am.* 1997;32:311–3239.

Additional Readings

Best T, Lobay G, Moysa G, Tredget E. A prospective randomized trial of absorbable staple fixation of skin grafts for burn wound coverage. *J Trauma.* 1995;38:915–919.

Blackburn JH II, Boemi L, Hall WW, et al. Negative pressure dressings as a bolster for skin grafts. *Ann Plast Surg.* 1998;40:453–457.

El Hadidy M, Tesauro P, Cavallini M, Colonna M, Rizzo F, Signorini M. Contraction and growth of deep burn wounds covered by non-meshed and meshed split thickness skin grafts in humans. *Burns.* 1994;20:226–228.

Mann R, Heimbach D. Prognosis and treatment of burns. *West J Med.* 1996;165:215–220.

McCain D, Sutherland S. Nursing essentials: skin grafts for patients with burns. *Am J Nurs.* 1998;98:34–38.

Monafo WW. Initial management of burns. *N Engl J Med.* 1997;335:1581–1586.

Ward CG. Burns. *J Am Coll Surg.* 1998;186:123–126.

Young T, Fowler A. Nursing management of skin grafts and donor sites. *Br J Nurs.* 1998;7:324–326, 328, 330.

PROCEDURE

118

Intracompartment Pressure Monitoring

P U R P O S E: Compartment syndrome results from increased pressure within a limited anatomic space. Compartment syndrome can affect any confined anatomic space where there is an increase in pressure. Most commonly, the upper and lower extremities are involved. Intracompartmental pressure monitoring detects pressure within the muscle compartments.

John J. Gallagher
Shawn McCabe

PREREQUISITE NURSING KNOWLEDGE

- Anatomy of the involved limb compartments (Fig. 118–1) should be understood.
- Knowledge of aseptic technique is essential.
- Two general factors may contribute to the development of compartment syndrome. First, there may be an increase in the contents of the compartment in excess of compartment size secondary to tissue edema or hemorrhage. Secondly, there may be restriction applied to the compartment from bandages, casts, or pneumatic antishock garment (PASG), reducing tissue expandability and thereby increasing compartment pressure.[1–10]
- The elevation of tissue pressure within the compartment causes compression or occlusion of arteriole flow resulting in ischemia and eventual necrosis of the tissues in the compartment.
- Tissue edema may be worsened, as venous outflow is compromised and additional tissue edema results. Interventions to relieve the pressure within the compartment, such as fasciotomy, should be initiated within 4 to 6 hours to prevent ischemia or severe complications.[10]
- Patients at risk for the development of limb compartment syndrome include those who have sustained vascular, soft-tissue, or orthopedic trauma; burns; shock; and those who have undergone massive fluid resuscitation (Table 118–1).

- In general, initial symptoms of compartment syndrome may be observed within 2 hours of the initial trauma or insult. Ischemia may result in 4 to 6 hours, with ischemic contractures and nerve injury resulting in permanent functional loss in 12 to 24 hours.[10]
- Intracompartmental pressures are monitored in patients who are at risk for the development of compartment syndrome.[4, 10] If left untreated, compartment syndrome results in tissue ischemia and necrosis, permanent nerve damage, limb contractures, and possibly, loss of the involved limb. The degree of tissue injury and functional loss depends on the severity and duration of compartment pressure elevation.
- Intracompartmental pressures are obtained from the muscle compartments in the upper and lower extremities using a variety of invasive measuring devices.[4, 12]
- Compartment pressure monitoring of the extremities is performed using a pressure monitoring device attached to a needle, wick, or slit catheter (Figs. 118–2 and 118–3).[4, 8, 11]
- Normal limb compartment pressure is 0 mm Hg. Compartment pressures that are within 10 to 30 mm Hg of the diastolic blood pressure may indicate the presence of compartment syndrome (eg, a compartment pressure increase to 40 to 45 mm Hg in a person with a diastolic blood pressure of 70 mm Hg may indicate compartment syndrome).[10]

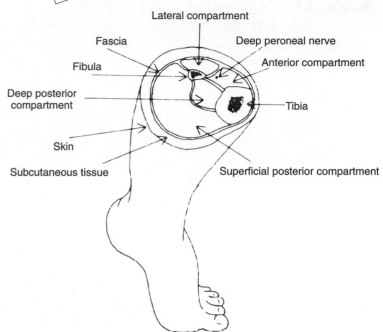

■ ● **FIGURE 118–1.** Muscle compartments of the lower extremity. (From Ross D. Acute compartment syndrome. *Orthop Nurs.* 1991; 10(2):33–38. Reprinted with permission of the publisher, the National Association of Orthopaedic Nurses.)

Table 118–1 ● ■ ■	**Etiology of Compartment Syndrome**

Trauma

> Fractures
> Surgery of the extremity
> Hematomas
> Postischemic swelling
> Crush injuries
> Electric injuries
> Vascular injuries

Factors Precipitating Edema Formation

> Prolonged use of tourniquets in surgery
> Vascular obstruction (arterial and venous)
> Replantation surgery
> Nephrotic syndrome
> Thermal injury (frostbite or burns)
> Excessive use (athletic injury)

Coagulopathies

> Anticoagulant therapy
> Hemophilia

Other

> Constrictive dressings, splints, or casts
> Premature or "tight" closure of a fascial defect
> Pneumatic antishock garment
> Hyperthermia or hypothermia
> Infiltration of intravenous infusions
> Intra-arterial injections
> Snake bite
> Legionnaire's disease
> Rocky Mountain spotted fever
> *Clostridium perfringens* infection
> Excessive pressure from prolonged immobility in one position

(Adapted from Ross D. Compartment syndrome. In: Swearingen PL, Sommers MS, Miller K. *Manual of Critical Care: Applying Nursing Diagnoses to Adult Critical Illness.* St Louis, Mo: C.V. Mosby; 1988.)

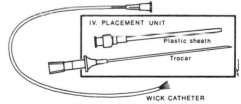

■ ● **FIGURE 118–2.** A wick catheter for intracompartmental pressure monitoring. (From Mubarak SJ, Hargens AR. *Compartment Syndromes and Volkmann's Contracture.* Philadelphia: WB Saunders; 1981:114.)

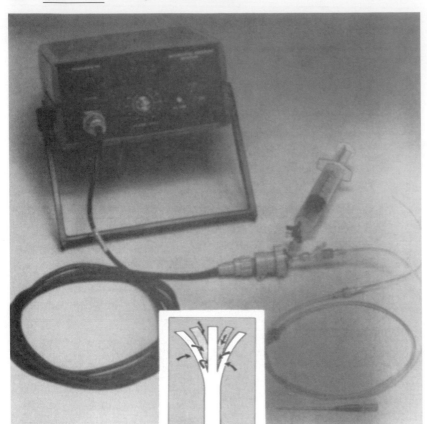

■ ● **FIGURE 118–3.** Slit catheter setup. Slit tip on catheter consists of five petals that allow a patent fluid path and prevent occlusion with material or tissue. (Courtesy of Howmedica, Inc.)

- Compartment syndrome in the extremities is heralded by the five "Ps": pain, paresthesia, pallor, pulselessness, and paralysis[3, 8–10]:
  - ❖ *Pain* is the earliest symptom of compartment syndrome; however, it may not be distinguishable from the pain related to injuries to the extremity. The pain is generally unremitting and is not responsive to therapeutic measures such as fracture stabilization or the administration of analgesic agents. Pain is generally exacerbated by passive flexion and extension of the hand or foot in the affected extremity.
  - ❖ *Paresthesia* is one of the earliest signs of impending, yet reversible, compartment syndrome. Paresthesia generally precedes motor dysfunction. Hypothesia of the nerves traversing the affected compartment may also occur (Fig. 118–4).
  - ❖ *Pallor* may be seen in the affected limb, which could also be mottled or cyanotic.
  - ❖ *Pulselessness* is an extremely late finding. Compromised arteriole flow may result in compartment syndrome while palpable pulses are still present.
  - ❖ *Paralysis* is a late sign and signals advanced compartment syndrome.

EQUIPMENT

- Introducer needle (angiocath), 16 G or larger
- Slit or wick catheter
- Electronic pressure monitoring device (bedside pressure monitor or a handheld monitoring device)
- Transducer and pressure tubing setup
- 30-mL syringe
- 50-mL sterile normal saline (NS)
- Sterile gloves
- Povidone pads, swabsticks, or solution
- Sterile dressing
- One roll of hypoallergenic tape
- 1% lidocaine without epinephrine

Additional equipment to have available as needed includes the following:

- Scissors

PATIENT AND FAMILY EDUCATION

- Explain the indication for compartment pressure monitoring to the patient and family. ➥*Rationale:* Improves patient and family understanding of why the procedure is needed.

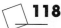

Peroneal Nerve
SENSATION
MOTION
☐ SENSATION
Prick the web space between the great toe and second toe
☐ MOTION
Have patient dorsiflex ankle and extend toes at the metatarsal phalangle joints
Tibial Nerve
SENSATION
MOTION
☐ SENSATION
Prick the medial and lateral surfaces of the sole of the foot
☐ MOTION
Have patient plantar flex ankle and toes
Radial Nerve
SENSATION
MOTION
☐ SENSATION
Prick the web space between the thumb and index finger
☐ MOTION
Have patient hyperextend thumb then wrist and hyperextend the four fingers at the MCP joints
Ulnar Nerve
SENSATION
MOTION
☐ SENSATION
Prick the distal fat pad of the small finger
☐ MOTION
Have patient abduct all fingers
Median Nerve
SENSATION
MOTION
☐ SENSATION
Prick the distal surface of the index finger
☐ MOTION
Have patient oppose thumb and small finger: note whether patient can flex wrist

■ ● **FIGURE 118–4.** Neurovascular assessment. (Courtesy of Howmedica, Inc.)

- Explain the procedure to the patient and family. ➻***Rationale:*** Explaining the procedure may decrease patient and family anxiety and assist in patient cooperation.

PATIENT ASSESSMENT AND PREPARATION

Patient Assessment

- Review the patient's health history for conditions predisposing the patient to compartment syndrome (see Table 118–1). ➻***Rationale:*** Patients with certain pathologies and injuries are at increased risk for compartment syndrome.
- Assess the patient's involved extremity for signs and symptoms that may indicate the onset of compartment syndrome. These include pain, paresthesia, changes in skin color and temperature, limitations in movement, change in the strength of distal pulses, tenseness of the tissue, and increase in the girth of the extremity.[8, 10] ➻***Rationale:*** These symptoms alone indicate the onset of compartment syndrome and the need for intracompartmental pressure measurement and therapeutic intervention.

Patient Preparation

- Ensure that the patient and family understand preprocedural teaching. Answer questions as they arise and reinforce information as needed. ➻***Rationale:*** Evaluates and reinforces understanding of previously taught information.
- Remove constricting dressings and bandages. Assist with the removal and modification of splints, casts, PSAGs, or other devices on the affected extremity.[4, 8, 10] ➻***Rationale:*** Reduces external pressure on the tissue of the affected extremity.
- Assist the patient to the supine position. ➻***Rationale:*** Provides access to the affected compartment.

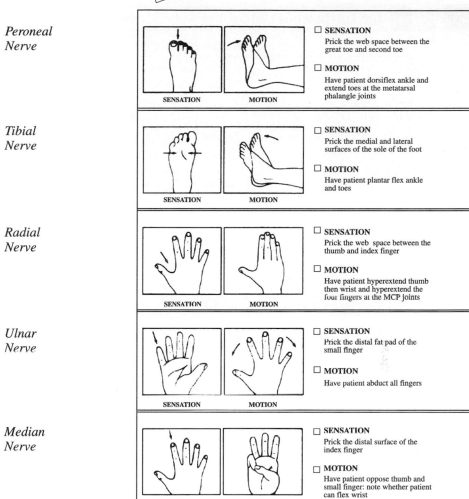

Procedure for Intracompartment Pressure Monitoring

Steps	Rationale	Special Considerations
1. Wash hands.	Reduces transmission of microorganisms; standard precautions.	
2. Assemble the pressure transducer and tubing system (Fig. 118–5).	Prepares the monitoring system.	
3. Fill the 30-mL syringe with normal saline and flush the tubing.	Ensures that there is no air in the system.	
4. Turn on the electronic monitoring device.	Establishes power to the monitoring system.	A portable bedside electonic monitoring device (see Fig. 118–5) designed for the purpose of monitoring compartment pressures can be used or a standard cardiac monitoring system with an available invasive pressure monitoring channel can be used. In addition, a handheld unit such as the Stryker Intracompartmental Pressure Monitor (Fig. 118–6) may be used.
5. Select the appropriate pressure scale on the monitor.	The 30 or 60 mm Hg scale will be sufficient to measure the majority of pressure ranges.	
6. Connect the transducer system to the monitoring device.	Prepares the monitoring system.	
7. Wash hands, and don clean gloves.	Reduces the transmission of microorganisms; standard precautions.	
8. Assist the physician with preparation of the intended site: A. Clip hairs in the area if necessary. B. Cleanse with povidone in a circular motion. C. Repeat the povidone cleansing.	Reduces the potential for infection.	
9. Remove gloves, and wash hands.	Reduces the transmission of microorganisms; standard precautions.	
10. Prepare the local anesthetic agent according to physician request or institutional protocol.	Local anesthetic agents may be used befor insertion of the introducer needle for patient analgesia.	Other concomitant analgesic or antianxiety agents may be indicated depending on patient need.

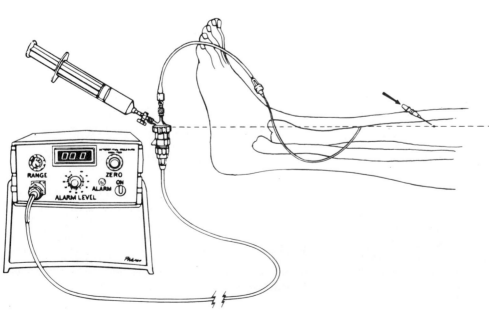

■ ● **FIGURE 118–5.** The open part of the venting stopcock is placed at the level of the tip of the intracompartmental catheter *(arrow).* Dashes show this level.

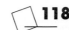

| Procedure | **for Intracompartment Pressure Monitoring** *Continued* |

Steps	Rationale	Special Considerations
11. Level the air–fluid interface (zeroing stopcock) with the planned insertion site of the catheter (see Fig. 118–5).	The intended insertion site of the catheter is the reference point.	
12. Set the system to zero.	Negates the effect of atmospheric system. Ensures accuracy of the system with the established reference point.	
13. Attach the sterile wick or slit catheter to the end of the pressure tubing (see Fig. 118–5).	Connects the monitoring system to the catheter.	
14. Check the responsiveness of the wick or slit catheter to changes in pressure by holding the catheter level with the air–fluid interface (monitor should read zero). Raise the catheter to eye level (monitor pressure should rise to 30 to 50 mm Hg).	Ensures the system is able to read changes in pressure.	Failure of the pressure to increase when the catheter is elevated or an increase in pressure with a rapid drop in pressure may indicate a system leak. A slow increase in pressure with elevation of the catheter may indicate air in the system.
15. Assist the physician as needed with insertion of the introducer needle and the wick or slit catheter (Figs. 118–7 and 118–8).	The introducer catheter is inserted first, then the wick or slit catheter is inserted through the introducer needle.	If only a single reading is being obtained, the pressure tubing may be attached directly to the introducer needle after insertion. A handheld device (see Fig. 118–6) equipped with a needle may be a better choice for single measurement use.
16. Measure the intracompartment pressure.	Determines presence or absence of pressure.	If measuring lower extremity pressure, the extremity can be resting on the bed, but the heel should be elevated to suspend the lower leg above the bed. This is important when the posterior compartments are measured because increased pressure is applied to the compartments resting on the bed.

Procedure continued on following page

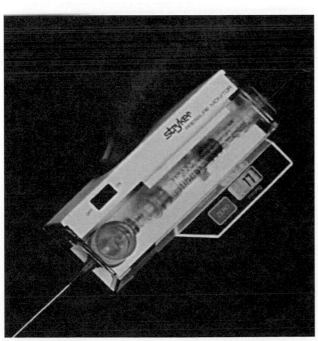

■ ● **FIGURE 118–6.** Stryker intracompartmental pressure monitor. (Courtesy of Stryker Instruments.)

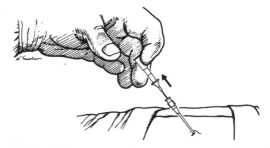

■ ● **FIGURE 118–7.** Jelco catheter used for insertion of wick catheter. (From Mubarak SJ, Hargens AR. *Compartment Syndromes and Volkmann's Contracture.* Philadelphia: WB Saunders; 1981:114.)

Procedure	**for Intracompartment Pressure Monitoring** *Continued*

Steps	Rationale	Special Considerations

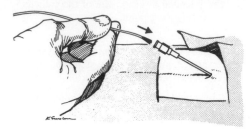

■ ● **FIGURE 118–8.** Threading wick catheter through Jelco catheter and into compartment to be measured. (From Mubarak SJ, Hargens AR. *Compartment Syndromes and Volkmann's Contracture.* Philadelphia: WB Saunders; 1981:114.)

Steps	Rationale	Special Considerations
17. Secure the wick or slit catheter to the patient (Fig. 118–9).	Prevents the catheter from becoming dislodged.	
18. Apply an occlusive sterile dressing to the catheter insertion site.	Reduces the risk of infection.	
19. Check the accuracy of the monitoring system by palpating the area over the catheter tip or by having the patient flex and extend the appropriate distal joint (Fig. 118–10).	Fluctuations in pressure should be noted with patient movement or palpation over the catheter tip. A rapid increase in pressure will be noted with applied pressure or contraction of the muscle.	Patients with normal compartment physiology will demonstrate a rapid rise in pressure during palpation or contraction of the muscle with a rapid return to baseline pressure. Patients with compartment syndrome will have a slow return to baseline pressure after relaxation of the muscle.
20. Assist with removal of the wick or slit catheter when monitoring is complete.	The catheter should not be left in place longer than 48 hours because there is an increased risk of infection.	
21. After removal, apply a dry sterile dressing secured with tape.	Protects the insertion site and assists in control of bleeding.	Do not apply dressing snugly, as this may further impede blood flow and raise compartment pressure.
22. Discard used supplies, and wash hands.	Reduces transmission of microorganisms; standard precautions.	

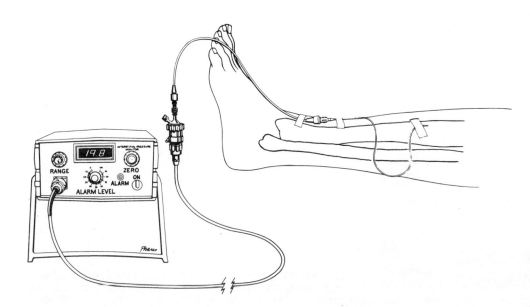

■ ● **FIGURE 118–9.** Tape and sutures are used to secure the catheter.

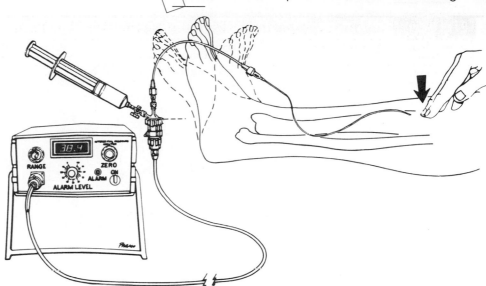

■ ● **FIGURE 118–10.** The system's response can be checked either by palpating the area over the catheter tip *(arrow)* or by having the patient flex-extend the appropriate distal joint; observe the scope for small, temporary elevations in the pressure pattern.

Expected Outcomes

- Insertion of the monitoring device is completed without complications and with minimal patient discomfort.
- Compartment pressure is within normal limits.
- If physical signs and symptoms of compartment syndrome are identified and compartment pressures are elevated, compartment syndrome is diagnosed and therapeutic interventions are initiated.
- The patient tolerates the procedure.

Unexpected Outcomes

- Inaccurate pressure readings obtained
- Excessive bleeding from the catheter insertion site
- Signs and symptoms of procedure-related infection

Patient Monitoring and Care

Patient Monitoring and Care	Rationale	Reportable Conditions
		These conditions should be reported if they persist despite nursing interventions.
1. Complete a neurovascular assessment of the affected extremity every hour and more often as needed.	Detects the onset of signs and symptoms associated with compartment syndrome.	• Onset of *pain* or worsening of pain despite administration of analgesic agents • *Paresthesia* or hypothesia of the affected extremity • Changes in extremity skin color (mottling, cyanosis, *pallor*) and skin temperature • Decrease or loss of peripheral *pulses* • *Paralysis* of the affected extremity • Increase in circumference and tenseness of the extremity

Continued on following page

Patient Monitoring and Care *Continued*

Patient Monitoring and Care	Rationale	Reportable Conditions
2. Assess the insertion site for signs and symptoms of infection.	The catheter insertion site may be a source of infection because of the presence of an invasive catheter.	• Erythema, swelling, or drainage around the insertion site • Increase in skin warmth surrounding the insertion site • Increased pain and tenderness at the insertion site • Increase in white blood cell (WBC) count on complete blood count • Fever
3. Measure compartment pressure every hour and more often if needed.	Assessment of compartment pressures along with physical assessment findings is necessary to detect the development of compartment syndrome.	• Elevations and changes in compartment pressure

Documentation

Documentation should include the following:

- Patient and family education
- Extremity assessment findings before compartment pressure measurement
- Identification of the compartments to be assessed
- Medications administered
- The compartment pressure measured
- The condition of the insertion site with the wick or slit catheter in place and after removal of the catheter or needle
- Postprocedure assessment of the limb
- Elevations in compartment pressure or physical assessment findings that are indicative of compartment syndrome onset
- Unexpected outcomes
- Additional interventions

References

1. Chan PS, Steinberg DR, Pepe MD, et al. The significance of the three volar spaces in forearm compartment syndrome: a clinical and cadaveric correlation. *J Hand Surg.* 1998; 23:1077–1081.
2. Childs SA. Musculoskeletal trauma: implications for critical care nursing practice. *Crit Care Nurs Clin North Am.* 1994;6:483–490.
3. Fecht-Gramley ME. Emergency: recognizing compartment syndrome. *Am J Nurs.* 1994;94:41.
4. Good LP. Compartment syndrome: a closer look at etiology, treatment. *AORN.* 1992;56:904–911.
5. Johansen K, Watson J. Compartment syndrome: new insights. *Semin Vasc Surg.* 1998;11:294–301.
6. Kracun MD, Wooten CL. Crush injuries: a case of entrapment. *Crit Care Nurs Q.* 1998;21:81–86.
7. Peck SA. Crush syndrome: pathophysiology and management. *Orthop Nurs.* 1990;9:33–40.
8. Ross D. Acute compartment syndrome. *Orthop Nurs.* 1991;10(2):33–38.
9. Csongradi JJ, Nagel DA. Complications of surgery on muscles, fasciae, tendons, tendon sheaths, ligaments and bursae. In: Epps CH, ed. *Complications in Orthopaedic Surgery.* 3rd ed, vol II. Philadelphia, Pa: J.B. Lippincott; 1994:1123.
10. Pelligrini VD, Reid JS, McCollister E. Complications. In: Bucholz RW, Green DP, Heckman JD, Rockwood CA, eds. *Rockwood and Green's Fractures in Adults.* 4th ed, vol 1. Philadelphia, Pa: Lippincott-Raven; 1996:487.
11. Mubarak SJ. Laboratory diagnosis of compartment syndromes. In: Mubarak SJ, Hargens AR, Akeson WH, eds. *Compartment Syndrome and Volkmann's Contractures.* Philadelphia, Pa: W.B. Saunders; 1981.
12. Wilson SC, Vrahas MS, Paul EM. A simple method to measure compartment pressures using an intravenous catheter. *Orthopedics.* 1997;20(5):403.

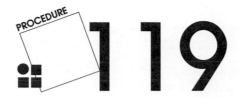

119

Pressure-Reducing Devices: Lateral Rotation Therapy

PURPOSE: The purpose of lateral rotation therapy is to provide dynamic pressure reduction to assist in preventing and treating complications of immobility, especially for patients who would benefit from chest percussion or continuous or regular turning from side to side, or both.

Nancy L. Tomaselli
Margaret T. Goldberg
Sandi Wind

PREREQUISITE NURSING KNOWLEDGE

- Principles of preventing pressure-induced injury should be understood.
- Understanding of the pathophysiology of tissue ischemia is needed.
- Knowledge is needed of the effects of immobility on the body systems, including factors contributing to impaired circulation, such as venous stasis and thrombosis, pulmonary stasis,[1] urinary stasis, pressure ulcers,[2] and friction and shear.
- Principles of wound healing should be understood.
- Understanding of the principles of lateral rotation therapy is needed.
- Indications for lateral rotation therapy include the following:
  - ❖ Coma
  - ❖ Trauma rehabilitation
  - ❖ Chronic neurologic disorders[3]
  - ❖ Stroke
  - ❖ Pulmonary conditions[4]
  - ❖ Spinal cord injury
  - ❖ Cervical traction
  - ❖ Skeletal traction
- Technical and clinical competence in caring for patients receiving lateral rotation therapy is essential.
- The surface below the patient and the positioning packs consist of pressure-reducing foam and a pad of nonliquid polymer gel with a low-friction, low-shear Gore-Tex fabric cover that does not absorb body fluids or odors.
- The gel pads prevent the patient from bottoming out, transfer body heat evenly, and are x-ray transparent.

- The bed provides continuous, slow, side-to-side turning of the patient by rotating the bed frame.
- The bed can turn more than 62 degrees on each side, either intermittently or constantly, providing either unilateral or bilateral rotation.
- The amount of time the patient is held at the rotation limit before rotating in the opposite direction can be adjusted from 7 seconds to 30 minutes.
- Head and shoulder packs provide cervical stability, and lateral arm and leg hatches facilitate range of motion.
- Hatches underneath the bed located in the cervical, thoracic, and rectal areas provide access for skin care, catheter maintenance, and bladder and bowel management.
- The bed has a built-in scale with a maximum patient weight of 300 lb.
- An optional vibrator pack is available to provide chest physiotherapy to further mobilize pulmonary secretions.

EQUIPMENT

- Lateral rotation therapy table (Fig. 119–1).

PATIENT AND FAMILY EDUCATION

- Explain to patient and family the effects of tissue compression. ➤*Rationale:* Encourages understanding and enables patient and family to ask questions.
- Explain how therapy achieves pressure relief. ➤*Rationale:* Increases understanding and cooperation.
- Evaluate the patient's need for long-term pressure reduction (eg, acute or chronic health problems remaining uncontrolled or chronic pressure ulcers or both). ➤*Rationale:* Allows the nurse to anticipate the need for patient discharge with pressure-reducing device.

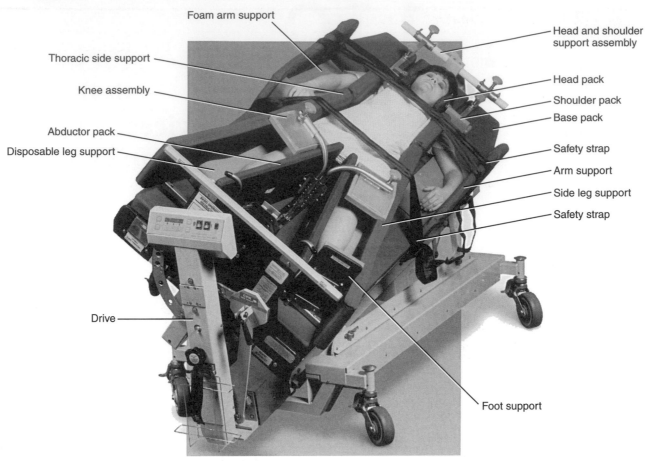

Foam arm support

Thoracic side support

Knee assembly

Abductor pack

Disposable leg support

Drive

Head and shoulder support assembly

Head pack

Shoulder pack

Base pack

Safety strap

Arm support

Side leg support

Safety strap

Foot support

■ ● **FIGURE 119–1.** Lateral rotation therapy table. (Courtesy of Kinetic Concepts, Inc.)

PATIENT ASSESSMENT AND PREPARATION

Patient Assessment

- Assess the patient's skin for evidence of pressure ulcer formation.   ➤*Rationale:* Provides baseline data.
- Assess the patient's wounds: type and amount of drainage, area of necrosis, surrounding skin for maceration and inflammation, and any pain on palpation of surrounding skin.   ➤*Rationale:* Provides baseline data. Relief of external pressure facilitates wound healing.
- Assess the patient's vascular system: ischemic rest pain, arterial pulses, condition of skin and hair of lower extremities, and presence of atrophic nails.   ➤*Rationale:* Provides baseline data. Lateral movement minimizes venous stasis.
- Assess the patient's pulmonary status: adventitious breath sounds, rate and depth of respirations, cough, cyanosis, dyspnea, nasal flaring, arterial blood gases, decreased mental acuity, and restlessness.   ➤*Rationale:* Provides baseline data. Lateral movement provides postural drainage and mobilizes secretions.
- Assess the patient's bladder: distended bladder, feeling of incomplete bladder emptying, or urinary infrequency.   ➤*Rationale:* Provides baseline data. Lateral movement decreases urinary stasis.

Patient Preparation

- Ensure that the patient and family understand preprocedural teaching. Answer questions as they arise, and reinforce information as needed.   ➤*Rationale:* Evaluates and reinforces understanding of previously taught information.
- Assist the patient to the supine position with the head of the bed flat or slightly elevated.   ➤*Rationale:* Eases transfer of the patient from one bed to another.

Procedure	for Lateral Rotation Therapy	
Steps	**Rationale**	**Special Considerations**

Placing a Patient on a Lateral Rotation Therapy Table

Steps	Rationale	Special Considerations
1. Wash hands.	Reduces transmission of microorganisms; standard precautions.	
2. Ensure that bed is locked in horizontal position and that the drive is disengaged.	Ensures patient safety.	The holes in the frame in which the side supports fit are near the surface of the base packs.
3. Check all hatches to be certain they are properly latched, and be sure castors are locked.	Prevents unplanned movement of bed.	
4. Slide the patient gently to the center of the bed while maintaining body alignment.	Bouncing of patient can result in skin abrasions.	May cover pillar bars with a towel or folded paper sheet to avoid possibility of abrasion.

Positioning a Patient on a Lateral Rotation Therapy Table

Steps	Rationale	Special Considerations
1. Center the patient on the bed by aligning the nose, umbilicus, and pubis with the center posts.	Facilitates proper balance. Rotating to one side indicates that the patient is not centered.	To initiate cardiopulmonary resuscitation (CPR), return the bed to the horizontal position and lock in place.
2. Place thoracic side supports in appropriate holes provided in the frame, and ensure that they are tightened securely.	These are the main supporting apparatus.	Packs and supports are labeled for patient's right and left sides. Maintain 1-in clearance between the end of the pack and the axilla.
3. Adjust the knee assembly to a position slightly above the patient's knee.	Provides support.	
4. Place the disposable leg support in a position under the thigh and calf so that it fits under the ankle and knee but not beneath the heel.	Decreases external pressure on the heels.	Leg supports should be changed when soiled.
5. Place the foot supports in the foot bracket assembly. The assembly should be positioned so that the footrest is in anatomic position. Tighten the foot assembly.	Maintains each foot in proper anatomic position.	The foot supports should not be left in place for longer than 2 hours at a time. A schedule of 2 hours on and 2 hours off should be maintained continuously. Side-to-side motion does not relieve pressure on the soles of the feet.
6. Install the abductor packs into the preset metal brackets.	Provides support.	
7. Place the side leg supports snugly against the patient's hips, and tighten securely.	Provides support.	
8. Install the knee pads in a position such that your hand just fits between the knee and the pack.	Prevents pressure on the knee.	Knee packs can be adjusted to allow for variation in abduction and flexion of the patient's legs. They maintain proper posture of the lower limbs in the patient with spasticity, discouraging contracture formation.
9. Adjust the head and shoulder support assembly.	Provides further support.	

Procedure continued on following page

Procedure **for Lateral Rotation Therapy** *Continued*

Steps	Rationale	Special Considerations
10. Place a hand on the patient's shoulder, and adjust the shoulder pack to lightly touch your hand.	Prevents pressure ulcers.	There should always be a 1 in (2.54 cm) clearance between the patient's shoulders and the shoulder packs. If cervical traction causes the patient to slide up on the bed during rotation, place the patient in the reverse Trendelenburg position.
11. Adjust the head pack so that it does not touch the patient's ears or come in contact with the tongs of cervical traction. Tighten head and shoulder assemblies securely.	Provides support.	To remove the head and shoulder packs, loosen the handle of the shoulder pack and slide to the side, or lift the entire assembly.
12. Tighten the clamps on the crossbar to secure the assemblies in correct lateral position.	Provides support.	
13. Install the disposable foam arm supports.	Ensures that the patient's hands are in a position of function and that the ulnar nerve and elbows are protected.	
14. Secure the arm supports in the holes provided on the frame.	Provides support.	
15. Safety straps are to be in place at all times. One safety strap is used to hold down the shoulder assembly. Place the other strap in proper position.	Prevents falls and patient injury.	
16. Wash hands.	Reduces transmission of microorganisms; standard precautions.	

Expected Outcomes

- Intact skin integrity
- Wound healing
- Absence of friction, shearing, and moisture on skin
- Improved peripheral circulation
- Improved urinary elimination
- Maximum pulmonary function achieved

Unexpected Outcomes

- Lateral movement of table may cause friction and shearing, motion sickness, agitation and disorientation, and falls if patient is not strapped in properly.
- Pressure ulcer formation or further deterioration of existing pressure ulcers occurs.

Patient Monitoring and Care

Patient Monitoring and Care	Rationale	Reportable Conditions
		These conditions should be reported if they persist despite nursing interventions.
1. Evaluate the patient's skin (particularly areas over bony prominences) for evidence of pressure necrosis every 4 to 8 hours.	Relief of external pressure prevents pressure ulcers.	• Development of pressure ulcers
2. Evaluate the patient's existing pressure ulcers, wounds, flaps, and grafts for evidence of healing at least every 8 hours.	Relief of external pressure facilitates healing.	• Deterioration or failure to heal
3. Evaluate the skin for evidence of friction, shearing, or moisture.	These factors contribute to pressure ulcer formation.	• Development of skin breakdown

Patient Monitoring and Care *Continued*

Patient Monitoring and Care	Rationale	Reportable Conditions
4. Evaluate the patient's peripheral vascular circulation.	Lateral movement discourages venous stasis.	• Edema, decreased or absent pulses, discoloration, pain
5. Evaluate the patient's pulmonary function.	Lateral movement provides continuous postural drainage and mobilization of secretions.	• Adventitious breath sounds, decreased respiratory rate and depth, cough, cyanosis, dyspnea, nasal flaring, decreased oxygen saturation, abnormal blood gases, decreased mental acuity, restlessness
6. Evaluate the patient for urinary retention.	Lateral movement decreases urinary stasis.	• Decreased urine output, bladder distention
7. Evaluate the patient's acceptance of and adaptation to the device (motion sickness, agitation, disorientation).	Increases cooperation and decreases anxiety.	• Intolerance to device
8. Maintain bed in motion for 18 hours of every 24-hour period.	Provides proper rotation and adequate mobility.	• Inability to rotate as per schedule
9. Maintain safety straps at all times.	Prevents falls and patient injury.	• Falls or injury
10. Maintain schedule for foot supports—2 hours on and 2 hours off continuously.	Side-to-side movement does not relieve pressure on soles of feet.	• Breakdown on soles of feet
11. Determine when therapy should be discontinued.	Lateral rotation therapy is no longer required.	• Discontinuing lateral rotation therapy

Documentation

Documentation in the patient record should include the following:

- Patient and family education
- Date and time therapy is instituted
- Rationale for use of lateral rotation therapy table
- Number of hours patient is in rotation mode
- Serial skin assessments
- Status of wound healing, if applicable
- Patient's response to therapy
- Any unexpected outcomes and interventions taken
- Phone number and name of company representative

References

1. Nelson LD, Choi SC. Kinetic therapy in critically ill trauma patients. *Clin Intensive Care.* 1992;3(6):248–252.
2. Collier M. Know how: kinetic therapy. *Nurs Times.* 1997;93(10):48–49.
3. Hartman MB, Chrin AM, Rechtine GR. Non-operative treatment of thoracolumbar fractures. *Paraplegia.* 1995;33(2):73–76.
4. Pape HC, Regel G, Borgmann W, Sturm JA, Tscherne H. The effect of kinetic positioning on lung function and pulmonary hemodynamics in post-traumatic ARDS: a clinical study. *Injury: Int J Care Injured.* 1994;25(1):51–57.

Additional Readings

Agency for Health Care Policy and Research (AHCPR). *Pressure ulcers in adults: prediction and prevention.* Rockville, Md: U.S. Department of Health and Human Services; 1992. AHCPR publication 92–0047.
Agency for Health Care Policy and Research (AHCPR). *Treatment of pressure ulcers.* Rockville, Md: U.S. Department of Health and Human Services; 1994. AHCPR publication 95–0652.
Centers for Disease Control and Prevention. Guideline for prevention of nosocomial pneumonia. *Respir Care.* 1994;39(12):1191–1236.
Kinetic Concepts, Inc. Roto-Rest Delta. *Operations and Maintenance Manual.* San Antonio, Tx: Kinetic Concepts; 1995.

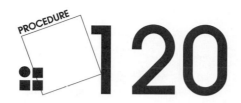

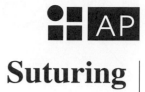

120

Suturing

P U R P O S E: Suturing is the process of placing threads to hold body tissues together. It is used to approximate tissues separated by a surgical or accidental trauma, expedite healing with minimal scarring and without infection, provide strength until the natural tensile strength of the healing wound is sufficient to maintain closure, and maintain appropriate positioning of tubes or drains.

Peggy Kirkwood

PREREQUISITE NURSING KNOWLEDGE

- The skin is the largest organ of the body and has two major tissue layers. The outermost layer, the epidermis, is made of stratified, squamous cells with keratin and melanin. This layer protects against environmental exposure, restricts water loss, and gives color. The inner layer, the dermis, is made of fibroelastic connective tissue with capillaries, lymphatics, and nerve endings, providing nourishment and strength. The layer beneath the dermis is the subcutaneous tissue, composed of areolar and fatty connective tissue to provide insulation, shock absorption, and calorie reserve.
- The natural components of wound healing include the following:
  - ❖ Inflammation—Vascular and cellular responses are designed to protect the body against alien substances. Blood loss is limited by immediate vasoconstriction of the small vessels that lasts 5 to 10 minutes, the initiation of the coagulation cascade, the tendency for leukocytes to "stick" to the endothelium, and the stimulation of red blood cell (RBC) adherence to each other to plug the cut ends of capillaries. Kinins and prostaglandins produce local vasodilation and increase permeability of the vasculature, thereby promoting development of inflammatory exudate. Wounds left open for 3 hours show a dramatic increase in vascular permeability that results in thick inflammatory exudate and limits the therapeutic value of antibiotics.[1]
  - ❖ Epithelization—After an incision, the divided parts of the epithelium are closed by cellular migration and mitosis, forming an epithelial bridge that protects the wound against bacteria. When the skin edges are slightly everted with suturing, epithelial bridging occurs within 18 to 24 hours. Wounds that have approximated skin edges may take 36 hours to epithelialize.

If the edges are inverted, it may take up to 72 hours to completely epithelialize.[1]
- The goals of primary wound closure are to stop bleeding, prevent infection, preserve function, and restore appearance.
- Principles of proper wound closure include the following:
  - ❖ Elimination of dead space where serum and blood can accumulate, thus decreasing the risk of infection
  - ❖ Accurate approximation of deep tissue layers to each other with minimal tension on the surrounding tissues
  - ❖ Avoidance of tissue ischemia and strangulation from tying sutures too tightly
  - ❖ Decreased risk of infection by closing clean wounds within 3 to 8 hours of injury and using aseptic technique in all aspects of wound management.
- Wounds with damage to the blood supply, nerves, or joint; wounds on the face; or wounds with extensive tissue damage or infection should be referred to an appropriate specialist (eg, vascular, orthopedic, plastic, or general surgeon).
- Wounds contaminated or infected with saliva, feces, or purulent exudate or that have been open longer than 8 hours may benefit from delayed closure on or after the fourth day in order to decrease risk of infection.[2, 3]
- Curved needles are either tapered or cutting. Needles used for skin closure have an angle of 135 degrees.
  - ❖ Tapered needles are used in soft tissues (intestine, blood vessels, muscle, and fascia) and produce minimal tissue damage.
  - ❖ Cutting needles are used to approximate tougher tissue, such as skin. Reverse cutting needles have a cutting edge on the outside of the curve and provide a wall of tissue, rather than an incision, for the suture to rest against. This resists suture cut-through and is, therefore, preferred.
- Most needles are swaged, or molded, around the suture, providing convenience, safety, and speed in placing sutures.
- Needles should be handled only with needle holders to prevent needle damage to surrounding tissue and to the user.

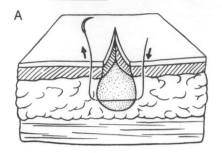

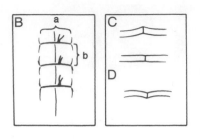

■ ● FIGURE 120–1. Interrupted dermal suture. *A,* Proper depth. *B,* Proper spacing (*a = b*). *C,* Proper final appearance. *D,* Improper final appearance. (From Pfenninger JL, Fowler GC, eds. *Procedures for Primary Care Physicians.* St. Louis: Mosby; 1994:15.)

- Suture material is characterized by tissue reactivity, flexibility, knot-holding ability, wick action, and tensile strength. Suture size is indicated by "0." More "0s" indicate smaller suture (4–0 < 3–0).
- Sutures are absorbable or nonabsorbable, braided or monofilament.
  - ❖ Absorbable suture (ie, natural gut, synthetic polymers) is used for layered closures. Gut suture is broken down by phagocytosis and induces a moderate inflammatory reaction. Chromic gut suture has increased strength and lasts longer in tissue, but is not used on the skin because it can cause a severe tissue reaction. Synthetic absorbable sutures are favored over gut because of decreased infection rates and increased strength and longevity.[4]
  - ❖ Nonabsorbable sutures are either natural fibers (ie, silk, cotton, linen) or synthetic (ie, nylon, Dacron, polyethylene) and are best for superficial lacerations because they are supple, easily handled, and facilitate knot construction.
  - ❖ Braided sutures are stronger, but the small spaces between the braids may harbor infection.
  - ❖ Monofilament is best suited for skin closure because it produces less of an inflammatory response; however, the knots are less dependable.
- Nonabsorbable synthetic monofilament sutures (ie, 4–0 or 5–0 nylon) are preferred for skin closure. Synthetic braided absorbable sutures provide the best closure for interrupted dermal sutures and ligating bleeding vessels.
- Preferred knotting technique involves a square knot or double loop followed by a square knot tie.
- Injured tissue will become edematous and the suture will tighten automatically within 12 to 24 hours. Therefore, the practitioner must avoid tying the suture too tightly, which could produce tissue necrosis.
- The number of sutures required is the minimum needed to hold the wound edges exactly opposed without crimp-

ing. Tension should be minimized but not eliminated on the wound edges. The more tension on a wound, the closer the sutures should be placed.

- Lacerations are approximated using a variety of suturing techniques.
  - ❖ Simple interrupted dermal suture (Fig. 120–1) is used when the skin margins are level or slightly everted. The needle should enter and exit the skin surface at a right angle. The stitch should be as wide as the suture is deep and no closer than 2 mm apart. The knot should be tied using an instrument tie and repeated four or five times. The first suture is placed in the midportion of the wound. Additional sutures are placed in bisected portions of the wound until it is appropriately closed.
  - ❖ Subcutaneous suture with inverted knot or buried stitch (Fig. 120–2) is used for deeper wounds or wounds under tension. Absorbable sutures are used with the knot inverted below the skin margin. Begin at the bottom of the wound, come up and go straight across the incision to the base again and tie.
  - ❖ Vertical mattress suture (Fig. 120–3) promotes eversion of the skin and is used when skin tension is present or where the skin is very thick (palms and soles of feet). Identical to a simple suture, but an additional suture is taken very close to the edge of each side of the wound.
  - ❖ Three-point or half-buried mattress suture (Fig. 120–4) is used to close an acute corner of a laceration without impairing blood flow to the tip. The needle is inserted into the skin on the nonflap portion of the wound, passed transversely through the tip, and returned on the opposite side of the wound, paralleling the point of entrance. The suture is then tied, drawing the tip snugly in place.
  - ❖ Subcuticular running suture (Fig. 120–5) is used for linear wounds under little or no tension, and allows for edema formation. Wound approximation may not

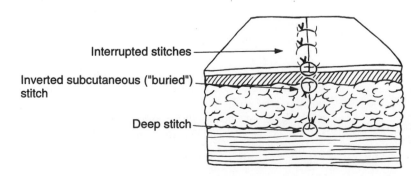

Interrupted stitches

Inverted subcutaneous ("buried") stitch

Deep stitch

■ ● FIGURE 120–2. Inverted subcutaneous suture. Also shown is layered closure. (From Pfenninger JL, Fowler GC, eds. *Procedures for Primary Care Physicians.* St. Louis: Mosby; 1994:16.)

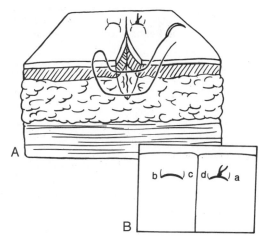

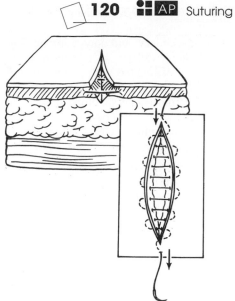

■ ● FIGURE 120–3. Vertical mattress suture. *A,* Cross-section. *B,* Overhead view. Begin at *a,* and go under skin to *b.* Come out, go in at *c,* and exit at *d.* (From Pfenninger JL, Fowler GC, eds. *Procedures for Primary Care Physicians.* St. Louis: Mosby; 1994:17.)

■ ● FIGURE 120–5. Intracuticular running suture. (From Pfenninger JL, Fowler GC, eds. *Procedures for Primary Care Physicians.* St. Louis: Mosby; 1994:17.)

be as meticulous as with an interrupted dermal suture. An anchor suture is placed at one end of the wound, then continuous sutures are placed at right angles to the wound <3 mm apart. The wound is pulled together and the other end secured with either another square knot or tape under slight tension.

- Lacerations that are not deep, have easily approximated edges, and are not in an area of tension or pressure may be closed with Steri-Strips rather than sutures.

- Sutures must be completely removed in a timely fashion to avoid further tissue inflammation and possible infection. Sutures on extremities and the trunk should be removed in 7 to 8 days; those on the face should be removed in 3 to 5 days; and those on the palms, soles, back, and skin over mobile joints should be removed in 10 to 14 days.

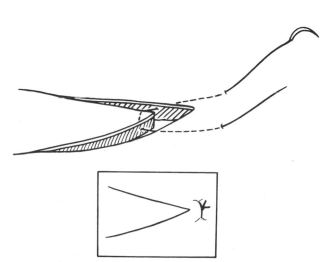

■ ● FIGURE 120–4. Three-point or half-buried mattress. (From Pfenninger JL, Fowler GC, eds. *Procedures for Primary Care Physicians.* St. Louis: Mosby; 1994:17.)

EQUIPMENT

- Local anesthetic (without epinephrine)
- Povidone-iodine and sterile normal saline (NS)
- Eight to ten 4 × 4 gauze sponges
- Sterile metal prep basin
- 30-mL or 60-mL syringe and 18-G needle
- Sterile drape
- Fenestrated drape
- Sterile gloves, mask, eye protection
- 6-inch needle holder
- Suture material and needle
- Curved dissecting scissors
- Two mosquito hemostats—one curved, one straight
- Suture scissors
- Tissue forceps
- Scalpel handle and no. 15 knife blade
- Skin hooks (for atraumatic tissue handling)

PATIENT AND FAMILY EDUCATION

- Explain the procedure and risks and reassure the patient and family. ➤*Rationale:* Decreases patient anxiety and encourages patient and family cooperation and understanding of procedure.
- As appropriate, instruct the patient and family on aftercare: pain medication, wound care, and observation for signs and symptoms of infection. ➤*Rationale:* Facilitates patient comfort, decreases risk of infection, and encourages prompt intervention to treat possible infection.

PATIENT ASSESSMENT AND PREPARATION
Patient Assessment

- History of present injury and past medical history. ➤*Rationale:* This allows a better understanding of the

⬛ AP This procedure should be performed only by physicians, advanced practice nurses, and other health care professionals (including critical care nurses) with additional knowledge, skills, and demonstrated competence per professional licensure or institutional standard.

nature of the injury and any complicating factors to wound healing. A delay in treatment of more than 3 hours often is associated with increased proliferation of bacteria and increased risk of infection.[5]

- Damage to peripheral nerve, blood supply, or motor function; x-rays may be needed to assess for bone injury. ➥*Rationale:* Determines the need for referral to a specialist.

Patient Preparation

- Ensure that patient understands preprocedural teaching. Answer questions as they arise and reinforce information as needed.   ➥*Rationale:* Evaluates and reinforces understanding of previously taught information.
- Administer tetanus prophylaxis, if necessary (Table 120–1).   ➥*Rationale:* Prevents possibility of tetanus from unclean wound.

Table 120–1 ● ■ ■   **Summary Guide to Tetanus Prophylaxis in Routine Wound Management**

History of Absorbed Tetanus Toxoid (Doses)	Clean, minor wounds		All other wounds*	
	Td[†]	TIG	Td[†]	TIG
Unknown or <three doses	Yes	No	Yes	Yes
≥Three doses‡	No§	No	No‖	No

Source: Centers for Disease Control. *MMWR.* 1991:40, No. Rr-10, 1-28.

*Such as, but not limited to, wounds contaminated with dirt, feces, soil, and saliva; puncture wounds; avulsions; and wounds resulting from missiles, crushing, burns, and frostbite.

†For children <7 years old; DTP (DT, if pertussis vaccine is contraindicated) is preferred to tetanus toxoid alone. For persons ≥7 years of age, Td is preferred to tetanus toxoid alone.

‡If only three doses of *fluid* toxoid have been received, then a fourth dose of toxoid, preferably an absorbed toxoid, should be given.

§Yes, if >10 years since last dose.

‖Yes, if >5 years since last dose. (More frequent boosters are not needed and can accentuate side effects.)

From Pfenninger JL, Fowler GC, eds. *Procedures for Primary Care Physicians.* St. Louis: Mosby; 1994:19.

Procedure   **for Suturing**

Steps	Rationale	Special Considerations
1. Wash hands, and don personal protective equipment.	Reduces transmission of microorganisms and body secretions; standard precautions.	
2. Anesthetize the wound. Use local anesthetic without epinephrine to infiltrate the area. *(Level IV: Limited clinical studies to support recommendations)*	Provides for maximum patient comfort and cooperation during suturing. Use of anesthetic with epinephrine produces local vasoconstriction, contributing to a decrease of white blood cells (WBCs), which may increase infection rate.[6]	Immobilization of site also aids in decreasing pain.
3. Examine wound thoroughly for foreign bodies, deep tissue layer damage, joint involvement, and injury to nerve, vessel, or tendon.	Prevents further damage. Assess need for referral.	Use aseptic technique to decrease contamination of wound.
4. Clean the wound. A. Mechanical—wiping, brushing, and irrigating with copious amounts of saline using a 30-mL or 60-mL syringe with 18-gauge needle.	Removes foreign substances and bacteria and prevents development of infection.	Mechanical cleaning is most important for prevention of infection. Wound must be properly scrubbed and irrigated with high pressure.
B. Chemical—antiseptic soaps.		Use a soap that is nontoxic to tissues.
C. If necessary, remove any hair in the area with an electric clipper. *(Level V: Clinical studies in more than one patient population and situation)*	Electric clippers (rather than razors) have been associated with significantly fewer infections.[7, 8]	
5. Apply sterile drapes over and under the area as necessary.	Creates a sterile field. Reduces risk of infection.	
6. Examine the wound again for devitalized tissue that needs removal or débridement.	Débridement may convert a jagged, contaminated wound into a clean surgical one and allow better approximation of tissues.	Use a scalpel or sharp tissue scissors, if necessary.
7. If needed, loosen the wound from the subcutaneous tissue beneath the dermis using scissors or scalpel.	Allows the skin to glide together easily.	

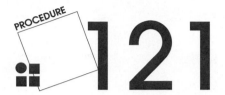

PROCEDURE

121

Cleansing, Irrigating, Culturing, and Dressing Open Wounds

P U R P O S E: Cleansing, irrigating, culturing, and dressing open wounds is performed to optimize healing. Wound culturing may be necessary to isolate and allow for treatment of organisms.

Mary Beth Flynn

PREREQUISITE NURSING KNOWLEDGE

- Goals of wound care must be clearly outlined so that proper wound care products are used. Coarse gauze debrides the wound bed and absorbs wound fluid; calcium alginates enhance wound absorption; hydrogels provide moisture to nondraining wounds; hydrocolloids provide wound moisture with minimal absorption.
- Wounds heal by either primary or secondary intention (Fig. 121–1). Most clean or clean/contaminated surgical wounds heal by primary intention. Suturing each layer of tissue approximates the wound edges. These wounds typically heal quickly and require minimal wound care. Contaminated surgical or traumatic wounds (open wounds) heal by secondary intention.
- Wounds healing by secondary intention granulate from the base of the wound to the skin surfaces; care must be taken to allow for uniform granulation and prevention of open pockets/tunneling.
- Open wounds must be clean and moist to promote effective and efficient wound healing. To that end, open wound care strives to maintain a clean, moist wound bed that allows for effective wound healing under the support of a dressing.
- Openly granulating wounds heal more slowly, must remain moist to enhance tissue granulation, and are more painful for the patient.
- Open wounds may have excessive wound drainage, requiring application of absorptive dressings or more frequent dressing changes to facilitate healing.

- Wound cleansing should be accomplished with minimal chemical and mechanical trauma. Cytotoxic cleaning agents should be avoided because they may delay healing and increase the risk of infection. Normal saline (NS) is the cleaning agent of choice for most wounds.[1]
- Wound infection is present if organisms are present at 10^5 colony-forming units per mL.
- Wound infections may be treated locally, systemically, or with combination therapy.
- Wound infections may delay wound healing; sterile wound cultures are obtained to isolate organisms and differentiate between colonization and active infection within a wound bed.

EQUIPMENT

- Nonsterile and sterile gloves (two pairs); sterile field
- Gowns and face protection
- Sterile gauze (4 × 4)
- Normal saline (NS)
- Sterile basin
- Waterproof barrier
- Sterile 35-mL slip-tip syringe and 19-G needle for irrigation (if necessary)

- Sterile gauze (4 × 4); ABD dressings may be needed (if the wound has excessive drainage, an absorptive dressing may be necessary or if the wound has minimal drainage, a moisture enhancing dressing may be needed)
- Hypoallergenic tape; one set of Montgomery straps
- Liquid skin barrier for applying Montgomery straps; hydrocolloid wafer

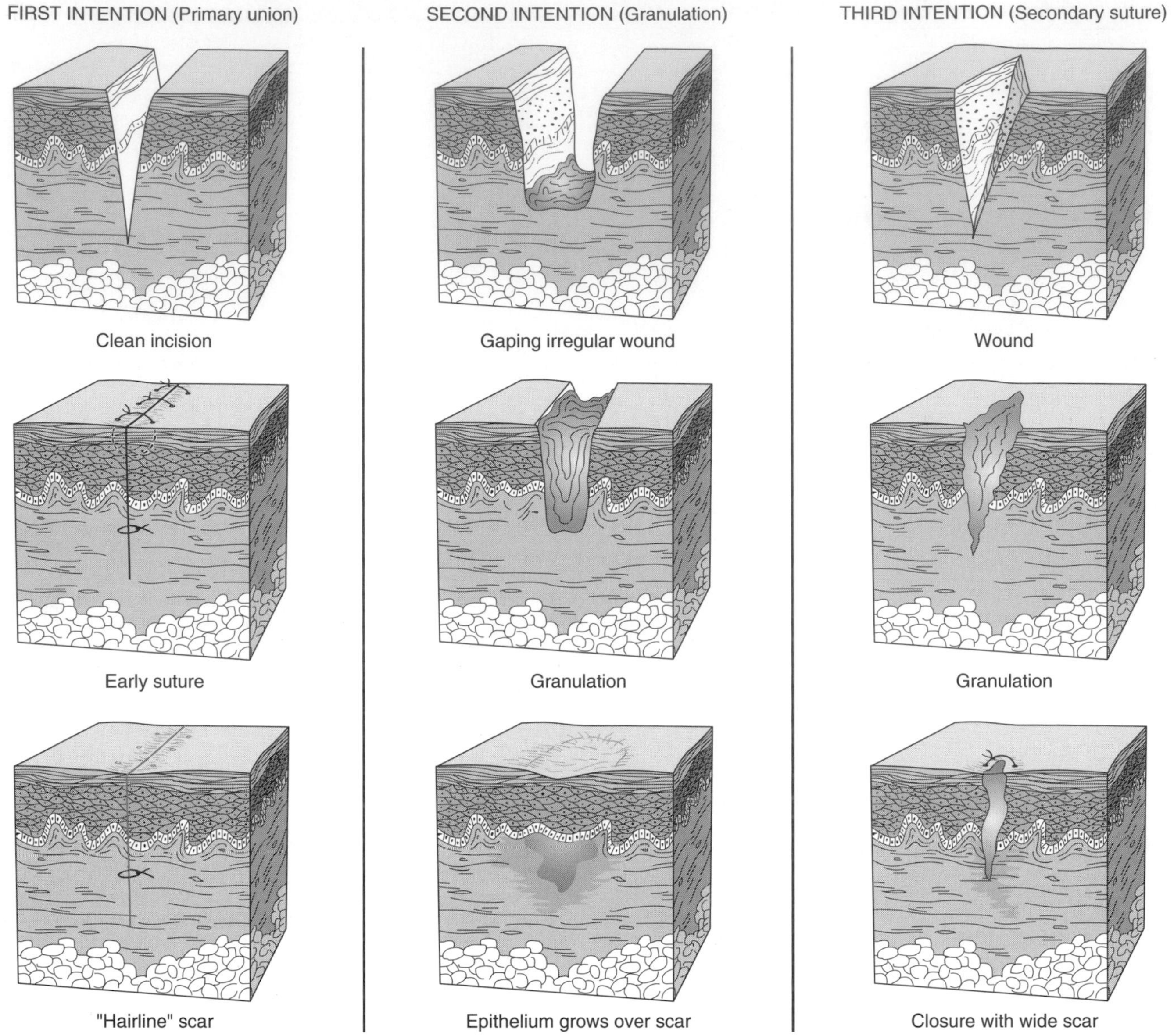

FIRST INTENTION (Primary union)   SECOND INTENTION (Granulation)   THIRD INTENTION (Secondary suture)

Clean incision   Gaping irregular wound   Wound

Early suture   Granulation   Granulation

"Hairline" scar   Epithelium grows over scar   Closure with wide scar

■ ● **FIGURE 121–1.** Wound healing by primary, secondary, and tertiary intention.

Additional equipment (to have available depending on patient need) includes the following:

- Swab culture: two sterile serum-tipped swabs
- Needle aspiration: 10-mL syringe and 22-G needle
- Tissue biopsy: scalpel, sterile forceps, and container

PATIENT AND FAMILY EDUCATION

- Explain the procedure and reason for wound cleansing, irrigation, culture, and dressing management.   ➤*Rationale:* Decreases patient anxiety and discomfort.
- Discuss patient's role in wound cleansing, irrigation, culturing, and dressing management.   ➤*Rationale:* Elicits patient cooperation; prepares patient for wound management on discharge (as appropriate).

- Explain the procedure and reason for obtaining a wound culture.   ➤*Rationale:* Decreases patient anxiety and discomfort.

PATIENT ASSESSMENT AND PREPARATION

Patient Assessment

- Assess for the following:
  ❖ Wound drainage
  ❖ Foul drainage or odor
  ❖ Darkened areas on tissue bed, pale red tissue bed
  ❖ Green or yellow wound bed
  ❖ Erythema
  ❖ Pain
  ❖ Change in wound drainage amount or color
  ❖ Elevated temperature

❖ Elevated white blood cell count

❖ Presence and depth of pocket/tunnel

➤*Rationale:* Assessment of the wound bed provides information about the healing process and assists in early identification of wound infection. True wound bed assessment cannot be completed until after the wound bed has been cleansed.

Patient Preparation

• Ensure that patient understands preprocedural teaching. Answer questions as they arise and reinforce information as needed. ➤*Rationale:* Evaluates and reinforces understanding of previously taught information.

• Place patient in position of optimal comfort and visualization for wound care procedures. ➤*Rationale:* Provides for effective wound visualization and enhances patient tolerance of procedure.

• Optimize lighting in room and provide privacy for patient. ➤*Rationale:* Allows for optimal wound assessment and patient comfort.

• Premedicate patient with prescribed analgesic. ➤*Rationale:* Decreases patient anxiety and increases comfort.

Procedure for Cleansing, Irrigating, Culturing, and Dressing Open Wounds		
Steps	**Rationale**	**Special Considerations**
Cleansing and Irrigating Wounds		
1. Wash hands; position patient to facilitate drainage and cleansing of wound.	Decreases contamination; use gravity to direct flow of solution away from wound bed.	
2. Position waterproof barrier to collect drainage.	Controls flow of cleansing solution and wound drainage; minimizes solution contact with intact skin.	
3. Position wound cleansing materials and soiled contamination container within reach of practitioner and patient; conform to principles of aseptic technique.	Decrease cross-contamination during wound cleansing process; enhances body mechanics for practitioner.	
4. Wash hands, and don personal protective equipment.	Reduces transmission of microorganisms; standard precautions.	
5. Remove soiled dressing and discard in appropriate container. Assess wound bed. Remove soiled gloves.	Assess wound upon dressing removal for type, odor, and amount of drainage.	True wound bed assessment cannot be completed until after the wound bed has been cleansed.
6. Establish sterile field; open sterile gauze; place sterile water or NS cleaning solution in sterile container. (*Level VI: Clinical studies in a variety of patient populations and situations*)	Decreases cross-contamination during the wound cleansing process. Cleansing solution should not be cytotoxic.[1, 4]	
7. If irrigation (Fig. 121–2) is necessary, attach 19-G needle to syringe for irrigation; draw up solution into syringe; don sterile gloves. Maintain needle 1 to 3 cm from wound surface; direct solution onto wound bed from area of least contamination to greatest. Continue with irrigation until return solution is clear. (*Level V: Clinical studies in more than one patient population and situation*)	Irrigation removes excess debris to enhance healing. A 35-mL syringe with a 19-G needle provides approximately 8 psi, which is sufficient force to remove debris without creating wound bed damage. The smaller the syringe, the greater the psi.[1, 2, 4] Too great a force during irrigation can create tissue damage, reinitiating the inflammatory process and delaying wound healing.	Not all open wound beds need irrigation with a needle. Gentle irrigation using a slip-tip 35-mL syringe is indicated for open wounds that are granulating well.[1, 2, 4]
8. Cleansing a closed wound: using moistened gauze, cleanse from top of wound to base (or center of wound to edges); discard gauze (Fig. 121–3A & B). Clean from area of least contamination to greatest.	Prevents wound contamination during the cleansing process.	If cleansing around a drain, clean from drain site outward in a circular motion; discard gauze with each circle.
9. Dry intact skin surrounding wound with gauze.	Limits maceration of healthy skin surrounding the wound.	

Procedure continued on page 855

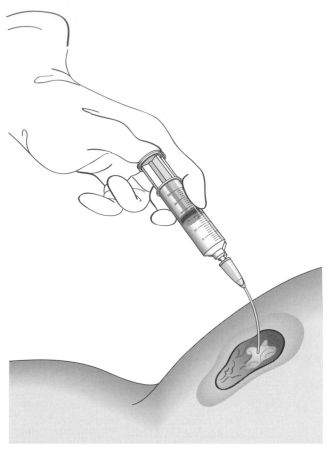

■ ● **FIGURE 121–2.** Irrigating a wound.

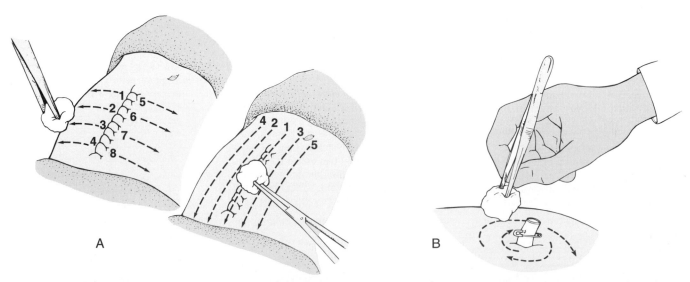

A

B

■ ● **FIGURE 121–3.** Cleaning a wound. (From Potter PA, Perry A. *Basic Nursing: Theory and Practice.* St. Louis, Mo: Mosby; 1995: 1143.)

Procedure	for Cleansing, Irrigating, Culturing, and Dressing Open Wounds *Continued*

Steps	Rationale	Special Considerations
Culturing Wounds		
Swab Culture		
1. Don clean gloves, and remove swab from culturette tube; maintain sterile technique. *(Level V: Clinical studies in more than one patient population and situation)*	Must clean wound before obtaining culture to ensure that debris contamination is not cultured.[2, 5, 6] Wound culturing is a sterile procedure.	
2. Swab across the surface of the wound in a zigzag manner, simultaneously rotating the swab between finger and thumb. *(Level IV: Limited clinical studies to support recommendations)*	Ensures collection of an adequate specimen.[5, 6]	
3. Carefully place swab into culturette tube without touching swab or inside of container.	Prevents contamination.	Swab center of wound and not wound edges. Culturing of wound edges may result in contamination from skin flora and wound debris.
4. Crush ampule of medium in culturette and close securely; observe that culture medium surrounds swab.	Keeps specimen from drying and provides growth-supporting medium for culture.	If collecting an anaerobic culture, ensure tube is maintained upright to prevent carbon dioxide from escaping.
5. Label specimen with patient name, date, wound site; transport to laboratory as soon as possible.		
Tissue Biopsy		
1. Don sterile gloves; using sterile scalpel and forceps, obtain a tissue sample approximately 1 to 2 cm in size (width and depth); apply pressure with sterile gauze to tissue sampling site. *(Level IV: Limited clinical studies to support recommendations)*	Ensures good sample size; provides for homeostasis of tissue bed.[1, 5, 6]	Caution must be exercised in obtaining a tissue biopsy; assess for excessive bleeding and damage to underlying and surrounding structures. Advanced training is encouraged for practitioners performing this skill.
2. Place tissue sample in sterile container and close tightly; sample may be placed on agar plate, if indicated.	Prevents contamination of sample.	
3. Label specimen with patient name, date, wound site; transport to laboratory as soon as possible. Proceed to "Dressing Open Wounds."		
Needle Aspiration		
1. Don clean gloves; insert sterile needle into drainage; aspirate approximtely 5 to 10 mL of drainge into sterile syringe. *(Level IV: Limited clinical studies to support recommendtions)*	Ensures good specimen collection. Use syringe method only when large amounts of drainage are present, or for collecting specimens from deep wounds.[1, 4]	
2. Express excess air out of syringe.		
3. Remove needle and replace with a needleless blunt end cap; maintain sterile technique.	Maintains standard precautions; prevents contamination.	
4. Label specimen with patient name, date, wound site; transport to laboratory as soon as possible.		

Procedure continued on following page

Procedure	**for Cleansing, Irrigating, Culturing, and Dressing Open Wounds** *Continued*

Steps	Rationale	Special Considerations
Dressing Open Wounds		
1. Open sterile gauze 4 × 4s and saturate with normal saline; don sterile gloves; wring out excessive moisture; apply 4 × 4s loosely over wound bed; gently pack gauze to wound edge but do not exceed wound edge. *(Level V: Clinical studies in more than one patient population and situation)*	Open, moist gauze protects wound bed, allows for placement of dressing without creating open areas or pockets; dressing must be moist but not wet to allow for absorption.[1, 7]	Moist dressing must stay within parameters of wound bed to prevent surrounding skin maceration. Dressings packed too firmly into wound will compromise perfusion and wound healing. Wound care dressing products that absorb drainage or provide moisture may also be used.
2. Place dry gauze 4 × 4s and ABDs over moist dressing.	Provides protection and absorption.	
3. Secure dressing with tape or Montgomery straps.		
A. Tape: apply tape across the wound dressing, extending approximately 2 in beyond dressing onto skin.	Hypoallergenic tape is less traumatic to noninjured skin; secures dressing in place.	
B. Montgomery straps (Fig. 121–4): ○ Apply a liquid or hydrocolloid barrier to surround skin where Montgomery straps will be applied.	Assists with providing a protective skin barrier and more effective anchoring of Montgomery straps.	
○ Peel paper backing off of Montgomery straps and apply to skin surface using gentle, even pressure.	Secures Montgomery straps to skin.	
○ Lace the cotton type (twill tape, umbilical tape, tracheotomies) through holes in the Montgomery straps in a criss-cross fashion.	Secures dressing in place beneath Montgomery strap.	

Expected Outcomes	Unexpected Outcomes
• Wound bed will be clean.	• Cross-contamination of wound
• Wound culture specimen obtained will confirm and identify causative organism of infection.	• Damage to wound bed (hemorrhage, dehiscence) from excessive force during irrigation
• Wound will heal uniformly without tunneling or tracking or infection.	• Maceration or inflammation of surrounding skin
• Surrounding skin is free of maceration and erosion.	• Hemorrhage from tissue biopsy culture technique
• Wound is free of signs of infection or compromised perfusion.	• Signs of infection; changes in amount and character of wound drainage
	• Wound healing (granulation and contraction) is not noticeably progressing on a weekly basis
	• Development of wound tunneling or tracking

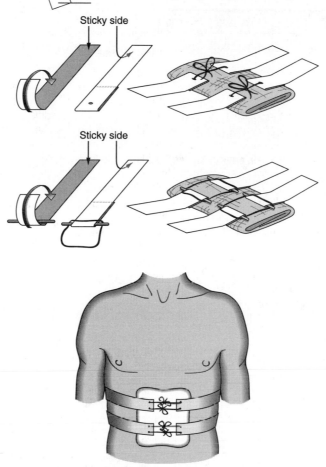

■ ● FIGURE 121–4. Montgomery straps.

Patient Monitoring and Care

Patient Monitoring and Care	Rationale	Reportable Conditions
		These conditions should be reported if they persist despite nursing interventions.
1. Assess patient, wound bed, and skin surrounding wound. *(Level V: Clinical studies in more than one patient population and situation)*	Continued assessment for wound infection is essential; wounds must be free of infection to heal. Wound colonization is the presence of bacteria in a wound in quantities that do not interfere with wound healing.[1] Infection is the presence of bacteria in a wound that elicits an inflammatory response and interferes with wound healing.[1-6] Healthy granulation tissue will be red in color. Discoloration may indicate infection, necrotic tissue, and poor perfusion or hypoxemia at the wound bed site.	• Foul drainage or odor • Darkened areas on tissue bed; pale red tissue bed • Green or yellow wound bed • Erythema • Pain • Change in wound drainage amount or color • Elevated temperature • Elevated white blood cell count
2. Monitor wound dressing site for bleeding.	Capillary bed of a healing wound is very fragile. Excessive stimulation created during the collection of a culture by tissue biopsy or needle aspiration may disrupt the capillary integrity, creating excessive bleeding.	• Bleeding that does not stop with mild pressure to wound bed • Excessive bleeding
3. Assess wound bed and edges for pockets or tunnels.	Wounds healing by secondary intention are at increased risk of developing pockets or tunnels.	• Presence and depth of pocket or tunnel

Documentation

Documentation should include the following:

- Patient and family education
- Premedication given, patient tolerance of procedure, and response to pain medication
- Wound cleansing and irrigation procedure completed, date, time
- Description of wound bed before and after cleansing or irritation; drainage and odors if appropriate; note presence of necrotic and granulation tissue
- Description of surrounding skin (color, moisture, integrity)
- Size of wound: measure or trace wound area and depth when appropriate
- Wound culture completed, date,

time; state type of culture obtained (swab, aerobic, anaerobic, needle aspiration, tissue biopsy)
- Description of approximate site where wound culture was obtained
- Description of wound drains, surrounding skin, and characteristics of wound drainage
- Type of dressing applied after wound care
- Unexpected outcomes
- Nursing interventions

References

1. Agency for Health Care Policy and Research. *Clinical Practice Guideline: Treatment of Pressure Ulcers.* Rockville, Md: US Department of Health and Human Services; 1994.
2. Thomson PD, Taddonio TE. Wound infection. In: Krasner D, Kane D, eds. *Chronic Wound Care: A Clinical Source Book for Healthcare Professionals.* 2nd ed. Wayne, Pa: Health Management Publications; 1997:84–88.
3. Crow S. Infection control perspectives. In: Krasner D, Kane D, eds. *Chronic Wound Care: A Clinical Source Book for Healthcare Professionals.* 2nd ed. Wayne, Pa: Health Management Publications; 1997:90–96.
4. Rodeheaver GT. Wound cleansing, wound irrigation, and wound disinfection. In: Krasner D, Kane D, eds. *Chronic Wound Care: A Clinical Source Book for Healthcare Professionals.* 2nd ed. Wayne, Pa: Health Management Publications; 1997:97–108.
5. Neil JA, Munro CL. A comparison of two culturing methods for chronic wounds. *Ostomy/Wound Management.* 1997;43:20–30.
6. Gilchrist B. Infection and culturing. In: Krasner D, Kane D, eds. *Chronic Wound Care: A Clinical Source Book for Healthcare Professionals.* 2nd ed. Wayne, Pa: Health Management Publications; 1997:109–114.
7. Maklebust J. Using wound care products to promote a healing environment. *Crit Care Nurs Clin North Am.* 1996;8:141–158.

Additional Readings

Bagley SM. Nutritional needs of the acutely ill with acute wounds. *Crit Care Nurs Clin North Am.* 1996;8:159–167.

Boynton PR, Paustian C. Wound assessment and decision making options. *Crit Care Nurs Clin North Am.* 1996;8:125–139.

Brylinsky CM. Nutrition and wound healing: an overview. *Ostomy/Wound Management.* 1995;41:14–24.

Flanigan KH. Nutritional aspects of wound healing. *Adv Wound Care.* 1997;10:48–52.

Flynn MB. Wound healing in critical illness. *Crit Care Nurs Clin North Am.* 1996;8:115–123.

Kane DP, Krasner D. Wound healing and wound management. In: Krasner D, Kane D, eds. *Chronic Wound Care: A Clinical Source Book for Healthcare Professionals.* 2nd ed. Wayne, Pa: Health Management Publications; 1997:1–4.

Kerstein MD. The scientific basis of healing. *Adv Wound Care.* 1997;10:30–36.

Rijswijk LV. The fundamentals of wound assessment. *Ostomy/Wound Management.* 1996;42:40–52.

Rijswik LV. Wound assessment and documentation. In: Krasner D, Kane D, eds. *Chronic Wound Care: A Clinical Source Book for Healthcare Professionals.* 2nd ed. Wayne, Pa: Health Management Publications; 1997:16–28.

Rook JL. Wound care pain management. *Adv Wound Care.* 1996;9:24–31.

122 Dressing Wounds with Drains

P U R P O S E: Dressing wounds with drains is performed to manage wound dressings in the presence of drains.

Mary Beth Flynn

PREREQUISITE NURSING KNOWLEDGE

- Goals of wound care must be clearly outlined so that proper wound care products are used. Coarse gauze will debride wound bed and absorb wound fluid; calcium alginates will enhance wound absorption; hydrogels will provide moisture to nondraining wounds; hydrocolloids will provide wound moisture with minimal absorption.[1]
- Drains are placed in wounds to facilitate healing by providing an exit for excessive fluid accumulating in or near the wound bed.
- Excessive wound fluid may create pressure in the wound bed and compromise perfusion.
- Excessive wound fluid may provide a source for proliferation of microorganisms.
- Wound drains may be ports of microorganism entry;[2, 3] aseptic techniques must be strictly observed.
- Most wound drains are surgically placed; drains may or may not be sutured in place.[3]

EQUIPMENT

- Nonsterile and sterile gloves; sterile field
- Gowns and face protection
- Sterile gauze (4 × 4); ABD dressings may be needed
- Sterile water or normal saline (NS) for cleansing
- Hypoallergenic tape; one set of Montgomery straps
- Liquid skin barrier for applying Montgomery straps; hydrocolloid wafer

PATIENT AND FAMILY EDUCATION

- Explain the procedure and the reason for changing wound dressing. ➟*Rationale:* Decreases patient anxiety and discomfort.

- Discuss patient's role in dressing change procedure and maintenance of wound drains. ➟*Rationale:* Elicits patient cooperation; prepares patient for wound management on discharge.

PATIENT ASSESSMENT AND PREPARATION
Patient Assessment

- Monitor for signs and symptoms of wound infection, including the following:
  ❖ Erythema at drainage site
  ❖ Heat
  ❖ Edema
  ❖ Pain
  ❖ Elevated temperature and white blood cell count
  ❖ Wound drainage becoming cloudy and foul smelling

- ➟*Rationale:* Drains assist with removal of excessive fluid but also provide a portal of entry for microorganisms.
- Assess patency of wound drainage system. ➟*Rationale:* Drains are frequently soft and pliable and thus can easily become kinked or blocked if wound drainage is fibrous in composition.

Patient Preparation

- Premedicate patient with prescribed analgesic. ➟*Rationale:* Decreases patient anxiety and discomfort.
- Place patient in position of optimal comfort and visualization for dressing the wound. ➟*Rationale:* Provides for effective wound visualization and enhances patient tolerance of procedure.
- Optimize lighting in room and provide privacy for patient. ➟*Rationale:* Allows for optimal wound assessment and patient comfort.

Procedure for Dressing Wounds with Drains

Steps	Rationale	Special Considerations
1. Wash hands, don gloves, and remove old dressing.	Maintains aseptic technique.	Use caution with dressing removal to ensure that drains are not dislodged.
2. Remove gloves, and wash hands		
3. Establish sterile field.	Maintains aseptic technique.	
4. Don personal protective equipment.	Standard precautions.	
5. Clean and irrigate wound (see Procedure 121) as indicated.	Removes contaminated drainage and debris from wound.	Irrigation of wound drains should be performed only if indicated by physician or nurse practitioner.[1, 3]
6. Change gloves; open 4 × 4 gauze pad and apply on top of wound and around drains (Fig. 122–1). Avoid wrapping gauze around drain site.	Gauze absorbs drainage to keep underlying skin dry; wrapping gauze around drain may result in inadvertent drain removal with future dressing changes.	Drains are placed to remove excessive wound fluid. Care must be taken to provide a dressing capable of absorbing wound drainage and preventing moisture accumulation on surrounding healthy skin.[4]
7. Apply gauze dressings from area of least contamination to area of greatest contamination.	Prevents cross-contamination of wound bed.	
8. If necessary, apply ABD or other absorptive dressing over 4 × 4 gauze pads.	Gauze 4 × 4 pads enhance removal of drainage away from skin; secondary dressing prevents contamination and protects clothing from drainage.	
9. Apply tape or Montgomery straps to secure dressing. Hydrocolloid wafers may be placed on skin, creating a protective barrier for application of tape or Montgomery straps.	When tape is used to secure dressings, frequent dressing changes may result in skin irritation or disruption from the adhesive tape. Hypoallergenic tape, Montgomery straps, and skin barriers help decrease mechanical irritation caused by frequent tape removal.	
A. Tape: Apply hypoallergenic tape across the wound dressing extending approximately 2 in beyond dressing onto skin.	Hypoallergenic tape is less traumatic to noninjured skin; it is necessary to extend tape beyond dressing edges to anchor and secure dressing well.	
B. Montgomery straps (see Fig. 121–4): ○ Apply a liquid or hydrocolloid barrier to surrounding skin when Montgomery straps are used.	Assists with providing protective skin barrier and more effective anchoring of Montgomery strap.	
○ Peel paper backing off Montgomery straps and apply to skin surface using gentle, even pressure.	Secures Montgomery straps to skin.	
○ Lace cotton tape (twill tape, umbilical tape, tracheostomy ties) through holes in the Montgomery straps in a crisscross fashion.	Secures dressing in place beneath Montgomery strap.	

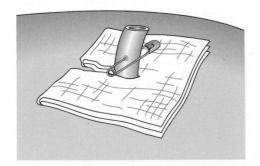

■ ● **FIGURE 122–1.** Dressing a wound with a drain.

Expected Outcomes	Unexpected Outcomes
• Drains remain intact and patent and effectively remove excessive wound fluid. • Surrounding skin is dry and free of excessive wound drainage moisture (maceration). • Wound drainage exit sites are clean and dry, without signs of infection or irritation. • Wound healing is enhanced because of effective wound drainage removal. • Wound drainage decreases in volume (over time) and is absent of foul odor or color.	• Wound drain becomes dislodged, blocked, or kinked. • Skin erosion or maceration occurs around wound drainage sites or skin sites or both.

Patient Monitoring and Care

Patient Monitoring and Care	Rationale	Reportable Conditions
		These conditions should be reported if they persist despite nursing interventions.
1. Observe for signs of wound infection.	Drains assist with removal of excessive fluid but also provide a portal of entry of microorganisms.[3]	• Erythema at drainage site • Heat • Edema • Pain • Elevated temperature and white blood cell count • Wound drainage becoming cloudy and foul smelling
2. Assess for patency of wound drainage system.	Drains are frequently soft and pliable and thus can easily become kinked or blocked if wound drainage is fibrous in composition.	• Wound drainage suddenly decreasing in amount or stopping
3. Monitor amount of wound drainage relative to patient intake and output.	If a wound produces excessive fluid, the patient may experience a fluid imbalance requiring intravenous or oral fluid replacements.	• Tachycardia • Hypotension • Oliguria • Increasing amounts of drainage

Documentation

Documentation should include the following:

- Patient and family education
- Premedication given, patient tolerance of procedure, and response to pain medication
- Wound cleansing and dressing change completed/date, time
- Description of wound bed, drains (suction if applied), surrounding skin, and characteristics of wound drainage
- Dressing applied after wound care
- Unexpected outcomes
- Nursing interventions

References

1. Faller NA. When a wound isn't a wound: tubes, drains, fistulae, and draining wounds. In: Krasner D, Kane D, eds. *Chronic Wound Care: A Clinical Source Book for Healthcare Professionals.* 2nd ed. Wayne Pa: Health Management Publications; 1997:202–208.

2. Dane DP. Surgical repair. In: Krasner D, Kane D, eds. *Chronic Wound Care: A Clinical Source Book for Healthcare Professionals.* 2nd ed. Wayne, Pa: Health Management Publications; 1997:235–244.

3. Hochberg J, Murray G. Principles of operative surgery: antisepsis, technique, sutures, and drains. In: Sabiston DC, ed. *Textbook of Surgery.* 5th ed. Philadelphia, Pa: WB Saunders; 1997:253–280.

4. Maklebust J. Using wound care products to promote a healing environment. *Crit Care Nurs Clin North Am.* 1996;8(2):141–158.

Additional Reading

Krasner D. Minimizing factors that impair wound healing: a nursing approach. *Ostomy/Wound Management.* 1995;41(1):22–30.

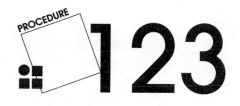

123 Drain Removal

PURPOSE: Drain removal is performed to safely remove a wound drain.

Mary Beth Flynn

PREREQUISITE NURSING KNOWLEDGE

- Goals of wound care must be clearly outlined so that proper wound care products are used. Coarse gauze debrides the wound bed and absorbs wound fluid; calcium alginates enhance wound absorption; hydrogels provide moisture to nondraining wounds; hydrocolloids provide wound moisture with minimal absorption.[1]
- Type of drain, location, and how the drain is secured must be known before drain removal. Competence should be demonstrated by the clinician performing drain removal, because significant tissue injury may result from an improperly removed drain.[2, 3]

EQUIPMENT

- Nonsterile gloves
- Gowns and face protection
- Sterile gauze (4 × 4)
- Suture removal kit or sterile scissors
- Hypoallergic tape

PATIENT AND FAMILY EDUCATION

- Explain the procedure and reason for drain removal. **➤Rationale:** Decreases patient anxiety and discomfort.
- Discuss patient's role in drain removal. **➤Rationale:** Elicits patient cooperation; prepares patient for wound management on discharge.

PATIENT ASSESSMENT AND PREPARATION

Patient Assessment

- Signs of wound infection at drain site include the following:
  - ❖ Erythema
  - ❖ Pain
  - ❖ Edema
  - ❖ Elevated temperature
  - ❖ White blood cell count
  - ❖ Foul drainage from exit site
  - ❖ Pressure or tenderness at exit site.

  ➤Rationale: Although drains are placed to remove excessive wound fluid and decrease the risk of infection, early detection of infection facilitates prompt, appropriate intervention.

Patient Preparation

- Ensure that patient understands preprocedural teaching. Answer questions as they arise and reinforce information as needed. **➤Rationale:** Evaluates and reinforces understanding of previously taught information.
- Premedicate patient with prescribed analgesic. **➤Rationale:** Although many patients do not require premedication for drain removal, all patients should be treated appropriately.

Procedure for Drain Removal

Steps	Rationale	Special Considerations
1. Don gloves and personal protective equipment.	Maintain aseptic technique; standard precautions.	
2. Open sterile scissors; cut any sutures.	Releases drain from tissue suture anchors.	
3. Open gauze 4 × 4; place gauze close to drain skin exit site; instruct patient to take a deep, easy breath; swiftly, evenly withdraw drain. *(Level IV: Limited clinical studies to support recommendations)*	Gauze is used to capture body fluids as you remove the drain. Deep breathing may decrease the pain the patient feels with drain removal.[2]	Do not force removal of drain. If resistance is felt, stop.
4. Place sterile dressing over drain exit site and secure with tape.	Provides protection of open wound site; prevents entrance of microorganisms.	

- Intact drain is removed without resistance.
- Wound drainage is minimal from drainage exit site.
- Wound drain exit site is free of signs of fluid accumulation, inflammation, or infection.
- Wound healing continues to progress without presence of excessive wound fluid.

- Resistance is felt on drain removal, creating tissue trauma beneath skin surface.
- Wound fluid accumulates beneath skin at drain exit site.[2]
- Infection of inflammation occurs at drain exit site.
- There is poor approximation of skin edges at drain exit site, requiring wound healing by secondary intention.
- A portion of the drain remains in the wound tract.

Patient Monitoring and Care

Patient Monitoring and Care	Rationale	Reportable Conditions
		These conditions should be reported if they persist despite nursing interventions.
1. Assess for presence of drainage from drain exit site.	Drainage should be minimal and potentially cease within 24 hours. Continued drainage from drain exit site may indicate accumulation of wound fluid beneath the skin that needs to be evacuated.	• Continued drainage
2. Monitor for signs of infection.	Drains are placed to remove excessive wound fluid and decrease risk of infection.	• Erythema • Pain • Edema • Elevated temperature and white blood cell count • Foul drainage from exit site • Pressure or tenderness at exit site

Documentation

Documentation should include the following:

- Patient and family education
- Type of drain removed, placement, date, time
- Amount of wound drainage documented in the last 24 hours prior to drain removal
- Premedication given, patient tolerance of procedure, and response to pain medication
- Dressing applied after drain removal
- Unexpected outcomes
- Nursing interventions

References

1. Hochberg J, Murray G. Principles of operative surgery: antisepsis, technique, sutures, and drains. In: Sabiston DC, ed. *Textbook of Surgery.* 5th ed. Philadelphia, Pa: W.B. Saunders, 1997:253–280.
2. Kane DP, Kranser D. Wound healing and wound management. In: Krasner D, Kane D, eds. *Chronic Source Book for Healthcare Professionals.* 2nd ed. Wayne, Pa: Health Management Publications; 1997:1–4.
3. Faller NA. When a wound isn't a wound: tubes, drains, fistulae, and draining wounds. In: Krasner D, Kane D, eds. *Chronic Wound Care: A Clinical Source Book for Healthcare Profes-* *sionals.* 2nd ed. Wayne, Pa: Health Management Publications; 1997:202–208.

Additional Readings

Dane DP. Surgical repair. In: Krasner D, Kane D, eds. *Chronic Wound Care: A Clinical Source Book for Healthcare Professionals.* 2nd ed. Wayne, Pa: Health Management Publications; 1997:235–244.
Krasner D. Minimizing factors that impair wound healing: a nursing approach. *Ostomy/Wound Management.* 1995;41:22–30.
Papantonio C. Alternative medicine and wound healing. *Ostomy/ Wound Management.* 1998;44:44–55.

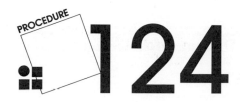

124

Dressing and Pouching Draining Wounds

P U R P O S E: Pouching a draining wound is performed to provide a method for dressing a heavily draining wound.

Mary Beth Flynn

PREREQUISITE NURSING KNOWLEDGE

- Goals for wound pouching must be clearly outlined; wound drainage to suction or collection must be defined.
- Excessive wound drainage is removed to allow for wound healing to occur without tissue congestion, microorganism proliferation, and skin maceration.

EQUIPMENT

- Nonsterile and sterile gloves; sterile field
- Gowns and face protection
- Sterile gauze (4 × 4)
- Normal saline (NS) for cleansing wound
- Drainage bag or pouch
- Skin barrier or wafer; paste; powder and sealant, if appropriate
- Clean scissors; forceps, if appropriate
- Tape

PATIENT AND FAMILY EDUCATION

- Explain the procedure and reason for changing wound dressing or pouch; educate regarding potential odor during procedure. ➤➤*Rationale:* Decreases patient anxiety and discomfort.
- Discuss patient's role in dressing/pouch change procedure and maintenance of wound drains/stomas. ➤➤*Rationale:* Elicits patient cooperation; prepares patient for wound management on discharge.

PATIENT ASSESSMENT AND PREPARATION
Patient Assessment

- Signs and symptoms of wound infection include the following:
  ❖ Erythema
  ❖ Pain
  ❖ Elevated temperature and white blood cell count
  ❖ Wound drainage changes in color, odor, or amount
  ❖ Pressure or tenderness at exit site

  ➤➤*Rationale:* Early detection of infection facilitates prompt, appropriate intervention.

Patient Preparation

- Ensure that patient understands preprocedural teaching. Answer questions as they arise and reinforce information as needed. ➤➤*Rationale:* Evaluates and reinforces understanding of previously taught information.
- Premedicate patient with prescribed analgesic. ➤➤*Rationale:* Decreases patient anxiety and discomfort.
- Place patient in position of optimal comfort and visualization for dressing the wound. ➤➤*Rationale:* Provides for effective wound visualization and enhances patient tolerance of procedure.
- Optimize lighting in room and provide privacy for patient. ➤➤*Rationale:* Allows for optimal wound assessment and patient comfort.

Procedure for Dressing and Pouching Draining Wounds

Steps	Rationale	Special Considerations
1. Wash hands, and don gloves and personal protective equipment.	Reduces transmission of microorganisms; standard precautions.	
2. If current drainage pouch has external opening, drain and measure content volume and discard.	Reduces transmission of microorganisms during dressing change; provides documentation of wound or fistula drainage.	Ensure that you have all needed supplies before removing old pouching system.
3. Gently remove old drainage pouch; support underlying skin with fingertips while drainage pouch is being removed; dispose of pouch.	Prevents tissue trauma to underlying skin.	A moist cloth may be applied to loosen edges of drainage pouch and assist with the removal process.
4. Using wet gauze 4 × 4s, gently clean wound site from area of least contamination to greatest (see Procedure 121); clean and dry surrounding intact skin.	Maintains clean wound environment; surrounding skin should be free of moisture.	
5. If ordered, irrigate wound/fistula (see Procedure 121) with NS until drainage is clear.	Cleans wound bed; decreases microorganism count.	
6. Using wrapper from wound drainage pouch or wafer, draw (measure) wound or fistula edge onto wrapper; cut out the center of the pattern on the wound skin barrier and drainage pouch (cut the pattern *slightly* larger than the tracing).	Irregular shapes and sizes of draining wounds are difficult to estimate; tracing wound onto wrapper will allow for a better seal to wound, with less moisture settling on intact surrounding skin.	
7. Apply skin barrier (wafer, liquid, paste, sealant).	Assists in providing a good seal for the drainage pouch.	
8. Remove adhesive paper from drainage pouch; apply drainage pouch over wound and, using gentle, even pressure, secure pouch edges to skin barrier. *(Level IV: Limited clinical studies to support recommendations)*	Gentle, even pressure helps ensure a better seal from the drainage pouch to skin barrier; care must be taken to avoid wrinkles from developing during pouch application; wrinkles in pouch barrier will create a leak and fluid will not be contained within drainage pouch.[1,2]	If wrinkles are present, sealant paste may be added to drainage pouch edges to fill spaces created by wrinkles. However, fluid may still track in the wrinkles, despite paste.
9. Close drainage pouch; wound drainage may be allowed to collect in pouch or suction may be attached to end of pouch to pull fluid away from wound into a more distant collection container. *(Level IV: Limited clinical studies to support recommendations)*	The type and amount of drainage coming from a wound determines whether or not suction is added to the drainage pouch.[1,2]	

Expected Outcomes

- Skin surrounding a draining wound remains intact.
- Wound drainage is effectively collected.
- Wound healing is enhanced because of removal of wound drainage into collection device.

Unexpected Outcomes

- Wound drainage is not effectively collected, and surrounding skin is macerated.
- Wound drain (if present) is dislodged during dressing or pouching procedure.
- Wound is not healing efficiently because management of wound drainage is not effective.

Patient Monitoring and Care

Patient Monitoring and Care	Rationale	Reportable Conditions
		These conditions should be reported if they persist despite nursing interventions.
1. Observe for signs of wound infection.	Wounds with unmanaged excessive drainage are at higher risk of infection. Wound drainage should slowly decrease as the wound is healing.	• Erythema • Pain • Elevated temperature and white blood cell count • Wound drainage changes in color, odor, or amount
2. Monitor amount of wound drainage relative to patient intake and output.	Excessive wound drainage may cause a fluid imbalance, requiring intravenous or oral fluid replacements.	• Tachycardia • Hypotension • Oliguria • Decreased filling pressures
3. Assess for continued adherence of drainage pouch (seal).	Leaking of the pouch may lead to maceration and skin breakdown in the area surrounding the wound.	• Leaking of drainage

Documentation

Documentation should include the following:

- Patient and family education
- Wound cleansing, irrigation (if performed), date and time dressing or pouch change was completed
- Description of wound, drainage, odors, presence of drains, suction, and surrounding skin
- Premedication given, patient tolerance of procedure, response to pain medication
- Type of dressing or pouch applied and sealant used
- Unexpected outcomes
- Nursing interventions

References

1. Maklebust J. Using wound care products to promote a healing environment. *Crit Care Nurs Clin North Am.* 1996;8:141–158.
2. Faller NA. When a wound isn't a wound: tubes, drains, fistulae, and draining wounds. In: Krasner D, Kane D, eds. *Chronic Wound Care: A Clinical Source Book for Healthcare Professionals.* 2nd ed. Wayne, Pa: Health Management Publications; 1997:202–208.

Additional Reading

Dane DP. Surgical repair. In: Krasner D, Kane D, eds. *Chronic Wound Care: A Clinical Source Book for Healthcare Professionals.* 2nd ed. Wayne, Pa: Health Management Publications; 1997:235–244.

125 Enteral Nutrition

PURPOSE: The purpose of enteral tube nutrition is to achieve the nutrition requirements, recommended daily allowance of vitamins and minerals, and the administration of free water in patients who cannot consume nutrients orally. The use of enteral feedings also maintains gastrointestinal (GI) function and integrity.

Deborah C. Stamps

PREREQUISITE NURSING KNOWLEDGE

- The first principle in providing nutrition for critically ill patients is to use the GI tract whenever possible. The absence of bowel sounds and stool or flatus does not preclude the use of the GI tract for feeding, particularly when feedings are administered distal to the pylorus. Increasing abdominal distention or severe GI disease may be reasons to administer parenteral nutrition (see Procedure 126).

- The goals of nutrition support include the provision of nutritional support consistent with the patient's available route of administration, nutritional status, and medical condition. They also include the prevention or treatment of macro- and micronutrient deficiencies, prevention of complications related to the technique of nutrition delivery, the improvement of patient outcomes, and enhanced recovery from illness.

- Use of the algorithm in Figure 125–1 can assist the nutritional support team in choosing the appropriate type of nutrition to best meet the patient's needs.

- Prior to administering enteral tube feedings, an individualized nutrition plan should be developed in collaboration with the multidisciplinary team. This would include a review of past medical history, current clinical status, laboratory values, and calculation of calorie and protein needs.

- The nurse should understand insertion, flushing, and confirmation of feeding tube placement (see Procedure 128).

EQUIPMENT

- Enteral feeding bag and administration set
- One 60-mL Luer-lok syringe
- One clean cup
- Prescribed enteral formula
- One enteral feeding pump
- 1-in roll of paper tape

PATIENT AND FAMILY EDUCATION

- Explain procedure for enteral nutrition to both patient and family. ➻*Rationale:* Decreases anxiety and promotes understanding of treatment regimen and possible length of therapy.

- If possible, teach patient to report signs and symptoms of nausea, abdominal cramping, and abdominal fullness. ➻*Rationale:* These symptoms indicate a potential intolerance to rate of infusion or type of formula and decrease the patient's comfort.

- Discuss patient's need for long-term enteral nutritional support. ➻*Rationale:* Allows for planning for long-term access, if needed.

PATIENT ASSESSMENT AND PREPARATION

Patient Assessment

- Fluid balance assessment includes the following:
  ❖ Patient's baseline weight
  ❖ Edema (pedal, sacral, generalized)
  ❖ Breath sounds
  ❖ Jugular venous distention

  ➻*Rationale:* Baseline weight and fluid balance assessment will promote evidence of effectiveness of enteral nutrition support after it has begun.

- Protein-calorie malnutrition assessment includes the following:
  ❖ Weight loss
  ❖ Muscle atrophy
  ❖ Edema
  ❖ Weakness or lethargy
  ❖ Failure to wean from ventilator support

  ➻*Rationale:* Physical signs and symptoms provide an indication of the severity of malnutrition and baseline for later evaluation.

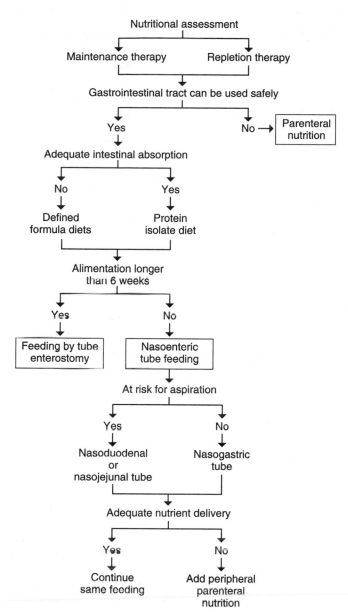

■ ● FIGURE 125–1. Patient selection for enteral feeding. (From Rombeau JL, Rolandelli RH, eds. *Enteral and Tube Feeding.* Philadelphia: WB Saunders; 1997:240.)

- Medical history for presence of chronic cardiac, hepatic, renal, or pulmonary disease. ➤*Rationale:* Chronic illness may dictate restrictions in volume of fluid or type of enteral formula administered.

- Serum proteins indicative of nutritional deficits include the following:
  - ❖ Albumin <3.5 g/dL
  - ❖ Total protein <7.0 mg/dL
  - ❖ Serum transferrin <150 g/dL
  - ❖ Prealbumin <200 g/dL

  ➤*Rationale:* Depressed levels indicate a patient with nutritional deficits.

- Past and current medication profile for use of catabolic steroids (eg, prednisone, dexamethasone). ➤*Rationale:* Catabolic steroids increase protein requirements.

- Medications. ➤*Rationale:* Note potential food and drug interactions and collaborate with the physician or nurse practitioner, as needed.

- GI tract function assessment includes the following:
  - ❖ Presence of bowel sounds
  - ❖ Abdomen soft and nondistended
  - ❖ Flatus or stool present

  ➤*Rationale:* Enteral feeding tolerance is improved when administered via a functioning GI tract.

- Baseline blood glucose, sodium, potassium, calcium, phosphate, magnesium, renal function, and liver function studies (Table 125–1). ➤*Rationale:* Baseline laboratory values provide data for decision making about the type and amount of enteral feedings, as well as the need for any supplementation of electrolytes.

- Skin integrity. ➤*Rationale:* Pressure wounds or large wounds require increased protein needs.

Patient Preparation

- Ensure that patient understands preprocedural teaching. Answer questions as they arise and reinforce information as needed. ➤*Rationale:* Evaluates and reinforces understanding of previously taught information.

- Assist the patient to a semi-Fowler's or high Fowler's position. The head of the bed should be at least 30 degrees during infusion of enteral feedings (in patients requiring prepyloric feedings). ➤*Rationale:* Decreases the risk of aspiration of gastric contents. Patients who must remain supine (eg, unstable neck fracture) must be monitored closely for aspiration during infusion of enteral feedings.

- Aspirate intestinal contents using a 60-mL syringe and assess pH (see Procedure 97). ➤*Rationale:* Verifies correct placement of feeding tube.

Table 125–1 ●■■	**Suggested Laboratory Monitoring**		
Baseline Tests	**Until on Stable Rate**	**When on Goal***
Body weight	Twice weekly	Weekly
Fluid intake/output	Daily	Daily
Glucose		
Nondiabetic	Daily	2–3 times/wk
Diabetic	Daily	Daily
Electrolytes	Daily	1–3 times/wk
Renal function	Daily	1–3 times/wk
Phosphorus	2–3 times/wk	Weekly
Liver function	1–2 times/wk	Weekly
Calcium/magnesium	2–3 times/wk	Weekly
Prealbumin	2 times/wk	Weekly
Albumin	Weekly	Monthly

*In the hospitalized patient. Patients at home or at long-term care facilities may require less frequent monitoring.

From Ideno KT: Enteral nutrition. *In*: Gottschlich MM, Matarese LE, Shronts EP, eds. *Nutrition Support: Dietetics Core Curriculum.* 2nd ed. Silver Spring, Md: American Society for Parenteral and Enteral Nutrition; 1993: 102.

Procedure for Enteral Nutrition Administration

Steps	Rationale	Special Considerations
1. Assemble all equipment and supplies at the bedside.	This ensures enteral feedings will be initiated quickly and efficiently.	
2. Wash hands, and don gloves. *(Level VI: Clinical studies in a variety of patient populations and situations)*	Decreases the transmission of microorganisms; standard precautions.[1–3]	
3. Check placement of feeding tube (see Procedure 128). *(Level VI: Clinical studies in a variety of patient populations and situations)*	Prevents delivery of feeding tube into the lungs.[1]	
4. Verify order for enteral feedings. *(Level VI: Clinical studies in a variety of patient populations and situations)*	Prescriber's order should include type of formula, volume to be delivered, and rate or length of infusion. Decreases the risk of error.[2]	
5. Elevate the head of the bed at least 30 degrees for patients receiving prepyloric feedings. *(Level V: Clinical studies in more than one patient population and situation)*	Decrease risk of aspiration of gastric contents during administration of feeding.[1–3]	If patient must be supine (eg, because of a neck fracture), extreme caution must be exercised to monitor for aspiration.
6. For continuous feeding: close the clamp on the enteral feeding bag, and pour up to 8 hours of formula into the bag; or hang prepackaged closed system container of prescribed formula. For intermittent feeding: hand 100 to 480 mL of formula in the bag at a time. *(Level V: Clinical studies in more than one patient population and situation)*	Hang no more than 8 hours worth of feeding to prevent bacterial overgrowth in formula. With the high-carbohydrate concentration and frequent exposure of formula to multiple personnel, bacterial growth can occur rapidly, leading to gastritis, nausea, vomiting, and diarrhea. Limit hang time or use a closed delivery system to reduce risk of contamination.[1, 2, 4]	
7. Hang bag on IV pole and prime tubing. For continuous enteral feeding, load administration set into enteral feeding pump. *(Level V: Clinical studies in more than one patient population and situation)*	Priming tubing will purge the system of air.[1–6]	
8. Evaluate for residual tube feeding. Attach a 60-mL syringe to the feeding tube. A. Nasogastric, nasoenteric, or gastrostomy tube: aspirate intestinal contents if greater than 60 mL, place returns in a clean cup at the bedside. B. Jejunostomy tube: unable to assess intestinal residual. *(Level V: Clinical studies in more than one patient population and situation)*	Determines the stomach's readiness for feeding. If gastric residual is more than 125 mL, feeding should be delayed 1 hour.[1–4, 6, 7] If unable to withdraw residual from small-bore feeding tube, some manufacturers recommend first instilling 30 to 60 mL of air through the tube. This helps to move the tube away from the gastric or intestinal wall and clear it of any residual water, formula, or medications.[3]	Gastric residual may be elevated because of formula intolerance, delayed gastric emptying, sepsis, or GI disease. Residual is also dependent on infusion rate and gastric emptying time. Notify the physician or nurse practitioner if the residual is greater than 125 mL after 2 hours.

Procedure **for Enteral Nutrition Administration** *Continued*

Steps	Rationale	Special Considerations
9. After determining the volume of residual, complete guaiac test. If guaiac is negative, return up to 125 mL of gastric aspirate to stomach using the same syringe. *(Level V: Clinical studies in more than one patient population and situation)*	If guaiac is positive, do not reinstill contents. Gastric aspirate contains enzymes and secretions essential for digestion of nutrients to be administered. Returning more than 125 mL of gastric aspirate may overfill the stomach when enteral feeding is started.[1–4]	
10. Flush feeding tube with 30 to 50 mL of water. *(Level V: Clinical studies in more than one patient population and situation)*	Prevents clogging of tube and provides additional free water to patient.[1–2, 5]	Patients on fluid restrictions (eg, renal failure, congestive heart failure) should have 10 to 20 mL of flush to clean the tube.
11. Connect feeding bag administration set to distal end of feeding tube with safety tape connection. *(Level II: Theory based, no research data to support recommendations: recommendations from expert consensus group may exist)*	Decreases risk of accidental disconnection.	
12. Remove gloves, and wash hands.	Decreases the transmission of microorganisms; standard precautions.	
13. Begin infusion. A. Feeding pump: set prescribed infusion flow rate for continuous feeding; begin infusion via pump. B. Gravity feeding: adjust roller clamp to infuse formula via gravity over 30 to 60 minutes for intermittent feeding. *(Level V: Clinical studies in more than one patient population and situation)* C. Syringe method: Remove the plunger from a 60-mL syringe. Pour the enteral formula to be administered slowly, trying not to introduce air into the GI system. Allow formula to flow in by gravity. *(Level V: Clinical studies in more than one patient population and situation)*	Initiates administration of feeding.[1, 2, 5]	For intermittent feeding, infuse 100 to 480 mL of formula every 4 to 6 hours (depending on total volume prescribed).
14. Label enteral feeding bag and administration set with date and time hung and type and amount of formula. Change bag and administration set every 24 hours. *(Level VI: Clinical studies in a variety of patient populations and situations)*	Changing enteral administration set every 24 hours prevents bacterial overgrowth in set.[1–5]	

Procedure continued on following page

Procedure	**for Enteral Nutrition Administration** *Continued*

Steps	Rationale	Special Considerations
15. Administer water boluses as prescribed. *(Level VI: Clinical studies in a variety of patient populations and situations)*	Enteral formulas do not contain sufficient water to meet some patient's needs. High-osmolality formulas could lead to dehydration.[1-5]	Adults require 25 to 35 mL/kg of water each day (ie, for a 70-kg patient receiving 2000 mL of an isotonic formula, 600 mL of additional water will need to be administered). Water boluses can be given with a syringe into feeding tube in 100-mL increments every 4 hours. The formula also could be diluted with necessary water and the infusion rate increased. The greater the formula's osmolarity, the less free water in the formula.
16. Remove gloves, and wash hands.	Decreases the transmission of microorganisms; standard precautions.	
17. Medication administration: prior to administration of medications via feeding tube, determine drug-nutrient incompatibilities[8] (Table 125–2). *(Level V: Clinical studies in more than one patient population and situation)*	Medications and enteral formulas may interact, reducing the effectiveness of the medication or causing enteral feeding side effects.[2, 9]	
18. To administer medications: stop feeding infusion. Flush feeding tube with 20 to 30 mL of water. Administer crushed tablets or liquid medications. Flush with 20 to 30 mL of water. Resume feeding. *(Level V: Clinical studies in more than one patient population and situation)*	Prevents clogging of tube and decreases GI upset.[2]	

Table 125–2 ● ■ ■ **Drug and Nutrient Interactions***

Drug	Interaction	Nursing Intervention
Phenytoin	Enteral feedings affect the absorption of phenytoin.	Phenytoin suspension is recommended. Shake the suspension well before measuring the dose from the bottle. Stop the tube feeding for 1 hour before and 2 hours after each dose. The rate of feeding administration may need to be adjusted to accommodate these changes and still meet the nutrition goals.
Warfarin	Enteral feedings containing vitamin K may inhibit anticoagulation, decreasing the effectiveness of warfarin therapy.	Select feedings with minimal or no vitamin K. If an enteral feeding with vitamin K is being used in a patient on warfarin therapy, close monitoring of the INR should be done if changes are made to the feeding formula, feeding rate, or warfarin dose.

*The two medications most commonly associated with drug and nutrient interactions are phenytoin and warfarin.
Abbreviation: INR, international normalized ratio.

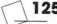

Procedure for Enteral Nutrition Administration *Continued*

Steps	Rationale	Special Considerations
Declogging the Tube		
1. Attach a 20- to 60-mL syringe to the end of the enteral tube and aspirate as much fluid as possible.	The key to maintaining a patent feeding tube is to flush frequently with water.	
2. Fill the syringe with 5 mL of warm water or carbonated beverage (ginger ale or cola). Instill using manual pressure for 1 minute; use a back-and-forth motion with the plunger.		
3. Clamp the tube for 5 to 15 minutes.		
4. Try to aspirate or flush the tube.		

Expected Outcomes

- Maintenance of baseline weight or weight gain of 0.5 to 1 pound every week
- Maintenance or elevation of serum visceral proteins, improved wound healing, maintenance of muscle mass, and positive nitrogen balance
- Fluid balance stable

Unexpected Outcomes

- Intolerance of enteral feeding formula
- Aspiration
- Dehydration
- Hyperosmolar hyperglycemic nonketotic dehydration or coma
- Persistent elevated glucose level
- Diarrhea
- Drug and nutrient interactions

Patient Monitoring and Care

Patient Monitoring and Care	Rationale	Reportable Conditions
		These conditions should be reported if they persist despite nursing interventions.
1. Monitor serum glucose levels daily (commonly by fingersticks).	High carbohydrate concentration of formula may exceed endogenous insulin therapy.	- Glucose >200 mg/dL
2. Weigh patient daily; compare with baseline weight. Document trends of weight gain or loss.	Evaluates patient's response to enteral feeding. Additionally, dehydration can occur as a result of hyperosmolar formulas, patient fluid losses, and inadequate water intake. Overhydration can occur in a patient with hepatic, cardiac, and renal failure. Fluid needs increase when a patient has an elevated temperature.	- Weight gain or loss - Poor skin turgor - Dry mucous membrane - Hypernatremia - Oliguria - Elevated blood urea nitrogen levels
3. Monitor intake and output every shift. Quantify diarrheal stool as output. Observe for a change in urine output.	Diarrhea can occur as a result of the use of hyperosmolar enteral formulas, lactose intolerance, prolonged use of antibiotics, bacterial contamination of formulas, or severe hypoalbuminemia (less than 2 mg/dL).	- Intake greater than output for more than 24 hours - More than three loose or liquid stools in 24 hours

Continued on following page

Patient Monitoring and Care	Rationale	Reportable Conditions
4. If persistent diarrhea occurs, send a stool culture to rule out *Clostridium difficile* and other pathogens.	*C. difficile* can be a cause of diarrhea.	
5. Assess patient's medications for ○ Potential cause or relationship to persistent diarrhea ○ Drug and nutrient interactions	Osmolarity of medications may cause diarrhea. Antibiotics cause bacterial overgrowth in GI tract, resulting in diarrhea. Elixir forms of medications may contain large amounts of sorbitol. Actions of medications alter GI tolerance of enteral feedings and may necessitate a change in administration regime.	
6. Administer antidiarrheal medications as indicated (if *C. difficile* is negative).	Narcotic antidiarrheal medications are an effective and appropriate treatment for many patients. Control of diarrhea prevents dehydration and improves absorption of nutrients. Banana flakes have been shown to be a successful natural way to firm up stool consistency.[2]	• More than three loose or liquid stools in 24 hours
7. Auscultate bowel sounds every 8 hours for GI mobility.	GI function will affect patient's tolerance to enteral feedings.	• Decreased or absent bowel sounds
8. Aspirate intestinal residuals before every feeding or at least every 8 hours.	Residuals greater than 150 mL indicate decreased gastric mobility or emptying. Continued feeds with high residuals increase the risk of vomiting and aspiration. Residuals may be increased because of intolerance to enteral formulas, indicating a need for reevaluation of the formula.	• Residual greater than 125 mL for more than 2 hours
9. Hold enteral feeding for 30 to 60 minutes before patient requires supine position (eg, transport, procedures).	Decreases the risk of aspiration.	
10. Administer mouth care every 2 hours, including brushing teeth or dentures at least daily. Moisten mouth with water-soaked sponge or gauze. Apply petroleum-based ointment to lips.	Decreases bacterial flora in the oral cavity, therefore reducing the risk of aspiration. Prevents drying and cracking of oral mucosa.	
11. Assess patency of feeding tube.	Feeding tubes that are not patent prevent the administration of nutrients, medications, and water.	• Inability to aspirate or flush feeding tube
12. Monitor laboratory values (see Table 125–1).	Baseline and ongoing laboratory values provide data for decision making about the type and amount of enteral feedings, as well as the need for any supplementation of electrolytes.	• Hyper/hypoglycemia • Hyper/hyponatremia • Hyper/hypokalemia • Hyper/hypocalcemia • Hyper/hypophosphatemia • Hyper/hypomagnesemia • Abnormal renal function or liver function studies

Documentation

Documentation should include the following:

- Patient and family teaching
- GI assessment
- Fluid balance (daily weight, intake and output, number of stools)
- Date and time enteral feeding was initiated
- Strength and type of enteral feeding
- Volumes of residuals
- Infusion rate
- Tolerance to feedings
- Total volume delivered
- Condition of oral cavity and mouth care completed
- Laboratory values
- Unexpected outcomes
- Nursing interventions

References

1. Bowers S. Tubes: a nurse's guide to enteral feeding devices. *Medsurg Nurs.* 1996;5:313 324.
2. Emery EA, Ahmad S, Koethe JD, et al. Banana flakes control diarrhea in enterally fed patients. *Nutr Clin Prac.* 1997;12:72–75.
3. Guenter P, Jones S, Ericson M. Enteral nutrition therapy. *Nurs Clin North Am.* 1997;32:651–667.
4. Goff KL. The nuts and bolts of enteral infusion pumps. *Medsurg Nurs.* 1997,6:9–15.
5. Lord LM, Lipp JS. Adult tube feeding formulas. *Medsurg Nurs.* 1996;5:407–419.
6. Lord LM. Enteral access devices. *Nurs Clin North Am.* 1997;32:685–703.
7. Ideno KT. Enteral nutrition formulas: an overview. *Medsurg Nurs.* 1996;5:264–268.
8. Doak KK, Haas CE, Dunnigan KJ, et al. Bioavailability of phenytoin acid and phenytoin sodium with enteral feedings. *Pharmacotherapy.* 1998;18:637–645.
9. Davis AE, Arrington K, Fields Ryan S, Pruitt JO. Preventing feeding-associated aspiration. *Medsurg Nurs.* 1995;4:111–119.

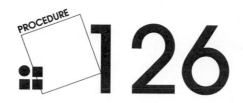

126

Parenteral Nutrition

PURPOSE: Parenteral nutrition (PN) is an important adjunctive therapy that provides macro- and micronutrients to patients who are unable to be adequately nourished via their gastrointestinal (GI) tracts.

Mary Donahue

PREREQUISITE NURSING KNOWLEDGE

- Principles of fluid and electrolyte balance.
- The goals of nutritional support include the provision of nutritional support consistent with the patient's available route of administration, nutritional status, and medical condition. They also include the prevention or treatment of macro- and micronutrient deficiencies, prevention of complications related to the technique of nutrition delivery, the improvement of patient outcomes, and enhanced recovery from illness.
- Use of the algorithm in Figure 125–1 can assist the nutritional support team in choosing the appropriate type of nutrition to best meet the patient's needs.
- Before administering PN, an individualized nutrition plan should be developed in collaboration with the multidisciplinary team. This would include a review of past medical history, current clinical status, laboratory values, and calculation of calorie and protein needs.
- There are two types of PN. Total parenteral nutrition (TPN) consists of a complex formulation of hyperosmolar dextrose, amino acids, lipids, minerals, vitamins, trace elements, and water. It is administered via a large-bore central catheter by an electronic infusion device. TPN formulations can meet the patient's complete or total nutritional needs. Peripheral parenteral nutrition (PPN) has a final concentration of dextrose of 10% or less. It is administered via a peripheral catheter. PPN does not provide enough carbohydrates to meet patient's daily nutritional needs. Instead, PPN is intended to supplement dietary intake or provide minimal support to uncompromised patients.
- The first principle in providing nutrition for critically ill patients is to use the GI tract whenever possible. The absence of bowel sounds and stool or flatus does not preclude the use of the GI tract for feeding, particularly when feedings are administered distal to the pylorus. Increasing abdominal distention or severe GI disease states may be reasons to administer PN.
- The indications for PN should be evaluated daily. The patient should receive oral or enteral nutrition once GI function returns. Clinical studies demonstrate that the use of the GI tract and enteral feedings are associated with preservation of GI tract integrity and immune function and a reduction in infections and complications.
- Prevention of the metabolic and infectious complications associated with the use of PN is accomplished by close monitoring and strict adherence to aseptic technique.
- Indications for PN include the following:
  - ❖ GI inflammation, obstruction, or ileus
  - ❖ High-output GI fistulas
  - ❖ Severe pancreatitis
  - ❖ Burns, trauma, sepsis
  - ❖ Extreme hemodynamic instability with decreased GI blood flow

EQUIPMENT

- Prescribed PN solution
- IV administration set for electronic infusion device
- In-line IV filter (ie, 0.22 μ for PN solutions without lipids; 1.2 μ for PN solution containing lipids)
- Nonsterile gloves
- Povidone-iodine preparation pads or swab sticks
- Alcohol preparation pads
- Syringes and needles or needleless injection cannula
- Normal saline (NS) for injection
- Heparin (100 μ/mL)
- Electronic infusion device

PATIENT AND FAMILY EDUCATION

- Assess patient and family understanding of PN therapy and the reason for its use. ➤**Rationale:** Clarification or reinforcement of information is an expressed family need during times of stress and anxiety.
- Explain standard care to the patient and family, including catheter site care and dressings, physical assessment and laboratory monitoring, infusion device function and alarms, and parameters for change in route of nutritional administration. ➤**Rationale:** Encourages patient and family to ask questions and voice concerns about PN therapy and patient's nutrition.

- Explain the procedure. ➤*Rationale:* Teaching provides information and may decrease anxiety and fear.

PATIENT ASSESSMENT AND PREPARATION

Patient Assessment

- Preadmission nutritional status (including history of weight loss), current nutritional status, including patient weight and lean body mass, if available. ➤*Rationale:* An individualized nutritional plan should be created to meet the patient's needs based on individual assessment. An evaluation by a nutrition support team member or dietitian may be very helpful in patients with sepsis, significant trauma, burns, multiple organ failure, and other conditions that require complex nutritional requirement evaluation.
- Current laboratory profile (Table 126–1). ➤*Rationale:* An individualized nutritional plan and nutritional formulas should be created to meet the patient's needs based on individual assessment.
- Patency of venous access. ➤*Rationale:* TPN is admin-

istered via a central venous line, PPN via a peripheral venous line.

Patient Preparation

- Ensure that patient understands preprocedural teaching. Answer questions as they arise and reinforce information as needed. ➤*Rationale:* Evaluates and reinforces understanding of previously taught information.

Table 126–1 ●■■	Suggested Weekly Laboratory Monitoring for PN Patients

Electrolytes (sodium, potassium, chloride, CO_2)*
Renal function tests (blood urea nitrogen, serum creatinine)*
Glucose, phosphate, magnesium*
Liver function tests (SGOT, alkaline phosphatase, total bilirubin)
Ionized and total calcium
Prealbumin/albumin
CBC

*These laboratory values should be done with initiation, daily for 5 days, and then weekly.
Abbreviations: CBC, complete blood count; SGOT, serum glutamic-oxalo-acetic transaminase.

Procedure	**for Parenteral Nutrition**

Steps	Rationale	Special Considerations
1. Verify orders with pharmacy label on PN bag. Remove PN bag from refrigeration 1 hour before initiation of infusion.	Reduces risk of error. The solution can be warmed to room temperature before infusion, increasing the patient's comfort.	Order should indicate volume to be infused, rate of delivery, and the number of hours of the PN infusion. If the rate is to be gradually increased or tapered, the length of time at each rate should be indicated. Note the expiration time and date of the PN solution.
2. Wash hands.	Reduces transmission of microorganisms; standard precautions.	
3. Compare patient's identification band with label on PN bag.	Prevents administration of PN to wrong patient.	
4. Aseptically spike PN bag with administration set for electronic infusion device.	Reduces transmission of microorganisms.	Volume-controlled electronic devices are preferred for PN solutions.
5. Add appropriate in-line filter, fill the drip chamber to the appropriate level, prime tubing so it is free of bubbles, and clamp tubing. *(Level V: Clinical studies in more than one patient population and situations)*	Traps particulate matter, bacteria, and endotoxins and vents air from intravenous tubing.[1, 2]	If using PN solution that contains lipids (three-in-one solutions), use a 1.2-µg filter to prevent clogging.
6. Don nonsterile gloves.	Reduces exposure to blood and body fluids.	
7. Clamp catheter port.	Prevents air embolism and blood backup.	
8. Cleanse catheter port or hub with povidone-iodine prep pad. If lipids are to be administered separately, that injection port also must be cleaned with povidone-iodine. *(Level IV: Limited clinical studies to support recommendations)*	Reduces microorganisms at catheter hub connection.[3, 4]	PN should be administered in a dedicated line or lumen. If the lumen has been previously used, the line should be changed over a guidewire before initiation of PN. Use of the catheter lumen for other IV fluids or medications increases the risk of contamination. Subsequent infusion of PN via the lumen may promote growth of microorganisms in the presence of high concentrations of dextrose.

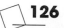

Procedure **for Parenteral Nutrition** *Continued*

Steps	Rationale	Special Considerations
9. Remove cap or IV tubing from catheter hub and attach PN administration set using Luer-Lok connection.	Luer-Lok connection prevents inadvertent disconnection of IV fluids.	Use of a needle or needleless injection cannula through an injection cap is not recommended. There is an increased risk of accidental disconnection, resulting in blood loss, air embolism, or hypoglycemia.
10. Place IV tubing into electronic infusion device. *(Level 1: Manufacturer's recommendation only)*	Use of an infusion device ensures accurate, consistent delivery of PN.	
11. Set prescribed rate of infusion and other parameters on infusion device.	Consistent delivery of PN decreases the risk of metabolic complications[5] (Table 126–2).	If PN needs to be suddenly interrupted, notify physician or nurse practitioner. $D_{10}W$ should be infused at the same rate as the PN to prevent hypoglycemia.
12. Open clamps on IV set and catheter; start pump.		
13. Assess patency of catheter or venous access device.		
14. Label PN bag and IV set with date and time and other required information.		Change set and filter every 24 hours to reduce risk of infection.

Separate Lipid Emulsion Infusion

1. If lipids are to be piggy-backed into PN line via injection site on the tubing, repeat steps 1 through 14 above. When spiking lipids bottle, remove metal cap from the top. Spike with administration set. Cleanse the rubber cap with povidone-iodine pad followed by an alcohol prep pad.	In-line filter used for lipids is 1.2 μ.	Lipid emulsions are available in 10% and 20% concentrations in 250-mL and 500-mL bottles. 1.2-μg filters are used on lipids to prevent clogging. If lipids are not filtered, introduce the line below the level of the PN filter. Lipids should be infused over 16 to 24 hours. Lipid administration sets are changed with each new bottle.

Cycled PN

1. Infuse PN at prescribed rate. Physician or nurse practitioner may order rate to be increased over 1 to 2 hours or to begin at full rate. *(Level II: Theory based, no research data to support recommendations: recommendations from expert consensus group may exist)*	Gradual increase in PN may improve patient tolerance to glucose.[5]	Cycled PN is infused over 10 to 14 hours. This may help to stimulate patient's appetite and supplement oral intake. Patients with hepatobiliary dysfunction may be able to clear excess glycogen during hours when PN is off.
2. Decrease rate of PN infusion as prescribed, typically decreasing in half 1 to 2 hours before end of cycle. *(Level II: Theory based, no research data to support recommendations: recommendations from expert consensus group may exist)*	Decreases glucose load, thus decreasing insulin secretion, to prevent rebound hypoglycemia.[5]	
3. At the end of PN infusion, turn off infusion device; disconnect PN from catheter.		
4. Flush catheter with NS or heparin per institutional standard (see Procedure 61).		

Table 126–2 ●■■ **Metabolic Complications of Parenteral Nutrition (PN)**

Complication	Etiology	Symptoms	Treatment
Carbohydrate Metabolism			
Hyperglycemia	Too-rapid administration of PN, diabetes mellitus, sepsis, stress, steroids	Elevated blood glucose levels, glycosuria, diuresis, thirst	Decrease PN infusion rate Add insulin to PN solution
Hypoglycemia	Abrupt decrease or discontinuance of PN infusion, too much insulin	Blood glucose <80 mg/dL, lethargy, diaphoresis, headache, pallor	Administer glucose by IV bolus or orally, depending on patient condition
Hyperglycemic hyperosmolar nonketotic (HHNK) dehydration/coma	Uncontrolled hyperglycemia	Blood glucose >500 mg/dL, increased BUN, increased serum osmolality/sodium levels, increased urine output, lethargy, coma	Decrease or stop PN, administer insulin to correct hyperglycemia, administer isotonic saline to rehydrate, administer potassium to correct hypokalemia
Respiratory compromise from excessive CO_2 production/retention	Overfeeding, excess calories, and total carbohydrate load	Respiratory quotient >1.0	Decrease total calorie load; decrease carbohydrates and fat
Protein Metabolism			
Azotemia	Excessive protein administration, impaired renal or liver function	Increased serum BUN	Decrease protein amounts in PN solution; current recommendation, 0.8 to 1.5 g/kg/day
Fat Metabolism			
Essential fatty acid deficiency	Lack of adequate fat intake or supplement	Dry, flaky skin, hair loss, coarse hair, impaired wound healing	Administer 10% to 20% lipid emulsion IV at a minimal rate of 4% of required daily calories per week
Hyperlipidemia	Overinfusion of lipid emulsions	Increased serum cholesterol, triglyceride, and phospholipid levels	Decrease amount or concentration of lipid emulsion administration
		Exacerbation of arteriosclerotic cardiovascular disease	Discontinue lipid infusions and monitor serum lipid levels
Volume Administration			
Hypovolemia	Inadequate free water administration or excessive glucose administration	Increased serum BUN and sodium levels, decreased urine output, dehydration, thirst	Increase free water in PN solution, administer additional free water IV, decrease glucose calories
Hypervolemia	Fluid volume overload in renal, cardiovascular, pulmonary, or hepatic disease	Jugular venous distention, dyspnea, pedal and sacral edema, increased right atrium/central venous pressures	Concentrate fluids in PN, decrease or concentrate other IV solutions; consider renal replacement in patients with renal impairment
Electrolyte Metabolism			
Hypokalemia	Inadequate administration or increased losses of potassium	Cardiac dysrhythmias, muscle weakness	Increase potassium in PN formula
Hyperkalemia	Excess administration or inadequate excretion of potassium, as in renal impairment	Cardiac dysrhythmias	Discontinue current PN infusion and decrease potassium amounts in subsequent formulas
Hypocalcemia	Inadequate calcium administration or excessive phosphorus administration	Paresthesias, positive Chvostek's sign	Increase calcium in PN
Hypomagnesemia	Inadequate magnesium administration	Tingling around the mouth, dizziness, paresthesias	Increase magnesium in PN
Hypophosphatemia	Inadequate phosphate administration	Lethargy, paresthesias, respiratory distress, coma	Add phosphates as potassium or sodium salts to PN
Anemia, iron deficiency	Excessive blood loss, inadequate iron, copper, B_{12}, folate replacement	Pallor, fatigue, exertional dyspnea	Addition of iron to PN; blood transfusion as indicated
Trace element deficiencies	Inadequate trace element administration, excessive losses	Dependent on specific element deficiency, impaired wound healing, glucose intolerance, hair loss	Appropriate replacement of trace elements Routine monitoring not helpful Measure individual element level when deficiency is clinically suspected
Acid-Base Metabolism			
Metabolic acidosis	Too rapid administration of PN, diabetes mellitus, sepsis	Arterial pH <7.35	Correct hyperglycemia, treat sepsis

Abbreviations: BUN, blood urea nitrogen; HHNK, hyperglycemic hyperosmolar nonketotic; IV, intravenous.

- Maintenance of baseline body weight or weight gain of 1 to 2 pounds per week in patients with weight loss
- Maintenance or repletion of serum proteins
- Normal or improved wound healing
- Positive nitrogen balance
- Maintenance of muscle mass
- Fluid balance slightly positive (=/+ 500 mL/24 h)
- Laboratory values within normal limits

- Fluid overload
- Dehydration
- Hyperglycemic hyperosmolar nonketotic (HHNK) coma
- Azotemia
- Hyperlipidemia
- Metabolic acidosis
- Refeeding syndrome
- Catheter site infection
- Systemic infection
- Venous access disruption or nonpatency of catheter/port

Patient Monitoring and Care

Patient Monitoring and Care	Rationale	Reportable Conditions
		These conditions should be reported if they persist despite nursing interventions.
1. Obtain serum glucose measurements; assess patient's insulin requirements every 6 hours.	High carbohydrate intake in PN solution may lead to glucose intolerance. Early treatment of hyperglycemia may prevent HHNK coma. Glycosuria may occur as a later symptom of hyperglycemia. Sudden increases in insulin requirements and glucose intolerance are early indicators of sepsis. Use of a bedside glucose monitor will facilitate measurement of patient's serum glucose level.	• Serum blood glucose >220 mg/dL • Glycosuria • Unexplained lethargy or coma

2. Evaluate patient's fluid status on a daily basis.
  ○ Daily weights
  ○ Skin turgor
  ○ Breath sounds
  ○ Jugular venous distention
  ○ Peripheral edema
  ○ Dyspnea
	Weight changes occurring within 24-hour periods are indicative of fluid imbalance. Dehydration may occur as a result of fluid loss and inadequate fluid intake. Fluid excess may occur, especially in patients with cardiac, hepatic, or renal compromise.	• Weight gain of 1 to 2 pounds in 24 hours
		• Changes in baseline breath sounds
		• Dyspnea
		• Peripheral edema
		• Jugular venous distention
		• Change in skin turgor

3. Monitor intake and output.	Intake and output is another indication of overall fluid balance. Trends over several days may indicate a positive or negative fluid balance, indicating need for adjustment in PN formula or volume.	• Positive or negative fluid balance of 1 to 2 L/24 hours
4. Monitor electrolytes, glucose, and renal function tests daily for first 5 days of PN therapy; weekly thereafter.	PN may alter electrolyte values if PN formulas are not adjusted to serum levels. Protein metabolism may elevate blood urea nitrogen (BUN), especially in patients with renal compromise.	• BUN >50 mg/dL, elevated serum creatinine • Hyper/hypoglycemia • Hyper/hypophosphatemia • Hyper/hypomagnesemia • Hyper/hypokalemia • Hyper/hyponatremia
5. Monitor liver function studies, albumin, and prealbumin at initiation of PN and weekly thereafter.	Infusion of PN may elevate liver function tests as a result of metabolism of amino acids, carbohydrates, or lipids.	• Total bilirubin >1 mg/dL • Alkaline phosphatase >130 mU/mL • Serum glutamic-oxalo-acetic transaminase (SGOT) >40 mU/mL • Albumin <3 g/dL • Prealbumin <20 mg/dL

Continued on following page

Patient Monitoring and Care *Continued*

Patient Monitoring and Care	Rationale	Reportable Conditions
6. Monitor complete blood count (CBC) weekly and iron, ferritin, vitamin B_{12}, and folate levels as necessary.	Excess blood loss and inadequate administration of iron, copper, and vitamins result in anemia and iron and vitamin deficiencies.	• Iron level <45 µg/dL • Hematocrit (Hct) <35% • Decreased vitamin B_{12} • Ferritin <10 µg/mL
7. Assess patient for signs of trace mineral deficiencies.	Deficiencies in trace minerals (eg, copper, zinc, chromium) may cause abnormalities in metabolism and impairment in skin integrity. Trace elements should be added to PN daily to prevent these deficiencies.	• Impaired wound healing • Glucose intolerance without signs of sepsis • Hair loss • Acne lesions • Anemia • Clotting abnormalities
8. Assess for hyperlipidemia.	Administration of lipids may cause increased serum lipid levels.	• Elevated total cholesterol, triglycerides, or phospholipids
9. Evaluate patient for evidence of refeeding syndrome.	Patients at risk include those with severely or moderately depleted nutritional states where efforts to provide nutritional support are too aggressive.	• Rapid decreases in serum phosphorus, potassium, and magnesium levels • Altered glucose metabolism • Altered cardiac function • Fluid shifts
10. Monitor temperature and vital signs every 4 hours. Monitor white blood cell count every 3 days.	Elevated temperature and white cell count may indicate the development of systemic infection. PN should be considered the cause of such infection until ruled out.	• Leukocytosis • Fever • Chills • Positive blood cultures
11. Monitor catheter insertion site daily or per institutional standard.	Local infection can progress to systemic infection if left untreated.	• Erythema • Pain/tenderness • Warmth • Purulent drainage

Documentation

Documentation should include the following:

- Patient and family education
- Laboratory assessment result
- Fluid balance assessment
- Temperature, vital signs, weights
- Observation of patient response to PN
- Unexpected outcomes
- Nursing interventions

References

1. ASPEN Board of Directors. Standards for nutrition support: hospitalized patients. *Nutr Clin Pract.* 1995;10:208–219.
2. ASPEN National Advisory Group on Standards and Practice Guidelines for Parenteral Nutrition. Safe practices for parenteral nutrition formulations. *J Parenteral Enteral Nutr.* 1997; 22:49–66.
3. Schwartz DB. Enhanced enteral and parenteral nutritional practice and outcomes in an intensive care unit with a hospital-wide performance improvement process. *J Am Diet Assoc.* 1996;5:484–489.
4. Skipper A. Nutrition Support Policies, Forms, and Formulas. Gaithersburg, Md: Aspen Publishers; 1995.
5. Goff K. Metabolic monitoring in nutrition support. *Nurs Clin North Am.* 1997;32:741–753.

Additional Readings

Alverdy JC, Burke D. Total parenteral nutrition: iatrogenic immunosuppression. *Nutrition.* 1992;8:359–365.
Cerra FB, Benitez MR, Blackburn GL, et al. Applied nutrition in ICU patients: a consensus statement of the American College of Chest Physicians. *Chest.* 1997;111:769–778.
Dark DS, Pingleton SK, Kerby GR. Hypercapnia during weaning: a complication of nutritional support. *Chest.* 1995;88:141–143.
Gallica LA. Parenteral nutrition. *Nurs Clin North Am.* 1997;32:704–717.
Moore FA, Feliciano DV, Andrassy RJ, et al. Early enteral feeding, compared with parenteral, reduces postoperative septic complications: the results of a meta-analysis. *Ann Surg.* 1992;216:172–183.

127

Gastrostomy or Jejunostomy Tube Care

PURPOSE: Gastrostomy, including percutaneous endoscopic gastrostomy (PEG), and jejunostomy tubes provide long-term access to the gastrointestinal (GI) tract for nutrition.

Margaret M. Ecklund

PREREQUISITE NURSING KNOWLEDGE

- Anatomy and physiology of the upper and lower GI system should be understood.
- Patients who cannot have enteral tubes passed orally or nasally secondary to anatomy or surgery and those who require supplemental enteral nutrition support for greater than 4 weeks should be considered as candidates for long-term enteral access.
- The most commonly used long-term enteral access is the PEG tube. The PEG tube is inserted without general anesthesia. A guidewire is threaded via endoscope through the oropharynx, esophagus, and stomach and brought out through the abdominal wall. The tube is then threaded over the guidewire and passed into the stomach. The tapered end of the tube is brought through a stab wound in the abdominal wall until the mushroomed end of the tube is set against the stomach wall. An adapter for infusion is attached to the end of the tube, and a disk on the tube is moved up to the abdominal wall to stabilize the tube in place.
- PEG tubes are large-bore catheters ranging from 18 French to 22 French, having a mushroom-shaped curved end in the stomach and a two-port distal end to instill enteral nutrition, medications, and fluid. PEG tubes have disks, perpendicular to the tube, to hold the device close to the skin and lessen shift of tube in and out of the skin (Fig. 127–1).
- Contraindications for PEG placement include the following:
  - ❖ Previous gastric resection
  - ❖ Tumors blocking the passage of the endoscope
  - ❖ Ascites
  - ❖ Morbid obesity
  - ❖ Esophageal or gastric varices
- Gastrostomy and jejunostomy tubes usually have a balloon in the intestinal lumen to prevent dislocation, which is inflated with sterile water. The distal end has an infusion port and a port for the balloon instillation (Fig.

127–2). A jejunostomy tube is indicated in those patients at risk of aspiration or who are unable to tolerate enteral feedings into the stomach (Fig. 127–3).
- If the tubes are removed, reinsertion of the tubes is a routine procedure after the tunnel and stoma are healed (approximately 2 weeks after insertion).
- Because these tubes all enter through the abdominal wall, skin care at the site of insertion is important for skin integrity and prevention of infection.
- Consult with the multidisciplinary team to individualize nutrition goals. The nutrition plan is developed based on the collaborative assessment of the nurse, dietitian, and physician or nurse practitioner.

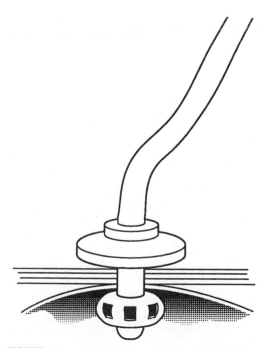

■ ● FIGURE 127–1. Percutaneous endoscopic gastrostomy.

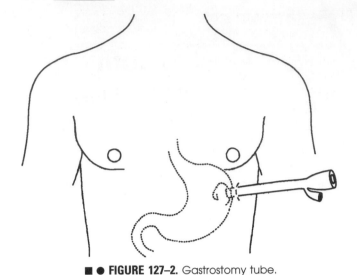

■ ● **FIGURE 127–2.** Gastrostomy tube.

EQUIPMENT

- Nonsterile gloves
- 4 × 4 gauze pads
- Cotton-tipped swabs
- 4 × 4 gauze pads—drain cut
- Protective skin barrier (eg, vitamin A and D ointment)
- Silk tape

Additional equipment (to have available depending on patient need) includes the following:

- Hydrogen peroxide
- Abdominal binder

PATIENT AND FAMILY EDUCATION

- Explain the purpose for the tube.   ➤**Rationale:** Knowledge decreases anxiety and fear of the unknown.
- Explain reason for skin care assessment and maintenance.   ➤**Rationale:** Knowledge decreases anxiety and fear of the unknown.
- Stress the importance of not pulling at the tube.   ➤**Rationale:** Avoids unnecessary pain and skin irritation.
- Oral nutrition is possible with the long-term enteral access catheter.   ➤**Rationale:** Knowledge decreases anxiety and fear of the unknown.
- Long-term enteral access catheters can be removed when oral intake meets the needs of the individual.   ➤**Rationale:** Knowledge decreases anxiety and fear of the unknown. This also may be a goal for the patient to consume more via the oral route.

PATIENT ASSESSMENT AND PREPARATION

Patient Assessment

- Gastrointestinal assessment.   ➤**Rationale:** A patient needs a functional gut to receive enteral nutrition.
- Skin condition at the feeding tube stoma; signs and symptoms of infection include the following:

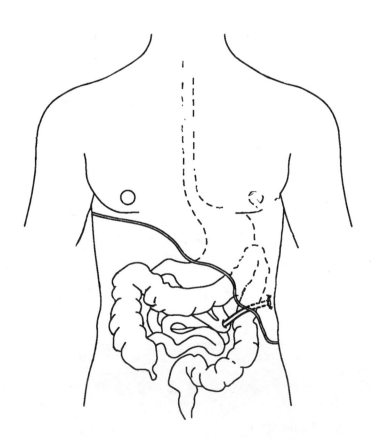

■ ● **FIGURE 127–3.** Jejunostomy tube placement.

❖ Site redness/edema
❖ Warmth
❖ Purulent drainage
❖ Pain or tenderness
❖ Fever

➙*Rationale:* Intact skin integrity is a defense against infection. Early assessment of signs of infection promotes early, appropriate intervention.

Patient Preparation

• Ensure that patient understands preprocedural teaching. Answer questions as they arise and reinforce information as needed. ➙*Rationale:* Evaluates and reinforces understanding of previously taught information.
• Assist patient to position of comfort. ➙*Rationale:* Stoma of tube is easily accessible.

Procedure	for Gastrostomy or Jejunostomy Tube Care

Steps	Rationale	Special Considerations
1. Wash hands, and don nonsterile gloves.	Prevent transmission of microorganisms; standard precautions.	
2. Use soap and warm water to moisten gauze pads and two cotton-tipped applicators. *(Level II: Theory based, no research data to support recommendations: recommendations from expert consensus group may exist)*	Soap and water will clean the skin surface at the stoma.	Hydrogen peroxide, diluted to half strength with water, should be reserved for use for situations in which wound cleansing is a goal. Hydrogen peroxide will dry skin at the stoma.[1,2]
3. Wipe the area closest to the tube (stoma) with the cotton-tipped applicators and proximal skin with the moistened gauze. Rinse with water. *(Level II: Theory based, no research data to support recommendations: recommendations from expert consensus group may exist)*		
4. Dry skin and stoma thoroughly with a dry gauze pad.	Prevents chafing and skin maceration.	
5. Using cotton-tipped applicator, apply protective skin barrier (eg, vitamin A and D ointment) in a circular motion around stoma. *(Level II: Theory based, no research data to support recommendations: recommendations from expert consensus group may exist)*	Protective barrier ointment provides a moisture barrier for skin and assists wound healing. If purulent drainage is persistent, collaborate with physician or nurse practitioner for an antimicrobial ointment after skin cleansing.[1-3]	
6. Apply a 4 × 4 split gauze sponge around tube and secure with tape along edges. Change gauze every 12 hours or when soiled or moist. *(Level II: Theory based, no research data to support recommendations: recommendations from expert consensus group may exist)*	If no drainage is evident, gauze pad may be left off.[1,2]	
7. Anchor tube to skin at adjacent spot on abdomen. *(Level II: Theory based, no research data to support recommendations: recommendations from expert consensus group may exist)*	Reduces tension on tube.	

- Intact skin at stoma of long-term enteral access device
- Patent long-term enteral access for enteral feeding and fluid

- Infection at stoma
- Tube removal by patient or accidental dislodgment with patient movement
- Migration of tube into intestinal lumen
- Peritonitis
- Aspiration

Patient Monitoring and Care

Patient Monitoring and Care	Rationale	Reportable Conditions
		These conditions should be reported if they persist despite nursing interventions.
1. Assess skin integrity and quality of drainage from stoma.	Intact skin is the first line of prevention against infection.	• Erosion of stoma • Change in drainage • Increased volume of foul-smelling, purulent drainage from around stoma • Redness or pain at stoma.
2. Ensure that PEG tube has disk aligned next to skin without pressure into skin.	Disk helps prevent excess movement of tube in and out of skin. If the disk pushes with excess pressure, tissue injury may occur.[4]	• Pressure injury adjacent to stoma
3. Ensure the patient does not remove long-term enteral access device. A loosely applied abdominal binder is helpful to deter a confused patient from pulling at the tube.	A tube removed before the tract is established is a surgical emergency and requires immediate return to the operating room for repair and replacement.[5] Consult with the physician or nurse practitioner to determine the urgency of replacement follow-up. Tubes with established tracts can be replaced by the nurse at the bedside.	
4. Note distance of tube from adapter to entrance into skin.	Evaluates whether tube has migrated inward or pulled outward. Emesis or nausea may indicate pyloric obstruction.	• Length has deviated significantly • Emesis or nausea
5. Evaluate wearing of tube with ongoing use.	No routine change is indicated. Change of tube is indicated with device failure.[5]	• Tube wearing

Documentation

Documentation should include the following:

- Patient and family education
- Condition of stoma
- Any treatment rendered related to site complications
- Tube patency
- Distance of tube from adapter to entrance into skin
- Unexpected outcomes
- Nursing interventions

References

1. Broscious SK. Preventing complications of PEG tubes. *DCCN.* 1995;14:37–41.
2. Lord LM. Enteral access devices. *Nurs Clin North Am.* 1997;32:685–702.
3. Holmes S. Percutaneous endoscopic gastrostomy: a review. *Nursing Times.* 1996;92:34–35.
4. Haslam N, Hughes S, Harrison RF. Peritoneal leakage of gastric contents, a rare complication of percutaneous endoscopic gastrostomy. *JPEN.* 1996;20:433–434.
5. Graham S, Sim G, Laughren R, et al. Percutaneous feeding tube changes in long-term care facility patients. *Infect Control Hosp Epidemiol.* 1996;17:732–736.

Additional Reading

Bowers S. Tubes: a nurse's guide to enteral feeding devices. *Medsurg Nurs.* 1996;5:313–324.

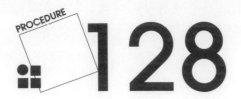

128

Small-Bore Feeding Tube Insertion

PURPOSE: A small-bore feeding tube is inserted to provide access to the gastrointestinal (GI) tract for the patient who is unable to consume adequate calories orally. The tube can be used for administration of nutrients, fluid, and medications.

Margaret M. Ecklund

PREREQUISITE NURSING KNOWLEDGE

- Anatomy and physiology of the upper and lower GI tract should be understood.
- The GI tract must be functioning (bowel sounds audible and active peristalsis) for enteral nutrition to be digested and absorbed.
- Small-bore feeding tubes are preferable over larger-bore nasogastric tubes over the course of critical illness, because the risk of tissue necrosis at the nares and sinusitis is lower.
- The small diameter of the tube allows simultaneous oral intake if the patient is able to consume orally without aspiration.
- Both weighted and unweighted small-bore nasogastric tubes are available. They typically are packaged with guidewires already in the lumen to assist passage of the tube. After successful placement, the guidewire is removed and discarded.
- Unweighted tipped tubes migrate post pylorically into the duodenum more often than tubes with weighted tips. Weighted-tip tubes are harder for the compromised patient to swallow; ultimately, the bolus-tip tube may be a more comfortable choice for the patient.
- Absolute contraindications for insertion of a nasoenteric feeding tube are basilar skull fracture and esophageal varices.
- Small-bore feeding tubes are not designed for drainage of gastric contents. If gastric decompression is desired, the small-bore nasogastric tube should be replaced with a large-bore tube (see Procedure 97).
- It is important to review institutional standards regarding insertion of small-bore feeding tubes. Some institutions

restrict insertion to physicians and advanced practice nurses.

EQUIPMENT

- Small-bore feeding tube (size range, 7 to 10 Fr—weighted or unweighted (bolus tip)
- Small glass of tap water
- 60-mL Luer-Lok tip syringe
- Skin preparation agent
- Pink plastic adhesive or clear tape
- Nonsterile gloves
- Water-soluble lubricant (if tube is not prelubricated)

PATIENT AND FAMILY EDUCATION

- Explain reason for insertion of tube and need for support of enteral nutrition. ➤*Rationale:* Knowledge decreases anxiety and fear of the unknown.
- Explain how patient can assist with passage of the tube, by positioning (eg, sitting upright, head tipped forward and swallowing) when cued. ➤*Rationale:* Tube passes easily with patient cooperation.
- Explain the risk of the gag reflex being stimulated during insertion. ➤*Rationale:* Knowledge decreases anxiety and fear of the unknown.
- Explain the reason for chest x-ray after insertion. ➤*Rationale:* Knowledge decreases anxiety and fear of the unknown.
- Discuss reasons for not pulling at tube once it has been placed and secured. ➤*Rationale:* Leaving the tube in place avoids the need for reinsertion and another x-ray for verification. Reinsertion increases risk of trauma to nares.

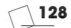

PATIENT ASSESSMENT AND PREPARATION

Patient Assessment

- Medical history of head and neck cancer and surgery, esophageal cancer, decreased pharyngeal reflexes. ➤➤*Rationale:* These conditions prohibit safe passage of a tube nasally through pharynx.
- Patency of the nares for potential obstructions to feeding tube passage. ➤➤*Rationale:* A tube cannot pass through occlusion.
- Gastrointestinal function. ➤➤*Rationale:* A functional gut is needed to administer enteral feedings.

Patient Preparation

- Ensure that patient understands preprocedural teaching. Answer questions as they arise and reinforce information as needed. ➤➤*Rationale:* Evaluates and reinforces understanding of previously taught information.
- If the patient has a large-bore nasogastric tube, it needs to be removed prior to placement of the small-bore nasogastric tube. ➤➤*Rationale:* Attempting to pass a small-bore tube will be extremely difficult with an oral or nasal NG tube already in place.

Procedure for Small-Bore Feeding Tube Insertion		
Steps	**Rationale**	**Special Considerations**
1. Wash hands.	Reduces transmission of microorganisms.	
2. Don nonsterile gloves.	Standard precautions.	
3. Sit patient upright and tip head forward. *(Level IV: Limited clinical studies to support recommendations)*	Facilitates passage of tube into esophagus. If patient cannot tolerate upright positioning, position laterally to the right side to insert tube.[1,2]	
4. Estimate depth of tube insertion by measuring tube from tip of nose to ear, then inferior to stomach (Fig. 97–3). *(Level IV: Limited clinical studies to support recommendations)*	Approximates length of tube to insert. If postpyloric placement is desired, add 10 to 15 cm to length of tube measured.[1]	
5. Lubricate tip of tube with water. *(Level I: Manufacturer's recommendation only)*	Water activates a lubricant on the surface of tube to facilitate passage through nares.	If tube does not have self-lubrication, a watersoluble lubricant can be applied to the tube.
6. Insert tip of tube into either nare; advance to posterior pharynx until resistance is met. *(Level IV: Limited clinical studies to support recommendations)*	Once tube is advanced through the nares, the oropharynx is reached, and the tube will stop.[2,3]	
7. At this point, ask patient to swallow. If the patient is able to cooperate, give sips of water to trigger swallow reflex and ease tube passage. *(Level IV: Limited clinical studies to support recommendations)*	Swallowing immediately assists passage of the tube into the esophagus.[3-5] If the patient is unable to cooperate with swallowing, neck positioning may facilitate passage.	If coughing begins immediately with advancing tube, immediately pull back to nares.
8. As patient swallows, advance tube to desired marking.	The initial swallow gets the tube into the esophagus, and the nurse can advance it to desired position without repeated swallowing.	If the patient is unconscious or unable to cooperate, do not attempt to use water orally to pass tube.
9. Apply skin preparation to nose and securing surface of face and allow to dry.	Prepares surface of skin to help with the tape adhering.	
10. Tape tube securely to nose, using one half of a 3-cm strip. The lower portion of the tape is then split up to the tip of the nose and wrapped around the tube (see Fig. 97–4). *(Level IV: Limited clinical studies to support recommendations)*	The tape needs to hold the tube to prevent slipping it out. Pink plastic tape has shown an ability to stay secure for a greater length of time compared to other methods.[4]	Tape the tube so it does not press against the skin. Excess pressure can cause breakdown.
11. Remove gloves, and wash hands.		

Procedure continued on following page

Procedure for Small-Bore Feeding Tube Insertion *Continued*

Steps	Rationale	Special Considerations
12. Leave guidewire in place and obtain chest x-ray (lower chest view) to verify placement. *(Level IV: Limited clinical studies to support recommendations)*	Chest x-ray verification is the safest way to ensure correct placement. Leaving the guidewire in allows the nurse to potentially reposition tube. Never reinsert guidewire into the tube once it has been removed from the tube. A lower chest view will ensure the tip is in stomach or intestine.[1-3, 5] Although chest x-ray is the gold standard for evaluating small-bore feeding tube placement, studies show that accurate placement also can be obtained via pH testing (see Procedure 97).	
13. When placement is verified in the stomach, hold tube at exit from nares and pull guidewire firmly and dispose.	Guidewire removal is necessary to allow enteral feeding to begin and is more comfortable because the tube becomes softer in the nose.	
14. If postpyloric placement is desired, allow 10 to 15 cm additional length when this tube is placed and tape tube to nose with slack. *(Level IV: Limited clinical studies to support recommendations)*	The extra length can allow the migration of tube past the pyloric valve. Extra tube length can be coiled off to the side of the face.[1]	
15. Position patient on right side.	This assists with peristalsis. If tube is in stomach, peristalsis should move it beyond the sphincter.	
16. Obtain abdominal x-ray; when tube tip is verified as postpyloric, remove guidewire.	Abdominal x-ray verification is the safest way to assure correct placement. Leaving the guidewire in allows the nurse to potentially reposition tube and visualization on x-ray.	Postpyloric placement is verified with abdominal film to ensure tip is visualized.
17. If tube has not migrated postpylorically, continue to position patient on right side and recheck x-ray after 12 hours. *(Level IV: Limited clinical studies to support recommendations)*	Right-side positioning potentially helps pass the tube post pyloric with the aid of peristalsis.[2-3]	
18. If tube remains in stomach, consult with physician or nurse practitioner to administer metoclopramide IV and repeat x-ray in 4 hours. *(Level IV: Limited clinical studies to support recommendations)*	Promotility agents have shown benefit in moving tube through pyloric valve.[1]	

Expected Outcomes

- Distal tip of tube is placed in either stomach or duodenum.
- Patent tube accepts enteral feedings, medications, and fluid.
- Patient is able to swallow oral foods and fluids while small-bore feeding tube is in place.

Unexpected Outcomes

- Coughing or dyspnea, indicating potential bronchial placement
- Pneumothorax from inadvertent pleural placement
- Tube coiled in esophagus or posterior pharynx
- Esophageal tear from trauma of tube passing
- Tube dislodging during therapy, necessitating removal and new tube placement
- Aspiration of stomach contents despite appropriate placement
- Clogging of enteral tube with medication fragments or enteral formula
- Skin irritation at nose

Patient Monitoring and Care

Patient Monitoring and Care	Rationale	Reportable Conditions
		These conditions should be reported if they persist despite nursing interventions.
1. Monitor tolerance to tube placement.	Agitation will inhibit successful placement.	• Self-extubation • Agitation and inability to cooperate with tube placement • Recurrent vomiting • Continued coughing and dyspnea
2. Assess oral cavity and perform oral care every 2 hours and prn.	Patients with orogastric or NG tubes in place tend to mouth breathe, drying their mouths, increasing the risk of mucosal breakdown and ulceration. Tube presence also may predispose a patient to sinusitis or oral infections.	• Ulceration, drainage, foul odor
3. Monitor insertion site of tube for redness, swelling, drainage, bleeding, or skin breakdown. Use only watersoluble lubricants at site.	Many critically ill patients have fragile skin and have associated conditions that predispose them to skin breakdown. Frequent monitoring and subsequent repositioning of the tube can prevent serious damage.	• Redness • Swelling • Drainage • Bleeding • Skin breakdown at insertion site
4. Reposition and retape tube every 24 hours or when tape is soiled.	Decreases risk of tissue damage to mouth or nares.	

Documentation

Documentation should include the following:

- Patient and family education
- Size and type of tube placed
- Patient response to insertion
- X-ray interpretation
- Unexpected outcomes
- Nursing interventions

References

1. Lord LM, Weiser-Maimone A, Pulhamus M, Sax HC. Comparison of weighted vs unweighted enteral feeding tubes for efficacy of transpyloric intubation. *JPEN.* 1993;17:271–273.
2. Welch SK. Certification of staff nurses to insert enteral feeding tubes using a research-based procedure. *Nutr Clin Prac.* 1996;11:21–27.
3. Lord LM. Enteral access devices. *Nurs Clin North Am.* 1997;32:685–702.
4. Burns SM, Martin M, Robbins V, et al. Comparison of nasogastric tube securing methods and tube types in medical intensive care patients. *AJCC.* 1995;4:198–203.
5. Fater KH. Determining nasoenteral feeding tube placement. *Medsurg Nurs.* 1995;4:27–32.

Additional Readings

Bowers S. Tubes: a nurse's guide to enteral feeding devices. *Medsurg Nurs.* 1996;5:313–324.
Zaloga GP. Bedside method for placing small bowel feeding tubes in critically ill patients. *Chest.* 1991;100:1643–1646.

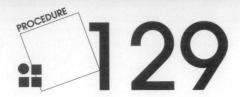

PROCEDURE

129

Advance Directives

P U R P O S E: Advance directives are designed to document patient's end-of-life medical decisions, as well as inform members of the health care team of those decisions.

Barbara B. Ott

PREREQUISITE NURSING KNOWLEDGE

- Documentation of an individual's wishes for future health care is called an advance directive and may include a living will or a health care proxy.
- A living will is a document that expresses a person's wishes for medical treatments when that person is terminally ill and unable to make his or her own decisions.[1] Using a living will, a patient can choose to accept or refuse specific life-sustaining medical treatments (eg, mechanical ventilation, cardiopulmonary resuscitation, tube feedings, blood products, dialysis, antibiotics).
- A health care proxy (also referred to as a durable power of attorney for health care) is a document that identifies a person who can make medical decisions for an individual if he or she becomes unable to make decisions in the future.[1] The patient's designated decision-maker is called a surrogate or proxy decision-maker.[2]
- Patients have the right to make treatment decisions.[3] The development of an advance directive encourages understanding, reflection, and discussion of treatment options by the patient, surrogate, family, and health care team.
- Treatment decisions differ from patient to patient because decisions are based on individual values.[4, 5]
- Both a living will and a health care proxy are easy to prepare, and both documents can be changed or revoked at any time. A patient can change or revoke a living will by telling the physician or nurse that he or she wishes to change or revoke it.
- The Patient Self-Determination Act[6, 7] is a federal law requiring hospitals to do the following:
  ❖ Ask patients if they have an advance directive
  ❖ Give patients and families information about advance directives
  ❖ Tell patients what state law says about advance directives
  ❖ Tell patients what hospital policies say about advance directives.

- The Joint Commission on Accreditation of Healthcare Organizations (JCAHO) requires hospitals to have clear standards on advance directives[1]; they may differ from institution to institution and state to state. Universally, patients are not required to have an advance directive, nor are institutions allowed to discriminate against patients based on whether or not they have an advance directive.
- Under most circumstances, the hospital is required to honor the patient's wishes when they are communicated to the hospital staff. A hospital's policy will explain any specific information or procedures.
- Most hospitals will not guarantee that a health care provider will follow advance directives in every circumstance. The physician should tell the patient or family if the physician cannot, in good conscience, honor the patient's wishes.
- Although not necessary in most states, specific forms may be available to make the preparation of an advance directive easier. Additionally, some states require an advance directive to be signed by two witnesses or notarized by a notary public. Hospitals have state-specific forms for both living wills and health care proxies. Typically, there are hospital employees (social workers, chaplains, patient services representatives) available to help patients prepare an advance directive. It is best if advance directive documents are prepared before a health care crisis occurs.
- Physicians, nurses, and other health care professionals can recommend various treatment options; the patient can choose among the various options or refuse all recommended treatments.[8]
- Patients make decisions regarding medical care with advice from their physician, nurse, and others.[9]
- If a person becomes too ill to make decisions about health care, a previously prepared advance directive can be used to help with those decisions.

- If a patient who does not have an advance directive becomes ill and is unable to make medical decisions, the physician asks a relative or close friend for guidance regarding what treatments the patient would want.[10]
- The hospital ethics committee may be consulted when concerns about patient care and medical decision making for patients are present.[11] The ethics committee also is available to provide additional information, answer questions, or address concerns about advance directives and the care of patients regarding end-of-life care.[12]
- It is best to keep a copy of the patient's living will or health care proxy on the patient's chart so that all individuals involved in patient care are aware of the patient's choices. It can be problematic if the only copy of the advance directive is locked in a safe deposit box or stored in a place without easy access.

EQUIPMENT

- State-specific advance directive forms (if required)
- Notary or witness (if required)

PATIENT AND FAMILY EDUCATION

- Give the patient and family the hospital's information about advance directives. ➤*Rationale:* Although patients are not required to have an advance directive, institutions have an obligation to inform patients about advance directives. This information should be provided in a manner that is not too difficult to read.[13]
- Answer any questions about advance directives. ➤*Rationale:* Advance directives are best prepared by well-informed patients.
- Encourage patients to think carefully about these important medical decisions with a focus on the goals of treatment. Discussions can help clarify values and desired treatments. ➤*Rationale:* An advance directive document should reflect an individual's values and beliefs.

PATIENT ASSESSMENT AND PREPARATION

Patient Assessment

- On admission, determine the existence of or interest in developing an advance directive. ➤*Rationale:* The Patient Self-Determination Act[6] requires that all patients

are asked, on admission, if they have an advance directive. Admission to a healthcare facility provides an opportunity for healthcare providers to open discussion with patients about their personal wishes for their health care.

- Confirm accuracy of the advance directive (if present). ➤*Rationale:* Verifies the accuracy of the document and its usefulness during the patient's stay.
- Assess decision-making capacity. ➤*Rationale:* Usually, the physician or advanced practice nurse determines decisional capacity with input from other sources, including nursing assessments, patient history, patient examination including mental status examination, conference with family, friends, or psychiatric consultation.[14] Decision-making capacity usually consists of three attributes:
  - ❖ Understanding: Can the patient understand information about his or her diagnosis and prognosis and information about the particular decision to be made (treatment options, risks, benefits, burdens)?
  - ❖ Evaluation: Can the patient determine how this information relates to his or her values, beliefs, and goals of treatment?
  - ❖ Reasoning: Can the patient analyze how health care decisions will affect him or her personally? This includes a basic understanding of probability and percentages.[11]
- Determine if the patient is 18 years of age or older. ➤*Rationale:* Persons over the age of 18 are assumed to be legally competent unless a court has determined otherwise. In the clinical setting, some legally competent individuals may have diminished capacity to make health care decisions.

Patient Preparation

- Ensure that patient and family understand preprocedural teaching. Answer questions as they arise and reinforce information as needed. ➤*Rationale:* Evaluates and reinforces understanding of previously taught information.
- If the patient wishes to develop an advance directive, arrange for a time and place for the patient, family, and health care provider to talk about advance directives. ➤*Rationale:* A quiet place, with comfortable seating, away from the noises of the critical care unit, for discussions to take place would be ideal for limiting distractions for these important discussions.

Procedure for Advance Directives		
Steps	**Rationale**	**Special Considerations**
1. Ask the patient if he or she has an advance directive (a living will or a health care proxy).	The Patient Self-Determintion Act requires that hospitals ask if patients have an advance directive.[6]	If the patient is unconscious or too ill to respond to the question, ask family members or friends if they know whether the patient has an advance directive.

Procedure continued on following page

Procedure for Advance Directives *Continued*

Steps	Rationale	Special Considerations
2. Document patient's response (yes or no—patient has or does not have an advance directive).	It is important to know if the patient has already prepared an advance directive.	It may be necessary to ask more than one family member or friend if the patient has an advance directive.
3. If the patient has an advance directive, place a copy of it on the current medical record.	Advance directive choices must be communicated to the health care team.	Some hospitals have special procedures for documenting the presence of an advance directive (eg, special sticker for the chart, designated placement in the medical record, special checklist). Advance directives can be changed or revoked by the patient verbally or in writing. The presence of an advance directive on the chart does not mean the patient has an order for Do Not Resuscitate.[15]
4. If the patient has an advance directive, but does not have a copy of it with him or her, make arrangements with a family member or friend to bring it to the hospital for incorporation into the medical record.	Copies of advance directives often are kept with other important papers in secure places (eg, bank safety deposit boxes and household safes). It is essential that the patient's advance directive is reviewed and is a part of the patient's chart.	Copies of advance directives can sometimes be found in medical records from the physician's office or from an old hospital record.
5. Assess that choices recorded on the advance directive document are accurate and up to date.	It is important to ensure that previously prepared documents reflect the patient's current choices.	
6. Confirm that medical treatments and nursing care are consistent with patient's advance directive choices.	Patients may change their minds regarding treatment choices. These changes must be communicated to the staff.	

Developing an Advance Directive

1. Assist the physician or advanced practice nurse with assessment of the patient's decision-making capacity.	Illness can cause a patient to have difficulty understanding information, relating the information to personal values, or communicating choices to the health care team.	
2. Provide the patient with information about advance directives and answer any questions about advance directives.	Federal law requires hospitals to give patients information about advance directives.[6]	
3. Provide the patient with appropriate resources (ie, hospital personnel who can assist with more information about advance directives) and with preparation of an advance directive document, if desired.	Provides assistance with the development of an advance directive.	
4. Encourage patients to discuss medical treatment decisions with their physician, surrogate, and family.	Providing information and encouraging discussion is important, so that patient treatment wishes are known.	Patients should not be pressured to sign an advance directive. Encourage discussion of all options.
5. Have a follow-up discussion with the patient about advance directives.	Upon admission, patients and family members may be quite stressed and overloaded with information. Patients and family members may need time to reflect on treatment wishes.	

Expected Outcomes	Unexpected Outcomes
• Patient treatment wishes are known.	• Patient treatment wishes are unknown.
• Patient treatment wishes are honored.	• Patient treatment wishes are not honored.

Patient Monitoring and Care

Patient Monitoring and Care	Rationale	Reportable Conditions
		These conditions should be reported if they persist despite nursing interventions.
1. Patients should be asked if they have a current advance directive and if it is accurate.	Advance directives can be prepared many months or years before a patient becomes sick. It is advisable to ask patients if their choices in their advance directives are still current. Sometimes, as a patient's physical condition changes through the course of an illness, the patient may want to modify decisions previously stated in the advance directive. Patients with decision-making capacity can revoke or change advance directives at any time.	• Patients' wishes to modify their advance directive
2. Ensure that the advance directive is communicated with members of the health care team and family.	It is possible that decisions made by a patient and reflected in an advance directive may not have been communicated to the patient's family or friends or the health care provider.	• Misunderstanding by health care professionals or family about the patient's choices for health care
3. Consult hospital ethics committee as needed.	The patient, family, or health care providers may need to consult the ethics committee if there are misunderstandings or disagreements about what treatment options should be pursued.	• Need and involvement of the ethics committee

Documentation

Documentation should include the following:

- Patient and family education
- Existence of an advance directive
- Location of the advance directive document, if the patient has one
- Name and phone number of individual who brought a copy of the advance directive to the hospital
- A copy of the living will or health care proxy in the front of the chart or in a location in the chart where it is easy to find
- Discussions with patient, surrogate, and family members regarding the advance directive
- Misunderstandings the patient or family may have about the law, institutional policy, or content of an advance directive
- Unexpected outcomes
- Additional nursing interventions

References

1. Monagler JF, Thomasma DC. *Health Care Ethics.* Gaithersburg, Md: Aspen Publications; 1998.
2. Ott BB. Advance directives: the emerging body of research. *Am J Crit Care.* 1999;8:514–519.
3. President's Commission for the Study of Ethical Problems in Medicine and Biomedical and Behavioral Research. *Making Health Care Decisions.* Washington, DC: US Government; 1982.
4. Beauchamp TL, Childress JF. *Principles of Biomedical Ethics.* New York, NY: Oxford University Press; 1994.

5. Davis AJ, Aroskar MA, Liaschenko J, Drought TS. *Ethical Dilemmas and Nursing Practice.* Stamford, Ct: Appleton & Lange; 1994.

6. Omnibus Budget Reconciliation Act of 1990 (OBRA-90), Patient Self-Determination Act. Pub L10-508:4206–4751.

7. American Nurses Association. *Position Statement on Nursing and the Patient Self-Determination Act.* Kansas City, Mo; American Nurses Association; 1992.

8. American Association of Critical Care Nurses. *Withholding and/or Withdrawing Life-Sustaining Treatment: A Position Statement.* Aliso Viejo, Ca: AACN; 1990.

9. SUPPORT. A controlled trial to improve care for seriously ill hospitalized patients. *JAMA.* 1995;274:1591–1598.

10. Buchanan AE, Brock DW. *Deciding for Others.* New York, NY: Cambridge University Press; 1989.

11. Devettere RJ. *Practical Decision Making in Health Care Ethics.* Washington, DC: Georgetown University Press; 1995.

12. Minogue B. *Bioethics: a Committee Approach.* Boston, Ma: Jones and Bartlett; 1966.

13. Ott BB, Hardie TL. Readability of advance directive documents. *Image.* 1997;29:53–57.

14. Molloy DW, Silberfeld M, Darzins P, et al. Measuring capacity to complete an advance directive. *J Am Geriatr Soc.* 1996; 44:660–664.

15. American Association of Critical-Care Nurses. *Clarification of Resuscitation Status in Critical Care Settings: Position Statement.* Aliso Viejo, Ca: AACN; 1985.

Additional Reading

American Association of Critical-Care Nurses. *Discovering Your Beliefs About Healthcare Choices.* Aliso Viejo, Ca: AACN; 1997.

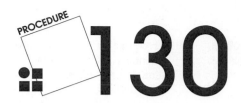

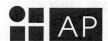

130

Determination of Death

P U R P O S E: Institutional policies and legislation governing declaration of death may vary across practice settings and states. However, standardized evidence-based criteria provide guidelines for practices involving determination of cardiopulmonary and brain death. Procedures used in death determination are described in this section.

Jacqueline Sullivan

PREREQUISITE NURSING KNOWLEDGE

- Death is determined when there is either (1) irreversible cessation of circulatory and respiratory functions or (2) irreversible cessation of all functions of the entire brain, including the brain stem.
- In cases of either cardiopulmonary or brain death, diagnosis of death requires both cessation of function and irreversibility.
- In cardiopulmonary death, cessation of function is determined by clinical examination.
- In cardiopulmonary death, irreversibility is confirmed by persistent cessation of functions during a period of observation.
- In brain death, cessation of function is determined when clinical evaluation discloses absence of both cerebral and brain stem function.
- In brain death, irreversibility is determined when (1) the etiology of coma sufficient to account for loss of brain functions is established, (2) the possibility of recovery of brain function is excluded, and (3) the cessation of all brain functions persists for a period of observation or therapy.
- Previously, death was solely described as the cessation of circulation and respiration (ie, cardiopulmonary death). However, the advent of mechanical ventilation and cardiovascular support modalities has presented new challenges for determining the end of life for patients with catastrophic cerebral insults who are able to be preserved using complex technology.[1, 2]
- Initial efforts to define death in this age of technologic advancement included development of the Harvard criteria released by an Ad Hoc Committee on Brain Death at Harvard Medical School.[3] These criteria described deter-

mination of a condition known as "irreversible coma," "cerebral death," or "brain death."[1]
- Since the initial introduction of the Harvard criteria, the Uniform Determination of Death Act (UDDA) was promulgated in 1980 and supported by the President's Commission for the Study of Ethical Problems in Medicine and Biomedical and Biobehavioral Research as a model statute for adopting state legislation that defines death.[1]
- UDDA asserts that "an individual, who has sustained either (1) irreversible cessation of circulatory and respiratory functions, or (2) irreversible cessation of all functions of the entire brain, including the brainstem, is dead. A determination of death must be made in accordance with accepted medical standards."[1]
- Since its initial inception, the concept of brain death continues to be the topic of international debate among medical clinicians, anthropologists, philosophers, and ethicists. Much of this discussion is the product of awareness of continuing technologic advances, neurodiagnostic developments, and clinical insight. This ongoing dialogue concerning determination of death is a process of developing multidisciplinary consensus responsive to continually changing technology.[4–6]
- Although conceptualization of death determination continues to evolve, clinical and scientific experts have generated clinical practice parameters for brain death diagnosis that are grounded in empirical knowledge, supported by sufficiently rigorous research, and substantiated by moderate to high degrees of clinical certainty.[7]
- Neuroscience experts continue to define brain death as irreversible cessation of all functions of the entire brain, including the brain stem. This definition remains consistent with the definition of brain death initially presented by the President's Commission for the Study of Ethical Problems in Medicine and Biomedical and Biobehavioral Research.[1, 7]
- Cardinal findings in brain death include coma or unresponsiveness, absence of cerebral motor responses to pain in all extremities, absence of brain stem reflexes

---

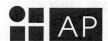

(including pupillary signs, ocular movements, facial sensory and motor responses, pharyngeal and tracheal reflexes), and apnea.

EQUIPMENT
Cardiopulmonary Death Determination

- Stethoscope
- Electrocardiogram (ECG) monitor
- ECG leads
- ECG electrodes

Brain Death Determination

Oculovestibular (Calorics) Test Equipment

- Iced saline or water solution
- 60-mL syringe with Luer-Lok end
- 18- or 20-G angiocatheter with needle removed
- Small basin (eg, emesis)
- Towels and protective bedding
- Nonsterile gloves

Apnea Test Equipment

- Oxygen delivery via endotracheal airway using nasal cannula or straight tubing for oxygen delivery
- Arterial blood gas kit supplies

FAMILY EDUCATION

- Assess family understanding of the death determination procedure and its purpose. **➤➤Rationale:** Clarification and repeat explanation may assist in allaying some stress and anxiety for grief-stricken family members.
- Assess family understanding of the concept of brain death. Give clear definition of brain death and death as synonymous and reinforce repeatedly with the family. **➤➤Rationale:** The concept of brain death may be confusing to family members, because the term may imply that only the brain is dead and that the rest of the body is alive. Brain death must be described as death. Brain death and death must be presented synonymously to the family to ensure clarity concerning death determination.
- Explain potential outcomes of the death determination procedure. **➤➤Rationale:** Awareness of duration and expectations of death determination procedures may allay some stress and anxiety in grief-stricken family members.
- When a patient has conclusively been declared brain dead, facilitate discussion of organ donation with family members by appropriate members of the health care team. **➤➤Rationale:** Brain-dead patients are potential candidates for organ donation. Most experts recommend separating the interaction involving declaration of death to the family from the interaction requesting consideration for organ donation (a process otherwise known as "decoupling"). In some institutions and states, request for organ donation is delegated to representatives of organ procurement organizations (OPOs) or to experts who have been specially trained by OPOs (see Procedure 133, "Request for Organ Donation").

PATIENT ASSESSMENT AND PREPARATION
Patient Assessment

- Assess baseline cardiopulmonary and neurologic status in preparation for clinical examination for death determination. **➤➤Rationale:** In cardiopulmonary death, clinical examination discloses absence of responsiveness, heartbeat, and respiratory effort. In brain death, clinical examination reveals an absence of both cerebral and brainstem function.
- For brain death determination, the following prerequisites must also be met:
  - ❖ Acquire clinical or neuroimaging evidence of an acute catastrophic cerebral event consistent with the clinical diagnosis of brain death
  - ❖ Exclude conditions that may confound clinical assessment of brain death (ie, acute metabolic or endocrine derangements, neuromuscular blockade)
  - ❖ Confirm the absence of drug intoxication or poisoning
  - ❖ Maintain core body temperature at greater than or equal to 32°C
  - **➤➤Rationale:** The brain death determination procedure must confirm both cessation of all brain function (including both cerebral and brainstem function) and irreversibility. These four criteria are required for confirmation of irreversible cessation of brain function.

Patient Preparation

- Ensure that the family understands preprocedural teaching. Answer questions as they arise and reinforce information as needed. **➤➤Rationale:** Evaluates and reinforces understanding of previously taught information.
- Place patient in supine position. **➤➤Rationale:** Facilitates patient assessment, oculovestibular testing, and arterial puncture.

Procedure for Determination of Death

Steps	Rationale	Special Considerations
Assisting with Determination of Cardiopulmonary Death		
1. Wash hands.	Reduces transmission of microorganisms; standard precautions.	
2. Assist the physician in conducting appropriate clinical examination.	Clinical examination in cardiopulmonary death reveals absence of responsiveness, heartbeat, and respiratory effort.	
3. Perform ECG, if required (see Procedures 51 and 54).	Medical circumstances may require a confirmatory test such as ECG monitoring or 12-lead ECG.	Physician legally is responsible to assess and declare patient's death.
4. Confirm irreversibility of cessation of cardiopulmonary function.	Irreversibility is confirmed by persistent cessation of functions, including pulselessness, apnea, and loss of consciousness.	In clinical situations, where death is expected and where the course has been gradual, the period of observation following cessation may be limited to the time required to complete the examination. If ventricular fibrillation and cardiac standstill develop in a monitored patient and resuscitation is not undertaken or is unsuccessful, the required period of observation may be limited to the time required to complete the examination. When a possible death is unobserved, unexpected, or sudden, the duration of the examination should be commensurate with continued resuscitative efforts. Declaration of death in patients who are first observed with rigor mortis may require only the period of observation necessary to establish that condition.
Assisting with Determination of Brain Death		
1. Wash hands.	Reduces transmission of microorganisms; standard precautions.	
2. Ensure that the patient's core body temperature is at least 32°C at the time of physician's clinical examination for brain death determination. *(Level V: Clinical studies in more than one or two different patient populations and situations to support recommendations)*	Hypothermia may artificially alter results of neurologic examination, leading to confounding results regarding irreversible cessation of all brain function.[5-7]	Physician legally is responsible to assess and declare patient's death.
3. Perform necessary endocrine screenings as required for the individual patient (eg, screen for conditions such as diabetic ketoacidosis [DKA], hyperglycemic hyperosmolar nonketotic coma [HHNK], thyroid disturbances). *(Level V: Clinical studies in more than one or two different patient populations and situations to support recommendations)*	Endocrine screening may exclude conditions that may confound clinical assessment of brain death (ie, acute metabolic or endocrine derangements).[7]	

Procedure continued on following page

■■ AP This procedure should be performed only by physicians, advanced practice nurses, and other health care professionals (including critical care nurses) with additional knowledge, skills, and demonstrated competence per professional licensure or institutional standard.

Procedure **for Determination of Death** *Continued*

Steps	Rationale	Special Considerations
4. Perform necessary toxicology screenings as required for the individual patient. *(Level V: Clinical studies in more than one or two different patient populations and situations to support recommendations)*	In cases where the possibility of excessive sedation is present, toxicology screening for all likely drugs should be considered.[7]	If exogenous intoxication of drugs is determined to exist, death should not be declared until the intoxicant is metabolized or until confirmatory testing for cessation of intracranial circulation is considered.
5. Assist in establishing evidence of coma or unresponsiveness. In brain death, intense stimulation evokes no verbal or voluntary motor responses. Spontaneous voluntary motor activity, shivering, or seizure activity are absent in brain death.	Coma is a cardinal finding consistent with brain death.	
6. Assess cerebral motor responses to pain using noxious stimulation (ie, nailbed pressure). *(Level V: Clinical studies in more than one or two different patient populations and situations to support recommendations)*	Absence of cerebral motor responses to pain is a cardinal finding consistent with brain death.[5–7]	Motor responses may occur sponta-neously during apnea testing with the occurrence of hypoxia or hypo-tension and are considered to be of spinal reflex origin. Respiratory aci-dosis and brisk neck flexion also may generate spinal cord reflexes. Spinal reflex responses occur more frequently in young adults and in-clude rapid spontaneous flexion and muscle stretch reflexes in arms and legs, with resulting grasplike walking-like movements. Spinal re-flex movements are not cerebrally modulated. Spinal reflex move-ments may occur in the presence of brain death. Involuntary posturing movements (ie, decorticate or decer-ebrate) are absent in brain death.
7. In the presence of neuromuscular blockade use, assessment with a bedside peripheral nerve stimulator is required before testing for cerebrally modulated motor responses (see Procedure 93). *(Level IV: Limited clinical studies to support recommendations)*	Neuromuscular blockade use may con-found motor testing in brain death due to pharmacologically induced motor weak-ness.[7]	In cases where neuromuscular blocking agents may have been pre-viously used, testing with a bedside peripheral nerve stimulator may de-termine whether adequate neuro-muscular function has returned, which is required for valid clinical brain death determination testing to proceed. Clinical brain death deter-mination procedures cannot be un-dertaken in the presence of active, ongoing neuromuscular blockade.
8. Assess pupillary size and response to light bilaterally. *(Level V: Clinical studies in more than one or two different patient populations and situations to support recommendations)*	Round, oval, or irregularly shaped pupils are compatible with brain death.[5–7] Pupillary light reflex must be absent in brain death. Absence of pupillary light reflexes, as a component of brain stem reflexes, is a cardinal finding consistent with brain death. Most pupils are midposition size (4 to 6 mm) in brain death.	Dilated pupils may occur even in the presence of brain death, because intact sympathetic cervical pathways connected to the pupillary dilator muscle may still be intact. Standard doses of atropine administered intravenously do not markedly affect pupillary response. Neuromuscular blocking agents do not significantly influence pupil size. Topical administration of medications and ocular trauma may influence pupillary size and reactivity. Preexisting ocular anatomic abnormalities may also confound pupillary assessment in brain death.

| Procedure | **for Determination of Death** *Continued* |

Steps	**Rationale**	**Special Considerations**
9. Assess oculocephalic (doll's eye) reflexes. Oculocephalic reflexes are elicited by rapidly and vigorously turning the head to 90 degrees laterally on both sides and normally results in eye deviation to the opposite side of head turning. *(Level V: Clinical studies in more than one or two different patient populations and situations to support recommendations)*	In brain death, oculocephalic reflexes are absent, with no eye movements occurring in response to head movements. Absence of oculocephalic reflexes, as a component of brain stem reflexes, is a cardinal finding consistent with brain death.[5-7]	Contraindications to performance of oculocephalic reflex testing include suspicion of cervical spine fracture or instability. In some institutions, nurses independently may assess oculocephalic reflexes.
10. Assist in assessment of oculovestibular (caloric) reflexes (see Procedure 84). Oculovestibular reflexes are tested with the head elevated 30 degrees during irrigation of both tympanic membranes with 50 mL of iced saline or water. Observation should persist for up to 1 minute after each ear irrigation, with a 5-minute waiting period between testing of each ear.	In brain death, oculovestibular reflexes are absent, with no deviation of the eyes in response to ear irrigation. Absence of oculovestibular reflexes, as a component of brain stem reflexes, is a cardinal finding consistent with brain death.	Contraindications to testing of oculovestibular reflexes include impaired integrity of tympanic membranes. Several medications may diminish oculovestibular reflexes, including sedatives, aminoglycosides, tricyclic antidepressants, anticholinergics, antiseizure agents, and neuromuscular blocking agents. Preexisting vestibular disease, preexisting cranial nerve disorders, and facial trauma involving the auditory canal and petrous bone also may inhibit oculovestibular reflex responses. In most institutions, oculovestibular reflex testing is reserved for physicians.
11. Assess corneal and jaw reflexes. Corneal reflexes should be tested with a cotton-tipped swab. Jaw reflexes are described as grimacing to pain and may be tested by application of deep pressure on nailbeds, the supraorbital ridge, or the temporomandibular joint. *(Level V: Clinical studies in more than one or two different patient populations and institutions to support recommendations)*	Absence of facial and motor responses, as a component of brain stem reflexes, is a cardinal finding consistent with brain death.[7] Corneal and jaw reflexes are absent in brain death.	Severe facial trauma may inhibit interpretation of facial brain stem reflexes.
12. Assess gag and cough reflexes. Gag reflex may be elicited by stimulating the posterior pharynx with a tongue blade. Cough reflex may be tested by bronchial suctioning. *(Level V: Clinical studies in more than one or two different patient populations and situations to support recommendations)*	Absence of pharyngeal and tracheal reflexes, as a component of brain stem reflexes, is a cardinal finding consistent with brain death.[5-7] Gag and cough reflexes are absent in brain death.	Gag reflex may be difficult to evaluate in orally intubated patients.

Procedure continued on following page

▪▪ AP This procedure should be performed only by physicians, advanced practice nurses, and other health care professionals (including critical care nurses) with additional knowledge, skills, and demonstrated competence per professional licensure or institutional standard.

Procedure **for Determination of Death** *Continued*

Steps	Rationale	Special Considerations
13. Prepare for performance of apnea test.	A cardinal finding and essential component in the clinical determination of brain death is the demonstration of apnea. Loss of brain stem function definitively results in loss of centrally controlled breathing function, with resultant apnea.	
14. Achieve conditions necessary for apnea test precautions.[7-13] A. Maintain core body temperature greater than or equal to 36.5°C. B. Maintain systolic blood pressure greater than or equal to 90 mm Hg. C. Achieve euvolemia. D. Achieve eucapnea (arterial $PaCO_2$ of greater than or equal to 40 mm Hg). E. Maintain/achieve normoxemia (arterial PaO_2 of greater than or equal to 200 mm Hg). *(Level V: Clinical studies in more than one or two different patient populations and situations to support recommendations)*	Maintenance of apnea test precautions assists in avoidance of cardiac dysrhythmias and systemic hypotension, which may occur during the apnea test.	Cardiac dysrhythmias and systemic hypotension may occur during apnea testing. Cardiac dysrhythmias usually result from hypercarbia and respiratory acidosis and occur most frequently in patients with hypoxia. Severe hypotension may occur in well-oxygenated patients whose arterial $PaCO_2$ rises to high levels with acidosis. It has been demonstrated that hemodynamic disturbances may be avoided during apnea testing when respiratory acidosis is limited to a pH of 7.17 (± 0.02) with an arterial $PaCO_2$ of 60 to 80 mm Hg.[8] Pretest hyperoxygenation and procedural administration of oxygen also have resulted in avoidance of significant hypoxemia in apnea testing.
15. Perform apnea test: A. Obtain baseline arterial blood gas (ABG). B. Disconnect the ventilator. C. Deliver 100% oxygen, 6 L/min. May place oxygen cannula at the level of carina. D. Observe closely for respiratory movements (ie, abdominal or chest excursions that produce adequate tidal volumes). E. Measure ABG for arterial PaO_2, $PaCO_2$, and pH after approximately 8 minutes and reconnect the ventilator.		In many institutions, a physician must be present during performance of apnea testing. The exact level of arterial $PaCO_2$ necessary to maximally stimulate the chemoreceptors of central respiratory centers remains unknown in conditions consistent with hyperoxygenation and brainstem destruction. Advisory guidelines for determination of death based on clinical and research data recommend achieving $PaCO_2$ levels of greater than 60 mm Hg for maximal stimulation of brainstem respiratory centers.[1] Target $PaCO_2$ levels for apnea tests in brain death determination may be higher in patients with chronic hypercapnia. Hypocarbia may also occur in patients with acute catastrophic cerebral insults and may result from therapeutic hyperventilation or hypothermia. Although correction of hypocarbia should precede apnea testing, use of carbon dioxide admixtures should probably be avoided due to associated consequences, including severe hypercarbia and respiratory acidosis.

Procedure	**for Determination of Death** *Continued*

Steps	Rationale	Special Considerations
16. Assist in interpretation of apnea test results. *(Level V: Clinical studies in more than one or two different patient populations and situations to support recommendations)*	Aids in determination of brain death.[7–13]	Apnea test results may be interpreted in the following four ways: (1) positive, (2) negative, (3) occurrence of cardiovascular/pulmonary instability, and (4) inconclusive. Table 130–1 provides a description of apnea test results.
17. Facilitate compliance with institutional recommendations regarding persistent observation in brain death determination. *(Level IV: Limited clinical studies to support recommendations)*	Persistent observation further confirms irreversibility in clinical determination of brain death.[7] A repeat clinical evolution of cardinal findings in brain death is recommended.	Most experts recommend an arbitrary interval of 6 hours between initial and repeat observations for clinical determination of brain death in adults; however, a firm recommendation based on scientific literature cannot be given.[7] All clinical tests of cardinal findings are equally essential in declaring brain death.
18. Assist in obtaining confirmatory tests for brain death determination as indicated. *(Level IV: Limited clinical studies to support recommendations)*	Confirmatory testing may aid diagnosis.[14–26] Although confirmatory tests are not mandatory in most situations, diagnostic testing may be necessary for declaring brain death with patients in whom specific components of clinical testing cannot be reliably evaluated.[7] Clinical experience with confirmatory tests mostly involves use of conventional angiography, electroencephalogram (EEG), transcranial Doppler ultrasonography (TCD), and cerebral blood flow studies (see Table 130–2).	Table 130–2 provides a review of described confirmatory tests and results expected in brain death.

Table 130–1 ● ■ ■ Apnea Test Results

Positive apnea test	Respiratory movements are absent Post-test arterial $PaCO_2$ is greater than or equal to 60 mm Hg Supports clinical determination of brain death
Negative apnea test	Respiratory movements are observed regardless of arterial $PaCO_2$ level Does *not* support clinical determination of brain death; apnea test may be repeated
Apnea test resulting in cardiovascular or pulmonary instability	Systolic blood pressure falls below 90 mm Hg Arterial oxygen desaturation occurs Cardiac dysrhythmia occurs Immediately draw an arterial blood gas sample and reconnect ventilator Confirmatory test to finalize clinical determination of brain death may be performed at discretion of physician
Inconclusive apnea test	No respiratory movements are observed Post-test arterial $PaCO_2$ is less than 60 mm Hg without significant cardiovascular instability Apnea test may be repeated with 10 minutes of apnea

Table 130–2 ● ■ ■ Confirmatory Brain Death Test Results

Cerebral angiography	No intracerebral filling at level of carotid bifurcation or circle of Willis External carotid circulation is patent
Electroencephalogram (EEG)	No electrical activity during a period of at least 30 minutes of recording
Transcranial Doppler ultrasonography	Absent diastolic or reverberating flow Flow only through systole or retrograde diastolic flow Small systolic peaks in early systole
Technetium 99m brain scan (cerebral blood flow scan)	No uptake of isotope in brain parenchyma ("hollow skull phenomenon")

■●■ AP This procedure should be performed only by physicians, advanced practice nurses, and other health care professionals (including critical care nurses) with additional knowledge, skills, and demonstrated competence per professional licensure or institutional standard.

Expected Outcomes	Unexpected Outcomes
• Clinical or diagnostic determination of death • Physician declaration of death and notification of family	• Indecisive results regarding determination of death

Patient Monitoring and Care

Patient Monitoring and Care	Rationale	Reportable Conditions
		These conditions should be reported if they persist despite nursing interventions.
1. Assess family understanding of and response to death determination procedure.	Family understanding of and response to death determination situations may vary based on religious beliefs and cultural practices. Adequate assessment of family's profile provides the necessary foundation for provision of support.	
2. Solicit family support provided by spiritual and psychological counselors.	Support of spiritual and psychological counselors may assist the family in the grieving process.	
3. Provide adequate private time for family members to visit with and grieve for the loss of their loved one.	Private visiting time provides family members with the opportunity for grieving and closure.	
4. In cases of brain death, facilitate discussion of organ donation options (see Procedure 133).	In most states, it is required to screen patients with brain death for organ donation.	
5. In cases where brain death has not been confirmed but where quality-of-life issues are being considered, be prepared to facilitate and provide support during discussions regarding possible withdrawal of therapy (see Procedure 134).	Indecisive results regarding brain death determination may lead to consideration of other treatment options, including withdrawal of therapy.	In cases of devastating neurologic insults without occurrence of brain death, the health care team, in collaboration with the patient's family, may make decisions regarding continuation or initiation of resuscitation measures, provision of supportive care, and withdrawal of therapy. These situations may require consultation with the hospital ethicist and pastoral counselor.

Documentation

Documentation should include the following:

- Family education and support
- Description of specific procedure(s) performed for death determination, results of such procedures, and patient's tolerance of procedures
- Documentation by the physician should include clinical examination components consistent with determination of death and exact time of death determination
- Time of death for cardiopulmonary death is documented as time of clinical or diagnostic confirmation of complete and irreversible cessation of circulatory and respiratory function; ECG strips, if obtained, should be interpreted and included in the patient's permanent medical record
- Time of death for brain death is documented as time of clinical diagnostic confirmation of complete and irreversible cessation of all brain function; time of death for brain death is *not* listed as time of removal of mechanical ventilation or time of organ donation

References

1. Guidelines for the determination of death: Report of the Medical Consultants on the Diagnosis of Death to the President's Commission for the Study of Ethical Problems in Medicine and Biomedical and Biobehavioral Research. *JAMA.* 1981;246:2184–2186.
2. *Practice Parameters for Determining Brain Death in Adults: Summary Statement.* Report of the Quality Standards Subcommittee of the American Academy of Neurology; 1995.
3. Report of the Ad Hoc Committee on Brain Death, Harvard Medical School. *JAMA.* 1968;205:337–340.
4. Kennedy M, Kiloh N. Drugs and brain death. *Drug Safety.* 1996;14:171–180.
5. Link J, Schaefer M, Lang M. Concepts and diagnosis of brain death. Forensic Sci Int. 1994;69:195–203.
6. Calliauw L. Brain death. *Acta Neurochir.* 1990;105(1–2):85–86.
7. Wijdicks EFM. Determining brain death in adults. *Neurology.* 1995;45:1003–1011.
8. Ebata T, Watanabe Y, Amaha K, Hosaka Y, Takagi S. Haemodynamic changes during the apnea test for diagnosis of brain deathy. *Can J Anesth.* 1991;38:436–440.
9. Gutmann DH, Marino PL. An alternative apnea test for the evaluation of brain death. *Ann Neurol.* 1991;30:852–853.
10. al Jumah M, McLean DR, al Rajeh S, Crow N. Balk diffusion apnea test in the dignosis of brain death. *Crit Care Med.* 1992;20:1564–1567.
11. Visram A, Marshall C. $PaCO_2$ and apnoea testing for brain stem death. *Anesthesia.* 1997;52:503.
12. Lang CJ. Blood pressure and heart rate changes during apnea testing with or without CO_2 insufflation. *Intens Care Med.* 1997;23:903–907.
13. Benzel EC, Mashburn JP, Conrad S, Modling D. Apnea testing for the determination of brain death: a modified protocol. Technical note. *J Neurosurg.* 1992;76:1029–1031.
14. Silverman D, Saunders MG, Schwab RS, Marana RL. Cerebral death and the electroencephalogram. Report of the Ad Hoc Committee of the American Electroencephalographic Society on EEG criteria for determination of cerebral death. *JAMA.* 1969;209:1505–1510.
15. Minimum technical standards for EEG recording in suspected cerebral death. *J Clin Neurophysiol.* 1994;11:10–13.
16. Payen DM, Lamer C, Pilorget A, et al. Evaluation of pulsed Doppler common carotid blood flow as a noninvasive method for brain death diagnosis: a prospective study. *Anesthesiology.* 1990;72:222–229.
17. Petty GW, Mohr JP, Pedley TA, et al. The role of transcranial Doppler in confirming brain death: sensitivity, specificity, and suggestions for performance and interpretation. *Neurology.* 1990;40:300–303.
18. Jalili M. Crade M, Davis AL. Carotid blood flow velocity changes detected by Doppler ultrasound in determination of brain death in children: a preliminry report. *Clin Pediatr.* 1994;33:669–674.
19. Newell DW. Transcranial Doppler measurements. *New Horizons.* 1995;3:423–430.
20. Ying Z, Schmid UD, Schmid J, Hess CW. Motor and somatosensory evoked potentials in coma: analysis and relation to clinical status and outcome. *J Neurol Neurosurg Psychiatry.* 1992;55:470–474.
21. Palma V, Guadagnino M. Evoked potentials in brain death: a critical review. *Acta Neurol.* 1992;14(4–6):363–368.
22. Machado C, Multimodality evoked potentials and electroretinography in a test battery for an early diagnosis of brain death. *J Neurol Sci.* 1993;37:125–131.
23. Goldie WD, Chiappa KH, Young RR, Brooks EB. Brainstem auditory and short-latency somatosensory evoked responses in brain death. *Neurology.* 1981;31:248–256.

▦ AP This procedure should be performed only by physicians, advanced practice nurses, and other health care professionals (including critical care nurses) with additional knowledge, skills, and demonstrated competence per professional licensure or institutional standard.

24. Erbengi A, Erbengi G, Cataltepe O, et al. Brain death: determination with brain stem evoked potentials and radionuclide isotope studies. *Acta Neurochir.* 1991;112(3–4):118–125.

25. Matsumura A, Meguro K, Tsurushima H, et al. Magnetic resonance imaging of brain death. *Neurol Med Chir.* 1996;36:166–171.

26. Ishii K, Onuma T, Kinoshita T, et al. Brain death: MR and MR angiography. *Am J Neuroradiol.* 1996;17:731–735.

Additional Readings

Black PM. Conceptual and practical issues in the declaration of death by brain critiera. *Neurosurg Clin North Am.* 1991;2:493–501.

Byrne PA, Nilges RG. The brain stem in brain death: a critical review. *Issues Law Med.* 1993;9:3–21.

Hanley DF. Brain death: an update on the North American viewpoint. *Anesth Intens Care.* 1995;23:24–25.

Lock M. Death in technological time: locating the end of meaningful life. *Med Anthropol Q.* 1996;10:575–600.

Machado C. Death on neurological grounds. *J. Neurosurg Sci.* 1994;38:209–222.

Nau R, Prange HW, Klingelhofer J, et al. Results of four technical investigations in fifty clinically brain dead patients. *Intens Care Med.* 1992;18:82–88.

Paolin A, Manuali A, DiPaola F, et al. Reliability in diagnosis of brain death. *Intens Care Med.* 1995;21:657–662.

Shann F. A personal comment: whole brain death versus cortical death. *Anesth Intens Care.* 1995;23:14–15.

Taylor RM. Rexamining the definition and criteria of death. *Semin Neurol.* 1997;17:265–270.

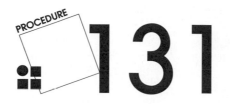

131

Care of the Organ Donor

PURPOSE: To preserve organ function until transplantation.

June Hinkle

PREREQUISITE NURSING KNOWLEDGE

- Knowledge of state, organ procurement organization (OPO), and hospital policies regarding organ donation from patients diagnosed with brain death and from patients who are non–heart-beating donors is essential.
- In brain death, cessation of function is determined when clinical evaluation discloses absence of both cerebral and brain stem function (see Procedure 130).
- Non–heart-beating donors are those who have experienced a cardiopulmonary arrest or are being removed from life support and the family or significant other wishes to donate organs.[1]
- The patient remains in the intensive care unit (ICU) until the organ donor matching process is completed.
- Hemodynamic instability may occur because of failure of the autonomic nervous system. Management goals should focus on maintenance of intravascular volume, normothermia, acid-base balance, and the optimization of oxygenation and perfusion.
- Costs associated with organ recovery are billed to the OPO.
- If organ recovery is occurring from a patient meeting brain death criteria, the donor remains on the ventilator until organ recovery is complete.
- If organ recovery is occurring from a non–heart-beating donor on a ventilator, the ventilator is stopped and death must be pronounced after the heart stops beating. Recovery of organs must occur quickly after the heart stops beating to ensure the organs are viable. All organs may be recovered from a non–heart-beating donor, but the kidney is the most frequently recovered organ.[1] OPO and hospital policies regarding non–heart-beating donors vary between institutions and states.
- If the donor experiences cardiac arrest, cardiopulmonary resuscitation (CPR) and advanced cardiac life support are initiated. If resuscitation is not successful, organ recovery is performed as soon as feasible. If the patient was designated as Do Not Resuscitate (DNR) before consent for organ donation, this usually is removed from the chart after consent is obtained for organ donation. Consent for removal of the DNR status needs to be approved by the patient's family.
- Organ donation is a cooperative effort between the family, critical care nurses, physicians, transplant coordinator, designated hospital requestor, OPO coordinator, operating room personnel, and the surgical recovery team.

EQUIPMENT

- Thermometer
- Electrocardiogram (ECG) monitor and electrodes
- Consent form
- Laboratory specimen containers and laboratory forms
- Prescribed intravenous fluids
- Urinary catheter
- Ventilator

Additional equipment may include the following:

- Arterial line and monitoring system

PATIENT AND FAMILY EDUCATION

- Evaluate the family's understanding of the organ recovery process. ➡️*Rationale:* Allows the critical care nurse to correct misunderstandings, clarify information, evaluate the efficacy of coping strategies, and reduce anxiety related to the care of the patient.
- Reinforce to the family that surgical removal of the organs takes place with respect and careful technique, similar to any operation. ➡️*Rationale:* Decreases the family's anxiety about the care of their loved one during the recovery.

PATIENT ASSESSMENT AND PREPARATION

Patient Assessment

- Assess oxygenation. ➡️*Rationale:* Provides baseline data.
- Assess vital signs and hemodynamic parameters. ➡️*Rationale:* Provides baseline data.

Patient Preparation

- Ensure that the family understands preprocedural teaching. Answer questions as they arise and reinforce information as needed. ➡️*Rationale:* Evaluates and reinforces understanding of previously taught information.

- An arterial catheter may be inserted, if not already in place. ➤*Rationale:* Facilitates assessment of blood pressure and ease of blood sampling.
- Communicate with the OPO coordinator to determine the timing and logistics of the recovery surgery. ➤*Rationale:* The OPO coordinator has the responsibility of organ placement and the coordination of the arriving surgical recovery teams.

- Determine a plan for communicating with the family during the recovery process. This should be developed with the critical care nurse, OPO coordinator, and the family. ➤*Rationale:* Each family has unique needs during the recovery process. Many families wish to leave the hospital as soon as the consent for donation is signed; others wish to see their deceased loved one after recovery has occurred.

Procedure for Care of the Organ Donor

Steps	Rationale	Special Considerations
1. Ensure that brain death criteria have been met.	Necessary criteria for organ donation.	Non–heart-beating donors also may donate organs in some states. Refer to institution guidelines for non–heart-beating donors.
2. Ensure that consent form for organ donation has been completed.	Necessary criteria for organ donation.	
3. Obtain blood samples for laboratory analysis as prescribed by the OPO coordinator.	Multiple laboratory analyses are needed before final placement of the patient's organs.	
4. Administer intravenous fluids and medications (including vasoactive agents) as prescribed by the OPO coordinator.	Therapies may be necessary to optimize organ function before recovery.	
5. Encourage family presence with the patient during the organ donation process.	Promotes family togetherness; prepares for family goodbyes and grieving.	
6. Transfer the patient to the operating room as directed by the OPO coordinator for organ donation.		
7. Provide family support.	Aids family coping.	
8. Provide a method for the family to obtain information about the recovery process.	Keeps family informed of recovered organs.	

Expected Outcomes

- Organ recovery is completed.
- Recovered organs are viable.

Unexpected Outcomes

- Inability to recover viable organs for transplantation
- Determination that the potential donor is medically unsuitable for organ donation

Patient Monitoring and Care

Patient Monitoring and Care	Rationale	Reportable Conditions
		These conditions should be reported if they persist despite nursing interventions.
1. Monitor the patient's cardiac and hemodynamic status continuously.	If the donor is unstable, it may compromise organ viability.	• Systolic blood pressure less than 90 mm Hg • Changes in heart rate or other parameters set by the OPO coordinator • Dysrhythmias
2. Monitor oxygenation status.	Determines presence of hypoxemia.	• PaO_2 less than or equal to 100 mm Hg • SaO_2 less than or equal to 96% or other parameter as set by the OPO coordinator
3. Maintain the patient's body temperature.	Hypothermia or hyperthermia may lead to coagulopathies.	• Temperature less than 96°F • Temperature greater than 99°F • Other parameters set by OPO coordinator
4. Monitor urine output.	Determines renal perfusion.	• Urine output less than 0.5 mL/kg/h
5. Monitor laboratory studies as determined by OPO coordinator.	Determines organ ischemia.	• Abnormal laboratory results
6. Provide family support. Incorporate grief counselor, social worker, and pastoral care.	Offers family resources during grieving.	

Documentation

Documentation should include the following:

- Family education
- Determination of brain death
- Completed consent form for organ donation and recovery
- Complete donor record, including vital signs, assessments, treatment, and the clinical status of the donor
- Communication with the family with summary of information provided and response of the family
- Preoperative checklist
- Unexpected outcomes
- Additional interventions

Reference

1. Herdman R, Potts JT. Non–heart-beating organ transplantation: medical and ethical issues in procurement. Washington, DC: National Academy Press; 1997.

Additional Readings

Coleman-Musser L. The physician's perspective: a survey of attitudes toward organ donor management. *J Trans Coor.* 1997;7:55–58.

Duckworth RM, Sproat GW, Morien M, Jeffrey TB. Acute bereavement services as a mechanism to increase donation. *J Trans Coor.* 1998;8:16–18.

Holmquist M. Organ donor care map: a multidisciplinary approach. *J Trans Nurs.* 1996;6:101–104.

McCoy J, Argue PC. The role of the critical care nurse in the donation process: a case study. *Crit Care Nurs.* 1999;19:48–52.

Novitzky D. Donor management: state of the art. *Trans Proc.* 1997;28:3773–3775.

Park KM, Lee SG, Lee YJ, et al. Proper donor management and multiorgan procurement: practical ways to cope with the organ shortage. *Trans Proc.* 1996;28:1869–1870.

Ptacek JT, Eberhardt, TL, Breaking bad news. *JAMA.* 1996:276:496–502.

Verbal M, Worth J. Reservations and preferences among procurement professionals concerning the donation of specific organs and tissues. *J Trans Coor.* 1997;7:111–115.

Wood RF. Donor management: multiorgan procurement and renal preservation. *J R Med.* 1996;89:23–24.

132

Identification of Potential Organ Donors

P U R P O S E: To maximize the availability of donor organs by early identification of potential donors.

June Hinkle

PREREQUISITE NURSING KNOWLEDGE

- Knowledge of state, organ procurement organization (OPO), and hospital policies regarding organ donation from patients diagnosed with brain death and from patients who are non–heart-beating donors is essential.
- Organ recovery takes place either from patients who have been declared brain dead or from non–heart-beating donors. Before the discussion of organ donation, the medical suitability of the patient should be determined.
- OPOs are nonprofit agencies that determine the medical suitability of potential donors and coordinate the recovery of organs.
- In brain death, cessation of function is determined when clinical evaluation discloses absence of both cerebral and brainstem function (see Procedure 130).
- Non–heart-beating donors are those who have experienced a cardiopulmonary arrest or are being removed from life support and the family or significant other wishes to donate organs.[1] OPO and hospital policies regarding non–heart-beating donors vary between institutions and states.
- As of August 1998, every death or imminent death in a hospital must be reported to an organ procurement agency to meet the federal rules of the U.S. Department of Health and Human Services.[2]
- The only persons who should approach the family about organ donation is the designated hospital requestor and the OPO coordinator.[2]
- Before caring for potential donors and their families, critical care nurses should explore personal values and beliefs about life, death, and ethical issues surrounding transplantation.[3]
- Organ transplantation is a viable therapeutic modality for patients with end-stage organ disease. Thousands of patients currently are waiting for the availability of an organ for their end-stage disease.
- The Joint Commission on Accreditation of Healthcare Organizations (JCAHO) established standards for accreditation related to organ donation in 1988. These standards are updated as federal regulations and rules change.

- A patient's driver's license may indicate the desire to be an organ donor. This information is helpful for the family when they make a decision about donation, but is not legally binding in most states.

EQUIPMENT

- Flashlight
- Neurologic checklist
- Tongue blade or suction catheter
- Cotton-tipped applicator or cotton ball
- Ventilator
- Arterial line or automatic blood pressure cuff
- Urinary catheter
- Electrocardiogram (ECG) monitor and electrodes

PATIENT AND FAMILY EDUCATION

- Explain the medical and nursing care being provided to the patient. ➨*Rationale:* Ensures that the family has some level of understanding about the therapies used to treat or support the patient, that they are confident that appropriate therapies are employed, and that they are reassured the patient is not experiencing increased discomfort because of these therapies.
- Inform the family of the patient's current condition. ➨*Rationale:* Keeps family informed and prepares the family for realistic expectations of patient outcome.

PATIENT ASSESSMENT AND PREPARATION

Patient Assessment

- Obtain a thorough medical and social history from the family about the patient that includes current age, injuries, chronic diseases, surgical history, familial history, and social habits. Of particular interest is a history of renal disease, hypertension, diabetes mellitus, malignant disease, hepatitis, and human immunodeficiency virus (HIV). ➨*Rationale:* Allows the OPO transplant coordinator to assess the medical suitability of the patient for organ donation.

- Perform a physical assessment, with emphasis on the following: old surgical scars, needle track marks, tattoos, body piercing, congenital anomalies, and injuries. ➤*Rationale:* Indicators of physical conditions or social behaviors that may influence organ suitability for transplantation. Patients with recent tattoos and body piercings or fresh needle tracks are considered high risk and may not be accepted as a donor by the transplant team.
- Assess the neurologic status hourly, including the response to pain, eye opening, communication attempts, pupillary response, gag reflex, cough reflex, corneal reflex, and observation of attempts to breath spontaneously at a rate greater than that set on the ventilator. ➤*Rationale:* Identifies changes in the neurologic status; implement treatment as appropriate.
- Monitor pertinent data, including urine output, liver function studies, renal function studies, electrolytes, serum osmolality, coagulation panel, urine studies including specific gravity, and culture results. ➤*Rationale:* Indicators that may influence organ suitability for transplantation.
- Determine an accurate measurement of height and weight. ➤*Rationale:* Provides information for matching organs to a recipient of corresponding body size.

Patient Preparation

- Ensure that the family understands preprocedural teaching. Answer questions as they arise and reinforce information as needed. ➤*Rationale:* Evaluates and reinforces understanding of previously taught information.
- "Any patient with a significant and potentially life-threatening injury to the head, whether caused by trauma, an intracerebral hemorrhage, or an anoxic event, should be referred to the OPO as early as possible for evaluation as a potential organ donor."[4] ➤*Rationale:* This allows the OPO coordinator to evaluate the patient and provides the critical care nurse with information about the patient's potential as an organ donor.
- When neurologic testing to determine clinical brain death begins, ensure that the patient is normothermic and that no sedating medications have been given (see Procedure 130). ➤*Rationale:* Necessary before determining brain death by clinical criteria.

Procedure **for Identification of Potential Organ Donors**

Steps	Rationale	Special Considerations
1. Discuss patient prognosis with the health care team.	Ensures that all members of the health care team have the same understanding of the patient's prognosis.	
2. Contact the OPO coordinator if the patient has a life-threatening illness.	Early referral provides information about the potential for organ donation.	
3. Obtain laboratory samples as prescribed.	Assesses organ function.	This information is used by the OPO coordinator to assess donor potential.
4. Monitor trends in vital signs.	Determines the presence of hemodynamic stability or instability. Decreased perfusion to organs may alter organ donor potential.	
5. Monitor fluid status.	Determines kidney perfusion or hypoperfusion. Decreased urine output may alter organ donor potential.	
6. Assist with brain death determination (see Procedure 130).	Facilitates process and assesses if the patient may be a possible organ donor.	
7. Assist the physician when he or she informs the family of the results of the brain death determination.	Facilitates the process and offers the opportunity to provide support.	This meeting is best done in a quiet, private setting.
8. Contact the OPO coordinator to discuss possible organ donation.	OPO coordinators will discuss possible organ donation with the family.	

Expected Outcomes	Unexpected Outcomes
• Timely determination of brain death occurs.	• The recognition and documentation of brain death does not occur.
• A representative of the OPO is notified of a patient determined to be brain dead.	• The organ procurement organization is not notified before the pronouncement of brain death or the discussion of organ donation.
• If the patient meets the criteria of brain death and is medically suitable to be a donor, the OPO coordinator is notified to help the health care team approach the family with the option of organ donation.	• The organ procurement organization is not notified when life support is removed from a patient who does not meet brain death criteria (institution and state specific).
• If a family decides to withdraw life support from a patient who does not meet brain death criteria, the OPO coordinator is notified of the imminent death; an assessment of medical suitability for organ donation prior to the withdraw of therapy occurs; refer to institution policies to determine if non–heart-beating donors are recovered.	• Family fails to comprehend patient status and prognosis.
• Family comprehends patient status and prognosis.	

Patient Monitoring and Care

Patient Monitoring and Care	Rationale	Reportable Conditions
		These conditions should be reported if they persist despite nursing interventions.
1. Monitor neurologic status and monitor intracranial pressure (if available) every hour and more frequently, as needed.	Determines changes in neurologic status so treatment can be initiated.	• Changes in neurologic function or sudden, sustained increase in intracranial pressure
2. Monitor vital signs every hour and more frequently, as needed.	Determines changes and needed treatment.	• Changes in vital signs
3. Continuously monitor cardiac rhythm.	Identifies dysrhythmias.	• Dysrhythmias
4. Monitor urinary output every hour.	Determines perfusion to the kidneys; may affect organ donation.	• Changes in urinary output; urinary output less than 0.5 mL/kg/h
5. Obtain laboratory samples for liver function tests, renal function tests, coagulation values, urine specific gravity, hemoglobin, white blood cell count, electrolytes, osmolality, and cultures.	Determines organ function; may affect organ donation.	• Abnormal laboratory results

Documentation

Documentation should include the following:

- Family education
- Patient history and physical findings
- Vital signs, neurologic findings and, if applicable, intracranial pressures
- Intake and output

- Communication with the physician about changes in the patient's physiologic status
- Communications with the OPO coordinators
- Unexpected outcomes
- Additional interventions

References

1. Herdman R, Potts JT. *Non–heart-beating Organ Transplantation: Medical and Ethical Issues in Procurement.* Washington, DC: National Academy Press; 1997.
2. Federal Register. Medicare and Medicaid programs: hospital condition of participation; identification of potential organ, tissue and eye donors. Health Care Financing Administration; June 22, 1998.
3. Heitman LK. Organ donation in community hospitals; a nursing perspective. *Curr Concepts Nurs.* 1987;1:2–5.
4. Ehrle RN, Shafer TJ, Nelson KR. Determination and referral of potential organ donors and consent for organ donation: best practices—a blueprint for success. *Crit Care Nurs.* 1999;19:21–36.

Additional Readings

Alleman K, Coolican M, Savaria D, et al. Public perceptions of an appropriate donor card/brochure. *J Trans Nurs.* 1996;6:105–108.

Flye MW. *Principles of Organ Transplantation.* Philadelphia Pa: W.B. Saunders; 1989.

Holmquist M. Organ donor care map: a multidisciplinary approach. *J Trans Nurs.* 1996;6:101–105.

Lewis DD, Valerius W. Non–heart beating organ donation: an answer to the organ shortage. *Crit Care Nurs.* 1999;19:70–75.

Olson L, Castro L, Ciancio G, et al. Twelve years' experience with non–heart beating donors. *J Trans Nurs.* 1996;6:196–199.

Summary statement: practice parameters for determining brain death in adults. *Neurology.* 1995;45:1012–1014.

Younger SL, Landefeld CS, Coulton CJ, et al. Brain death and organ retrieval: a cross-sectional survey of knowledge and concepts among health care professionals. *JAMA.* 1989;261:2205–2210.

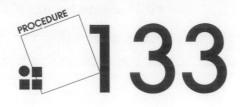

133

Request for Organ Donation

P U R P O S E: To facilitate an informed decision about organ donation. The focus of the discussion should be the best decision for the family, and that decision may not be organ donation.

June Hinkle

PREREQUISITE NURSING KNOWLEDGE

- Knowledge of state, organ procurement organization (OPO), and hospital policies regarding organ donation from patients diagnosed with brain death and from patients who are non–heart-beating donors is essential.
- Every death or imminent death in a hospital must be reported to an OPO to meet the federal rules of the U.S. Department of Health and Human Services.[1]
- Only a designated requestor approved by the hospital and trained by the OPO may approach the family about the possible organ donation. The designated requestor must complete an OPO-approved program.
- Consent rates for organ donation increase when families are given time to accept their relative's death, when the request for donation is made by a member of the OPO with the hospital designated requestor, and when the request is made in a quiet, private setting.[2]
- According to a Gallup survey done in 1993, only 52% of people wishing to be an organ donors have told their families of their desire and only 28% have signed a donor card or designated their wishes on their driver's license.[3] If the family does not know the patient's desire related to organ donation, it is sometimes helpful to locate the patient's driver's license. Most states use some form of designation for organ donation on the driver's license.
- Knowledge about state advance directives and laws related to organ donation is essential. The health care proxy may be the decision-maker for organ donation, or the decision related to organ donation may revert to the nearest next-of-kin.

EQUIPMENT

- Brain death information materials for the family
- Donor information materials for the family
- Forms needed for consent for organ donation

PATIENT AND FAMILY EDUCATION

- Assess the family's understanding of brain death. ➤*Rationale:* The diagnosis may be difficult for the family to understand and frequently requires multiple explanations before the diagnosis is understood.
- Allow a designated, trained requestor to provide information to the family regarding organ donation in conjunction with the OPO staff. ➤*Rationale:* Meets the federal mandates and provides family with accurate, complete information about the organ donation process.

PATIENT ASSESSMENT AND PREPARATION

Patient Assessment

- Before assessing if a family is interested in organ donation, determine if the patient is a potential organ donor. ➤*Rationale:* The transplant coordinator from the OPO determines the appropriateness of potential organ donors. Donation should not be offered to family members as an option unless the OPO has determined that the patient is a potential donor.
- Assess the family's ability to verbalize and understand brain death. ➤*Rationale:* The family is more likely to donate organs if they accept the diagnosis of brain death.[2]

Patient Preparation

- Ensure that the family understands preprocedural teaching. Answer questions as they arise and reinforce information as needed. ➤*Rationale:* Evaluates and reinforces understanding of previously taught information.
- Consult the designated requestor and OPO coordinator to determine when and how they will approach the family about organ donation. ➤*Rationale:* Coordinates the request process.

Procedure for **Request for Organ Donation**

Steps	Rationale	Special Considerations
1. Assist with determination of brain death (see Procedure 130).	Facilitates process and assesses if the patient may be a possible organ donor.	
2. Consult the OPO when brain death testing begins.	Early assessment by the OPO coordinator determines whether the family is offered the option of donation.	
3. Ensure that patient meets brain death criteria.		
4. Coordinate a meeting between the family, designated requestor, and OPO coordinator.	Facilitates the process.	This meeting is best done in a quiet, private setting.
5. The designated requestor or the OPO coordinator will determine if the patient had the desire to be an organ donor.	If a discussion about organ donation had occurred, the family is more likely to donate organs.	According to the Gallup survey, 93% of family members would donate organs if the loved one had requested it, whereas 47% of family members would donate organs if no discussion had taken place.[3]
6. The designated requestor or the OPO coordinator will determine if the family will consider organ donation.	Determines family willingness to consider organ donation.	
7. If the family decides to donate, the OPO will coordinate the donation process.	The OPO coordinator becomes responsible for prescribing care for the patient until recovery occurs.	All laboratory values and changes in patient condition should be reported to the OPO coordinator.
8. If the patient is brain dead and the family decides not to donate, discuss with the physician, family, and health care team when and how to discontinue therapy.	Coordinates end of life care.	Ensure that the family understands what will happen when therapy is withdrawn.
9. Provide the emotional support the family needs to cope with the death of their loved one.	Supports grieving family.	
10. Involve pastoral care, social workers, or grief counselors.	Provides additional support to the grieving family.	

Expected Outcomes

- The family receives accurate, timely information about organ donation provided by the designated hospital requestor in conjunction with the OPO coordinator.
- The family makes a decision about organ donation based on the prior expressed desires of the patient, cultural and religious beliefs, and the information provided about the organ donation process.

Unexpected Outcomes

- The family is approached about organ donation before the determination of brain death.
- An untrained staff member approaches the family about organ donation.
- The family are not kept informed as to the care of their loved one.

Patient Monitoring and Care

Patient Monitoring and Care	Rationale	Reportable Conditions
		These conditions should be reported if they persist despite nursing interventions.
1. Encourage the family to be at the bedside and to be involved as much as possible with patient care.	Promotes patient and family time together. Facilitates family and health care provider relationship.	• Changes in family preferences for care
2. The OPO will coordinate the care of the patient if the family decides to donate organs.	Facilitates patient management and the donation process.	• Changes in patient condition
3. If the family of a patient who is brain dead decides not to donate, coordinate a plan for removal of therapy.	Facilitates the removal of therapy.	• Removal of therapy wishes
4. Support the family decision whether the family decides for or against organ donation.	Organ donation is a personal decision for each family. The family needs to make the decision they feel is correct for their loved one and their family.	
5. Encourage family involvement in end of life care.	Promotes family involvement, family presence, family control, and family time together.	

Documentation

Documentation should include the following:

- Family education
- Date and time of brain death determination
- Notification of the OPO
- Presentation of organ donation options to the family; include the date, time, and location, name of requestor, summary of information provided, and response of family
- If family requests organ donation, completion of appropriate donation consent forms
- Unexpected outcomes
- Additional interventions

References

1. Federal Register. Medicare and Medicaid programs: hospital condition of participation; identification of potential organ, tissue and eye donors. Health Care Financing Administration; June 22, 1998.
2. Beasley CL, et al. The impact of a comprehensive, hospital-focused intervention to increase organ donation. *J Trans Coor.* 1997;7:6–13.
3. The Gallup Organization. The American public's attitudes toward organ donation and transplantation. The Partnership for Organ Donation; 1993.

Additional Readings

Cuter JA, et al. Increasing the availability of cadaveric organs for transplantation: maximizing the consent rate. *Transplantation.* 1993;56:225–228.
DeJong W, Franz HG. Requesting organ donation: an interview study of donor and nondonor families. *Am J Crit Care.* 1998;7:13–23.

Duckworth RM, Sproat GW, Morien M, Jeffrey TB. Acute bereavement services and routine referral as a mechanism to increase donation. *J Trans Coor.* 1998;8:16–18.
Ehrle RN, Shafer TJ, Nelson KR. Referral, request, and consent for organ donation: best practice—a blueprint for success. *Crit Care Nurs.* 1999;19:21–33.
Frants HG, DeJong W, Wolfe M, et al. Explaining brain death: a critical feature of the donation process. *J Trans Coor.* 1997;7:14–21.
Holmquist M, Chabaleewski F, Blount T, et al. A critical pathway: guiding care for organ donors. *Crit Care Nurs.* 1999;19:84–98.
Klieger J, Nelson K, Davis R, et al. Analysis of factors influencing organ donation consent rates. *J Trans Coor.* 1994; 4:132–134.
Riley LP, Collican MB. Needs of families of organ donors: facing death and life. *Crit Care Nurs.* 1999;19:53–59.
Schaefdfer MJ, Johnson E, Suddaby EC. Analysis of donor versus non-donor demographics. *J Trans Coor.* 1998;8:9–15.
Sullivan H, Blakely D, Davis K. An in-house coordinator program to increase organ donation in public teaching hospitals. *J Trans Coor.* 1998;8:40–42.

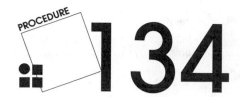

134

Withholding/ Withdrawing Life-Sustaining Treatment

PURPOSE: To assist patients and family members with the process of withholding or withdrawing life-sustaining treatment. Life-sustaining treatment may include nutrition, hydration, antibiotics, dialysis, ventilatory therapy, vasoactive therapy, and additional therapies.

Debra J. Lynn-McHale
Margaret M. Mahon

PREREQUISITE NURSING KNOWLEDGE

- Withholding and withdrawing life-sustaining treatments are end-of-life decisions that commonly result in the death of the patient.
- Knowledge of state regulations regarding end-of-life decision making is necessary.
- Knowledge of hospital policies or procedures regarding end-of-life decision making is needed.
- Hospitals should have policies that direct the process to withhold or withdraw life-sustaining treatment.[1]
- As much information as possible should be obtained from the patient and the patient's family regarding the patient's desired wishes regarding life-sustaining treatment. This information may be ascertained from an advance directive or from verbal conversations with family, friends, or health care providers.
- Advance directives (see Procedure 129):
  - ❖ May exist in the form of a living will or a health care proxy
  - ❖ A living will is a document that identifies treatments that a patient would or would not want under specific end-of-life situations (eg, most are specific to terminal illness)
  - ❖ A health care proxy or a durable power of attorney for health care is a document that identifies a predetermined person who has been given the authority to make health care decisions for the patient if he or she is unable to make decisions (eg, comatose state)
- Patients have a moral and legal right and responsibility to make decisions about their health care and the use of life-sustaining treatment.[1]
- Decision-making capacity is determined by an individual's ability to[2]:

  - ❖ Understand relevant information
  - ❖ Make a judgment about the information in light of his or her values
  - ❖ Intend a certain outcome
  - ❖ Communicate his or her decision to health care providers
- If the patient no longer has decision-making capability, decisions should be made by the patient's health care proxy. Decisions made by the health care proxy should be based on the patient's previously stated wishes.
- Usually the patient's family is very involved in the process of withholding or withdrawing life-sustaining treatment. On occasion, the patient prefers that the family not be involved. If the patient does not want the family to be involved, the health care team should work with the patient to identify another person who can serve as his or her health care proxy in the event that the patient loses decision-making capacity.
- Dialogue regarding end-of-life care should be comprehensive. Discussions should include what treatments are going to be withheld or withdrawn. Discussions should focus on patient wishes and goals of care. If the goal of care is a peaceful death, then all treatments that do not contribute toward this goal should be considered for discontinuation, including cessation of vasoactive agents, intravenous fluids, nutrition, laboratory studies, x-rays, extubation, etc. Treatments that support the goal of a peaceful death should be continued, such as pain management, frequent skin and mouth care, family presence, etc.
- Health care providers are responsible for knowing how their personal beliefs affect interactions and decisions about withholding and withdrawing of life-sustaining treatment.
- Patients, families, and health care providers often have different values.

- Patients and their families should be actively involved in all health care decisions, including end-of-life decisions.
- Family members involved in end-of-life decision making should be guided by their knowledge of what the patient wants or would want.
- If a critical care nurse cannot support the patient and family in the process of withholding or withdrawing life-sustaining treatment, the critical care nurse should proceed through the appropriate channels to transfer care to another critical care nurse.[1]
- Paralyzing agents must be discontinued and cleared from the patient's body before withdrawal of life-sustaining treatment.
- Maintaining patient dignity and comfort is essential at all times and especially at the end of life.
- Medications given to relieve pain often have sedative or respiratory depressant side effects, yet this should not be an overriding consideration in their use for dying patients, as long as such use is consistent with the patient's wishes.[3]
- Pain medication titrated to achieve adequate symptom control is ethically justified, even at the expense of maintaining life or hastening death secondarily.[3]
- Family meetings can be very helpful in aiding patients, families, and health care providers in planning end-of-life care.
- Hospital ethics committees can be very helpful in aiding patients, families, and health care providers when conflicts arise with decision making or during the process of withholding or withdrawing life-sustaining therapy.

PATIENT AND FAMILY EDUCATION

- In collaboration with the physician, inform the patient or family of the patient's current condition and prognosis. ➦*Rationale:* Informs and prepares the patient or family of anticipated outcomes.
- Explain resources available to aid with end-of-life decision making (eg, nurses, physicians, social workers, pastoral care, grief counselors, palliative care team, ethics consultation, ethics committee). ➦*Rationale:* Offers additional resources and support to assist the patient or family with end-of-life decisions.
- Describe how the patient is likely to respond to withholding or withdrawing of therapies, including expected outcomes and unexpected outcomes. ➦*Rationale:* Prepares the patient and the family for the process. If death is anticipated, the dying process may progress quickly or slowly. Although rare, death may not ensue after life-sustaining treatment is withheld or withdrawn.
- Explain that analgesia or sedatives will be administered to relieve discomfort that may be experienced during withholding or withdrawing life-sustaining treatment. In addition, explain that although only enough medication to relieve discomfort will be administered, at times pain medication may hasten the dying process by lowering blood pressure or decreasing respirations. This response to pain medication is normal and expected. ➦*Rationale:* Decreases patient and family anxiety to know that patient comfort will be promoted. Allows patient and family the opportunity to verbalize any concerns related to pain or pain management.

PATIENT ASSESSMENT AND PREPARATION

Patient Assessment

- Assist the physician or advanced practice nurse to assess the patient's decision-making capacity (see also Procedure 129). ➦*Rationale:* Patients with decision-making capacity should make their own treatment decisions.
- If patients do not have decision-making capacity, determine if the patient has a designated health care proxy. ➦*Rationale:* The patient's health care proxy should make decisions for the patient if he or she no longer has decision-making capacity.
- If patients do not have decision-making capacity or a health care proxy, identify key individuals who will be active participants in treatment decisions. ➦*Rationale:* It is essential that family members are able to communicate patient wishes for end-of-life care or are able to determine to the best of their knowledge what treatments the patient would or would not want. The patient may also have communicated treatment wishes to primary care providers.

Patient Preparation

- Ensure that the patient or family understands preprocedural teaching. Answer questions as they arise and reinforce information as needed. ➦*Rationale:* Evaluates and reinforces understanding of previously taught information.
- Plan the day and time that life-sustaining care will be withheld or withdrawn. ➦*Rationale:* Allows family and friends to spend time with the patient before treatment changes. Allows health care team time to plan their availability to be present during treatment changes.
- Identify family or friends whom the patient or family would like present during the withholding or withdrawal process. ➦*Rationale:* Involves patient or family in planning of the withholding or withdrawal of care.
- In addition to nursing, medicine, and possibly respiratory therapy, identify additional members of the health care team whom the patient or family would like present during the withholding or withdrawal process (eg, clergy, social worker, grief counselor, etc). ➦*Rationale:* Provides control to the patient or family as they determine essential members of the health care team who should be involved with the withholding or withdrawing of care process.
- Encourage the patient and family to personalize the environment by bringing in music or other items that will make the room as the patient would want it to be. ➦*Rationale:* Promotes a peaceful, caring environment.

Procedure for Withholding/Withdrawing Life-Sustaining Treatment

Steps	Rationale	Special Considerations
1. With the patient, family, and health care team coordinate a comprehensive plan for the process of withholding and/or withdrawing life-sustaining treatment.	Ensures that key individuals are aware of the plan of end-of-life care. Addresses what aspects of care will be withheld and what aspects of care will be withdrawn.	The patient, family, and health care providers need to work together to facilitate the process. Thorough preplanning facilitates the process of end-of-life care.
2. Ensure that the patient, health care proxy, or family understand and agree to the process of withholding and/or withdrawing life-sustaining treatment.	Ensures the understanding of what will be withheld or withdrawn, when it will be withheld or withdrawn, and in what order or all at once.	
3. Ensure that the patient, health care proxy, or family understand the probable outcome of withholding and/or withdrawing life-sustaining treatment.	Ensures that there are no misperceptions regarding what will happen after treatment is withheld or withdrawn.	
4. Allow the patient and family time to complete family affairs, communicate with each other, spend time together, and say goodbyes.	Facilitates family functioning and grief process.	
5. Ensure that key members of the health care team are actively involved in the process of withholding and/or withdrawing life-sustaining treatment.	Presents a team approach to support the patient, family, and each other.	Predetermine who will withdraw treatment (eg, endotracheal tube, pacing wires, central lines, etc).
6. In collaboration with the physician, determine the type, route of administration, dosage, and time that analgesia or sedatives will be initiated.	Allows time to ensure intravenous access, obtain and prepare medication.	Continuous intravenous infusion of pain medication (eg, morphine sulfate) facilitates constant administration and ease of dosage adjustment.
7. In collaboration with the physician, determine how the pain medication will be titrated to signs of patient discomfort.	Provides a pain management plan to promote patient comfort.	Pain medication should be titrated to increasing dosages only if signs of patient discomfort are present. Signs of discomfort might include verbalization of pain, moaning, facial grimacing, increase in heart rate, increase in blood pressure, or labored respirations.
8. Assist or place patient in preferred position of comfort.	Promotes comfort.	Supine position with the head of bed elevated may facilitate comfort and ease of respirations.
9. Lower the side rails.	Allows family easier access to be close to the patient, hold his or her hand, or sit on the bed.	Side rails may need to be raised if the patient is moving, experiencing a seizure, etc.
10. Turn off all monitors.	Eliminates "monitor watching" and alarms.	Pulse can be checked by palpation. Blood pressure can be checked manually, if necessary, to assess if additional pain medication is necessary.
11. Ensure that the family is present.	Ensure that significant family members are there to support the patient and each other.	Some family members may choose to be close by but not in the room when life-sustaining treatment is withheld or withdrawn.
12. Ensure that the environment is as the patient or family wants it.	Promotes patient and family involvement.	
13. Ensure that key members of the health care team are present (critical care nurse, attending physician, respiratory therapy, pastor, etc).	Presents a team approach to support the patient, family, and each other.	There may be health care providers who the patient or family specifically request to be present.
14. Initiate pain medication as prescribed (eg, low dose of pain medication; <5 mg/hr of morphine).	Promotes comfort.	If the patient was already receiving pain medication at a constant infusion, the same rate of infusion would continue.

Procedure continued on following page

| Procedure | **for Withholding/Withdrawing Life-Sustaining Treatment** *Continued* |

Steps	Rationale	Special Considerations
15. Withhold or withdraw treatment.	Discontinues unwanted treatment.	
16. Titrate intravenous pain medication to signs of patient distress.	Minimizes distress and promotes comfort.	Large dosages of pain medication may be necessary to promote comfort.
17. Support the patient and the family.	Aids comfort.	
18. Provide time for the patient and the family to be alone, if so desired.	Aids grief process.	
19. Assist the family with the grief process.	Aids family coping.	

Expected Outcomes	Unexpected Outcomes
• Patient wishes regarding end-of-life care are honored. • Treatments that are not wanted by the patient or family or both are withheld or withdrawn. • Patient dignity and comfort are achieved. • Family is actively involved in end-of-life care. • Patient and family receive needed support. • Patient death occurs (time frame may vary from minutes to hours to days).	• Patient receives unwanted treatments. • Patient has discomfort. • Family members are not involved in end-of-life care. • Family conflicts arise regarding end-of-life treatment decisions. • Patient survives withholding or withdrawing of life support, necessitating consideration of a new plan of care and the possibility of long-term care.

Patient Monitoring and Care

Patient Monitoring and Care	Rationale	Reportable Conditions
		These conditions should be reported if they persist despite nursing interventions.

1. Assess the patient for discomfort:
  ○ Verbalization of pain
  ○ Moaning
  ○ Facial grimacing
  ○ Increase in heart rate
  ○ Increase in blood pressure
  ○ Labored respirations
  ○ Restlessness
  ○ Delirium
	Signs of discomfort indicate ineffective management of comfort.	• Discomfort

2. Titrate analgesia or sedatives to comfort.	Promotes patient dignity and comfort.	• Unrelieved pain
3. Assess vital signs before withholding or withdrawing life-sustaining treatment, then only as necessary to ensure that the patient is not experiencing pain.	Promotes patient dignity and comfort. Minimizes unnecessary data.	• Decreasing values of vital signs are normal and expected as life-sustaining treatment is being withheld or withdrawn, and thus should only be reported to keep the health team informed. • Increasing values of vital signs may indicate that pain medication is insufficient.
4. Support the patient and the family through the entire process.	Provides additional emotional support, promotes family functioning, aids in the grief process.	• Ineffective family functioning or need for additional support services

Documentation

Documentation should include the following:

- Patient and family education
- Patient, health care proxy, or family wishes regarding end-of-life care
- Coordination of the end-of-life process
- Patient, health care proxy, or family understanding of the withholding or withdrawing process and anticipated outcome

- Involved family and health care team members
- When and how life-sustaining treatment was withheld or withdrawn
- Patient level of comfort
- How comfort was promoted
- Time of patient death
- Unexpected outcomes
- Additional interventions

References

1. American Association of Critical-Care Nurses. *Withholding and/or Withdrawing Life-sustaining Treatment.* Laguna Niguel, Ca: AACN; 1990.
2. Beauchamp TL, Childress JF. *Principles of Biomedical Ethics.* 4th ed. New York, NY: Oxford University Press; 1994.
3. American Nurses Association. *Position Statement on Promotion of Comfort and Relief in Dying Patients.* Kansas City, Mo: ANA; 1991.

Additional Readings

American Nurses Association. *Position Statement on Nursing Care and Do-not-resuscitate Decisions.* Washington, DC: ANA; 1992.

American Nurses Association. *Position Statement on Foregoing Artificial Nutrition and Hydration.* Washington, DC: ANA; 1992.

American Nurses Association. *Position Statement on Nursing and the Patient Self-determination Act.* Kansas City, MO: ANA; 1991.

Campbell ML. *Forgoing Life-sustaining Therapy.* Laguna Niguel, Ca: AACN; 1998.

President's Commission for the Study of Ethical Problems in Medicine and Biomedical and Behavioral Research. Washington, DC: Government Printing Office; 1983.

The Hasting Center. *Guidelines on the Termination of Life Sustaining Treatment and the Care of the Dying.* Briarcliff Manor, NY: The Hastings Center; 1987.

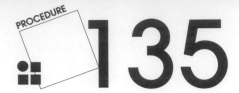

PROCEDURE

135

Calculating Doses, Flow Rates, and Administration of Continuous Intravenous Infusions

P U R P O S E: The critical care nurse calculates dosages and flow rates for continuous intravenous (IV) infusions to ensure delivery of the correct amount of medication. Many of the medications delivered by continuous IV infusion have narrow margins of safety; therefore, accuracy in calculating and administering these agents is imperative.

Barbara A. Brown

PREREQUISITE NURSING KNOWLEDGE

* Knowledge of aseptic technique is important.
* Many different types of medications are delivered as continuous IV infusions in critical care. These are potent medications including, but not limited to, vasoactive, inotropic, and antidysrhythmic agents. The critical care nurse must possess knowledge about the actions, indications, desired patient response, dosage, and adverse effects of the medication being administered.
* Hemodynamic assessment and electrocardiographic (ECG) monitoring are frequently necessary to evaluate the patient response to the infusion. The critical care nurse must be familiar with monitoring equipment such as noninvasive blood pressure cuffs, cardiac monitors, arterial lines, and pulmonary artery catheters.
* Titration is adjustment of the dose, either increasing or decreasing, to attain the desired patient response. Weaning is a gradual decrease of the dose when the medication is being discontinued.
* Volume-controlled infusion devices are required to precisely deliver and titrate continuous infusions. Alterations or interruptions of the flow rate can significantly affect

the dose of medication being delivered and adversely affect the patient.
* There are three factors involved in the calculations for continuous IV infusions:
  ❖ The concentration is the amount of medication diluted in a given volume of IV solution (eg, 400 mg dopamine diluted in 250 mL normal saline (NS), or 2 g lidocaine diluted in 500 mL 5% dextrose in water [D_5W]).
  ❖ The dose of the medication is the amount of medication to be administered over a certain length of time (eg, dopamine 5 μg/kg/min, or lidocaine 2 mg/min). The units of measure for the dose will differ for various medications. The length of time is 1 minute or 1 hour. If the medication is weight based, the dose of the medication is per kilogram of patient weight.
  ❖ The flow rate is the rate of delivery of the IV fluid solution (eg, 20 mL/hr). The units of measure of the flow rate are always mL/hr.
* All units of measure in the formula must be the same. It frequently is necessary to perform some conversions on the concentration prior to entering it into the formula. The units of measure of the concentration must be converted to the same units of measure of the dose (eg, the

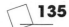

concentration of dopamine is measured in mg, but the dose of dopamine is measured in μg). Additionally, the mathematical calculations are simplified if the concentration is expressed per milliliter of fluid, rather than the total volume of the IV container.

- The mathematical formula for continuous IV infusions contains the three factors involved in continuous infusions (Table 135–1). When two factors are known, the third can be calculated by using the basic formula. Therefore, when the concentration of the solution and the prescribed dose are known, the flow rate can be determined. When the concentration of the solution and the flow rate are known, the dose can be determined. The two known factors are entered into the formula, and the mathematical computations are solved to determine the third factor. Variations on the basic formula are used to allow for medications delivered per hour or per minute, and for medications that are weight based (Tables 135–2 and 135–3).

EQUIPMENT

- Prepared IV solution with medication to be administered
- IV tubing
- IV infusion device
- Nonsterile gloves
- Alcohol pads
- Calculator (optional)

PATIENT AND FAMILY EDUCATION

- Explain the indications and expected response to the pharmacologic therapy. **→Rationale:** Patients and families need explanations of the plan of care and interventions.
- Instruct the patient to report adverse symptoms, as indicated. Reportable symptoms include, but are not limited to pain, burning, itching, or swelling at the IV site, dizziness, shortness of breath, palpitations, and chest pain. **→Rationale:** Assists the nurse to evaluate response to the pharmacologic therapy and to identify adverse reactions.

Table 135–1 **Basic Formula**

To determine an unknown flow rate

$$\frac{\text{Dose (mg/hr or } \mu\text{/hr)}}{\text{Concentration (mg/mL or } \mu\text{/mL)}} = \text{Flow rate (mL/hr)}$$

To determine an unknown dose

$$\text{Flow rate (mL/hr)} \times \text{Concentration (mg/mL or } \mu\text{/mL)} = \text{Dose (mg/hr or } \mu\text{/hr)}$$

Example when flow rate is unknown: diltiazem 125 mg/125 mL D5W to be administered at 10 mg/hr.

A. Calculate concentration of drug in 1 mL of fluid:

$$\frac{125 \text{ mg}}{125 \text{ mL}} = \frac{1 \text{ mg}}{1 \text{ mL}}$$

B. Enter known factors into the formula and solve:

$$\frac{10 \text{ mg/hr}}{1 \text{ mg/mL}} = 10 \text{ mL/hr}$$

Example when dose is unknown: diltiazem 125 mg/125 mL D5W is infusing at 15 mL/hr.

A. Calculate concentration of drug in 1 mL of fluid:

$$\frac{125 \text{ mg}}{125 \text{ mL}} = \frac{1 \text{ mg}}{1 \text{ mL}}$$

B. Enter known factors into the formula and solve:

$$15 \text{ mL/hr} \times 1 \text{ mg/mL} = 15 \text{ mg/hr}$$

Table 135–2 **Variation for Medication Doses Measured per Minute (mg/min or μg/min)***

To determine unknown flow rate

$$\frac{\text{Dose (mg/min or } \mu\text{g/min} \times 60 \text{ min/hr}}{\text{Concentration (mg/mL or } \mu\text{g/mL)}} = \text{Flow rate (mL/hr)}$$

To determine unknown dose

$$\frac{\text{Flow rate (mL/hr)} \times \text{Concentration (mg/mL or } \mu\text{g/mL)}}{60 \text{ min/hr}} = \text{Dose (mg/min or } \mu\text{g/min)}$$

Example when flow rate is unknown: nitroglycerin 50 mg/250 mL D5W to be administered at 30 μg/min.

a. Convert the concentration to like units of measure:

$$\frac{50 \text{ mg}}{250 \text{ mL}} \times \frac{1000 \ \mu\text{g}}{1 \text{ mg}} = \frac{50{,}000 \ \mu\text{g}}{250 \text{ mL}}$$

b. Calculate concentration of drug in 1 mL of fluid:

$$\frac{50{,}000 \ \mu\text{g}}{250 \text{ mL}} = \frac{200 \ \mu\text{g}}{1 \text{ mL}}$$

c. Enter known factors into the formula and solve:

$$\frac{30 \ \mu\text{g/min} \times 60 \text{ min/hr}}{200 \ \mu\text{g/mL}} = 9 \text{ mL/hr}$$

Example when dose is unknown: lidocaine 2 g/500 mL D5W is infusing at 30 mL/hr.

a. Convert the concentration to like units of measure:

$$\frac{2 \text{ g}}{500 \text{ mL}} \times \frac{1000 \text{ mg}}{1 \text{ g}} = \frac{2000 \text{ mg}}{500 \text{ mL}}$$

b. Calculate concentration of drug in 1 mL of fluid:

$$\frac{2000 \text{ mg}}{500 \text{ mL}} = \frac{4 \text{ mg}}{1 \text{ mL}}$$

c. Enter known factors into formula and solve:

$$\frac{30 \text{ mL/hr} \times 4 \text{ mg/mL}}{60 \text{ min/hr}} = 2 \text{ mg/min}$$

*The time factor of 60 min/hr must be added to the basic formula.

PATIENT ASSESSMENT AND PREPARATION

Patient Assessment

- Assess medication allergies. **→Rationale:** Identification and prevention of allergic reactions.
- Obtain vital signs and hemodynamic parameters. **→Rationale:** Provides baseline data and the need for vasoactive agents.
- Assess the ECG. **→Rationale:** Provides baseline data and the need for antidysrhythmic therapy.

Patient Preparation

- Ensure that the patient and family understand preprocedural teaching. Answer questions as they arise and reinforce information as needed. **→Rationale:** Evaluates and reinforces understanding of previously taught information.

Table 135–3 ● ■ ■   **Variation for Weight-Based Medication Doses Measured per Minute (µg/kg/min)***

To determine unknown flow rate

$$\frac{\text{Dose (µg/kg/min)} \times 60 \text{ min/hr} \times \text{pt. weight (kg)}}{\text{Concentration (µg/mL)}} = \text{Flow rate (mL/hr)}$$

To determine unknown dose

$$\frac{\text{Flow rate (mL/hr)} \times \text{Concentration (µg/mL)}}{60 \text{ min/hr} \times \text{Patient weight (kg)}} = \text{Dose (µg/kg/min)}$$

Example when flow rate is unknown:

Dopamine 400 mg/250 mL D5W to infuse at 5 µg/kg/min. Patient weighs 100 kg.

a. Convert the concentration to like units of measure

$$\frac{400 \text{ mg}}{250 \text{ mL}} \times \frac{1000 \text{ µg}}{1 \text{ mg}} = \frac{400,000 \text{ µg}}{250 \text{ mL}}$$

b. Calculate concentration of drug in 1 mL of fluid

$$\frac{400,000 \text{ µg}}{250 \text{ mL}} = \frac{1600 \text{ µg}}{1 \text{ mL}}$$

c. Enter known factors into the formula and solve

$$\frac{5 \text{ µg/kg/min} \times 60 \text{ min/hr} \times 100 \text{ kg}}{1600 \text{ µg/mL}} = 18.75 \text{ mL/hr}$$

Example when dose is unknown: dobutamine 500 mg/250 mL D5W is infusing at 15 mL/hr. Patient weighs 70 kg.

a. Convert the concentration to like units of measure:

$$\frac{500 \text{ mg}}{250 \text{ mL}} \times \frac{1000 \text{ µg}}{1 \text{ mg}} = \frac{500,000 \text{ µg}}{250 \text{ mL}}$$

b. Calculate concentration of drug in 1 mL of fluid

$$\frac{500,000 \text{ µg}}{250 \text{ mL}} = \frac{2000 \text{ µg}}{1 \text{ mL}}$$

c. Enter known factors into the formula and solve

$$\frac{15 \text{ mL/hr} \times 2000 \text{ µg/mL}}{60 \text{ min/hr} \times 70 \text{ kg}} = 7.14 \text{ µg/kg/min}$$

---

*The patient's weight in kilograms and the time factor of 60 min/hr must be added to the basic formula.

- Weigh the patient, if the medication is weight based.
  ➻*Rationale:* Permits calculation of the correct dose based on patient weight.
- Verify patency or obtain patent, appropriate IV access.

➻*Rationale:* Ensures delivery of the medication into the IV space. Some continuous infusion medications require central line access to prevent irritation or damage to smaller peripheral veins.

| Procedure | for Calculating Doses, Flow Rates, and Administration of Continuous IV Infusions |

Procedure for Calculating Doses, Flow Rates, and Administration of Continuous IV Infusions

Steps	Rationale	Special Considerations
1. Verify the physician or the advanced practice nurse prescription.	Prevents errors in medication administration.	The prescription should include the medication, dose, concentration of the solution, type of solution diluted in, and the prescribed parameters for titration of the dose.
2. Wash hands, and don gloves.	Reduces transmission of microorganisms; standard precautions.	
3. Connect and flush the IV solution (with prescribed medication) through the tubing system.	Prepares the infusion system.	
4. Place the IV infusion in the infusion device.	The infusion device controls the consistent and accurate delivery of the flow rate.	Infusion devices are electrical equipment and may malfunction. Monitor the infusion for accuracy in flow rate.
5. Connect the infusion system to the intended IV line or catheter.	Prepares the infusion.	Alcohol is used to cleanse the IV port before connecting the infusion, or the infusion system may be connected into a stopcock port.
6. Convert the concentration of the solution to the same units of measure as the dose.	All units of measure must be the same to perform the mathematical functions.	
7. Calculate the concentration of the medication per mL of fluid.	Necessary for medication calculation.	
8. Enter the concentration and the dose into the formula and solve for the flow rate.	Necessary for medication calculation.	Use alternate formulas if medication dose is per minute or is weight based.
9. Double-check the calculations.	Prevents mathematical errors.	
10. Set the flow rate on the infusion pump, and initiate the infusion	Initiates therapy.	
11. Discard used supplies, and wash hands.	Reduces transmission of microorganisms; standard precautions.	

Expected Outcomes	**Unexpected Outcomes**
• Desired patient response is achieved. • Correct dose of medication is administered. • Dose is titrated to desired patient response.	• Adverse reactions to the medication occur. • Incorrect dose of medication is administered. • Desired patient response is not achieved. • Infiltration or extravasation of medication occurs.

Patient Monitoring and Care

Patient Monitoring and Care	Rationale	Reportable Conditions
		These conditions should be reported if they persist despite nursing interventions.
1. Evaluate patient response by monitoring the indicated parameters for the medication being infused.	Medications given as continuous infusions often have potent effects and potentially serious adverse effects. Most medications given as continuous infusions have a quick onset of action. Frequent monitoring of parameters is necessary during initiation of the infusion.	• Adverse reactions, hemodynamic instability, and cardiac dysrhythmias
2. If the patient response is inadequate, titrate the infusion as prescribed until the prescribed parameters are met.	Patient response to many continuous infusions is dose dependent. To achieve the desired response, titration of the dose is necessary.	• Desired response not achieved within an acceptable dosage
3. Asssess IV access for placement and patency every 1 to 4 hours and as needed.	Ensures delivery of the medication into the venous system. Prevents interruptions in delivery of the medication.	

Documentation

Documentation should include the following:

• Patient and family education
• Name of the medication and the type of solution diluted in, concentration of the solution, dose, flow rate, and administration times
• Assessment of the IV access and site
• Parameters monitored and patient response
• Adverse reactions and interventions to treat the reaction
• Titration

Additional Readings

Burns C, Crawford M. A method for rapidly calculating intravenous drip rates. *Focus Crit Care.* 1988;15:46–48.

Curren A, Munday L. Critical care IV calculations. In: *Math for Meds: A Programmed Text of Dosages and Solutions.* San Diego, Ca: Wallcur, Inc., 1988.

Guiliano K, Richards N, Kaye W. A new strategy for calculating medication infusion rates. *Crit Care Nurs.* 1993;13:77–82.

Robison J, Coleman R. A pocket guide for critical care drug dosing. *Crit Care Nurs* 1991;11:90–96.

Index

Note: Page numbers in *italics* refer to illustrations, page numbers followed by a t refer to tables.

A

Abdominal compartment syndrome (ACS), 674, 674t. See also
    Compartment syndrome.
  monitoring of, 675–679, *676–677*
  physiologic response to, 675t
Abdominal paracentesis, 689–693, *690, 692*
  albumin intravenous solution in, 691
  assistance in, 694–697
  contraindications to, 689
  x-rays in, 690
Abiomed 5000 BVS, 321, *322*, 325, 326, 327
Absorption, 717
Acceleration contractility index (ACI), 421, 422t, 428
Acetate, in dialysate solutions, 720
Acidosis, body rewarming and, 593, 768
  cardiac contractility and, 389
  metabolic, 880t
    end-tidal carbon dioxide and, 68
  reperfusion injury and, 768
  shivering and, 592
Acute respiratory distress syndrome (ARDS), 83
  arterial blood gas analysis and, 496
  compliance and, 161
  intrapulmonary shunt and, 175
  mechanical ventilation and, positive end-expiratory pressure in, 183
  partial pressure of oxygen ratio to inspired oxygen and, 170
  prone positioning for, 83–84
  pulmonary artery catheter insertion for, 432, 439
  pulmonary artery wedge pressure and, 441
Adams Micro-Hematocrit Reader, *802*
α-Adrenergic agonists, for epidural analgesia, 639
β-Adrenergic blockers, and cardiac pacing, 253, 272, 278
  pacing with, 285
Advance directives, 892–895
  vs. Do Not Resuscitate, 894
Airway, nasopharyngeal, 27–30, 27t, *28*
    contraindications to, 27
  oropharyngeal, 31–33, 31t, *32, 34*, 35
    seizure and, 31
Airway obstruction, end-tidal carbon dioxide and, 67, 68, 69
  nasopharyngeal airway for, 27
Airway resistance, 161
  manual resuscitation and, 165
Albumin solutions, 777
Alcohol, as sclerosing agent, 711t
  povidone-iodine solutions and, 525, 546
  thermoregulation and, 591, 592
Alkalosis, metabolic, end-tidal carbon dioxide and, 67
Allen test, 361–362, 498, *499*
Alveolar ventilation, end-tidal carbon dioxide and, 67
  prone positioning and, 83
Alveolar–arterial oxygen difference, 170, 171t
American Heart Association, cardioversion energy recommendations of,
  215t
  defibrillator energy recommendations of, 221
Aminoglycosides, and oculovestibular reflexes, 599, 901

Analgesia, epidural, 639, 640–645, *640–641*
  contraindications to, 640
  equipment for, 640
  local anesthetic toxicity and, 644
  opiate reactions and, 645
  patient positioning for, 641, *641*
  sedation score and, 643
Anemia, iron deficiency, 880t
Anesthesia, general, thermoregulation and, 592
  local, epinephrine and, 846
  pulmonary artery catheter insertion following, 432
  recovery from, nasopharyngeal airway in, 27
  oropharyngeal airway in, 33
Anesthetic(s), local, for epidural analgesia, 639, 642
  malignant hyperthermia and, 593
  thermoregulation and, 592
Aneurysm, aortic, cerebrospinal fluid monitoring and, 613
    intra-abdominal hypertension and, 674t
    intra-aortic balloon pump therapy and, 299, 313
    transcranial Doppler monitoring and, 586
Angina, intra-aortic balloon pump therapy for, 299
  intra-aortic balloon pump timing and, *306*
  pulmonary artery catheter insertion for, 432
  ST segment monitoring for, 349
Angiography, brain death and, 903t
  catheter removal procedure following, 375
Angioplasty, coronary artery, intra-aortic balloon pump therapy and, 299
  electrocardiogram lead placement with, 332
Antacids, for gastrointestinal bleeding, 671
  scleral therapy and, 715
Anticholinergics, and oculovestibular reflexes, 599, 901
Anticoagulants, arterial puncture and, 497
  in autotransfusion, 96
  with cardioversion, 211
Antidepressants, tricyclic, and oculovestibular reflexes, 599, 901
Antidysrhythmic agents, cardiac pacing and, 272–273, 288
  following cardioversion, 217
Antihistamines. See also *Histamine blockers.*
  for transfusion reaction, 760, 787t
Antimicrobials, for burns, 814, 815t
Antipyretics, for transfusion reaction, 760, 787t
Antiseizure agents, and oculovestibular reflexes, 599, 901
Antiseptic solutions, 518
Aortic dissection, and intra-aortic balloon pump placement, 313
Aortic systolic pressure, *367*
Apheresis, 753
Apnea, and brain death, 902–903, 903t
Apnea test equipment, 898
Arterial blood gas (ABG) analysis, 496
  equipment for, 497
  nebulizer therapy and, 497, 498
Arterial catheter. See also *Catheter(s).*
  insertion of, 361–365. See also *Allen test.*
    assistance in, 367, 368–369, 371–372, 376–377
    brachial artery in, 361, 362, 364, *496*, 497
    complications with, 361, 362

Arterial catheter *(Continued)*
contraindications to, 362, 368
dressing for, 375, 405
equipment for, 362
femoral artery in, 362, 364, *497*
heparin flush for, 371
radial artery in, 361, 362, 363, 364, *496*
ulnar artery in, 362, 363
removal of, 375
hemostasis after, 484–488
Arterial partial pressure of oxygen. See *Pao₂ (arterial partial pressure of oxygen).*
Arterial pressure monitoring, 367–368, *367–368*, 472. See also *Hemodynamic monitoring; Pulmonary artery wedge pressure (PAWP).*
arterial line care in, 376, 377, 481
assistance in, 376–377
complications of, 368
dynamic response test in, *369–370*, 377
indications for, 361
transducer for, 472, *476*
Arterial pressure waveform, 361, 367, *367–368*, 368. See also *Transcranial Doppler (TCD) monitoring.*
in intra-aortic balloon pump therapy, 301, 303, *303–304*, 304, 307, *308*
in intra-aortic balloon pump timing errors, 305–306, *305–307*
overdamping in, *370*, 372, *373*, 374, 376
underdamping in, *370*, 374, 376
Arterial puncture, 496–502, *500*. See also *Allen test; Arterial sheath removal; Venipuncture.*
brachial artery in, 496, *496*, 497, 498, 500, *500*
central venous catheter insertion and, 516t
femoral artery in, 496, 497, *497*, 498, 500, *500*
radial artery in, 496–497, *496*, 498, 500, *500*
ulnar artery in, 496, *496*
Arterial sheath removal, 484–488
Arterial-venous oxygen difference (a-vDO₂), 155–157
Arteriovenous jugular oxygen content difference (AVjDO₂), 570, 571, 571t, 572t, 577
Arteriovenous rewarming, continuous, 768–772, 773–776
contraindications to, 768
equipment for, 769, *769–770*
patient transportation and, 772
reperfusion injury and, 768, 775
Ascitic fluid, 689
Assist/Control (A/C) ventilation, 179t
Assisted Mandatory Ventilation (AMV), 179t
Asthma, auto positive end-expiratory pressure and, 159
mechanical ventilation and, expiratory times for, 182
Asystole, from overdrive atrial pacing, 254
Atelectasis, compliance and, 161
intrapulmonary shunt and, 175
signs of, 181
Atrial electrogram (AEG), 243–249, *244–248*
Atrial fibrillation, cardioversion for, 211
energy recommendations for, 215t
hypothermia and, 592t, 594
Atrioventricular (AV) heart block, hypothermia and, 594
transcutaneous pacing for, 271
transvenous pacing for, 278
Atropine, for right ventricular myocardial infarction, 346
in esophagogastric tamponade therapy, 658
in gastric lavage, 666
in scleral therapy, 712
in thoracentesis, 146
pupillary response and, 900
Automated external defibrillators (AED), 205–209, *206–207*
Auto-PEEP (positive end-expiratory pressure), 158, *158*
calculation of, 158–160, *158*
volume mode ventilation and, 183
Autotransfusion, 95–98
anticoagulants in, 96
contraindications to, 95
Azotemia, 880t

B

Bagging, 164–169, *164*
complications with, 168–169
equipment for, 164, *165*
lung compliance and, 165
Barbiturates, oculovestibular reflex and, 599
thermoregulation and, 591, 592
Barotrauma, 180
auto positive end-expiratory pressure and, 158
positive pressure ventilation and, 180
signs of, 181
static pressure and, 161
Benzoin, and external cardiac pacing, 273
Berman airway, 31, *32*
Beta blockers. See *β-Adrenergic blockers.*
Bicarbonate, in dialysate solutions, 720
Biopsy, bone marrow, 791–796
assistance in, 797–800
contraindications to, 791
equipment for, 791–792
indications for, 791
wound tissue, 855
Bladder pressure, monitoring of, 676–677, *676*
Bleeding. See *Hemorrhage.*
Blood, transfusion of, 757–764, 758t, 761t, 777
citrate and, 786
complications with, 778
component storage for, 760
filters for, 758, *779*
hypervolemia and, 786
transfusion reaction and, 763
transfusion reaction premedication for, 760, 787t
urine output and, 784
Blood flow, cerebral, brain death and, 903t
by transcranial Doppler, 580–582, *581–582*, 581t, 583t, 584–586
hypercarbia and, 580, 581
intrapulmonary shunt calculation of, 175–177, 176t
pulmonary, *432*
wasted, 175
Blood group compatibility, 761t
Blood pressure, 367–368, 390t
continuous monitoring of, 361. See also *Hemodynamic monitoring; Mean arterial blood pressure (MAP).*
Blood pump, 765–767
ventricular fibrillation and, 765
Blood sampling, *548*. See also *Arterial puncture; Butterfly set; Venipuncture.*
for hematocrit, 801–804
from arterial pressure lines, 379–384, *380–382*
from peripheral intravenous line, *528*
from pulmonary artery catheter, 385–387
Body temperature, 591–593, 591t–592t
afterdrop and, 592
blood pump and, 765
brain death and, 898, 899
cardiac output measurement and, 392
overshoot and, 593
Bone marrow aspirate, 791–796
assistance in, 797–800
bone marrow core biopsy for, 795
Brain death, 897–898
apnea and, 902–903, 903t
body temperature and, 898, 899
determination of, 899–903, 903t, 905
jugular venous oxygen saturation and, 575
oculocephalic reflexes and, 901
oculovestibular reflexes and, 901
pain and, 900, 901
prerequisites for, 898
pupillary light reflex and, 900
shivering and, 900
spinal reflex movements and, 900
time of, 905
British Pacing and Electrophysiology Group (BPEG), ICD defibrillator code of, 258, 258t
pacemaker code of, 265t

Bronchitis, suction for, 41–42
Bronchodilators, auto positive end-expiratory pressure and, 158
  end-tidal carbon dioxide monitoring and, 69
Bronchospasm, auto positive end-expiratory pressure and, 158
  end-tidal carbon dioxide and, 69
  high-pressure ventilator alarms and, 185t
Bundle branch block, right, pulmonary artery catheter insertion and, 433
Burn care facility criteria, 813t
Burns, 811–815. See also *Graft(s)*.
  central venous catheters and, 533
  chemical, 815
  electrical, 815, *815*
  emergent treatment of, 815
  infection with, 813–814
  inflammatory response and, 813
  Lund-Browder size chart for, 812–813, *813*
  metabolic rate and, 806, 814
  mixed venous oxygen saturation monitoring for, 73
  pain control and, 814
  thermoregulation and, 592
  types of, 811–812, 811t, *812*
  wound management for, 806–810, 816–820. See also *Wound management*.
    alternative pain therapies for, 816, 819
    antimicrobials for, 814, 815t
    autografts for, 814
    closed method for, 814
    donor sites in, 805, 806, *806*
    dressings for, 805–806, 817–818
    equipment for, 815–816
    escharotomy in, *812*, 813, *814*
    open method for, 814
Burns Weaning Assessment Program (BWAP), 197t
Butterfly set, 522, *524*, 529, 548
  VACUTAINER, *545*, *547–549*

C
Calcium alginate, 851
Calcium channel blockers, and cardiac pacing, 253, 272
Caloric testing, for vestibular function, 598–601, *598–599*
  contraindications to, 599
Capnograph, 64–65, *65*, *67–69*
Carbon dioxide (CO₂), 64
  arterial partial pressure of, brain death and, 902, 903t
    oxygen saturation and, 77
    ventilation adequacy and, 199
  partial pressure of end-tidal, 64
  patient consciousness and, 39
Carbon dioxide monitoring, continuous end-tidal, 64–69, *65*, *67–69*
  equipment for, 65
  indications for, 64, 65
  medications and, 69
  hyperthermia and, 67, 593
Carbon monoxide, and pulse oximetry, 79
Cardiac arrest. See also *Heart failure*.
  pulse oximetry and, 79
  transcutaneous pacing for, 271
  transvenous pacing for, 278
Cardiac catheterization. See *Hemodynamic monitoring*.
Cardiac dysrhythmias, cardiac output measurement and, 395
  cardioversion for, 211, 212
    energy recommendations for, 215t
  cardioverter-defibrillator pacing for, 258, 258t
  central venous catheter insertion and, 517t
  digitalis and, 212
  electrolytes and, 212, 222
  following cardioversion, 217
  from overdrive atrial pacing, 252
  hypothermia and, 592t, 594, 768
  intra-aortic balloon pump therapy for, 299
  peripherally inserted central catheters and, 536, 541
  reperfusion injury and, 768, 775
  transcutaneous pacing for, 271
  transvenous pacing for, 278

Cardiac index (CI), 390, 390t, 422t, 427
Cardiac monitoring. See *Electrocardiogram (ECG); Impedance cardiography (ICG)*.
Cardiac output (CO), 389–390, *390*, 390t, 422t, 427
  afterload in, 389, 390t
  end-tidal carbon dioxide and, 68
  heart rate and, 389, 390
  intra-abdominal hypertension and, 675, 675t
  intra-aortic balloon pump therapy and, 299, *299*, 310, 312
  measurement of, *391*, 392, 394–399
    body temperature and, 392
    closed system delivery sets for, *393*
    dysrhythmias and, 395
    equipment for, *391*, 392, *393*
    thermodilution, 390, *391*, 392, 394–397
  preload in, 389, 390t
  sinus rhythm in, 251
  venous oxygen content and, 71, 155, 385
Cardiac pacing. See *Pacing therapy*.
Cardiac tamponade, central venous catheter insertion and, 517t
  chest tube placement and, 110
  left atrial catheter removal and, 420
  pericardial effusion and, 238
  pulmonary artery catheter insertion for, 432, 439
  signs of, 230, 238
Cardiopulmonary arrest, end-tidal carbon dioxide and, 68
  ventilation weaning and, 203
Cardiopulmonary bypass, brain emboli and, 586
  end-tidal carbon dioxide and, 68
  intra-aortic balloon pump therapy and, 299
  thermoregulation and, 592
  ventricular assist devices and, 320
Cardiopulmonary death, 897, 898
  determination of, 899
Cardiopulmonary resuscitation (CPR), arterial blood gas analysis and, 496
  automated external defibrillation with, 205, 207
Cardiovascular depression, auto positive end-expiratory pressure and, 158, 159
  intra-abdominal hypertension and, 674, 675t
  signs of, 181
  static pressure and, 161
Cardioversion, 211–217, *214*
  anticoagulants and, 211
  cerebral emboli and, 217
  digitalis and, 212
  dysrhythmias following, 217
  electrolytes and, 212
  energy recommendations for, 215t
  for atrial fibrillation, 211
  implantable cardioverter-defibrillators and, 215
  oxygenation and, 212
  pacemakers and, 215, 257, 258, 265
  paddle placement in, 214–215, *214*
  R wave and, 212–213, *213*
  ventricular fibrillation and, 216
Catheter(s). See also *Left atrial pressure (LAP); Right atrial/central venous pressure (RA/CVP)*.
  angiocatheter, in bladder pressure monitoring, *676*, 677, 678
  arterial, 361. See also *Arterial catheter*.
  central, peripherally inserted, 533, *534–535*, 535–542, *537–540*
    complications of, 536, 540, 541–542
    contraindications to, 533
    equipment for, 535
    sizes of, 533
  central venous, 503, 514. See also *Central venous pressure (CVP)*.
    jugular venous oxygen saturation monitoring with, 570
    removal of, 401–404
  dressings for, 405, 528, *528*
  epidural, 639
  for continuous arteriovenous rewarming, 768, 770
  for rapid infusers, 777
  heat-exchange cardiac output, 392
  internal jugular. See *Catheter(s), jugular venous oxygen saturation*.
  intrathecal, 613
  intraventricular, 552, *552*, 561, 562

Catheter(s) *(Continued)*
  contraindications to, 562
  insertion of, 563–565
  monitoring of, 567–569
  removal of, 566
  troubleshooting for, 566
 Jelco, *833–834*
 jugular venous oxygen saturation, 570, 571–578
  fiberoptic limitations with, 574
  insertion of, 571–574
   equipment for, 571
  removal of, 575–576
   intracranial pressure and, 576
  troubleshooting of, 574–575
  vessel wall artifact and, 575
 left atrial, 415
  removal of, 418, 420
 long-term enteral access, 883, *883–884*, 884
 lumbar subarachnoid, 613
  insertion of, *603*, 614–616, 617–619
   complications of, 617
  removal of, 616
 over-the-needle, 522, *523*
  insertion of, 526, *526–527*
  sizes of, 522
 pericardial, 490–493, *490*, 494–495
  medication infusion by, 493–494
 pressure line site care for, 405–407
 pulmonary artery. See *Pulmonary artery catheter(s)*.
 removal of, hemostasis after, 484–488
 Seldinger technique placement of, 506, *507*, 533
 septicemia and, 401, 405
 slit, 828, *830*
 suction, sizes of, 42t
 Swan-Ganz, *393*, *440*, *475*
 Tenckhoff, *746*
 thoracic, 109
 through-the-needle, 522
 transvenous pacing, *286*
 wick, 828, *829*
Central nervous system (CNS), infection of, meningeal signs of, 589
Central venous pressure (CVP), 390t, 408, 408t, 503, *515*
 impedance cardiography and, 426
 monitoring of, 408–409, *410*, 411, *412*, 413, 479
  access sites for, 504t
  arm veins in, 510–512, *511*
  catheter insertion for, 504–507, *505*, *507*, 512–513
   assistance in, 514–515, 518–521
   complications of, 516t–518t
  contraindications to, 503
  equipment for, 504
  femoral vein in, 510
  indications for, 503
  internal jugular vein in, *505*, 505–507, *508*
  pulmonary artery line care in, 454, 482
  subclavian vein in, *505*, 507–509, *508–509*
  waveform in, 514, *515*
 pacemakers and, 503
 pulmonary artery pressure in, 447–448, *447*. See also *Hemodynamic monitoring*.
 pulmonary artery wedge pressure in, 448–450, *449–450*
 pulmonary artery wedge pressure waveforms and, 441, *441*
 right atrial waveforms in, 441, *441*, 445–446, *446*
Cerebral autoregulation, 551–553, 552t
Cerebral circulatory arrest, by transcranial Doppler monitoring, 583t
Cerebral extraction of oxygen (CeO$_2$), 570, 571, 571t, 572t, 577
Cerebral oxygen extraction ratio (O$_2$ER), global, 570, 571t, 572t, 577
Cerebral perfusion pressure (CPP), 552, 559
Cerebrospinal fluid (CSF), 551, 588, 602
 drainage of, 588, 589, 613
 glucose and, 588
 halo sign and, 588
 laboratory tests of, 602
 monitoring of, 610, 613
Cervical fixation, 620, 622–624, 625
Cervical traction devices, 620, *621*, 625, *625*

Cervical traction devices *(Continued)*
 care of, 625, 627–630, 631–633
 skin assessment guide for, 637t
Chest drainage system(s). See also *Wound management, drains in*.
 closed, 127, 129–140
  disposable, 127, *128–129*, 131
   waterless, 127
  double-bottle, 127, 129, 132–134, *133*
  four-bottle, 127, 129, 136–137, *136*
  single-bottle, 127, 129, 131, *132*
  triple-bottle, 127, 129, *129*, 134–136, *135*
 milking of, 139
 pressure relief valve in, 127
 water seal in, 127
Chest tube(s), 99–100, 109–110, 117. See also *Wound management, drains in*.
 complications from, 120
 drainage connections for, *110*, 112
  milking of, 114
 indications for, 99, 109, 110
 insertion of, 99–107, *100*, *103–105*
  anesthetic for, 102, *102*
  assistance in, 109–115, *110*
  dressing for, 105, *110*, 113
  equipment for, 100
  signs for, 100–101
 multiple, 110
 removal of, 117–120, *118*
  assistance in, 123–126
  equipment for, 117–118
  indications for, 117
 sizes of, 99
 x-rays and, 105, 117, 119
Chest x-ray. See also *Radiography*.
 in feeding tube insertion, 888, 890
 in intra-aortic balloon placement, 303
 in intubation, 9
 in peripherally inserted central catheter placement, 540
 in thoracentesis, 146, 149
 in transvenous cardiac pacing, 281, 283
 pleural effusions on, 146
Chronic obstructive pulmonary disease (COPD), arterial blood gas analysis and, 496
 auto positive end-expiratory pressure and, 158
 central venous catheters and, 533
 pulmonary artery catheter insertion for, 432
 pulmonary artery wedge pressure and, 441
Cirrhosis, and intra-abdominal hypertension, 674t
Cisternal puncture, 608–612
 contraindications to, 608
 indications for, 608
 meningeal irritation and, 609
 patient position for, 608, *608*, 609
 patient preparation for, 609, 610
Citrate, 753
 in autotransfusion, 96
 in continuous renal replacement therapies, 720, 726
 in plasmapheresis, 753, 754
Coagulopathy(ies), chest tubes and, 99
 fluid resuscitation and, 768, 777–778
 hypothermia-induced, 592t, 768, 777–778
  continuous arteriovenous rewarming for, 768, 775
 intra-aortic balloon pump therapy and, 299, 312–313
 transfusion reaction and, 789
COBE Spectra Apheresis System, *754*
Colloid fluids, 777
Coma, brain death and, 897, 899, 900
 hepatic, hypothermia and, 592
 vestibular function in, caloric testing for, 599, *599*
Compartment syndrome, 828, 829t, 830. See also *Abdominal compartment syndrome (ACS)*.
 pressure monitoring of, 828, 830–836, *832–835*
  equipment in, *829–830*, 830
Compliance, 161
 dynamic, 161, 163

Compliance (*Continued*)
measurement of, 162
intracranial, 551
manual resuscitation and, 165
mechanical ventilation and, positive end-expiratory pressure in, 183
Compliance, Rate, Oxygenation, and Pressure (CROP) index, 197t
Congestive heart failure, cardioversion in, 211
pulmonary artery catheter insertion for, 432
Continuous arteriovenous rewarming (CAVR), 768–772, 773–776
contraindications to, 768
equipment for, 769, *769–770*
patient transportation and, 772
reperfusion injury and, 768, 775
Continuous positive airway pressure (CPAP), 179t
in ventilation weaning, 197–198, 198t, 201
Continuous renal replacement therapies (CRRT), 717, 718t–719t, 720, 722–723, 729–731
complications of, 720, 731
equipment for, 720
replacement fluid amounts in, 731
vs. hemodialysis, 720
Control Ventilation (CV), 179t
Controlled Mandatory Ventilation (CMV), 179t
Convective transport, 717
Cooling devices, 591, 593
procedure for, 593–595, 596
Coughing, and airway management, 22
CPAP (continuous positive airway pressure) protocol, 198t
Cricoid pressure, in intubation, 1, *1*
Crutchfield tongs, 620, *621*
skin assessment guide for, 637t
Cryoprecipitate, administration of, 757, 758t, 760, 762
Crystalloid fluids, 777
Cycler machine, for peritoneal dialysis, 746, *747*
Cystic fibrosis, central venous catheters and, 533
closed pneumothorax and, 99
suction for, 41–42

D
Dantrolene, 593
Death, determination of, 897–905
Decannulation, 21–23
assistance in, 24–26
complications from, 22
indications for, 21
Defibrillation, 205, 219
external, 219–222
energy recommendations for, 221
internal, 224–228, 226
energy recommendations for, 224
pacemakers and, 207, 220. See also *Implantable cardioverter-defibrillator (ICD).*
pharmacologic agents for, 219
Defibrillators, 219
automated external, 205–209, *206–207*
electrodes of, 220
placement of, *207*, 220
implantable cardioverter-defibrillator, *207*, 257–262, *257*, 258t
deactivation of, 260–261
electromagnetic interference and, 259
external defibrillation and, *207*, 260
reactivation of, 261
ventricular fibrillation and, 226, 257
Dermis, 811, *812*, 843
Dextran solutions, 777
Diabetes mellitus, arterial catheter insertion and, 362
dialysis and, 752
thermoregulation and, 591, 592
Diabetic ketoacidosis (DKA), and brain death, 899
Dialysate solutions, 733, 735
glucose in, 720, 752
Dialysis, peritoneal, 746–752, *746*
Dialysis therapies, 719t
Dialyzer(s), 733

Dialyzer(s) (*Continued*)
hollow-fiber, 733
parallel-plate, 733
Diastole, 367
Diazepam, in scleral therapy, 712
Dicrotic notch, 367, *367*
Diffusion, 717
Digitalis, cardioversion and, 212
ischemia and, 339
Digoxin, and cardiac pacing, 272
Disseminated intravascular coagulopathy (DIC), and transfusion reaction, 789
Diuretics, for infusion-induced hypervolemia, 786
right ventricular myocardial infarction and, 346
Do Not Resuscitate (DNR), organ donation and, 907
vs. advance directives, 894
Dobutamine, as intermittent inotropic agent, 533
Doll's eyes, 901
Drug(s). See also specific drug or drug group.
brain death and, 900
concentration of, 922–923
enteral nutrition and, 872, 872t, 874
for epidural analgesia, 639, 640, 642
intravenous, dosage of, 922, 923t, 924t, 925
patient weight and, 922, 924, 924t
intravenous infusion rates and, 922–923, 923t, 924t, 925
oculovestibular reflexes and, 599, 901
plasmapheresis and, 756
Dynamic compliance (Cdyn), 161, 163
measurement of, 162
Dynamic response test, *369–370*, 377
Dysphagia, and scleral endoscopic therapy, 715

E
Edema. See also *Intra-abdominal hypertension (IAH).*
burn wound management and, 814
compartment syndrome and, 828, 829t
grafts and, 823
preeclampsia-induced, pulmonary artery catheter insertion for, 432
pulmonary, colloid solutions and, 777
compliance and, 161
high-pressure ventilator alarms and, 185t
intrapulmonary shunt and, 175
thoracic fluid status and, 422t, 427
Edetate calcium disodium, for bone marrow biopsy, 791, 793
Effusion(s), pericardial, 238, 490
pleural, 145, 146
Electrocardiogram (ECG), 329–330, *329–330*, 335, *335*, 338–339. See also *Myocardial infarction (MI); QRS complex; ST segment monitoring.*
body shivering and, 592
electrical artifact in, 336, *336*, 345, 592
electrode placement for, 332–334, *333–334*, 350
gastric lavage and, 665
implantable cardioverter-defibrillators and, 259–260
in atrial electrogram, 243, 244–248, *245–248*, 249
in cardioversion, 212–213, *213*, 214
in central venous pressure monitoring, 503, *515*, 520
in left atrial pressure monitoring, 416–417, *417*
in pericardiocentesis, 239, 240, *240*, 241
in permanent pacing, 264, 265, *265–266*, 267
in transcutaneous pacing, 272, 273, 275, *275*, 276
in transvenous pacing, 280, 281–282, *282*, 290, 294, *294*
interference with, 336, *336*, 345, 592
intra-aortic balloon pump therapy and, 299, 301
lead wire placement for, 290, 331–332, *332*, 341, *350*
transvenous, 290
left bundle branch block on, *340*
left posterior leads in, 338, 342, *343*, 344, *345*
indications for, 339
multiple-channel, 344, 356, *357*
overdrive atrial pacing on, *252*
pad polarity of, 207
patient monitoring during, 336–337

Electrocardiogram (ECG) *(Continued)*
  precordial leads in, 338
    right, 342, *342–343*, 344
      indications for, 339
  procedure for, 341, 344–346
  pulmonary artery pressure and, 447–448, *447*
  pulmonary artery wedge pressure and, 449, *449–450*
  R wave in, 335
    cardioversion and, 212–213, *213*
  respiratory artifact in, 357
  right atrial/central venous pressure and, *441*, 446, *446*
  ST segment monitoring by, 349–352, *350–351*
  twelve-lead, 354–359, *354, 356–359*
    electrode placement in, 355–356, *356*
  wandering baseline in, *336*
Electroencephalogram (EEG), and brain death, 903t
Electrogram, atrial, 243–249, *244–248*
Electrolytes, in dialysate solutions, 720
  postconversion dysrhythmias and, 212
  ventricular dysrhythmias and, 222
Electrophysiologic monitoring, 329–335, *329–330, 332–335*. See also
  QRS complex; ST segment monitoring.
  interference with, 336, *336*
  patient monitoring during, 336–337
  telemetry in, 329, *330*, 335
Embolism, air, 401, 402, 409, 530
  central venous catheter insertion and, 517t
    venous access and, 530
  catheter-induced, 415, 530
  cerebral, cardiopulmonary bypass and, 586
    cardioversion and, 217
  intra-aortic balloon pump therapy and, 302, 310, 312, 313
  left atrial pressure monitoring and, 415
  pulmonary, 530
    central venous catheter insertion and, 518t
    end-tidal carbon dioxide and, 68
    intravenous catheters and, 530
    pleural effusion and, 145
    pulmonary artery pressure and, 441
  ventricular assist devices and, 324, 325
Emphysema, central venous pressure lines and, 504
  closed pneumothorax and, 99
  compliance and, 161
  mechanical ventilation and, expiratory times for, 182
End-of-life decisions, 917–921
Endoscopic therapy, scleral, 711–715, *713*
  agents in, 711t
Endotracheal intubation. See *Intubation.*
Endotracheal (ET) tube(s), 1–2, *2*, 41
  auto positive end-expiratory pressure and, 158
  care of, 17–19
    indications for, 17, 19. See also *Tracheal tube cuff.*
  malpositioned, signs of, 181
  oropharyngeal airways and, 31
  sizes of, 1–2, 42t
  suction of, 41–47, 42t
    chest tube removal and, 117
    complications from, 41, 46
    indications for, 41
End-tidal carbon dioxide monitoring, 64–69, *65, 67–69*
  equipment for, 65
  indications for, 64, 65
  malignant hyperthermia and, 593
  medications and, 69
Epidermis, 811, *812*, 843
Epinephrine, as sclerosing agent, 711t
  for anaphylactic transfusion reaction, 787t
  local anesthesia and, 846
Epithelization, 843
Eschar, 813
Escharotomy, *812*, 813, *814*
Esophagogastric tamponade therapy, 655–659, *656, 660*, 661–663
  contraindications to, 655
Esophagogastric tamponade tubes, 655, *656*
Essential fatty acid deficiency, 880t
Ethanol, as sclerosing agent, 711t

Ethanolamine oleate, 711t
Ethics committee, healthcare facility, 893, 895
  end-of-life decisions and, 918
Ethyl alcohol, as sclerosing agent, 711t
Euthermia, 591t
Extubation, 21–23. See also *Standard weaning criteria (SWC).*
  assistance in, 24–26
  complications from, 22
  inadvertent, signs of, 181
  indications for, 21

F

Feeding tubes. See also *Gastrostomy tubes; Nasogastric (NG) tube(s);*
  Nutrition.
  small bore, 888
    complications of, 891
    insertion of, 888–891
    postpyloric, 889, 890
Femostop mechanical compression device, *485*
Fentanyl, in scleral therapy, 712
Fever, 591t, 593
Fick equations, for blood oxygen content, 156
Fixation, external, cervical, 620, 622–624, 625
    devices for, 620, *621*, 625, *625*
      care of, 625, 627–630, 631–633
    skin assessment guide for, 637t
Fluid resuscitation, 757, 777, 779–785
  blood products in, 757–764, 758t, 761t, 777
  blood pump for, 765–767
  citrate and, 786
  coagulopathy and, 768, 777–778
  colloids in, 777
  complications with, 778
  crystalloids in, 777
  hypervolemia and, 786
  hypothermia and, 768, 777–778
  infusion devices for, 765, 777, *778–779*
    troubleshooting of, 783
  transfusion reaction and, 763, 786, 787t
  urine output and, 784
Fluoroscopy, in intra-aortic balloon placement, 300
  transvenous cardiac pacing on, 282
    lead wire placement in, 290
Fractures, external cervical devices for, 620, *621*
  pneumatic antishock garments for, 315, *316*
Frank-Starling law, 389, *428*
Fresh frozen plasma (FFP), transfusion of, 757, 758t, 759, 761t, 762, 763
Furosemide (Lasix), and right ventricular myocardial infarction, 346

G

Gardener-Wells tongs, 620, *621*
  skin assessment guide for, 637t
Gastric lavage, 664
  contraindications to, 664
  equipment for, 664–665
  for esophageal varices, 664
  for hemorrhage, 664, 665, 666, 667, 668–669, *668*, 670–671, 672, *682*
  for overdose, 664–672, *668, 682*
  indications for, 664
  tube removal in, 669
Gastrostomy tubes, 883, *884*
  care of, 884–886
  percutaneous endoscopic, 883, *883*
Gentle Work Protocol, for ventilation weaning, 198t
Glucagon, in gastric lavage, 669
Glucose, cerebrospinal fluid and, 588
  in dialysate solutions, 720, 752
Graft(s), 822–827, *823*
  cultured autografts as, 822
  for burn wound management, 814, 822

Graft(s) *(Continued)*
  meshed, 822, *822–823*
  sheet, 822
Granulocytes, administration of, 757, 758t, 760, 762
Guedal airway, 31, *32*

H
Halo ring device, 620, *621*, 625, *625*, 627
  care of, 627–630
  skin assessment guide for, 637t
Health care, power of attorney for, 892, 917
Health care proxy, 892, 917
Heart. See also *Cardiac; Cardio*-entries.
Heart failure, malignant hyperthermia and, 594
  mixed venous oxygen saturation monitoring for, 73
  pericardial effusion and, 490
  pulmonary artery catheter insertion for, 432, 439
  thoracic fluid status and, 422t, 427
Heart rate, 389–390, 390t
Heat and moisture exchanges (HMEs), 185, 186
Heat stroke, 593, 594
Hematocrit, 801–802
  blood sampling for, 801–804
Hematocrit linear scale, *802*
Hematoma, 501
  central venous catheter insertion and, 516t, 517t
  venipuncture and, 550
Hemodiafiltration, continuous arteriovenous, 717, 719t, 720, 721, *721*, 723–725
  continuous venovenous, 717, 719t, 721–722, 725–728, *721*
    dialysate solution in, 726, 727
    vs. slow continuous ultrafiltration, 721
Hemodialysis, 733, *734*, 735–745
  arteriovenous access for, 733, *734*
  arteriovenous fistula for, 733, 735, 736–737
  catheter for, 733, 735, 737–739
  complications of, 744
  continuous arteriovenous, 717, 719t, 720, *720*, 721, 723–725
  continuous venovenous, 717, 719t, 721–722, 725–728, *721*
    vs. slow continuous ultrafiltration, 721
  equipment for, 735
  thermoregulation and, 592
  transmembrane pressure for, 741
Hemodynamic monitoring, 471, 472–474, 475–480, 479–482. See also
    Blood sampling; Impedance cardiography (ICG); Mean arterial blood pressure (MAP); Pulmonary artery catheter(s).
  arterial pressure monitoring as, 367–368, *367–368*, 472
    arterial line care in, 376, 377, 481
    complications of, 368
    dynamic response test in, *369–370*, 377
    indications for, 361
  central venous pressure in, 390t, 408, 408t, 461
    monitoring of, 408–409, *410*, 411, *412*, 413
      pulmonary artery line care in, 454, 482
  flush solution for, 473
  hemostasis after, 484–488
  heparin solution for, contraindications to, 473
  left atrial pressure monitoring as, 415–418, *415*, *417*, 419–420
  pressure monitoring scale for, 473
  pulmonary artery catheter pressure monitoring as, 445–451, *446–447*, *449–452*, 453–454, 461
    pulmonary artery line care in, 454, 482
  reference points for, 479–480, *479–480*
  right atrial waveforms in, 441, *441*, 445–446, *446*, 461
  right ventricle waveforms in, 467–468, *468*
  transducers for, 472, 473, 474, *475–476*, 478
    calibration of, 480–481
    leveling of, 479–480, *479–480*
Hemofiltration, continuous arteriovenous, 717, 718t, 720–721, 723–725, *720*
  continuous venovenous, 717, 719t, 721–722, 725–728, *721*
    vs. slow continuous ultrafiltration, 721
Hemoglobin, activities of daily living and, 759
  hypothermia and, 768

Hemoglobin *(Continued)*
  oxygen affinity and, 77
Hemolysis, and hematocrit, 801
Hemoperitoneum, signs of, 700
Hemopneumothorax, chest tube sizes for, 99
Hemorrhage, gastric lavage for, 664, 665, 666, 667, 668–669, *668*, 670–671, 672, *682*
  pneumatic antishock garments for, 315
  signs of, 665
  subarachnoid, red blood cells and, 610
    thermoregulation and, 591
    transcranial Doppler monitoring and, 586
Hemothorax, central venous catheter insertion and, 516t
  chest tube sizes for, 99
Heparin, arterial catheter insertion and, 371, 433, 443
  epidural analgesia and, 640
  for bone marrow biopsy, 792, 793
  for catheter irrigation, 520
  in arterial puncture, 499
  in continuous renal replacement therapies, 720, 723
  in hemodynamic monitoring flush solution, 473
  in intra-aortic balloon catheter removal, 310
  in intra-aortic balloon placement, 300
  in plasmapheresis, 753, 754
  in thoracentesis, 145, 147, 148
  peripheral intravenous lines and, 528
  thrombocytopenia and, 443
Hetastarch solutions, 777
Histamine blockers, for gastrointestinal bleeding, 671
  scleral therapy and, 715
Histoacryl, 711t
Hydrocolloid(s), 851
Hydrocolloid membrane, in intubation, 8
Hydrocortisone, for transfusion reaction, 760
Hydrogels, 851
Hydrostatic pressure, 717
Hydrothorax, and central venous catheter insertion, 516t
Hypercapnia, cerebral blood flow and, 581
  mean blood flow velocity and, 580
Hypercarbia, cerebral blood flow and, 581
  intra-abdominal hypertension and, 675
  mean blood flow velocity and, 580
  permissive, 160, 182
    contraindications to, 182
    respiratory muscle fatigue with, 178
Hyperglycemia, 880t
  dialysis and, 752
Hyperglycemic hyperosmolar nonketotic dehydration/coma, 880t
  brain death and, 899
Hyperinflation, dynamic, 164
Hyperkalemia, 880t
  cardiac contractility and, 389
Hyperlipidemia, 880t
Hypernatremia, and gastric lavage, 667
Hypertension, arterial catheter insertion and, 362
  intra-abdominal, 674, 674t, 675t
  intracranial, intracranial pressure and, 570, 577
  pulmonary, pulmonary artery pressure and, 441
  stroke volume and, 389
Hyperthermia, 591t, 593
  compartment syndrome and, 829t
  end-tidal carbon dioxide and, 67, 593
  malignant, 593, 594
  seizure and, 594
Hypertonic saline, as sclerosing agent, 711t
Hypervolemia, 880t
  pulmonary artery pressure and, 441
Hypocalcemia, 880t
Hypoglycemia, 880t
Hypokalemia, 880t
  postconversion dysrhythmias and, 212
Hypomagnesemia, 880t
Hypoperfusion, signs of, 95
Hypophosphatemia, 880t
Hypotension, arterial-venous oxygen difference and, 155

Hypotension (*Continued*)
    auto positive end-expiratory pressure and, 158, 159
    epidural analgesia and, 644
    manual resuscitation and, 164
    pneumatic antishock garments for, 315
    positive pressure ventilation and, 155
    pulmonary artery catheter insertion for, 432, 439
    reperfusion injury and, 768
Hypothermia, 591t, 592, 594, 768
    coagulopathy and, 592t, 768, 777–778
    compartment syndrome and, 829t
    end-tidal carbon dioxide and, 68
    fluid resuscitation and, 768, 777–778
    physiologic response to, 592t, 594, 768, 786
Hypothyroidism, and body temperature, 592
Hypoventilation, and end-tidal carbon dioxide, 67
Hypovolemia, 880t
    cardiac stroke volume and, 427, *428*
    end-tidal carbon dioxide and, 68
    positive pressure ventilation and, 181
    signs of, 95, 427, *428*
Hypoxemia, 176, 178
    intrapulmonary shunt and, 171, 172, 175, 176, 177
    positive end-expiratory pressure and, 158, *158*
Hypoxia, and lactic acid, 155

I

ICP (intracranial pressure) waveforms, 552, *552–554*, 553
    calibration for, 556
    dampening of, 557, 558
Immobility, physiologic response to, 636t
    skin assessment guide for, 637t
Impedance cardiography (ICG), 421–429, *421*, 422t
    central venous pressure and, 426
    contraindications to, 422–423
    electrocardiography and, *421–422*, 424, 425
        R wave in, 425
    electrode placement for, 424, *424*
    equipment for, 423
    indications for, 422
Implantable cardioverter-defibrillator (ICD), *207*, 257–262, *257*, 258t
    deactivation of, 260–261
    electromagnetic interference and, 259
    external cardioversion and, 215
    external defibrillation and, *207*, 260
    for ventricular fibrillation, 226, 257
    reactivation of, 261
Infection, chest tubes and, 117, 120
    meningeal signs of, 589
    pericardial effusion and, 490
    peripheral intravenous line and, 530, 542
    wound healing and, 851, 857
Inflammation, 843
Infusion device(s), 925
    blood pump as, 765–767
    butterfly set as, 522, *524*, 529. See also *Butterfly set.*
    rapid, 777, *778–779*
        patient transport with, 783
        troubleshooting of, 783
Inspiratory flow, 182
Intermittent mandatory ventilation (IMV), 179t, 182
    hemodynamic pressure monitoring with, 451, *452*, 453
    in ventilation weaning, 201–202
Intra-abdominal hypertension (IAH), 674, 674t
    monitoring of, 675–679, *676–677*
    physiologic response to, 675t
Intra-aortic balloon pump (IABP) therapy, 299–305, *299–300*, *303–305*
    balloon pressure waveform in, 307, *307–308*
    catheter removal procedure in, 310, 375
    contraindications to, 299
    during asystole, 308
    during atrial fibrillation, 308
    during defibrillation, 309
    during tachycardia, 308

Intra-aortic balloon pump (IABP) therapy (*Continued*)
    embolism and, 302, 310, 312, 313
    femoral artery in, 300, 301, 304, *304*
    patient monitoring during, 311–314
    platelet dysfunction with, 312, 313
    pulmonary artery catheter insertion with, 432
    radial artery in, 301, 304, *304*, 312
    thrombus formation and, 302, 308, 310, 311, 313
    timing errors with, 305–306, *305–307*
    troubleshooting for, 308–309
    urine output and, 301, 310, 312
    weaning parameters for, 310, 313
Intracranial bolts, 551, 552, *552*, 554–560
    contraindications to, 553
    equipment for, 554
    removal of, 557
Intracranial pressure (ICP), 551–553. See also *Catheter(s), intraventricular.*
    intra-abdominal hypertension and, 675, 675t
    intracranial hypertension and, 570, 577
    jugular venous oxygen saturation catheter and, removal of, 576
        thrombosis and, 577
    jugular venous oxygen saturation monitoring of, 570, 577
    transcranial Doppler monitoring of, 583t
    waveform of, 552, *552–554*, 553
        calibration for, 556
        dampening of, 557, 558
Intrapulmonary shunt. See *Pulmonary shunt.*
Intravenous (IV) line, insertion of, 522, 524–531, *526–527*
    equipment for, 522, 524
    patient assessment for, 524
    medication by, 922–926
    peripheral, 522
        complications of, 522, 530
        embolism and, 530
        heparin flush and, 528
        infection and, 530
Intraventricular catheters. See *Catheter(s), intraventricular.*
Intubation, 1–10, *1*, *3*, *5–6*. See also *Extubation; Standard weaning criteria (SWC).*
    assistance in, 11–16
    complications from, 9
    equipment for, 2
    gastric, 681–686, *682*
        tube removal for, 685
    indications for, 1
    intravenous access in, 3
    nasal, 2, 9
    nasogastric, 681, 682, 683
    orogastric, 681, 682, 683
    patient positioning for, 2, 3, *3*
    spinal cord injury and, 2, 3, 4
    tube stabilization in, 8, *8*
Ischemia, compartment syndrome and, 828
    global cerebral, jugular venous oxygen saturation and, 570, 571
    myocardial, *345*, 349
        cardioversion for, 211
        digitalis and, 339
Isoproterenol, for right ventricular myocardial infarction, 346

J

Jamshidi needle, for bone marrow biopsy, 793, 794
Jejunostomy tubes, 883, *884*
    care of, 884–886
Joint Commission on Accreditation of Healthcare Organizations (JCAHO), 892, 910
Jugular venous oxygen saturation (SjvO$_2$), 570–571, 571t, 572t
    clinical intervention and, 571, 572t
    desaturation and, 571, 571t, 576
    intracranial pressure monitoring by, 570, 577
    monitoring of, 576–578

K

Kidney(s). See *Renal* entries.
Kinetic therapy, *635*
Kinins, in inflammation, 843
Kyphoscoliosis, and lung compliance, 161

L

Lactate dehydrogenase (LDH), and pleural effusion, 145
Lactic acid, in hypoxia, 155
Laryngoscope, blade types of, 1
Lasix (furosemide), and right ventricular myocardial infarction, 346
Lateral rotation therapy, 837–841, *838*. See also *Pronation therapy.*
  indications for, 837
Lateral rotation therapy table, *838*
Lavage. See *Gastric lavage; Peritoneal lavage.*
Left atrial pressure (LAP), 415
    monitoring of, 415–418, *417*, 419–420
      cardiac tamponade and, 420
      embolism and, 415
    waveforms in, 415, *415*, 417
      overdampening of, 418
Left cardiac work index (LCWI), 422t
Leukapheresis, 753
Leukocytes, in inflammation, 843
  local anesthetics and, epinephrine in, 843
Level 1 rapid infuser, 777, *778–779*
Levin tube, 681, *681*
Lidocaine, for abdominal paracentesis, 689, 691
  for chest tube insertion, 102, *102*
  for chest tube removal, 118
  for intra-aortic balloon placement, 300
  for peritoneal lavage, 699, 700
  in arterial catheter insertion, 363–364
  in arterial puncture, 499
  in central venous catheter insertion, 506
  in lumbar puncture, 602, 604, 605
  in thoracentesis, 145, 147
  with peripherally inserted central catheters, 538
Linton-Nachlas esophagogastric tamponade tube, 655
Lipid emulsion infusion, 879
Living will, 892, 917
Luer-Lok adapter needle, *380*
Lumbar drains, 613
Lumbar puncture, 602–607, *604*, 608–612
  contraindications to, 602, 608
  indications for, 602, 608
  mass herniation effect and, 603, 606, 607
  meningeal irritation and, 602, 603, 609
  patient position for, *603*, 608, 609
Lund-Browder chart, 812–813, *813*
Lungs. See also *Pulmonary* entries.
  physiologic zones of, *432*

M

Macintosh laryngoscope blade, 1
Mafenide acetate (Sulfamylon), for burns, 814, 815t
Manometer, water, 408, *410*
Manual resuscitation, 164–169, *164*
  complications with, 168–169
  equipment for, 164, *165*
Maximal inspiratory pressure (MIP), 191
Mean arterial blood pressure (MAP), *367–368*, 368, 390t
  cerebral autoregulation and, 552, 552t
  intra-aortic balloon pump therapy and, 301, 310
Mechanical ventilation, 178–181, 179t, 186–188. See also *Bagging; Standard weaning criteria (SWC); Ventilation.*
  alarms in, 185t
  chest tube removal and, 117
  emergent sternotomy and, 229
  end-tidal carbon dioxide and, 67, 68–69
  equipment for, 180
  for transfusion reaction, 788

Mechanical ventilation *(Continued)*
  hemodynamic pressure monitoring with, 451, *452*, 453
  humidified gases in, 185–186
  long-term, 196
    weaning and, 200
  positive pressure, 155. See also *Ventilation, pressure mode in.*
    closed pneumothorax and, 99
    hemodynamics and, 155, 157
    venous return and, 181
  pressure-controlled inverse ratio, 179t, 184
    auto-PEEP and, 158, 184
  short-term, 196
    weaning and, 200
  weaning from. See *Ventilation, weaning from.*
Mediastinal tubes, 100, 109, 117
Medications. See also named drug or drug group.
  brain death and, 900
  concentration of, 922–923
  enteral nutrition and, 872, 872t, 874
  for epidural analgesia, 639, 640, 642
  intravenous, dosage of, 922, 923t, 924t, 925
    patient weight and, 922, 924, 924t
    intravenous infusion rates and, 922–923, 923t, 924t, 925
  oculovestibular reflexes and, 599, 901
  plasmapheresis and, 756
Meningitis, signs of, 589
Meperidine, in scleral therapy, 712
Mercury transducers, 408
Metabolism, body temperature and, 592
  burn management and, 806, 814
  end-tidal carbon dioxide and, 67
Metoclopramide, in feeding tube placement, 890
Microhematocrit, 801
  via centrifuge, 801–804, *802–803*
Midazolam, in scleral therapy, 712
Miller laryngoscope blade, 1
Minimum leak volume (MLV), for tracheal tube cuff inflation, 49, 51
Minimum occlusion volume (MOV), for tracheal tube cuff inflation, 49, 51
Minnesota esophagogastric tamponade tube, 655, *656*
Mixed venous oxygen saturation (Svo₂), 71–76, 71t
  blood sampling for, 385–387
  cardiac output and, 71, 71t, 385
  shivering and, 596
  spectrophotometry components in, 72, *72*
Montgomery straps, 856, *857*
Morphine, for chest tube removal, 118
  for epidural analgesia, 642
Muscle, strength assessment of, 627t
Muscle compartments, lower extremity, *829*
Muscle relaxants. See also *Neuromuscular blockade.*
  mechanical ventilation and, 181, 182
Myocardial infarction (MI), *340*, *343*
  electrocardiogram lead placement with, 332. See also *Electrocardiogram (ECG), left posterior leads in,* and *precordial leads in.*
  mixed venous oxygen saturation monitoring for, 73
  pericardial effusion and, 490
  pulmonary artery catheter insertion following, 432, 439
  right ventricular involvement in, 339, 346
    atrioventricular node conduction disturbance and, 339, 346
  transvenous pacing for, 278
Myocardial ischemia, *345*, *349*
  cardioversion for, 211
  digitalis and, 339
Myoglobinuria, 815
Myxedema, and pericardial effusion, 490

N

Naloxone (Narcan), for opioid sedation, 643
  in scleral therapy, 712
Narcotics. See also *Morphine.*
  auto positive end-expiratory pressure and, 158
  for epidural analgesia, 639, 642

Narcotics *(Continued)*
  mechanical ventilation and, 181
Nasogastric (NG) tube(s), 681, *681–682*. See also *Feeding tubes.*
Nasotracheal intubation. See *Intubation, nasal.*
Needle(s), 843, *847*
  for bone marrow biopsy, 793, 794
  Vacutainer Luer-Lok adapter, *380*
  venipuncture VACUTAINER, *545*
Negative inspiratory pressure (NIP), 191, *192*, 194
Neoplasm, intra-abdominal hypertension and, 674t
  pericardial effusion and, 490
  thermoregulation and, 591
Neuromuscular blockade. See also *Muscle relaxants.*
  brain death motor testing and, 900
  end-tidal carbon dioxide and, 67
  oculovestibular reflex and, 599
Neuromuscular blocking agents (NMBAs), 647
  end-tidal carbon dioxide monitoring and, 67, 69
  in peripheral nerve stimulation assessment, 651
  oculovestibular reflexes and, 901
  pupillary response and, 900
  thermoregulation and, 592
Neurovascular assessment, *831*
Nitroglycerin, cardiac pacing and, 273
  right ventricular myocardial infarction and, 346
Norepinephrine, and cardiac contractility, 389
North American Society of Pacing and Electrophysiology (NASPE),
    ICD defibrillator code of, 258, 258t
  pacemaker code of, 265t
Nutrition. See also *Gastrostomy tubes.*
  assessment of, 868–869, *869*, 869t
  burn care and, 806, 810
  drug interactions with, 872t
  enteral, 868, 869–875
    diarrhea and, 873–874
    medications and, 872, 872t, 874
    patient transport and, 874
  parenteral, 877–879, 878t, 881–882
    metabolic complications of, 880t
Nystatin, mafenide acetate with, 814

O
Obesity, and lung compliance, 161
Obstructive pulmonary disease, chronic. See *Chronic obstructive
    pulmonary disease (COPD).*
  intrapulmonary shunt and, 175
Octreotide, and scleral therapy, 715
Oculocephalic reflexes, 901
Oculovestibular reflexes, 598, *598*
  brain death and, 901
  medications and, 599, 901
  testing of, 598–601, *598–599*
Oculovestibular test equipment, 599, 898
Omeprazole, for gastrointestinal bleeding, 671
  scleral therapy and, 715
Oncotic pressure, 717
Opiates. See *Narcotics.*
Organ donation, 907–909
  designated requestor for, 914
  Do Not Resuscitate order and, 907
  donor identification for, 910–912, 914, 915
  initiation of, 898, 914
Organ procurement organizations (OPOs), 898, 907, 910
Orogastric tube(s), 681, *681–682*
Orotracheal intubation. See *Intubation.*
Orthopedic frame, *635*
Osmosis, 717
Oximetry, fiber optic spectrophotometric, 72, *72*
  pulse, 77, *77–78*, 79–82
    carbon monoxide and, 79
    in intubation, 1, 7
Oxygen, cerebral extraction of, 570, 571, 571t, 572t, 577
  hemoglobin affinity and, 77, 768, 778
Oxygen consumption, 155

Oxygen content, of blood, 71, 155. See also *Oxygen saturation; Pao₂
    (arterial partial pressure of oxygen).*
Oxygen cylinders, 37, 38
Oxygen delivery, 155
Oxygen saturation, 71, 77, 155. See also *Venous oxygen saturation.*
  hypothermia and, 768, 778
Oxygen tank setup, 37–40
Oxygen therapy, intrapulmonary shunt and, 171, 172, 175
  portable tank in, 37–40
Oxygenation, arterial blood gas analysis and, 496
  cardioversion and, 212
  hypothermia and, 768, 778
  indices of, 170–173
  signs of, 175, 199
  ventilation and, 83–84, *84*

P
Pacemaker(s), 264, *264*
  asynchronous mode of, 279, 287. See also *Pacing therapy, asynchro-
    nous.*
  capture by, 265, 287, 294
  cardioversion and, 215, 257, 258, 265
  central venous pressure lines and, 503
  failure of, 265, *266*, 269
  firing of, 265, *265*, 287
    R on T phenomenon and, 292, 293
  generic code for, 265t
  lead wire connections for, 290, *291*
  myocardial depolarization and, 287–288
  permanent pulse generator in, 264, *264*
  sensing by, 264–265, 286, 294
  synchronous mode of, 279, 287
  temporary pulse generator of, 251, *251–252*, 275, 279, 287, *287–288*
  temporary transcutaneous, 271, *271*, 275
Pacing therapy, 264–265, 267, 271–272, 278, 279
  assessment of, 267–269
  asynchronous, 292
  bipolar, 264
  capture in, 265, 287, 294
  code for, 265t
  contraindications to, 264
  defibrillation and, *207*, 220. See also *Implantable cardioverter-
    defibrillator (ICD).*
  dual-chamber, 265, *266*, 287, *287–288*
  electromagnetic interference and, 265
  epicardial, 286, *286*, 292
  implantable cardioverter-defibrillator in, 257, 258, 258t
  indications for, 264
  invasive. See also *Pacing therapy, temporary.*
    indications for, 285
  medications and, 253, 272–273, 278, 280, 285
  myocardial depolarization and, 287–288
  on electrocardiogram, *252*, 264, 265, *265–266*, 287, 294, *294*
  on fluoroscopy, 290
  overdrive atrial, 251–256, *251–252*, 287
  oversensing in, 265, *266*
  pacemaker firing in, 265, *265*, 287
    R on T phenomenon and, 292, 293
    threshold determination for, 293
  patient identification in, 267
  pulmonary artery catheter, 286, *286*, 291–292
  rate-responsive, 265
  sensing in, 264–265, 286, 294
    threshold determination for, 293
  single-chamber, *265*, 287, *287*
  temporary, 285, 288–289, *289*, 292–297
    equipment for, 288
    patient monitoring in, 296–297
  transcutaneous, 271–277, *274–275*
  transvenous, 278–284, *279*, 285–286
    atrial, 290–291, 294
    equipment for, 279–280, 282, 286
    ventricular, 289–290
  undersensing in, 265, *266*

Pacing therapy (Continued)
  unipolar, 264
PACO₂ (alveolar partial pressure of carbon dioxide), 64
PaCO₂ (arterial partial pressure of carbon dioxide), brain death and, 902, 903t
  oxygen saturation and, 77
  ventilation adequacy and, 199
Pain, and brain death, 900, 901
Pain management, 639
  alternative, 816, 819
  compartment syndrome and, 830
  end-of-life care and, 918, 919, 920
  epidural, 639, 640–645, 640–641
    contraindications to, 640
    equipment for, 640
    local anesthetic toxicity and, 644
    opiate reactions and, 645
    patient positioning for, 641, 641
    sedation score and, 643
  for burns, 814
Pain score, 643
PaO₂ (arterial partial pressure of oxygen), 77
  alveolar oxygen partial pressure ratio to, 170, 171t
  fraction of inspired oxygen ratio to, 170, 171t
  oxygenation adequacy and, 199
Paracentesis. See also Pericardiocentesis; Thoracentesis.
  abdominal, 689–693, 690, 692
    albumin intravenous solution in, 691
    assistance in, 694–697
    contraindications to, 689
    x-rays in, 690
Parenteral nutrition (PN), 877–879, 878t, 881–882
  metabolic complications of, 880t
Patient breathing, and hemodynamic pressure monitoring, 450–451, 451–452, 453
Patient decision-making capacity, 893
Patient instruction, wound dressing care for, 849
Patient Self-Determination Act, 892, 893
Patient transport, continuous arteriovenous rewarming and, 772
  enteral nutrition and, 874
  rapid infusion devices and, 783
  to burn care facility, 813t
Peak inspiratory pressure (PIP), 161, 162
  intra-abdominal hypertension and, 675, 675t
PEEP. See Positive end-expiratory pressure (PEEP).
Percutaneous endoscopic gastrostomy (PEG) tubes, 883, 883
Pericardial effusion, 238, 490
Pericardiocentesis, 238–242, 240
  pericardial catheter with, 491
Peripheral nerve stimulation, 647–653, 647t
  facial nerve in, 649–650, 650
  in brain death determination, 900
  posterior tibial nerve in, 650–651, 650
  supramaximal stimulation level in, 648, 651
  ulnar nerve in, 648–649, 649
Peripheral nerve stimulators (PNSs), 647
Peritoneal automated cycler machine, 746, 747
Peritoneal dialysis (PD), 746–752, 746
Peritoneal lavage, 698–703, 701
  assistance in, 705–709
  contraindications to, 698
PETCO₂ (partial pressure of end-tidal carbon dioxide), 64
pH, and oxygen saturation, 77
Pharmacologic therapy. See Medications.
Phenothiazines, and thermoregulation, 591
Phenytoin, enteral feeding and, 872t
  oculovestibular reflex and, 599
Phlebitis, and intravenous access, 530
Phlebostatic axis, 479–480, 479–480
Plasma, fresh frozen, transfusion of, 757, 758t, 759, 761t, 762, 763
Plasma exchange, 753
Plasmapheresis, 753–754, 754
  assistance in, 755–756
  complications of, 753, 754, 755
Plateau pressure, 161

Platelet function, mechanical trauma and, 322, 325
Platelets, left atrial catheter removal and, 420
  transfusion of, 757, 758t, 760, 762, 763
Pleural effusions, 145, 146
Pleural tubes, 117
Pneumatic antishock garments (PASGs), 315–319, 316
  compartment syndrome and, 829t
    abdominal, 674t
  contraindications to, 315
  weaning parameters for, 318
Pneumocephalus, signs of, 590
Pneumonia, arterial blood gas analysis and, 496
  compliance and, 161
  intrapulmonary shunt and, 175
  necrotizing, closed pneumothorax and, 99
Pneumothorax, 99
  central venous pressure lines and, 504, 504t, 516t
  chest tube sizes for, 99
  high-pressure ventilator alarms and, 185t
  lung compliance and, 165
  signs of, 181
  tension, 99, 141–142
Polidocanol, 711t
Positive end-expiratory pressure (PEEP), 155, 179t
  auto-, 158, 158
  closed pneumothorax and, 99
  pulmonary artery wedge pressure and, 449
Positive expiratory pressure (PEP), 191, 192, 194
Positive pressure ventilation (PPV), 155. See also Mechanical ventilation, positive pressure.
Post-surgical patients, pulmonary artery catheter insertion for, 432
Power of attorney for health care, 892, 917
Preejection period (PEP), 422t
Pregnancy, abdominal paracentesis and, 689
  peritoneal lavage and, 698
  pulmonary artery catheter insertion for, 432
  transfusion reactions and, 786
Pressure infusion cuff, external, 765–767. See also Fluid resuscitation.
  ventricular fibrillation and, 765
Pressure support ventilation (PSV), 179t, 182, 183, 184
  in ventilation weaning, 198, 198t, 202
Pressure-Controlled/Inverse Ratio Ventilation (PC/IRV), 179t, 184
  auto-PEEP and, 158, 184
Pronation therapy, 83–89, 87, 91–93. See also Immobility; Lateral rotation therapy.
  contraindications to, 84
  hemodynamic status and, 85
  hydrocolloid dressings in, 92
  positioner device in, 85, 87–88, 89, 90
Prostaglandins, in inflammation, 843
PROTECTIV PLUS IV Catheter Safety System, 523, 527
PROTECTIV valved safety introducer system, 538–540
Pseudotumor cerebri, 613
PSV (pressure support ventilation) protocol, for ventilation weaning, 198t
Pulmonary artery catheter(s), 393, 431, 440
  blood sampling from, 385–387
  continuous arteriovenous rewarming and, 768, 769
  contraindications to, 432–433, 439
  fiber optic, 72, 72. See also Catheter(s), jugular venous oxygen saturation.
  indications for, 422, 431, 432, 439
  insertion of, 433–437, 435, 440
    assistance in, 442–445, 444, 447, 453–455
    heparin and, 433, 443
    right bundle branch block and, 433
    waveforms during, 439, 441, 441–442. See also Central venous pressure (CVP).
  pulmonary artery pressure and, 447–448, 447
  removal of, 457–460
    contraindications to, 457
    dysrhythmias and, 459
    indications for, 457
    transvenous pacemaker and, 457, 458

Pulmonary artery catheter(s) *(Continued)*
  right ventricle waveform and, 467–468, *468*
  temporary pacing, *286*
  troubleshooting of, 461–464, *462, 464–465,* 466–470, *468*
  wedge pressure and, 431–432, 439. See also *Pulmonary artery wedge pressure (PAWP).*
    overinflated balloon and, 462, *462*
Pulmonary artery wedge pressure (PAWP), 390t, *435,* 439, *440,* 441, *442,* 461
  cardiac preload by, 389
  catheterization and, 431–432, 439. See also *Hemodynamic monitoring.*
  intra-aortic balloon pump therapy and, 301, 310
  monitoring of, 448–450, *449–450,* 461
  overwedged balloon and, 462–463, 467, *462*
  positive end-expiratory pressure and, 449
  pulmonary artery diastolic pressure and, 461
  right ventricular failure and, 503
Pulmonary disease, obstructive, chronic. See *Chronic obstructive pulmonary disease (COPD).*
  mechanical ventilation and, expiratory times for, 182
  patient ventilation and, 77, 79
  prone positioning for, 83–84, 85
  pulmonary artery catheter insertion for, 432
Pulmonary edema, colloid solutions and, 777
  compliance and, 161
  high-pressure ventilator alarms and, 185t
  intrapulmonary shunt and, 175
  preeclampsia-induced, pulmonary artery catheter insertion for, 432
  thoracic fluid status and, 422t, 427
Pulmonary embolism, 530
  central venous catheter insertion and, 518t
  end-tidal carbon dioxide and, 68
  intravenous catheters and, 530
  pleural effusion and, 145
  pulmonary artery pressure and, 441
Pulmonary fibrosis, and compliance, 161
Pulmonary hypoperfusion, and end-tidal carbon dioxide, 68
Pulmonary shunt, 170–171, *172,* 175
  calculation of, 175–177, 176t
Pulsatility index (PI), 580, *582*
Pulse generator(s), atrial pacing, 251, *251*
  permanent, 264, *264*
  temporary, 251, *251–252,* 275, 279, 287, *287–288*
Pulse oximetry, 77, *77–78,* 79–82
  carbon monoxide and, 79
  hypothermia and, 594
  in intubation, 1, 7
Pulse pressure, 367, *367*
Pupillary light reflex, and brain death, 900

Q

QRS complex, 338–339, *351*
  defibrillation and, 207, 220
  in temporary cardiac pacing, 294
  intra-aortic balloon pump therapy and, 299, 301
Queckenstedt test, 605, 610

R

Radiography, atelectasis on, 181
  brain death and, 903t
  chest tubes removal and, 117, 119
  in abdominal paracentesis, 690
  in chest tube insertion, 105
  in esophagogastric tamponade tube placement, 658
  in feeding tube insertion, 888, 890
  in intra-aortic balloon placement, 300, 303
  in intubation, 9
  in jugular venous oxygen saturation catheter placement, 574
  in peripherally inserted central catheter placement, 540
  in thoracentesis, 145, 146, 147, 149
  mediastinal blood on, 230

Radiography *(Continued)*
  pleural effusions on, 146
  pneumothorax on, 181
  transvenous cardiac pacing on, 281, 282, 283
    lead wire placement in, 290
Rapid shallow breathing index (fx/VT), 191, 197t
Red blood cells (RBCs), in inflammation, 843
  in subarachnoid hemorrhage, 610
Renal failure, acute hemolytic reactions and, 788
  metabolic abnormalities of, medications for, 751
  myoglobin in, 815
  pericardial effusion and, 490
Renal replacement therapies, continuous, 717, 718t–719t, 720, 722–723, 729–731
  complications of, 722, 731
  equipment for, 722
  replacement fluid amounts in, 731
  vs. hemodialysis, 720
Resuscitation, manual, 164–169, *164*
  complications with, 168–169
  equipment for, 164, *165*
  lung compliance and, 165
Resuscitation bag(s), 164, *165*
Right atrial/central venous pressure (RA/CVP), 390t, 408, 503
  monitoring of, 408–409, *410,* 411, *412,* 413
  waveforms in, 441, *441,* 445–446, *446,* 461, 503
    overdampened, 464, *465,* 466–467
Rigor mortis, and cardiopulmonary death, 899
Ringer's lactated solution, 777
  in continuous renal replacement therapies, 731
Romazicon, in scleral therapy, 712
Rotating Kinetic Treatment Table, *635*

S

Salem sump tube, 681, *682*
Scleral endoscopic therapy, 711–715, *713*
  agents in, 711t
Sedation score, 643
Sedatives, auto positive end-expiratory pressure and, 158
  end-tidal carbon dioxide monitoring and, 69
  mechanical ventilation and, 181, 182
  oculovestibular reflexes and, 599, 901
Seizure, and hyperthermia, 594
Seldinger technique, 506, *507,* 533
Sellick maneuver, 1, *1*
Sengstaken-Blakemore esophagogastric tamponade tube, 655, *656*
Sensory dermatomes, *627*
Sepsis, arterial-venous oxygen difference and, 155
  end-tidal carbon dioxide and, 67
  hypothermia and, 592
  transcutaneous pacing and, 271
Septicemia, catheter-related, 401, 405
Shock. See also *Pneumatic antishock garments (PASGs).*
  arterial blood gas analysis and, 496, 497
  hypovolemic, body rewarming and, 593
  intra-aortic balloon pump therapy for, 299
Shunt, pulmonary, 170–171, *172,* 175
  calculation of, 175–177, 176t
Silver nitrate, for burns, 814, 815t
Silver sulfadiazine (Silvadene), for burns, 814, 815t
Sinus rhythm, 251
Skin, 811, *812,* 843
Skin preparation, antiseptic, 518, *519*
Sodium morrhuate, 711t
Sodium tetradecyl sulfate, 711t
Somatostatin, and scleral therapy, 715
Spinal cord injury. See also *Cervical fixation; Traction.*
  intubation and, 2, 3, 4
  physiologic response to, 636t
  thermoregulation and, 591
Spinal cord injury assessment form, *626*
Spinal reflex movements, 900
SpO₂ (oxygen saturation by pulse oximetry), 77

Spontaneous tidal volume (SV$_t$), 191, 193
Sprint Protocol, for ventilation weaning, 198t
Square wave test, *369–370*, 377
ST segment monitoring, 349–352, *350–351*
   hypothermia and, 594
Standard weaning criteria (SWC), 191, *192*, 193–195, 196t
Static compliance (C$_{stat}$), 161, 163
   measurement of, 162–163
Static pressure, 161
Status asthmaticus, and auto-positive end-expiratory pressure, 159
Sternotomy, emergent, 229–233
    assistance in, 234–237
Stroke, heat, 593, 594
Stroke volume (SV), 389, 390t, 422t, 427, *428*
   hypertension and, 389
Stryker Intracompartmental Pressure Monitor, 832, *833*
Succinylcholine, and malignant hyperthermia, 593
Sucralfate, for gastrointestinal bleeding, 671
   scleral therapy and, 715
Suction, 41
   chest tube removal and, 117
   closed-suction technique of, 41, *42*, 43, 44–46
     equipment for, 42
   complications of, 41
   for endotracheal tube, 41–47, 42t
   for tracheostomy tube, 41–47, 42t
   gastric intubation and, 681
   indications for, 41
   nasopharyngeal airway in, 27
   open-suction technique of, 41, 43–46
     equipment for, 42
   oropharyngeal airway in, 31
Sulfamylon (mafenide acetate), for burns, 814, 815t
Suture(s), 844–845
   half-buried mattress, 844, *845*
   interrupted dermal, 844, *844*
   purse-string, 117, *118*
   subcutaneous, 844, *844*
   subcuticular running, 844–845, *845*
   vertical mattress, 844, *845*
Suturing, 843, *844–845*, 846–850, *847*
   equipment for, 845, *847*
SV index (SVI), 390t, 422t
SVR index (SVRI), 422t
Swan-Ganz catheter, *393*, 440, 475
Synchronized intermittent mandatory ventilation (SIMV), 179t
   in ventilation weaning, 201–202
Systemic inflammatory response syndrome, and hypothermia, 592
Systemic vascular resistance (SVR), 422t, 428. See also *Cardiac output (CO), afterload in.*

T
Tachydysrhythmias, 219–220
   cardioversion for, 211
     energy recommendations for, 215t
   hyperthermia and, 594
   pulmonary artery wedge pressure and, 441
Tenckhoff catheter, *746*
Tetanus prophylaxis, 846t
ThermoCardiosystems Heartmate, 320–321, 325, 326, 327, *320*
Thermoregulation, 591
Thoracentesis, 145–149, *146*
   assistance in, 151–154
   complications from, 148–149
   contraindications to, 145
   diagnostic, 145
Thoracic fluid status (Zo), 421, 422t, 427
Thoracoabdominal aortic aneurysm (TAAA), cerebrospinal fluid monitoring and, 613
Thoracostomy, needle, 141–144, *142*
     complications from, 143
   tube, 99–107, *100*, *103–105*
Thoratec biventricular assist device, 321, *321*, 325, 326, 327
Thrombin, as sclerosing agent, 711t

Thrombocytopenia, and heparin, 443
Thrombophlebitis, central venous catheter insertion and, 518t
   intravenous access and, 530
   peripherally inserted central catheters and, 541
Thrombosis, arterial catheter insertion and, 362, 443
   ventricular assist devices and, 323, 324, 325
Tissue oxygenation, 77. See also *Oxygen* entries.
Titration, of medication, 922
Total parenteral nutrition (TPN), 877
Tracheal tube cuff, 49, *50*
   care of, 49–51, 53–55
   complications with, 49
   emergent inflation for, 52–53, *53*
   pressure measurement for, 52, *52*
Tracheostomy, 56, *57*
   indications for, 56t
Tracheostomy tubes, 41, 56, *57*
   cannula of, 56, *57*
   care of, 58–62, *60*
   complications from, 61
   cuff of, 56, *57*
   sizes of, 42t
   suction of, 41–47, 42t
     chest tube removal and, 117
     complications from, 41, 46
     indications for, 41
Traction, 634–638
   cervical, 620, 622–624, 625. See also *Halo ring device.*
   immobility of, physiologic response to, 636t
   skin assessment guide for, 637t
Train-of-four (TOF) stimulation, 647, 647t
Transcranial Doppler (TCD) monitoring, 580–582, *581–582*, 581t, 583t, 584–586
Transducer(s), hemodynamic pressure, 472, 473, 474, *475–476*, *478*, 479
   calibration of, 480–481
   leveling of, 479–480, *479–480*
   multiple, 475, 479
   reusable, 474, *478*
beta-2-Transferrin, in cerebrospinal fluid, 588
Transfusion reaction, 763, 786
   acute, 786, 787t
   acute tubular necrosis as, 789
   disseminated intravascular coagulopathy and, 789
   management of, 760, 787t, 788–790
Transfusion therapy, 757–764, 758t, 761t, 777. See also *Fluid resuscitation; Infusion device(s).*
   blood filters for, 758, *779*
   citrate and, 786
   complications with, 778
   component storage for, 760
   hypervolemia and, 786
   transfusion reaction and, 763, 786, 787t
     premedication for, 760, 787t
   urine output and, 784
Transplantation, 910
   donor care in, 907–909
   organ donation and, 907
   transcutaneous pacing and, 271
Trauma. See also *Burns.*
   autotransfusion for, 95
   central venous catheters and, 533
   chest tube sizes for, 99
   compartment syndrome and, 828, 829t
   facial, brain death and, 901
   intra-abdominal hypertension and, 674t
   jugular venous oxygen saturation and, 571
   oculovestibular reflexes and, 599, 901
   pericardial effusion and, 490
   pneumatic antishock garments for, 315
   pupillary reactivity and, 900
   spinal cord, physiologic response to, 636t
   thermoregulation and, 591
   volu-pressure, 179
Tuberculosis, and closed pneumothorax, 99
Tubular necrosis, and acute hemolytic reactions, 788

Turning frame, *635*
Type O negative blood, 761t, 777

U

Ultrafiltration, 717
   slow continuous, 717, 718t, 720–721, 723–725, *720*
Ultrasonography, brain death and, 903t
   in thoracentesis, 145, 146, 147
   transcranial Doppler, 580–582, *581–582*, 581t, 583t, 584–586
Urokinase, dialysis catheter cleaning by, 752

V

Vacutainer Luer-Lok adapter needle, *380*
VACUTAINER system, *528*, *545*, *547–549*
Varices, esophagogastric tamponade therapy for, 655
   scleral endoscopic therapy for, 711
Vascular disease, and transcutaneous pacing, 271
Vasoconstrictors, for nasopharyngeal airway insertion, 29
Vasospasm, arterial, transcranial Doppler monitoring and, 583t
Venipuncture, *538*, 543–550, *543–544*, *547–548*. See also *Arterial puncture.*
   collection tube order in, 547
   complications of, 550
   indications for, 543
   postpuncture hematoma and, 550
   tourniquet in, 544, 545, *546*
Venous admixture, 175
Venous oxygen saturation. See also *Oxygen saturation.*
   cardiac output and, 71, 71t, 385
   jugular, 570–571, 571t, 572t
      clinical intervention and, 571, 572t
      desaturation and, 571, 571t, 576
      intracranial pressure monitoring by, 570, 577
      monitoring of, 576–578
   mixed, 71–76, 71t
      blood sampling for, 385–387
      shivering and, 596
      spectrophotometry components in, 72, *72*
Venous sheath removal, 484–488
Ventilation, 83. See also *Mechanical ventilation; Resuscitation, manual.*
   alarms in, 185t
   for transfusion reaction, 788
   humidified gases in, 185–186
   inspiratory times and, 184
   maintenance, 167–169
      complications with, 168–169
      equipment for, 164
   oxygenation and, 83–84, *84*
   patient monitoring in, 186–188
   pressure mode in, 178, 179–180, 179t, 183–185
      closed pneumothorax and, 99
      complications with, 179–180
      hemodynamic pressure monitoring with, 451, *452*
      hemodynamics and, 155, 157
      volume guaranteed, 185

Ventilation *(Continued)*
   volume, 178–179, 179t, 182–183
   weaning from, 191, 196–203, *196*, 196t, 197t, 198t
      continuous positive airway pressure in, 197–198, 198t, 201
      equipment for, 191, 199
      intermittent mandatory ventilation in, 201–202
      intolerance criteria for, 198, 198t
      pressure support ventilation in, 198, 198t, 202
      synchronized intermittent mandatory ventilation in, 201–202
Ventilators, 178, 179
   with volume-assured pressure option, 183, 185
Ventilatory failure, 178, 180
Ventricular assist devices (VADs), 320–327, *320–322*
   contraindications to, 320
   filling and emptying signs with, 325
   platelet function and, 325
   weaning parameters for, 326
Ventricular dysfunction, and hyperthermia, 594
   left, cardiac stroke volume and, 427, *428*
Ventricular ejection time (VET), 422t
Ventricular fibrillation (VF), 205, 219
   cardioversion and, 216
   continuous arteriovenous rewarming and, 775
   external pressure infusion cuffs and, 765
   hypothermia and, 594, 786
Ventricular hypertrophy, cardioversion for, 211
Vinke tongs, 620, *621*
   skin assessment guide for, 637t
Vital capacity (VC), 191, 193
Vollman Prone Positioner, *85*, 87–88, 89, *90*

W

Warfarin, and enteral feeding, 872t
Warming devices, 591, 593, 768, *769*
   procedure for, 593–596
Water manometer, 408, *410*
Weaning Continuum Model, *196*
West's lung zones, *432*
Winged infusion set, *522*, *524*, 529, 548. See also *Butterfly set.*
Withdrawing treatment, 917–921
   death and, 918
Withholding therapy, 917–921
   death and, 918
Wound management, 843, 851–853, *852*, 855–858. See also *Burns, wound management for.*
   biopsy in, 855
   cleansing in, 851, 853, *854*
   culturing in, 855
   drains in, 859
      dressings for, 859–861, *860*
      removal of, 863–864
   dressing for, 856, *857*
   infection and, 851, 857
   needle aspiration in, 855
   pouching in, 865–867
   tetanus prophylaxis for, 846t